About This Treatment Guide

The Oncology Group, a division of CMPMedica, publisher of the journal *ONCOLOGY* and the news magazine *Oncology News International,* as well as the comprehensive cancer website, cancernetwork.com, is pleased to bring you the 10th annual edition of *Cancer Management: A Multidisciplinary Approach.*

The fundamental principle behind this treatment guide is the importance of a truly integrated, multidisciplinary approach to the management of the patient with cancer. Accordingly, the discussion of each disease site combines the perspectives of medical oncology, surgical oncology, and radiation oncology, as appropriate. This 10th edition of our easy-to-use handbook features the efforts of over 100 contributors from approximately 50 different institutions.

The background of this text's cover should be familiar to readers. It is identical to that of *ONCOLOGY,* our flagship publication, which has provided important medical information to oncology professionals for the past 20 years. This cover symbolizes our ongoing commitment to oncology education. To further this commitment, we are pleased to continue to provide you with selected chapters of this 10th edition, and all of the articles published in *ONCOLOGY* since 1995, online, at our website www.cancernetwork.com.

We have produced this 10th edition in an effort to keep pace with the rapidly changing field of oncology. We are committed to providing readers with the newest information on cancer therapeutics and patient care. As in earlier editions, our goal with this newest edition is to provide readers with up-to-date, practical, and authoritative information on patient management.

We at The Oncology Group would like to thank everyone involved in the development and production of this handbook. In particular, we thank the book's principal editors, Richard Pazdur, MD, of the Center for Drug Evaluation and Research, US Food and Drug Administration; Lawrence R. Coia, MD, of Southern Ocean County Radiation Oncology, in Manahawkin New Jersey; William J. Hoskins, MD, Director of the Curtis and Elizabeth Anderson Cancer Institute at the Memorial Health University Medical Center in Savannah, Georgia; and Lawrence D. Wagman, MD, of City of Hope National Medical Center. We also thank the staff of The Oncology Group and in particular wish to recognize the efforts of Angela Cibuls and Susan Reckling.

Your thoughts are important. Please let us know how you use this book, and how we can make it even more valuable. Contact Angela Cibuls at acibuls@cmp.com or Cara Glynn at cglynn@cmp.com. We hope you find this comprehensive and multidisciplinary guide helpful in the day-to-day care of your patients with cancer.

Cara H. Glynn
Sr. Editorial Director

Melissa Warner
Group Vice President/
General Manager

About This Treatment Guide

[illegible]

10TH EDITION, 2007–2008

Cancer Management: A Multidisciplinary Approach

Medical, Surgical, & Radiation Oncology

Edited by

Richard Pazdur, MD
Director, Office of Oncology Drug Products
Center for Drug Evaluation and Research
US Food and Drug Administration

Lawrence R. Coia, MD
Medical Director, Southern Ocean County Radiation Oncology
Manahawkin, New Jersey

William J. Hoskins, MD
Director, Curtis and Elizabeth Anderson Cancer Institute
at Memorial Health University Medical Center
Savannah, Georgia

Lawrence D. Wagman, MD
Chairman, Division of Surgery
City of Hope National Medical Center

And the publishers of the journal ONCOLOGY

CMPMedica
United Business Media

Note to the reader

The information in this volume has been carefully reviewed for accuracy of dosage and indications. Before prescribing any drug, however, the clinician should consult the manufacturer's current package labeling for accepted indications, absolute dosage recommendations, and other information pertinent to the safe and effective use of the product described. This is especially important when drugs are given in combination or as an adjunct to other forms of therapy. Furthermore, some of the medications described herein, as well as some of the indications mentioned, had not been approved by the US Food and Drug Administration at the time of publication. This possibility should be borne in mind before prescribing or recommending any drug or regimen.

> The views expressed are the result of independent work and do not necessarily represent the views or findings of the US Food and Drug Administration or the United States.

Library of Congress Catalog Card Number 2006937481
ISBN Number 9781891483486

For information on purchasing additional copies of this publication, contact us at this address, Cancer Management Handbook, CMP Media LLC, 4601 W. 6th St., Ste. B, Lawrence, KS 66049. Phone: 1-800-444-4881 or 1-785-838-7576; fax: 1-785-838-7566, or e-mail: orders@cmp.com.

CMPMedica
United Business Media

Publishers of
ONCOLOGY
ONCOLOGY: Nurse Edition
Oncology News International
cancernetwork.com

Contents

PREFACE
Richard Pazdur, Lawrence R. Coia, William J. Hoskins, and Lawrence D. Wagman

PRINCIPLES OF MULTIDISCIPLINARY THERAPY

Ch 1 **Principles of surgical oncology** 1
Lawrence D. Wagman

Ch 2 **Principles of radiation therapy** 11
Michael J. Gazda and Lawrence R. Coia

Ch 3 **Principles of oncologic pharmacotherapy** 23
Chris H. Takimoto and Emiliano Calvo

CANCERS OF THE HEAD AND NECK REGION

Ch 4 **Head and neck tumors** 35
John Andrew Ridge, Bonnie S. Glisson, Eric M. Horwitz, and Miriam N. Lango

Ch 5 **Thyroid and parathyroid cancers** 83
Gilbert G. Fareau, Rena Vassilopoulou-Sellin, Robert Lustig, and Jeffrey P. Lamont

LUNG CANCER

Ch 6 **Non–small-cell lung cancer** 103
Benjamin Movsas, Fadlo R. Khuri, and Kemp Kernstine

Ch 7 **Small-cell lung cancer, mesothelioma, and thymoma** 145
Bonnie S. Glisson, Benjamin Movsas, and Walter Scott

BREAST CANCER

Ch 8 **Breast cancer overview** 163
Risk factors, screening, genetic testing, and prevention
Lori Jardines, Bruce G. Haffty, Paul Fisher, Jeffrey Weitzel, and Melanie Royce

Ch 9 **Stages 0 and I breast cancer** 193
Lori Jardines, Bruce G. Haffty, and Melanie Royce

Ch 10 **Stage II breast cancer** 211
Lori Jardines, Bruce G. Haffty, and Melanie Royce

Ch 11 **Stages III and IV breast cancer** 229
Lori Jardines, Bruce G. Haffty, Melanie Royce, and Ishmael Jaiyesimi

GASTROINTESTINAL CANCERS

Ch 12 **Esophageal cancer** 251
I. Benjamin Paz, Jimmy J. Hwang, and Rajesh Iyer

Ch 13 **Gastric cancer** 273
Charles D. Blanke, Lawrence R. Coia, and Roderich E. Schwarz

Ch 14 **Pancreatic, neuroendocrine GI, and adrenal cancers** 287
Al B. Benson III, Robert J. Myerson, and John Hoffman

Ch 15 **Liver, gallbladder, and biliary tract cancers** 319
Lawrence D. Wagman, John M. Robertson, and Bert O'Neil

Ch 16 **Colon, rectal, and anal cancers** 339
Joshua D. I. Ellenhorn, Carey A. Cullinane, Lawrence R. Coia, and Steven R. Alberts

GENITOURINARY MALIGNANCIES

Ch 17 **Prostate cancer** 373
Judd W. Moul, Brent K. Hollenbeck, Kathleen W. Beekman, Joseph Lattanzi, and Maha Hussain

Ch 18 **Testicular cancer** 401
Patrick J. Loehrer, Thomas E. Ahlering, Mark Buyyounouski, and Douglas Skarecky

Ch 19 **Urothelial and kidney cancers** 423
Bruce G. Redman, Mark Hurwitz, Philippe E. Spiess, and Louis L. Pisters

GYNECOLOGIC MALIGNANCIES

Ch 20 **Cervical cancer** **441**
Dennis S. Chi, Carlos A. Perez, Rachelle M. Lanciano, and John Kavanagh

Ch 21 **Uterine corpus tumors** **471**
Kathryn M. Greven, Maurie Markman, and David Scott Miller

Ch 22 **Ovarian cancer** **499**
Stephen C. Rubin and Paul Sabbatini

SKIN CANCERS

Ch 23 **Melanoma and other skin cancers** **523**
Eric H. Jensen, Kim A. Margolin, and Vernon K. Sondak

The ABCDs of moles and melanomas **555**

A color atlas of skin lesions **559**

SARCOMAS

Ch 24 **Bone sarcomas** **565**
Alan W. Yasko and Warren Chow

Ch 25 **Soft-tissue sarcomas** **577**
Peter W. T. Pisters, Mitchell Weiss, Robert Maki, and Gary N. Mann

BRAIN TUMORS

Ch 26 **Primary and metastatic brain tumors** **609**
Lisa M. DeAngelis, Jay S. Loeffler, and Adam N. Mamelak

OTHER SOLID TUMORS

Ch 27 **AIDS-related malignancies** **631**
Ronald T. Mitsuyasu and Jay S. Cooper

Ch 28 **Carcinoma of an unknown primary site** **657**
John D. Hainsworth and Lawrence M. Weiss

HEMATOLOGIC MALIGNANCIES

Ch 29 **Hodgkin lymphoma** 667
Joachim Yahalom and David Straus

Ch 30 **Non-Hodgkin lymphoma** 689
Steven T. Rosen, Jane N. Winter, Leo I. Gordon, Andrew M. Evens, and Nicos Nicolaou

Ch 31 **Multiple myeloma and other plasma cell dyscrasias** 741
Sundar Jagannath, Paul Richardson, and Nikhil C. Munshi

Ch 32 **Acute leukemias** 761
Margaret R. O'Donnell

Ch 33 **Chronic myelogenous leukemia** 789
Jorge E. Cortes, Richard T. Silver, and Hagop Kantarjian

Ch 34 **Chronic lymphocytic leukemia** 805
William G. Wierda, Nicole Lamanna, Jorge E. Cortes, and Mark A. Weiss

Ch 35 **Myelodysplastic syndromes** 821
Jorge E. Cortes, Alan List, and Hagop Kantarjian

Ch 36 **Hematopoietic cell transplantation** 839
Stephen J. Forman

PALLIATIVE AND SUPPORTIVE CARE

Ch 37 **Pain management** 859
Sharon M. Weinstein, Penny R. Anderson, Alan W. Yasko, and Lawrence Driver

Ch 38 **Management of nausea and vomiting** 873
Steven M. Grunberg and Marisa Siebel

Ch 39 **Depression, anxiety, and delirium** 885
Alan Valentine

Ch 40 **Hematopoietic growth factors** 901
Sally Yowell Barbour and Jeffrey Crawford

Ch 41 **Fatigue and dyspnea** **917**
Sriram Yennurajalingam and Eduardo Bruera

Ch 42 **Anorexia and cachexia** **929**
Charles Loprinzi and Aminah Jatoi

Ch 43 **Long-term venous access** **935**
Stephen P. Povoski

COMPLICATIONS

Ch 44 **Prevention and management of radiation toxicity** **947**
Nicos Nicolaou

Ch 45 **Oncologic emergencies and paraneoplastic syndromes** **979**
Carmen P. Escalante, Ellen Manzullo, and Mitchell Weiss

Ch 46 **Infectious complications** **1003**
James Ito, Jr.

Ch 47 **Fluid complications** **1035**
Frederic W. Grannis, Jr., Carey A. Cullinane, and Lily Lai

APPENDICES

Appendix 1: Performance scales **1053**

Appendix 2: Cancer information on the Internet **1055**
J. Sybil Biermann

Appendix 3: Cancer Drugs and Indications Newly Approved by U.S. Food and Drug Administration **1060**

Appendix 4: Chemotherapeutic agents and their uses, dosages, and toxicities **1062**
Chris H. Takimoto and Emiliano Calvo

INDEX **1073**

Ch 41 [illegible]

Ch 42 [illegible]

Ch 43 [illegible]

COMPLICATIONS

Ch 44 [illegible]

Ch 45 [illegible]

Ch 46 [illegible]

Ch 47 [illegible]

APPENDICES

Appendix 1: Performance scales [illegible]

Appendix 2: Cancer information on the Internet [illegible]

Appendix 3: Cancer Drugs and Biologic [illegible] approved by U.S. Food and Drug Administration [illegible]

Appendix 4: Chemotherapeutic agents and their uses, dosages, and toxicities [illegible]

INDEX

Contributors

Thomas E. Ahlering, MD
Urology Division
University of California,
Irvine Medical Center

Steven R. Alberts, MD
Department of Medical Oncology
Mayo Clinic

Penny R. Anderson, MD
Department of Radiation Oncology
Fox Chase Cancer Center

Kathleen W. Beekman, MD
Division of Hematology/Oncology
University of Michigan
Comprehensive Cancer Center

Al B. Benson III, MD
Division of Hematology/Oncology
Northwestern University

J. Sybil Biermann, MD
Department of Orthopaedic Surgery
University of Michigan
Comprehensive Cancer Center

Charles D. Blanke, MD
Department of Medicine
Oregon Health Sciences University

Eduardo Bruera, MD
Department of Palliative Care
and Rehabilitation Medicine
M. D. Anderson Cancer Center

Mark Buyyounouski, MD
Department of Radiation Oncology
Fox Chase Cancer Center

Emiliano Calvo, MD, PhD
Division of Medical Oncology
The Institute for Drug Development
Cancer Therapy and Research Center

Dennis S. Chi, MD
Gynecology Service
Memorial Sloan-Kettering
Cancer Center

Warren Chow, MD
Department of Medical Oncology
City of Hope National Medical Center

Lawrence R. Coia, MD
Southern Ocean County
Radiation Oncology
Manahawkin, New Jersey

Jay S. Cooper, MD
Division of Radiation Oncology
Maimonides Medical Center

Jorge E. Cortes, MD
Department of Leukemia
M. D. Anderson Cancer Center

Jeffrey Crawford, MD
Department of Medical Oncology
Duke University Medical Center

Carey A. Cullinane, MD
Department of Surgical Oncology
Long Beach Memorial Medical Center
Long Beach, California

Lisa M. DeAngelis, MD
Department of Neurology
Memorial Sloan-Kettering
Cancer Center

Lawrence Driver, MD
Pain Symptom Management Section
M. D. Anderson Cancer Center

Joshua D. I. Ellenhorn, MD
Division of Surgery
City of Hope National Medical Center

Carmen P. Escalante, MD
Department of General Internal Medicine, Ambulatory Treatment, and Emergency Care
M. D. Anderson Cancer Center

Andrew M. Evens, DO
Division of Hematology/Oncology
Robert H. Lurie Comprehensive Cancer Center, Feinberg School of Medicine/ Northwestern University

Gilbert G. Fareau, MD
Department of Endocrine Neoplasia and Hormonal Disorders
M. D. Anderson Cancer Center

Paul Fisher, MD
Department of Radiology
Stony Brook University Hospital and Medical Center

Stephen J. Forman, MD
Division of Hematology and Bone Marrow Transplantation
City of Hope National Medical Center

Michael J. Gazda, MS
Department of Radiation Oncology
Radiation Physics, Inc.
Coral Gables, Florida

Bonnie S. Glisson, MD
Department of Thoracic/ Head and Neck Medical Oncology
M. D. Anderson Cancer Center

Leo I. Gordon, MD
Division of Hematology/Oncology
Robert H. Lurie Comprehensive Cancer Center, Feinberg School of Medicine/ Northwestern University

Frederic W. Grannis, Jr., MD
Section of Thoracic Surgery
City of Hope National Medical Center

Kathryn M. Greven, MD
Department of Radiation Oncology
Wake Forest University School of Medicine

Steven M. Grunberg, MD
Division of Medical Oncology
University of Vermont

Bruce G. Haffty, MD
Department of Radiation Oncology
UMDNJ - Robert Wood Johnson Medical School
The Cancer Institute of New Jersey

John D. Hainsworth, MD
Department of Clinical Research
Sarah Cannon Research Institute
Nashville, Tennessee

John Hoffman, MD
Department of Surgical Oncology
Fox Chase Cancer Center

Brent K. Hollenbeck, MD
Department of Medicine/Urology
University of Michigan Comprehensive Cancer Center

Eric M. Horwitz, MD
Department of Radiation Oncology
Fox Chase Cancer Center

William J. Hoskins, MD
Curtis and Elizabeth Anderson Cancer Institute at Memorial Health
University Medical Center
Savannah, Georgia

Mark Hurwitz, MD
Department of Radiation Oncology
Brigham and Women's Hospital

Maha Hussain, MD
Division of Hematology/Oncology
University of Michigan Comprehensive Cancer Center

Jimmy J. Hwang, MD
Division of Hematology/Oncology
Lombardi Cancer Center
Georgetown University Medical Center

James Ito, Jr., MD
Department of Infectious Diseases
City of Hope National Medical Center

Rajesh V. Iyer, MD
Department of Radiation Oncology
Community Medical Center
Toms River, New Jersey
An Affiliate of Saint Barnabas
Health Care System

Sundar Jagannath, MD
Myeloma and Transplant
St. Vincent's Comprehensive
Cancer Center

Ishmael Jaiyesimi, DO
Division of Hematology/Oncology
William Beaumont Hospital
Royal Oak, Michigan

Lori Jardines, MD
Department of Surgery
Albert Einstein Medical Center

Aminah Jatoi, MD
Department of Medical Oncology
Mayo Clinic

Eric H. Jensen, MD
Department of Surgical Oncology
H. Lee Moffitt Cancer Center and
Research Institute

Hagop Kantarjian, MD
Department of Leukemia
M. D. Anderson Cancer Center

John J. Kavanagh, MD
Department of Gynecologic Oncology
M. D. Anderson Cancer Center

Kemp H. Kernstine, MD, PhD
Department of Thoracic Surgery
City of Hope National Medical Center

Fadlo R. Khuri, MD
Department of Hematology/Oncology
Winship Cancer Institute of
Emory University

Lily Lai, MD
Division of Surgery
City of Hope National Medical Center

Nicole Lamanna, MD
Department of Medicine/
Leukemia Service
Memorial Sloan-Kettering Cancer Center

Jeffrey P. Lamont, MD
Department of Surgery
Baylor University Medical Center

Rachelle M. Lanciano, MD
Department of Radiation Oncology
Delaware County Memorial Hospital
Drexel Hill, Pennsylvania

Miriam N. Lango, MD
Department of Surgical Oncology
Fox Chase Cancer Center

Joseph Lattanzi, MD
Southern Ocean County
Radiation Oncology
Manahawkin, New Jersey

Alan List, MD
Department of Hematologic
Malignancies
H. Lee Moffitt Cancer Center and
Research Institute

Jay S. Loeffler, MD
Department of Radiation Oncology
Massachusetts General Hospital

Patrick J. Loehrer, MD
Division of Hematology/Oncology
Indiana University Cancer Center

Charles Loprinzi, MD
Department of Medical Oncology
Mayo Clinic

Robert Lustig, MD
Department of Radiation Oncology
University of Pennsylvania

Robert Maki, MD, PhD
Department of Medicine
Memorial Sloan-Kettering Cancer Center

Adam N. Mamelak, MD
Division of Neurosurgery
Cedars-Sinai Medical Center

Gary N. Mann, MD
Department of Surgical Oncology
University of Washington

Ellen Manzullo, MD
Department of General Internal Medicine, Ambulatory Treatment, and Emergency Care
M. D. Anderson Cancer Center

Kim A. Margolin, MD
Department of Medical Oncology
City of Hope National Medical Center

Maurie Markman, MD
Department of Clinical Research
M. D. Anderson Cancer Center

David Scott Miller, MD
Division of Gynecologic Oncology
University of Texas Southwestern Medical Center

Ronald T. Mitsuyasu, MD
Department of Medicine
UCLA Center for Clinical AIDS Research and Education

Judd W. Moul, MD
Division of Urologic Surgery
Duke University Medical Center

Benjamin Movsas, MD
Department of Radiation Oncology
Henry Ford Health System

Nikhil C. Munshi, MD
Department of Adult Oncology
Dana-Farber Cancer Institute

Robert J. Myerson, MD, PhD
Department of Radiation Oncology
Washington University

Nicos Nicolaou, MD
Department of Radiation Oncology
Fox Chase Cancer Center

Margaret R. O'Donnell, MD
Department of Hematology/Hematopoietic Stem Cell Transplantation
City of Hope National Medical Center

Bert O'Neil, MD
Department of Medicine
University of North Carolina at Chapel Hill

I. Benjamin Paz, MD
Division of Surgery
City of Hope National Medical Center

Richard Pazdur, MD
Office of Oncology Drug Products
Center for Drug Evaluation and Research
US Food and Drug Administration

Carlos A. Perez, MD
Department of Radiation Oncology
Washington University School of Medicine

Louis L. Pisters, MD
Department of Urology
M. D. Anderson Cancer Center

Peter W. T. Pisters, MD
Division of Surgery
M. D. Anderson Cancer Center

Stephen P. Povoski, MD
Department of Surgery
The Ohio State University

Bruce G. Redman, DO
Division of Hematology/Oncology
University of Michigan Comprehensive Cancer Center

Paul Richardson, MD
Department of Medical Oncology/Hematologic Malignancies
Dana-Farber Cancer Institute

John Andrew Ridge, MD, PhD
Department of Surgical Oncology
Fox Chase Cancer Center

John M. Robertson, MD
Department of Radiation Oncology
William Beaumont Hospital

Steven T. Rosen, MD
Division of Hematology/Oncology
Robert H. Lurie Comprehensive Cancer Center, Feinberg School of Medicine/ Northwestern University

Melanie Royce, MD, PhD
Division of Hematology/Oncology
University of New Mexico Cancer Research and Treatment Center

Stephen C. Rubin, MD
Division of Gynecologic Oncology
Hospital of the University of Pennsylvania

Paul Sabbatini, MD
Gynecologic Section
Solid Tumor Division
Memorial Sloan-Kettering Cancer Center

Roderich E. Schwarz, MD, PhD
Department of Surgery
UMDNJ - Robert Wood Johnson Medical School
The Cancer Institute of New Jersey

Walter Scott, MD
Department of Thoracic Surgical Oncology
Fox Chase Cancer Center

Marisa Siebel, MD
Department of Hematology/Oncology
University of Vermont

Richard T. Silver, MD
Department of Medicine
Weill Cornell Medical College

Douglas Skarecky, BS
Department of Urology
University of California, Irvine Medical Center

Vernon K. Sondak, MD
Department of Surgical Oncology
H. Lee Moffitt Cancer Center and Research Institute

Philippe E. Spiess, MD
Department of Urology
M. D. Anderson Cancer Center

David Straus, MD
Department of Medicine
Memorial Sloan-Kettering Cancer Center

Chris H. Takimoto, MD, PhD
Division of Medical Oncology
The Institute for Drug Development
Cancer Therapy and Research Center

Alan Valentine, MD
Department of Neuro-Oncology
M. D. Anderson Cancer Center

Rena Vassilopoulou-Sellin, MD
Department of Endocrine Neoplasia and Hormonal Disorders
M. D. Anderson Cancer Center

Lawrence D. Wagman, MD
Division of Surgery
City of Hope National Medical Center

Sharon M. Weinstein, MD
Department of Anesthesiology
Huntsman Cancer Institute
University of Utah

Lawrence M. Weiss, MD
Division of Pathology
City of Hope National Medical Center

Mark A. Weiss, MD
Department of Medicine/ Leukemia Service
Memorial Sloan-Kettering Cancer Center

Mitchell Weiss, MD
Department of Radiation Oncology
Monmouth Medical Center

Jeffrey Weitzel, MD
Department of Clinical Cancer Genetics
City of Hope National Medical Center

William G. Wierda, MD, PhD
Department of Leukemia
M. D. Anderson Cancer Center

Jane N. Winter, MD
Division of Hematology/Oncology
Robert H. Lurie Comprehensive Cancer Center, Feinberg School of Medicine/ Northwestern University

Joachim Yahalom, MD
Department of Radiation Oncology
Memorial Sloan-Kettering Cancer Center

Alan W. Yasko, MD
Department of Orthopaedic Oncology
M. D. Anderson Cancer Center

Sriram Yennurajalingam, MD
Department of Palliative Care and Rehabilitation Medicine
M. D. Anderson Cancer Center

Sally Yowell Barbour, PHARMD
Department of Medical Oncology
Duke University Medical Center

Publishing Staff

Cara H. Glynn	*Sr. Editorial Director*
Angela Cibuls	*Project Manager*
Susan Reckling	*Managing Editor*
Stacey Cuozzo	*Production Editor*
Terri Gelfand	*Sr. Editorial Coordinator*
Lisa Katz	*Creative Director*
Jeannine Coronna	*Publishing Operations Director*
Beth Scholz	*Publisher*
Melissa Warner	*Group Vice President/General Manager*

Preface

The concept for *Cancer Management: A Multidisciplinary Approach* arose more than 10 years ago. This 10th edition reflects the ongoing commitment of the authors, editors, and publishers to rapidly disseminate to oncologists the most current information on the clinical management of cancer patients.

Important updates and revisions have been made throughout this newest edition. Substantial revisions have been made to a number of chapters, including those on non–small-cell lung cancer, prostate cancer, cervical cancer, Hodgkin lymphoma, and non-Hodgkin lymphoma. And throughout all of the book chapters, updates have been made to reflect the latest information about cancer treatment and data on ongoing and new clinical trials.

This 10th volume also provides information on some of the oncology drugs that are listed below, which are newly approved or that have newly approved indications since the last edition was published, including anastrozole (Arimidex), bevacizumab (Avastin), bortezomib (Velcade), capecitabine (Xeloda), cetuximab (Erbitux), dasatinib (Sprycel), decitabine (Dacogen), docetaxel (Taxotere), erlotinib (Tarceva), exemestane (Aromasin), gefitinib (Iressa), gemcitabine (Gemzar), lapatinib (Tykerb), lenalidomide (Revlimid), letrozole (Femara), nelarabine (Arranon), panitumumab (Vectibix), pegaspargase (Oncaspar), rituximab (Rituxan), sorafenib (Nexavar), sunitinib (Sutent), thalidomide (Thalomid), topotecan (Hycamtin), trastuzumab (Herceptin), and vorinostat (Zolinza).

The 47 chapters and 4 Appendices in this newest edition represent the efforts of over 100 contributors from approximately 50 institutions in the United States and Canada.

Three consistent goals continue to guide our editorial policies:

- To provide practical information for physicians who manage cancer patients
- To present this information concisely, uniformly, and logically, emphasizing the natural history of the malignancy, screening and diagnosis, staging and prognosis, and treatment
- To emphasize a collaborative multidisciplinary approach to patient management that involves surgical, radiation, and medical oncologists, as well as other health care professionals, working as a cohesive team.

As with all previous annual editions, each chapter (as appropriate) in the current volume has been authored jointly by practicing medical, surgical, and radiation oncologists. In some cases, other specialists have been asked to contribute their expertise to a particular chapter.

All of our contributors personally manage patients using a multidisciplinary approach in their respective institutions. Thus, these chapters reflect the recommendations of practitioners cognizant that decisions and recommendations regarding therapies must be founded on evidence-based research directed at practical patient care in a cost-effective manner.

To write, edit, and publish this 1,000+-page text requires the dedication of all of the authors, as well as a professional publication staff to coordinate the technical aspects of editing and publishing. We, the authors and editors, acknowledge the following individuals: especially Angela Cibuls, Project Manager for the book; Susan Reckling, Managing Editor of the volume; Stacey Cuozzo, Production Editor; Cara Glynn, Senior Editorial Director; Jeannine Coronna, Publishing Operations Director; Beth Scholz, Publisher; and Melissa Warner, Group Vice President/General Manager of the Oncology Publishing Group of CMP Healthcare Media. We also thank Andrea Bovee, Christina Fennessey, Terri Gelfand, Lisa Katz, Claudine Kiffer, Anne Landry, Andrew Nash, and Ronald Piana for their efforts.

Richard Pazdur, MD
Office of Oncology Drug Products
Center for Drug Evaluation and Research
US Food and Drug Administration

Lawrence R. Coia, MD
Southern Ocean County Radiation Oncology
Manahawkin, New Jersey

William J. Hoskins, MD
Curtis and Elizabeth Anderson Cancer Institute
Memorial Health University Medical Center
Savannah, Georgia

Lawrence D. Wagman, MD
Division of Surgery
City of Hope National Medical Center
Duarte, California

CHAPTER 1

Principles of surgical oncology

Lawrence D. Wagman, MD

Surgical oncology, as its name suggests, is the specific application of surgical principles to the oncologic setting. These principles have been derived by adapting standard surgical approaches to the unique situations that arise when treating cancer patients.

The surgeon is often the first specialist to see the patient with a solid malignancy, and, in the course of therapy, he or she may be called upon to provide diagnostic, therapeutic, palliative, and supportive care. In each of these areas, guiding paradigms that are unique to surgical oncology are employed.

In addition, the surgical oncologist must be knowledgeable about all of the available surgical and adjuvant therapies, both standard and experimental, for a particular cancer. This enables the surgeon not only to explain the various treatment options to the patient but also to perform the initial steps in diagnosis and treatment in such a way as to facilitate and avoid interfering with future therapeutic options.

Invasive diagnostic modalities

As the surgeon approaches the patient with a solid malignancy or abnormal nodal disease or the rare individual with a tissue-based manifestation of a leukemia, selection of a diagnostic approach that will have a high likelihood of a specific, accurate diagnosis is paramount. The advent of high-quality invasive diagnostic approaches guided by radiologic imaging modalities has limited the open surgical approach to those situations where the disease is inaccessible, a significant amount of tissue is required for diagnosis, or a percutaneous approach is too dangerous (due, for example, to a bleeding diathesis, critical intervening structures, or the potential for unacceptable complications, such as pneumothorax).

Lymph node biopsy

The usual indication for biopsy of the lymph node is to establish the diagnosis of lymphoma or metastatic carcinoma. Each situation should be approached in a different manner.

Lymphoma The goal of biopsy in the patient with an abnormal lymph node and suspected lymphoma is to make the general diagnosis and to establish the lymphoma type and subtype. Additional analyses of the cells in the node, its internal architecture, and the subpopulations of cells are critical for subsequent treatment. Although advances in immunocytochemical and histochemical analyses have been made, adequate tissue is the key element in accurate diagnosis.

Consequently, the initial diagnosis of lymphoma should be made on a completely excised node that has been minimally manipulated to ensure that there is little crush damage. When primary lymphoma is suspected, the use of needle aspiration does not consistently allow for the complete analyses described above and can lead to incomplete or inaccurate diagnosis and treatment delays.

When recurrent lymphoma is the primary diagnosis, the analysis of specific cell type is important for assessing changes in the type of lymphoma and whether a transformation has occurred. In the rare situation in which recurrent Hodgkin lymphoma is suspected, a core biopsy may be adequate if the classic Reed-Sternberg cells are identified. However, in the initial and recurrent settings, biopsy of an intact node is often required.

Carcinoma The diagnosis of metastatic carcinoma often requires less tissue than is needed for lymphoma. Fine-needle aspiration (FNA), core biopsy, or subtotal removal of a single node will be adequate in this situation. For metastatic disease, the surgeon will use a combination of factors, such as location of the node, physical examination, and symptoms, to predict the site of primary disease. When this information is communicated to the pathologist, the pathologic evaluation can be focused on the most likely sites so as to obtain the highest diagnostic yield. The use of immunocytochemical analyses can be successful in defining the primary site, even on small amounts of tissue.

Head and neck adenopathy The head and neck region is a common site of palpable adenopathy that poses a significant diagnostic dilemma. Nodal zones in this area serve as the harbinger of lymphoma (particularly Hodgkin lymphoma) and as sites of metastasis from the mucosal surfaces of the upper aerodigestive tract; nasopharynx; thyroid; lungs; and, occasionally, intra-abdominal sites, such as the stomach, liver, and pancreas.

Since treatment of these nodal metastases varies widely, and since subsequent treatments may be jeopardized by inconveniently placed biopsy incisions, the surgical oncologist must consider the most likely source of the disease prior to performing the biopsy. FNA or core biopsy becomes a valuable tool in this situation, as the tissue sample is usually adequate for basic analysis (cytologic or histologic), and special studies (eg, immunocytochemical analyses) can be performed as needed.

Biopsy of a tissue-based mass

Several principles must be considered when approaching the seemingly simple task of biopsying a tissue-based mass. As each of the biopsy methods has unique risks, yields, and costs, the initial choice can be a critical factor in the timeliness and expense of the diagnostic process. It is crucial that the physician charged with making the invasive diagnosis be mindful of these factors.

Mass in the aerodigestive tract In the aerodigestive tract, biopsy of a lesion should include a representative amount of tissue taken preferably from the periphery of the lesion, where the maximum amount of viable malignant cells will be present. Since the treatment of in situ and invasive disease varies greatly, the biopsy must be of adequate depth to determine penetration of the tumors. This is particularly true for carcinomas of the oral cavity, pharynx, and larynx.

Breast mass Although previously a common procedure, an open surgical biopsy of the breast is rarely indicated today. Palpable breast masses that are highly suspicious (as indicated by physical findings and mammography) can be diagnosed as malignant with close to 100% accuracy with FNA. However, because the distinction between invasive and noninvasive disease is often required prior to the initiation of treatment, a core biopsy, performed either under image guidance (ultrasonography or mammography) or directly for palpable lesions, is the method of choice.

An excellent example of the interdependence of the method of tissue diagnosis and therapeutic options is the patient with a moderate-sized breast tumor considering breast conservation who chooses preoperative chemotherapy for downsizing of the breast lesion. The core biopsy method establishes the histologic diagnosis, provides adequate tissue for analyses of hormone-receptor levels and other risk factors, causes little or no cosmetic damage, does not perturb sentinel node analyses, and does not require extended healing prior to the initiation of therapy. In addition, a small radio-opaque clip can be placed in the tumor to guide the surgical extirpation. This step is important because excellent treatment responses can make it difficult for the surgeon to localize the original tumor site.

Mass in the trunk or extremities For soft-tissue or bony masses of the trunk or extremities, the biopsy technique should be selected on the basis of the planned subsequent tumor resection. The incision should be made along anatomic lines in the trunk or along the long axis of the extremity. When a sarcoma is suspected, FNA can establish the diagnosis of malignancy, but a core biopsy will likely be required to determine the histologic type and plan neoadjuvant therapy.

Preoperative evaluation

As with any surgical patient, the preoperative evaluation of the cancer patient hinges primarily on the individual's underlying medical condition(s). Because most new cancers occur in older patients, careful attention must be paid to evaluation of cardiovascular risks. Adequate information can usually be obtained from a standard history, physical examination, and electrocardiogram (ECG), but any concerns identified should be subjected to a full diagnostic work-up.

The evaluation should also include a detailed history of current and previous therapies. Many patients will be on anticoagulation, aspirin, or analgesics, all of which may impact on their perioperative management. Previous use of doxorubicin may be associated with cardiac dysfunction and the use of bleomycin with severe lung sensitivity to oxygen concentrations > 30%. Due to the association of bowel anastomotic perforation with the use of bevacizumab (Avastin), the timing of colonic surgery should be modified.

Prior radiation therapy is associated with fibrosis and delayed healing. An appreciation of potential postoperative problems secondary to these factors is important in planning the surgical extirpation and reconstruction. For example, in a patient who requires mastectomy after failed breast-conserving surgery, the zone of tissue damage from the original radiation therapy can be assessed by reviewing the port and boost site films or by examining the irradiated site for tattoo marks used to align the radiation field. Plans for resection of heavily irradiated tissues should be made preoperatively in concert with the reconstructive surgeon, and the relative increased risk of postoperative problems should be discussed with the patient. This evaluation should include the type of tissue to be transferred, analysis of potential donor and recipient sites and vessels, and assurance that the appropriate microvascular equipment is available, in the event that it is needed during surgery.

Pathologic confirmation of the diagnosis

The treatment of cancer is based almost exclusively on the organ of origin and, to a lesser degree, on the histologic subtype. Unless the operative procedure is being performed to make a definitive diagnosis, review of the pathologic material is needed to confirm the diagnosis preoperatively.

There are few exceptions to this doctrine, and it behooves the surgeon to have a confirmed diagnosis, including the in situ or invasive nature of the cancer, prior to performing an operation. This tenet assumes paramount importance when one is performing procedures for which there is no recourse once the specimen is removed, eg, laryngectomy, mastectomy, removal of the anal sphincter, and extremity amputation.

Ironically, in some situations, a preoperative or intraoperative diagnosis cannot be confirmed, despite the fact that the preoperative and intraoperative physical findings, laboratory data, and radiologic studies (pre- and intraoperative) overwhelmingly suggested the cancer diagnosis. The classic example of this dilemma is the jaundiced patient with a firm mass in the pancreatic head. The Whipple procedure (pancreaticoduodenectomy) causes significant morbidity but is required to make the diagnosis and treat the cancer. In any of these situations, the preoperative discussion with the patient must include the possibility that the final diagnosis may be a benign lesion.

Resection

The principles of resection for malignant disease are based on the surgical goal (complete resection vs debulking), functional significance of the involved organ or structure, and the ability to reconstruct the involved and surrounding structures. Also important are the technical abilities of the surgeon or availability of a surgical team, adequacy of neoadjuvant and adjuvant therapies, and the biologic behavior (local and systemic) of the disease. Although "operable" is used to describe the physiologic status of the patient, the definition of "resectable" varies, and this term can be defined only in the context of the aforementioned modifying parameters.

Wide excision

A wide excision includes the removal of the tumor itself and a margin of normal tissue, usually exceeding 1 cm in all directions from the tumor. The margin is variable in a large, complex (multiple tissue compartments) specimen, and the limiting point of the resection is defined by the closest approximation of cancerous tissue to the normal tissue that is excised.

Wide margins are recommended for tumors with a high likelihood of local recurrence (eg, dermatofibrosarcoma protuberans) and for tumors without any reliable adjuvant therapeutic options.

Breast The use of adjuvant radiation therapy has permitted the use of breast-conserving surgery, which limits the excision of wide margins of normal breast tissue.

Colon and rectum For carcinoma of the colon and rectum, the width of excision is defined by the longitudinal portion of the bowel and the inclusion of adjacent nodal tissue. The principles of wide resection require removal of normal bowel (including at least 5 cm of uninvolved tissue), the associated mesenteric leaf, and adjacent rectal soft tissue (mesorectum).

This general principle has been modified in the distal rectum, where lateral margins are maintained using the principles of mesorectal excision, and longitudinal bowel margins of 2 cm are accepted. This modification reflects the emphasis on functional results (ie, maintenance of anal continence) and the availability of neoadjuvant (preoperative chemotherapy and irradiation) therapy to reduce the tumor size and resectability and postoperative adjuvant radiation therapy and chemotherapy to improve local control.

No touch technique

This principle is based on the concept that direct contact with and manipulation of the tumor during resection can lead to an increase in local implantation and embolization of tumor cells, respectively. Theoretically, the metastatic potential of the primary lesion would be enhanced by the mechanical extrusion of tumor cells into local lymphatic and vascular spaces. There may be some validity to this theory with respect to tumors that extend directly into the venous system (eg, renal cell tumors with extension to the vena cava) or those that extensively involve local venous drainage (eg, large hepatocellular carcinomas).

Extensive palpation and manipulation of a colorectal primary have been shown to result in direct shedding of tumor cells into the lumen of the large bowel. The traditional strategy to lessen this risk was to ligate the proximal and distal lumen of the segment containing the tumor early in the resection. These areas were then included in the resection, limiting the contact of shed tumor cells with the planned anastomotic areas.

Neither of the previous theoretical situations (ie, manipulation of the tumor and direct contact of the tumor with the anastomotic area) has been definitively tested in controlled, prospective, randomized trials. Therefore, the risk-benefit ratio should favor adherence to the general principles of minimal tumor manipulation, protection of the anastomotic areas, and exclusion of the resection bed from potential implantation with tumor cells.

The minimally invasive surgical techniques introduced approximately 20 years ago were incorporated into the surgical procedures for a non-oncologic scenario–cholecystectomy, hiatal and inguinal hernia repair, and treatment of benign diseases of the female reproductive tract. Transfer of the technology to the oncologic setting was met with resistance, as questions of technical (number of nodes resected and less tactile input during resection) and therapeutic (local control, disease-free survival, and overall survival) equivalence were raised.

Careful clinical research has answered these initial reservations for colon cancer. Results from a prospective randomized trial reported by the Laparoscopic Colectomy (LC) trial group documented that although the laparoscopic operations took longer than the open procedures (150 vs 95 minutes), there was no difference in the margins obtained, the 30-day mortality, or the complication rate. LC resulted in a shorter overall hospital stay (4 vs 5 days) and less use of parenteral narcotics (3 vs 4 days) than the open procedure. There was no difference identified for the oncologic outcomes of disease-free recurrence or overall survival.

Examples in colon cancer will serve as paradigms for the study of other tumors. The introduction of the da Vinci robotic system has opened new areas for technical investigation and evaluation of operative outcomes. Expansion of minimally invasive techniques (laparoscopic and robotic-assisted), with preservation of oncologic principles and improvement in patients' quality-of-life outcomes, will drive surgical interventions.

Lymphadenectomy

Early surgical oncologic theory proposed that breast cancer progressed from the primary site to the axillary lymph nodes to the supraclavicular nodes and nodes of the neck. This theory led to the radical surgical approach that included resection of all of the breast tissue and some or all of the above-noted draining nodal basins (ie, modified radical, radical, or extended radical mastectomy).

Absent from this approach was an appreciation of the nodes not only as a deposit of regional metastatic disease but also as a predictor of systemic disease. Modern treatment approaches view nodal dissection as having a triple purpose: the surgical removal of regional metastases, the prediction of prognosis, and the planning of adjuvant therapy.

The surgical technique and boundaries for lymphadenectomy are based on nodal basins that are defined by consistent anatomic structures. For example, dissection of the neck is defined by the mandible, anterior strap muscles of the neck, clavicle, trapezius muscle, carotid artery, vagus nerve, brachial plexus, and fascia overlying the deep muscles of the neck.

Modifications of classic techniques Each of the classic anatomic lymphadenectomies has been modified along lines that consider the predicted positivity and functional impact of the dissection. To use the example of radical neck dissection, the modifications include supraomohyoid dissection for tumors of the floor of the mouth (a high-risk zone) and sparing of the spinal accessory nerve (functional prevention of shoulder drop and loss of full abduction of the shoulder).

Sentinel node biopsy

As alluded to in the previous paragraphs, lymph node dissection has therapeutic value only in patients with positive nodes. In individuals with pathologically negative nodes, the benefit is limited to prediction of prognosis and documentation of pathologic negativity. Therefore, in the pathologically negative nodal basin, there is minimal benefit to outweigh the risks and untoward sequelae of the dissection.

Technique The technique of sentinel node identification has been developed to address clinically negative nodal basins. With this technique, the node or nodes that preferentially drain a particular primary tumor are identified by mapping and then surgically excised. The mapping agents include radiolabeled materials and vital dyes that are specifically taken up by, and transported in, the lymphatic drainage systems. These mapping and localizing agents, used alone or in combination, are critical in defining the unique flow patterns to specific lymph node(s) and ambiguous drainage patterns (eg, a truncal melanoma that may drain to the axilla, supraclavicular, or inguinal spaces).

Unresolved issues As this field of directed diagnostic node biopsy and dissection develops, many technical issues related to the timing and location of the injection sites are being evaluated. In addition, the type of pathologic evaluation (ie, the number of sections examined per node and the use of immunohistochemical analysis) is undergoing intense scrutiny.

A study of 200 consecutive patients who had sentinel lymph node biopsies performed for breast cancer examined the concepts of injecting dye and radioactive tracer into either the breast or the overlying dermis. The authors believed that the technical aspects of intradermal injection were simpler and more easily reproduced than those of injections into the breast. Injections were performed in group 1 intraparenchymally and in group 2 intradermally. The combination of blue dye and isotope localization produced a 92% success rate in group 1 and a 100% success rate in group 2. The authors concluded that dermal and parenchymal lymphatics of the breast drain to the same lymph node and that the more simple approach of dermal injection may simplify and optimize sentinel lymph node localization.

For melanoma, for which these techniques were originally developed, researchers are studying the feasibility and clinical relevance of evaluating nodal material with polymerase chain reaction (PCR) techniques. These techniques are also being studied in breast cancer, where the clinical relevance (indication for adjuvant therapy) of the presence of micrometastases or PCR-only metastases is highly controversial and, therefore, questions the need for this intense level of pathologic scrutiny.

Elective lymph node dissection has limited value in intermediate-thickness melanoma. In clinically node-negative patients, the use of the sentinel node technique can avoid postoperative complications, increase confidence about the better prognosis, and avoid the significant side effects of adjuvant immunologic therapy. However, the identification of histologically positive nodes via sentinel node biopsy is expected to have significant benefit in consideration of therapeutic node dissection and systemic therapies. In contrast, for patients with sentinel node–positive breast cancer, the value of completing a level I, II axillary node dissection is uncertain. This important question is being examined in two national, prospective clinical trials.

Palliation

In the continuum of care for the cancer patient, aspects of palliation, or the reduction of suffering, are delegated to the surgeon. This text includes many examples of palliative surgical procedures: venous access, surgical relief of ascites with shunt procedures, neurosurgical intervention for chronic pain, fixation of pathologic fractures, and placement of feeding tubes to deliver food and medications. The surgeon must be versed in the techniques of and indications for such interventions and discuss their risks and benefits with the patient, caregivers, and referring physician. The barriers to the initiation and practice of palliative surgery include the reluctance of patients, family, and referring physicians; health care system administrative obstacles; and cultural factors. A "therapeutic index" (time spent receiving treatment for symptoms vs time symptom free) should be constructed and discussed during the benefit/risk, informed consent process.

Resuscitation issues An ethical issue of resuscitation must be addressed when considering palliative surgical intervention. Some may take the position that if a patient is to have surgery, he or she must be willing to undergo full resuscitation if required. That tenet may be set aside in the palliative setting, in which the operative intervention is planned only to relieve suffering. In such a case, a frank discussion with the patient and appropriate family members can avoid the distressing situation of the patient being placed on unwanted, fruitless life support. Again, the surgeon is called upon not only to provide a technical service but also to achieve a comprehensive understanding of the disease process and how it affects each individual cancer patient.

SUGGESTED READING

Fortner JG: Inadvertent spread of cancer at surgery: Incidence and outcomes. J Surg Oncol 53:191–196, 1993.

Krouse RS, Nelson RA, Farrell BR, et al: Surgical palliation at a cancer center. Arch Surg 136:773–778, 2001.

McCahill LE, Krouse R, Chu D, et al: Indications and use of palliative surgery–results of Society of Surgical Oncology survey. Ann Surg Oncol 9:104–112, 2002.

McIntosh SA, Purushotham AD: Lymphatic mapping and sentinel node biopsy in breast cancer. Br J Surg 85:1347–1356, 1998.

The Clinical Outcomes of Surgical Therapy Study Group: A comparison of laparoscopically assisted and open colectomy for colon cancer. N Engl J Med 350:2050–2059, 2004.

CHAPTER 2

Principles of radiation therapy

Michael J. Gazda, MS, and Lawrence R. Coia, MD

RADIATION THERAPY

This chapter provides a brief overview of the principles of radiation therapy. The topics to be discussed include the physical aspects of how radiation works (ionization, radiation interactions) and how it is delivered (treatment machines, treatment planning, and brachytherapy). Recent relevant techniques of radiation oncology, such as conformal and stereotactic radiation therapy, also will be presented. These topics are not covered in great technical detail, and no attempt is made to discuss the radiobiological effects of radiation therapy. It is hoped that a basic understanding of radiation treatment will benefit those practicing in other disciplines of cancer management. This chapter does not address principles of radiobiology, which guide radiation oncologists in determining issues of treatment time, dose, and fractionation or in combining radiation with sensitizers, protectors, and chemotherapy or hormones.

How radiation works

IONIZING RADIATION

Ionizing radiation is energy sufficiently strong to remove an orbital electron from an atom. This radiation can have an electromagnetic form, such as a high-energy photon, or a particulate form, such as an electron, proton, neutron, or alpha particle.

High-energy photons By far, the most common form of radiation used in practice today is the high-energy photon. Photons that are released from the nucleus of a radioactive atom are known as gamma rays. When photons are created electronically, such as in a clinical linear accelerator, they are known as x-rays. Thus, the only difference between the two terms is the origin of the photon.

Inverse square law The intensity of an x-ray beam is governed by the inverse square law. This law states that the radiation intensity from a point source is inversely proportional to the square of the distance away from the radiation source. In other words, the dose at 2 cm will be one-fourth of the dose at 1 cm.

Electron volt Photon absorption in human tissue is determined by the energy of the radiation, as well as the atomic structure of the tissue in question. The basic unit of energy used in radiation oncology is the electron volt (eV); 10^3 eV = 1 keV, 10^6 eV = 1 MeV.

PHOTON-TISSUE INTERACTIONS

Three interactions describe photon absorption in tissue: the photoelectric effect, Compton effect, and pair production.

Photoelectric effect In this process, an incoming photon undergoes a collision with a tightly bound electron. The photon transfers practically all of its energy to the electron and ceases to exist. The electron departs with most of the energy from the photon and begins to ionize surrounding molecules. This interaction depends on the energy of the incoming photon, as well as the atomic number of the tissue; the lower the energy and the higher the atomic number, the more likely that a photoelectric effect will take place.

An example of this interaction in practice can be seen on a diagnostic x-ray film. Since the atomic number of bone is 60% higher than that of soft tissue, bone is seen with much more contrast and detail than is soft tissue. The energy range in which the photoelectric effect predominates in tissue is about 10–25 keV.

Compton effect The Compton effect is the most important photon-tissue interaction for the treatment of cancer. In this case, a photon collides with a "free electron," ie, one that is not tightly bound to the atom. Unlike the photoelectric effect, in the Compton interaction both the photon and electron are scattered. The photon can then continue to undergo additional interactions, albeit with a lower energy. The electron begins to ionize with the energy given to it by the photon.

The probability of a Compton interaction is inversely proportional to the energy of the incoming photon and is independent of the atomic number of the material. When one takes an image of tissue using photons in the energy range in which the Compton effect dominates (~25 keV–25 MeV), bone and soft-tissue interfaces are barely distinguishable. This is a result of the atomic number independence.

The Compton effect is the most common interaction occurring clinically, as most radiation treatments are performed at energy levels of about 6–20 MeV. Port films are films taken with such high-energy photons on the treatment machine and are used to check the precision and accuracy of the beam; because they do not distinguish tissue densities well, however, they are not equal to diagnostic films in terms of resolution.

Pair production In this process, a photon interacts with the nucleus of an atom, not an orbital electron. The photon gives up its energy to the nucleus and, in the process, creates a pair of positively and negatively charged electrons. The positive electron (positron) ionizes until it combines with a free electron. This generates two photons that scatter in opposite directions.

The probability of pair production is proportional to the logarithm of the energy of the incoming photon and is dependent on the atomic number of the material. The energy range in which pair production dominates is $\geq$ 25 MeV. This interaction occurs to some extent in routine radiation treatment with high-energy photon beams.

ELECTRON BEAMS

With the advent of high-energy linear accelerators, electrons have become a viable option in treating superficial tumors up to a depth of about 5 cm. Electron depth dose characteristics are unique in that they produce a high skin dose but exhibit a falloff after only a few centimeters.

Electron absorption in human tissue is greatly influenced by the presence of air cavities and bone. The dose is increased when the electron beam passes through an air space and is reduced when the beam passes through bone.

Common uses The most common clinical uses of electron beams include the treatment of skin lesions, such as basal cell carcinomas, and boosting of areas that have previously received photon irradiation, such as the postoperative lumpectomy or mastectomy scar in breast cancer patients, as well as select nodal areas in the head and neck.

MEASURING RADIATION ABSORPTION

The dose of radiation absorbed correlates directly with the energy of the beam. An accurate measurement of absorbed dose is critical in radiation treatment. The deposition of energy in tissues results in damage to DNA and diminishes or eradicates the cell's ability to replicate indefinitely.

Gray The basic unit of radiation absorbed dose is the amount of energy (joules) absorbed per unit mass (kg). This unit, known as the gray (Gy), has replaced the unit of rad used in the past (100 rads = 1 Gy; 1 rad = 1 cGy).

Exposure To measure dose in a patient, one must first measure the ionization produced in air by a beam of radiation. This quantity is known as exposure. One can then correct for the presence of soft tissue in the air and calculate the absorbed dose in Gy.

Percentage depth dose The dose absorbed by tissues due to these interactions can be measured and plotted to form a percentage depth dose curve. As energy increases, the penetrative ability of the beam increases and the skin dose decreases.

How radiation is delivered

TREATMENT MACHINES

Linear accelerators

High-energy radiation is delivered to tumors by means of a linear accelerator. A beam of electrons is generated and accelerated through a waveguide that increases their energy to the keV to MeV range. These electrons strike a tungsten target and produce x-rays.

X-rays generated in the 10–30-keV range are known as grenz rays, whereas the energy range for superficial units is about 30–125 keV. Orthovoltage units generate x-rays from 125–500 keV.

Orthovoltage units continue to be used today to treat superficial lesions; in fact, they were practically the only machines treating skin lesions before the recent emergence of electron therapy. The maximum dose from any of these low-energy units is found on the surface of patients; thus, skin becomes the dose-limiting structure when treating patients at these energies. The depth at which the dose is 50% of the maximum is about 7 cm. Table 1 lists the physical characteristics of several relevant x-ray energies.

Megavoltage units The megavoltage linear accelerator has been the standard radiotherapy equipment for the past 20 to 30 years. Its production of x-rays is identical to that of lower-energy machines. However, the energy range of megavoltage units is broad–from 4 to 20 MeV. The depth of the maximum dose in this energy range is 1.5–3.5 cm. The dose to the skin is about 30%-40% of the maximum dose.

Most megavoltage units today also have electron-beam capabilities, usually in the energy range of about 5–20 MeV. To produce an electron beam, the tungsten target is moved away from the path of the beam. The original electron beam that was aimed at the tungsten target is now the electron beam used for treatment. Unlike that of photons, the electron skin dose is high, about 80%–95% of the maximum dose. A rule of thumb regarding the depth of penetration of electrons is that 80% of the dose is delivered at a depth (in cm) corresponding to one-third of the electron energy (in MeV). Thus, a 12-MeV beam will deliver 80% of the dose at a depth of 4 cm.

Altering beam intensity and field size When measurements are made at the point just past the target, the beam is more intense in the center than at the edges. Optimal treatment planning is obtained with a relatively constant intensity across the width of the beam. This process is accomplished by placing a flattening filter below the target.

For the radiation beam to conform to a certain size, high atomic number collimators are installed in the machine. They can vary the field size from 4 × 4 cm to 40 × 40 cm at a distance of 100 cm from the target, which is the distance at which most treatments are performed.

TABLE 1: Depth dose characteristics for clinical radiotherapy beams

Nominal energy	Depth of maximum dose (cm)	Skin dose (%)
240 kV(p)	Surface	100
Cobalt-60	0.500	50
6 MeV	1.500	35
10 MeV	2.500	25
18 MeV	3.000	15

kV(p) = kilovolt (peak)

If it is decided that a beam should be more intense on one side than the other, high atomic number filters, known as wedges, are placed in the beam. These filters can shift the dose distribution surrounding the tumor by 15°–60°. Wedges can also be used to optimize the dose distribution if the treatment surface is curved or irregular.

Shielding normal tissue Once the collimators have been opened to the desired field size that encompasses the tumor, the physician may decide to block out some normal tissue that remains in the treatment field. This is accomplished by placing blocks (or alloy), constructed of a combination of bismuth, tin, cadmium, and lead, in the path of the beam. In this way, normal tissues are shielded, and the dose can be delivered to the tumor at a higher level than if the normal structures were in the field. These individually constructed blocks are used in both x-ray and electron treatments. A more modern technique involves multileaf collimators mounted inside the gantry. They provide computerized, customized blocking instead of having to construct a new block for each field. (See section on "Intensity-modulated radiation therapy.")

PRETREATMENT PROCEDURES

Certain imaging procedures must be performed before radiation therapy is begun.

Pretreatment CT Before any treatment planning can begin, a pretreatment CT scan is often performed. This scan allows the radiation oncologist to identify both the tumor and surrounding normal structures.

Simulation The patient is then sent for a simulation. The patient is placed on a diagnostic x-ray unit that geometrically simulates an actual treatment machine. With use of the CT information, the patient's treatment position is simulated by means of fluoroscopy. A series of orthogonal films are taken, and block templates that will shield any normal structures are drawn on the films. These films are sent to the mold room, where technicians construct the blocks to be used for treatment. CT simulation is a modern alternative to "conventional" simulation and is described later in this chapter.

Guides for treatment field placement Small skin marks, or tattoos, are placed on the patient following proper positioning in simulation. These tattoos will guide the placement of treatment fields and give the physician a permanent record of past fields should the patient need additional treatment in the future.

It is imperative that the patient be treated in a reproducible manner each day. To facilitate this, Styrofoam casts that conform to the patient's contour and place the patient in the same position for each treatment are constructed. Lasers also help line up the patient during treatment.

TREATMENT PLANNING AND DELIVERY

Determining optimal dose distribution The medical physicist or dosimetrist uses the information from CT and simulation to plan the treatment on a computer. A complete collection of machine data, including depth dose and beam profile information, is stored in the computer. The physics staff aids the radiation oncologist in deciding the number of beams (usually two to four) and angles of entry. The goal is to maximize the dose to the tumor while minimizing the dose to surrounding normal structures.

Several treatment plans are generated, and the radiation oncologist chooses the optimal dose distribution. The beam-modifying devices discussed earlier, such as blocks and wedges, may be used to optimize the dose distribution around the tumor.

Establishing the treatment plan The planning computer will calculate the amount of time each beam should be on during treatment. All pertinent data, such as beam-on time, beam angles, blocks, and wedges, are recorded in the patient's treatment chart and sent to the treatment machine. The radiation therapist will use this information, as well as any casts, tattoos, and lasers, to set up and treat the patient consistently and accurately each day.

Taking weekly port films As part of departmental quality assurance, weekly port films are taken for each beam. They ensure that the beams and blocks are consistently and correctly placed for each treatment. Port films are images generated by the linear accelerator at energies of 6–20 MeV. Because of the predominance of the Compton effect in this energy range, these images are not as detailed as those at diagnostic film energies (as mentioned earlier), but they still provide important information on treatment accuracy and ensure the quality of setup and treatment.

BRACHYTHERAPY

Brachytherapy is the term used to describe radiation treatment in which the radiation source is in contact with the tumor. This therapy contrasts with external-beam radiotherapy, in which the radiation source is 80–100 cm away from the patient.

In brachytherapy, dose distribution is almost totally dependent on the inverse square law because the source is usually within the tumor volume. Because of this inverse square dependence, the proper placement of radiation sources is crucial.

Isotopes Table 2 lists commonly used isotopes and their properties. In the past, radium was the primary isotope used in brachytherapy. Recently, because of its long half-life and high energy output, radium has been replaced with cesium (Cs), gold (Au), and iridium (Ir). These isotopes have shorter half-lives than radium and can be shielded more easily because of their lower energies.

Types of implants Brachytherapy procedures can be performed with either temporary or permanent implants. Temporary implants usually have long half-lives and higher energies than permanent implants. These sources can be manufactured in several forms, such as needles, seeds, and ribbons.

All temporary sources are inserted into catheters that are placed in the tumor during surgery. A few days after surgery, the patient is brought to the radiation clinic and undergoes pretreatment simulation. Wires with nonradioactive metal

TABLE 2: Physical characteristics of commonly used radioisotopes

Isotope	Energy (MeV)	Half-life
Radium-226	0.830	1,600 yr
Cesium-137	0.662	30 yr
Cobalt-60	1.250	5.26 yr
Iridium-192	0.380	74.2 d
Iodine-125	0.028	60.2 d
Gold-198	0.412	2.7 d
Palladium-103	0.210	17d

seeds are threaded into these catheters. Several films are taken, and the images of the seed placement can be digitized into a brachytherapy treatment planning computer.

Once the treatment plan is complete and the physician has chosen the optimal dose rate (usually 50–60 cGy/h), the sources can be implanted. The actual implantation takes place in the patient's private room. The duration of treatment is usually 1 to 3 days. The majority of temporary implants are loaded interstitially.

Common uses Interstitial low-dose–rate (LDR) brachytherapy is commonly used for cancer of the oral cavity and oropharynx and sarcoma. Prostate cancer is probably the most common site for which LDR brachytherapy "seeds" are used today. Intracavitary LDR brachytherapy is frequently used in gynecologic applications. High-dose–rate (HDR) brachytherapy is used with remote afterloading techniques, as described below.

Remote afterloading brachytherapy

Because brachytherapy requires numerous safety precautions and entails unnecessary exposure of personnel and family members to radiation, remote afterloading of temporary implants has become popular in recent years. The two types of remote afterloading that can be used for treatment are LDR and HDR sources. The most popular LDR source used today is Cs-137, which has a dose rate of about 1 cGy/min. The most widely used HDR source is Ir-192. This isotope has a dose rate of about 100 cGy/min.

General procedures The pretreatment brachytherapy procedures outlined above are also implemented in remote afterloading brachytherapy. Once the treatment plan has been approved by the physician, the patient is brought into the treatment room. The LDR cesium source or HDR iridium source is connected to the end of a cable inside its respective afterloading unit. This unit is programmed with the data from the planning computer. The cable is sent out from the unit into one of the patient's catheters. Several catheters can be connected to the unit. Each catheter is irradiated, one at a time, until the prescribed dose has been delivered.

The motor that drives the source out of the treatment unit is connected electronically to the door of the treatment room. If the treatment must be stopped for any reason, simply opening the door triggers an interlock that draws the source back into the unit. Because of this device, oncology personnel will not be exposed to any radiation should they need to see the patient during treatment. This interlock is the main safety advantage of remote afterloading over manual afterloading.

LDR treatment Uterine cancer is the most popular application for intracavitary treatment with LDR remote afterloading brachytherapy. These procedures are performed in the patient's room. The interlock is connected to the patient's door so that nurses can take vital signs and give medication and family members can visit the patient without risk of radiation exposure.

HDR treatment The most common applications of HDR brachytherapy are for tumors of the vaginal apex, esophagus, lungs, and, most recently, breasts and prostate. Most HDR treatments are performed on an outpatient basis. Allowing the patient to return home the same day after therapy is one advantage of HDR afterloading brachytherapy. Patients with prostate cancer are the exception. They may remain in the hospital for 2 to 3 days during treatment.

Recent advances in planning and treatment

CT SIMULATION

Until recently, CT and simulation were separate pretreatment procedures. Within the past decade, many cancer centers have combined CT and simulation into a single diagnostic-treatment planning unit, known as a CT simulator. The major advantage of this combination is that both procedures can be performed by one unit, and, thus, the patient does not have to make two separate visits to the clinic. Also, CT simulation is bringing the radiation clinic into the digital age, with hospitals reporting an increase in speed, efficiency, and accuracy of treatment planning and delivery.

Procedure In brief, in the first step of this new procedure, the patient is placed on the CT simulator table and undergoes a normal CT study. The physician has the capability of outlining the tumor and any normal structures on each CT slice. A computer performs a three-dimensional (3D) transformation of the CT slices and creates a digitally reconstructed radiograph (DRR).

The DRR resembles a normal diagnostic film, except that it is digital and can be manipulated to achieve better contrast and detail than regular film. The outlines of the tumor and organs are displayed on the DRR for any viewing angle. The physician can then draw blocks on the DRR with a more accurate idea of where the tumor and normal tissues actually are.

The DRR is digitized into the treatment planning computer, and any CT slices and their contours drawn by the physician are transferred as well. This DRR is either sent to the mold room for block construction or is transferred to the treatment planning software for multileaf collimator optimization. Treatment plans are generated as discussed earlier.

At the time of the patient's first treatment, DRRs and port films are digitized and saved on a local area network (LAN). Physicians can then call up these images on their desktop computers for weekly patient quality assurance.

CONFORMAL RADIATION THERAPY

Conformal radiation therapy is a geometric shaping of the radiation beam that conforms with the beam's eye view of the tumor. Conformal therapy utilizes the outlining capabilities of the CT simulator. The physician outlines the tumor volume, generates DRRs, and draws an appropriate margin from 1–2 cm around the tumor. These fields conform closely to the shape of the tumor and, thus, shield more critical structures than do normal blocks. The margin allows for setup errors of a few millimeters each day. Appropriate immobilization of the target volume must be achieved in each patient through the use of devices that constrain movement ("casts"), so that the target is accurately localized.

Films are sent to the mold room for block construction. Since the fields are "tighter" around the tumor, the prescribed dose can be increased. By increasing the dose to the tumor, local control will be improved.

INTENSITY-MODULATED RADIATION THERAPY (IMRT)

Intensity-modulated radiation therapy (IMRT), an extension of conformal therapy, allows for shaping of the intensity of the radiation beam. This is an important improvement, especially when the target is not well separated from normal tissues.

A uniform dose distribution can be created around the tumor by either modulating the intensity of the beam during its journey through the linear accelerator or using multileaf collimators. Multileaf collimators consist of 80 or more individual collimators, or "leaves," located at the head of the linear accelerator, which can be adjusted to the shape of the tumor. (For a technical description, the reader is referred to the text by Khan; see "Suggested Reading.")

Both of these methods alter the fluence (the number of x-rays per unit area) of radiation exiting the accelerator. The final result is a uniform dose distribution around the tumor and minimal dose to the surrounding normal tissues, often below tolerance levels. This improves the risk-benefit ratio.

The clinical use of IMRT has grown as computer power increases and costs decline. Preliminary clinical data have shown that prostate doses can be increased significantly without increasing the complication rate. IMRT must be administered within a closely monitored program with rigorous quality assurance, since it can potentially cause significant injury if not appropriately applied.

Several types of IMRT delivery are now becoming standard in radiation oncology clinics. Dynamic conformal therapy with multileaf collimators is being used routinely in hospitals around the country. With this approach, collimators conform to the tumor volume with the beam on while the treatment unit is rotating around the patient. This is an example of totally computer-controlled radiation delivery.

TOMOTHERAPY

Serial tomotherapy is an enhancement of the method previously described. An accelerator is equipped with mini-multileaf collimators that form a "slit" of radiation (normally 2 × 20 cm). The gantry is rotated through an entire arc around the patient while the mini-multileaf collimators are driven in and out of the field, thus modulating the intensity of the beam. The treatment couch is advanced by a few millimeters and the next arc is treated. An entire treatment is given once all the adjoining arcs have been delivered.

Instead of treating the patient on a normal linear accelerator, with helical tomotherapy the patient travels continuously through a modified CT ring. This CT ring has the capability of administering 6-mV x-rays, as in a standard linear accelerator, while at the same time performing a conventional diagnostic CT scan. Any anatomic or position changes that might require replanning can be performed before that day's treatment. Following treatment, a daily, real-time image of the dose distribution can be obtained.

PROTON THERAPY

Protons, a form of particulate radiation, have been investigated recently as a means to improve tumor control. A proton has a charge of +1, is a stable particle, and, together with the neutron, makes up the atomic nucleus.

Protons are delivered to the tumor in the same manner as are photons and electrons. The dose deposited by protons remains relatively constant as they travel through the normal tissues proximal to the target.

The kinetic energy of the protons is transferred to the tumors by electrons knocked out of atoms. These electrons ionize DNA, and their biologic effectiveness resembles that of megavoltage photons.

Bragg peak At the end of the path, biologic effectiveness increases sharply as the protons slow down and eventually stop. This increase in dose is called the Bragg peak. The size of the Bragg peak is usually smaller than the tumor, however. This problem can be resolved by scanning the Bragg peak through the tumor volume by sequentially irradiating the target with lower energies. The dose falloff of the Bragg peak is sharp enough that the normal tissues distal to the tumor receive a negligible radiation dose.

Current clinical applications Uveal melanomas and skull-base sarcomas adjacent to CNS tissues, as well as prostate cancer, are areas in which proton therapy has been under clinical study, with promising results. Clinical studies are also examining its use in non–small-cell lung, hepatocellular, and paranasal sinus carcinomas.

STEREOTACTIC RADIOSURGERY

Stereotactic radiosurgery is a 3D technique that delivers the radiation dose in one fraction. Specially designed collimators are attached to a linear accelerator, which delivers a high dose of radiation to a small volume, usually about 3 cm in diameter. Several stationary beams or multiple arc rotations concentrate the radiation dose to the lesion while sparing surrounding normal tissue.

Although it is most often used to treat lesions within the brain, it can be used for selected extracranial sites (in which case it may be referred to as "**body radiosurgery**").

Use in treating arteriovenous malformations Stereotactic radiosurgery is used to treat certain patients with arteriovenous malformations. These intracranial lesions arise from the abnormal development of arteries and venous sinuses. Surgical excision is the standard treatment of choice for operable lesions, but stereotactic radiosurgery has become a viable option for inoperable malformations.

Use in treating brain tumors As with conformal radiotherapy, clinical trials involving stereotactic radiosurgery for brain tumors are being conducted at major cancer centers. However, based on positive early results, many community centers have begun instituting a stereotactic radiosurgery program, either with a dedicated cobalt unit (gamma knife) or a linear accelerator-based system. Small (< 4 cm) tumors of the brain, whether primary, metastatic, or recurrent, may benefit from this treatment technique. The gamma knife is a form of stereotactic radiosurgery that uses multiple focused cobalt beams to treat lesions in the brain.

SUGGESTED READING

Chao KSC: Practical Essentials of Intensity Modulated Radiation Therapy, 2nd edition. Philadelphia, Lippincott Williams & Wilkins, 2004.

Coia LR, Schultheiss TE, Hanks GE: A Practical Guide to CT Simulation. Madison, Wisconsin, Advanced Medical Publishing, 1995.

IMRT CWG: Intensity modulated radiotherapy: Current status and issues of interest. Int J Radiat Oncol Biol Phys 51:880–914, 2001.

Khan FM: Treatment Planning in Radiation Oncology. Baltimore, Maryland, Williams & Wilkins, 1998.

Perez CA, Brady LW: Principles and Practice of Radiation Oncology. Philadelphia, Lippincott-Raven, 1998.

Suit H: The Gray Lecture: Coming technical advances in radiation oncology. Int J Radiat Oncol Biol Phys 53:798–809, 2002.

Van Dyk J: The Modern Technology of Radiation Oncology. Madison, Wisconsin, Medical Physics Publishing, 1999.

CHAPTER 3

Principles of oncologic pharmacotherapy

Chris H. Takimoto, MD, PhD, and Emiliano Calvo, MD, PhD

PHARMACOTHERAPY

The effective use of cancer chemotherapy requires a thorough understanding of the principles of neoplastic cell growth kinetics, basic pharmacologic mechanisms of drug action, pharmacokinetic and pharmacodynamic variability, and mechanisms of drug resistance. Recent scientific advances in the field of molecular oncology have led to the identification of large numbers of potential targets for novel anticancer therapies. This has resulted in a tremendous expansion of the drug development pipeline, and in the present era, the diversity of clinically useful novel anticancer therapeutic agents is growing at an unprecedented rate. However, the great enthusiasm that surrounds these new agents must be tempered by the challenges they present in optimizing their clinical use and in rationally integrating them with existing anticancer therapies. This discussion focuses on the basic principles underlying the development of modern combination chemotherapy, and it is followed by a description of the major classes of chemotherapeutic drugs and their mechanisms of action.

The cell cycle and tumor growth pattern

The growth pattern of individual neoplastic cells may greatly affect the overall biologic behavior of human tumors and their responses to specific types of cancer therapy. Tumor cells can be subdivided into three general populations: (1) cells that are not dividing and are terminally differentiated; (2) cells that continue to prolife rate; and (3) nondividing cells that are currently quiescent but may be recruited into the cell cycle. The kinetic behavior of dividing cells is best described by the concept of the cell cycle.

The cell cycle is composed of four distinct phases during which the cell prepares for and undergoes mitosis. The G_1 phase consists of cells that have recently completed division and are committed to continued proliferation. After a variable period, these cells begin to synthesize DNA, marking the beginning of the S phase. After DNA synthesis is complete, the end of the S phase is followed by the premitotic rest interval called the G_2 phase. Finally, chromosome condensation occurs and the cells divide during the mitotic M phase. Resting diploid cells that are not actively dividing are described as being in the G_0 phase. The transition between cell-cycle phases is strictly regulated by specific signaling proteins; however, these cell-cycle checkpoints may become aberrant in some tumor types.

Some anticancer agents induce their cytotoxic effects during specific phases of the cell cycle. Antimetabolites, such as fluorouracil (5-FU) and methotrexate, are more active against S-phase cells, whereas the vinca alkaloids, epipodophyllotoxins, and taxanes are relatively more M-phase specific. These kinetic properties may have clinically important consequences for cancer chemotherapy. For example, cell-cycle–nonspecific agents, such as the alkylating agents and platinum derivatives, generally have linear dose-response curves (ie, increasing the dose increases cytotoxicity). In contrast, cell-cycle–specific agents will often plateau in their concentration-dependent effects because only a subset of proliferating cells remain fully sensitive to drug-induced cytotoxicity. These cell-cycle–specific agents tend to be schedule dependent, because the only way to increase the total cell kill is by extending the duration of exposure, not by increasing the dose.

In clinical practice, solid tumors typically have low growth fractions and heterogeneous doubling times; as they increase in size, tumors may outgrow their blood and nutrient supply, leading to slower growth rates. In real life, most tumors display a sigmoid-shaped Gompertzian growth pattern in which growth rates decline as tumors expand. The most rapid growth occurs at small tumor volumes, whereas larger tumors may harbor higher numbers of nonproliferating cells, potentially making them less sensitive to agents that selectively target dividing cells. This understanding of tumor growth kinetics has been used to support the development of novel clinical strategies for optimizing cancer chemotherapy. This includes the use of adjuvant chemotherapy to treat small volumes of tumor cells during times of high growth rates and the sequential administration of non–cross-resistant drug combinations.

Principles of combination chemotherapy

Based upon cell kinetic and pharmacologic principles, a set of guidelines for designing modern combination chemotherapy regimens has been derived. Multiagent therapy has three important theoretical advantages over single-agent

TABLE 1: Principles for selecting agents for use in combination chemotherapy regimens

Drugs known to be active as single agents should be selected for use in combinations; preferentially drugs that induce complete remission should be included.
Drugs with different mechanisms of action and with additive or synergistic cytotoxic effects on the tumor should be combined.
Drugs with different dose-limiting toxicities should be combined, so full or nearly full therapeutic doses can be utilized.
Drugs should be used at their optimal dose and schedule.
Drugs should be given at consistent intervals, and the treatment-free period should be as short as possible to allow for recovery for the most sensitive normal tissues.
Drugs with different patterns of resistance should be used to minimize cross-resistance.

therapy. First, it can maximize cell kill while minimizing host toxicities by using agents with nonoverlapping dose-limiting toxicities. Second, it may increase the range of drug activity against tumor cells with endogenous resistance to specific types of therapy. Finally, it may also prevent or slow the development of newly resistant tumor cells. Specific principles for selecting agents for use in combination chemotherapy regimens are listed in Table 1.

DEFINITION OF RESPONSE

In clinical studies, formal response criteria have been developed and have gained wide acceptance. The National Cancer Institute (NCI) has proposed and implemented newer standard response criteria called Response Evaluation Criteria in Solid Tumors (RECIST). In contrast, the World Health Organization (WHO) has a different standard for assessing response. Major differences between these guidelines are listed in Table 2.

DRUG RESISTANCE

Drug resistance to chemotherapy may arise from a variety of different mechanisms, including anatomic, pharmacologic, and genetic processes. Some of the common factors that may broadly affect tumor cell sensitivity to different classes of agents include the failure of drugs to penetrate into specific sanctuary sites, such as the brain and testes, or the development of mutations in the target proteins that render them less sensitive to specific molecular inhibitors. Another factor may be decreased drug accumulation resulting from the increased expression of drug efflux pumps in the cell membrane, such as *p*-glycoprotein, which is encoded for by the multidrug resistance (MDR-1) gene. This 170-kDa glycoprotein normally removes toxins or xenobiotic metabolites from cells via

TABLE 2: Comparison of RECIST and WHO guidelines

Characteristic	RECIST	WHO
Objective response (OR) (LD is the longest diameter)	**Target lesions** (change in sum of LDs, maximum 5 per organ up to 10 total [more than one organ])	**Measurable disease** (change in the sum of the products of LDs and greatest perpendicular diameters, no maximum number of lesions specified)
Complete response (CR)	Disappearance of all target lesions, confirmed at ≥ 4 weeks	Disappearance of all known disease, confirmed at ≥ 4 weeks
Partial response (PR)	≥ 30% decrease from baseline, confirmed at ≥ 4 weeks	≥ 50% decrease from baseline, confirmed at ≥ 4 weeks
Progressive disease (PD)	≥ 20% increase over smallest sum observed or appearance of new lesions	≥ 25% increase in one or more lesions or appearance of new lesions
Stable disease (SD)	Neither PR nor PD criteria met	Neither PR nor PD criteria met (no change)

an energy-dependent process. High levels of MDR-1 expression in tumor cells correlate with resistance to a wide range of cytotoxic agents. Other drug efflux pumps that have been implicated in the development of broad resistance to cancer chemotherapy include the MDR-associated protein (MRP) and breast cancer resistance protein (BCRP).

Pharmacokinetic and pharmacodynamic variability

VARIABILITY IN CLEARANCE

The rational clinical use of cancer chemotherapy requires a thorough understanding of the variability in human response to drug therapy. One of the major goals of the field of clinical pharmacology is to precisely define the processes responsible for this variability in drug action. Pharmacokinetic variability can arise from interindividual differences in drug adsorption, distribution, metabolism, and excretion. All of these processes result in differences in drug delivery to its ultimate site of action. In contrast, pharmacodynamic variability arises from inherent differences in the sensitivity of target tissues to drug effects. Both kinetic and dynamic factors can complicate the treatment of individual cancer patients and must be addressed by the practicing oncologist on a daily basis. Although a formal review of drug pharmacokinetics and pharmacodynamics is not possible here, a brief discussion of the most clinically relevant points is warranted.

The most clinically useful parameter in drug therapy is clearance, because clearance reflects all the processes in the body that contribute to drug elimination. In oncology, the importance of clearance is enhanced because clearance is the only parameter that relates dose to the measured area under the concentration vs time curve (AUC), which is a useful measure of systemic drug exposure. Mathematically, clearance is defined as dose/AUC. Clearance is not a rate of drug elimination; instead it is defined as a volume of drug cleared per unit of time.

Overcoming interindividual variation in clearance is a fundamental goal of pharmacokinetic analyses. Because they tend to be highly toxic with low efficacy, anticancer drugs may have the narrowest therapeutic index of any class of agents used in clinical medicine. Thus, the ability to administer an individualized dose of drug to achieve a uniform target AUC and a uniform clinical result is often a high priority for cancer therapeutics. Because clearance defines the relationship between dose and AUC, estimating clearance prior to anticancer drug administration is extremely important. A common attempt to individualize cancer chemotherapy is to dose a drug based upon the body surface area (BSA) expressed in mg/m^2 to achieve a uniform AUC in patients with different body sizes. Inherent in this approach is the fundamental assumption that clearance is strongly correlated with BSA. However, when studied formally, the relationship between clearance and BSA is often weak and does not consistently justify the routine use of this dosing approach. Nonetheless, although the application of BSA-based dosing has been widely criticized, it still remains a common practice.

Recognizing clinical situations in which drug clearance is commonly altered, such as in patients with hepatic or renal dysfunction, is important for agents that are eliminated by these routes. For example, carboplatin is extensively cleared by glomerular filtration, and its systemic AUC in plasma ultrafiltrates is strongly correlated with pharmacodynamic effects, such as thrombocytopenia. Thus, dosing strategies that estimate the glomerular filtration rate (GFR) to achieve a targeted AUC and thereby minimize excessive toxicity in individual patients have gained wide clinical acceptance. Likewise, for hepatically metabolized drugs, doses must be adjusted in patients with liver dysfunction. However, accurately assessing hepatic drug-metabolizing capacity is more difficult than estimating the GFR. Nonetheless, guidelines for dose-adjusting agents metabolized in the liver, such as doxorubicin, have been established.

PHARMACOGENOMIC VARIABILITY

Variability in drug action may also be caused by genetic factors. The new field of pharmacogenomics attempts to define the impact of genetic differences on drug kinetics and dynamics. McLeod and Evans have defined pharmacogenomics as the field of study of "the inherited nature of interindividual differences in drug disposition and effects." Clinically relevant genetic variations have been characterized in specific drug-metabolizing enzymes, such as the cytochrome P-450 isoforms CYP2D6 and CYP2C9.

In the field of medical oncology, well-defined examples of clinically relevant pharmacogenetic differences are relatively few; however, this is an important area of ongoing research. Perhaps the best characterized example in clinical oncology is the inherited deficiency of the thiopurine methyltransferase (TPMT) enzyme that results in severe intolerance to thiopurine therapy. Another example is the inherited variation in dihydropyrimidine dehydrogenase (DPD) activity, the rate-limiting catabolic enzyme responsible for clearance of 5-FU. Genetic alterations associated with DPD deficiency have been identified in rare patients experiencing severe and fatal toxicity after treatment with standard doses of 5-FU. Finally, interindividual variation in irinotecan (Camptosar)-induced toxicities may be partially explained by genetic polymorphisms in the gene encoding the UDP-glucuronosyltransferase (UGT) 1A1 enzyme that is involved in the clearance of the active metabolite SN-38. Also, the identification of somatic mutations in the tyrosine kinase domain of the epidermal growth factor receptor (EGFR) in non-small-cell lung cancer (NSCLC) and their correlation with response to EGFR inhibitors has become an important event in the fields of cancer genomics and therapeutics. The issue of ethnic diversity in the pathogenesis of given tumors was raised by the initial observation of a higher response to gefitinib (Iressa) and erlotinib (Tarceva) in patients of Asian origin, together with the discovery that they harbor more frequent EGFR mutations in NSCLC.

Pharmacodynamic polymorphisms that directly affect target tissue sensitivity to drug effects are also clinically important. For example, polymorphisms in the promoter region of the thymidylate synthase gene have been correlated with tumor response to 5-FU–based chemotherapy that targets this enzyme. In the near future, our understanding of how genetics affects a drug's pharmacokinetics may ultimately allow for the optimization of specific treatment regimens for individual patients. Likewise, our understanding of how genetics affects pharmacodynamic variation may be enhanced by powerful new technologies that can characterize the expression of literally thousands of genes within the tumor itself. The molecular profiling of tumor cells by DNA microarray techniques and other advances in biotechnology offer tremendous hope for improving our ability to treat cancer in the near future.

Molecularly targeted therapies

At the beginning of the 21st century, important and meaningful advances in anticancer therapeutics are being discovered at an unparalleled rate. Much of this progress is driven by the explosion of knowledge in the field of molecular oncology. The sequencing of the entire human genome has dramatically increased the number of promising molecular targets for new and novel anticancer treatment strategies. These advances hold great promise for developing a new generation of agents with high specificity for tumor cells (see discussion later in this chapter).

Chemotherapeutic agents classified by mechanism of action

Alkylating agents

The alkylating agents impair cell function by forming covalent bonds with the amino, carboxyl, sulfhydryl, and phosphate groups in biologically important molecules. The most important sites of alkylation are DNA, RNA, and proteins. The electron-rich nitrogen at the 7 position of guanine in DNA is particularly susceptible to alkylation.

Alkylating agents depend on cell proliferation for activity but are not cell-cycle-phase–specific. A fixed percentage of cells are killed at a given dose. Tumor resistance probably occurs through efficient glutathione conjugation or by enhanced DNA repair mechanisms. Alkylating agents are classified according to their chemical structure and mechanism of covalent bonding; this drug class includes the nitrogen mustards, nitrosoureas, and platinum complexes, among other agents (Table 3).

Nitrogen mustards The nitrogen mustards, which include such drugs as mechlorethamine (Mustargen), cyclophosphamide, ifosfamide, and chlorambucil (Leukeran), are powerful local vesicants; as such, they can cause problems ranging from local tissue necrosis to pulmonary fibrosis to hemorrhagic cystitis. The metabolites of these compounds are highly reactive in aqueous

TABLE 3: Chemotherapeutic agents[a]

Alkylating agents

- **Nitrogen mustards:** chlorambucil, cyclophosphamide, estramustine, ifosfamide, mechlorethamine, melphalan
- **Aziridine:** thiotepa
- **Alkyl sulfonate:** busulfan
- **Nitrosoureas:** carmustine, lomustine, streptozocin
- **Platinum complexes:** carboplatin, cisplatin, oxaliplatin
- **Nonclassic alkylators:** altretamine, dacarbazine, procarbazine, temozolomide

Antimetabolites

- **Folate analog:** methotrexate, pemetrexed
- **Purine analogs:** fludarabine, mercaptopurine, thioguanine
- **Adenosine analogs:** cladribine, pentostatin
- **Pyrimidine analogs:** capecitabine, cytarabine, floxuridine, fluorouracil, gemcitabine
- **Substituted urea:** hydroxyurea

Natural products

- **Antitumor antibiotics:** bleomycin, dactinomycin, daunorubicin, doxorubicin, epirubicin, idarubicin, mitoxantrone, mitomycin, valrubicin
- **Epipodophyllotoxins:** etoposide, teniposide
- **Microtubule agents:** docetaxel, paclitaxel, vinblastine, vincristine, vinorelbine
- **Camptothecin analogs:** irinotecan, topotecan
- **Enzyme:** asparaginase

Targeted agents

- **Monoclonal antibodies:** alemtuzumab, bevacizumab, cetuximab, panitumumab, rituximab, trastuzumab,
- **Molecularly targeted therapies:** bortezomib, dasatinib, erlotinib, gefitinib, imatinib, lapatinib, sorafenib, sunitinib

[a]For a comprehensive table of drug information including dosages and toxicities, see Appendix 4.

solution, in which an active alkylating moiety, the ethylene immonium ion, binds to DNA. The hematopoietic system is especially susceptible to these compounds.

Nitrosoureas The nitrosoureas are distinguished by their high lipid solubility and chemical instability. These agents rapidly and spontaneously decompose into two highly reactive intermediates: chloroethyl diazohydroxide and isocyanate. The lipophilic nature of the nitrosoureas enables free passage across membranes; therefore, they rapidly penetrate the blood-brain barrier, achieving effective CNS concentrations. As a consequence, these agents are used for a variety of brain tumors.

Platinum agents Cisplatin is an inorganic heavy metal complex that has activity typical of a cell-cycle-phase–nonspecific alkylating agent. The compound produces intrastrand and interstrand DNA cross-links and forms DNA adducts, thereby inhibiting the synthesis of DNA, RNA, and proteins. Carboplatin has the same active diamine platinum moiety as cisplatin, but it is bonded to an organic carboxylate group that allows increased water solubility and slower hydrolysis to the alkylating aqueous platinum complex, thus altering toxicity profiles. Oxaliplatin (Eloxatin) is distinguished from the other platinum compounds by a di-amino-cyclohexane ring bound to the platinum molecule, which interferes with resistance mechanisms to the drug.

Antimetabolites

Antimetabolites are structural analogs of the naturally occurring metabolites involved in DNA and RNA synthesis. As the constituents of these metabolic pathways have been elucidated, a large number of structurally similar drugs that alter the critical pathways of nucleotide synthesis have been developed.

Antimetabolites exert their cytotoxic activity either by competing with normal metabolites for the catalytic or regulatory site of a key enzyme or by substituting for a metabolite that is normally incorporated into DNA and RNA. Because of this mechanism of action, antimetabolites are most active when cells are in the S phase and have little effect on cells in the G_0 phase. Consequently, these drugs are most effective against tumors that have a high growth fraction.

Antimetabolites have a nonlinear dose-response curve, such that after a certain dose, no more cells are killed despite increasing doses (5-FU is an exception). The antimetabolites can be divided into folate analogs, purine analogs, adenosine analogs, pyrimidine analogs, and substituted urea.

Natural products

A wide variety of compounds possessing antitumor activity have been isolated from natural substances, such as plants, fungi, and bacteria. Likewise, selected compounds have semisynthetic and synthetic designs based on the active chemical structure of the parent compounds, and they, too, have cytotoxic effects.

Antitumor antibiotics Bleomycin preferentially intercalates DNA at guanine-cytosine and guanine-thymine sequences, resulting in spontaneous oxidation and formation of free oxygen radicals that cause strand breakage.

Anthracyclines The anthracycline antibiotics are products of the fungus *Streptomyces percetus* var *caesius.* They are chemically similar, with a basic anthracycline structure containing a glycoside bound to an amino sugar, daunosamine. The anthracyclines have several modes of action. Most notable are intercalation between DNA base pairs and inhibition of DNA–topoisomerases I and II. Oxygen free radical formation from reduced doxorubicin intermediates is thought to be a mechanism associated with cardiotoxicity.

Epipodophyllotoxins Etoposide is a semisynthetic epipodophyllotoxin extracted from the root of *Podophyllum peltatum* (mandrake). It inhibits topoisomerase II activity by stabilizing the DNA–topoisomerase II complex; this process ultimately results in the inability to synthesize DNA, and the cell cycle is stopped in the G_1 phase.

Vinca alkaloids The vinca alkaloids are derived from the periwinkle plant *Vinca rosea.* Upon entering the cell, vinca alkaloids bind rapidly to the tubulin. The binding occurs in the S phase at a site different from that associated with paclitaxel and colchicine. Thus, polymerization of microtubules is blocked, resulting in impaired mitotic spindle formation in the M phase.

Taxanes Paclitaxel and docetaxel (Taxotere) are semisynthetic derivatives of extracted precursors from the needles of yew plants. These drugs have a novel 14-member ring, the taxane. Unlike the vinca alkaloids, which cause microtubular disassembly, the taxanes promote microtubular assembly and stability, therefore blocking the cell cycle in mitosis. Docetaxel is more potent than paclitaxel in enhancing microtubular assembly and also induces apoptosis.

Camptothecin analogs include irinotecan and topotecan (Hycamtin). These semisynthetic analogs of the alkaloid camptothecin, derived from the Chinese ornamental tree *Camptotheca acuminata,* inhibit topoisomerase I and interrupt the elongation phase of DNA replication.

Targeted agents

Monoclonal antibodies Although monoclonal antibodies (MAbs) have been used in cancer therapeutics since the late 1990s, the number of new agents in this class is growing exponentially. Several unconjugated MAbs have established utility in medical oncology as highly targeted therapies. The earliest therapeutic MAb to show convincing utility in medical oncology was rituximab (Rituxan), approved in 1997 for the treatment of non-Hodgkin lymphoma. This antibody targets the CD20 antigen found on B-cell lymphocytes and can be used clinically as a single agent or in association with combination chemotherapy. Another MAb, trastuzumab (Herceptin), has shown excellent activity in combination with chemotherapy in breast cancer patients whose tumor cells overexpress the HER2 protein. Finally, alemtuzumab (Campath) is a MAb that recognizes the CD52 antigen expressed on both B-cell and T-cell lymphocytes. This agent is useful in the treatment of chemotherapy-refractory B-cell chronic lymphocytic leukemia.

In 2004, two new MAbs were approved by the US Food and Drug Administration (FDA) for the treatment of patients with advanced colorectal cancer: bevacizumab (Avastin) and cetuximab (Erbitux). Bevacizumab binds to the vascular endothelial growth factor (VEGF) and prevents ligand-induced VEGF receptor activation, which blocks the stimulation of endothelial cell growth and inhibits new blood vessel formation in tumors that secrete VEGF. Cetuximab binds the epidermal growth factor receptor (EGFR) on the surface of tumor cells, ultimately leading to down-regulation of this signaling pathway. This process blocks tumor growth and proliferation and can reverse tumor resistance to chemotherapeutic agents such as irinotecan.

Panitumumab (Vectibix), approved by the FDA in 2006, is another monocloncal antibody that targets EGFR and is approved for use in colorectal cancer that has metastasized following standard chemotherapy.

A recent randomized trial found that the addition of bevacizumab to irinotecan- and 5-FU–based chemotherapy in newly diagnosed patients with advanced colorectal cancer significantly improved the response rate (45% vs 35%; P = .0029), duration of response (10.4 vs 7.1 months; P = .0014), and median survival (20.3 vs 15.6 months; P = .0003) compared with placebo. Grade 3 hypertension (10.9% vs 2.3%) and GI perforations (1.5% vs 0%) were more common in the bevacizumab arm, but overall, the bevacizumab therapy was thought to be well tolerated. This was the first randomized clinical trial demonstrating a survival benefit for antiangiogenic therapy.

Molecularly targeted therapies

Molecularly targeted therapies are designed to selectively interact with specific molecular pathways within cells to achieve a rational antitumor effect. The classic rationally designed molecularly targeted agent is imatinib (Gleevec), which was identified in screening studies designed to detect inhibitors of the Bcr-Abl tyrosine kinase, present in virtually all cases of chronic myelogenous leukemia. Originally synthesized as an inhibitor of platelet-derived growth factor receptor, it is also a potent inhibitor of the c-*kit* tyrosine kinase. Imatinib binds to the ATP binding site and inhibits the tyrosine kinase's ability to phosphorylate its substrates.

Gefitinib is another small-molecule–targeted therapy that is a signal transduction inhibitor of the EGFR tyrosine kinase. It binds noncovalently to the ATP binding site of the intracellular domain of the EGFR protein and blocks the kinase activity. Its anticancer effects arise from the ability to interfere with EGFR-mediated signaling, which is associated with cell proliferation, angiogenesis, and cell motility.

Erlotinib is an HER1/EGFR-targeted therapy that has demonstrated a significant survival benefit as second-line therapy for patients with advanced non–small-cell lung cancer (NSCLC). A randomized phase III study performed by the National Cancer Institute of Canada compared erlotinib with best supportive care in patients with recurrent or refractory non–small-cell lung cancer following treatment with either one or two lines of prior chemotherapy. As reported by Shepherd et al, erlotinib was significantly better than best supportive care in terms of response rate (8.9% vs < 1%, $P < .001$), disease progression-free survival (2.23 vs 1.84 months, $P < .001$), and median survival (6.7 vs 4.7 months, $P = .001$). Rash and diarrhea were the most frequent side effects, although only 5% of patients discontinued erlotinib due to drug-related toxicities. This is the first randomized trial of an EGFR inhibitor in lung cancer demonstrating a significant survival benefit.

Temsirolimus is a specific inhibitor of mTOR, a signaling protein that regulates cell growth and angiogenesis. It has been evaluated in a phase III, randomized, 3-arm study versus interferon-alpha or the combination of both agents in the treatment of first-line, poor-risk patients with advanced renal cell carcinoma. Recently reported results show this agent to be the first to produce a significant increase in overall survival with an acceptable safety profile *(Hudes G, Carducci M, Tomczak P, et al: Proc Am Soc Clin Oncol 24:LBA4, 2006).*

Another targeted therapy is the 26S proteasome inhibitor bortezomib (Velcade). The 26S proteasome is a ubiquitous multiprotein complex responsible for degrading a variety of regulatory proteins involved in cancer cell proliferation. In multiple myeloma cells, bortezomib induces apoptosis by mechanisms that are not precisely defined. One hypothesis is that the inhibition of the proteasomal degradation of I-κB, an inhibitor of the transcription factor NF-κB, prevents the constitutive activation of NF-κB. In multiple myeloma cells, NF-κB is thought to be necessary for cell proliferation and survival.

Sunitinib malate (SUD011248, Sutent) is an oral small molecule multitargeted tyrosine kinase inhibitor with antiproliferative and antiangiogenic activity attributed to the inhibition of PDGFR, VEGFR, KIT, and FLT_3. In a phase II study by Motzer et al, involving 63 patients with metastatic renal cell carcinoma, sunitinib resulted in a 33% partial response rate (95% confidence interval [CI], 22% to 46%), a 37% rate of stable disease lasting at least 3 months, and a 1-year median survival of 65% (95% CI, 50% to 76%). Treatments were well tolerated, with major grade 3 or 4 toxicities consisting of lymphopenia, neutropenia, elevated amylase/lipase levels without associated pancreatitis, and fatigue or asthenia. If the results are confirmed, this study will have produced one of the highest response rates reported for single-agent therapy for patients with renal cell carcinoma.

Sunitinib and sorafenib (Nexavar) are two new oral small multitargeted molecules with antiproliferative and antiangiogenic activity attributed to the inhibition of PDGFR, VEGFR, KIT, and FLT3 and, in the case of sorafenib, RAF-1. Both agents show significant activity in advanced renal cell cancer patients, frequently producing prolonged stabilization of disease, and in the case of sunitinib, objective remissions. These targeted therapies have displaced cytokines as the gold standard for treating advanced-stage renal cell tumors.

Other newer molecularly targeted therapies include dasatinib (Sprycel), approved by the FDA for treatment of chronic myelogenous leukemia and Philadelphia-positive acute lymphoblastic leukemia, and lapatinib (Tykerb), approved by the FDA for treatment of advanced or metastatic Her2-positive breast cancer in combination with capecitabine (Xeloda).

The relevance of pharmacogenomics to molecularly targeted therapies was highlighted by the impressive finding that specific somatic mutations localizing to the ATP-binding site of the EGFR tyrosine kinase in lung tumors were associated with clinical response. In eight of nine patients with NSCLC who responded to gefitinib therapy, specific mutations were identified, whereas none was found in seven matched nonresponders. This landmark finding, coupled with what is already known about c-kit mutations that "drive" the proliferation of gastrointestinal stromal cell tumors in response to imatinib therapy, suggests that it may ultimately be possible to prospectively select patients with NSCLC who have a high probability of responding to EGFR tyrosine kinase inhibitors. Further studies are under way to confirm these findings and to extend the observation to other tumor types.

See Appendix 3 for a list of drugs and/or new indications recently approved for treatment of cancer and Appendix 4 for the uses, dosages, and toxicities of the chemotherapeutic agents discussed in this chapter.

SUGGESTED READING

Cunningham D, Humblet Y, Siena S, et al: Cetuximab monotherapy and cetuximab plus irinotecan in irinotecan-refractory metastatic colorectal cancer. N Engl J Med 351:337–345, 2004.

Hurwitz H, Fehrenbacher L, Novotny W, et al: Bevacizumab plus irinotecan, fluorouracil, and leucovorin for metastatic colorectal cancer. N Engl J Med 350:2335–2342, 2004.

Lynch TJ, Bell DW, Sordella R, et al: Activating mutations in the epidermal growth factor receptor underlying responsiveness of non-small-cell lung cancer to gefitinib. N Engl J Med 350:2129–2139, 2004.

McLeod HL, Evans WE: Pharmacogenomics: Unlocking the human genome for better drug therapy. Annu Rev Pharmacol Toxicol 41:101–121, 2001.

Morabito A, De Maio E, Di Maio M, et al: Tyrosine kinase inhibitors of vascular endothelial growth factor receptors in clinical trials: current status and future directions. Oncologist 11:753-764, 2006.

Motzer RJ, Rini BI, Michaelson MD, et al: SU011248, a novel tyrosine kinase inhibitor, shows antitumor activity in second-line therapy for patients with metastatic renal cell carcinoma: Results of a phase 2 trial. J Clin Oncol [abstract] 22[suppl]:14s, 2004.

Olopade OI, Schwartsmann G, Saijo N, et al: Disparities in cancer care: a worldwide perspective and roadmap for change. J Clin Oncol 24:2135-2136, 2006.

Paez JG, Janne PA, Lee JC, et al: EGFR mutations in lung cancer: Correlation with clinical response to gefitinib therapy. Science 304:1497–1500, 2004.

Shepherd FA, Pereira J, Ciuleanu TE, et al: A randomized placebo-controlled trial of erlotinib in patients with advanced non-small cell lung cancer (NSCLC) following failure of first-line or second-line chemotherapy. A National Cancer Institute of Canada Clinical Trials Group (NCIC CTG) trial. J Clin Oncol [abstract] 22[suppl]:14s, 2004.

Weinshilboum R: Inheritance and drug response. N Engl J Med 348:529–537, 2003.

CHAPTER 4

Head and neck tumors

John Andrew Ridge, MD, PhD, Bonnie S. Glisson, MD, Eric M. Horwitz, MD, and Miriam N. Lango, MD

In 2006, it was estimated that head and neck cancers comprised 2%–3% of all cancers in the United States and accounted for 1%–2% of all cancer deaths. This total includes 22,040 cases of oral cavity cancer, 9,510 cases of laryngeal cancer, and 8,950 cases of pharyngeal cancer. Most patients with head and neck cancer have metastatic disease at the time of diagnosis (regional nodal involvement in 43% and distant metastasis in 10%).

Head and neck cancers encompass a diverse group of uncommon tumors that frequently are aggressive in their biologic behavior. Moreover, patients with a head and neck cancer often develop a second primary tumor. These tumors occur at an annual rate of 3%–7%, and 50%–75% of such new cancers occur in the upper aerodigestive tract or lungs.

The anatomy of the head and neck is complex and is divided into sites and subsites (Figure 1). Tumors of each site have a unique epidemiology, anatomy, natural history, and therapeutic approach. This chapter will review these lesions as a group and then individually by anatomic site.

Epidemiology

Gender Head and neck cancer is more common in men; 66%–95% of cases occur in men. The incidence by gender varies with anatomic location and has been changing as the number of female smokers has increased. The male-female ratio is currently 3:1 for oral cavity and pharyngeal cancers. In patients with Plummer-Vinson syndrome, the ratio is reversed, with 80% of head and neck cancers occurring in women.

Age The incidence of head and neck cancer increases with age, especially after 50 years of age. Although most patients are between 50 and 70 years old, head and neck cancer does occur in younger patients. There are more women and fewer smokers in the younger patient group.

It is controversial whether head and neck cancer is more aggressive in younger patients or in older individuals. This "aggressiveness" probably reflects the common delay in diagnosis in the younger population, since, in most studies, younger patients do not have a worse prognosis than their older counterparts.

Race The incidence of laryngeal cancer is higher in African Americans relative to the white, Asian, and Hispanic populations.

Additionally, in African Americans, head and neck cancer is associated with lower survival for similar tumor stages. The overall 5-year survival rate is 56% in whites and 34% in African Americans.

Geography There are wide variations in the incidence of head and neck cancer among different geographic regions. The risk of laryngeal cancer, for example, is two to six times higher in Bombay, India, than in Scandinavia. The higher incidence of the disease in Asia is thought to reflect the prevalence of risk factors, such as betel nut chewing and use of smokeless tobacco. In the United States, the high incidence among urban males is thought to reflect ex-

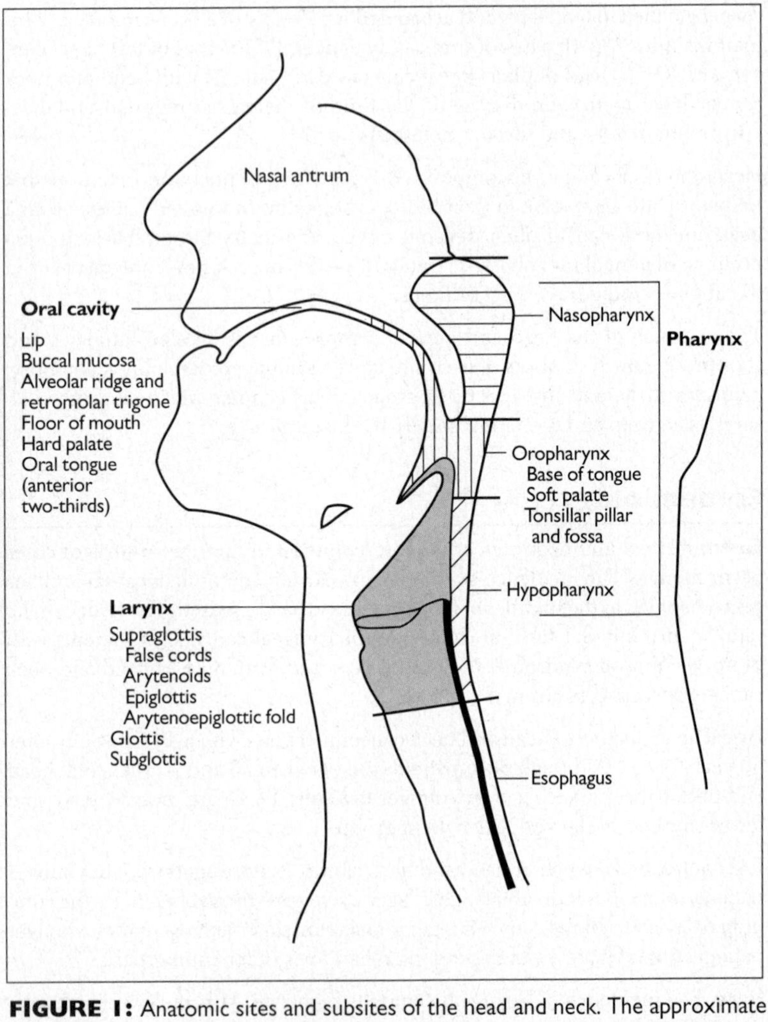

FIGURE 1: Anatomic sites and subsites of the head and neck. The approximate distribution of head and neck cancer is oral cavity, 44%; larynx, 31%; and pharynx, 25%.

HEAD AND NECK

posure to tobacco and alcohol. Among rural women, there is an increased risk of oral cancer related to the use of smokeless tobacco (snuff).

Nasopharyngeal carcinoma is another head and neck tumor with a distinct ethnic predilection. Endemic areas include southern China, northern Africa, and regions of the far Northern Hemisphere—areas in which the diet of inhabitants includes large quantities of salted meat and fish. When people from these regions migrate to areas with a lower disease incidence, their risk falls but remains elevated. Cancer of the nasopharynx in these geographic areas also has been associated with Epstein-Barr virus (EBV) infection (see section on "Etiology and risk factors").

Etiology and risk factors

Risk factors for head and neck cancer include tobacco and alcohol use, ultraviolet (UV) light exposure, viral infection, and environmental exposures.

Tobacco The incidence of head and neck tumors correlates most closely with the use of tobacco.

Cigarettes Head and neck tumors occur six times more often among cigarette smokers than nonsmokers. The age-standardized risk of mortality from laryngeal cancer appears to rise linearly with increasing cigarette smoking. For the heaviest smokers, death from laryngeal cancer is 20 times more likely than for nonsmokers. Furthermore, active smoking by head and neck cancer patients is associated with significant increases in the annual rate of second primary tumor development (compared with former smokers or those who have never smoked). Use of unfiltered cigarettes or dark, air-cured tobacco is associated with further increases in risk.

Cigars Total cigar smoking increased by nearly 50% in the United States in the 1990s. Often misperceived as posing a lower health risk than cigarette smoking, cigar smoking results in a change in the site distribution for aerodigestive tract cancer, according to epidemiologic data. Although the incidence of cancer at some sites traditionally associated with cigarette smoking (eg, larynx, lungs) is decreased in cigar smokers, the incidence of cancer is actually higher at other sites where pooling of saliva and associated carcinogens tends to occur (oropharynx, esophagus).

Smokeless tobacco Use of smokeless tobacco also is associated with an increased incidence of head and neck cancer, especially in the oral cavity. Smokeless tobacco users frequently develop premalignant lesions, such as oral leukoplakia, at the site where the tobacco quid rests against the mucosa. Over time, these lesions may progress to invasive carcinomas. The use of snuff has been associated with an increase in cancers of the gum and oral mucosa.

Alcohol Alcohol consumption, by itself, is a risk factor for the development of pharyngeal and laryngeal tumors, although it is a less potent carcinogen than tobacco. For individuals who use both tobacco and alcohol, these risk factors appear to be synergistic and result in a multiplicative increase in risk.

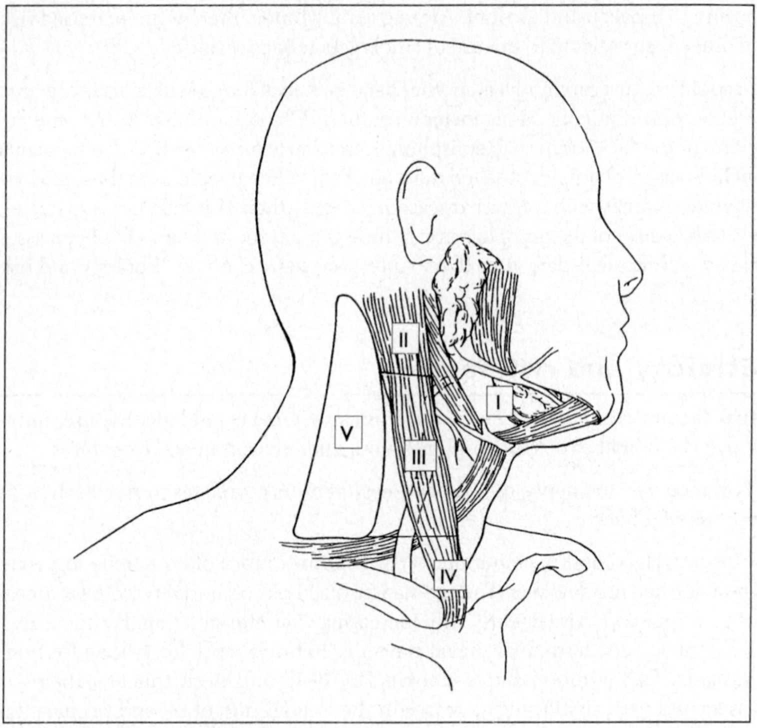

FIGURE 2: Levels of the neck as determined by lymphatic drainage patterns

UV light exposure is a risk factor for the development of cancer of the lips. At least 33% of patients with lip cancer have outdoor occupations.

Occupational exposures A small group of head and neck cancers may be attributable to occupational exposures. Nasal cancer has been associated with wood dust exposure, and squamous cell cancer of the maxillary sinus, with nickel exposure. Petroleum exposure may be associated with pharyngeal cancer, but the relationship has not been proven.

Radiation exposure Exposure to radiation is clearly an important risk factor for thyroid cancer and has been associated with cancer of the salivary glands.

Viruses There is a strong link between EBV exposure and the development of nasopharyngeal cancer. The relationship between human papillomavirus and some head and neck cancers is increasingly recognized.

Diet Epidemiologic studies suggest that dietary intake of vitamin A, β-carotene, and α-tocopherol may reduce the risk of developing head and neck cancer.

Marijuana Smoking marijuana is associated with the development of head and neck cancer, but the degree of risk is unknown.

Anatomy

As mentioned previously, the anatomy of the head and neck region is complex. The anatomic sites are illustrated in Figure 1. More detailed descriptions are included below in the discussions of specific sites and subsites.

Levels of the neck

The anatomy of the neck is relevant to the treatment of all head and neck cancers. The neck may be divided into levels (Figure 2). The lymphatic drainage of the unmanipulated neck is systematic and predictable; knowledge of these drainage patterns assists the clinician in locating the primary tumor that has given rise to a neck metastasis (Table 1).

Level I includes the submental and submandibular triangles.

Level II includes the superior jugular chain nodes extending from the mandible down to the carotid bifurcation and posteriorly to the posterior border of the sternocleidomastoid muscle.

Level III consists of the jugular nodes from the carotid bulb inferiorly to the omohyoid muscle.

Level IV continues from the omohyoid muscle inferiorly to the clavicle.

Level V represents the posterior triangle bounded by the posterior border of the sternocleidomastoid anteriorly, the anterior border of the trapezius posteriorly, and the clavicle inferiorly.

Signs and symptoms

Head and neck cancer typically produces symptoms referable to the upper aerodigestive tract, including alterations in deglutition, phonation, hearing, and respiration. In particular, patients should be questioned about dysphagia, odynophagia, globus sensation, hoarseness, a change in the ability to form words, epistaxis, epiphora, otalgia, hemoptysis, stuffiness of the ears, and trismus. (Signs and symptoms of cancer at specific anatomic sites and subsites can be found in the respective discussions of these tumors.)

It is important to ascertain the duration and course (progression or improvement) of symptoms. Progression of disease is often noted during the evaluation and worsens the prognosis.

Screening and diagnosis

SCREENING

Molecular diagnostic techniques have shown promise as screening tools to identify neoplastic cells in saliva and sputum specimens. Nevertheless, since patients with head and neck cancer are unlikely to be engaged in the health care system, the means by which patient screening would be achieved remains a fundamental problem.

TABLE 1: Lymphatic drainage of the head and neck and associated sites of primary tumors

Lymphatic drainage	Likely primary sites
Level I	
Submental	Lower lip, chin, anterior oral cavity (including anterior one-third of the tongue and floor of the mouth)
Submandibular	Upper and lower lips, oral tongue, floor of the mouth, facial skin
Level II	Oral cavity and pharynx (including soft palate, base of the tongue, and piriform sinus)
Level III	Larynx, hypopharynx, and thyroid
Level IV	Larynx, hypopharynx, thyroid, cervical esophagus, and trachea
Level V	Nasopharynx, thyroid, paranasal sinuses, and posterior scalp
Supraclavicular	Infraclavicular sites (including lungs, esophagus, breasts, pancreas, GI tract, GU and gynecologic sources)

DIAGNOSIS

The need for expeditious diagnosis of head and neck cancer and referral to a skilled head and neck specialist cannot be overemphasized, as early diagnosis can lead to a reduction in mortality. One study suggested that in the 24 months prior to the diagnosis of head and neck cancer, patients had a median of 10.5 health-care visits. These visits provide an opportunity to evaluate patients' symptoms and underscore the important role of dentists and primary care physicians in the early diagnosis of head and neck cancer.

History

Risk factors as outlined previously, including a history of tobacco and alcohol use and environmental exposures, should be reviewed. Any adult patient with symptoms referable to the upper aerodigestive tract that have lasted longer than 2 weeks or with an asymptomatic neck mass should undergo a thorough examination with a high index of suspicion for carcinoma.

Physical examination

The physical examination is the best means for detecting lesions of the upper aerodigestive tract. Frequently, the initial assessment also will indicate the severity and chronicity of the disease. Due to the frequent occurrence of multiple primary tumors in patients with a head and neck tumor, careful evaluation of the entire upper aerodigestive tract is necessary at the time of diagnosis. The examination should always follow a systematic approach.

Skin/scalp A search should be made for ulcers, nodules, and pigmented or other suspicious lesions. This part of the evaluation is frequently overlooked.

Cranial nerves A cranial nerve evaluation is essential for any patient with a head and neck tumor or neck mass (which may be a manifestation of occult cancer). This evaluation should include assessing eye motion (cranial nerves [CN] III, IV, and VI); testing sensation of the face (CN V); examining the muscles of facial expression by having the patient grin, grimace, raise eyebrows, close eyes tightly, show teeth, and puff out the cheeks (CN VII); testing of hearing (CN VIII); assessing gag reflex (CN IX); evaluating vocal cord mobility (CN X); and having the patient fully abduct the shoulder (CN XI) and protrude the tongue (CN XII). Even the slightest abnormality may be helpful in identifying a primary tumor.

Eyes/ears/nose The eyes, ears, and nose should be evaluated for any sign of mass effect, abnormal drainage/discharge, bleeding, or effusion.

Oral cavity Halitosis may be the first indication of a lesion in the upper aerodigestive tract. The teeth, gingivae, and entire mucosal surface should be inspected. (Dentures should be removed.) The lymphoid tissue of the tonsillar pillars should be inspected and any asymmetry noted. Tongue mobility also should be evaluated.

The floor of the mouth, tongue, and cheeks should be palpated using a bimanual technique (one gloved finger inside the mouth and the second hand under the mandible). Palpation should be the last step of the examination due to stimulation of the gag reflex. Worrisome lesions should be biopsied.

Neck A systematic examination of the neck consistently documents the location of any mass. Palpation is the cornerstone of the examination. It is performed by grasping the tissue and feeling the nodes between the thumb and index and long fingers. The relationship of a mass to major structures, such as the salivary gland, thyroid, and carotid sheath, should be considered.

Important qualities of a mass include location, character, tenderness, size, mobility, and associated thrill or bruit. The thyroid should be palpated.

Indirect laryngoscopy The nasopharynx, hypopharynx, and larynx should all be examined with care. The vocal cords should be visualized and their mobility evaluated. Mirror examination provides an overall impression of mobility and asymmetry, which may point to a hidden tumor.

Direct laryngoscopy Nasopharyngoscopes permit a thorough inspection of the upper aerodigestive tract in the office setting. Attention should be focused individually on the piriform sinuses, tongue base, pharyngeal walls, epiglottis, arytenoids, and true and false vocal cords. Also, any pooling of secretions should be noted.

Endoscopy Approximately 5% of patients with head and neck cancer have a synchronous primary squamous cell cancer of the head and neck, esophagus, or lungs. Examination with the patient under anesthesia with endoscopy (which may include direct laryngoscopy, esophagoscopy, and bronchoscopy) and directed biopsy should be performed in all patients with an occult primary squamous cell cancer and in many patients with a *known* head and neck primary. Examination with the patient under anesthesia also can provide information regarding the extent of the tumor.

The most common sites of silent primary tumors are the tonsils, base of the tongue, and piriform sinuses. Tumors of the nasopharynx have become easier to identify with the increased use of flexible nasopharyngoscopy. Biopsies should be performed in common areas of silent primaries in addition to the primary anatomic sites associated with lymphatic drainage of any neck mass.

Laboratory evaluation

There are no specific screening laboratory tests other than preoperative studies performed in the diagnostic evaluation of most head and neck carcinomas. EBV, anticapsid antibodies, and serum IgG are tumor markers for nasopharyngeal carcinomas.

Diagnostic imaging

Plain x-rays PA and lateral chest x-rays should be obtained in all adult patients to eliminate the possibility of occult lung metastasis or a second primary. A Panorex film may be helpful in delineating bony involvement in some cases of oral cavity lesions.

CT The CT scan is probably the single most informative test in the assessment of a head and neck tumor. It may delineate the extent of disease and the presence and extent of lymphatic involvement. CT scans of the chest, abdomen, and pelvis sometimes may identify the site of an occult primary tumor presenting with a node low in the neck. CT offers high spatial resolution and discriminates among fat, muscle, bone, and other soft tissues and surpasses MRI in the detection of bony erosion.

MRI may provide accurate information regarding the size, location, and soft-tissue extent of tumor. It provides limited information regarding bony involvement, unless there is gross involvement of the marrow space. Relatively greater sensitivity of MRI in relation to CT is offset by its decreased specificity. The main disadvantage of MRI is movement artifact, which is a particular problem in the larynx and hypopharynx. Gadolinium-enhanced MRI is probably superior to CT for imaging tumors of the nasopharynx and oropharynx.

PET has been evaluated in both primary and recurrent squamous cell carcinomas of the head and neck. ^{18}Fluorodeoxyglucose (FDG) is the most commonly used PET radiotracer. It enters the cell and undergoes the first step in glycolysis to produce ^{18}FDG-6-phosphate, which reflects the metabolic rate of the tissue. The metabolic rate of malignancies is higher than that of most benign tumors or normal tissues. ^{18}FDG imaging therefore has the potential to distinguish between benign and malignant processes, grade tumors, identify metastases, and diagnose tumor recurrence. In head and neck cancer,

^{18}FDG imaging has been useful in detecting clinically occult recurrences, although it has proved less useful in identifying an occult primary site for metastatic cervical disease.

Biopsy

Biopsies of the primary tumor often can be performed in an outpatient setting.

Punch or cup forceps biopsy is important in the diagnosis of mucosal lesions. The biopsy should be obtained at the border of the lesion away from areas of obvious necrosis.

Fine-needle aspiration (FNA) is a useful diagnostic modality. Multiple passes are made through the lesion with a fine-gauge (22-gauge) needle while suction is applied. Suction should be released before withdrawing the needle through surrounding soft tissue of the neck. FNA has an associated false-negative rate as low as 7%. The diagnostic accuracy depends on the physician's skill and the cytopathologist's experience.

Cytology is particularly useful in distinguishing a metastatic squamous cell carcinoma from other malignant histologies. However, a negative result should not be interpreted as "absence of malignancy."

Core biopsy should not be performed on a neck mass, with the rare exception of a proven lymphoma.

Open biopsy should be performed only when a diagnosis has not been made after extensive clinical evaluation and FNA is nondiagnostic. The operation should be performed only by a surgeon prepared to conduct immediate definitive surgical treatment at that time (which may entail radical neck dissection).

Pathology

Squamous cell carcinoma

More than 90% of all head and neck cancers are squamous cell carcinomas.

Histologic grade There are three histologic grades based on the amount of keratinization: A well-differentiated tumor is characterized by > 75% keratinization; a moderately differentiated tumor, by 25%–50%; and a poorly differentiated tumor, by < 25%.

In general, the more poorly differentiated a lesion, the higher is the incidence of regional metastases and the poorer the prognosis. Histologic grade has not been a consistent predictor of clinical behavior, however. Features that predict aggressive behavior include perineural spread, lymphatic invasion, and tumor spread beyond the lymph node capsule.

Morphologic growth patterns Four morphologically distinct growth patterns have been recognized. The ulcerative type is the most common form and begins as a round or oval ulcer that is friable. Ulcerative lesions progress toward infiltration. Infiltrative lesions extend deeply into underlying tissues. The exophytic type tends to grow more superficially and metastasize later than the other types. It begins as an area of thickened epithelium.

Verrucous cancer is an uncommon variant that, in the United States, typically occurs in elderly patients with poor oral hygiene or ill-fitting dentures. It is characterized by a warty, bulky, elevated, fungating appearance. Verrucous cancers seldom metastasize.

Other tumor types

Other less common head and neck cancers include mucoepidermoid carcinoma, adenoid cystic carcinoma, and adenocarcinoma, all of which may arise in the salivary glands. Head and neck cancers with neuroendocrine features include small-cell undifferentiated cancer and esthesioneuroblastoma (olfactory neuroblastoma). Both Hodgkin lymphoma and non-Hodgkin lymphoma may also be diagnosed as head and neck tumors, often involving the lymph nodes of the neck or Waldeyer's ring.

Sequence of disease progression

There is a sequence of disease progression from atypia/dysplasia through carcinoma in situ to frankly invasive cancer. Leukoplakia and erythroplakia are terms applied to clinically identifiable lesions that may harbor invasive cancer or undergo malignant transformation.

Leukoplakia results from chronic irritation of mucous membranes by carcinogens; this irritation stimulates the proliferation of white epithelial and connective tissue. Histopathologic examination reveals hyperkeratosis variably associated with underlying epithelial hyperplasia. In the absence of underlying dysplasia, leukoplakia rarely (< 5%) is associated with progression of disease to malignancy.

Erythroplakia is characterized by superficial, friable, red patches adjacent to normal mucosa. It is commonly associated with underlying epithelial dysplasia and has a much greater potential for malignancy than leukoplakia. Carcinoma is found in nearly 40% of erythroplakia.

Dysplasia is characterized by cellular atypia, loss of normal maturation, and loss of normal epithelial stratification. It is graded as mild, moderate, or severe, based on the degree of nuclear abnormality present. In the transition from mild to severe dysplasia, nuclear abnormalities become more marked, mitoses become more apparent, and these changes involve increasing depth of epithelium. The likelihood of developing a carcinoma relates to the degree of dysplasia. In the case of severe dysplasia, as many as 24% of patients may develop invasive squamous cell cancer.

Carcinoma in situ is characterized by the presence of atypical changes throughout the epithelium with complete loss of stratification. It is estimated that approximately 75% of invasive squamous cell carcinomas have an associated in situ component. Specific DNA mutations have also been identified in the sequence of disease progression from mild dysplasia to atypia to carcinoma in situ to invasive carcinoma.

Regional and distant metastases

The incidence of lymph node metastases is related to the size and thickness of the primary tumor. If the primary site is near the midline, contralateral or bilateral metastases should be anticipated. In the presence of lymph node metastases, extracapsular spread of tumor is an important prognostic factor.

Staging and prognosis

Staging system The TNM staging system of the American Joint Committee on Cancer (AJCC) maintains uniformity in the staging of head and neck tumors. The staging of primary mucosal tumors of the head and neck varies with the anatomic location and will be covered later by site. However, the staging system for metastases and stage groupings are nearly uniform for all mucosal sites.

Prognosis correlates strongly with stage at diagnosis. For many head and neck cancer sites, survival for patients with stage I disease exceeds 80%. For patients with locally advanced disease at the time of diagnosis, stages III and IV disease, survival drops below 40%. Development of nodal metastases reduces survival of a patient with a small primary tumor by ~50%. Involvement of even a single lymph node is associated with a marked decline in survival. Most patients with head and neck cancer have stage III or IV disease at diagnosis.

Pattern of relapse Despite aggressive primary treatment, the majority of relapses that occur following a head and neck cancer are within the head and neck. Locoregional relapse accounts for ~80% of primary treatment failures. Distant metastases increase as the disease progresses and most often involve the lungs, bones, and liver. By the time of death, 10%–30% of patients will have clinically detected distant metastases.

Field cancerization is an important concept related to the natural history of head and neck cancer. This term describes the diffuse epithelial injury throughout the head and neck, lungs, and esophagus that results from chronic exposure to carcinogens.

Clinically, field cancerization is manifested by the frequent occurrence of (1) mucosal abnormalities, such as leukoplakia and dysplasia, beyond the margins of a head and neck cancer and (2) second primary tumors within this exposed field. The lifetime risk of a patient with head and neck cancer developing a new cancer is 20%–40%. Over time, as the risk of relapse of the initial cancer declines, the development of a new cancer represents the greatest risk for these patients.

Treatment approaches

Head and neck tumors may be treated with curative intent using surgery, radiation therapy, or a combination of the two modalities. Chemotherapy may be combined with irradiation (chemoradiation therapy) in the management of advanced (stage III/IV) lesions of the oral cavity, oropharynx, hypopharynx, and larynx and for nasopharyngeal cancers more advanced than stage T2b.

Stages I and II disease at most sites may be treated with either resection or radiation therapy. The best therapeutic approach for the primary tumor depends on the anatomic site. The approach to treatment of the neck also varies with the site and treatment of the primary tumor. When the primary tumor is treated with irradiation, the "at-risk" regional lymphatics are incorporated into the treatment fields. Neck dissections should remain standardized (ie, complete anatomic dissections, as opposed to "berry picking" or random biopsy) in these settings so as to avoid incomplete surgery.

Preoperative assessment Before surgical resection, preoperative assessment of the extent of disease is essential. Complete physical examination and appropriate radiologic evaluation are necessary. Direct laryngoscopy and esophagoscopy are frequently performed to determine tumor extent and to rule out the presence of a second primary tumor. A chest x-ray or CT scan may be obtained to screen for distant metastases or a primary lung cancer.

Surgical principles Classic principles of surgical oncology apply to head and neck cancer. Complete resection is necessary. Securing sufficient margins may be challenging due to the many structures in this area. Reconstruction is complex after resection of head and neck tumors, as the surgery may have an impact on appearance, speech, and swallowing. Decisions regarding the extent of resection should be made by experienced surgeons.

Surgery plus radiation therapy

The combination of radical surgery and radiation therapy has been used for several decades to treat patients with advanced head and neck cancers.

Postoperative vs preoperative radiation therapy Postoperative radiation therapy (60–70 Gy in 6–7 weeks) reduces the rate of locoregional recurrence from ~50% to 15% for tumors with pathologic features predictive of locoregional recurrence. The indications for postoperative radiation therapy are well established and include a large primary tumor (T4), close or positive margins, an involved lymph node > 3 cm or multiple involved lymph nodes, extracapsular extension, tumor fixation, and connective tissue invasion. The addition of postoperative radiation therapy reduces the risk of locoregional failure but does not decrease the risk of developing distant metastases.

Preoperative radiotherapy (45–50 Gy in 4–5 weeks) has been used for patients with advanced primary tumors, but rates of locoregional recurrence appear to be lower and complications fewer with postoperative radiation therapy. Preoperative radiotherapy is indicated for marginally resectable tumors, such as those with fixed cervical lymph nodes. In this setting, preoperative irradiation often permits resection of an otherwise unresectable tumor.

Postoperative chemotherapy/radiation therapy Two randomized clinical trials were launched to determine whether the addition of concurrent chemotherapy to radiation therapy enhanced locoregional control and survival in high-risk patients with head and neck cancer following definitive surgical resection. The results of these trials were published in 2004. In the Radiation Therapy Oncology Group (RTOG) 95-01/intergroup trial, patients with high-risk features including two or more involved lymph nodes, extracapsular extension, or positive margins following definitive surgical resection were randomized to receive 6,000–6,600 cGy of postoperative irradiation with or without cisplatin (given on days 1, 22, and 43). With a median follow-up of 45.9 months, the estimated 2-year rate of local and regional tumor control was 82% in the combined-therapy group vs 72% in the radiotherapy group ($P = .01$). The disease-free ($P = .04$) but not overall ($P = .19$) survival was significantly longer in the combined-treatment group. The incidence of acute adverse effects (grade 3 or greater) was higher in the combined-treatment relative group, 77% vs 34% ($P < .001$).

In the EORTC (European Organization for Research on the Treatment of Cancer) trial 22931, similar conclusions were reported. In this study, however, the overall survival rate was found to be significantly improved in the combined-therapy group compared with the radiotherapy group. After a mean of 60 months, the overall survival of 334 randomized patients was 53% in the combined-treatment group vs 40% in the radiation-alone group ($P = .02$). The discrepancy in effect on overall survial was thought to be related to different entry criteria used in the RTOG and EORTC trials.

In a recently published comparative analysis of the two trials, extracapsular extension and/or microscopically involved surgical margins were the only risk factors for which the impact of chemoradiation therapy was significant for survival in both trials. Patients with two or more histopathologically involved lymph nodes without the presence of extracapsular extension as their only risk factor did not benefit from the addition of chemotherapy.

Curative radiation therapy

Radiation therapy with curative intent usually involves daily treatment for 6–7 weeks (total dose, 60–70 Gy). Although there is no tissue loss with radiation therapy, complications include dry mouth, tissue fibrosis, trismus, bone necrosis, and hypothyroidism. Some problems are common and sufficiently debilitating to warrant significant concern in treatment planning for head and neck cancer. Surgery often produces less morbidity.

Radiation fractionation

The RTOG 90-03 trial was conducted to determine the efficacy of various fractionation schemes in the treament of locally advanced head and neck cancer. Four schedules were tested: (1) standard fractionation at 2 Gy/fraction/day, 5 days/week, to 70 Gy/35 fractions/7 weeks; (2) hyperfractionation at 1.2 Gy/fraction, twice daily, 5 days/week to 81.6 Gy/68 fractions/7 weeks; (3) accelerated fractionation with split at 1.6 Gy/fraction, twice daily, 5 days/week, to 67.2 Gy/42 fractions/6 weeks, including a 2-week rest after 38.4 Gy; or (4) accelerated fractionation with concomitant boost at 1.8 Gy/fraction/day, 5 days/week, and 1.5 Gy/fraction/day to a boost field as a second daily treatment for the last 12 treatment days to 72 Gy/42 fractions/6 weeks. A total of 1,113 patients were entered in the study, with a median follow-up of 23 months.

Patients treated with both hyperfractionation and accelerated fractionation with a concomitant boost had significantly increased locoregional control rates compared with patients on the other two arms. All three groups treated with the altered fractionation schemes had more acute, but not late, side effects. The study concluded that hyperfractionation and accelerated fractionation with a concomitant boost are the optimal treatment schemes.

Intensity-modulated radiation therapy

Intensity-modulated radiation therapy (IMRT) is a more sophisticated approach for obtaining highly conformal radiation dose distributions needed to irradiate complex targets positioned near sensitive normal structures. Treatment planning for IMRT (also known as inverse planning) is different from that of conventional or three-dimensional cranial radiation therapy planning. The starting point with IMRT is a description of the desired dose distribution rather than the application of traditional fields and beam modifiers to generate an acceptable plan. Conventional radiation treatment utilizes relatively uniform beams of radiation (typically between 2 and 4 beams), whereas IMRT, instead of using 4 beams of 50 cGy each, could use 50 beams of 4 cGy each. Each beam direction is divided into multiple segments to modulate the radiation dose.

The role of IMRT continues to be defined, although its widespread use should not be considered standard for all head and neck tumors. IMRT in head and neck cancer is ideal in the setting of a unilateral tumor adjacent to a critical structure (eyes, optic nerve, spinal cord, brainstem, optic chiasm), which would not otherwise be treatable with conventional planning.

Various groups have examined dosimetric and quality-of-life differences between IMRT and conventional radiation techniques. The group at Memorial Sloan-Kettering Cancer Center compared its IMRT planned treatment for nasopharyngeal cancer with conventional treatment with a conformal boost. Locoregional control was 97%, vs 78%, at 2 years. The University of Michigan and Washington University have reported reductions in xerostomia with IMRT.

Chemotherapy

Induction (neoadjuvant) chemotherapy vs concomitant chemotherapy and radiation therapy A rationale for using induction chemotherapy for treating advanced-stage laryngeal cancer involves using chemotherapy as a marker of radiation sensitivity to select potentially radiocurable patients. In the VA

Laryngeal Cancer Cooperative Study, the major benefit for the patients in the experimental arm was laryngeal preservation in two-thirds of patients. In this study, lack of substantial tumor response to induction chemotherapy was not associated with reduced survival. In addition, patients who failed to respond to induction chemotherapy underwent surgery, which had the advantage of not being performed in an irradiated field.

This use of induction chemotherapy has recently been challenged by data from the RTOG, which has revealed that concurrent treatment using chemotherapy and irradiation is associated with an increased likelihood of locoregional tumor control. When used concurrently with radiotherapy, the function of chemotherapy is thought to "radiosensitize" the tissue in the radiation field, rather than to function as a selection marker of radiation response. The recently published results of the RTOG 91-11 trial demonstrated improved locoregional tumor control as well as an increased rate of laryngeal preservation in patients with stage III and IV resectable laryngeal cancer who underwent concurrent chemoradiation therapy (for details, see discussion later in chapter). However, the rate of mucosal toxicity in those receiving concomitant chemotherapy was double the rate in either of the other two arms. One year following treatment, 23% of patients in the concurrent treatment group tolerated only a soft or liquid diet, and 3% could not swallow at all. Patients with extensive T4 primaries, such as those with cartilage invasion or those with involvement of the tongue base, were not included in the study.

Due to the toxicity of chemoradiation therapy, there is much interest in the potential for molecular-targeted agents to radiosensitize tumor more selectively than chemotherapy. Intriguing results from a randomized trial testing the addition of cetuximab (Erbitux), a humanized monoclonal antibody to the epidermal growth factor receptor (EGFR), to irradiation vs irradiation alone for intermediate-stage squamous cell cancer have been reported. At a 2-year time point, locoregional tumor control (56% vs 48%) and survival (62% vs 55%) were both improved with the addition of cetuximab. Unlike the combination of chemotherapy and irradiation, the benefit of cetuximab was not offset by any increase in mucosal toxicity.

Chemotherapy and survival Numerous clinical trials have shown an improvement in locoregional control using concurrent chemoradiation therapy, but a survival benefit has been more challenging to demonstrate. In a randomized clinical trial published by Brizel et al, the addition of chemotherapy or hyperfractionated radiotherapy to treat locally advanced head and neck cancer improved locoregional control. At 3 years, overall survival was 34% vs 55% in favor of the chemoradiation therapy arm ($P = .07$), and the relapse-free survival rate was 41% vs 65% ($P = .08$).

In the 91-11 randomized clinical trial, chemotherapy given concurrently with irradiation, or sequentially prior to irradiation, was found to suppress the incidence of distant metastases and to improve disease-specific survival relative to irradiation alone. Overall survival, however, was not affected, likely due to the effectiveness of surgical salvage, competing causes of death, and the toxicity of chemotherapy.

Concurrent chemoradiation therapy has been found to have greater efficacy than irradiation alone in the setting of unresectable squamous cell cancer, based on a head and neck intergroup study. In this study, 295 patients with stages III and IV head and neck cancer were randomized to participate in one of three arms: (A) radiotherapy alone to 70 Gy in 35 fractions; (B) 70 Gy in 35 fractions plus concurrent cisplatin on days 1, 22, and 43; and (C) split-course radiotherapy and 3 cycles or concurrent cisplatin/5-FU (fluorouracil) chemotherapy, with 30 Gy given with cycle 1 and 30–40 Gy given with cycle 3. Grade 3 or worse toxicity occurred in 53% of arm A patients, 86% of arm B patients, and 77% of arm C patients. The 2- and 3-year Kaplan-Meier projected survivals for arm A are 30% and 20%, compared with 43% and 37% for arm B ($P = .016$) and 40% and 27% for arm C ($P = .13$). Median survival is 12.6 months for arm A, 19.1 months for arm B, and 14.0 months for arm C. The addition of concurrent high-dose single-agent cisplatin to conventional radiotherapy significantly improved survival with acceptable toxicity. Additionally, concurrent multiagent chemotherapy did not offset the loss of efficacy resulting from split-course irradiation.

The impact of adjuvant concomitant chemotherapy and radiotherapy on survival was assessed in two similarly designed trials in high-risk postoperative head and neck cancer patients testing adjuvant chemoradiation therapy against standard postoperative radiotherapy. In the RTOG 95-01 trial, disease-free survival was significantly increased in patients treated with adjuvant chemoradiation therapy relative to those treated with radiotherapy alone, but overall survival was not affected. In the EORTC trial published at the same time as the RTOG trial, the 5-year overall survival was also significantly improved in the concomitant chemotherapy and radiotherapy group.

Adjuvant chemotherapy following surgery or irradiation Adjuvant chemotherapy has been given following initial surgery or radiation therapy in an attempt to eliminate microscopic residual disease and distant metastases. Although this approach has resulted in a reduced rate of distant metastasis, it has not been associated with improved locoregional control or survival. As concomitant approaches evolve and locoregional control for advanced disease becomes the rule rather than the exception, the value of additional chemotherapy (as induction or adjuvant therapy) will need to be reexplored to address the problem of distant metastasis.

Locally advanced head and neck cancer Data from prospective trials continue to support the use of altered fractionation and concurrent chemotherapy and irradiation as an alternative to surgery or conventionally fractionated irradiation alone for locally advanced cancers of the head and neck. The long-term results of RTOG 90-03, which randomized 1,113 patients with stages III and IV squamous cell carcinoma of the oral cavity, oropharynx, or supraglottic larynx and stages II–IV squamous cell carcinoma of the base of the tongue or hypopharynx to receive one of four different schedules of irradiation alone, were recently reported. They included 72 Gy/42 fractions (1.8 Gy/fraction initially, followed by 1.5 Gy/fraction to a boost field for the last 12 fractions bid).

Locoregional control and disease-free survival were superior for the hyperfractionated arm and accelerated fractionation with the concomitant boost (AFX-C; 49.8% and 30.7% for the hyperfractionated arm and 49.3% and 28.9% for the AFX-C arm, respectively) compared with the other two arms. The hyperfractionated arm demonstrated a trend toward improved overall survival (37.1% vs 29.5%, 30.8% and 33.5%, respectively, $P = .06$) compared with the other three arms.

Updated results for RTOG 99-14, a phase II prospective study designed to integrate the altered fractionated radiation regimen from RTOG 90-03 with chemotherapy, were also reported in 2005. Cisplatin was given during weeks 1, 3, and 5. Longer term results for 76 of 84 patients were reported, and the 3-year disease free, overall, and cause-specific survival rates were 45.8%, 57.7%, and 61.2%, respectively. The 3-year local recurrence and distant metastases rates were 38.7% and 23.3%, respectively. Of 35 patients who were alive, 22 had a temporary feeding tube, and 17% (6 patients) still required a feeding tube at the time of their last follow-up.

RTOG 97-03, the most recent study to support the use of concurrent chemotherapy and irradiation for treating locally advanced head and neck cancer, has been reported. In this study, three different regimens of chemotherapy were used with irradiation (70 Gy/35 fractions) for oral cavity, oropharyngeal, and hypopharyngeal cancers. Patients randomized to arm 1 received cisplatin, 10 mg/m^2, and 5-FU, 400 mg/m^2 continuous infusion daily, for the final 10 days of radiation treatments. Treatment on arm 2 consisted of hydroxyurea, 1 g/d, and 5-FU, 800 mg/m^2 continous infusion delivered concurrently, with each daily fraction of radiation. Patients randomized to arm 3 received paclitaxel, 30 mg/m^2, and cisplatin, 20 mg/m^2, weekly. The 2-year rates of overall survival were 57.4% , 69.4%, and 66.2%, respectively.

Experience incorporating biologic agents continues to grow, and more results were reported in 2005. Preliminary results of a multi-institutional, multinational randomized prospective study was presented at the American Society of Clinical Oncology (ASCO) 2004 meeting. It compared irradiation alone with irradiation plus the EGFR-blocking antibody cetuximab. A total of 424 patients were randomized between the arms. The median survival was 28 months in the irradiation-alone arm, vs 54 months with cetuximab. The 2-year survival rate was 55%, vs 62%, respectively, for irradiation alone and irradiation with cetuximab ($P = .02$). Results of a subgroup of 171 patients with laryngeal and hypopharyngeal primaries were analyzed, and a nonsignificant improvement in laryngeal preservation was observed in the group of patients who were treated with cetuximab (92% vs. 83%).

Chemotherapy for recurrent or metastatic disease The combination of cisplatin/5-FU produces overall response rates of approximately 30% and survival rates of 6 months. In randomized trials comparing this combination with single-agent cisplatin, 5-FU, or methotrexate, response rates with the single agents are lower, but survival is equivalent. However, because many practitioners believe response is a surrogate for palliation,

In March 2006, cetuximab (Erbitux) received FDA approval for use in combination with radiotherapy (RT) for patients with squamous cell cancer of the head and neck as well as monotherapy for metastatic disease. In a recent study, 424 patients with locoregionally advanced head and neck cancer were randomly assigned to treatment with high-dose RT alone or with weekly cetuximab. The primary endpoint was the duration of control of locoregional disease; secondary endpoints included overall and progression-free survival. The median duration of locoregional control was 24.4 months among patients treated with cetuximab plus RT and 14.9 months among those given RT alone (hazard ratio [HR] for locoregional progression or death, 0.68; *P* = .005). With a median follow-up of 54.0 months, the median duration of overall survival was 49.0 months among patients treated with combined therapy and 29.3 months among those treated with RT alone (HR for death, 0.74; *P* = .03). RT plus cetuxuimab significantly prolonged progression-free survival (HR for disease progression or death, 0.70; *P* = .006) (*Bonner JA, Harari PM, Giralt J, et al: N Engl J Med 354:567-578, 2006*).

cisplatin/5-FU has been used widely in this setting.

The taxanes are the most active cytotoxins yet identified in head and neck cancer, with overall response rates of approximately 35% in patients with recurrent or incurable disease. In a recent randomized trial, the combination of paclitaxel/cisplatin has been compared with cisplatin/5-FU in patients with recurrent disease. ECOG (Eastern Cooperative Oncology Group) 13-93 randomized patients with recurrent squamous cell cancer of the head and neck to receive cisplatin (100 mg/m^2 on day 1) and 5-FU (1 g/m^2 on days 1–4; arm 1) or cisplatin (75 mg/m^2 on day 1) and paclitaxel (75 mg/m^2 on day 1; arm 2). Patients could have had no prior treatment for recurrent disease and were required to have an ECOG performance status of 0 or 1. A total of 194 patients were studied, with 96 and 92 patients eligible on arms 1 and 2, respectively.

Overall response and median survival rates were equivalent (arm 1: 22% and 8 months; arm 2: 28% and 9 months). The toxicity analysis favored arm 2, which was associated with fewer cases of stomatitis, diarrhea, myelosuppression, and infection. Quality of life did not favor either arm. Paclitaxel/cisplatin was less toxic overall and can now be considered a safer, more convenient alternative to cisplatin and infusional 5-FU in recurrent disease.

Other drugs receiving recent attention are those targeting growth factors and their receptors. The EGFR is particularly notable, since nearly 100% of head and neck tumors overexpress this receptor. A number of EGFR inhibitors are currently being evaluated alone and in combination with other drugs.

The monoclonal antibody to EGFR, cetuximab, as well as the EGFR tyrosine kinase inhibitors gefitinib (Iressa) and erlotinib (Tarceva) have single-agent response rates of 5%–10% in patients with recurrent disease. A randomized trial testing the addition of cetuximab to cisplatin vs cisplatin alone in patients with recurrent disease showed additive effects for response but no impact on survival for the cetuximab-cisplatin arm. These agents are being studied in combination with chemotherapy and irradiation in the curative-intent setting.

Photodynamic therapy

Photodynamic therapy may have some promise in the treatment of mucosal dysplasia and small head and neck tumors.

Small studies of photodynamic therapy, performed at several institutions, suggest that widespread areas of carcinoma in situ or severe dysplasia, as well as cancer, are often extirpated after photodynamic therapy. Although some patients have experienced durable remissions, the long-term efficacy of this modality remains uncertain.

Pulsed dye laser therapy for early laryngeal lesions

The pulsed dye laser initially used to treat vascular lesions has recently been investigated in the treatment of respiratory papillomatosis, dysplastic, and early invasive glottic carcinomas. The efficacy of the laser is mediated through its antiangiogenic properties. The treatment is nontoxic, preserves the laryngeal microarchitecture, and preserves or restores near-normal vocal quality. Additionally, this modality can be utilized in an outpatient clinic setting. Preliminary findings are favorable. At this time, however, pulsed dye laser therapy should be considered investigational.

Chemoprevention

The area of chemoprevention has received a great deal of attention in recent years, and the concept of field cancerization is important in this context. As mentioned previously, this concept refers to the diffuse epithelial injury incurred by upper aerodigestive tract mucosa due to chronic exposure to carcinogens (most commonly alcohol and tobacco). These mucosal changes increase the risk of developing premalignant lesions (leukoplakia and erythroplakia), as well as multiple primary lesions.

Retinoids (vitamin A analogues) have been investigated as chemopreventive agents in the aerodigestive tract based on their efficacy in tumor models, such as the hamster buccal pouch. Retinoids mediate changes in gene expression through interaction with nuclear retinoic acid receptors, which function as transcription factors. Nutritional epidemiology studies also have indicated that low serum levels of both carotenoids and retinoids contribute to the risk of cancer development in the epithelium of the upper aerodigestive tract.

The role of retinoids in the prevention of second primary tumors in patients treated with curative intent for an early-stage index squamous cell cancer of the head and neck has been investigated in three randomized trials. The initial study was a small, single-center phase III trial of *cis*-retinoic acid (1–2 mg/kg/d) by Hong et al. Although this study demonstrated decreased second primary tumors in the experimental arm, compliance and morbidity with this high dose were problematic. A second study using a low dose of *cis*-retinoic acic (10 mg/d) was performed by ECOG and was negative. Results from a third large, multicenter trial with an intermediate dose of 30 mg/d have been reported in abstract form and are also negative in regard to second primary prevention.

Rehabilitation

Rehabilitation also is very important in the perioperative care of patients with head and neck cancer. It includes physical and occupational therapy, speech and swallowing rehabilitation, and nutritional support. For example, resection of the spinal accessory nerve, which innervates the trapezius muscle, leads to scapular winging, inability to abduct the arm fully, and, eventually, severe pain around the shoulder. These symptoms may be ameliorated with appropriate physical therapy.

Adapting to the loss of the larynx also requires intensive rehabilitation and patient motivation. Voice rehabilitation options include esophageal speech, artificial larynges (portable, battery-operated devices), and tracheoesophageal shunts.

Nutritional support is facilitated by temporary nasoduodenal tubes or gastrostomy tubes (which impose added morbidity but are more socially acceptable and ease the patient's transition to normal activities).

Management of symptoms and treatment side effects

Eating problems At the time of diagnosis, many patients with head and neck cancer will have lost a significant amount of weight. Maintaining adequate nutrition is a major problem for these patients, as both the tumor and treatment side effects, such as mucositis from chemotherapy and radiation therapy, may be contributory. For patients who are unable to eat or who are being treated with aggressive concomitant chemotherapy and radiation therapy protocols, placement of a gastrostomy tube is often desirable to maintain caloric intake and adequate hydration.

Pain Clinicians must also be aware of the significant pain associated with these lesions and use narcotic analgesics appropriately to relieve discomfort.

Mucositis The use of chemotherapy concomitantly with radiation therapy increases the occurrence of mucositis.

Nephrotoxicity and ototoxicity For patients treated with cisplatin-containing regimens, renal insufficiency and ototoxicity are potential serious side effects.

Xerostomia Following radiation therapy of a head and neck cancer, xerostomia may be a significant long-term side effect. In some patients, pilocarpine (Salagen) has been useful in stimulating the production of saliva.

The use of organic thiophosphates, such as amifostine (Ethyol), in patients undergoing radiotherapy for head and neck cancer may reduce the severity of acute and late xerostomia without compromising the antitumor activity of the irradiation.

Gastroesophageal reflux Often asymptomatic or "silent" gastroesophageal reflux disease (GERD) is a common finding in patients treated for pharyngolaryngeal squamous cell carcinoma. In addition, cisplatin-containing chemotherapy may aggravate GERD.

Treatment of the neck

Either irradiation alone or radical neck dissection will control metastatic squamous cell cancer to a single small neck node more than 90% of the time if there is no extracapsular tumor spread. Hence, radiation treatment may easily provide prophylactic treatment of the neck if control of the primary tumor is undertaken with irradiation. Traditionally, if the tumor in the neck was N2 or greater, or if there was tumor beyond the confines of a node, neck dissection and irradiation were combined for optimal control of the neck tumor. More recently, evidence suggests that N2–N3 disease that has a complete clinical and radiologic response to induction chemoradiotherapy may not require a complete neck dissection.

Types of dissection

There are several approaches to the surgical treatment of the neck nodes in patients with head and neck cancer (Table 2). This discussion will be limited to two types of neck dissection: comprehensive and selective.

Comprehensive neck dissection entails complete removal of all lymphatic tissue from the neck (levels I–V). A radical neck dissection includes comprehensive node dissection with removal of the sternocleidomastoid muscle, jugular vein, and spinal accessory nerve. Modified radical neck dissection was developed to diminish the morbidity of the classic operation. The most important structure to preserve is the spinal accessory nerve.

Selective neck dissection consists of the removal of lymph node groups at highest risk of containing metastases from a primary cancer. In such procedures, the lymph nodes removed correspond to the most significant drainage basins of specific head and neck tumor sites. These are staging operations usually performed in patients with clinically N0 neck cancer. If metastases are identified, further treatment to the neck will be required. A selective neck dissection should not be employed as the sole treatment of clinically palpable disease.

Sentinel lymph node biopsy for oral cavity lesions has been evaluated. Forty patients with clinically N0 neck cancer underwent sentinel lymph node biopsy followed by complete neck dissection. A sentinel node was identified in 90% of necks, with a 97% accuracy rate in predicting the nodal status of the remainder of the neck. This finding corresponded to a sensitivity of 94% and a specificity of 100%. Although these results are encouraging, they need to be validated in a larger trial. An ongoing American College of Surgeons Oncology Group study (Z0360) is examining this technique in patients with T1 or T2, N0 oral cavity cancer. Sentinel lymph node biopsy may prove useful in small lesions without deep penetration, but it remains investigational.

Follow-up of long-term survivors

As mentioned, head and neck cancers are aggressive tumors. The majority (80%) of recurrences will develop within 2 years. Since many recurrences are

TABLE 2: Types of neck dissection and structures removed in the treatment of head and neck cancer

Type of neck dissection	Structures removed
Comprehensive neck dissection	
"Classic" radical neck dissection	All lymph-bearing tissue (levels I-V), spinal accessory nerve (cranial nerve [CN] XI), sternocleidomastoid muscle, and internal jugular vein
Modified radical neck dissection	Neck dissection with sparing of one or more of the above structures
Type I	CN XI spared
Type II	CN XI and internal jugular vein spared
Type III (functional neck dissection)	All three structures spared (CN XI, internal jugular vein, and sternocleidomastoid muscle)
Selective neck dissection	Removal of lymph-bearing tissue from:
Lateral	Levels II-IV
Posterolateral	Levels II-V
Supraomohyoid	Levels I-III

From Medina JE, Rebual NM: Neck dissection, in Cummings CW, Fredrickson J, Harker LE, et al (eds): Otolaryngology: Head and Neck Surgery, pp 1649–1672. St. Louis, Mosby Yearbook, 1993.

treatable with curative intent, patients should be followed closely during the months following their treatment. This period coincides with the time of greatest need from the standpoint of rehabilitation.

After 2 years, second primary tumors of the head and neck and lungs become important causes of death and morbidity. Late complications of treatment such as radionecrosis, radiation-induced fibrosis, and hypothyroidism, as well as sequelae of spinal accessory nerve sacrifice or injury, may develop even after years. Complications and second primary cancers are more common in patients who continue to smoke.

Timing of follow-up evaluations Follow-up evaluations at regular intervals should be complete and should include a focused history and examination, as outlined previously. Physicians who are able to perform a head and neck examination (including laryngoscopy) should direct follow-up. After surgical treatment, this evaluation will usually require visits with the head and neck surgeon. Patients treated with irradiation should be followed by both their radiation oncologist and a head and neck surgeon or otolaryngologist.

Evaluations should be scheduled every 1–2 months during the first year after treatment, every 2–4 months during the second year, every 3–6 months during the third year, and every 6 months thereafter for several more years.

Imaging and laboratory studies Any mucosal abnormality should be biopsied. There are no tumor markers or other useful laboratory studies to follow. Chest x-rays should be obtained yearly. There is little justification for performing CT scans or MRI in the follow-up of asymptomatic patients. Thyroid-stimulating hormone (TSH) should be measured yearly in patients who have received irradiation to the larynx or nasopharynx.

HEAD AND NECK TUMOR REGIONS

As mentioned previously, tumors occurring at different anatomic sites and subsites of the head and neck vary considerably with regard to epidemiology, risk factors, anatomy, natural history, staging of the primary tumor, and therapy. The following sections highlight these differences.

ORAL CAVITY

Sites of the oral cavity include the lips, hard palate, floor of the mouth, buccal mucosa, and tongue. Cancers at these sites comprise < 5% of all malignancies in the United States.

Anatomy

The oral cavity extends from the cutaneous vermilion junction of the lips to the junction of the hard and soft palates above and to the line of the circumvallate papillae below. It includes the lips, buccal mucosa, upper and lower alveolar ridges, retromolar trigone, floor of the mouth, hard palate, and anterior two-thirds of the tongue (the "oral" tongue). The primary lymphatic drainage is to the submental triangle, submandibular nodes, and upper deep jugular nodes.

Natural history

The most common presenting complaint is a sore in the mouth or on the lips. One-third of patients present with a neck mass.

The differential diagnosis includes other malignancies and benign diseases or lesions. Other malignancies to be considered include salivary gland tumors, sarcoma, lymphoma, and melanoma. Benign diseases include pyogenic granuloma, tuberculous disease, aphthous ulcers, and chancres.

Benign mucosal lesions include papillomas and keratoacanthomas, which may be exophytic or infiltrative. The exophytic lesions are less aggressive. The infiltrative papillomas and keratoacanthomas are more often associated with destruction of surrounding tissues and structures. These lesions may progress to malignancy. The TNM staging system for cancers of the lips and oral cavity is outlined in Table 3. T4 lesions have been divided into T4a (resectable) and T4b (unresectable) in the sixth edition of the *AJCC Cancer Staging Manual.*

TABLE 3: TNM staging system for cancers of the lips and oral cavity

Primary tumor (T)	
Tx	Primary tumor cannot be assessed
T0	No evidence of primary tumor
Tis	Carcinoma in situ
T1	Tumor 2 cm or less in greatest dimension
T2	Tumor more than 2 cm but not more than 4 cm in greatest dimension
T3	Tumor more than 4 cm in greatest dimension
T4	(lip) Tumor invades through cortical bone, inferior alveolar nerve, floor of mouth, or skin of face, ie, chin or nose[a]
T4a	(oral cavity) Tumor invades adjacent structures (eg, through cortical bone, into deep [extrinsic] muscle of the tongue, maxillary sinus, or skin of face); resectable lesions
T4b	Tumor involves masticator space, pterygoid plates, or skull base and/or encases internal carotid artery; unresectable lesions
Regional lymph nodes (N)	
Nx	Regional nodes cannot be assessed
N0	No regional lymph node metastasis
N1	Metastasis in a single ipsilateral lymph node, 3 cm or less in greatest dimension
N2	Metastasis in a single ipsilateral lymph node, more than 3 cm but not more than 6 cm in greatest dimension; or in multiple ipsilateral lymph nodes, none more than 6 cm in greatest dimension; or in bilateral or contralateral lymph nodes, none more than 6 cm in greatest dimension
N2a	Metastasis in a single ipsilateral lymph node, more than 3 cm but not more than 6 cm in greatest dimension
N2b	Metastasis in multiple ipsilateral lymph nodes, none more than 6 cm in greatest dimension
N2c	Metastasis in bilateral or contralateral lymph nodes, none more than 6 cm in greatest dimension
N3	Metastasis in a lymph node, more than 6 cm in greatest dimension

Treatment

Management of cancers of the oral cavity involves surgery or radiotherapy for T1 or T2 lesions or combined-modality treatment that includes surgical resection and postoperative radiation therapy (60–70 Gy in 6–7 weeks) for advanced disease. For early-stage disease, surgery and radiotherapy are considered to have equivalent efficacy. Supraomohyoid neck dissection is performed in surgically treated patients with N0 necks, although surgery is associated with less morbidity. Bilateral neck dissection is performed if the tumor approaches the midline or if tumor thickness is at least 4 mm.

Distant metastases (M)

Mx	Distant metastasis cannot be assessed
M0	No distant metastasis
M1	Distant metastasis

Stage grouping

Stage 0	Tis	N0	M0
Stage I	T1	N0	M0
Stage II	T2	N0	M0
Stage III	T3	N0	M0
	T1	N1	M0
	T2	N1	M0
	T3	N1	M0
Stage IVA	T4a	N0	M0
	T4a	N1	M0
	T1	N2	M0
	T2	N2	M0
	T3	N2	M0
	T4a	N2	M0
Stage IVB	Any T	N3	M0
	T4b	Any N	M0
Stage IVC	Any T	Any N	M1

From Greene FL, Page DL, Fleming ID, et al (eds): AJCC Cancer Staging Manual, 6th ed. New York, Springer-Verlag, 2002.

[a] Superficial erosion alone of bone/tooth socket by gingival primary is not sufficient to classify a tumor as T4.

ORAL CAVITY SITE: LIPS

The lips are the most common site of oral cavity cancer. There are approximately 4,000 new cases per year in the United States. The lower lip is affected most often. The vast majority of patients (90%) with lip cancer are men, and 33% have outdoor occupations.

Natural history

The most frequent presentation is a slow-growing tumor of the lower lip that may bleed and hurt. Physical examination must include assessment of hypoesthesia in the distribution of the mental nerve (cutaneous sensation of the chin area). Currently, fewer than 10% of American patients with squamous cell carcinoma of the lower lip have cervical metastases.

Treatment

The primary tumor Patients with early-stage lip cancers are usually treated with surgery. Radiation therapy may be utilized in patients who are medically unsuited for surgery or who refuse surgical resection.

Resection involves excision with at least 0.5 cm of normal tissue circumferentially beyond the recognized border of the tumor. After the resection of larger lesions, reconstruction may pose a major challenge. Small tumors are excised with a V incision.

Patients with advanced disease (stage III or IV) are usually managed with a combination of surgery and postoperative radiation therapy (60–70 Gy in 6–7 weeks).

The neck Elective treatment of the neck is seldom recommended for patients with squamous cell carcinoma of the lower lip and a clinically negative neck because few of these patients have cervical metastases. Neck dissection is recommended only in patients with palpable cervical metastases. Neck dissection is followed by postoperative radiation therapy.

Results The cure rate for T1–T3 tumors is 90% with surgical excision alone. Smaller lesions (T1–T2) may be treated equally well with radiation therapy. Survival rates for patients with T1 and T2 lesions are 90% and 80%, respectively. Overall, younger patients have a poorer prognosis, as do those with involvement of the mandible and extension of the tumor within the oral cavity.

ORAL CAVITY SITE: TONGUE

The oral tongue (anterior two-thirds) is the site of 75% of all tongue cancers. There are approximately 7,320 new cases of oral tongue cancer each year in the United States.

Natural history

The most common presenting symptom in patients with cancer of the tongue is a persistent, nonhealing ulcer with or without associated pain. Other symptoms include difficulty with deglutition and speech. There may be a history of leukoplakia, especially in younger women.

Rate of growth Cancer of the tongue seems to grow more rapidly than other oral cavity cancers. Tongue cancers may grow in an infiltrative or exophytic fashion. The infiltrative tumors may be quite large at presentation.

Lesion thickness Thicker lesions have a worse prognosis than thin cancers, and lesion thickness is a more important prognostic factor than is simple tumor stage. The incidence of clinically occult cervical metastases to the neck is significantly higher when the tumor thickness exceeds 4 mm.

Cervical metastases occur more frequently from tongue cancer than from any other tumor of the oral cavity. At initial evaluation, 40% of patients have node metastases.

Treatment

Early-stage disease Treatment usually entails partial glossectomy. Margins should be assessed at the time of resection, as the disease spreads along muscle bundles, leading to more extensive tumor than is appreciated grossly.

Radiation therapy (60–70 Gy in 6–7 weeks) is a suitable option for small or minimally infiltrating tumors. Large, infiltrative lesions should be treated with combined-modality therapy (radiation therapy and surgical resection).

Advanced disease More advanced tumors with mandibular involvement require composite resection, including a partial glossectomy, mouth floor resection, and mandibulectomy.

The neck A selective neck dissection is often recommended for clinically N0 neck cancer. Comprehensive neck dissection is required in the presence of palpable cervical metastases.

Results Control of disease closely correlates with the extent of the primary tumor and the presence of metastases. Rates of local control using radiation therapy or surgery are similar for T1 (~85%) and T2 (~80%) tumors. T3 tumors should be treated using surgery and radiation therapy. Only 10%–15% of local recurrences are amenable to repeat resection.

Overall survival is approximately 50%. Rates of survival at 5 years by stage follow: stage I, 80%; stage II, 60%; and stages III–IV, 15%–35%. For equivalent primary cancers, the presence of lymph node metastases decreases the survival rate by 50%.

ORAL CAVITY SITE: FLOOR OF THE MOUTH

There are approximately 4,000 cases of floor of the mouth cancer in the United States annually. Mouth floor cancer accounts for 10%–15% of all oral cavity cancers.

Pathology

Most lesions are moderately differentiated to well-differentiated squamous cell cancers and are exophytic.

Natural history

Patients usually present with a painful mass located near the oral tongue. Since these lesions do not cause pain until they are deep, they are frequently advanced at presentation.

Extension of disease into the soft tissues of the submandibular triangle is not uncommon. Fixation of the tumor to bone suggests possible mandibular involvement. A Panorex film of the mandible may reveal invasion of the mandible via direct extension (through a tooth socket) or via perineural invasion spreading along the mental nerve through the mental foramen. Changes in the mental foramen can be distinct or demonstrate slight asymmetry when compared with the contralateral anatomy. Restricted tongue mobility reflects invasion into the root of the tongue. Palpation demonstrates the depth of infiltration much better than does inspection alone.

Tumors near the midline may obstruct the duct of the submandibular gland, leading to swelling and induration in the neck, which may be difficult to distinguish from lymph node metastases. Level I nodes are the first-echelon metastatic sites.

Multifocality Multifocal cancers are more common in the floor of the mouth than in other oral cavity sites. Approximately 20% of patients with mouth floor tumors have a second primary tumor, half of which are in the head and neck.

Treatment

Early invasive lesions (T1–T2) involving the mucosa alone may be treated with either surgery or irradiation (60–70 Gy in 6–7 weeks) alone, with comparable results. Primary tumors with mandibular involvement should be surgically resected.

Cancer invades the mandible through tooth sockets. Hence, if the tumor merely abuts the mandible, a marginal mandibulectomy (which removes the bone margin but preserves continuity) may be performed. Otherwise, a segmental resection is needed. Selective neck dissection for treatment planning is advisable for thick stage I or II cancers.

Advanced disease The treatment of choice for advanced disease is combined-modality therapy with surgery and radiation therapy. Complete surgical resection may require a composite resection of the mandible, including a partial glossectomy and neck dissection for advanced primary cancers. Lesions near the midline with a clinically positive lymph node require ipsilateral comprehensive neck dissection with a contralateral selective (supraomohyoid) neck dissection. Otherwise, both sides of the neck should be treated with irradiation.

Results Overall, ~40% of patients are cured of their disease; 80% of recurrences appear within the first 2 years. Survival rates at 5 years by stage follow: stage I, 85%; stage II, 75%; stage III, 66%; and stage IV, 30%. Signs of poor prognosis include involvement of both the tongue and mandible and extension of the tumor beyond the oral cavity.

OROPHARYNX

Carcinoma of the oropharynx affects 4,000 patients in the United States annually.

Anatomy and pathology

The opening to the oropharynx is a ring bounded by the anterior tonsillar pillars (faucial arch), extending upward to blend with the uvula and inferiorly across the base of the tongue (behind the circumvallate papillae). The walls of the oropharynx are formed by the pharyngeal constrictor muscles, which overlie the cervical spine posteriorly. The superior boundary is the soft palate, which separates the oropharynx from the nasopharynx.

Inferiorly, the oropharynx is divided conceptually from the hypopharynx (laryngopharynx) at the level of the epiglottis. Subsites include the base of the tongue, soft palate, tonsillar area, and posterior pharyngeal wall. The extent of a primary tumor may be difficult to assess due to its location.

The jugulodigastric nodes (levels II and III) constitute the first echelon of lymphatic drainage. Metastases may also appear in the parapharyngeal and retropharyngeal nodes and may be detected only through imaging studies.

Premalignant lesions occur in the oropharynx but are less common than in the oral cavity.

Treatment

Radiation therapy External-beam radiation therapy (65–70 Gy over 7 weeks) and interstitial irradiation have been used in the curative treatment of oropharyngeal carcinomas for over 70 years. Radiation therapy represents a reasonable alternative to surgery and may also be required following radical resection of tumors with poor pathologic features to reduce the likelihood of local recurrence.

Altered fractionation schedules (accelerated and/or hyperfractionated) have gained interest in the past several years based on both theoretical grounds and the results of mainly retrospective data. One prospective, randomized trial in patients with oropharyngeal cancer (excluding base of the tongue cancer) documented a 20% increase in locoregional control and a 14% survival benefit at 5 years in patients who received 8,050 cGy in a hyperfractionated schedule, as opposed to 7,000 cGy in a conventionally fractionated schedule. This improvement in outcome was not offset by any significant increase in acute or late tissue toxicity.

Local control rates with radiation therapy for all primary sites (including the tonsil, soft palate, base of the tongue, and posterior oropharyngeal wall) follow: T1, 90%; T2, 80%; T3, 65%; and T4, 55%. Cancers of the tonsillar fossa are better controlled with irradiation than are cancers arising in other subsites of the oropharynx.

Chemoradiation therapy Recent studies support the use of concurrent chemoradiation therapy as an alternative to surgery or irradiation alone for locally advanced cancers of the oropharynx or for disease deemed unresectable. Most of these trials, with the exception of one, have included diverse primary sites in the head and neck. However, oropharyngeal primary tumors predominate in all.

The most recent of the phase III trials is reported by Adelstein et al. This trial, performed via the intergroup mechanism, lends support to a growing body of evidence that suggests therapy with cisplatin (100 mg/m^2) given every 3 weeks with standard irradiation is reasonably safe and effective in this setting.

A second study by the RTOG compared three different chemotherapy/radiation therapy regimens for patients with stage III/IV squamous cell carcinoma of the head and neck. RTOG 97-03 randomized patients to receive 70 Gy in 7 weeks with cisplatin and 5-FU during the last 10 days of treatment, hydroxyurea and 5-FU with radiation therapy delivered on alternating weeks, or weekly cisplatin and paclitaxel. Two-year survival rates for all three arms ranged from 60%–67%.

Surgery Excision through the open mouth of all but small palatal and tonsillar lesions is generally inadequate. Substantial dissection is needed to provide exposure, and reconstruction is often required. A mandibulotomy, composite resection of the mandible, and/or total laryngectomy are occasionally required.

OROPHARYNGEAL SITE: BASE OF THE TONGUE

Cancer of the base of the tongue is far less common than that of the oral tongue.

Anatomy

The base of the tongue is bordered anteriorly by the circumvallate papillae and posteriorly by the epiglottis. There is a rich lymphatic network, with metastases frequently seen in levels II–V.

Natural history

The base of the tongue is notorious for lesions that infiltrate deeply into muscle and are advanced at diagnosis. This finding is probably due to the relatively asymptomatic anatomic location. Thus, bimanual oral examination with digital palpation is a critical part of the physical examination.

Most patients present with pain and dysphagia. Other symptoms include a neck mass, weight loss, otalgia, and trismus.

All oropharyngeal cancers have a strong propensity to spread to the lymph nodes, and base of the tongue tumors are no exception. Approximately 70%

of patients with T1 primary base of the tongue tumors have clinically palpable disease in the neck, and 20%–30% have palpable, bilateral lymph node metastases. The risk of nodal metastases increases with increasing T stage and approaches 85% for T4 lesions.

Treatment

Early-stage disease Stage I or II cancers may be treated equally effectively with either surgical resection or radiation therapy (65–70 Gy in 6–7 weeks) alone. Radiation therapy often results in less of a functional deficit.

With surgery, lymphadenectomy is recommended due to the high frequency of metastatic spread. If irradiation of the primary tumor is employed, both sides of the neck should be treated, even if the nodes do not seem to be involved.

Advanced disease More advanced disease may require total resection of the tongue base with or without laryngectomy to ensure complete removal of disease. Total resection of the tongue base is associated with severe oropharyngeal dysphagia with aspiration, but even subtotal resection of the base of the tongue may result in significant aspiration, which is exacerbated by postoperative radiotherapy. Total laryngectomy may be the only way to isolate the airway from oral secretions and eliminate the risk of aspiration. Chemoradiation therapy via external-beam irradiation or irradiation alone combined with an implant can be curative for patients with advanced tumors of the tongue base.

Results In general, the prognosis of cancers of the tongue base is poor due to their advanced stage at presentation. The extent of nodal disease predicts survival. For T1 and T2 cancers, local control rates approach 85%. The major determinant of treatment failure is the tumor's growth pattern, with a high local control rate for exophytic lesions and a far worse rate for infiltrative tumors.

OROPHARYNGEAL SITE: TONSIL AND TONSILLAR PILLAR

The tonsil and the tonsillar pillar are the most common locations for tumors of the oropharynx.

Natural history

Tonsillar fossa tumors tend to be more advanced and more frequently metastasize to the neck than do tonsillar pillar cancers. At presentation, 55% of patients with fossa tumors have N2 or N3 disease, and contralateral metastases are common. Symptoms include pain, dysphagia, weight loss, a mass in the neck, and trismus.

Treatment

Single-modality therapy (irradiation or surgery alone) is acceptable for T1 and T2 tumors. Irradiation alone (60–70 Gy in 6–7 weeks) may be curative for more advanced tumors, although many of these lesions will require surgery combined with irradiation. The neck should always be included in treatment planning. More advanced disease usually requires surgery combined with irradiation (60–70 Gy in 6–7 weeks).

HYPOPHARYNX

Hypopharyngeal cancers are approximately one-third as common as laryngeal cancers.

Anatomy

The hypopharynx (or laryngopharynx) is the entrance to the esophagus. The superior aspect (above the plane of the hyoid bone) communicates with the oropharynx, and the inferior border is situated in the plane of the lowest part of the cricoid cartilage (the esophageal inlet). The anterior surface (postcricoid area) is contiguous with the posterior surface of the larynx, adjacent to the lamina of the cricoid cartilage. The pharyngeal musculature forms the lateral and posterior walls. The piriform sinuses are within the hypopharynx on each side of the larynx.

The hypopharynx contains three subsites: the paired piriform sinuses (lateral, pear-shaped funnels); the posterior pharyngeal wall, from the level of the vallecula to the level of the cricoarytenoid joints; and the postcricoid area (pharyngoesophageal junction), which begins just below the arytenoids and extends to the inferior border of the cricoid cartilage. The piriform sinuses are composed of a medial wall, which abuts the aryepiglottic fold, and a lateral wall. Seventy percent of hypopharyngeal cancers occur in the piriform sinuses.

Natural history

Hypopharyngeal tumors produce few symptoms until they are advanced (~70% are stage III at presentation). They may cause a sore throat, otalgia, a change in voice, odynophagia, or an isolated neck mass. Subtle changes on physical examination, including pooling of secretions, should be regarded with concern.

Nodal metastases Diffuse local spread is common and is due to tumor extension within the submucosa. Abundant lymphatic drainage results in a higher incidence of lymph node metastases than with other head and neck tumors. At presentation, 70%–80% of patients with hypopharyngeal tumors have palpable cervical lymph node metastases; in half of these patients, palpable cervical nodes are the presenting complaint. Levels II and III are most commonly involved. Bilateral metastases are seen in only 10% of patients with piriform sinus cancers but in 60% of those with postcricoid tumors.

Synchronous lesions are common. Overall, 20%–25% of patients with hypopharyngeal cancer develop a second primary tumor within 5 years, usually in the head and neck.

Chemotherapy and external-beam radiotherapy Similar in design to the VA Cooperative Laryngeal Cancer Study, a randomized EORTC trial has shown that initial therapy with cisplatin and 5-FU, followed by definitive irradiation in patients with complete remissions (or, alternatively, surgical salvage), results in at least equivalent survival relative to immediate pharyngolaryngectomy. Of patients treated with initial chemotherapy, 28% retained a functional larynx at 3 years.

Though directed to laryngeal cancers (rather than hypopharyngeal cancers), the RTOG 91-11 trial results have been widely interpreted as applying to hypopharyngeal cancer, increasing enthusiasm for concomitant chemoradiation therapy for patients with advanced cancers of the hypopharynx.

Transoral laser surgery for piriform sinus carcinoma Organ-sparing approaches such as transoral laser microsurgery for piriform sinus carcinomas have been used in several institutions for the past 25 years. Long-term follow-up in a retrospective review of 129 previously untreated patients has been published (Steiner et al). In this series, which included mostly advanced-stage disease, the reported 5-year local control rate was 82% for patients with stages I and II cancers and 69% for those with stages III and IV cancers. Laryngeal preservation rates were comparable to the local control rates. The 2-year overall survival rates were 91% for patients with stages I and II cancer and 75% for patients with stages III and IV cancer. These oncologic and functional results compare favorably with those obtained with either nonsurgical or surgical approaches requiring opening the neck and pharynx.

LARYNX

Laryngeal cancers constitute approximately 1.2% of all new cancer diagnoses in the United States. Approximately 10,270 new cases are expected in the year 2006.

Anatomy and pathology

Laryngeal anatomy is complex and includes cartilages, membranes, and muscles. The three subsites of the larynx are the glottis, or true vocal cords; the supraglottis, which includes the false cords, epiglottis, and aryepiglottic folds; and the subglottis, which is the region below the glottis and within the cricoid cartilage. The TNM staging system for cancers of the larynx is outlined in Table 4.

Treatment

Surgery Surgical treatment for laryngeal cancer includes transoral or open approaches. Treatment is dictated by the site and extent of the lesion. All or part of the larynx may need to be removed to achieve surgical control of laryn-

TABLE 4: TNM staging system for cancers of the larynx

Primary tumor (T)	
Tx	Primary tumor cannot be assessed
T0	No evidence of primary tumor
Tis	Carcinoma in situ
Glottis	
T1	Tumor limited to the vocal cord(s) (may involve anterior or posterior commissure) with normal mobility
T1a	Tumor limited to one vocal cord
T1b	Tumor involves both vocal cords
T2	Tumor extends to the supraglottis and/or subglottis or with impaired vocal cord mobility
T3	Tumor limited to the larynx with vocal cord fixation
T4a	Tumor invades through the thyroid cartilage and/or invades tissues beyond the larynx (eg, trachea, soft tissues of the neck, including deep extrinsic muscle of the tongue, strap muscles, thyroid, or esophagus [resectable])
T4b	Tumor invades prevertebral space, encases carotid artery, or invades mediastinal structures (unresectable)
Supraglottis	
T1	Tumor limited to one subsite of the supraglottis with normal vocal cord mobility
T2	Tumor invades mucosa of more than one adjacent subsite of the supraglottis or glottis or region outside the supraglottis (eg, mucosa of base of the tongue, vallecula, medial wall of piriform sinus) without fixation of the larynx
T3	Tumor limited to the larynx with vocal cord fixation and/or invades any of the postcricoid area or pre-epiglottic tissues
T4a	Tumor invades through the thyroid cartilage and/or invades tissues beyond the larynx (eg, trachea, soft tissues of neck [resectable], including deep extrinsic muscle of the tongue, strap muscles, thyroid, or esophagus)
T4b	Tumor invades prevertebral space, encases carotid artery, or invades mediastinal structures (unresectable)
Subglottis	
T1	Tumor limited to the subglottis
T2	Tumor extends to vocal cord(s) with normal or impaired mobility
T3	Tumor limited to the larynx with vocal cord fixation
T4a	Tumor invades cricoid or thyroid cartilage and/or invades tissues beyond the larynx (eg, trachea, soft tissues of the neck, including deep extrinsic muscles ofthe tongue, strap muscles, thyroid, or esophagus [resectable])
T4b	Tumor invades prevertebral space, encases carotid artery, or invades mediastinal structures (unresectable)

geal cancer. Decision-making for partial laryngectomy is complex and depends on the patient's overall health, the extent of local disease, the skill of the surgeon, and patient preference.

Regional lymph nodes (N)

Nx	Regional lymph nodes cannot be assessed
N0	No regional lymph node metastasis
N1	Metastasis in a single ipsilateral lymph node, 3 cm or less in greatest dimension
N2	Metastasis in a single ipsilateral lymph node, more than 3 cm but not more than 6 cm in greatest dimension; or in multiple ipsilateral lymph nodes, none more than 6 cm in greatest dimension; or in bilateral or contralateral lymph nodes, none more than 6 cm in greatest dimension
N2a	Metastasis in a single ipsilateral lymph node, more than 3 cm but not more than 6 cm in greatest dimension
N2b	Metastasis in multiple ipsilateral lymph nodes, none more than 6 cm in greatest dimension
N2c	Metastasis in bilateral or contralateral lymph nodes, none more than 6 cm in greatest dimension
N3	Metastasis in a lymph node(s), more than 6 cm in greatest dimension

Distant metastases (M)

Mx	Distant metastasis cannot be assessed
M0	No distant metastasis
M1	Distant metastasis

Stage grouping

Stage 0	Tis	N0	M0
Stage I	T1	N0	M0
Stage II	T2	N0	M0
Stage III	T3	N0	M0
	T1	N1	M0
	T2	N1	M0
	T3	N1	M0
Stage IVA	T4a	N0	M0
	T4a	N1	M0
	T1	N2	M0
	T2	N2	M0
	T3	N2	M0
	T4a	N2	M0
Stage IVB	T4b	Any N	M0
	Any T	N3	M0
Stage IVC	Any T	Any N	M1

From Greene FL, Page DL, Fleming ID, et al (eds): AJCC Cancer Staging Manual, 6th ed. New York, Springer-Verlag, 2002.

External-beam radiation therapy and chemoradiation therapy With improvements in techniques and fractionation schedules, external-beam radiation therapy, which allows for laryngeal preservation, is an option for all but the most advanced tumors.

Results As in other head and neck sites, patients with early laryngeal cancer may be treated with surgery or radiation therapy, and those with advanced-stage disease require multimodal therapy, including surgery and postoperative radiation therapy or chemotherapy and radiation therapy. For T1 and T2 tumors of the glottic or supraglottic larynx, radiation therapy is associated with local control rates of 75%–95%. Open partial laryngectomy for early laryngeal cancer is associated with local control rates of 84%–98% but requires a temporary tracheotomy and may be associated with postoperative vocal and swallowing dysfunction. Transoral laser surgery for early laryngeal cancer has yielded local control rates of 82%–100%, without significant dysphagia or need for a temporary tracheotomy. However, transoral laser surgery requires technical expertise limited to a small number of institutions.

Select patients with T3 or T4 laryngeal cancers may be candidates for laryngeal preservation surgery, but most require total laryngectomy, as the surgical option. The VA Cooperative Laryngeal Cancer Study was the first trial to test the efficacy of chemotherapy and radiation therapy in the management of stages III and IV laryngeal cancer, assess the possibility for laryngeal preservation using such a regimen, and compared its efficacy against the historic standard of surgery and postoperative radiation therapy. The VA Cooperative Laryngeal Cancer Study randomized patients with resectable squamous cell carcinoma of the larynx to receive either total laryngectomy followed by radiation therapy or neoadjuvant therapy with cisplatin and 5-FU followed by radiation therapy for those achieving a good response to chemotherapy.

Approximately two-thirds of patients survived 2 years following the combination of either chemotherapy plus irradiation or resection plus irradiation. Of those patients initially treated with chemotherapy and irradiation, one-third required total laryngectomy because of a lack of response to treatment; the larynx was successfully preserved in two-thirds of these patients. In this study, the increased local recurrence rate in the chemoradiation therapy group was offset by the decreased incidence of distant metastases and second primary tumors, and the 2-year survival rate was comparable between the groups. Advanced T stage was a risk factor for local failure in this study. The rate of salvage total laryngectomy was required for 56% of T4 laryngeal cancers, suggesting patients with bulky primary tumors may not be optimal candidates for organ-preservation therapy.

Data from the RTOG 91-11 trial demonstrated an improvement in locoregional control using concurrent chemoradiation therapy relative to induction chemotherapy followed by radiotherapy or radiotherapy alone. There was no primarily surgical arm in this study. This three-armed study randomized 517 patients with stages III and IV laryngeal cancer to receive one of the following regimens: induction chemotherapy (with cisplatin/5-FU) followed by radiation therapy or concurrent chemoradiotherapy (with cisplatin given on days 1, 22, and 43). Locoregional control for the three arms was 61%, 78%, and 56%, respectively. The laryngeal preservation rate was 75%, 88%, and 70%, respectively. Notably, patients with T4 laryngeal cancers comprised only

10% of patients in this study, compared with 25% in the original VA Cooperative Laryngeal Cancer Study, accounting for the improved local control and laryngeal preservation achieved in the RTOG 91-11 study.

The cure rate for early cancers of the larynx approaches 80% or more. Half of patients with T3 cancer are cured, whereas more than two-thirds of patients with T4 cancer will die of the disease.

LARYNGEAL SITE: SUPRAGLOTTIS

Supraglottic tumors occur less frequently than tumors of the true vocal cords. The epiglottis is the most common location for supraglottic cancers.

Natural history

Tumors close to the glottis produce symptoms earlier than tumors at other subsites. In contrast, nearly 60% of patients with supraglottic tumors have T3 or T4 primary tumors at presentation.

The supraglottis has a rich lymphatic network. There is an associated high incidence of lymph node metastases in early-stage tumors (40% for T1 tumors). The incidence of metastases in patients with clinically N0 neck cancer is about 15%. The incidence of bilateral cervical lymph node involvement is about 10%, and this rate increases to 60% for anterior tumors. The neck is a frequent site of recurrence in patients with supraglottic malignancies.

Treatment

The primary tumor Appropriate cancers may be treated with partial laryngectomy. Supraglottic laryngectomy removes the upper portion of the thyroid cartilage and its contents, including the false vocal cords, as well as the epiglottis and aryepiglottic folds. This approach preserves speech and swallowing, but more extensive resections are not well tolerated by patients with impaired lung function who are not able to tolerate the inevitable postoperative aspiration. Supracricoid partial laryngectomy is suitable for supraglottic tumors that cross the ventricle to involve the glottis. Select T3 tumors with limited pre-epiglottic space involvement may be approached with this procedure. Patients must have sufficient pulmonary reserve to be able to tolerate the chronic aspiration associated with this procedure. The local control rates of transoral laser supraglottic laryngectomy are between 75% and 100% for T1 and T2 lesions in recent series and are associated with less postoperative dysphagia than open approaches. Significant technical expertise is needed, and patients must have the proper habitus to assure adequate exposure. Supraglottic laryngectomy is seldom appropriate as salvage therapy following irradiation due to complications, including swelling, difficulty swallowing, and poor wound healing. The usual salvage operation for persistent supraglottic cancer following radiation therapy is total laryngectomy. Advanced disease requires multimodal therapy, as previously discussed.

More advanced disease requires combined-modality treatment and often requires total laryngectomy. Radiation therapy may be employed with curative intent, as may induction chemotherapy followed by irradiation, as described earlier.

The neck The high incidence of cervical metastases makes treatment of the neck a necessity. About one-third of cases of clinically negative neck cancer contain involved nodes, and the incidence of recurrence in untreated patients is high. For patients undergoing surgical treatment of T1–T2 primary tumors, bilateral selective neck dissection is advisable.

Preservation of the larynx Mature data from RTOG 91-11 have been published, confirming preliminary results. A total of 547 patients were randomly assigned to undergo one of three treatments: induction cisplatin plus 5-FU followed by radiotherapy, radiotherapy with concurrent administration of cisplatin, or radiotherapy alone. The rate of locoregional tumor control was significantly better with radiotherapy and concurrent cisplatin (78% vs 61% with induction cisplatin plus 5-FU followed by radiotherapy and 56% with radiotherapy alone). Both regimens with chemotherapy had lower rates of distant metastases and resulted in better disease-free survival than radiotherapy alone. Overall survival rates were similar in all three groups.

At 2 years, the proportion of patients in whom the larynx was preserved after irradiation and concurrent cisplatin (88%) differed significantly from the proportion in the groups given induction chemotherapy followed by irradiation (75%, $P = .005$) or irradiation alone (70%, $P < .001$). The authors concluded that the combination of irradiation and concurrent cisplatin was superior to induction chemotherapy followed by irradiation or irradiation alone for laryngeal preservation and locoregional control.

LARYNGEAL SITE: GLOTTIS

The glottis is the most common location of laryngeal cancer in the United States, comprising more than half of all cases.

Natural history

The cure rate for tumors of the true vocal cords is high. These cancers produce symptoms early, and, thus, most are small when detected. Approximately 60% are T1 and 20% are T2. Normal cord mobility implies invasion of disease limited to the submucosa. Deeper invasion results in impaired vocal cord motion; this finding is most common in the anterior two-thirds of the vocal cord.

The true vocal cords have very little lymphatic drainage. Cervical metastases are infrequent with T1 and T2 tumors.

Treatment

The primary tumor Carcinoma in situ is highly curable and may be treated equally well with microexcision, laser vaporization, or radiation therapy. Treatment decisions should be based on the extent of local disease. Serial recurrences should heighten suspicion of an invasive component, and a more aggressive approach, such as partial or total laryngectomy or irradiation, should be employed. Local control for T1 using surgery or irradiation is comparable, usually greater than 90%. Local control for T2 glottic lesions is reported between 70% and 85% with radiotherapy and 85% and 95% with open partial laryngectomy. Partial laryngectomy can be performed in selected patients after irradiation failure of some T1–T2 glottic cancers.

Advanced T4 disease is best treated with total laryngectomy. Most T3 lesions are now being treated with concomitant chemoradiotherapy, with salvage laryngectomy required in ~20% of patients for residual/recurrent disease or laryngeal dysfunction.

The neck Due to the sparse lymphatic network and low incidence of cervical metastases, elective neck dissection is indicated only for transglottic lesions.

Results Cure rates by tumor size alone follow: T1, 90%; T2, 80%; T3, 50%; and T4, 40%. Neck involvement worsens the prognosis dramatically.

LARYNGEAL SITE: SUBGLOTTIS

Subglottic cancer is unusual, accounting for fewer than 10% of all laryngeal cancers.

Natural history

These cancers tend to be poorly differentiated, and, as the region is clinically "silent," most present as advanced lesions (~70% are T3–T4). The subglottis also has rich lymphatic drainage, and the incidence of cervical metastases is 20%–30%.

Treatment

Partial laryngectomy is not practical for the treatment of tumors in the subglottis, and, thus, therapy usually includes total laryngectomy plus neck dissection. Combination therapy (surgery plus radiation therapy [60–65 Gy in 6–7 weeks]) is recommended for more advanced disease.

Results The cure rate for the uncommon T1 and T2 tumors is ~70%. Most failures occur in the neck. The cure rate for more advanced lesions is ~40%.

UNKNOWN HEAD AND NECK PRIMARY SITE

The cervical lymph nodes are the most common metastatic site at which squamous cell carcinoma is found.

Natural history

Most patients who present with squamous cell carcinoma involving cervical lymph nodes, especially in the upper or middle portion of the cervical chain, will have a primary site within the head and neck. When the lower cervical or supraclavicular lymph nodes are involved, a primary lung cancer should be suspected.

In the overwhelming majority of these cases, the primary lesion will be discovered based on history, physical examination, proper radiographic evaluation (CT and/or MRI), and examination with the patient under anesthesia with endoscopy (direct laryngoscopy and nasopharyngoscopy), targeted biopsies, and tonsillectomy. Esophagoscopy and bronchoscopy seldom yield a diagnosis in patients with upper cervical lymph node involvement. "Silent" primary tumors are most often discovered in the base of the tongue or within tonsillar crypts.

Treatment

A substantial percentage of patients achieve long-term disease-free survival after treatment of the involved side of the neck. Locoregional control and survival are diminished by multiple lymph nodes and the presence of extracapsular extension of disease in the involved neck.

Irradiation alone Patients with early-stage neck disease (N1 disease or small, mobile N2a disease) can often be treated with radiotherapy alone. Radiation therapy dosages and techniques should be similar to those used in patients with advanced primary head and neck cancer. The nasopharynx, oropharynx, and hypopharynx should be included in the irradiated field.

Surgery alone When neck dissection is used at the initial treatment, a primary tumor in the head and neck subsequently becomes obvious in about 20% of patients.

Irradiation alone or combined with surgery Combination therapy (surgery plus radiation therapy [60–65 Gy in 6–7 weeks]) is recommended for patients found at surgery to have multiple involved nodes or extracapsular extension or who have suspected residual microscopic disease in the neck without a clinically detectable tumor. Open nodal biopsy does not appear to compromise outcome as long as adequate radiotherapy is delivered subsequently.

In most modern series utilizing predominantly combination therapy, 5-year survival rates exceed 50%. The volume of tumor in the involved neck influences outcome, with N1 and N2 disease having a significantly higher cure rate than N3 disease or massive neck involvement. Regional relapse is usually predicted by extranodal disease.

Chemotherapy The role of chemotherapy in treating patients with unknown primary metastatic squamous carcinoma in cervical lymph nodes remains undefined. The benefit of concurrent chemoradiation therapy of these patients is uncertain (because their primary sites are small or absent), and neck control after resection followed by irradiation, or after irradiation alone, is excellent in patients with cancers of an unknown primary site.

NASOPHARYNX

Nasopharyngeal carcinoma is uncommon in most of the world. Endemic areas include southern China, northern Africa, and regions of the far Northern Hemisphere. The incidence (per 1,000 population) ranges from 25.6 in men and 10.2 in women in Hong Kong to 0.6 in men and 0.1 in women in Connecticut.

Epidemiology and risk factors

Gender and age The incidence of nasopharyngeal cancer peaks in the fourth to fifth decades of life, and the male-female ratio is 2.2:1.0. Both patient age at disease onset and male-female ratio are lower for nasopharyngeal cancer than for other head and neck malignancies.

Risk factors Nasopharyngeal carcinoma (most notably WHO [World Health Organization] types 2 and 3 [see section on "Anatomy and pathology") appears to have different determinants than other head and neck cancers. They include diet, viral agents, and genetic susceptibility. Populations of endemic areas have a diet characterized by high consumption of salt-cured fish and meat. Studies reveal an association between EBV and nasopharyngeal carcinoma. Anti-EBV antibodies have been found in the sera and saliva of patients with this type of carcinoma. Major histocompatibility (MHC) profiles associated with increased relative risk include H2, BW46, and B17 locus antigens.

Anatomy and pathology

The nasopharynx communicates anteriorly with the nasal cavity and inferiorly with the oropharynx. The superior border is the base of the skull. The lateral and posterior pharyngeal walls are composed of muscular constrictors. Posteriorly, the nasopharynx overlies the first and second cervical vertebrae. The eustachian tubes open into the lateral walls. The soft palate divides the nasopharynx from the oropharynx.

Cancers arising in the nasopharynx are classified using WHO criteria: type 1 denotes differentiated squamous cell carcinoma; type 2, nonkeratinizing carci-

TABLE 5: TNM staging system for cancers of the pharynx (including base of tongue, soft palate, and uvula)

Primary tumor (T)	
Tx	Primary tumor cannot be assessed
T0	No evidence of primary tumor
Tis	Carcinoma in situ
Nasopharynx	
T1	Tumor confined to the nasopharynx
T2	Tumor extends to the soft tissue of the oropharynx and/or nasal fossa
T2a	Without parapharyngeal extension[a]
T2b	With parapharyngeal extension[a]
T3	Tumor invades bony structures and/or paranasal sinuses
T4	Tumor with intracranial extension and/or involvement of cranial nerves, infratemporal fossa, hypopharynx, or orbit
Oropharynx	
T1	Tumor 2 cm or less in greatest dimension
T2	Tumor more than 2 cm but not more than 4 cm in greatest dimension
T3	Tumor more than 4 cm in greatest dimension
T4a	Tumor invades the larynx, deep/extrinsic muscle of the tongue, medial pterygoid, hard palate, or mandible (resectable)
T4b	Tumor invades lateral pterygoid muscle, pterygoid plates, lateral nasopharynx, or skull base or encases carotid artery (unresectable)
Hypopharynx	
T1	Tumor limited to one subsite of the hypopharynx and 2 cm or less in greatest dimension
T2	Tumor involves more than one subsite of the hypopharynx or an adjacent site or measures more than 2 cm but not more than 4 cm in greatest dimension without fixation of the hemilarynx
T3	Tumor measures more than 4 cm in greatest dimension or with fixation of the hemilarynx
T4a	Tumor invades thyroid/cricoid cartilage, hyoid bone, thyroid gland, esophagus, or central compartment soft tissue[b] (resectable)
T4b	Tumor invades prevertebral fascia, encases carotid artery, or involves mediastinal structures (unresectable)

noma; and type 3, undifferentiated carcinoma. The TNM staging system for cancers of the pharynx is outlined in Table 5.

Natural history

A mass in the neck is the presenting complaint in 90% of patients. Other presenting symptoms include a change in hearing, sensation of ear stuffiness, tinnitus, nasal obstruction, and pain.

Regional lymph nodes (N): Nasopharynx	
Nx	Regional lymph nodes cannot be assessed
N0	No regional lymph node metastasis
N1	Unilateral metastasis in lymph node(s), 6 cm or less in greatest dimension, above the supraclavicular fossa[c]
N2	Bilateral metastasis in lymph node(s), 6 cm or less in greatest dimension, above the supraclavicular fossa[c]
N3	Metastasis in a lymph node(s) > 6 cm and/or to the supraclavicular fossa
N3a	Greater than 6 cm in dimension
N3b	Extension to the supraclavicular fossa[c]
Regional lymph nodes (N): Oropharynx and hypopharynx	
Nx	Regional lymph nodes cannot be assessed
N0	No regional lymph node metastasis
N1	Metastasis in a single ipsilateral lymph node, 3 cm or less in greatest dimension
N2	Metastasis in a single ipsilateral lymph node, more than 3 cm but not more than 6 cm in greatest dimension; or in multiple ipsilateral lymph nodes, none more than 6 cm in greatest dimension; or in bilateral or contralateral lymph nodes, none more than 6 cm in greatest dimension
N2a	Metastasis in a single ipsilateral lymph node, more than 3 cm but not more than 6 cm in greatest dimension
N2b	Metastasis in multiple ipsilateral lymph nodes, none more than 6 cm in greatest dimension
N2c	Metastasis in bilateral or contralateral lymph nodes, none more than 6 cm in greatest dimension
N3	Metastasis in a lymph node, more than 6 cm in greatest dimension
Distant metastases (M)	
Mx	Distant metastasis cannot be assessed
M0	No distant metastasis
M1	Distant metastasis

[a] Parapharyngeal extension denotes posterolateral infiltration of tumor beyond the pharyngobasilar fascia.

[b] Central compartment soft tissue includes prelaryngeal strap muscles and subcutaneous fat.

[c] Midline nodes are considered ipsilateral nodes.

continued on following page

Cranial nerve involvement Invasion of disease into the base of the skull is seen in ~25% of cases and may lead to cranial nerve involvement. CN VI is the first cranial nerve to be affected, followed by CN III and CN IV. Deficits are manifested by changes in ocular motion. Involvement of CN V may also occur; this is manifested by pain or paresthesia high in the neck or face.

Level V metastases Unlike malignancies of the oral cavity and oropharynx, nasopharyngeal cancers often metastasize to level V lymph nodes. Bilateral metastases are common.

TABLE 5: TNM staging system for cancers of the pharynx (including base of tongue, soft palate, and uvula) *(continued)*

Stage grouping: Nasopharynx			
Stage 0	Tis	N0	M0
Stage I	T1	N0	M0
Stage IIA	T2a	N0	M0
Stage IIB	T1	N1	M0
	T2	N1	M0
	T2a	N1	M0
	T2b	N0	M0
	T2b	N1	M0
Stage III	T1	N2	M0
	T2a	N2	M0
	T2b	N2	M0
	T3	N0	M0
	T3	N1	M0
	T3	N2	M0
Stage IVA	T4	N0	M0
	T4	N1	M0
	T4	N2	M0
Stage IVB	Any T	N3	M0
Stage IVC	Any T	Any N	M1
Stage grouping: Oropharynx and hypopharynx			
Stage 0	Tis	N0	M0
Stage I	T1	N0	M0
Stage II	T2	N0	M0
Stage III	T3	N0	M0
	T1	N1	M0
	T2	N1	M0
	T3	N1	M0
Stage IVA	T4a	N0	M0
	T4a	N1	M0
	T1	N2	M0
	T2	N2	M0
	T3	N2	M0
	T4a	N2	M0
Stage IVB	T4b	Any N	M0
	Any T	N3	M0
Stage IVC	Any T	Any N	M1

From Greene FL, Page DL, Fleming ID, et al (eds): AJCC Cancer Staging Manual, 6th ed. New York, Springer-Verlag, 2002.

Treatment

Treatment of nasopharyngeal cancer usually involves radiation therapy (65-70 Gy) for the primary tumor and draining lymph nodes. Overall survival is 50% at 5 years. Surgical resection has high morbidity and is seldom entertained.

Nasopharyngeal cancer is distinguished from other sites of head and neck cancer by its radiosensitivity and chemosensitivity. Although advanced nodal disease can be controlled by irradiation alone in ~50% of patients, eventual distant metastasis remains a problem.

The final report of the intergroup trial 0099 confirmed that for patients with locally advanced nasopharyngeal cancer, concurrent cisplatin chemotherapy with radiation therapy (followed by systemic chemotherapy) provided a clear survival benefit compared with treatment with irradiation alone. At 5 years, patients who received combined-modality therapy had an overall survival rate of 67%, compared with 37% with radiation therapy alone ($P = .001$). Disease-free survival at 5 years was 74% for the chemoradiation therapy arm vs 46% for the radiation therapy-alone arm.

RECURRENT HEAD AND NECK CANCER

As mentioned previously, surveillance after treatment of head and neck cancer is mandatory, as early detection of second primary cancers or locoregional recurrence affords the best chance for disease control. Nearly two-thirds of patients whose head and neck cancer recurs develop a tumor at (or near) the primary site or in the neck nodes. Eighty percent of head and neck cancer recurrences eventuate within 2 years. Development of a recurrent tumor in the neck is the single most common type of treatment failure in patients with squamous cell carcinoma of the upper aerodigestive tract.

Differentiating recurrence from late complications of irradiation Differentiating between recurrent carcinoma and significant sequelae of radiotherapy is a difficult clinical problem at all sites within the head and neck. Any suspicious mucosal changes, enlarged nodes in the neck, or discrete subcutaneous nodules warrant prompt biopsy.

Candidates for surgery Different choices of first treatment (ie, surgery or radiation therapy) and the intensity of follow-up influence success in treating recurrence. Aggressive surgical intervention should be offered to two groups of patients with recurrent local or regional disease: those whose therapy is chosen with curative intent and those who have the prospect for significant palliation.

The types of recurrence that may be approached surgically with the greatest likelihood of success include (1) metastases in the neck after initial treatment limited to the primary tumor alone and (2) reappearance or persistence of cancer at a site previously treated with radiotherapy alone. Salvage resection may also be considered in other situations, however. They include the appearance of cancer in the neck after prior irradiation or neck dissection, at the margins after previous resection, and even at the base of the skull.

Although surgery is the standard of care for the treatment of recurrent disease, there is a growing body of evidence suggesting that reirradiation with concurrent chemotherapy can save selected patients when resection is not possible. Several institutions have reported experiences retreating patients, and these results led to the development of the first multi-institution reirradiation study.

A single-arm, phase II study (RTOG 96-10) evaluated toxicity and therapeutic results for patients with recurrent squamous cell carcinoma of the head and neck. Eighty-six patients received four weekly courses of 1.5-Gy fractions twice daily with concurrent 5-FU and hydroxyurea. Each cycle was separated by 1 week of rest. The median survival was 8.1 months and the 1- and 2-year survival rates were 41.7% and 16.2%, respectively. Compared with patients who experienced early recurrences, patients whose disease recurred 3 years after the original irradiation fared better, with 1- and 2-year survival rates of 48.1% and 32.1%, respectively.

The first results for the entire cohort of patients for RTOG 99-11, the successor trial to RTOG 96-10, were presented in 2005. In this study, patients previously irradiated, with locally recurrent or second primary head and neck tumors were treated with split-course hyperfractionated radiotherapy (60 Gy total; 1.5 Gy/fraction twice daily for 5 days every 2 weeks for 4 cycles), in combination with cisplatin (15 mg/m^2 IV daily) x 5 and paclitaxel (20 mg/m^2 IV daily x 5)every 2 weeks for 4 cycles. G-CSF support was administered on days 6 through 13 of each 2-week cycle. Of the 105 patients enrolled, 99 were eligible for analysis, and 23% of the patients had second primary head and neck tumors. The median prior dose of radiotherapy was 65.4 Gy (range 45–75 Gy), and the median time from prior radiotherapy was 40 months.

Of eight patients with grade 5 (fatal) toxicities, five occurred during the acute period (dehydration, pneumonitis, neutropenia [2 cases], and cerebrovascular accident) and three during the late period (two of three attributable to carotid hemorrhage). Other acute toxicities included leukopenia (30% grade 3/4), anemia (21% grade 3/4), and gastrointestinal toxicity (48% grade 3/4). The median follow-up for alive patients was 23.6 months, and the median survival was 12.1 months.

The estimated 1- and 2-year overall survival rates were 50.2% and 25.9%, respectively. The median and 1-year progression-free survival rates were 7.8 months and 35%, respectively. Overall survival was significantly better ($P = .044$) than for the historic control RTOG 96-10 (estimated 1- and 2-year overall survival rates 41.7% and 16.7%, respectively).

Despite significant toxicity and high mortality, hyperfractionated split-course re-irradiation with concurrent cisplatin and paclitaxel chemotherapy proved feasible in this select patient population. This approach will be tested in an RTOG 04-21, a phase III trial, which randomizes patients between this arm and chemotherapy alone.

Unless a patient cannot tolerate an operation, resection of discrete local or regional recurrent tumors should be entertained as the first course of treatment. Management of recurrences involves complex decision-making and requires familiarity with multidisciplinary care.

SUGGESTED READING

Adelstein DJ, Li Y, Adams GL, et al: An Intergroup phase III comparison of standard radiation therapy and two schedules of concurrent chemoradiotherapy in patients with unresectable squamous cell head and neck cancer. J Clin Oncol 21:92–98, 2003.

Al-Sarraf M, LeBlanc M, Giri PGS, et al: Superiority of 5-year survival with chemoradiotherapy (CR-RT) vs radiotherapy in patients (pts) with locally advanced nasopharyngeal cancer (NPC). Intergroup (0099) (SWOG 8892, RTOG 8817, ECOG 2388) phase III study: Final report (abstract). Proc Am Soc Clin Oncol 20:227, 2001.

Ang KK, Harris J, Garden AS, et al: Concomitant boost radiation and concurrent cisplatin for advanced head and neck carcinomas: Preliminary results of a phase II trial of the RTOG (99-14). Int J Radiat Oncol Biol Phys 54:2–3, 2002.

Bernier J, Cooper JS Pajak TF, et al: Defining risk levels in locally advanced head and neck cancers: A comparative analysis of concurrent postoperative radiation plus chemotherapy trials of the EORTC (#22931) and RTOG (#9501). Head Neck 27:843–850, 2005.

Bernier J, Domenge C, Ozsahin M, et al: Postoperative irradiation with or without concomitant chemotherapy for locally advanced head and neck cancer. N Engl J Med 350:1945–1952, 2004.

Bonner JA, Giralt J, Harari PM, et al: Cetuximab prolongs survival in patients with locoregionally advanced squamous cell carcinoma of the head and neck: A phase III study of high dose radiation with or without cetuximab (abstract). J Clin Oncol 22(suppl):489S, 2004.

Bonner JA, Harari PM, Giralt J, et al: Radiotherapy plus cetuximab for squamous-cell carcinoma of the head and neck. N Engl J Med 354:567–578, 2006.

Cooper JS, Pajak TF, Forastiere AA, et al: Postoperative concurrent radiotherapy and chemotherapy for high-risk squamous-cell carcinoma of the head and neck. N Engl J Med 350:1937–1944, 2004.

Corry J, Smith JG, Peters LJ: The concept of a planned neck dissection is obsolete. Cancer J 7:472–474, 2001.

Forastiere AA, Goepfert H, Maor M, et al: Concurrent chemotherapy and radiotherapy for organ preservation in advanced laryngeal cancer. N Engl J Med 349:2091–2098, 2003.

Garden AS, Harris J, Jones CU, et al: Concomitant boost radiation and concurrent cisplatin for advanced head and neck carcinomas: Update of a phase II trial of the RTOG (99-14). Int J Radiat Oncol Biol Phys 63:S71–S72, 2005.

Garden AS, Harris J, Vokes EE, et al: Preliminary results of Radiation Therapy Oncology Group 97-03: A randomized phase II trial of concurrent radiation and chemotherapy for advanced squamous cell carcinomas of the head and neck. J Clin Oncol 22:2856–2864, 2004.

Horwitz EM, Harris J, Langer CJ, et al: Combination with split course concomitant hyperfractionated re-irradiation in patients with recurrent squamous cell cancer of the head and neck: Results of RTOG 99-11. Int J Radiat Oncol Biol Phys 63(suppl 1):S72–S73, 2005.

Hu YC, Sidransky D, Ahrendt SA: Molecular detection approaches for smoking associated tumors. Oncogene 21:7289–7297, 2002.

Lin A, Kim HM, Terrell JE, et al: Head and neck cancer-specific quality of life (HN-QOL) and its correlation with xerostomia following parotid-sparing irradiation (RT) of head and neck cancer. Int J Radiat Oncol Biol Phys 54:167, 2002.

Parliament MB, Scrimger R, Kurien E, et al: Preservation of oral health-related quality of life and salivary flow rates after inverse-planned intensity modulated radiotherapy (IMRT) for head and neck cancer (HNC). Int J Radiat Oncol Biol Phys 54:165–166, 2002.

Pradier O, Christiansen H, Schmidberger H, et al: Adjuvant radiotherapy after transoral laser microsurgery for advanced squamous carcinoma of the head and neck. Int J Radiat Oncol Biol Phys 63:1368–1377, 2005.

Shoaib T, Souta DS, MacDonald DG, et al: The accuracy of head and neck carcinoma sentinel lymph node biopsy in the clinically N0 neck. Cancer 91:2077–2083, 2001.

Spencer SA, Harris J, Wheeler RH, et al: RTOG 96-10: Reirradiation with concurrent hydroxyurea and 5-fluorouracil in patients with squamous cell cancer of the head and neck. Int J Radiat Oncol Biol Phys 51:1299–1304, 2001.

Steiner W, Ambrosch P, Hess CF, et al: Organ preservation by transoral laser microsurgery in piriform sinus carcinoma. Otolaryngol Head Neck Surg 124:58–67, 2001.

Trotti A, Fu KK, Pajak TF, et al: Long-term outcomes of RTOG 90-03: A comparison of hyperfractionation and two variants of acclerated fractionation to standard fractionation radiotherapy for head and neck squamous carcinoma. Int J Radiat Oncol Biol Phys 63:S70–S71, 2005.

Vermorken JB, Remenar E, Van Herpen C, et al: Standard cisplatin/infusional 5-fluorouracil vs. docetaxel plus PF as neoadjuvant chemotherapy for nonresectable locally advanced squamous cell carcinoma of the head and neck: A phase III trial of the EORTC Head and Neck Cancer Group (EORTC 24971; late-breaking abstract). Proc Am Soc Clin Oncol 23:#5508, 2004.

Wolden S, Pfister D, Zelefsky M, et al: Intensity modulated radiation therapy improves locoregional control for nasopharyngeal carcinoma (abstract). Proc Am Soc Clin Oncol 21:240a, 2002.

Yom SA, Machtay M, Biel MA, et al: Survival impact of planned restaging and early surgical salvage following definitive chemoradiation for locally advanced squamous cell carcinomas of the oropharynx and hypopharynx. Am J Clin Oncol 28:385–392, 2005.

Zeitels SM, Franco RA Jr, Dailey SH, et al: Office-based treatment of glottal dysplasia and papillomatosis with the 585-nm pulsed dye laser and local anesthesia. Ann Otol Rhinol Laryngol 113:265–276, 2004.

CHAPTER 5

Thyroid and parathyroid cancers

Gilbert G. Fareau, MD, Rena Vassilopoulou-Sellin, MD, Robert Lustig, MD, and Jeffrey P. Lamont, MD

Endocrine malignancies, although relatively uncommon, are often difficult to diagnose and treat effectively. According to American Cancer Society (ACS) estimates, more than 32,000 new cases of endocrine neoplasms will be diagnosed in the United States in 2006, and approximately 2,290 deaths will result from these cancers. This chapter will focus on thyroid and parathyroid cancers. (A discussion of carcinoid tumors, insulinomas, gastrinomas, and other gastrointestinal neuroendocrine tumors, as well as adrenocortical cancer, can be found in chapter 14.)

THYROID CANCER

Thyroid cancer is the most common endocrine cancer. The number of deaths from thyroid cancer projected for the year 2006 is 1,500, or 7% of all new thyroid cancer cases.

The prevalence rate for occult thyroid cancers found at autopsy is 5%–10%, except in Japan and Hawaii, where the rate can be as high as 28%. Autopsy rates do not correlate with clinical incidence.

The incidence of thyroid nodules in the general population is 4%–7%, with nodules being more common in females than males. The prevalence of thyroid cancer in a solitary nodule or in multinodular thyroid glands is 10%–20%; this increases with irradiation of the neck in children and older men (see section on "Etiology and risk factors").

Tumor types

Thyroid cancer is classified into four main types according to its morphology and biologic behavior: papillary, follicular, medullary, and anaplastic. Differentiated (papillary and follicular) thyroid cancers account for > 90% of thyroid malignancies and constitute approximately 0.8% of all human malignancies. Medullary thyroid cancers represent 5%–10% of all thyroid neoplasms. About 80% of patients with medullary cancer have a sporadic form of the disease, whereas the remaining 20% have inherited disease. Anaplastic carcinoma represents ≤ 5% of all thyroid carcinomas.

> With use of polymerase chain reaction (PCR) in 17 surgical specimens containing multifocal papillary carcinoma, 5 specimens had tumors with unique genetic signatures. This finding suggests that multifocal papillary cancer can arise as independent tumors (*Shattuch TM, Westra WH, Ladenson PW, et al: N Engl J Med 352:2406-2412, 2005*).

Papillary thyroid carcinoma is the most common subtype and has an excellent prognosis. Most papillary carcinomas contain varying amounts of follicular tissue. When the predominant histology is papillary, the tumor is considered to be a papillary carcinoma. Because the mixed papillary-follicular variant tends to behave like a pure papillary cancer, it is treated in the same manner and has a similar prognosis.

Papillary tumors arise from thyroid follicular cells, are unilateral in most cases, and are often multifocal within a single thyroid lobe. They vary in size from microscopic to large cancers that may invade the thyroid capsule and infiltrate into contiguous structures. Papillary tumors tend to invade the lymphatics, but vascular invasion (and hematogenous spread) is uncommon.

Up to 40% of adults with papillary thyroid cancer may present with regional lymph node metastases, usually ipsilateral. Distant metastases occur, in decreasing order of frequency, in the lungs, bones, and other soft tissues. Older patients have a higher risk for locally invasive tumors and for distant metastases. Children may present with a solitary thyroid nodule, but cervical node involvement is more common in this age group; up to 10% of children and adolescents may have lung involvement at the time of diagnosis.

Follicular thyroid carcinoma is less common than papillary thyroid cancer, occurs in older age groups, and has a slightly worse prognosis. Follicular thyroid cancer can metastasize to the lungs and bones, often retaining the ability to accumulate radioactive iodine (which can be used for therapy). Metastases may be appreciated many years after the initial diagnosis.

Follicular tumors, although frequently encapsulated, commonly exhibit microscopic vascular and capsular invasion. Microscopically, the nuclei tend to be large and have atypical mitotic figures. There is usually no lymph node involvement.

Follicular carcinoma can be difficult to distinguish from its benign counterpart, follicular adenoma. This distinction is based on the presence or absence of capsular or vascular invasion, which can be evaluated after surgical excision but not by fine-needle aspiration (FNA).

Thyroglobulin, normally synthesized in the follicular epithelium of the thyroid, is present in well-differentiated papillary and follicular carcinomas and infrequently in anaplastic carcinomas but not in medullary carcinomas. Therefore, thyroglobulin immunoreactivity is considered to be indicative of a follicular epithelial origin.

Hürthle cell carcinoma Hürthle cell, or oxyphil cell, carcinoma is a variant of follicular carcinoma. Hürthle cell carcinoma is composed of sheets of Hürthle cells and has the same criteria for malignancy as does follicular carcinoma. Hürthle cell carcinoma is thought to have a worse outcome than follicular carcinoma and is less apt to concentrate radioactive iodine.

Medullary thyroid carcinoma originates from the C cells (parafollicular cells) of the thyroid and secretes calcitonin. On gross examination, most tumors are firm, grayish, and gritty.

Sporadic medullary thyroid carcinoma usually presents as a solitary thyroid mass; metastases to cervical and mediastinal lymph nodes are found in half of patients and may be present at the time of initial presentation. Distant metastases to the lungs, liver, bones, and adrenal glands most commonly occur late in the course of the disease. Secretory diarrhea, related to calcitonin secretion, can be a clinical feature of advanced medullary thyroid carcinoma.

Familial medullary thyroid carcinoma presents as a bilateral, multifocal process. Histologically, familial medullary carcinoma of the thyroid does not differ from the sporadic form. However, the familial form is frequently multifocal, and it is common to find areas of C-cell hyperplasia in areas distant from the primary carcinoma. Another characteristic feature of familial medullary carcinoma is the presence of amyloid deposits.

Anaplastic carcinoma Anaplastic tumors are high-grade neoplasms characterized histologically by a high mitotic rate and lymphovascular invasion. Aggressive invasion of local structures is common, as are lymph node metastases. Distant metastases tend to occur in patients who do not succumb early to regional disease. Occasional cases of anaplastic carcinoma have been shown to arise from preexisting differentiated thyroid carcinoma or in a preexisting goiter.

Other tumor types Lymphomas of the thyroid account for < 5% of primary thyroid carcinomas. Other tumor types, such as teratomas, squamous cell carcinomas, and sarcomas, may also rarely cause primary thyroid cancers.

Genetic factors In addition to sporadic medullary thyroid cancer, which represents the majority of cases, there are three hereditary forms: familial medullary thyroid carcinoma; multiple endocrine neoplasia type 2A (MEN-2A), characterized by medullary thyroid cancer, pheochromocytomas, and hyperparathyroidism; and multiple endocrine neoplasia type 2B (MEN-2B), characterized by medullary thyroid cancer, marfanoid habitus, pheochromocytomas, and neuromas. These syndromes are associated with germ-line mutations of the *RET* proto-oncogene, which codes for a receptor tyrosine kinase (RTK). Familial medullary thyroid carcinoma is inherited as an autosomal-dominant trait with high penetrance and variable expression. (For a discussion of genetic testing to screen for *RET* mutations in MEN-2A kindreds, see section on "Staging and prognosis.")

Epidemiology

Age and gender Most patients are between the ages of 25 and 65 years at the time of diagnosis of thyroid carcinoma. Women are affected more often than men (2:1 ratio for the development of both naturally occurring and radiation-induced thyroid cancer).

Etiology and risk factors

Differentiated thyroid cancer

Therapeutic irradiation External low-dose radiation therapy to the head and neck during infancy and childhood, frequently used between the 1940s and 1960s for the treatment of a variety of benign diseases, has been shown to predispose an individual to thyroid cancer. The younger a patient is at the time of radiation exposure, the higher is the subsequent risk of developing thyroid carcinoma. Also, as mentioned previously, women are at increased risk of radiation-induced thyroid cancer. There is a latency period ranging from 10–30 years from the time of low-dose irradiation to the development of thyroid cancer.

As little as 11 cGy and as much as 2,000 cGy of external radiation to the head and neck have been associated with a number of benign and malignant diseases. It was once thought that high-dose irradiation (> 2,000 cGy) to the head and neck did not increase the risk of neoplasia. However, recently it has been shown that patients treated with mantle-field irradiation for Hodgkin lymphoma are at increased risk of developing thyroid carcinoma compared with the general population, although they are more likely to develop hypothyroidism than thyroid cancer.

Radiation-associated thyroid cancer has an identical natural history and prognosis as sporadic thyroid cancer.

Other factors Besides radiation-induced thyroid cancer, there are only sparse data on the etiology of differentiated thyroid cancer.

Signs and symptoms

Most thyroid cancers present as asymptomatic thyroid nodules. Patients may feel pressure symptoms from nodules as they begin to increase in size. A change in the voice can be caused by a thyroid cancer or benign goiter. The voice change usually occurs when there is compression of the larynx or invasion of the recurrent laryngeal nerve.

On physical examination, a thyroid nodule that is hard or firm and fixed may represent a cancer. The presence of palpable enlarged nodes in the lateral neck, even in the absence of a palpable nodule in the thyroid gland, could represent metastases to the lymph nodes.

Diagnostic work-up

As mentioned previously, thyroid nodules are present in 4%–7% of the general population and in a higher percentage of individuals who have had irradiation to the head and neck region. Most thyroid nodules are benign (colloid nodules or adenomas); therefore, it is important for the work-up to lead to surgical resection for malignant nodules and to avoid unnecessary surgery for benign lesions. Although most solid nodules are benign, thyroid carcinomas usually present as solid nodules. A cystic nodule or a "mixed" (cystic-solid) lesion is less likely to represent a carcinoma and more likely to be a degenerated colloid nodule.

History The history is very important in the evaluation of thyroid nodules. If there is a history of irradiation to the head and neck, the risk of there being cancer in the nodule is higher (as great as 50%) than in non-irradiated patients (10%–20% risk).

A panel of genes that regulate cell invasion and metastases were evaluated in fine-needle aspiration (FNA) specimens using PCR. ECM1 and TMPRSS4 were independent predictors of thyroid malignancy and may be used to improve the diagnostic accuracy of FNA (*Kebebew E, Peng M, Reiff E, et al: Ann Surg 242:353-363, 2005*).

Age also is important in the evaluation of thyroid nodules. Nodules that occur in either the very young or the very old are more likely to be cancerous, particularly in men.

A new nodule or a nodule that suddenly begins to grow is worrisome as well.

FNA has become the initial diagnostic test for the evaluation of thyroid nodules. First, FNA can determine whether the lesion is cystic or solid. For solid lesions, cytology can yield one of three results: benign, malignant, or indeterminate. The accuracy of cytologic diagnosis from FNA is 70%–80%, depending on the experience of the person performing the aspiration and the pathologist interpreting the cytologic specimen.

In a series of 98 "suspicious" FNAs, findings of cellular atypia (pleomorphism, enlarged nuclei, nuclear grooves, coarse or irregular chromatin, prominent or multiple nucleoli, or atypical or numerous mitotic figures) or follicular lesions with atypia were associated with malignancy 20% and 44% of the time, respectively. Follicular lesions without atypia have a 6.7% risk of malignancy.

Imaging modalities Ultrasonographic and radionuclide (radioiodine and technetium) scans are also used in the evaluation of thyroid nodules.

Ultrasonography can be used to determine whether a nodule is cystic or solid. It cannot differentiate a benign solid nodule from a malignant one but can be used to assess the number of nodules present and their size. A nodule in a gland with multiple other nodules of similar size is unlikely to be malignant. A dominant nodule in a multinodular gland carries a risk of malignancy similar to that of a true solitary nodule. Ultrasonographically guided FNA can be performed, increasing the diagnostic efficacy; it also allows evaluation of cervical lymph nodes.

Thyroid isotope scans cannot differentiate absolutely a benign from a malignant nodule but can, based on the functional status of the nodule, assign a probability of malignancy. "Hot" thyroid nodules (ie, those that concentrate radioiodine) represent functioning nodules, whereas "cold" nodules are nonfunctioning lesions that do not concentrate the isotope. Most thyroid carcinomas occur in cold nodules, but only 10% of cold nodules are carcinomas. It is not necessary to operate on all cold thyroid nodules. CT or MRI scan of

A total of 50 patients (19 years old or younger) were surgically treated based on RET mutation analysis. Thirty-three patients had carcinoma identified in the surgical specimen and 44 patients are without disease, based on basal and stimulated calcitonin levels (*Skinner MA, Moley JA, Dilley WG, et al: N Engl J Med 353:1105-1113, 2005*).

the neck may be appropriate in some cases.

Calcitonin level Medullary thyroid carcinomas usually secrete calcitonin, which is a specific product of the thyroid C cells (parafollicular cells). In patients who have clinically palpable medullary carcinoma, the basal calcitonin level is almost always elevated. In patients with smaller tumors or C-cell hyperplasia, the basal calcitonin level may be normal, but administration of synthetic gastrin (pentagastrin) or calcium results in marked elevation of calcitonin levels. The use of calcitonin levels as a tumor marker and stimulation screening in familial forms of medullary cancers has been largely replaced by genetic testing (see below).

Carcinoembryonic antigen (CEA) Serum CEA levels are elevated in patients with medullary thyroid cancer.

Ruling out pheochromocytoma Medullary thyroid carcinoma can be associated with MEN-2A, MEN-2B, or familial non-MEN. Both the MEN-2A and MEN-2B syndromes are characterized by medullary thyroid cancer and pheochromocytoma. Thus, in any patient with familial medullary thyroid carcinoma, it is imperative that the preoperative work-up include a determination of 24-hour urinary catecholamine levels (metanephrine and vanillylmandelic acid) to rule out the presence of a pheochromocytoma. Fractionated plasma metanephrine levels have been demonstrated to have a high sensitivity and may be included in the initial assessment.

Genetic testing Germ-line mutations in the *RET* proto-oncogene are responsible for familial non-MEN medullary thyroid carcinoma in addition to MEN-2A and MEN-2B. DNA analysis performed on a peripheral blood sample is a highly reliable method for identifying the presence of a *RET* mutation. Approximately 95% of patients with *RET* mutation will eventually develop medullary carcinoma of the thyroid, thus prophylactic surgical treatment is recommended. The specific mutated codon of *RET* may correlate with the aggressiveness of medullary carcinoma of the thyroid. This should be considered when counseling affected individuals and their families regarding prophylactic thryoidectomy and the age at which to perform such surgery. Recommended ages for prophylactic surgery range from within the first 6 months of life to 10 years of age depending on the mutation. The prophylactic surgical procedure of choice is total thyroidectomy with or without central lymph node dissection. Although this approach reflects general recommendations, there remain significant concerns about the ethics and safety of surgery based on genetic testing for this and many other diseases.

Periodic determinations of stimulated calcitonin levels may help make the early diagnosis of medullary thyroid carcinoma in those who do not undergo surgery but will not always prevent the development of metastatic medullary thyroid carcinoma.

TABLE 1: UICC staging of thyroid cancer

Primary tumor (T)

Tx	Primary tumor cannot be assessed
T0	No evidence of primary tumor
T1	Tumor ≤ 1 cm in greatest dimension, limited to the thyroid
T2	Tumor > 1 cm but not > 4 cm in greatest dimension, limited to the thyroid
T3	Tumor > 4 cm in greatest dimension, limited to the thyroid
T4	Tumor of any size extending beyond the thyroid capsule

Note: All categories may be subdivided: (a) solitary tumor, (b) multifocal tumor (the largest determines the classification).

Regional lymph nodes (N)

Nx	Regional lymph nodes cannot be assessed
N0	No regional lymph node metastasis
N1	Regional lymph node metastasis
N1a	Metastasis in ipsilateral cervical lymph node(s)
N1b	Metastasis in bilateral, midline, or contralateral cervical or mediastinal lymph node(s)

Distant metastasis (M)

Mx	Presence of distant metastasis cannot be assessed
M0	No distant metastasis
M1	Distant metastasis

Stage grouping: Papillary or follicular							**Stage grouping: Medullary**			
	< 45 years old			**≥ 45 years old**						
Stage I	Any T	Any N	M0	T1	N0	M0	Stage I	T1	N0	M0
Stage II	Any T	Any N	M1	T2	N0	M0	Stage II	T2	N0	M0
				T3	N0	M0		T3	N0	M0
Stage III				T4	N0	M0		T4	N0	M0
				Any T	N1	M0	Stage III	Any T	N1	M0
Stage IV				Any T	Any N	M1	Stage IV	Any T	Any N	M1

Stage grouping: Undifferentiated[a]

Stage IV	Any T	Any N	Any M

UICC = International Union Against Cancer

[a] For undifferentiated cancers (eg, anaplastic carcinoma), all cases are classified as stage IV.

Screening

At this time, no organization recommends periodic screening for thyroid cancer using neck palpation or ultrasonography in average-risk, asymptomatic adults. However, the ACS recommends examination of the thyroid during a routine checkup, since this surveillance can result in case findings.

Staging and prognosis

Unlike most other cancers, in which staging is based on the anatomic extent of disease, the International Union Against Cancer (UICC) staging of thyroid cancer also takes into consideration patient age at the time of diagnosis and tumor histology (Table 1).

Differentiated thyroid cancers Recurrence and death following initial treatment of differentiated thyroid cancer can be predicted using a number of risk classification schemes. The most commonly used systems are the AMES (age, metastases, extent, and size) and AGES (age, grade, extent, and size) classifications.

Low-risk patients are generally those < 45 years of age with low-grade nonmetastatic tumors that are confined to the thyroid gland and are < 1–5 cm. Low-risk patients enjoy a 20-year survival rate of 97%–100% after surgery alone.

High-risk patients are those ≥ 45 years old with a high-grade, metastatic, locally invasive tumor in the neck or with a large tumor. Large size is defined by some authors as > 1 cm and by other authors as > 2 or > 5 cm. The 20-year survival rate in the high-risk group drops to between 54% and 57%.

Intermediate-risk patients include young patients with a high-risk tumor (metastatic, large, locally invasive, or high grade) or older patients with a low-risk tumor. The 20-year survival rate in this group of patients is ~85%.

Medullary thyroid carcinoma is associated with an overall 10-year survival rate of 40%–60%. When medullary carcinoma is discovered prior to becoming palpable, the prognosis is much better: Patients with stage I medullary tumors (ie, tumors < 1 cm or nonpalpable lesions detected by screening and provocative testing) have a 10-year survival rate of 95%.

Stage II medullary cancers (tumors > 1 but < 4 cm) are associated with a survival rate of 50%–90% at 10 years. Patients who have lymph node involvement (stage III disease) have a 10-year survival rate of 15%–50%.

When there are distant metastases (stage IV), the long-term survival rate is compromised. In patients with metastatic medullary thyroid cancer, the disease often progresses at a very slow rate, and patients may remain alive with disease for many years.

Anaplastic thyroid cancer does not have a generally accepted staging system, and all patients are classified as having stage IV disease. Anaplastic carcinoma is highly malignant and has a poor 5-year survival rate (0%–25%). Most patients die of uncontrolled local disease within several months of diagnosis.

Treatment

As most thyroid nodules are not malignant, it is important to differentiate malignant from benign lesions to determine which patients should undergo surgery. If the cytologic result from FNA indicates that the nodule is benign, which is the case most of the time, the nodule can be safely followed. The patient may be placed on thyroxine therapy to suppress thyroid-stimulating hormone (TSH) and reevaluated in 6 months. Adequate suppression is considered to be a TSH level of 0.2–0.4 μU/mL for 6 months.

SURGERY

Malignant or indeterminate cytologic features are the main indications for surgery.

Malignant nodule

Differentiated thyroid cancer If the cytologic result shows a malignant lesion, thyroidectomy should be performed. There is significant debate in the literature regarding the extent of thyroid surgery for primary tumors confined to one lobe. The surgical options include total lobectomy, total lobectomy with contralateral subtotal lobectomy (subtotal thyroidectomy), or total thyroidectomy. The decision about which procedure to perform should be based on the risk of local recurrence and the anticipated use of radioactive iodine (see section on "Radioactive I-131").

Most authorities agree that a good-risk patient (age < 45 years) with a 1-cm or smaller papillary thyroid cancer should undergo ipsilateral total lobectomy alone. Most experts also agree that total thyroidectomy (or at least subtotal thyroidectomy) is appropriate for high-risk patients with high-risk tumors. Intermediate-risk patients are treated with total lobectomy alone or total (or subtotal) thyroidectomy plus postoperative radioactive iodine. Preoperative neck imaging may help plan the surgery. Patients with radiation-induced thyroid malignancies can be treated similarly, as their cancers have a similar prognosis; however, a total thyroidectomy may be preferable in these patients because of the increased risk of multicentric tumors.

> In a review of locally advanced differentiated thyroid cancer invading the airway, most authors recommend surgical resection, including either en bloc or shave resection of the involved respiratory tract (*Kim AW, Maxhimer JB, Quiros RM, et al: J Am Coll Surg 201:619-627, 2005*).

The neck should be palpated intraoperatively. If positive nodes are found, a regional lymph node dissection should be performed.

Medullary carcinoma Patients with medullary thyroid cancer should be treated with total thyroidectomy and a sampling of the regional nodes. If there is involvement of the nodes, a modified neck dissection should be performed (see section on "Lymph node dissection"). If the cancer is confined to the thyroid gland, the patient is usually cured. Postoperative adjuvant external irradiation may be used in certain circumstances (see section on "External radiation therapy").

Anaplastic carcinoma A tracheostomy often is required in patients with anaplastic thyroid cancer because of compression of the trachea. If the tumor is confined to the local area, total thyroidectomy may be indicated to reduce local symptoms produced by the tumor mass. Radiation therapy is used to improve locoregional control, often together with radiosensitizing chemotherapy.

Indeterminate or suspicious nodule

The nodule that yields indeterminate or suspicious cytologic results and is cold on thyroid scanning should be removed for histologic evaluation. The initial operation performed in most patients should be total lobectomy, which entails removal of the suspicious nodule, hemithyroid, and isthmus. There is no role for nodulectomy or enucleation of thyroid nodules. The specimen can be sent for frozen-section analysis during surgery. If the diagnosis is a colloid nodule, no further resection of the thyroid is required.

Follicular lesion If frozen-section biopsy results indicate a follicular lesion in a patient who is a candidate for total thyroidectomy, and a decision cannot be made as to whether the lesion is benign or malignant, two options are available: (1) stop and wait for final confirmation of the diagnosis, which may require a future operation; or (2) proceed with subtotal or total thyroidectomy, which obviates the need for a later operation. The diagnosis of follicular carcinoma requires identification of vascular or capsular invasion, which may not be evident on frozen-section biopsy.

Hürthle cell carcinoma If the nodule is diagnosed as a Hürthle cell carcinoma, total thyroidectomy is generally recommended for all large (> 4 cm) invasive lesions. Small lesions can be managed with total lobectomy. However, controversy remains over the optimal treatment approach for this cancer.

Lymph node dissection

Therapeutic dissection Therapeutic central neck node dissection should be performed for medullary carcinomas and other thyroid neoplasms with nodal involvement. The dissection should include all the lymphatic tissue in the pretracheal area and along the recurrent laryngeal nerve and anterior mediastinum. If there are clinically palpable nodes in the lateral neck, a modified neck dissection is performed.

Prophylactic dissection There is no evidence that performing prophylactic neck dissection improves survival. Therefore, aside from patients with medullary thyroid cancer, who have a high incidence of involved nodes, only therapeutic neck dissection is indicated.

Removal of individual abnormal nodes ("berry picking") is not advised when lateral neck nodes are palpable because of the likelihood of missing involved nodes and disrupting involved lymphatic channels.

Metastatic or recurrent disease

Survival rates from the time of the discovery of metastases (lung and bone) from differentiated thyroid cancer are less favorable than those associated with local recurrence (5-year survival rates of 38% and 50%, respectively). Survival also depends on whether the metastatic lesions take up I-131.

Surgery, with or without I-131 ablation (discussed below), can be useful for controlling localized sites of recurrence. Approximately half of patients who undergo surgery for recurrent disease can be rendered free of disease with a second operation.

RADIOACTIVE I-131

Uses in papillary or follicular thyroid carcinoma

There are two basic uses for I-131 in patients diagnosed with papillary or follicular thyroid carcinoma: ablation of normal residual thyroid tissue after thyroid surgery and treatment of thyroid cancer, either residual disease in the neck or metastasis to other sites in the body. It should be emphasized that patients with medullary, anaplastic, and most Hürthle cell cancers do not benefit from I-131 therapy.

Postoperative ablation of residual thyroid tissue should be considered in high-risk patients and patients with high-risk tumors. Ablation of residual normal thyroid tissue allows for the use of I-131 scans to monitor for future recurrence, possibly destroys microscopic foci of metastatic cancer within the remnant, and improves the accuracy of thyroglobulin monitoring.

Ablation must also be accomplished in patients with regional or metastatic disease prior to the use of I-131 for treatment, as the normal thyroid tissue will preferentially take up iodine compared to the cancer. Some states permit the use of I-131 for ablation and treatment on an outpatient basis, but administration is strictly governed by national guidelines, which minimize the risk of radiation exposure to the public.

Following surgery, the patient should not be given thyroid hormone replacement. The TSH level should be determined approximately 4–6 weeks after surgery; in patients who undergo total or subtotal thyroidectomy, TSH levels will generally be > 50 μU/mL. A postoperative iodine scan can then be performed. If this scan documents residual thyroid tissue, an ablative dose of I-131 should be given. The patient should be advised not to undergo any radiographic studies with iodine during ablation therapy and to avoid seafood and vitamins or cough syrups containing iodine. Patients are prepared with a specific diet prior to the I-131 therapy. Iodine-123 may also be used in the postoperative setting. It may produce a better image quality than I-131 scans.

Iodine-131 dose In general, doses of I-131 up to 75–100 mCi will ablate residual thyroid tissue within 6 months following ingestion. In some patients, it may take up to 1 year for complete ablation to occur. Patients should be monitored following ablation, and when they become hypothyroid, hormone replacement therapy should be given until they are clinically euthyroid and TSH is suppressed. Recently, lower doses have been found to be effective,

> Verburg et al have reported that patients with a successful ablation had a better prognosis than those with an unsuccessful ablation, with a disease-free survival of 87% vs 49% at 10 years and a thyroid cancer survival of 93% vs 78% (*Verburg FA, de Keizer B, Lips CJ, et al: Eur J Endocrinol 152:33-37, 2005*).

and some authors have recommended doses between 25 and 50 mCi, assuming they achieve euthyroid levels with TSH suppression to < 0.1 μU/mL.

Follow-up I-131 scan Approximately 6–12 months after ablation of the thyroid remnant, a follow-up I-131 scan should be performed. Recombinant human thyrotropin alpha (Thyrogen) is now available. Patients may continue on thyroid replacement and receive two doses of thyrotropin prior to I-131 scanning; this approach can prevent the symptoms of hypothyroidism.

Treatment of residual cancer For disease in the tumor bed or lymph nodes that was not surgically resectable, an I-131 dose of 100–150 mCi is given. For disease in the lungs or bone, the I-131 dose is 200 mCi. Following this therapy, the patient is again put on thyroid hormone replacement, and adequate suppression is maintained by monitoring TSH levels.

Follow-up Some clinicians advocate obtaining a repeat scan in 1 year, along with a chest x-ray, and repeating this procedure yearly until a normal scan is obtained. However, the frequency of repeat scans and the dose of I-131 are rather controversial and should be guided by the individual's risk profile.

Following thyroid remnant ablation, serum thyroglobulin measurements are useful in monitoring for recurrence. Since thyroglobulin in a patient receiving thyroid hormone replacement may be suppressed, a normal test may be incorrect ~ 10% of the time. In general, the presence of disease is accurately predicted by a thyroglobulin value > 5 ng/mL while the patient is in the suppressed state and by a value > 10 ng/mL in the hypothyroid state. However, measurable disease may not be identified in many patients. Whether or not they should be treated on the basis of the thyroglobulin value if the I-131 scan is normal is a subject of current debate. Any rise in the thyroglobulin level from the previous value should increase the suspicion of recurrent disease.

Chest x-rays should continue to be performed at yearly intervals for at least 10 years. Neck ultrasonography is also useful to evaluate locoregional recurrence. Continued monitoring is necessary, as late recurrence can occur. It should be pointed out that certain aggressive tumors may neither be radioactive iodine–avid nor synthesize thyroglobulin. PET scanning may contribute to localization of disease in some cases and may even carry prognostic value. PET/CT may be more useful than other imaging techniques; in a recent study, additional information was obtained with PET/CT in up to 67% of cases.

Side effects and complications

Acute effects The acute side effects of I-131 therapy include painful swelling of the salivary glands and nausea. Ibuprofen or other pain relievers are usually used to decrease salivary gland discomfort. Nausea may be treated with standard antiemetics.

Rarely, in patients with significant residual thyroid tissue, radioactive iodine may cause acute thyroiditis, with a rapid release of thyroid hormone. This problem can be treated with steroids and β-blockers.

Patients must also be cautioned not to wear contact lenses for at least 3 weeks following ingestion of I-131, as the tears are radioactive and will contaminate the lenses and possibly lead to corneal ulceration.

Bone marrow suppression and leukemia are potential long-term complications of I-131 therapy but are poorly documented and appear to be extremely rare. Patients should have a CBC count performed prior to ingestion of an I-131 dose to ensure adequate bone marrow reserve. They should also have yearly blood counts. Leukemia occurs rarely with doses of I-131 < 1,000 mCi.

Pulmonary fibrosis may be seen in patients with pulmonary metastases from papillary or follicular thyroid cancer who are treated with I-131. Those with a miliary or micronodular pattern are at greater risk, as a portion of normal lung around each lesion may receive radiation, leading to diffuse fibrosis.

Effects on fertility Recent data have documented an increase in follicle-stimulating hormone (FSH) levels in one-third of male patients treated with I-131. Changes in FSH after one or two doses of I-131 are generally transitory, but repeated doses may lead to lasting damage to the germinal epithelium. Sperm banking should be considered in male patients likely to receive cumulative doses of I-131 higher than 500 mCi.

The effects of I-131 on female fertility have been investigated. A recently published article showed no significant difference in the fertility rate in women receiving radioactive iodine. However, it is generally recommended to avoid pregnancy for 1 year after therapeutic I-131 administration.

No ill effects have been noted in the offspring of treated patients.

EXTERNAL RADIATION THERAPY

Papillary or follicular thyroid cancer

There are a number of indications for external irradiation of papillary or follicular thyroid carcinoma. Surgery followed by radioactive iodine may be used for disease that extends beyond the capsule. However, if all gross disease cannot be resected, or if residual disease is not radioactive iodine–avid, external irradiation is used as part of the initial approach for locally advanced disease in older patients.

Unresectable disease External irradiation is useful for unresectable disease extending into the connective tissue, trachea, esophagus, great vessels, and anterior mediastinum. For unresected disease, doses of 6,000–6,500 cGy are recommended. The patient should then undergo I-131 scanning, and, if uptake is detected, a dose of I-131 should be administered.

Recurrence after resection External irradiation may also be used after resection of recurrent papillary or follicular thyroid carcinoma that no longer shows uptake of I-131. In this situation, doses of 5,000–6,000 cGy are delivered to the tumor bed to prevent local recurrence. Multiple-field techniques and extensive treatment planning are necessary to deliver high doses to the target volume without the risk of significant complications.

Palliation of bone metastases External radiation therapy is useful in relieving pain from bone metastasis. If the metastasis shows evidence of I-131 uptake, the patient should be given a therapeutic dose of I-131 followed by local external radiation therapy to the lesion of up to 4,000–5,000 cGy. The use of intravenous bisphosphonate therapy has been shown to decrease the pain of bone metastasis and improve reported quality of life.

Anaplastic thyroid carcinoma

Anaplastic carcinoma of the thyroid is an exceptionally aggressive disease. It often presents as a rapidly expanding mass in the neck and may not be completely resected. External irradiation to full dose (6,000–6,500 cGy) may slow the progress of this disease but rarely controls it.

Chemoradiation therapy There are reports of the use of accelerated fractionation regimens of external irradiation (160 cGy twice daily to 5,700 cGy) with weekly doxorubicin in patients with anaplastic thyroid cancer, as well as reports of the combination of doxorubicin and cisplatin with external irradiation. These regimens have improved local control but at the expense of increased toxicity. Unfortunately, the majority of patients die of progressive disease.

Medullary thyroid carcinoma

External irradiation has been used for medullary thyroid cancer in the postoperative setting. Indications include positive surgical margins, gross residual disease, or extensive lymph node metastasis. The recommended dose is 5,000 cGy in 5 weeks.

ROLE OF MEDICAL THERAPY

Differentiated thyroid cancer

Thyroid hormone replacement As mentioned previously, thyroid hormone replacement is used to suppress TSH in most patients with differentiated thyroid cancer after surgery and prior to I-131 scanning and (as appropriate) treatment.

Systemic chemotherapy is used for widespread disease, although reproducibly effective regimens have not been identified to date.

Medullary thyroid carcinoma

In patients with medullary thyroid carcinoma, the usual treatment is surgery. In patients with familial medullary carcinoma who have a coexisting pheochromocytoma, appropriate control of catecholamine hypersecretion should precede thyroid surgery.

Anaplastic thyroid carcinoma

As mentioned previously, the usual treatment for patients with resectable or localized anaplastic thyroid cancer is surgery. Like radiotherapy, chemotherapy is an important alternative approach, but further evaluation is needed to optimize its effectiveness.

PARATHYROID CARCINOMA

Parathyroid carcinoma is a rare cause of hypercalcemia, accounting for < 2% of cases with primary hyperparathyroidism.

Epidemiology and etiology

The disease presents in midlife and occurs with similar frequency in both genders. The etiology of parathyroid carcinoma is obscure; an association with prior neck irradiation is not apparent. Treatment of parathyroid carcinoma is primarily surgical.

Signs and symptoms

Most patients with parathyroid cancer have symptomatic moderate to severe hypercalcemia (mean serum calcium level, 15 mg/dL) and high parathyroid hormone levels. They often present with a palpable neck mass. Unlike benign hyperparathyroidism, renal and bone abnormalities are more common in patients with parathyroid cancer.

Rarely, nonfunctioning tumors may present as neck masses; their clinical course is similar to that of functioning tumors. Clinical concern about parathyroid cancer should be raised in the presence of a palpable neck mass and severe hypercalcemia, recurrent hyperparathyroidism, or associated vocal cord paralysis.

Pathology

The principal features of parathyroid cancer include a trabecular pattern, mitotic figures, thick fibrous bands, and capsular or vascular invasion of disease. Other important features include lymphatic or hematogenous metastases and histologic evidence of tumor infiltration into the surrounding tissues (including macroscopic adherence or vocal cord paralysis).

Although cytologic evidence of mitoses is necessary to establish the diagnosis of carcinoma, mitotic activity alone is an unreliable indicator of malignancy. The only reliable microscopic finding of malignancy is invasion of surrounding structures or metastasis to lymph nodes or other organs.

Treatment

Surgical treatment of primary hyperparathyroidism

The diagnosis of parathyroid carcinoma is sometimes made during surgical exploration for primary hyperparathyroidism. Most surgeons advocate identification of all four parathyroid glands. In most cases, the upper glands can be found on the posterior aspect of the upper third of the thyroid lobe, just cephalad to the inferior thyroid artery and adjacent to the recurrent laryngeal nerve as it enters the larynx.

The inferior parathyroid glands are more variable in location. Most are found on the posterior or lateral aspect of the lower pole of the thyroid gland, but the inferior parathyroid glands may be ectopically placed in the superior or true mediastinum, often within the thymus.

The inferior and, less commonly, superior glands can be located in an ectopic location in the upper or lateral neck, adjacent to the esophagus, or within the carotid sheath.

Surgical exploration for primary hyperparathyroidism Most cases of primary hyperparathyroidism are caused by a single hyperfunctioning parathyroid adenoma. If the surgeon finds one (or occasionally two) enlarged abnormal gland(s) and the remaining glands are normal, the enlarged gland should be removed.

If four enlarged glands are found, indicating the rare case of primary parathyroid hyperplasia, subtotal parathyroidectomy including 3.5 glands should be performed. Consideration should be given to transplanting the remaining gland remnant to an ectopic location that would be easily accessible to the surgeon if hyperparathyroidism recurs.

If only normal glands are found at exploration, a missed adenoma in an ectopic location should be suspected. Thorough intraoperative neck and superior mediastinal exploration should be performed, and if the missing gland cannot be found, thymectomy and hemithyroidectomy should be performed to exclude an intrathymic or intrathyroidal adenoma. Localization studies, including CT/MRI or radionuclide imaging, should precede reexploration for a missed adenoma.

Intraoperative parathyroid hormone (ioPTH) levels are increasingly used to guide surgery for primary hyperparathyroidism. A 50% or greater decrease in ioPTH level from the preexcision value to the 10-minute postexcision value is used as a predictor of successful surgery. The advent of ioPTH monitoring, coupled with preoperative localization studies (sestamibi scanning), has facilitated less invasive surgical techniques, such as minimally invasive parathyroidectomy. This has resulted in shorter average hospitalization stays and reduced postoperative recovery times.

The use of ioPTH with parathyroid hyperplasia requires more strict evaluation of ioPTH levels. Siperstein et al performed a prospective evaluation of ioPTH and bilateral neck exploration and found that up to 15% of cases will have additional "abnormal" glands that were not predicted by ioPTH or preoperative imaging. This study demonstrates the need for long-term follow-up of patients undergoing focused parathyroid surgery.

If parathyroid carcinoma is suspected, based on the severity of hyperparathyroidism or invasion of surrounding tissues by a firm parathyroid tumor, aggressive wide excision is indicated. This procedure should include ipsilateral thyroidectomy and en bloc excision of surrounding tissues as necessary.

Patterns of recurrence of cancer The average time from initial surgery to the first recurrence of cancer is approximately 3 years but may be as long as 10 years. The thyroid gland is the usual site of involvement, with disease "seeding" in the neck a common pattern. Other sites of involvement include the recurrent nerve, strap muscles, esophagus, and trachea.

Distant metastases can be present at the time of initial surgery, or local spread to contiguous structures in the neck may be followed subsequently by distant metastases to the lungs, bone, and liver.

In a recent analysis, 85% of patients with parathyroid carcinoma were alive 5 years after diagnosis; death usually results from complications of the hypercalcemia rather than from the tumor burden.

Treatment of isolated metastases Isolated metastases should be aggressively resected to enhance survival and control hypercalcemia.

Medical therapy

Morbidity and mortality are generally caused by the effects of unremitting hypercalcemia rather than tumor growth. Medical treatment provides temporary palliation of hypercalcemia. Drugs used include bisphosphonates, such as pamidronate (60–80 mg q4-6d) or zoledronic acid (Zometa); calcitonin, 4-8 IU/kg q6-12h; mithramycin (plicamycin [Mithracin]), 25 μg/kg q4–6d; and gallium nitrate (Ganite), 100–200 mg/m^2/d IV for 5 days.

SUGGESTED READING

ON THYROID CARCINOMA

Alsanea O, Clark OH: Familial thyroid cancer. National Library of Medicine. Curr Opin Oncol 13:44–51, 2001.

Bal CS, Kumar A, Pant GS: Radioiodine dose for remnant ablation in differentiated thyroid carcinoma: A randomized clinical trial in 509 patients. J Clin Endocrinol Metab 89:1666–1673, 2004.

Berg G, Lindstedt G, Suurkula M, et al: Radioiodine ablation and therapy in differentiated thyroid cancer under stimulation with recombinant human thyroid-stimulating hormone. J Endocrinol Invest 25:44–52, 2002.

Chow SM, Law SC, Mendenhall WM, et al: Prognostic factors and the role of radioiodine and external radiotherapy. Int J Radiat Oncol Biol Phys 52:784–795, 2002.

David A, Blotta A, Rossi R, et al: Clinical value of different responses of serum thyroglobulin to recombinant human thyrotropin in the follow-up of patients with differentiated thyroid carcinoma. Thyroid 15:267–273, 2005.

Goldstein RE, Netterville JL, Burkey B, et al: Implications of follicular neoplasms, atypia, and lesions suspicious for malignancy diagnosed by fine-needle aspiration of thyroid nodules. Ann Surg 235:656–662, 2002.

Guiffrida D, Gharib H: Anaplastic thyroid carcinoma: Current diagnosis and treatment. National Library of Medicine. Ann Oncol 11:1083–1089, 2000.

Haigh PI, Ituarte PH, Wu HS, et al: Completely resected anaplastic thyroid carcinoma combined with adjuvant chemotherapy and irradiation is associated with prolonged survival. Cancer 91:2335–2342, 2001.

Haugen BR, Lin EC: Isotope imaging for metastatic thyroid cancer. Endocrinol Metab Clin North Am 30:469–492, 2001.

Krassas GE, Pontikides N: Gonadal effect of radiation from 131I in male patients with thyroid carcinoma. Arch Androl 51:171–175, 2005.

Kuriakose MA, Hicks Jr WL, Loree TR, et al: Risk group-based management of differentiated thyroid carcinoma. J R Coll Surg Edinb 46:216–223, 2001.

Larson SM, Robbins R: Positron emission tomography in thyroid cancer management. Semin Roentgenol 37:169–174, 2002.

Luster M, Lassmann M, Haenscheid H, et al: Use of recombinant human thyrotropin before radioiodine therapy in patients with advanced differentiated thyroid carcinoma. J Clin Endocrinol Metab 85:3640–3645, 2000.

Mazzaferri EL, Kloos RT: Clinical review 128: Current approaches to primary therapy for papillary and follicular thyroid cancer. National Library of Medicine. J Clin Endocrinol Metab 86:1447–1463, 2001.

Mazzaferri EL, Robbins RJ, Spencer CA, et al: A consensus report of the role of serum thyroglobulin as a monitoring method for low-risk patients with papillary thyroid carcinoma. J Clin Endocrinol Metab 88:1433–1441, 2003.

Nahas Z, Goldenberg D, Fakhry C, et al: The role of positron emission tomography/computed tomography in the management of recurrent papillary thyroid carcinoma. Laryngoscope 115:237–243, 2005.

Pacini F, Capezzone M, Elisei R, et al: Diagnostic 131-iodine whole-body scan may be avoided in thyroid cancer patients who have undetectable stimulated serum Tg levels after initial treatment. J Clin Endocrinol Metab 87:1499–1501, 2002.

Pacini F, Elisei R, Romei C, et al: *RET* proto-oncogene mutations in thyroid carcinomas: Clinical relevance. National Library of Medicine. J Endocrinol Invest 23:328–338, 2000.

Pacini F, Molinaro E, Lippi F, et al: Prediction of disease status by recombinant human TSH-stimulated serum Tg in the postsurgical follow-up of differentiated thyroid carcinoma. J Clin Endocrinol Metab 86:5686–5690, 2001.

Sautter-Bihl ML, Raub J, Hetzel-Sesterheim M, et al: Differentiated thyroid cancer: Prognostic factors and influence of treatment on the outcome in 441 patients. Strahlenther Onkol 177:125–131, 2001.

Sawka AM, Jaeschke R, Singh RJ, et al: Comparison of biochemical tests for pheochromocytoma: Measurement of fractionated plasma metanephrines compared with the combination of 24-hour urinary metanephrines and catecholamines. J Clin Endocrinol 88:553–558, 2003.

Tennvall J, Lundell G, Wahlberg P, et al: Anaplastic thyroid carcinoma: Three protocols combining doxorubicin, hyperfractionated radiotherapy, and surgery. Br J Cancer 86:1848–1853, 2002.

Torlontano M, Attard M, Crocetti U, et al: Follow-up of low risk patients with papillary thyroid cancer: Role of neck ultrasonography in detecting lymph node metastases. J Clin Endocrinol Metab 89:3402–3407, 2004.

United States Nucler Regulatory Commission: Medical, industrial, and acdemic uses of nuclear materials: Regulations, guidance, and communications. Available at: www.nrg.gov. Accessed September 6, 2005.

Verburg FA, de Keizer B, Lips CJ, et al: Prognostic significance of successful ablation with radioiodine of differentiated thyroid cancer patients. Eur J Endocrinol 152:33–37, 2005.

Vitale G, Caraglia M, Ciccarelli A, et al: Current approaches and perspectives in the therapy of medullary thyroid carcinoma. Cancer 91:1797–1808, 2001.

Wang W, Larson SM, Fazzari M, et al: Prognostic value of [18F]fluorodeoxyglucose positron emission tomographic scanning in patients with thyroid cancer. J Clin Endocrinol Metab 85:1107–1113, 2000.

Wu HS, Young MT, Ituarte PH, et al: Death from thyroid cancer of follicular cell origin. J Am Coll Surg 191:600–606, 2000.

ON PARATHYROID CARCINOMA

Busaidy N, Jimenez C, Habra MA, et al: Parathyroid carcinoma: A 22-year experience. Head Neck 26:716–726, 2004.

Dackiw AP, Sussman JJ, Fritsche HA Jr, et al: Relative contributions of technetium Tc 99m sestamibi scintigraphy, intraoperative gamma probe detection, and the rapid parathyroid hormone assay to the surgical management of hyperparathyroidism. Arch Surg 135:550–557, 2000.

Dotzenrath C, Goretzki PE, Sarbia M, et al: Parathyroid carcinoma: Problems in diagnosis and the need for radical surgery even in recurrent disease. Eur J Surg Oncol 27:383–389, 2001.

Grant CS, Thompson G, Farley D, et al: Primary hyperparathyroidism surgical management since the introduction of minimally invasive parathyroidectomy: Mayo Clinic experience. Arch Surg 140:472–479, 2005.

Rawat N, Khetan N, Williams DW, et al: Parathyroid carcinoma. Br J Surg 92:1345–1353, 2005.

Rolighed L, Heickendorff L, Hessov I, et al: Primary hyperparathyroidism: Intraoperative PTH measurements. Scand J Surg 93:43–47, 2004.

Sheehan JJ, Hill AD, Walsh MF, et al: Parathyroid carcinoma: Diagnosis and management. Eur J Surg Oncol 27:321–324, 2001.

Siperstein A, Berber E, Mackey R, et al: Prospective evaluation of sestamibi scan, ultrasonography, and rapid PTH to predict the success of limited exploration of sporadic primary hyperparathyroidism. Surgery 136:872–880, 2004.

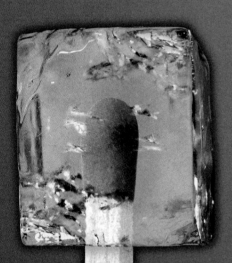

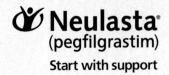

ADVERSE REACTIONS

(See **WARNINGS**, **Splenic Rupture**, **Adult Respiratory Distress Syndrome (ARDS)**, **Allergic Reactions**, and **Sickle Cell Disease**.)

Because clinical trials are conducted under widely varying conditions, adverse reaction rates observed in the clinical trials of Neulasta® cannot be directly compared to rates in the clinical trials of other drugs and may not reflect the rates observed in practice. The adverse reaction information from clinical trials does, however, provide a basis for identifying the adverse events that appear to be related to Neulasta® use and for approximating rates.

The data described below reflect exposure to Neulasta® in 932 patients. Neulasta® was studied in placebo- and active-controlled trials (n = 467, and n = 465, respectively). The population encompassed an age range of 21 to 88 years. Ninety-two percent of patients were female. The ethnicity of the patients was as follows: 75% Caucasian, 18% Hispanic, 5% Black, and 1% Asian. Patients with solid tumors (breast [n = 823], lung and thoracic tumors [n = 53]) or lymphoma (n = 56) received Neulasta® after nonmyeloablative cytotoxic chemotherapy. Most patients received a single 100 mcg/kg (n = 259) or a single 6 mg (n = 546) dose per chemotherapy cycle over 4 cycles.

In the placebo-controlled trial, bone pain occurred at a higher incidence in Neulasta®-treated patients as compared to placebo-treated patients. The incidence of other commonly reported adverse events were similar in the Neulasta®- and placebo-treated patients, and were consistent with the underlying cancer diagnosis and its treatment with chemotherapy. The data in Table 1 reflect those adverse events occurring in at least 10% of patients treated with Neulasta® in the placebo-controlled study.

TABLE 1. Adverse Events Occurring in ≥10%[a] of Patients in The Placebo-Controlled Study

Event	Neulasta® (n = 467)	Placebo (n = 461)
Alopecia	48%	47%
Bone Pain[b]	31%	26%
Diarrhea	29%	28%
Pyrexia (not including febrile neutropenia)	23%	22%
Myalgia	21%	18%
Headache	16%	14%
Arthralgia	16%	13%
Vomiting	13%	11%
Asthenia	13%	11%
Edema Peripheral	12%	10%
Constipation	10%	6%

[a]*Events occurring in ≥ 10% of Neulasta®-treated patients and at a higher incidence as compared to placebo-treated patients*

[b]*Bone pain is limited to the specified adverse event term, "bone pain"*

In the active-controlled studies, common adverse events occurred at similar rates and severities in both treatment arms (Neulasta®, n = 465; Filgrastim, n = 331). These adverse experiences occurred at rates between 72% and 15% and included: nausea, fatigue, alopecia, diarrhea, vomiting, constipation, fever, anorexia, skeletal pain, headache, taste perversion, dyspepsia, myalgia, insomnia, abdominal pain, arthralgia, generalized weakness, peripheral edema, dizziness, granulocytopenia, stomatitis, mucositis, and neutropenic fever.

Bone Pain

The analysis of bone pain described below is based on a composite analysis using multiple, related, adverse event terms.

In the placebo-controlled study, the incidence of bone pain was 57% in Neulasta®-treated patients compared to 50% in placebo-treated patients. Bone pain was generally reported to be of mild-to-moderate severity.

Among patients experiencing bone pain, approximately 37% of Neulasta®- and 31% of placebo-treated patients utilized non-narcotic analgesics and 10% of Neulasta®- and 9% of placebo-treated patients utilized narcotic analgesics.

In the active-controlled studies, the use of non-narcotic and narcotic analgesics in association with bone pain was similar between Neulasta®- and Filgrastim-treated patients. No patient withdrew from study due to bone pain.

Laboratory Abnormalities

In clinical studies, leukocytosis (WBC counts > 100 x 10^9/L) was observed in less than 1% of 932 patients with nonmyeloid malignancies receiving Neulasta®. Leukocytosis was not associated with any adverse effects.

In the placebo-controlled study, reversible elevations in LDH, alkaline phosphatase, and uric acid that did not require treatment occurred at similar rates in Neulasta®- and placebo-treated patients.

Immunogenicity

As with all therapeutic proteins, there is a potential for immunogenicity. The incidence of antibody development in patients receiving Neulasta® has not been adequately determined. While available data suggest that a small proportion of patients developed binding antibodies to Filgrastim or pegfilgrastim, the nature and specificity of these antibodies have not been adequately studied. No neutralizing antibodies have been detected using a cell-based bioassay in 46 patients who apparently developed binding antibodies. The detection of antibody formation is highly dependent on the sensitivity and specificity of the assay, and the observed incidence of antibody positivity in an assay may be influenced by several factors, including sample handling, concomitant medications, and underlying disease. Therefore, comparison of the incidence of antibodies to Neulasta® with the incidence of antibodies to other products may be misleading.

Cytopenias resulting from an antibody response to exogenous growth factors have been reported on rare occasions in patients treated with other recombinant growth factors. There is a theoretical possibility that an antibody directed against pegfilgrastim may cross-react with endogenous G-CSF, resulting in immune-mediated neutropenia, but this has not been observed in clinical studies.

OVERDOSAGE

The maximum amount of Neulasta® that can be safely administered in single or multiple doses has not been determined. Single subcutaneous doses of 300 mcg/kg have been administered to 8 healthy volunteers and 3 patients with non-small cell lung cancer without serious adverse effects. These patients experienced a mean maximum ANC of 55 x 10^9/L, with a corresponding mean maximum WBC of 67 x 10^9/L. The absolute maximum ANC observed was 96 x 10^9/L with a corresponding absolute maximum WBC observed of 120 x 10^9/L. The duration of leukocytosis ranged from 6 to 13 days. Leukapheresis should be considered in the management of symptomatic individuals.

DOSAGE AND ADMINISTRATION

The recommended dosage of Neulasta® is a single subcutaneous injection of 6 mg administered once per chemotherapy cycle. Neulasta® should not be administered in the period between 14 days before and 24 hours after administration of cytotoxic chemotherapy (see **PRECAUTIONS**).

The 6 mg fixed-dose formulation should not be used in infants, children, and smaller adolescents weighing less than 45 kg.

No dosing adjustment is necessary for renal dysfunction (see **CLINICAL PHARMACOLOGY, Special Populations**).

Rx Only

This product, its production, and/or its use may be covered by one or more US Patents, including US Patent Nos. 5,824,784; 4,810,643; 4,999,291; 5,582,823; 5,580,755, as well as other patents or patents pending.

Reference

*Heil G, Hoelzer D, Sanz MA, et al. A randomized, double-blind, placebo-controlled, phase III study of Filgrastim in remission induction and consolidation therapy for adults with de novo Acute Myeloid Leukemia. *Blood.* 1997;90:4710-4718.

Issue Date: 01/03/2007

AMGEN®

Manufactured by:
Amgen Manufacturing Limited,
a subsidiary of Amgen Inc.
One Amgen Center Drive
Thousand Oaks, CA 91320-1799

CHAPTER 6

Non–small-cell lung cancer

Benjamin Movsas, MD, Fadlo R. Khuri, MD, and Kemp H. Kernstine, MD, PhD

Lung cancer has been the leading cause of cancer death among men in the United States for years, and since 1988, it has become the number-one cause of cancer death among women. An estimated 213,380 new cases of lung cancer are expected in 2007, and 160,390 deaths due to this disease are expected to occur. This exceeds the combined number of deaths from the leading causes of cancer (breast, prostate, and colon cancers). It accounts for 6% of all deaths in the United States.

Lung cancer develops from pulmonary parenchymal or bronchial supportive tissues. Although multiple cell types are often found within a single lung tumor, one type usually predominates. Based on the therapeutic approach, there are two major subdivisions of lung cancer: small-cell lung cancer (SCLC), for which chemotherapy is the primary treatment, and non–small-cell lung cancer (NSCLC), which in its early stages (I and II) is treated primarily with surgery.

This chapter provides basic information on the epidemiology, etiology, screening, prevention, and signs and symptoms of lung cancer in general, and then focuses specifically on the diagnosis, staging, pathology, and treatment of NSCLC and carcinoid tumors of the lungs, as well as the pulmonary evaluation of lung cancer patients and follow-up of long-term survivors.

Chapter 7 provides information on the staging, pathology and pathophysiology, and treatment of the far less common SCLC and concludes with brief discussions of mesothelioma and thymoma.

Epidemiology

Gender In the United States, the estimated number of new lung cancer cases for 2005 was 93,010 for men and 79,560 for women. Although the incidence of lung cancer had been rising in women, the rate of increase has begun to slow recently. The incidence is decreasing in men.

Age The age at which lung cancer patients are diagnosed varies widely, but the median age at diagnosis is approximately 70 years.

Race In the United States, the highest incidence of lung cancer in men and women is found in African-Americans (117.2/100,000 for men and 54.5/100,000 for women) followed by Caucasians (77.9/100,000 for men and 51.3/100,000 for women).

Geography There are geographic variations in the incidence of lung cancer, with the highest rates worldwide observed in North America and Eastern Europe; in the United States, the highest rates are found in northern urban areas and along the southern coast from Texas to Florida.

Survival The overall 5-year survival rate for lung cancer is 15%, of which there has been a 1% improvement each decade for the past 30 years.

Etiology and risk factors

Cigarette smoking Approximately 87% of all cases of lung cancer are related to cigarette smoking. There is a relatively strong dose-response relationship between cigarette smoking and the development of this cancer. The greater the number of cigarettes smoked on a daily basis and the greater the number of years of smoking, the greater is the risk of lung cancer. An individual who smokes one pack of cigarettes daily has a 20-fold increased risk of lung cancer compared to a nonsmoker.

The overall incidence of cigarette smoking decreased from 1974 through 1992. Smoking cessation decreases the risk of lung cancer, but a significant decrease in risk does not occur until approximately 5 years after stopping, and the risk remains higher in former smokers than in nonsmokers for at least 25 years. The benefit of smoking cessation is greater if it occurs at a younger age.

Smoking cessation is difficult. Recent data have suggested that a variety of hereditary factors increase the risk of addiction to nicotine among some individuals. Nevertheless, millions of former smokers have quit successfully. Smoking cessation programs that address both physical withdrawal from nicotine and psychological dependence appear to be more effective than either of these approaches alone. In addition, continued efforts are needed to prevent adolescents and preadolescents from beginning to smoke or to encourage them to quit after a brief period of experimentation.

Several cancer centers have recently reported that more than half of their patients with newly diagnosed lung cancer are former smokers, having quit more than 1 year before diagnosis. Healthy ex-smokers represent a large group of individuals who may benefit from effective tools for early detection and/or chemoprevention of lung cancer.

Secondhand smoke Not only is smoking risky for those who smoke, but it also poses a hazard to nonsmokers who either live or work with smokers. It is estimated that approximately 3,000 lung cancer deaths per year in the United States are due to secondhand smoke. Individuals who live in a household with a smoker have a 30% increase in the incidence of lung cancer compared to nonsmokers who do not live in such an environment.

Asbestos exposure is another risk factor for lung cancer. Cigarette smokers who are exposed to asbestos develop lung cancer at an extremely high rate. There is a 90-fold increase compared with unexposed individuals. Exposure to asbestos is also a major risk factor for the development of mesothelioma (see discussion of this cancer in the following chapter).

Radioactive dust and radon exposure Uranium miners who have been exposed to radioactive dust and radon gas also have an increased incidence of lung cancer. Although there has been some controversy about the risk posed by exposure to residential radon gas, a study conducted in Sweden showed an increased incidence of lung cancer in individuals who were exposed to a high level of radon in their homes.

Screening and prevention

Screening

Currently, screening for lung cancer among asymptomatic individuals at elevated risk due to smoking history or occupational exposures is not recommended. An unfortunate result of this policy is that most patients present in advanced stage, and cure rates have improved little over the past 30 years. Only 7% of NSCLC patients are diagnosed in stage IA.

Three randomized screening trials conducted in the United States in the 1970s failed to show a reduction in lung cancer mortality among the smokers who were screened by sputum cytology and chest x-ray for lung cancer. Despite the fact that these American trials were not designed to evaluate chest x-ray as a screening tool, the results led most experts to conclude that screening for lung cancer was not worthwhile. In addition, most investigators recommended that research efforts and resources be allocated to the *prevention* of lung cancer. A more recent, randomized, prospective trial from Czechoslovakia showed that screening with a chest x-ray increased the diagnosis of early-stage lung cancer but failed to reduce the mortality from lung cancer.

The potential to screen for lung cancer has received renewed interest due to the superior performance of low-dose helical CT compared with chest radiography in detecting small lesions. Although there is insufficient evidence to establish policy related to routine screening for lung cancer with spiral CT, there is a growing trend toward promoting screening with this new technology to individuals at increased risk for lung cancer.

Numerous studies are currently under way to evaluate chest CT scan for lung cancer screening. Several recent reports from Japan, Germany, and the United States have documented the ability of low-dose spiral CT scans to detect lung cancer at an early stage. In some recent trials, more than 80% of lung cancers detected by screening were diagnosed in stage I.

Kaneko screened male smokers > 50 years of age. Of the 15 cancers detected by CT scan, only 4 were seen on chest x-ray; 14 of the 15 cancers were stage I, with an average diameter of 1.6 cm. Ohmatsu found 35 lung cancers (0.37% detection rate) with 9,452 CT scans. Of these cancers, 27 were stage IA. These patients had a 3-year survival rate of 83%.

The International Early Lung Cancer Action Project (I-ELCAP, http://www.ielcap.org/professionals.htm) is a single-arm prospective study that has accrued more than 35,000 study subjects in 30 sites and documented that a high percentage of lung cancers are detected in stage I, a stage in which long-term survival can reasonably be anticipated in more than 60% of patients. These studies provide early evidence to suggest that CT lung cancer population screening has the potential to reduce lung cancer mortality in the near future.

Henschke et al have reported encouraging results from ELCAP of screening with spiral CT scan. Included in the initial report were 1,000 symptom-free volunteers, aged 60 years or older, with at least 10 pack-years of cigarette smoking and no previous cancer who were medically fit to undergo thoracic surgery. Noncalcified pulmonary nodules were detected in 233 participants (23% [95% confidence interval (CI): 21–26]) by low-dose CT at baseline, compared with 68 (7% [95% CI: 5–9]) by chest radiography. Lung cancer was detected by CT in 27 patients (2.7% [95% CI: 1.8–3.8]) and by chest radiography in 7 patients (0.7% [95% CI: 0.3–1.3]).

Of the 27 CT-detected cancers, 26 were resectable. Stage I cancers were diagnosed in 23 of 27 patients (85%) by CT and 4 of 7 patients (57%) by chest radiography. In addition, low-dose CT detected four more nonparenchymal cases of lung cancer: two with endobronchial lesions and two in the mediastinum. These cases show an added benefit of low-dose CT over chest radiography, although the data were not included in the analysis. (The study primarily focused on malignant disease in noncalcified pulmonary nodules detected by low-dose CT or radiography.) It remains to be seen, however, whether lung cancer screening with low-dose spiral CT will reduce the lung cancer mortality of the study population or only improve the 5-year survival rate of the patients diagnosed with lung cancer.

Based on growing evidence that spiral CT may truly provide for a successful early detection strategy, the National Cancer Institute (NCI) launched the National Lung Screening Trial (NLST, http://www.nci.nih.gov/NLST) in September 2002. NLST has accrued 50,000 current and former smokers (aged 55–74) into a prospective trial, randomizing participants to receive annual spiral CT or annual chest x-rays. Survival data will not be available for a number of years.

The efficacy of lung cancer screening is also being evaluated as part of the Prostate, Lung, Colorectal, and Ovarian Cancer Screening Trial (PLCO). Men and women were randomized to receive annual chest x-ray vs usual care. Eligibility was not based on risk of lung cancer, because given the large size of the study (> 100,000 participants), it was expected that there would be appreciable numbers of current and former smokers among the participants.

The lack of demonstrated benefit for the older screening approaches should not be misinterpreted as nihilism about the early detection of patients with lung cancer. Individuals at risk (current and former smokers) who present with symptoms consistent with lung cancer deserve appropriate evaluation. The lack of resolution of radiographic abnormalities on a chest x-ray obtained after the completion of empiric antibiotic therapy for pneumonia should prompt further evaluation for possible lung cancer.

Chemoprevention

The concept of field carcinogenesis was originally developed for the aerodigestive tract in the early 1950s. Reducing the exposure of the epithelial mucosa to carcinogens, predominately cigarette smoke, has the greatest impact on reducing the incidence of cancer in high-risk individuals.

The Finnish Alpha-Tocopherol Beta Carotene Study evaluated 29,133 male smokers over 5 to 8 years and there was an 18% increased incidence of lung cancer in the group taking beta-carotene. Other chemopreventative agents studied include aspirin, retinyl palmitate, etretinate, isotretinoin, 4-hydroxyphenyl retinamide, anethole dithiolethione, and N-acetylcysteine. There has been no clear benefit of beta carotene identified in any of the studies.

Second primary lung tumors develop at a rate of 1%–3% annually for the first 5 years following resection of stage I NSCLC. The retinoid 13-*cis*-retinoic acid (isotretinoin [Accutane]) has reduced the incidence of second primary cancer in head and neck cancer patients in one small randomized trial.

The intergroup randomized trial that assessed the ability of 13-*cis*-retinoic acid to prevent the occurrence of a second primary cancer in patients with completely resected stage I NSCLC showed no impact of treatment on the incidence of second primary tumors. Furthermore, patients who continued to smoke and who received isotretinoin had a higher risk of recurrence of the index cancer. The early findings have demonstrated a higher-than-expected recurrence rate in patients with early-stage lung cancer who received 13-*cis*-retinoic acid and continued to smoke. Also, there was no reduction in second primary tumors in the 13-*cis*-retinoic acid-treated group. Trials using cyclooxygenase-2 (COX-2) inhibition are yet to be reported in former and current smokers. Tyrosine kinase inhibition is currently being studied to reverse bronchial premalignant lesions and Ki-67 levels in the Lung Cancer Biomarkers Chemoprevention Consortium trial.

Selenium as L-selenomethionine has been shown to inhibit cell growth, induce apoptosis in vitro, and retard carcinogenesis at higher dose levels in animal models. Epidemiologic data suggest an inverse relationship between selenium intake and lung cancer.

In a study by Clark et al designed to determine the effects of selenium on the incidence of basal or squamous cell carcinomas, nutritional supplementation with this agent showed no consequences on the incidence of skin cancer; however, secondary analyses revealed that it was associated with significantly fewer cases of lung cancer.

A phase III intergroup selenium prevention trial has been designed to follow the lung cancer isotretinoin prevention trial. To reduce the incidence of second primary tumors, this double-blind design is randomizing patients by a 2:1 ratio to receive either selenomethionine (200 μg/d) vs placebo daily for 48 months. Patients will be monitored for safety, development of second primary tumors, and recurrence.

Educational programs Although the information from the intergroup randomized chemoprevention study is being collected, it is important to continue educational efforts to prevent adolescents from starting to smoke cigarettes and to advocate smoking cessation in active smokers. Some experts believe that educational programs must begin during childhood, probably between the ages of 6 and 10 years. Targeting children and young adults is a significant priority of any lung cancer reduction program.

Signs and symptoms

The clinical manifestations of lung cancer depend on the location and extent of the tumor. In patients who have localized disease, the most common symptoms are related to obstruction of major airways, infiltration of lung parenchyma, and invasion of surrounding structures, including the chest wall, major blood vessels, and viscera.

Cough is a major manifestation of lung cancer and is present in nearly 80% of patients with symptomatic lung cancer. It is important to remember, however, that most lung cancer patients are current or former smokers and may have a cough related to chronic irritation of the upper and/or lower airways from cigarette smoke. Therefore, smokers should be asked whether there has been a change in their cough, such as an increase in frequency or severity.

Dyspnea and hemoptysis Increasing dyspnea and hemoptysis may be signs of lung cancer, although in the case of hemoptysis, 70% of patients bleed from nonmalignant causes, mostly infection and more frequently bronchitis. In patients who present with hemoptysis, are older than age 40, and have a history of smoking and chronic obstructive pulmonary disease without abnormality on chest radiograph, lung cancer should be considered in the differential diagnosis.

Pneumonia Postobstructive pneumonia secondary to partial or complete bronchial obstruction occurs relatively frequently in association with lung cancer. It is important to obtain repeat chest x-rays in adults who have been treated for pneumonia to be certain that the radiographic abnormalities have cleared completely.

Pleural effusion Lung cancer may spread to the pleural surface or may obstruct segmental or lobar lymphatics, resulting in pleural effusion and increased dyspnea.

Chest pain Approximately 5% of lung tumors invade the chest wall. The resultant pain is a better predictor of chest wall invasion than are chest CT findings. An individual who complains of persistent chest pain should have a chest x-ray to exclude the presence of peripheral lung cancer that has invaded the chest wall.

Shoulder and arm pain Apical tumors that infiltrate surrounding structures (also called Pancoast tumors) produce shoulder and/or arm pain as a result of brachial plexus compression. Tumors in the apical lung segments may be difficult to detect on a routine chest x-ray; therefore, a person who complains of persistent shoulder pain, particularly with signs of neurologic involvement, should have a CT scan of the chest to look for an apical tumor. An MRI scan of the chest apex may be beneficial. It is also important to examine the lung apex in bone films obtained to evaluate shoulder pain.

Horner's syndrome Invasion of the sympathetic ganglion by an apical lung tumor causes Horner's syndrome (ptosis, myosis, and ipsilateral anhidrosis).

Hoarseness secondary to vocal cord paresis or paralysis occurs when tumors and lymph node metastases compress, cause dysfunction in, or invade the recurrent laryngeal nerve. This situation is more common on the left side, where the recurrent laryngeal nerve passes under the aortic arch, but it may also occur with high lesions on the right side of the mediastinum.

Other symptoms of tumor compression Lung tumors may also cause dysphagia by compression or invasion of the esophagus or superior vena cava syndrome by compression or invasion of this vascular structure.

Some tumors may result in wheezing or stridor secondary to compression or invasion of the trachea and may also cause signs of cardiac tamponade secondary to involvement of the pericardial surface and subsequent accumulation of pericardial fluid.

Signs and symptoms of metastatic disease Lung cancer can metastasize to multiple sites, most commonly to bone, liver, brain, lungs (contralateral or ipsilateral), and adrenal glands.

A lung cancer patient who has brain metastases may complain of headaches or specific neurologic symptoms, or family members may notice a decrease in the patient's mental acuity. Also, metastatic lung cancer may cause spinal cord compression, resulting in a characteristic sequence of symptoms: pain, followed by motor dysfunction, and then sensory symptoms. The patient may have any or all of these symptoms.

Patients who complain of band-like pain encircling one or both sides of the trunk may have spinal cord compression. In addition, coughing and sneezing may cause significant exacerbation of pain from spinal cord compression.

Bone x-rays and/or a bone scan are warranted in lung cancer patients who complain of persistent pain in the trunk or extremities. If performed in the evaluation of lung cancer, ^{18}fluorodeoxyglucose (FDG)-PET supplants the need for a bone scan in most patients. PET appears to be more sensitive but less specific for bone metastases. If plain films are normal or equivocal for metastases, CT and/or MRI may be helpful to evaluate suspicious areas. MRI of the spine is the most effective way to evaluate suspected spinal cord compression.

Systemic paraneoplastic symptoms Lung cancer is commonly associated with systemic manifestations, including weight loss (with or without anorexia). In addition, patients frequently complain of fatigue and generalized weakness. SCLC is associated with hormone production, which causes endocrine syndromes in a subset of patients, such as SIADH (syndrome of inappropriate antidiuretic hormone secretion) and via secretion of ACTH (adrenocorticotropic hormone) hypercortisolism.

Specific neurologic syndromes, such as Lambert-Eaton syndrome (see chapter 45), cortical cerebellar degeneration, and peripheral neuropathy, may occur in lung cancer patients but are relatively rare.

Clubbing Although clubbing may occur in a variety of conditions, it is important for the clinician to evaluate a patient's hands. If clubbing is noted, obtaining a chest x-ray may result in the early diagnosis of lung cancer.

Hypertrophic osteoarthropathy A relatively small percentage of patients with lung cancer may present with symptomatic hypertrophic osteoarthropathy. In this syndrome, periosteal inflammation results in pain in affected areas, most commonly the ankles and knees.

Carcinoid syndrome is extremely uncommon in patients who have a bronchial carcinoid tumor. Most of these patients are asymptomatic (tumors are found by x-ray), and a few have cough from an endobronchial lesion.

TUMOR BIOLOGY

Non–small-cell tumors account for approximately 85% of all lung cancers. The three major tumor types included under this category are adenocarcinoma, squamous cell carcinoma, and large-cell carcinoma.

Staging and prognosis

Staging

The staging of lung cancer must be conducted in a methodical and detailed manner. The TNM staging system, updated by Mountain (Table 1), applies equally well to all histologies of NSCLC, but TNM for SCLC is less helpful. Most patients have advanced disease at the time of presentation.

Stage is commonly reported as either clinical or pathologic, designated as c or p, respectively. Clinical stage is based on noninvasive (or minimally invasive) tests, whereas pathologic stage is based on tissue obtained during surgery (see section on "Diagnosis and staging evaluation").

Prognostic factors

Stage The most important prognostic factor in lung cancer is the stage of disease.

Performance status and weight loss Within a given disease stage, the next most important prognostic factors are performance status and recent unexplained weight loss. The two scales used to define performance status are the Eastern Cooperative Oncology Group (ECOG) performance status system and the Karnofsky system (see Appendix 1). Simply, patients who are ambulatory have a significantly longer survival than those who are nonambulatory. Similarly, patients who have lost > 5% of body weight during the preceding 3–6 months have a worse prognosis than patients who have not lost a significant amount of weight.

Molecular prognostic factors Several studies published over the past decade have indicated that mutations of *ras* proto-oncogenes, particularly K-*ras*, por-

TABLE 1: TNM staging of lung cancer

Primary tumor (T)

Tx	Tumor proven by the presence of malignant cells in bronchopulmonary secretions but not visualized roentgenographically or bronchoscopically or any tumor that cannot be assessed, as in pretreatment staging
T0	No evidence of primary tumor
Tis	Carcinoma in situ
T1	Tumor ≤ 3.0 cm in greatest dimension, surrounded by lung or visceral pleura, and without evidence of invasion proximal to a lobar bronchus at bronchoscopy
T2	Tumor > 3.0 cm in greatest dimension; or tumor of any size that either invades the visceral pleura or has associated atelectasis or obstructive pneumonitis extending to the hilar region (but involving less than the entire lung). At bronchoscopy, the proximal extent of demonstrable tumor must be within a lobar bronchus or at least 2.0 cm distal to the carina
T3	Tumor of any size with direct extension into the chest wall (including superior sulcus tumors), diaphragm, or mediastinal pleura or pericardium without involving the heart, great vessels, trachea, esophagus, or vertebral body; or tumor in the main bronchus within 2 cm of, but not involving, the carina
T4	Tumor of any size with invasion of the mediastinum or involving the heart, great vessels, trachea, esophagus, vertebral body, or carina; or presence of exudative pleural effusion (whether cytology positive or negative)

Regional lymph nodes (N)

Nx	Regional lymph nodes cannot be assessed
N0	No demonstrable metastasis to regional lymph nodes
N1	Metastasis to lymph nodes in the peribronchial and/or ipsilateral hilar region, including direct extension
N2	Metastasis to ipsilateral mediastinal and subcarinal lymph nodes
N3	Metastasis to contralateral mediastinal, contralateral hilar, ipsilateral or contralateral scalene, or supraclavicular lymph nodes

Distant metastasis (M)

Mx	Distant metastasis cannot be assessed
M0	No distant metastasis
M1	Distant metastasis

Stage grouping

Occult carcinoma	Tx	N0	M0
Stage 0	Tis	N0	M0
Stage IA	T1	N0	M0
Stage IB	T2	N0	M0
Stage IIA	T1	N1	M0
Stage IIB	T2	N1	M0
	T3	N0	M0
Stage IIIA	T3	N1	M0
	T1-3	N2	M0
Stage IIIB	Any T	N3	M0
	T4	Any N	M0
Stage IV	Any T	Any N	M1

From Mountain CF: Revisions in the International System for Staging Lung Cancer. Chest 111:1710–1717, 1997.

tend a poor prognosis in NSCLC and in the case of adenocarcinomas are more frequently found in smokers. Accordingly, selective research has focused on developing molecularly targeted therapeutic approaches to the *ras* proto-oncogenes, in particular, the farnesyl transferase inhibitors as well as epidermal growth factor receptor (EGFR) inhibitors and antiangiogenic approaches (see section on "Novel and promising agents").

Of equal relevance was the completion of large studies by Pastorino et al and Kwiatowski et al evaluating the prognostic importance of immunocytochemical and molecular pathologic markers in stage I NSCLC. The findings of these two studies suggest that pathologic invasion and extent of surgical resection may yield the most critical prognostic information, but mutation of the K-*ras* oncogene and absence of expression of the H-*ras* p21 proto-oncogene may augment the pathologic information. Further data indicate that a molecular prognostic model differentiating patients with lung cancer may be possible using proteomics or other molecular biology techniques.

Molecular profiling has been described as a means to molecularly characterize tumors and to identify the metastatic potential and regional growth character. Other molecular markers that portend a poor prognosis include reduced expression of RASSF1A and FHIT (fragile histidine triad); reduced expression of catenins and E-cadherin; reduction in tumor suppressor genes p53, retinoblastoma gene, p16INK4A and p15INK4B; increased telomerase activity; overexpression of EGFR (c-erbB-1), matrix metalloproteinase, HER2/*neu* (c-erb-2), and vascular endothelial growth factor (VEGF); c-Met overexpression; overexpression of mutated p53; urokinase plasminogen activator overexpression; promoters of angiogenesis; reduced expression of nm23 gene; and low KAI1/CD82.

Diagnosis and staging evaluation

History and physical examination

The diagnosis and preoperative staging of lung cancer begin with a good history and physical examination. When obtaining the history, the clinician should keep in mind the tendency for lung cancer to involve major airways and other central structures. Similarly, the patterns of metastatic dissemination and systemic manifestations must be considered when conducting the physical examination.

Patients should be questioned specifically about the presence of palpable masses, dysphagia, bone pain, headache, or changes in vision. Careful auscultation and percussion may suggest the presence of atelectasis or pleural effusion. Auscultation of the chest also may provide evidence of large airway obstruction and pulmonary consolidation. Ronchi and wheezing may provide some helpful treatment planning information. An enlarged liver may indicate hepatic metastases.

Palpation of the neck and supraclavicular fossa Discovery of adenopathy of the neck and supraclavicular fossa may allow both diagnosis and staging, by needle or open biopsy.

Imaging studies

Chest x-rays provide initial helpful information in patients with new respiratory symptoms. Posteroanterior (PA) and lateral chest x-rays are fundamental in assessing the local extent of the primary tumor and also may provide valuable information regarding metastatic disease.

The chest x-ray should be inspected for the presence of a pleural effusion or synchronous pulmonary nodules, and the bones should be examined for evidence of osseous metastases. A widened mediastinum usually indicates metastatic disease within the mediastinal lymph nodes. Comparison with previous x-rays is helpful and well worth the effort expended in their retrieval.

Chest CT from the lower neck to the mid level of the kidneys, including the entire liver and adrenal glands with 5–10 mm slices, is performed routinely to further define the primary tumor and to identify lymphatic or parenchymal metastases. In a review of 20 studies that assessed the value of CT scan to determine mediastinal lymph node involvement, with an average prevalence of 28%, CT had a pooled sensitivity of 57%, a specificity of 82%, and a negative predictive value (NPV) of 83%. Benign enlargement of mediastinal nodes is more common in patients with postobstructive infection. Histologic confirmation of the presence or absence of tumor within the mediastinal lymph nodes is necessary whenever this information will change treatment recommendations. In patients who are considered surgical candidates, metastatic tumor is found in approximately 15%–20% of mediastinal lymph nodes < 1 cm in greatest diameter.

It is important to remember that patients with persistent symptoms, such as cough and dyspnea, who have a normal chest x-ray may be harboring a central lesion that is not obvious on chest x-ray but can be easily detected by chest CT. Also, as previously mentioned, apical tumors (Pancoast tumors) may be difficult to detect on a chest radiograph but are usually readily apparent on a CT scan.

PET For lung masses, FDG accumulation on PET implies a significant likelihood of malignancy.

Standardized uptake value (SUV) of 2.5 optimizes the sensitivity and specificity of PET in assessing suspicious lung lesions larger than 1 cm. An FDG-avid lesion on PET should never be assumed to be malignant, and a PET-negative lesion is not absolutely benign. Bronchioalveolar and carcinoid are two cell types that do not readily accumulate FDG. Furthermore, higher SUV lesions do not imply a greater likelihood of cancer; the highest SUVs have been found in inflammatory lesions, such as granulomas and infections.

A review of 18 studies of the utility of PET to assess the mediastinal lymph nodes demonstrated a pooled sensitivity of 84% and a specificity of 89%, with a positive predictive value (PPV) of 79% and an NPV of 93%. Combining the results of CT and PET, the PPV and NPV were 83%–93% and 88%–95%, respectively. Thus, FDG-PET is superior to CT scanning in staging the mediastinal lymph nodes. An estimated 15% to 20% of patients with a known or suspected diagnosis benefit from a preoperative FDG-PET, because previously unrecognized metastatic disease will be discovered.

TABLE 2: Selective indications for mediastinoscopy

Enlarged N1, N2, or N3 lymph nodes on chest CT scan
FDG-PET–positive mediastinal disease
Centrally located tumors
T2-T4 tumors

Several trials have evaluated the prognostic significance of FDG uptake on PET scan in NSCLC. Utilizing multivariate Cox analysis, these studies noted that SUV, particularly when > 7–10, was an independent prognostic factor.

PET scanning may also prove a valuable tool for staging and evaluating patients undergoing radiation therapy and patients with NSCLC treated with chemoradiotherapy or irradiation. In a study by MacManus et al, the PET response was found to be a powerful predictor of survival.

Adrenal gland The adrenal gland may be the sole site of metastatic disease in as many as 10% of patients with NSCLC, though patients with adrenal masses should not be assumed to have metastatic disease and denied a potentially curative surgery on the basis of a scan alone. Less than 1% of adrenal masses at least 1 cm in size that are negative on FDG-PET are malignant. Contrast-enhanced MRI-weighted images may assist in achieving a diagnosis. Suspicious adrenal masses should be either biopsied or resected in potentially operable patients to confirm the stage of disease.

Obtaining a tissue diagnosis

The next step is to obtain a histologic or cytologic diagnosis of the radiologically revealed lesion, although preoperative histologic diagnosis need not be obtained in a highly suspicious lung mass without evidence of distant or locoregional metastases (see below).

Central lesions Collecting sputum cytologies for 3 consecutive days provides a cytologic diagnosis for central lesions 71% of the time and for peripheral lesions 49% of the time. In clinically suspicious lung nodules/masses, a negative sputum cytology result warrants further clinical investigation. Flexible bronchoscopy is commonly required to achieve a diagnosis. For central lesions that are exophytic, at least three direct forceps biopsies should be performed to achieve a 74% sensitivity. Washings and brushings add to the sensitivity but by themselves have a sensitivity of 48% and 59%, respectively. Further improved sensitivity is obtained with bronchoscopic fluoroscopically directed transbronchial needle aspiration biopsies. For central lesions, the overall sensitivity for flexible bronchoscopy is 88% in experienced hands.

In addition, bronchoscopy may provide important staging information, such as whether the tumor involves the distal trachea or carina, and may help plan the appropriate operation (lobectomy or sleeve resection vs pneumonectomy). Determining the degree of bronchial involvement assists surgical planning. Bronchoscopy-directed biopsies should be performed to assist in determining the intended line of resection, especially when evaluating for submucosal involvement.

Peripheral lesions Bronchoscopy is less likely to yield a diagnosis in patients with peripherally located lesions. Bronchoscopic ability to make a diagnosis of malignancy in peripheral lesions is dependent upon size; for those less than 2 cm, the sensitivity is 33%, and for lesions greater than 2 cm, it is 62%. If a bronchiole is seen traversing or extending to the mass on CT, the sensitivity is reported to be twice as high, nearly 60%.

A CT-guided needle biopsy may diagnose up to 90% of peripheral lung cancers but is dependent on the quality of the CT scan and the experience of the radiologist performing the procedure. The false-negative rate is 20%–30%. Needle biopsy is usually reserved for patients who are not candidates for an operation due to distant metastatic disease or poor health or performance status. If the patient is a candidate for surgery, resection is generally recommended for any suspicious mass whether the result of needle biopsy is positive or nondiagnostic. Therefore, for patients with a suspicious peripheral lesion that is not associated with pleural effusion, mediastinal adenopathy, or other evidence of metastatic disease, it is reasonable to proceed directly to surgery.

Mediastinoscopy Mediastinoscopy is a time-tested technique whereby the middle (cervical mediastinoscopy) and the anterior mediastinum may be assessed for direct or metastatic lymph node involvement. In the hands of a specialist, the risk of biopsy trauma to local structures (great vessels, trachea, or esophagus), bleeding, recurrent nerve paresis, infection, or death is minimal. Whole-node biopsies may be taken, achieving a great deal of information about the location, degree of nodal involvement, and lymph node capsular invasion. There is no evidence that mediastinoscopic biopsy spreads tumor within the mediastinum, worsens the prognosis, or renders eventual surgical mediastinal dissection difficult.

Selective indications for mediastinoscopy are listed in Table 2. To assess response to therapy, repeat mediastinoscopy has been performed with few complications. Patients with N2 disease may potentially benefit from neoadjuvant treatment. Patients with N3 disease are considered to be stage IIIB and less likely to benefit from surgical resection. There have been a few retrospective reports that have demonstrated survival from induction therapy in patients with microscopic N3 involvement.

Thoracentesis and thoracoscopy Individuals who have pleural effusions should undergo thoracentesis. Video-assisted thoracoscopic surgery (VATS) should be used to assess patients who have cytology-negative effusions. Sixty percent of patients with known pleural disease and effusions will have cytology-negative effusions. However, lung cancer patients with exudative cytology-negative effusions and their cytology-positive counterparts appear to have equally poor survival. VATS permits direct visualization of the pleural surface, enables one to directly biopsy pleural nodules, and also may facilitate biopsy of ipsilateral mediastinal lymph nodes. The role of VATS to assess effusions remains to be elucidated.

Measurement of serum tumor-associated antigens has no current role in the staging of NSCLC.

Diagnosis and evaluation of suspected carcinoid tumor

A carcinoid tumor of the lungs may be suspected in a patient with a slowly enlarging pulmonary mass and a prolonged history of respiratory symptoms. Patients usually have no symptoms. Most tumors are located centrally and exist endobronchially. When they occur, symptoms may include wheezing, recurrent pneumonia, dyspnea, and potentially paraneoplastic syndromes. Bronchoscopy frequently assists in diagnosing the lesion. The finding of a polypoid, pale, firm mass should not lull the bronchoscopist into taking a large-forceps biopsy. First, these masses are frequently vascular, and massive bleeding has been reported; second, the entire mass can be accidentally removed, making it difficult to identify the site of the original location of the polyp.

Given the bleeding potential, rigid bronchoscopy may be a better way to assess these lesions. Especially with cytology, carcinoid tumors may be difficult to differentiate from small-cell and atypical carcinoid tumors. Carcinoid tumor should be suspected when a small-cell tumor diagnosis by fine-needle aspiration does not respond to therapy. True carcinoids will have metastatic nodal disease in 5%–10% of patients and have an excellent prognosis with surgical resection. Atypical carcinoid tumors are differentiated from typical tumors in that they have more than two mitotic figures per high-powered field, and areas of necrosis.

Unlike its infradiaphragmatic counterpart, pulmonary carcinoid tumors rarely present with paraneoplastic syndromes, including carcinoid, acromegaly, and Cushing syndromes. Therefore, it is only necessary to measure urinary 5-hydroxyindoleacetic acid (5-HIAA) excretion prior to surgery in symptomatic patients. Less than 3% of all patients with pulmonary carcinoid tumors can be found to have any detectable urinary 5-HIAA.

Intraoperative staging

Intraoperative staging is an integral part of any operation for lung cancer. In addition to the thorough visual and tactile inspection of the lungs, diaphragm, and pleura, the ipsilateral mediastinal lymph nodes must be either completely removed or at least sampled.

The American Thoracic Society has assigned numbered levels to locations in which lymph nodes are regularly found, defined by their relation to constant anatomic structures. A complete mediastinal lymph node dissection is associated with little morbidity and lengthens the operation only slightly.

Pulmonary evaluation

To determine the volume of lung that can be removed without rendering the patient a pulmonary cripple and to identify those individuals at risk for postoperative complications, each patient may undergo pulmonary function testing, spirometry, and potentially a diffusing capacity. The results of pulmonary testing should be referenced to the normal values for ethnicity, height, age, and sex rather than the absolute value.

Forced expiratory volume in 1 second Postoperative respiratory failure rarely occurs if the postresection forced expiratory volume in 1 second (FEV_1) is > 30% of predicted. Regardless of the extent of the scheduled resection, if the preoperative FEV_1 is < 60% of predicted, a split-function perfusion scan should be obtained to determine the contribution of each lung region to overall pulmonary function. This information may be critical when an unplanned pneumonectomy is required to achieve complete tumor resection.

Other pulmonary function tests A diffusing capacity of the lung for carbon monoxide (D_LCOa; a = adjusted for the patient's hemoglobin) < 60% of the predicted value or a maximum voluntary ventilation (MVV) < 35% is associated with increased postoperative morbidity. Patients with a baseline oximetry saturation of less than 90% and those who desaturate with exercise more than 4% have a greater likelihood of postoperative complications. Arterial blood gas pCO_2 > 45 mm Hg is an independent risk factor for increased operative morbidity and mortality.

In patients with borderline lung function, further physiologic testing may be required to better estimate pulmonary reserve prior to and after surgery. Quantitative pulmonary effusion scanning may assist in this endeavor. The perfusion portion is used to calculate the percentage of lung to be removed and the estimated postoperative percentage of normal. An additional test is exercise pulmonary function testing. Patients are monitored for heart rate, rhythm, blood pressure, and oxygen consumption. Patients who reach their target heart rate and exercise capacity and who have a maximal oxygen consumption > 15 mL/kg/min are less likely to have a postoperative complication.

Pathology

The World Health Organization and the International Association for the Study of Lung Cancer have devised guidelines for the histologic classification of lung cancer, which are revised as necessary (Table 3). The different cell-type classifications are performed using light microscopy and do not require electron microscopy or immunohistochemistry. There are variations in the natural history of the different cell types and potential differences in response to treatment and survival. Overall, 90%–95% of NSCLC is adenocarcinoma, squamous, or large cell, with 3%–4% being mixed tumors, such as adenosquamous carcinoma. Three major types of tumors are included under the NSCLC category: adenocarcinoma, squamous cell carcinoma, and large-cell carcinoma.

Adenocarcinoma is the most common type of NSCLC, accounting for approximately 30%–40% of cases. Of all the types of lung cancer, adenocarcinoma is most likely to occur in nonsmokers or former smokers. It is also the most common tumor in women.

Typically, adenocarcinoma presents as a small peripheral lesion that has a high propensity to metastasize to both regional lymph nodes and distant sites. Because of the tendency of the primary tumor to occur in peripheral locations, it frequently produces no symptoms. In contrast with their metastatic lesions, the primary adenocarcinoma tumor is histologically heterogeneous in 80% of patients, consisting of numerous histologic subtypes, and is classified as "mixed-" or "indeterminate-adenocarcinoma."

Bronchioloalveolar adenocarcinoma (BAC) During the past decade, it has become apparent that the incidence of BAC is increasing. This tumor originates from type II pneumocytes, and it may present as a pneumonic infiltrate, as multiple nodules scattered throughout the lungs, and, occasionally, as a single nodule.

Squamous cell tumors comprise approximately 30% of all cases of lung cancer. These tumors tend to occur in a central location and tend to spread to regional lymph nodes; they are the most likely of all lung cancers to remain localized and to cavitate. In fact, autopsy studies have shown that about 15%–30% of patients with squamous cell carcinoma may die of local disease without evidence of distant metastases.

Large-cell carcinoma accounts for approximately 10%–15% of all lung cancers. It tends to present as a relatively large peripheral lesion and, like adenocarcinoma, has a high propensity to metastasize to regional lymph nodes and distant sites.

Treatment

In operable candidates, clinically staged IA, IB, IIA, and IIB NSCLC should undergo anatomic complete surgical resection. Primarily, patients with stage IIIB and IV disease are treated nonoperatively. Although multimodality therapy is routinely recommended for stage IIIA disease, it is recommended that it be performed within a clinical trial.

SURGICAL APPROACH

The appropriate treatment of NSCLC is resection of the lobe containing the tumor. Occasionally, a bilobectomy or pneumonectomy is required. Mortality approximates 3% following lobectomy and 7% following pneumonectomy. A wedge or segmental resection has a three to five times higher incidence of local recurrence and a lower 5-year survival than a lobectomy. Therefore, if the patient can tolerate the procedure, the standard operation should be a lobectomy, rather than a wedge resection or segmentectomy. Segmentectomy, though, was not studied separately from wedge resection, and more recent evaluation demonstrates that in selected tumors, when the bronchus and vascular supply are individually ligated with a regional node resection, survival appears to be comparable and salvages lung parenchyma.

VATS Traditionally, lung cancers have been resected through a posterolateral thoracotomy incision. Muscle-sparing incisions may reduce pain. The current trend is toward an even less invasive approach: lobectomy and lymph node

TABLE 3: WHO and IASLC guidelines for the histologic classification of lung cancer

I	**Adenocarcinoma**
	i. Adenocarcinoma with mixed subtypes
	1. Well-differentiated fetal adenocarcinoma
	2. Mucinous adenocarcinoma
	3. Mucinous cystadenocarcinoma
	4. Clear cell adenocarcinoma
	5. Signet ring adenocarcinoma
	ii. Acinar
	iii. Papillary
	iv. Bronchioloalveolar carcinoma
	1. Mucinous
	2. Nonmucinous
	3. Mixed mucinous and nonmucinous
	v. Solid adenocarcinoma with mucin
II	**Squamous**
	i. Papillary
	ii. Small-cell
	iii. Clear cell
	iv. Basaloid
III	**Large-cell**
	i. Large cell neuroendocrine carcinoma
	ii. Basaloid carcinoma
	iii. Lymphoepithelioma-like carcinoma
	iv. Mixed large-cell neuroendocrine carcinoma
	v. Clear cell carcinoma with rhabdoid phenotype
IV	**Adenosquamous carcinoma**
V	**Carcinomas with pleomorphic, sarcomatous characteristics**
	i. Carcinosarcoma
	ii. Pulmonary blastoma
	iii. Carcinomas with spindle and/or giant cells
	1. Giant cell carcinoma
	2. Spindle cell carcinoma
	3. Pleomorphic carcinoma
	iv. Other
VI	**Carcinoid**
	i. Typical carcinoid
	ii. Atypical carcinoid
VII	**Carcinomas of salivary gland origin**
	i. Adenoid cystic carcinoma
	ii. Mucoepidermoid carcinoma
	iii. Others
VIII	**Unclassified**

Adapted from the World Health Organization (WHO): Histologic typing of lung tumors. In: International Classification of Tumors. Geneva, Switzerland: WHO, 1991; Travis WD, Colby TV, Corrin B, et al: World Health Organization: Histological Typing of Lung and Pleural Tumours, 3rd ed. Berlin: Springer-Verlag, 1999.
IASLC = International Association for the Study of Lung Cancer

dissection with VATS. This approach appears to offer the same cancer operation and survival with perhaps lower morbidity.

Two VATS methods have been described: the mass hilar ligation technique and individual ligation of the vasculature and airway. Patients with peripheral tumors up to 4–6 cm without clinical hilar or mediastinal adenopathy appear to be good candidates for a VATS procedure. Conversion rates to open thoracotomy are 10%, and hospital stays are usually 3–5 days.

The results of several VATS series show lower complication rates than reported series for thoracotomy, granted a selection bias may have occurred. One small randomized trial showed a significant benefit favoring VATS. Patients have better shoulder function, better performance on the 6-minute walk, and less impairment of vital capacity after VATS than after thoracotomy. A VATS approach may be better tolerated than other approaches for older patients.

Patients with pathologic stage IA disease have a 70%–80% 5-year survival rate after resection, whereas 5-year survival rates are 60% in those with stage IB disease and 40%–50% in those with stage IIA/IIB disease. Patients found to have N2 (stage IIIA) disease located at a single nodal level have a 25%–30% 5-year survival rate.

Mediastinal lymph node involvement The standard lung cancer operation should include sampling or dissection of mediastinal lymph nodes. The presence of metastases in any of the mediastinal lymph nodes (N2 and/or N3 disease) is indicative of advanced disease and is thought by some to represent a contraindication to surgery. Resection of mediastinal disease may have prognostic significance, implications for postoperative care, and potential therapeutic value. Some series of patients with N2 disease have shown a 5-year survival rate of 20%–30%, but patients in these series are highly selected.

Patients with N2 disease may potentially benefit from neoadjuvant treatment. Patients with N3 disease are considered to be stage IIIB and less likely to benefit from surgical resection. There have been a few retrospective reports that have demonstrated survival from induction therapy in patients with microscopic N3 involvement. The American College of Surgeons has completed accrual to a randomized, prospective study comparing survival following mediastinal lymph node sampling vs dissection. Complications and operative mortality appear equivalent between the sampling and dissection groups. Long-term survival is under investigation. Also, clinical trials are currently testing preoperative chemotherapy and chemoradiation therapy in patients with mediastinal node involvement.

Preoperative histologic assessment of the mediastinal lymph nodes is essential if multilevel metastases are suspected, as there have been few long-term survivors among patients with metastatic disease at more than one level. Nonsurgical treatment appears preferable, or patients should be offered participation in a trial designed to assess the benefits of neoadjuvant therapy. Although patients with stage IIIB tumors are usually treated with irradiation and chemotherapy (see later discussions), the occasional patient with isolated involvement of the vena cava or atrium can undergo resection.

Carcinoid tumors Although the majority of carcinoid tumors remain localized, regional lymph node metastases are identified in 5%–15% of patients. The surgical approach, therefore, should be similar to that used in NSCLC. If a small tumor in a proximal airway is identified and there is no histologic evidence of lymph node disease, a bronchoplastic procedure with preservation of lung tissue can sometimes be performed. Rates of survival at 10 years are > 90% for patients with stage I disease and 60% for patients with stage II disease.

ADJUVANT THERAPY

Chemotherapy

Classic postoperative adjuvant chemotherapy has been tested in three randomized trials conducted by the Lung Cancer Study Group (LCSG). For almost 20 years, the relative value of adjuvant chemotherapy for resectable NSCLC has been disputed and debated. In a randomized, prospective study involving 488 patients, Keller et al showed no benefit to adjuvant chemotherapy. The ALPI (Adjuvant Lung Project Italy) study of 1,209 patients also showed no survival benefit. In contrast, the International Adjuvant Lung Cancer Trial (IALT) randomized 1,867 patients to receive cisplatin-based, adjuvant chemotherapy or no treatment. At 5 years, the treatment arm showed a survival advantage of 4.1% ($P = .003$), compared with the observation arm.

Two recently presented trials, the Canadian BR-10 and Cancer and Leukemia Group B (CALGB) 9633, both demonstrated clinically significant improvement in survival, with minimal chemotherapy side effects; cisplatin and vinorelbine were used in the BR-10 trial and carboplatin (Paraplatin) and paclitaxel were used in CALGB 9633. These results, in combination with the recent positive findings of the adjuvant trial of UFT (a drug composed of tegafur and uracil mixed at the ratio of 1:4) in patients with stage IB NSCLC, increase the likelihood of adjuvant platinum-based therapy becoming the standard of treatment for patients with stages IB–IIIB NSCLC.

Further data from two subsequent positive adjuvant chemotherapy trials support this new standard. Based on these data, the standard of practice has shifted to chemotherapy for operable NSCLC, either adjuvant or in the induction setting. The potential benefits are higher efficacy of chemotherapy early in the natural history of disease, facilitation of subsequent local therapy, and early eradication of distant micrometastases. Despite these positive data, not all patients benefit from adjuvant chemotherapy.

Stage I disease In one trial, adjuvant therapy with 6 courses of CAP (cyclophosphamide, Adriamycin [doxorubicin], and Platinol [cisplatin]) failed to produce a significant survival advantage in patients with stage I lung cancer. The IALT demonstrated that modern adjuvant chemotherapy could be provided with a survival advantage. In patients with stage IB disease, CALGB 9335 compared postoperative carboplatin and paclitaxel with surgery alone and found a clinically significant survival advantage, with minimal morbidity. The Canadian BR-10 trial demonstrated similar results using cisplatin and vinorelbine; patients with stage II disease were included as well.

The current trend is to provide involvement in a chemopreventive clinical trial for stage IA patients. For patients with stage IB disease, platinum-based adju-

The Adjuvant Navelbine International Trialist Association (ANITA) trial randomized 840 patients with early-stage (IB, II, or IIIA) NSCLC to either observation (433) or 4 cycles of chemotherapy (407) with cisplatin (100 mg/m^2) or vinorelbine (30 mg/m^2) per week. With a median follow-up of 70 months, the toxic death rate on the chemotherapy arm was 1.7% and the rate of febrile neutropenia was 12%. Five-year survival significantly favored the chemotherapy arm (51% vs 43%; *P* = .013), as did progression-free (36.3 vs 20.7 months; *P* = .002) and median overall survival (65.8 vs 43.8 months; *P* = .013). This improvement was seen primarily in patients with higher stage disease (*Douillard J-Y, Rosell R, Delena M, et al: J Clin Oncol [abstract] 23[suppl]:624s, 2005*).

vant chemotherapy (cisplatin or carboplatin combined with a taxane or vinorelbine) should be strongly considered.

Stage II/III disease In two earlier trials, postoperative adjuvant chemotherapy with 6 courses of CAP, given alone in one study and following postoperative radiation therapy in the other, resulted in a modest improvement in median survival but had no impact on long-term survival. In contrast, the IALT, ANITA (Adjuvant Navelbine International Trialist Association), CALGB 9623, and Canadian BR-10 trials demonstrated a clinically significant survival advantage, justifying consideration for adjuvant chemotherapy. There does not appear to be any survival advantage to adding adjuvant mediastinal radiotherapy to chemotherapy, unless there are particularly high risk factors for local recurrence.

Radiation therapy

A trial conducted by the LCSG showed that in patients with squamous cell carcinoma of the lungs and resected N1/N2 disease, administration of postoperative radiation reduced the risk of recurrence in the chest from 20% to 1%. Although there was no improvement in overall survival, postoperative irradiation was associated with a significant improvement in disease-free survival for patients with N2 disease. A trial by the British Medical Research Council reached similar conclusions.

A meta-analysis of nine randomized trials assessing postoperative radiation therapy in lung cancer reported a 21% increase in mortality in patients receiving this therapy. However, many of the patients in these trials had N0 disease, for whom few would advocate radiation therapy. Also, most of the patients were treated with cobalt-60 beams and technically limited treatment planning, not with modern radiation therapy techniques.

These results created a lack of consensus about treatment recommendations, with some experts advocating the use of postoperative radiation therapy to reduce local recurrence, and others avoiding it because of the absence of an effect on survival.

At present, therefore, the appropriate role of postoperative radiation therapy remains controversial. Such therapy should be seriously considered, however, in patients at high risk for locoregional relapse (ie, those with hilar or mediastinal disease, squamous histology, multiple positive lymph nodes or lymph node stations, extracapsular extension, bulky nodal disease, or close or microscopically positive margins). In patients who are receiving adjuvant chemotherapy, it is reasonable to administer the chemotherapy first (as it has been associated with a survival benefit) followed by radiation therapy (for enhanced local control).

Moreover, in a randomized trial by Keller et al, no benefit was shown for concurrent chemoradiation over radiation therapy when in the adjuvant setting for completely resected patients with stage II/IIIA NSCLC. An exception may be in patients with microscopic residual disease (ie, positive margins or extracapsular extension), for whom a delay in radiation therapy may be detrimental.

> The results of the intergroup trial 0139 (RTOG 93-09) have been reported. In this trial, 396 eligible patients with pathologic N2 (stage IIIA) disease were randomized to receive either induction chemoradiation therapy (cisplatin and etoposide and 45 Gy) followed by surgical resection vs definitive chemoradiation therapy without surgery (cisplatin and etoposide and 61 Gy). The pathologic nodal complete response rate on the surgical arm was 46%. More treatment-related deaths occurred on the surgical arm (8% vs 2% on the chemoradiation arm). The 5-year disease progression-free survival was superior on the surgical arm (22% vs 5%, $P = .02$). There were more early noncancer deaths on the surgical arm, but overall survival curves crossed so that at year 5, overall survival was trending to be better on the surgical arm (absolute: 27% vs 20%). The greatest benefit was seen in the nonpneumonectomy and pathologic N0 patients. *(Albain KS, Swann RS, Rusch VR, et al: J Clin Oncol [abstract] 23[suppl]:624s, 2005).*

NEOADJUVANT CHEMOTHERAPY OR CHEMORADIATION THERAPY

During the past decade, numerous phase II trials showed that, in general, it is feasible to perform pulmonary resection following chemotherapy or chemoradiation therapy. Although surgery can be more difficult after preoperative treatment, morbidity and mortality were acceptable.

Stage IIIA/IIIB disease The greater effectiveness of current chemotherapeutic regimens to reduce disease bulk suggested that their use prior to surgery, either alone or in combination with radiation therapy, might increase both resectability and survival in patients with stage IIIA NSCLC. Multiple phase II trials have shown such an approach to be feasible; however, it is not clear that such a strategy improves median or long-term survival over best nonsurgical chemoradiotherapy among patients who initially have more than minimal N2 disease.

Current recommendations In selected patients, preoperative treatment may have a favorable effect on outcome in surgically resectable stage IIIA NSCLC. Although aggressive neoadjuvant approaches may have increased treatment-associated mortality, in experienced institutions, potential benefits seem to outweigh the risks. The results of the intergroup randomized trial (see box) comparing preoperative chemoradiation therapy with definitive chemoradiation therapy (in pathologic N2 disease) showed a significant improvement in disease progression–free survival (but not overall survival) in the surgical arm ($P = .02$). This approach, however, may not be optimal if a pneumonectomy is required, as this procedure was associated with a high rate of treatment-related deaths (> 20%). It is not clear whether patients with persistently positive N2 disease after neoadjuvant therapy will benefit from surgical resection.

The Neoadjuvant Trial of Chemotherapy Hope (NATCH) is currently being conducted to compare neoadjuvant chemotherapy with carboplatin and paclitaxel vs the same chemotherapy given in the adjuvant setting vs surgery alone for resectable NSCLC. Patients with resectable disease are eligible, and to date, 530 of 600 planned patients (200 per arm) have enrolled in this study.

Stage I–IIIA disease Neoadjuvant chemotherapy may even play a role in early-stage disease. A multicenter trial from France randomized 373 stage I–IIIA NSCLC patients to undergo either surgery alone or chemotherapy (mitomycin [Mutamycin, 6 mg/m^2 on day 1], ifosfamide [Ifex, 1.5 g/m^2 on days 1–3], and cisplatin [30 mg/m^2 on days 1–3]) at 3-week intervals for 3 cycles followed by surgery. Disease-free survival was significantly longer in the patients randomized to receive neoadjuvant chemotherapy than in those treated with surgery alone (P= .02). The most striking benefit of chemotherapy was seen in patients who had minimal lymphadenopathy (either N0 or N1, P= .008). No excessive complications were seen in the chemotherapy-treated patients.

A phase III trial comparing neoadjuvant chemotherapy with paclitaxel/carboplatin vs surgery alone in early-stage NSCLC (the Bimodality Lung Oncology Team [BLOT] or KNOT study) closed prematurely, based on the reported positive adjuvant data. Preliminary results suggest similar morbidity and mortality in both arms. Complete (R0) resections were achieved in 95% of the BLOT arm vs 88% of the KNOT arm (P= .03).

TREATMENT OF PATIENTS WITH MEDICALLY INOPERABLE STAGE I/II DISEASE

Some patients with resectable stage I or II NSCLC are high-risk operative candidates because of poor cardiopulmonary function or other medical problems. Other patients refuse to undergo surgery despite the recommendation of their treating physicians. In such patients, an attempt should be made to optimize pulmonary function by encouraging smoking cessation and initiating vigorous treatment with bronchodilators, corticosteroids, and antibiotics.

Radiation therapy

Several institutions have reported their experience with definitive radiation therapy for such patients. Although the results are not as good as those reported in patients selected for surgery (possibly due to differences in patient selection and between clinical vs pathologic staging), patients with medically inoperable early-stage NSCLC clearly should be offered radiation therapy, with reasonable expectation of cure.

Onishi et al reviewed the clinical outcomes of 245 patients treated in Japan using hypofractionated stereotactic radiation therapy (SRT) for stage I NSCLC. A total dose of 18–75 Gy at the isocenter was administered in 1–22 fractions. With a median follow-up of 24 months, the local control rate was 85%, and the NCI–CTC (Common Toxicity Criteria) pulmonary complication rate (grade > 2) was only 2.4%. Interestingly, the 3-year overall survival rate for medically operable patients was 88% for those treated with a biologically equivalent dose (BED) ≥ 100 Gy vs 69% for those receiving a BED < 100 Gy(P < .05).

Timmerman et al reported the results of a phase I study of extracranial SRT in patients with medically inoperable stage I NSCLC. SRT was delivered in 3 fractions over 2 weeks, with a starting dose of 800 cGy per fraction. The dose was escalated to 2,000 cGy per fraction for 3 fractions (6,000 cGy total). Of 36 patients, 1 developed grade 3 hypoxemia and another, symptomatic radiation pneumonitis. The maximum tolerated dose was not reached in the T1 patients.

Radiofrequency ablation

Patients who are not operative candidates may be treated with radiofrequency ablation (RFA). There is considerable experience with RFA for cancer in other organs, and its use for lung cancer is growing. It can be performed either intraoperatively or percutaneously with CT guidance. The preliminary findings show these radiologic results: complete response (0%), partial response (50%), stable disease (30%), and disease progression (20%). In a recent study in which more than 300 intrathoracic lesions were treated in 211 sessions, pneumothoraces developed in 51% of the sessions, of which 17% required aspiration and 22% required chest tube placement.

TREATMENT OF PATIENTS WITH STAGE IIIA/IIIB DISEASE

Radiation therapy

In the past, radiation therapy was considered the standard therapy for patients with stage IIIA or IIIB disease. Long-term survival was poor, in the range of 5%, with poor local control and early development of distant metastatic disease.

Altered fractionation schedules A randomized trial compared standard daily radiation therapy (66 Gy) with a continuous hyperfractionated accelerated radiation therapy regimen [CHART] that delivered 54 Gy over 2.5 weeks. The altered fractionation schedule resulted in improved 2-year survival.

Various efforts are under way to look at combining altered fractionation schema with chemotherapy. Although the preliminary results of Radiation Therapy Oncology Group (RTOG) 94-10 do not favor altered fractionation (see section on "Concurrent vs sequential chemoradiation therapy"), the long-term results of another study support this strategy.

Jeremic et al compared hyperfractionated radiation therapy (bid to 69.6 Gy) and concurrent low-dose daily carboplatin/etoposide with or without weekend carboplatin/etoposide in a randomized trial of approximately 200 patients. Although investigators found no benefit with the addition of weekend carboplatin/etoposide, both arms demonstrated promising median survival times of 20 and 22 months and excellent 5-year survival rates of 20% and 23%.

Conformal radiation therapy

Hayman et al reported updated results of the Michigan phase I dose-escalation trial of three-dimensional (3D) conformal radiation therapy for NSCLC. In this study, the radiation dose was escalated based on the effective volume of irradiated lung (up to 102.9 Gy). Such doses produced acceptable toxicity and no cases of isolated failures in purposely nonirradiated, clinically uninvolved nodal regions. This strategy is now being integrated with chemotherapy.

Socinski et al reported a dose-escalation radiotherapy (from 60 Gy up to 74 Gy) trial, using 3D computer-assisted planning techniques, in patients receiving induction carboplatin and paclitaxel and concurrent weekly carboplatin/paclitaxel. Ninety-seven percent (31 of 32) of the patients completed therapy to 74 Gy, as planned. The grade 3/4 esophagitis rate overall was relatively low at only11%. Moreover, the results found a promising median survival of 26 months and 3-year survival of 47%.

Chemoradiation therapy

Chemoradiation vs radiation therapy alone At least 11 randomized trials have compared thoracic irradiation alone with chemoradiation therapy in patients with stage III NSCLC. Several meta-analyses have demonstrated a small, but statistically significant, improvement in survival with the combined-modality regimens. Indeed, six randomized trials have demonstrated a statistically significant survival advantage favoring chemoradiation therapy: Three of these trials employed sequential chemoradiation therapy and the other three employed concurrent chemoradiation therapy.

Analyses of these positive randomized trials favoring chemoradiation over radiation therapy alone suggest a difference in the patterns of failure that relates to the method of combining chemotherapy with thoracic radiotherapy. In the three trials employing sequential chemoradiation therapy, the improvement in survival rates over irradiation alone appeared to be linked to a decrease in the development of distant metastases. In contrast, in the three positive trials employing concurrent chemoradiation therapy, the survival advantage appeared to be associated with an improvement in locoregional control.

Concurrent vs sequential chemoradiation therapy Furuse et al evaluated mitomycin, vindesine, and Platinol (MVP), administered either concurrently or prior to thoracic irradiation (56 Gy), in patients with unresectable stage III NSCLC. With over 300 patients randomized, survival favored concurrent over sequential therapy (median survival, 16.5 vs 13.3 months, and 5-year survival rates, 15.8% vs 8.9%; $P = .04$). Furuse et al also reported the patterns of failure, which demonstrated a benefit of concurrent chemoradiotherapy in improving the local relapse-free survival ($P = .04$) but not the distant relapse-free survival ($P = .6$).

Curran et al presented the long-term results of a larger randomized trial (> 600 patients) comparing sequential vs concurrent chemoradiotherapy (RTOG 9410). The 4-year survival with concurrent cisplatin/vinblastine and once-daily irradiation was 21% vs 12% with sequential treatment ($P = .04$). The third treatment arm (concurrent cisplatin/oral etoposide and hyperfractionated irradiation) was intermediate, with a 4-year survival of 17%.

The role of altered radiation therapy fractionation, though, deserves further study. ECOG 2597 randomized patients after induction chemotherapy (with carboplatin and paclitaxel) to receive either standard radiation therapy (64 Gy/

2 Gy fraction) vs hyperfractionated accelerated radiation therapy (HART), 57.6 Gy delivered 1.5 Gy tid over 2.5 weeks. Although the study closed prematurely due to poor accrual (only 111 patients were eligible), the median survival in the investigational arm appeared promising (22 months).

Several randomized phase II trials also appear to support the use of concurrent chemoradiation therapy for locally advanced NSCLC. For example, Belani et al performed a randomized phase II study in 276 patients of three chemoradiation therapy regimens with paclitaxel, carboplatin, and thoracic irradiation in their locally advanced multimodality protocol (LAMP). They found that concurrent chemoradiation therapy followed by adjuvant chemotherapy appeared to have the best therapeutic outcome, with a median survival of 16.3 months, compared with either induction chemotherapy followed by concurrent chemoradiation therapy (median survival, 12.7 months) or sequential chemotherapy followed by irradiation (median survival, 13 months).

Similarly, in another randomized phase II study, Zatloukal et al studied 102 patients treated with concurrent chemoradiation therapy and sequential chemotherapy followed by irradiation. The chemotherapy consisted of 4 cycles of cisplatin and vinorelbine. The investigators reported a median survival in the concurrent arm of ~20 months, vs ~13 months in the other arm ($P = .02$).

Movsas et al reported the results of the first Patterns of Care Study (PCS) for lung cancer, which was conducted to determine the national patterns of radiation therapy practice in patients treated for nonmetastatic lung cancer. As supported by clinical trials, the PCS for lung cancer demonstrated that patients with clinical stage III NSCLC received chemotherapy plus radiation therapy more than radiation therapy alone ($P < .0001$). In clinical stage I NSCLC, though, radiation therapy alone was the primary treatment ($P < .0001$). Factors correlating with increased use of chemotherapy included lower age ($P < .0001$), histology (SCLC > NSCLC, $P < .0001$), increasing clinical stage ($P < .0001$), increasing Karnofsky performance status ($P < .0001$), and lack of comorbidities ($P = .0002$) but not academic vs nonacademic facilities ($P = .81$). Of all patients receiving chemotherapy, approximately three-quarters received it concurrently with radiation therapy. Only 3% of all patients were treated on Institutional Review Board–approved trials, demonstrating the need for improved accrual to clinical trials.

New chemotherapeutic agents plus irradiation Several phase I/II trials evaluated carboplatin and paclitaxel given concurrently with thoracic irradiation. These studies showed acceptable toxicity and relatively high response rates, and in one of the studies, the 3-year survival rate was quite high (39%).

In addition to paclitaxel and carboplatin, many other chemotherapeutic agents with activity in NSCLC have emerged, including docetaxel (Taxotere), vinorelbine, gemcitabine (Gemzar), UFT, and irinotecan (CPT-11, Camptosar). A trial from Japan tested induction chemotherapy with irinotecan and cisplatin followed by radiation therapy with weekly irinotecan (30 mg/m^2 during radiation therapy). The study reported a response rate of 65% and a median survival rate of 16.5 months, with a grade 3/4 esophagitis rate of only 4%.

Typically, it can be difficult to deliver systemic doses of chemotherapy following concurrent chemoradiotherapy. However, the Southwest Oncology Group (SWOG) has reported a phase II study of concurrent chemoradiation therapy (cisplatin/etoposide) followed by consolidation docetaxel (75–100 mg/m^2 q21d × 3). This group of patients with pathologically documented stage IIIB NSCLC (pleural effusion excluded) had a promising median survival of 27 months. Toxicity during consolidation consisted primarily of neutropenia (56% grade 4).

Current treatment recommendations

At present, it is reasonable to consider concurrent chemoradiation therapy (with once-daily radiation therapy) as a new treatment paradigm in stage III (inoperable) lung cancer patients with an ECOG performance status of 0/1 who have not lost more than 5% of their usual body weight.

TREATMENT OF PATIENTS WITH STAGE IV DISEASE

Until recently, there was considerable controversy over the value of treating stage IV NSCLC patients with chemotherapy. Treatment with older cisplatin-containing regimens, such as cisplatin/etoposide, showed only a modest effect on survival, improving median survival by approximately 6 weeks, according to a meta-analysis, and yielding a 1-year survival rate of approximately 20% (as compared with a rate of approximately 10% for supportive care).

However, several newer chemotherapeutic agents have produced response rates in excess of 20% in NSCLC (Table 4). The potentially useful new agents include the taxanes (paclitaxel and docetaxel), vinorelbine, gemcitabine, and irinotecan. Several of these new drugs have unique mechanisms of action. Paclitaxel and docetaxel increase polymerization of tubulin; gemcitabine is an antimetabolite; and irinotecan is a topoisomerase I inhibitor.

Furthermore, randomized trials demonstrated that a combination of a newer agent plus cisplatin significantly improves the response rate over cisplatin monotherapy (historically considered the most active agent for NSCLC). This increase in response rate translates into significant, although modest, improvement in survival (Table 5).

Optimal chemotherapy for advanced NSCLC

Until the early 1990s, regimens of cisplatin plus a vinca alkaloid or etoposide were most common. More recently, regimens that employ newer agents are more widely used. However, choosing one regimen from many options is a difficult task because there is no survival advantage documented for one regimen over another or standard regimen vs regimens containing newer agents.

Table 6 summarizes the results of selected randomized trials in which combination regimens containing a newer agent are compared with old "standard" regimens or regimens containing another newer agent. Subtle differences in the eligibility criteria (eg, inclusion of patients with stage III tumors or those with poor performance status) make it difficult to directly compare the trial results.

TABLE 4: Active newer agents for NSCLC chemotherapy

Agent	Number of studies	Number of patients	Response rate (%) (range)
Irinotecan	3	150	34 (32-37)
Docetaxel	7	257	33 (21-54)
Paclitaxel	4	151	22 (10-24)
Gemcitabine	7	566	21 (20-26)
Vinorelbine	4	501	21 (12-32)

Nevertheless, there is a trend indicating that regimens containing newer agents show higher response rates and also better survival outcomes in some series than do older regimens.

Vinorelbine plus cisplatin combination Vinorelbine was the first agent that demonstrated improved activity against NSCLC in combination with cisplatin. The European multicenter trial reported by LeChevalier showed the results favoring a cisplatin plus vinorelbine combination (vinorelbine, 30 mg/m^2 weekly; cisplatin, 120 mg/m^2 on days 1 and 29, then every 6 weeks) over a vindesine plus cisplatin combination (vindesine, 3 mg/m^2 weekly; cisplatin, 120 mg/m^2 on days 1 and 29, then every 6 weeks) and vinorelbine alone (30 mg/m^2 weekly). The median survival duration of 40 weeks in the vinorelbine/cisplatin treatment arm was significantly longer than the 32 weeks in the vindesine/cisplatin arm ($P = .04$) and 31 weeks in the vinorelbine monotherapy arm ($P < .001$). This trial, however, did not confirm the role of vinorelbine in NSCLC therapy, even though it confirmed the role of cisplatin.

To address this issue, SWOG conducted a study comparing cisplatin alone (100 mg/m^2 every 4 weeks) with the vinorelbine/cisplatin combination (cisplatin, 100 mg/m^2 every 4 weeks; vinorelbine, 25 mg/m^2 weekly × 3 every 4 weeks). Survival outcome was analyzed for 415 patients, 92% with stage IV tumors. The vinorelbine/cisplatin treatment significantly improved the disease progression-free (median, 2 vs 4 months; $P = .0001$) and overall survival (median, 6 vs 8 months; 1-year survival 20% vs 36%; $P = .0018$).

Comella et al reported interim analysis results of a phase III trial of the Southern Italy Cooperative Oncology Group. A three-drug regimen (cisplatin, gemcitabine, and vinorelbine) was associated with a substantial survival gain over the cisplatin and vinorelbine regimen (median survival time, 51 and 35 weeks, respectively).

Paclitaxel plus platinum compound A number of studies demonstrate promising results with paclitaxel in combination with cisplatin or carboplatin and other agents. Two large randomized trials compared paclitaxel plus cisplatin with standard regimens. In a three-arm, randomized ECOG trial (ECOG 5592) reported by Bonomi et al, 600 eligible patients with chemotherapy-naive stage IIIB to IV NSCLC were randomly assigned to receive a combination of

TABLE 5: Results of selected randomized trials of chemotherapy comparing cisplatin alone vs cisplatin plus a newer agent in advanced NSCLC

Investigator	Chemotherapy regimen	Pts (n)	Response rate (%)	Median survival (mo)	1-yr survival (%)
Klastersky (1989)	Cisplatin	81	19	6.0	NA
	Cisplatin + etoposide	81	26[a]	5.0	NA
Wozniak (1998)	Cisplatin	209	12	6	20
	Cisplatin + vinorelbine	206	26	8[a]	36[a]
Gatzemeier (1998)	Cisplatin	206	17	8.6	NA
	Cisplatin + paclitaxel	202	26[a]	8.1	NA
Sandler (1998)	Cisplatin	262	10	7.6	28
	Cisplatin + gemcitabine	260	26[a]	9.0[a]	39[a]
Von Pawel (1998)	Cisplatin	219	13.7	6.3	21
	Cisplatin + tirapazamine	218	27.5[a]	8.5[a]	33[a]

[a] The difference between the groups was statistically significant ($P < .05$).

NA = data not available

cisplatin (75 mg/m²) plus etoposide (100 mg/m² daily on days 1 to 3) vs either low-dose (135 mg/m² over 24 hours) or high-dose (250 mg/m² over 24 hours with growth factor) paclitaxel plus cisplatin (75 mg/m²). The response rates for the low-dose and high-dose paclitaxel arms were 26.5% and 32.1%, respectively, significantly better than the cisplatin/etoposide arm (12.0%). Superior survival was observed with the combined paclitaxel regimens (median survival time, 9.99 months; 1-year survival rate, 39.1%) compared with etoposide plus cisplatin (median survival time, 7.69 months; 1-year survival rate, 31.6%; $P = .048$). Comparing survival rates for the two dose levels of paclitaxel revealed no significant differences.

In a European trial of similar design reported by Giaccone et al, cisplatin/paclitaxel improved the response rate and quality-of-life parameters. There was no improvement in overall survival, however, compared with a standard regimen of cisplatin/teniposide (Vumon).

Paclitaxel/carboplatin has been the most widely favored regimen for first-line chemotherapy in all NSCLC stages among US medical oncologists, mainly due to promising phase II trial results and the ease of administration as outpatients, with manageable toxicity profiles compared with cisplatin-containing regimens. One of the early phase II trials, for example, reported a response rate of 62%, a median survival duration of 53 weeks, and a 1-year survival rate of 54%. However, a randomized trial sponsored by the manufacturer of paclitaxel failed to demonstrate a survival advantage over the standard cisplatin plus

TABLE 6: Results of selected randomized trials evaluating chemotherapy regimens of newer agents in advanced NSCLC

Investigator	Chemotherapy regimen	No. of patients	Response rate (%)	Median survival	1-yr survival rate (%)
LeChevalier (1994)	Vinorelbine + cisplatin	206	30	40 wk	35
	Vindesine + cisplatin	200	19	32 wk	27
	Vinorelbine	206	14	31 wk	30
Bonomi (1996)	Etoposide + cisplatin	600 (total)	12.0	7.69 mo	31.6
	Paclitaxel + cisplatin		26.5	9.56 mo	36.9
	Paclitaxel + cisplatin + G-CSF		32.1	9.99 mo	39.1
Giaccone (1997)	Teniposide + cisplatin	157	28	9.9 mo	41
	Paclitaxel + cisplatin	152	41	9.7 mo	43
Belani (1998)	Etoposide + cisplatin	179	14.0	9.9 mo	37
	Paclitaxel + carboplatin	190	21.6	9.5 mo	32
Crino (1998)	Mitomycin + ifosfamide + cisplatin	152	28	38 wk	NA
	Gemcitabine + cisplatin	154	40	35 wk	NA
Georgoulias (1999)	Docetaxel + cisplatin	152	32	10 mo	42
	Docetaxel + gemcitabine	144	34	9 mo	34
Masuda (1999)	Irinotecan + cisplatin	378 (total)	43	50.3 wk	47.5
	Vindesine + cisplatin		31	47.4 wk	37.9
	Irinotecan		21	46.1 wk	40.7
Kelly (1999)	Paclitaxel + carboplatin	184	27	8 mo	36
	Vinorelbine + cisplatin	181	27	8 mo	33
Schiller (2000)	Paclitaxel + cisplatin	1,163 (total)	21.3	7.8 mo	31
	Gemcitabine + cisplatin		21.0	8.1 mo	36
	Docetaxel + cisplatin		17.3	7.4 mo	31
	Paclitaxel + carboplatin		15.3	8.2 mo	35
Frasci (2000)	Gemcitabine + vinorelbine	60	22	29 wk	30
	Vinorelbine	60	15	18 wk	13
Lilenbaum (2002)	Paclitaxel + carboplatin	292	29	10 mo	NA
	Paclitaxel	290	17	8.6 mo	NA

G-CSF = granulocyte colony-stimulating factor; NA = data not available

etoposide regimen. Nevertheless, paclitaxel plus carboplatin may remain a community standard because a recently completed SWOG trial reported results equivalent to the time-tested vinorelbine/cisplatin regimen (see Table 6).

Combination vs single-agent chemotherapy A randomized phase III study conducted by the CALGB further supported the superiority of combination chemotherapy over single-agent therapy. Previous trials had indicated that a platinum plus a novel agent was superior to a platinum alone. Lilenbaum et al demonstrated that for patients with stage IIIB–IV NSCLC, carboplatin and paclitaxel are superior to paclitaxel alone, even for patients with a performance status of 2. This randomized trial showed a median survival advantage for the combination therapy.

Gemcitabine plus cisplatin Gemcitabine has also been approved by the FDA for use against NSCLC based on a series of successful phase II trials of cisplatin/gemcitabine and three major phase III trials. The Hoosier Oncology Group study, reported by Sandler et al, compared gemcitabine/cisplatin with cisplatin alone and showed a modest improvement in median and 1-year survival comparable to that seen in the vinorelbine trials (Table 5). The Spanish and Italian trials, reported by Cardenal et al and Crino et al, compared gemcitabine plus cisplatin with standard-regimen cisplatin plus etoposide and mitomycin plus ifosfamide plus cisplatin, respectively. Although there was a significant improvement in overall response, these two studies failed to demonstrate a survival benefit.

Since gemcitabine is relatively well tolerated without dose-limiting myelosuppression, it is being evaluated for use as a single agent or in combination with other agents in older or medically compromised patients. Italian investigators report that gemcitabine combined with the vinorelbine regimen is associated with significantly better survival than single-agent vinorelbine in elderly patients with NSCLC.

Other combination regimens that contain cisplatin plus newer agents, such as docetaxel or irinotecan, also showed similar results when compared with other two-drug regimens of either two newer or two older agents (Table 6).

Major randomized trials comparing cytotoxic regimens

To identify a better chemotherapy regimen for advanced-stage NSCLC, the US cooperative study groups conducted large phase III trials. The SWOG investigators compared paclitaxel/carboplatin with vinorelbine/cisplatin (the time-tested regimen in previous European and SWOG trials). A total of 404 evaluable patients were randomized to receive either paclitaxel (225 mg/m^2 over 3 hours) plus carboplatin (at an area under the curve [AUC] of 6 mg/mL/min on day 1) every 21 days or vinorelbine (25 mg/m^2 weekly) plus cisplatin (100 mg/m^2 on day 1) every 28 days. Overall response rates were 27% for both groups. The median survival times were also identical (8 months), with virtually identical 1-year survival rates (35% and 33%, respectively). Although both regimens provided effective palliation for advanced NSCLC, the investigators identified paclitaxel/carboplatin for future studies because of a favorable toxicity profile and better tolerability and compliance.

The ECOG 1594 trial compared three platinum-based regimens containing new agents in the treatment of NSCLC with a control arm of cisplatin and paclitaxel. The regimens were gemcitabine (1,000 mg/m^2 on days 1, 8, and 15) plus cisplatin (100 mg/m^2 on day 1) every 4 weeks, docetaxel (75 mg/m^2) plus cisplatin (75 mg/m^2 on day 1) every 3 weeks, and paclitaxel (225 mg/m^2 over 3 hours) plus carboplatin (at AUC of 6 mg/mL/min on day 1) every 21 days; the reference regimen was paclitaxel (175 mg/m^2 over 24 hours) plus cisplatin

(75 mg/m^2 on day 1) every 21 days.

Analysis of 1,163 eligible patients showed no statistically significant differences in overall response, median survival, and 1-year survival rates when compared with the control arm, paclitaxel and cisplatin. Gemcitabine plus cisplatin was associated with a statistically significant prolongation of time to disease progression when compared with the control arm (4.5 vs 3.5 months, $P = .002$) but was also associated with a higher percentage of grade 4 thrombocytopenia, anemia, and renal toxicity.

Since all the regimens showed similar efficacy, quality of life becomes a critical issue in choosing a particular regimen. The decision to use one regimen over another will depend not only on ease of administration and side effects, but also on the personal preference and experience of the treating oncologist.

> Movsas et al reported the results of RTOG 98-01, a phase III study of amifostine (Ethyol, 500 mg IV 4×/wk) in patients with locally advanced NSCLC receiving chemotherapy and hyperfractionated radiation therapy. Seventy-three percent received amifostine per protocol or with minor deviation. On the amifostine arm, there were significantly higher rates of low-grade acute nausea and vomiting, acute cardiovascular toxicity, mostly transient hypotension, and episodes of acute infection/febrile neutropenia. The rate of grade ≥ 3 esophagitis was 30% with amifostine vs 34% without amifostine ($P = .9$). Based on daily patient diaries, though, the swallowing dysfunction area under the curve was lower with amifostine ($P = .03$). Overall, amifostine did not reduce grade ≥ 3 esophagitis per the NCI-CTC. However, direct patient assessment suggests a possible advantage to amifostine that is being explored with modified dosing/route strategies *(Movsas B, Scott C, Langer C, et al: J Clin Oncol 23:2145-2154, 2005).*

Second-line chemotherapy for NSCLC

Before the new generation of more effective agents became available, few, if any, significant benefits were expected from second-line chemotherapy. As a result, reports in the literature seldom address this issue specifically or systematically. The most experience with second-line chemotherapy in NSCLC is with docetaxel, which has received FDA approval for this indication based on two randomized phase III trials confirming the promising phase II results of docetaxel monotherapy in patients with advanced NSCLC previously treated with platinum-based chemotherapy.

In a multicenter US trial reported by Fossella et al, 373 patients were randomized to receive either docetaxel, 100 mg/m^2 (D100) or 75 mg/m^2 (D75) vs a control regimen of vinorelbine (30 mg/m^2/wk) or ifosfamide (2 g/m^2 × 3 days) every 3 weeks. Overall response rates were 10.8% with D100 and 6.7% with D75, each significantly higher than the 0.8% response of the control arm ($P = .001$ and $P = .036$, respectively). Although overall survival was not significantly different among the three groups, the 1-year survival was significantly higher with D75 than with the control treatment (32% vs 19%; $P = .025$).

The second trial reported by Shepherd et al compared single-agent docetaxel with best supportive care. The initial docetaxel dose was 100 mg/m^2, which was changed to 75 mg/m^2 midway through the trial because of toxicity. A total of 204 patients were enrolled; 49 received D100, 55 received D75, and 100 received best supportive care. Treatment with docetaxel was associated with significant prolongation of survival (7.0 vs 4.6 months; log-rank test, $P = .047$) and time to disease progression (10.6 vs 6.7 weeks, $P < .001$).

Hanna et al conducted a noninferiority trial to test whether pemetrexed (Alimta) was equivalent to docetaxel in the second-line setting. They randomized 571 patients to receive 500 mg/m^2 of pemetrexed or 75 mg/m^2 of docetaxel preceded by a vitamin B_{12} injection every 2 cycles. The median survival on the two arms was equivalent, but the pemetrexed arm had significantly less grade 3/4 neutropenia and fewer hospitalizations overall. On the basis of this study, the FDA approved pemetrexed for second-line therapy for NSCLC.

Duration of chemotherapy

The American Society of Clinical Oncology (ASCO) has recommended that no more than 8 cycles of chemotherapy be administered to patients with stage IV NSCLC. However, therapy should be individualized depending on the quality of tumor response and the patient's tolerance.

Novel and promising agents

Several novel agents are being developed for the treatment of solid tumors, including lung cancer. For example, farnesyl transferase inhibitors target prenylation of the *ras* family of proto-oncogenes. Farnesylation causes the *ras* oncogene to be constitutively active.

Other novel agents include signal transduction inhibitors, such as tyrosine kinase inhibitors (eg, erlotinib [Tarceva], gefitinib [Iressa]), antiangiogenic agents, and monoclonal antibodies (C225 [antiepidermal growth factor receptor antibody] and trastuzumab [Herceptin]). Many of these novel agents are being tested in combination with chemotherapeutic agents, as their mechanisms of action suggest that they may be far more effective as chronic inhibitors of cancer progression than as classic cytotoxics.

To date, most phase I studies of these various compounds have suffered from a difficulty in developing pharmacologically or molecularly driven endpoints that will serve as reasonable intermediate biomarkers of efficacy or even surrogates for toxicity. Further research has focused on the novel small molecule tyrosine kinase inhibitors erlotinib and gefitinib. Two phase II trials of gefitinib in the second- and third-line settings were conducted in Europe and Japan. Patients were randomized to receive either 250 or 500 mg/d. The drug was found to be active, with an 11%–18% response rate, and there was no superiority for the higher dose. Similar data were seen for erlotinib.

Unfortunately, randomized combination trials of gefitinib at 250 and 500 mg/d with cytotoxic chemotherapy, either paclitaxel and carboplatin in one trial or gemcitabine and cisplatin in the other study vs placebo in front-line therapy, failed to demonstrate any survival advantage. These results have cast a pall over the development of tyrosine kinase inhibitors in combination with chemotherapy. Regardless, the question of whether or not to approve these new agents for third-line therapy of lung cancer in cisplatin/docetaxel-refractory patients remains open for debate.

The activity demonstrated by gefitinib and erlotinib as single agents in advanced NSCLC generated much optimism, including a recent trial indicating that erlotinib improved survival (by a median of 2 months) in the second- and third-line treatment of NSCLC, with a substantial increase in 1-year survival ($P <$ .001). After the initial successes with chemotherapy and promising results from targeted tyrosine kinase inhibitors in stages IIIB and IV NSCLC, several large phase III trials of either gefitinib or erlotinib in combination with conventional platinum-based chemotherapy were conducted as the INTACT 1 and INTACT 2 trials or the TALENT and TRIBUTE trials.

The phase III trials of single-agent erlotinib and gefitinib, when compared with best supportive care in the second- and third-line settings, had dramatically different results. Shepherd et al conducted a randomized trial of erlotinib (150 mg/d) vs placebo in 723 patients previously treated with front- or second-line chemotherapy for NSCLC. A total of 488 patients received erlotinib and 243 received placebo.

The median overall survival significantly favored the erlotinib arm (6.7 vs 4.7 months), with a reduction in the hazard ratio of 0.73 ($P > 0.001$), as did the 1-year survival rate (31% vs 21%; $P > 0.01$). Quality of life and median time to deterioration also significantly favored erlotinib. On the other hand, the phase III trial of gefitinib vs best supportive care in more than 1,600 patients was reported and showed no significant advantage to gefitinib at 250 mg/d in a patient population with a significant number of active smokers.

Unfortunately, these large trials indicated no benefit to adding the tyrosine kinase inhibitors to conventional chemotherapy. A phase III trial combining the farnesyl transferase inhibitor lonafarnib (Sarasar) with paclitaxel and carboplatin in unselected, untreated patients with stage IIIB/IV NSCLC also failed to yield a survival advantage, despite promising phase I and II data. There was evidence that the combination of chemotherapy and the signal transduction inhibitors was potentially detrimental. The placebo plus chemotherapy results initially showed a survival benefit over the first 6 months in two of these four trials. Survival data after 6 months from the INTACT 2 and the TRIBUTE trials indicate that from that point forward, patients who remained on erlotinib or gefitinib appeared to have a significant survival benefit when compared with placebo.

In general, there appears to be little to favor triplet cytotoxic drug combinations vs doublet combinations in NSCLC. An area of great excitement, however, has been the addition of novel biologically or molecularly targeted agents to cytotoxic chemotherapy combinations. Several recent trials have failed to demonstrate the potential advantages of adding a small molecule targeted to either the epidermal growth factor receptor (EGFR) or *ras* (namely the farnesyl transferase inhibitors). The interest in these agents in advanced NSCLC appears to have superseded the new cytotoxic agents with activity in other diseases, such as oxaliplatin (Eloxatin), tirapazamine, and UFT. A phase III com-

A phase III trial of 731 patients conducted by the National Cancer Institute of Canada Clinical Trials Group sought to determine whether erlotinib (Tarceva) prolonged survival in patients with advanced NSCLC whose disease had progressed after first- or second-line chemotherapy. The overall response rate to erlotinib was 8.9% ($P < .001$), with a median response duration of 34.3 weeks. Overall (6.7 vs 4.7 mo, $P =$ .001) and disease progression–free survival rates (2.23 vs 1.84 mo, $P < .001$) were significantly higher in the erlotinib arm than in the placebo arm (*Shepherd FA, Pereira J, Ciuleanu TE, et al: J Clin Oncol [abstract] 22 [suppl]:14s, 2004).*

bination of farnesyl transferase with paclitaxel and carboplatin failed to show superiority over paclitaxel and carboplatin.

When combined with chemotherapy, bevacizumab appears to result in a significant survival advantage for patients with advanced NSCLC. Based on promising phase II data of bevacizumab in combination with carboplatin and paclitaxel, Sandler et al randomized 878 patients to receive either bevacizumab with carboplatin and paclitaxel or carboplatin and paclitaxel alone.

There was a significant increase in the response rate for the combination (27.2%) with bevacizumab vs paclitaxel and carboplatin alone (10%; $P < .0001$), and both median and progression-free survival significantly favored the bevacizumab combination arm (overall survival: 12.5 vs 10.2 months; $P =$ .007; hazard ratio = 0.77; 95% confidence interval = 0.65–0.93; progression-free survival: 6.4 vs 4.5 months; $P < .0001$; hazard ratio = 0.62; 95% confidence interval = 0.53–0.72). As in the phase II trial, this study reported a total of eight treatment-related deaths on the bevacizumab arm vs two on the paclitaxel and carboplatin arm.

The mechanisms of action of these new small molecules are widely divergent, and their combinations with the cytotoxics may not necessarily lead to an enhanced response rate. Khuri and colleagues demonstrated, however, that the combination of cisplatin, vinorelbine, and bexarotene (Targretin, a retinoid-X-receptor [RXR]-specific novel retinoid) resulted in substantial median and 2-year survival rates in patients with stage IIIB NSCLC with malignant pleural effusion or stage IV NSCLC. Median survival in this multicenter study was 14 months in the phase II portion; 2-year survival was 32%; and 3-year survival was 18%. The combination yielded modest response rates (25%), not markedly superior to what was expected with cisplatin and vinorelbine alone. Two phase III trials adding bexarotene to standard chemotherapy failed to show a significant overall difference in median survival. Some survival benefit was seen in those patients who developed grade 3/4 hypertriglyceridemia as a result of the bexarotene, accounting for 35%–40% of all patients enrolled in this study.

This finding has led to an uncoupling of the requirement for higher response rates when adding cytotoxic agents to one another in the belief that doing so may lead to enhanced survival. There now appears to be a great deal of promise associated with several small molecules, either alone or combined with chemotherapy. Novel agents such as gefitinib or lonafarnib have shown promising efficacy in small trials that have included patients with NSCLC; gefitinib alone resulted in an 18% response rate in second- or third-line therapy for NSCLC in a study population recruited across several continents.

Current treatment recommendations It is important to note that patients who have lost significant amounts of weight or who have poor performance status are at greater risk for toxicity, including a higher likelihood of lethal toxicity, when they are treated with modest doses of chemotherapy. Based on currently available data, a reasonable approach for patients with stage IV NSCLC who have good performance status (ECOG performance status 0/1) and have not lost a significant amount of weight (< 5% of usual weight) would be to encourage them to participate in a clinical trial. However, it would also be appropriate to treat this group of patients with etoposide plus cisplatin or with one of the newer combination regimens, such as gemcitabine/cisplatin, vinorelbine/cisplatin, paclitaxel/cisplatin, paclitaxel/carboplatin, or docetaxel/cisplatin (Tables 7 and 8).

In a phase III trial led by Hanna et al, 572 previously treated patients were randomized to receive pemetrexed (Alimta) with vitamin B_{12}, folic acid, and dexamethasone or docetaxel (Taxotere) with dexamethasone. The overall response rate in the pemetrexed arm was higher, 9.1% vs 8.8%. The median disease progression–free survival was 2.9 months for each arm, and the median survival favored pemetrexed (8.3 vs 7.9 mo). The 1-year survival for each arm was 29.7%. Adverse reactions (grade 3/4) were more severe with docetaxel (*Hanna N, Shepherd FA, Fossella FV, et al: J Clin Oncol 22:1589-1597, 2004*).

ROLE OF PHOTODYNAMIC THERAPY

Photodynamic therapy (PDT), which combines Photofrin (a hematoporphyrin derivative in which the less active porphyrin monomers have been removed) with an argon-pumped dye laser, has been explored in a variety of different tumors, with varying results. Several investigators have reported excellent results with PDT in early-stage head and neck cancers as well as intrathoracic tumors. However, initial studies have involved a limited number of patients.

Although this novel technique seems to be extremely promising, it appears to be applicable to only a small minority of patients with NSCLC. Nevertheless, PDT appears to be particularly useful for the treatment of early-stage lung cancer for a variety of reasons. First, it appears to preserve lung function and can be repeated as additional tumors appear–an important consideration since such patients appear to be at high risk for developing other new tumors. Second, this technique does not preclude ultimate surgical intervention when deemed necessary.

Results in early-stage NSCLC Perhaps most striking are the results reported by Furuse et al, who treated 54 patients with 64 early-stage lung cancers using Photofrin (2.0 mg/kg) and 630-nm illumination of 100–200 J/cm^2. Of 59 accessible tumors, 50 responded completely and 6 showed partial responses. Five of the complete responders developed recurrences 6–8 months after treatment.

The major predictor of response in this study was tumor length. The likelihood of achieving a complete response was 97.8% if the tumor was < 1 cm, as opposed to only 42.9% if the lesion was > 1 cm. The overall survival rate in these patients was 50% at 3 years.

TABLE 7: Single-agent chemotherapy regimens for NSCLC

Drug	Dose and schedule
Vinorelbine	30 mg/m^2 IV weekly
LeChevalier T, Brisgand D, Douillard J-Y, et al: J Clin Oncol 12:360–367, 1994.	
Vinorelbine	For patients 70 years old or older: 30 mg/m^2 IV on days 1 and 8, every 21 days
Gridelli C, Perrone F, Cigolari S, et al: Proc Am Soc Clin Oncol [abstract] 20:308a, 2001.	
Docetaxel	75 mg/m^2 IV on day 1 every 3 weeks
Shepherd FA, Dancey J, Ramlau R, et al: J Clin Oncol 18:2095–2103, 2000.	
Pemetrexed	500 mg/m^2 IV piggyback every 3 weeks
Dexamethasone (4 mg by mouth twice daily) should be started a day before and a day after pemetrexed. All patients should also receive folic acid (350-1,000 mg/d) started about a week before and thereafter while taking pemetrexed. Vitamin B_{12} (1,000 mg IM) should be started about 1 to 2 weeks before pemetrexed and every 9 weeks while taking pemetrexed.	
Hanna N, Shepherd F, Fossella FV, et al: J Clin Oncol [abstract] 22:1589–1597, 2004.	
Gefitinib	250 mg orally once a day
Kris MG, Natale RB, Herbst RS, et al: JAMA 290:2149–2158, 2003.	
Gemcitabine	1,000 mg/m^2 IV on days 1, 8, and 15 every 4 weeks
Vansteenkiste J, Vandebroek J, Nackaerts K, et al: Proc Am Soc Clin Oncol [abstract] 19:1910a, 2000.	

Table prepared by Ishmael Jaiyesimi, DO

A similar study by Kato et al also indicated a 96.8% complete response rate for tumors < 0.5 cm but only a 37.5% rate for tumors > 2 cm. The overall 5-year survival rate for the 75 patients treated in this study was 68.4%, which is acceptable by current standards.

Further work by Lam et al supported these promising results of PDT in early-stage NSCLC.

Results in advanced-stage NSCLC Two prospective, randomized trials (European; US/Canadian) compared PDT with the neodymium:yttrium-aluminum-garnet (Nd:YAG) laser for partially obstructive, advanced NSCLC. Investigators analyzed results from the two trials both individually and collectively. Collective analysis included data from 15 centers in Europe and 20 centers in the United States and Canada and involved a total of 211 patients. In the European trial, 40% of the patients had received prior therapy, whereas in the US/Canadian trial, all of the patients had received previous treatment.

Tumor response was similar for both therapies at 1 week. However, at 1 month, 61% and 42% of the patients treated with PDT in the European and US/Canadian trials, respectively, were still responding, compared with 36% and 19% of patients who underwent laser therapy in the two trials.

TABLE 8: Combination chemotherapy regimens recommended for NSCLC

Regimen	Agents	Dose and schedule	Treatment interval
PE	Platinol	60 mg/m^2 IV on day 1	3 weeks
	Etoposide	120 mg/m^2 IV on days 1-3	
MIC	Mitomycin	6 mg/m^2 IV on day 1	4 weeks
	Ifosfamide	3 g/m^2 IV on day 1	
	Cisplatin	100 mg/m^2 IV on day 2	
PT	Platinol	75 mg/m^2 IV on day 2	3 weeks
	Taxol	135 mg/m^2 IV on day 1 (24-h infusion)	
CP	Carboplatin	AUC of 6 mg/mL/min IV on day 1	
	Paclitaxel	225 mg/m^2 IV on day 1 (3-h infusion)	3 weeks
PG	Platinol	100 mg/m^2 IV on day 1	4 weeks
	Gemcitabine	1,000 mg/m^2 IV on days 1, 8, and 15	
PD	Platinol	75 mg/m^2 IV on day 1	3 weeks
	Docetaxel	75 mg/m^2 IV on day 1	
PV	Platinol	100 mg/m^2 IV on day 1	4 weeks
	Vinorelbine	25 mg/m^2 IV on days 1, 8, 15, and 22	
PCB	Paclitaxel	200 mg/m^2 IV on day 1 (3-hr infusion)	3 weeks
	Carboplatin	AUC of 6 mg/mL/min IV on day 1	
	Bevacizumab	15 mg/kg IV	
GV	Gemcitabine	1,200 mg/m^2 IV on days 1 and 8	3 weeks
	Vinorelbine	30 mg/m^2 IV on days 1 and 8	

AUC = area under the curve

PDT also produced more dramatic improvements in dyspnea and cough than did Nd:YAG therapy in the European trial, but the two treatments had similar effects on these symptoms in the US/Canadian trial. Both sets of investigators concluded that PDT appears to be superior to laser therapy for the relief of dyspnea, cough, and hemoptysis. Also, the overall incidence of adverse reactions was similar with the two therapies (73% for PDT vs 64% for Nd:YAG therapy). Early-stage lung cancer, most specifically endobronchial squamous cell carcinoma smaller than 1 cm, is effectively treated, with a complete response rate of 75% and a recurrence rate of 30% over 5 years.

PALLIATION OF LOCAL AND DISTANT SYMPTOMS

Radiation therapy

Many patients with lung cancer experience distressing local symptoms at some time. They may arise from airway obstruction by the primary tumor, compression of mediastinal structures by nodal metastases, or metastatic involvement of distant organs. Radiation therapy is effective in palliating most local symptoms, as well as symptoms at common metastatic sites, such as bone and brain. For selected patients with a solitary brain metastasis and controlled disease in other sites, resection followed by irradiation appears to be superior to radiation therapy alone in improving both survival and quality of life. (For more information regarding management of brain metastases, see chapter 26.)

Doses In the United States, radiation oncologists often use doses of ~30 Gy in 10 fractions for palliative thoracic treatment in lung cancer. Data from the United Kingdom suggest that similar efficacy without greater toxicity may be achieved with more abbreviated schedules, such as 17 Gy in 2 fractions 1 week apart or single fractions of 10 Gy (see Table 9). Such schedules may facilitate the coordination of irradiation and chemotherapy and also reduce patient travel and hospitalization.

Recently, just over 400 patients with inoperable NSCLC (stage III/IV) were randomized to receive three different fractionation regimens (8.5 Gy × 2, 2.8 Gy × 15, or 2.0 Gy × 25). Using the EORTC (European Organization for Research on the Treatment of Cancer) Quality-of-Life Questionnaire (QLQ) C-30 with the lung cancer-specific module (LC-13), Sundstrom et al found the effect of hypofractionated irradiation (17 Gy in 2 fractions) was comparable to that with longer fractionation schemes with regard to symptom relief and survival.

Endobronchial irradiation with cobalt-60 or iridium-192 has been used to palliate symptoms arising from partial airway obstruction, including cough, dyspnea, and hemoptysis. The dosimetric advantage of being able to deliver a high radiation dose to the obstructing endobronchial tumor while sparing adjacent normal structures, such as the lungs, spinal cord, and esophagus, has clear appeal, particularly in the patient whose disease has recurred following prior external-beam irradiation. Although good rates of palliation have been reported with endobronchial irradiation, significant complications, including fatal hemoptysis, are seen in 5%–10% of patients. It remains unclear, however, how often this complication is actually due to the irradiation vs the underlying disease itself.

Endobronchial irradiation should be considered as one of several approaches (including laser excision, cryotherapy, and stent placement) used in the management of patients with symptomatic airway obstruction, and management should be individualized. All of these approaches are more suitable for partial than for complete airway obstruction.

Chemotherapy

Several recent trials have explored the use of chemotherapy to palliate specific symptoms in patients with lung cancer. In general, these trials have found that rates of symptomatic improvement were considerably higher than objective response rates and were not dissimilar to symptomatic response rates with local radiation therapy.

A randomized phase II study suggests that rhuMAb vascular endothelial growth factor (VEGF; 15 mg/kg) in combination with carboplatin/paclitaxel chemotherapy may increase response rates and prolong time to disease progression in patients with previously untreated NSCLC when compared with carboplatin/paclitaxel chemotherapy alone. Patients with progressive disease who received carboplatin/paclitaxel alone were allowed to cross over to receive rhuMAb VEGF. The median survival time was 7.7 months with high-dose rhuMAb VEGF (15 mg/kg q3wk) and 4.9 months with carboplatin/paclitaxel alone. Although sudden and life-threatening hemoptysis occurred in six rhuMAb VEGF–treated subjects and was fatal in four, survival data are encouraging, and a phase III trial is in progress without crossover to rhuMAb VEGF.

> A large prospective trial of gefitinib (Iressa) in patients with bronchioloalveolar carcinoma (BAC) conducted by the Southwest Oncology Group (SWOG S0126) found that 19% of 102 previously untreated patients with measurable disease responded to the drug. Among 67 chemotherapy-naive patients with measurable disease, the response rate was 21%. In 21 previously treated patients, the response rate was 10%. The median survival was 12 months and 10 months for chemotherapy-naive and previously treated patients, respectively. The 1-year survival in each group was about 50%. Adverse events included acneiform rash and diarrhea (*West H, Franklin WA, Gumerlock PH, et al: J Clin Oncol [abstract] 22 [suppl]:14s, 2004*).

Thus, although radiation therapy remains the most appropriate modality for the treatment of such problems as superior vena cava obstruction, spinal cord compression, brain metastases, or localized bone pain, patients who have more extensive disease without these local emergencies may be considered for palliative chemotherapy, which may relieve local symptoms and prolong survival.

Bisphosphonates

Approximately 30%–65% of patients with advanced lung cancer develop bone metastases. The median survival following development of bone metastases is 6 months. Bone disease is associated with significant morbidity, including severe pain, hypercalcemia of malignancy, pathologic fracture, and spinal cord or nerve root compression. Treatment of bone metastases may include surgical intervention, radiation therapy, and chemotherapy. Bisphosphonate treatment can decrease skeleton-related complications, delay progressive disease, and relieve bone pain.

Bisphosphonates such as clodronate, pamidronate, and zoledronic acid (Zometa) exhibit strong affinity for the hydroxyapatite crystal of bone and preferentially accumulate at sites of active bone remodeling, where they prevent bone resorption. They provide effective treatment for hypercalcemia of malignancy and have been shown to delay the onset of progressive bone disease and relieve bone pain in studies largely performed in patients with metastases secondary to breast cancer, multiple myeloma, and prostate cancer. Nitrogen-containing bisphosphonates, such as pamidronate and zoledronic acid, appear to exert antitumor effects. Zoledronic acid has also been found to have pronounced antinociceptive effects, which have been absent with other bisphosphonates in preclinical studies. Zoledronic acid is the only bisphosphonate shown to be effective in reducing skeletal complications in patients with bone metastases from lung cancer and solid tumors other than breast and prostate cancers.

TABLE 9: Percentage of patients with symptoms of NSCLC palliated by external-beam irradiation

Symptom	Standard RT (24-30 Gy in 6-10 fractions)	17 Gy in 2 fractions (first trial/second trial)	1 fraction of 10 Gy
Cough	56	65/48	56
Hemoptysis	86	81/75	72
Chest pain	80	75/59	72
Anorexia	64	68/45	55
Depression	57	72/NA	NA
Anxiety	66	71/NA	NA
Breathlessness	57	66/41	43

NA = data not available; RT = radiation therapy

Data from Bleehen NM, Girling DJ, Fayers PM, et al: Br J Cancer 63:265–270, 1991; Bleehen NM, Bolger JJ, Hasleton PS, et al: Br J Cancer 65:934–941, 1992.

Follow-up of long-term survivors

At present, no standard follow-up protocol exists for patients with cured NSCLC or SCLC. However, long-term follow-up should at least include serial physical examinations once the patient has reached the 5-year mark. Controversy currently exists about the value of utilizing CT scanning or even chest x-rays for the long-term follow-up of these patients.

In this vein, retrospective reviews of the literature have revealed that patients with SCLC appear to have the highest rate of second primary tumor development–as high as 30%–over the course of their lifetime, with some studies reporting annual second primary tumor rates of 5%–10%. Therefore, the concept of chemoprevention appears to have particular merit in these patients.

A randomized chemoprevention study of patients with stage I NSCLC showed a surprisingly high annual recurrence rate of 6.5% in patients with T1 tumors, as opposed to 11.2% in patients with T2 tumors. Whether retinoids are effective chemopreventive agents remains to be seen. Nevertheless, there is clearly a need for effective chemoprevention for both of these tumor subsets, as well as the establishment of consistent guidelines for routine long-term follow-up. Given the current controversy over lung cancer screening, however, it is unlikely that this issue will be resolved without the performance of another prospective screening trial.

SUGGESTED READING

American College of Chest Physicians; Health and Science Policy Committee: Diagnosis and management of lung cancer: ACCP evidence-based guidelines. Chest 123(1 suppl):D-G, 1S–337S, 2003.

Arriagade R, Bergman B, Dunant A, et al: Cisplatin-based adjuvant chemotherapy in patients with completely resected non-small-cell lung cancer. N Engl J Med 350:351–360, 2004.

Bach PB, Jett JR, Pastorino, et al: Computed tomography screening and lung cancer outcomes. JAMA 297(9):953–961, 2007.

Belani CP, Wang W, Johnson DH, et al: Induction chemotherapy followed by either standard thoracic radiotherapy or hyperfractionated accelerated radiotherapy for patients with unresectable stage IIIA and B NSCLC. J Clin Oncol 23:3760–3767, 2005.

Fukuoka M, Yano S, Giaccone G, et al: Multi-institutional randomized phase II trial of gefitinib for previously treated patients with advanced non-small-cell lung cancer. J Clin Oncol 21:2237–2246, 2003.

Gandara DR, Chansky K, Albain KS, et al: Consolidation docetaxel after concurrent chemoradiotherapy in stage IIIB non–small-cell lung cancer: Phase II Southwest Oncology Group Study S9504. J Clin Oncol 21:2004–2010, 2003.

Giaccone G, Herbst RS, Manegold C, et al: Gefitinib in combinaton with gemcitabine and cisplatin in advanced non-small-cell lung cancer: A phase III–INTACT 1. J Clin Oncol 22:777–84, 2004.

Herbst RS, Giaccone G, Schiller JH, et al: Gefitinib in combination with paclitaxel and carboplatin in advanced non-small -cell lung cancer: A phase III trial–INTACT 2. J Clin Oncol 22:785–794, 2004.

I-ELCAP; Henschke CI, Yankelevitz DF, et al: Survival of patients with stage I lung cancer detected on CT screening. N Engl J Med 355(17):1763–1771, 2006.

Jemal A, Siegel R, Ward E, et al: Cancer statistics, 2006. CA Cancer J Clin 56:106–130, 2006.

Kato H, Ichinose Y, Ohta M, et al: A randomized trial of adjuvant chemotherapy with uracil-tegafur for adenocarcinoma of the lung. N Engl J Med 350:1713–1721, 2004.

Kawahara M: Irinotecan in the treatment of small cell lung cancer: A review of patient safety considerations. Expert Opin Drug Saf 5:303–312, 2006.

Keller SM, Adak S, Wagner H, et al: A randomized trial of postoperative adjuvant therapy in patients with completely resected stage II or IIIA non-small-cell lung cancer. Eastern Cooperative Oncology Group. N Engl J Med 343:1217–1222, 2000.

Kris MG, Natale RB, Herbst RS, et al: Efficacy of gefitinib, an inhibitor of the epidermal growth factor receptor tyrosine kinase, in symptomatic patients with non-small cell lung cancer: A randomized trial. JAMA 290:2149–2158, 2003.

Lilenbaum RC, Herndon J, List M, et al: Single-agent versus combination chemotherapy in advanced NSCLC: The Cancer and Leukemia Group B (study 9730). J Clin Oncol 23:190–196, 2005.

Martelli M, Clerici M, Cognetti F, et al: Adjuvant Lung Project Italy/European Organisation for Research Treatment of Cancer–Lung Cancer Cooperative Group Investigators: Randomized study of adjuvant chemotherapy for completely resected stage I, II, or IIIA non–small-cell lung cancer. J Natl Cancer Inst 95:1453–1461, 2003.

Movsas B, Moughan J, Komaki R, et al: Radiotherapy (RT) Patterns of Care Study (PCS) in lung carcinoma. J Clin Oncol 21:4553–4559, 2003.

Movsas B, Scott C, Langer C, et al: Randomization of amifostine in locally advanced NSCLC patients receiving chemotherapy and hyperfractionated radiation. Radiation Therapy Oncology Group 98-01. J Clin Oncol 23:2145–2154, 2005.

Pisters K, Vallieres E, Bunn P, et al: S9900: A phase III trial of surgery alone or surgery plus preoperative paclitaxel/carboplatin chemotherapy in early stage non-small cell lung cancer: Preliminary results. Proc Am Soc Clin Oncol 23:LBA7012, 2005.

Rosen LS, Bordon D, Tchekmedyian S, et al: Zoledronic acid versus placebo in the treatment of skeletal metastases in patients with lung cancer and other solid tumors: A phase III, double-blind, randomized trial–The Zoledronic Acid Lung Cancer and Other Solid Tumors Study Group. J Clin Oncol 21:3150–3157, 2003.

Sandler AB, Gray R, Brahmer J, et al: Randomized phase II/III trial of paclitaxel plus carboplatin with or without bevacizumab in patients with advanced non-squamous non-small-cell lung cancer: An Eastern Cooperative Oncology Group trial. N Engl J Med In press.

Schiller JH, Harrington D, Belani CP, et al: Comparison of four chemotherapy regimens for advanced non–small-cell lung cancer. N Engl J Med 2:92–98, 2002.

Shepherd FA, Rodrigues Pereira J, Ciuleanu T, et al: Erlotinib in previously treated non-small-cell lung cancer. N Engl J Med 353:123–132, 2005.

Strauss GM: Adjuvant chemotherapy of lung cancer: Methodologic issues and therapeutic advances. Hematol Oncol Clin North Am 19:263–281, 2005.

Strauss GM, Herndon JE II, Maddaus MA, et al: Adjuvant chemotherapy in stage IB non-small cell lung cancer: Update of Cancer and Leukemia Group B protocol 9633 (abstract). J Clin Oncol 24:365s, 2006.

Sundstrom S, Bremnes RM, Aasebo U, et al: Hypofractionated palliative radiotherapy (17 Gy/2 fractions) in advanced NSCLC is comparable to standard fractionation for symptom control and survival: A national phase III trial. J Clin Oncol 22:801–810, 2004.

Swann RS, Machtay M, Komaki R, et al: Impact of overall treatment time during concurrent chemoradiotherapy for locally advanced NSCLC: An RTOG secondary analysis (abstract). Proc Am Soc Clin Oncol 23:7061, 2005.

Timmerman R, Papiez L, McGarry R, et al: Extracranial stereotactic radioablation: Results of a phase I study in medically inoperable stage I non–small-cell lung cancer patients. Chest 124:1946–1955, 2003.

Winton T, Livingston R, Johnson D, et al: Vinorelbine plus cisplatin vs. observation in resected non-small cell lung cancer. N Engl J Med 352:2589–2597, 2005.

CHAPTER 7

Small-cell lung cancer, mesothelioma, and thymoma

Bonnie S. Glisson, MD, Benjamin Movsas, MD, and Walter Scott, MD

As discussed in chapter 6, there are two major subdivisions of lung cancer: small-cell lung cancer (SCLC), for which chemotherapy is the primary treatment, and non–small-cell lung cancer (NSCLC). SCLC is decreasing in frequency in the United States, with recent data showing it represents only 14% of lung cancers. This chapter provides information on the staging and prognosis, pathology and pathophysiology, treatment, and follow-up of long-term survivors of SCLC and concludes with brief discussions on mesothelioma and thymoma.

Chapter 6 provides information on the epidemiology, etiology, screening and prevention, and diagnosis of lung cancer in general and covers NSCLC and carcinoid tumors of the lungs.

SMALL-CELL LUNG CANCER

Staging and prognosis

The TNM staging system, used for all NSCLC patients, does not predict well for survival in SCLC patients and is generally not utilized in SCLC, except for surgical staging (see chapter 6, Table 1). Rather, SCLC is usually described as either limited (M0) or extensive (M1), although these general terms are inadequate when evaluating the role of surgery. Patients with SCLC who have stages I–III disease, excluding those with a malignant pleural effusion, are classified as having limited disease. These patients constitute approximately one-third of all SCLC patients. The remaining SCLC patients fall into the extensive-disease category, which includes any patient with a malignant pleural effusion or any site of distant disease, such as the brain, liver, adrenal gland, bone, and bone marrow.

The staging of lung cancer must be conducted in a methodical and detailed manner to permit appropriate therapeutic recommendations and to allow comparison of treatment results from different institutions.

Stage is commonly reported as either clinical or pathologic. The former is based on noninvasive (or minimally invasive) tests, whereas the latter is based on tissue obtained during surgery (see chapter 6).

The most important prognostic factor in lung cancer is the stage of disease. Within a given disease stage, the next most important prognostic factors are performance status and recent weight loss. The two scales used to define performance status are the Eastern Cooperative Oncology Group (ECOG) performance status system and the Karnofsky performance index (see Appendix 1). In short, patients who are ambulatory have a significantly longer survival. Those who have lost ≥ 5% of body weight during the preceding 3–6 months have a worse prognosis.

Pathology and pathophysiology

SCLC tends to present with a large central lung mass and associated extensive hilar and mediastinal lymphadenopathy. Clinically evident distant metastases are present in approximately two-thirds of patients at diagnosis. Additionally, data from autopsy examination indicate micrometastatic disease in 63% of patients who died within 30 days of attempted curative resection of SCLC. Thus, it is a systemic disease at presentation in the majority of patients.

SCLC is a small, blue, round cell tumor that is primitive and undifferentiated at the light microscopic level. Electron microscopy demonstrates its neuroendocrine derivation by the presence of dense core granules. The immunohistochemical evidence of neuroendocrine derivation includes positive staining for chromogranin, synaptophysin, and other proteins. The APUD (amine precursor uptake and decarboxylation) machinery present in the dense core granule leads to the production of biologically active amines and promotes the synthesis of polypeptide hormones such as ADH and ACTH. Paraneoplastic syndromes due to hormone excess result. The most common of these syndromes, syndrome of inappropriate antidiuretic hormone secretion (SIADH), occurs in approximately 10% of patients with SCLC. Hypercortisolism and a Cushing's-like syndrome are more rare, seen in only 1%–2% of patients.

Treatment

TREATMENT OF DISEASE LIMITED TO LUNG PARENCHYMA

Surgery

The majority of patients with SCLC present with advanced-stage disease. In the 5%–10% of patients whose tumor is limited to the lung parenchyma, very often the diagnosis is established only after the lung mass has been removed. If, however, the histology has been determined by bronchoscopic biopsy or fine-needle aspiration and there is no evidence of metastatic disease following extensive scanning, examination of the bone marrow, and biopsy of the mediastinal lymph nodes, resection should be performed. Adjuvant chemotherapy is recommended because of the high likelihood of the development of distant metastases following surgery.

The surgical approach in SCLC is similar to that used in NSCLC: A lobectomy or pneumonectomy should be followed by a thorough mediastinal lymph node dissection. Tumor resection in SCLC should be limited to patients who have no evidence of mediastinal or supraclavicular lymph node metastases. Recent data suggest that patients with SCLC, presenting as a solitary pulmonary nodule and proven pathologically to be stage I, have a 5-year survival rate of ~70% when treated with resection and adjuvant chemotherapy.

TREATMENT OF DISEASE LIMITED TO THE THORAX

Approximately one-third of SCLC patients present with disease that is limited to the thorax and can be encompassed within a tolerable radiation portal. In early studies in which either radiation therapy or surgery alone was used to treat such patients, median survival was only 3–4 months, and the 5-year survival rate was in the range of 1%–2%. The reason for the failure of these therapies was both rapid recurrence of intrathoracic tumor and development of distant metastasis.

Chemotherapy

During the 1970s, it became apparent that SCLC was relatively sensitive to chemotherapy. Various combination chemotherapy regimens were used to treat limited SCLC. Although none of the regimens was clearly superior, median survival was approximately 12 months, and the 2-year survival rate was approximately 10%–15%. It appears that maintenance chemotherapy adds little to survival in patients with limited SCLC.

Chemotherapy plus thoracic irradiation

One of the major advances in treating SCLC in the past 15 years is the recognition of the value of early and concurrent thoracic chemoradiation therapy. This advance was clearly facilitated by the increase in therapeutic index when PE (cisplatin [Platinol]/etoposide) chemotherapy is given with thoracic irradiation, as opposed to older anthracycline or alkylator-based regimens. Although the major impact from this approach is improved locoregional control, there are also hints from randomized trials that early control of disease in the chest can also reduce the risk of distant metastasis.

An intergroup trial directly compared once-daily with twice-daily fractionation (45 Gy/25 fractions/5 weeks vs 45 Gy/30 fractions/3 weeks) given at the beginning of concurrent chemoradiation therapy with PE. Initial analysis showed excellent overall results, with median survival for all patients of 20 months and a 40% survival rate to 2 years. With a minimum follow-up of 5 years, survival was significantly better in the twice-daily than in the once-daily irradiation group

(26% vs 16%). The only difference in toxicity was a temporary increase in grade 3 esophagitis in patients receiving twice-daily radiation therapy.

Outcomes for patients with limited-stage SCLC have improved significantly over the past 20 years. In an analysis of phase III trials during this period, median survival was 12 months in the control arm in 26 phase III studies initiated between 1972 and 1981, compared with 17 months in studies between 1982 and 1992 ($P < .001$). Five studies demonstrated a statistically significant improvement in survival in the experimental arm compared with the control arm. Interestingly, all five studies involved some aspect of thoracic radiation therapy (three trials compared chemotherapy alone vs chemoradiation therapy; one compared early with late radiation therapy; and one compared daily vs twice-daily thoracic radiation therapy). Similarly, data from the Surveillance, Epidemiology, and End Results (SEER) database demonstrate that the 5-year survival rate has more than doubled from 1973 to 1996 (5.2% vs 12.2%, $P = .0001$).

Current recommendations Although important questions remain as to the optimal radiation doses, volumes, and timing with regard to chemotherapy, a reasonable standard is to deliver thoracic irradiation concurrently with PE chemotherapy (cisplatin [60 mg/m^2 IV on day 1] and etoposide [120 mg/ m^2 IV on days 1–3]). An attempt is made to integrate thoracic irradiation as early as possible, during cycle 1 (or 2). Fried et al performed a meta-analysis evaluating early vs late timing of radiation therapy in limited-stage SCLC. Earlier radiation therapy was defined as prior to 9 weeks after initiation of chemotherapy vs late radiation therapy (≥ 9 weeks). Seven trials (n = 1,542 patients) were included in the analysis. They reported a small but significant improvement in 2-year overall survival for early vs late radiation therapy (5.2%, $P = .03$). This finding is similar to the benefit of adding radiation therapy or prophylactic cranial irradiation to chemotherapy. A greater difference was evident for the subset of patients receiving early rather than late hyperfractionated radiation therapy and platinum-based chemotherapy. Hyperfractionated accelerated fractionation should be considered, given the results of the intergroup 0096 trial. The data extant do not indicate that chemotherapy beyond 4 cycles has a favorable impact on long-term outcome.

Irradiation can be incorporated sequentially with chemotherapy; however, this approach appears to be inferior to early concurrent therapy and should be reserved for use in those for whom concurrent approaches are predicted to be excessively toxic. Takada et al reported on a randomized trial of concurrent vs sequential thoracic radiotherapy in combination with PE (Platinol/etoposide) in over 200 patients with limited-stage SCLC demonstrated a benefit to concurrent therapy, with a median survival of 27.0 months (30%; concurrent arm) vs 19.7 months (20%; sequential arm, $P = .097$). Thoracic radiation therapy consisted of 45 Gy over 3 weeks, starting either with the first cycle of PE in the concurrent arm or after the fourth cycle in the sequential arm.

Results of an intergroup trial indicate that radiation therapy strategies that increase biologic dose can improve local control and survival. Further exploration of accelerated fractionation or conventional doses > 45 Gy is warranted and is currently being investigated in prospective trials.

Komaki et al recently reported on a phase I dose-escalation trial of thoracic radiotherapy with concurrent chemotherapy (Radiation Therapy Oncology Group [RTOG] 9712). In this regimen, the initial (larger) radiation field was treated once a day, and the smaller boost field was treated twice daily, to a maximum tolerated dose of 61.2 Gy.

Movsas et al reported the results of the first Patterns of Care Study (PCS) for lung cancer in the United States. This study was conducted to determine the national patterns of radiotherapy practice in patients treated for nonmetastatic lung cancer in 1998–1999. As supported by clinical trials, patients with limited-stage SCLC received chemotherapy plus radiotherapy more often than radiotherapy alone (92% vs 5%, $P < .0001$). However, the median radiotherapy dose was 50 Gy, 80% at 1.8–2.0 Gy per fraction. Only 6% of patients received hyperfractionated (twice-daily) radiotherapy. A total of 22% received prophylactic cranial irradiation (PCI), with a median dose of 30 Gy in 15 fractions. As key studies supporting twice-daily radiotherapy in PCI and NSCLC were published in 1999, the penetration of these trials will be assessed in the next PCS lung survey.

Interestingly, Choi et al reported long-term survival data from their phase I trial assessing chemotherapy with either standard daily radiotherapy or accelerated twice-daily radiotherapy as from the Cancer and Leukemia Group B (CALGB) 8837 trial. They previously reported that the maximum tolerated dose was 45 Gy in 30 fractions for twice-daily radiotherapy and > 70 Gy in 35 fractions for once-daily radiotherapy. The 5-year survival estimated (from this phase I trial) for the twice-daily arm was 20%, vs 36% for the once-daily radiotherapy arm. They suggest a phase III randomized trial to compare standard daily radiotherapy (to 70 Gy) vs twice-daily radiotherapy (to 45 Gy). Indeed, the long-term results of a phase III trial comparing once-daily irradiation (to 50.4 Gy in 28 fractions) vs twice-daily irradiation (to 48 Gy in 32 fractions via a split course) demonstrated similar outcomes in either arm. The median and 5-year survival rates of patients in this study (21 months and 20%, respectively) were similar to those reported by Turrisi et al.

Surgery

Although surgical resection is not usually part of the standard therapy for SCLC, the Japanese Clinical Oncology Lung Cancer Study Group reported the results of a phase II trial of postoperative adjuvant cisplatin/etoposide in patients with completely resected stages I–IIIA SCLC. The 5-year survival rates (in a cohort of 62 patients) for pathologic stages I, II, and IIIA SCLC were 69%, 38%, and 40%, respectively.

Prophylactic cranial irradiation

Recognition that patients with SCLC were at high risk for the development of brain metastases led to the suggestion that they be given PCI to prevent the clinical manifestation of previously present but occult CNS disease. The role of PCI has been controversial. Most trials have shown a reduction in CNS relapse

Based on promising data from a phase II trial, patients with extensive SCLC (aged 70 years or younger) were randomized to receive irinotecan/cisplatin vs etoposide/cisplatin in a phase III trial completed in Japan. Results of this trial demonstrated a 17% increase in response rate and 3.4-month improvement in median survival for the patients receiving irinotecan/cisplatin. Grade 3/4 diarrhea (16%) was more common on the irinotecan arm, whereas grade 3/4 neutropenia was more common with etoposide/cisplatin (92% vs 65%). Preliminary results of a confirmatory trial in the United States indicated no response rate or survival benefit for irinotecan/cisplatin using a schedule that was slightly different from that in the Japanese study. In this study, the median overall survival was 9.3 months for irinotecan/cisplatin and 10.2 months for etoposide/cisplatin. A second confirmatory trial with the schedule of irinotecan/cisplatin used by Noda et al is ongoing in the United States. *(Noda K, Nishiwaki Y, Kawahara M, et al: N Engl J Med 346:85-91, 2002; Hanna NH, Einhorn L, Sandler A, et al: J Clin Oncol [abstract] 23[suppl]:622s, 2005).*

rates but little effect on survival with PCI. There also has been concern about the contribution of PCI to the late neurologic deterioration seen in some patients with SCLC, although recent studies show neurologic impairment in many patients with SCLC prior to any treatment.

A meta-analysis of all randomized trials of PCI in patients with SCLC who achieved a complete or near-complete response to induction chemotherapy (alone or combined with thoracic irradiation) showed a statistically significant improvement in survival in patients treated with PCI (20.7% at 3 years vs 15.3% in those not given PCI). The survival improvement with PCI was seen in all patient subgroups, regardless of age, stage of disease, type of induction treatment, or performance status.

Model calculations from data on patterns of failure in patients achieving a systemic complete response suggest that the greatest gain in survival to be expected with PCI is in the range of 5%. To demonstrate this convincingly would require randomized trials of about 700 patients–substantially larger than trials conducted to date. However, the recent meta-analysis of randomized trials of PCI in SCLC patients achieving complete or near-complete response of systemic disease showed a survival improvement of this magnitude with PCI.

Current recommendations Patients should be offered PCI if they have achieved a complete or near-complete remission of disease outside the CNS. Use of chemotherapeutic agents with known CNS toxicity (eg, methotrexate, procarbazine [Matulane], and nitrosoureas) should be avoided, and chemotherapy should not be given during or after irradiation.

Radiation doses for PCI should probably be in the range of 25–30 Gy, with a daily fraction size of 2.0–2.5 Gy, although recent data suggest that such doses delay and reduce rates of CNS relapse but may not eliminate it; thus, higher doses may warrant exploration. Larger fraction sizes would be expected to produce greater toxicity. Smaller fractions given twice daily may reduce toxicity, and trials of this approach are under way.

TABLE 1: Common chemotherapy regimens for SCLC

Drug/combination	Dose and schedule
Etoposide + cisplatin or carboplatin	
Etoposide	100-120 mg/m^2 IV on days 1-3
Cisplatin	60-75 mg/m^2 IV on day 1
	or
Etoposide	100 mg/m^2 IV on days 1-3
Carboplatin	Area under the curve of 5 mg/mL/min IV on day 1
Repeat cycle every 3 weeks.	
Irinotecan + cisplatin	
Irinotecan	60 mg/m^2 on days 1, 8, and 15
Cisplatin	60 mg/m^2 IV on day 1
Repeat cycle every 4 weeks for 4 cycles.	

Noda K, Nishiwaki Y, Kawahara M, et al: N Engl J Med 346:85–91, 2002.

Table prepared by Ishmael Jaiyesimi, DO

TREATMENT OF EXTENSIVE DISEASE

As mentioned previously, two-thirds of SCLC patients have extensive disease at diagnosis. Without treatment, median survival in this group of patients is 6–8 weeks. Treatment with combination chemotherapy increases the median survival duration to approximately 8–10 months.

Combination chemotherapy

The combination of cisplatin or carboplatin (Paraplatin)/etoposide (see Table 1 for common dose ranges) is considered the standard of care in the United States at this time. This standard is primarily based on therapeutic index, as randomized trials have not demonstrated a survival benefit for this combination relative to the older regimen of cyclophosphamide, doxorubicin, and vincristine. The regimen is repeated at 3-week intervals for 4 to 6 courses. Randomized trials of maintenance chemotherapy, either with other drugs or reduced doses of the induction regimen, show improvement in the duration of remission but no impact on overall survival.

New agents

A variety of novel agents have been investigated in SCLC. Of these agents, the taxanes and topoisomerase I inhibitors, particularly topotecan (Hycamtin), have demonstrated the greatest efficacy.

Taxanes Because of their novel mechanism of action and clinical activity in other solid tumors, including NSCLC, the taxanes–paclitaxel and docetaxel (Taxotere)–are particularly attractive agents for evaluation in the treatment of SCLC.

Paclitaxel Ettinger et al reported that single-agent paclitaxel produces an overall response rate of 34% in untreated patients with SCLC. This taxane is currently being evaluated in combination with a variety of different agents, including etoposide and cisplatin (or carboplatin), in SCLC patients.

Docetaxel Compared with paclitaxel, docetaxel appears to have a slightly lower response rate of 26% (12 of 46 patients), even when administered at a dose of 100 mg/m^2, as reported by the Southwest Oncology Group (SWOG). This lower response rate with docetaxel was offset somewhat by the fact that median survival was promising at 9 months, similar to that obtained with combination chemotherapy. Disturbingly, however, the median time to disease progression was only 3 months.

Topoisomerase I inhibitors The topoisomerase I inhibitors–topotecan and irinotecan (CPT-11 [Camptosar])–are clearly active in SCLC, with single-agent response rates of 40%–60%. The topoisomerase I inhibitors have been studied in patients with recurrent and refractory SCLC, as many of these patients have been previously exposed to topoisomerase II inhibitors (epipodophyllotoxins/anthracyclines) during the induction phase of therapy. Furthermore, preclinical data suggest that topoisomerase I levels are upregulated in cells resistant to topoisomerase II inhibitors, via downregulation of topoisomerase II levels.

Topotecan A randomized, phase III trial compared topotecan vs CAV (cyclophosphamide, doxorubicin [Adriamycin], vincristine) in patients who had a response to initial therapy and a minimum drug-free interval of 60 days. Overall response rates were 24% for topotecan alone vs 18% for CAV ($P > .05$). Time to disease progression and median survival also were similar in the two arms. However, topotecan offered superior palliation for many disease-related symptoms, including dyspnea, fatigue, and hoarseness, and also improved patients' ability to perform daily tasks. Moreover, topotecan had toxicities similar to those of CAV, with the exception of a slight increase in grade 4 thrombocytopenia.

Oral topotecan and cisplatin were compared with etoposide/cisplatin in a randomized phase III trial in patients with previously untreated extensive-stage SCLC. Preliminary results show that the median survival was 39.3 weeks for the topotecan arm vs 40.3 weeks for the etoposide/cisplatin arm. There were also no significant differences in response, time to disease progression, or toxicity profile for the two regimens.

Irinotecan also has been investigated in recurrent or refractory SCLC in a limited number of patients. Like topotecan and other new agents, irinotecan produced a disappointingly low response rate among patients with SCLC resistant to primary chemotherapy, with only 1 of 27 patients exhibiting a response. In contrast, the response rate to irinotecan among patients with initially sensitive disease that later recurred was 29%.

Data from Japan suggest a 4-month overall survival benefit for irinotecan and cisplatin combined as induction therapy for patients with extensive disease. The data await confirmation; a randomized American trial is ongoing.

Other agents, such as gemcitabine (Gemzar) and vinorelbine, have shown activity in SCLC, but it has been less impressive than that reported for the taxanes and topoisomerase I inhibitors.

Phase II trials of new combinations, such as PET (cisplatin [Platinol]/etoposide/paclitaxel [Taxol]) and topotecan/paclitaxel, have yielded promising median and 2-year survival estimates in patients with extensive disease. Three phase III trials testing PET vs PE have, however, shown only excessive toxicity in the experimental arms without improvement in efficacy. Final data from similar trials with topotecan/paclitaxel are awaited.

Experimental approaches

A variety of experimental approaches have been tested in SCLC. They include high doses of chemotherapy and autologous bone marrow transplantation (BMT), alternating regimens of chemotherapy, and weekly administration of chemotherapy.

High-dose chemotherapy plus BMT Most phase II trials using high doses of chemotherapy plus BMT appear to show no advantage to the high-dose approach over standard doses of chemotherapy.

Alternating chemotherapy regimens have been used to overcome drug resistance. In randomized trials, alternating chemotherapy regimens have shown a slight improvement in terms of median survival (4–6 weeks) when compared with a single chemotherapeutic regimen but no improvement in long-term survival.

PALLIATION OF LOCAL AND DISTANT SYMPTOMS

Radiation therapy

Many patients with lung cancer have distressing local symptoms at some point in their disease course. These symptoms may arise from airway obstruction by the primary tumor, compression of mediastinal structures by nodal metastases, or metastatic involvement of distant organs. Radiation therapy is effective in palliating most local symptoms as well as symptoms at common metastatic sites, such as bone and brain.

Doses In the United States, most radiation oncologists use doses in the range of 30 Gy in 10 fractions for palliative treatment. Data from the United Kingdom suggest that similar efficacy without greater toxicity may be achieved with more abbreviated schedules, such as 17 Gy in 2 fractions 1 week apart or single fractions of 11 Gy (see chapter 6, Table 5). Such schedules may facilitate the coordination of irradiation and chemotherapy and also reduce patient travel and hospitalization.

Endobronchial irradiation with cobalt-60 or iridium-192 has been used to palliate symptoms arising from partial airway obstruction, including cough, dyspnea, and hemoptysis. The dosimetric advantage of being able to deliver a high radiation dose to the obstructing endobronchial tumor while sparing adjacent normal structures, such as the lungs, spinal cord, and esophagus, has clear appeal, particularly in the patient whose disease has recurred following prior external-beam irradiation. Although good rates of palliation have been reported with endobronchial irradiation, significant complications, including fatal hemoptysis, are seen in 5%–10% of patients. Whether this represents a true treatment complication vs the underlying disease remains unclear.

Other local approaches

Endobronchial irradiation should be considered as only one of several approaches (including laser excision, cryotherapy, and stent placement) in the treatment of patients with symptomatic airway obstruction, and management should be individualized. All of these approaches are more suitable for partial than for complete airway obstruction.

Chemotherapy

Several recent trials have explored the use of chemotherapy to palliate specific symptoms in patients with lung cancer. In general, these trials have found that rates of symptomatic improvement were considerably higher than objective response rates and were not dissimilar to symptomatic response rates with local radiation therapy. Chemotherapy in the newly diagnosed patient is highly palliative for relief of symptoms related to superior vena cava syndrome, obstructive lung disease, and painful bony metastases. In the patient with recurrent disease, irradiation is more commonly associated with symptomatic relief from these localized problems. Radiation therapy remains the standard of care for even chemotherapy-naive patients with spinal cord compression or symptomatic brain metastasis.

Follow-up of long-term survivors

At present, no standard follow-up protocol exists for patients with cured SCLC or NSCLC. However, at least long-term follow-up should include serial physical examinations once the patient has reached the 5-year mark. Controversy currently exists about the value of utilizing CT scanning or even chest x-rays for the long-term follow-up of these patients.

In this vein, retrospective reviews of the literature have revealed that patients with SCLC appear to have the highest rate of second primary tumor development, as high as 30% over the course of their lifetime, with some studies reporting annual second primary tumor rates of 5%–10%. Therefore, the concept of chemoprevention appears to have particular merit in these patients.

MESOTHELIOMA

Mesotheliomas are uncommon neoplasms derived from the cells lining the pleura and peritoneum. Currently, 2,000–3,000 new cases are diagnosed in the United States each year.

Epidemiology

Gender Men are affected five times more commonly than women.

Age The median age at diagnosis is 60 years.

Etiology and risk factors

Asbestos exposure The relationship between asbestos exposure and diffuse pleural mesothelioma was first reported by Wagner, who documented 33 pathologically confirmed cases from an asbestos mining region in South Africa. Selikoff and colleagues documented a 300-fold increase in mortality from mesothelioma among asbestos insulation workers in the New York metropolitan region when compared with the general population. The interval between asbestos exposure and tumor formation is commonly 3–4 decades.

Asbestos fibers are generally divided into two broad groups: serpentine and amphibole. The latter includes crocidolite, the most carcinogenic form of asbestos. The inability of phagocytic cells to digest the fiber appears to initiate a cascade of cellular events that results in free-radical generation and carcinogenesis.

Diagnosis

Patients with mesothelioma usually seek medical attention while the disease is limited to a single hemithorax and commonly complain of dyspnea and pain. Dyspnea results from diffuse growth of the tumor on both the parietal and visceral pleurae, which encases the lung in a thick rind. Pain is caused by direct tumor infiltration of intercostal nerves.

Chest x-ray and CT Chest x-ray demonstrates pleural thickening, pleura-based masses, or a pleural effusion. Chest CT scan more accurately portrays the extent of disease and frequently reveals chest wall invasion, as well as pericardial and diaphragmatic extension.

Thoracentesis and thoracoscopy Thoracentesis and pleural biopsy usually are sufficient to establish the diagnosis of malignancy, but a thoracoscopic or open biopsy is often required to provide enough tissue to make an accurate histologic diagnosis of mesothelioma.

Distinguishing mesothelioma from other neoplasms Light microscopy is often insufficient for differentiating among mesothelioma, metastatic adenocarcinoma, and sarcoma. Immunohistochemistry and electron microscopy are frequently necessary to establish the diagnosis.

Although adenocarcinomas stain positive for carcinoembryonic antigen (CEA), Leu-M1, and secretory component, mesotheliomas stain negative for these markers. Mesotheliomas stain positive for cytokeratin, whereas sarcomas do not. Mesotheliomas have characteristically long microvilli that are well demonstrated by the electron microscope; adenocarcinomas have short microvilli.

Pathology

Mesotheliomas may contain both epithelial and sarcomatoid elements and are classified by the relative abundance of each component. Epithelial mesotheliomas are most common (50%), followed by mixed (34%) and sarcomatoid (16%) tumors. Survival for the epithelial type is 22 months, compared with patients with only 6 months for patients with other types.

Staging and prognosis

The most commonly utilized staging system for mesothelioma, that of Butchart, is based on inexact descriptions of the extent of local tumor growth or distant metastases (Table 2). Other, more detailed staging systems based on TNM criteria have been proposed.

The median survival following diagnosis ranges from 9–21 months. Although autopsy series have demonstrated distant metastases in as many as 50% of patients with mesothelioma, death usually results from local tumor growth.

PET scanning may prove to be a viable prognostic tool for malignant pleural mesothelioma.

Treatment

Treatment rarely results in cure and should be considered palliative.

Combined-modality treatment options include chest tube insertion and pleurodesis to control the pleural effusion. Currently, there is renewed interest in aggressive treatment that includes extrapleural pneumonectomy with concomitant resection of the diaphragm and pericardium, followed by chemotherapy and radiotherapy. Recent studies are exploring the role of postoperative intensity-modulated radiotherapy in this setting. Subtotal pleurectomy is a less extensive surgical procedure that debulks the majority of tumor, permits reexpansion of the lung, and prevents recurrence of the pleural effusion.

Chemotherapy The benefit of chemotherapy for patients who have unresectable mesothelioma was clarified in a recent randomized trial. This study was a single-blind, multicenter, two-arm trial with cisplatin alone in the control arm and cisplatin combined with the multitargeted antifolate pemetrexed (Alimta) in the experimental arm. The study was based on the observation that pemetrexed produced a 16% objective response rate in previous phase II evaluation. In the randomized trial, patients treated with pemetrexed and cisplatin had an estimated median survival of 12.1 months, as compared with 9.3 months in those treated with cisplatin alone. On the basis of this improvement in survival, the combination of pemetrexed and cisplatin has received an FDA indication for the treatment of unresectable mesothelioma. The same combination is undergoing further evaluation in a neoadjuvant approach in patients with resectable disease.

TABLE 2: Staging of mesothelioma according to Butchart

Stage	Description
I	Tumor confined within the "capsule" of the parietal pleura, ie, involving only the ipsilateral pleura, lungs, pericardium, and diaphragm
II	Tumor invading the chest wall or involving mediastinal structures, eg, the esophagus, heart, opposite pleura; lymph node involvement within the chest
III	Tumor penetrating the diaphragm to involve the peritoneum; involvement of opposite pleura; lymph node involvement outside the chest
IV	Distant blood-borne metastases

THYMOMA

Thymoma is a rare mediastinal tumor that occurs mainly in the anterosuperior mediastinum.

Epidemiology

Gender The tumor affects both sexes equally.

Age Thymoma is most often seen in people in the fourth and fifth decades of life.

Etiology and associated syndromes

The etiology of thymoma is unknown, and the risk factors have not been identified. Thymoma is a tumor originating within the epithelial cells of the thymus. One-third to one-half of patients present with an asymptomatic anterior mediastinal mass, one-third present with local symptoms (eg, cough, chest pain, superior vena cava syndrome, and/or dysphagia), and one-third of cases are detected during the evaluation of myasthenia gravis. Distant metastases are distinctly uncommon at initial presentation of this tumor.

In addition to myasthenia gravis, which occurs in approximately 30% of patients with thymoma, a host of paraneoplastic syndromes have been seen in association with thymoma. These other syndromes, which occur in less than 5% of patients, include pure red cell aplasia, hypogammaglobulinemia, and a variety of other autoimmune disorders.

Diagnosis

The most commonly described symptoms are pleuritic chest pain or discomfort, dry cough, and dyspnea. Physical examination may reveal adenopathy, wheezing, fever, superior vena cava syndrome, vocal cord paralysis, and other paraneoplastic syndromes.

Chest x-ray and CT scan A chest x-ray provides an initial basis for diagnosis. The location, size, density, and presence of calcification within the mass can all be determined. Comparison of the film to previously obtained films is usually helpful.

Following identification of a mediastinal mass on conventional radiography, contrast-enhanced CT scanning should be performed. CT scanning can differentiate the cystic form from a solid lesion as well as the presence of fat, calcium, or fluid within the lesion. MRI is increasingly available for use in the evaluation of mediastinal pathology, but it is less frequently utilized than CT. MRI is superior to CT scanning in defining the relationship between mediastinal masses and vascular structures and is useful in the assessment of vascular invasion by the tumor.

Invasive diagnostic tests CT-guided percutaneous needle biopsy specimens are obtained using fine-needle aspiration techniques and cytologic evaluation or with larger-core needle biopsy and histologic evaluation. Fine-needle specimens are usually adequate to distinguish carcinomatosis lesions, but core biopsies may be necessary to distinguish most mediastinal neoplasms. Immunohistochemical techniques and electron microscopy have greatly improved the ability to differentiate the cell of origin in mediastinal neoplasms. Most series reported diagnostic yields for percutaneous needle biopsy of 70%–100%.

Mediastinoscopy is a relatively simple surgical procedure accomplished with the patient under general anesthesia. It is an adequate approach to the superior, middle, and upper posterior mediastinum, and most series report a diagnostic accuracy of 80%–90%. Anterior mediastinotomy (Chamberlain approach) provides for direct biopsy of tissue and has a diagnostic yield of 95%–100%. Thoracotomy is occasionally necessary to diagnose mediastinal neoplasms, but its indications have been largely supplanted by video-assisted thoracoscopic techniques, which yield 100% accuracy.

The most common tumors in the differential diagnosis of an anterior mediastinal tumor are lymphomas and germ-cell tumors. Immunohistochemical markers are helpful to differentiate thymoma from tumors originating from other cell types.

Pathology

Three of the most common classification schemes for thymoma are listed in Table 3. Verley and Hollman propose a classification system based on tumor architecture, cellular differentiation, and predominant cell type. Bernatz et al describe a simpler classification by presenting thymoma based on the percentage of epithelial cells and lymphocytes. In both of these systems, thymoma with a predominance of epithelial cells is associated with a greater increased incidence of invasion and a subsequently worse prognosis.

TABLE 3: Clinicopathologic correlates of thymoma

Authors	Number of patients	Subgroups (percentage)
Verley and Hollman	200	Type I: Spindle and oval cells (30)
		Type II: Lymphocyte rich (30)
		Type III: Differentiated epithelial rich (33)
		Type IV: Undifferentiated epithelial rich (equivalent to thymic carcinoma) (7)
Bernatz et al	283	Predominantly lymphocytic (25)
		Mixed lymphoepithelial (43)
		Predominantly epithelial (25)
		Spindle cell (6)
Muller-Hermelink et al	58	Cortical (43)
		Mixed: Predominantly cortical (8)
		Mixed: Common (36)
		Medullary (5)
		Mixed: Predominantly medullary (8)

Staging and prognosis

The staging system proposed by Masaoka et al has been widely adopted (Table 4). Stage is an independent predictor of recurrence and long-term survival. The 5-year survival rates are 96% for stage I thymoma, 86% for stage II, 69% for stage III, and 50% for stage IV.

Treatment

SURGICAL TREATMENT

All patients whose tumors are potentially resectable should undergo surgery. If the patient has evidence of myasthenia gravis, a preoperative consultation with a clinical neurologist should be considered. The incision of choice is almost always a median sternotomy, which is quick and easy to make and provides excellent exposure to the anterior mediastinum and neck. Although the surgeon is considered the best judge of a tumor's invasiveness, it is often difficult to grossly separate invasion from adherence to surrounding tissue. Experience with minimally invasive approaches (such as transcervical thymectomy) is growing; however, until longer term data become available, sternotomy should still be considered the standard surgical approach.

Complete resection of thymoma has been found to be the most significant predictor of long-term survival. Several studies have examined the extent of surgical resection on survival and disease-free survival rates. In 241 operative cases, Maggi and colleagues found an 82% overall survival rate in those whose tu-

TABLE 4: Thymoma staging system of Masaoka et al

Stage	Description
I	Macroscopically completely encapsulated Microscopically no capsular invasion
II	Macroscopic invasion into surrounding fatty tissue or mediastinal pleura Microscopic invasion into the capsule
III	Macroscopic invasion into neighboring organs (pericardium, great vessels, lungs)
IVA	Pleural or pericardial dissemination
IVB	Lymphogenous or hematogenous metastasis

Masaoka A, Monden Y, Nakahara K, et al: Cancer 48:2485, 1981.

mors underwent complete resection and a 26% survival rate at 7 years in those undergoing biopsy alone. Other investigators reported similar results in surgical patients. Therefore, regardless of stage, tumor resectability is one of the important predictors of treatment outcome.

RADIATION TREATMENT

Thymomas are generally radiosensitive tumors, and the use of radiation therapy in their treatment is well established. It has been used to treat all stages of thymoma, either before or after surgical resection. General agreement exists regarding the postoperative treatment of invasive thymoma (stages II and III). The value of adjuvant radiation therapy for invasive thymomas is well documented and should be included in the treatment regimen regardless of the completeness of tumor resection.

CHEMOTHERAPY

Chemotherapy has been used in the treatment of invasive thymomas with increasing frequency during the past decade (Table 5). The most active agents appear to be cisplatin, doxorubicin, ifosfamide (Ifex), and corticosteroids. Combination chemotherapy has generally shown higher response rates and has been used in both neoadjuvant and adjuvant settings and in the treatment of metastatic or recurrent thymomas. CAP or CAPPr (cyclophosphamide, Adriamycin [doxorubicin], Platinol [cisplatin], and prednisone) regimens have been used in neoadjuvant and/or adjuvant settings. These regimens have also been used for recurrent thymoma.

Unresectable thymoma

Advanced-stage (III/IVA) thymomas are usually difficult to remove completely. Multidisciplinary approaches, including induction chemotherapy followed by surgical resection, postoperative radiation therapy, and consolidation chemotherapy, have been reported.

TABLE 5: Common chemotherapy regimens for thymoma

Regimen	Dose and schedule
CAPPr	
Cyclophosphamide	500 mg/m^2 IV on day 1
Adriamycin (doxorubicin)	20 $mg/m^2/d$ infused continuously on days 1-3
Platinol (cisplatin)	30 $mg/m^2/d$ IV on days 1-3
Prednisone	100 mg/d PO on days 1-5
Repeat cycle every 3-4 weeks.	
Adapted from Shin DM, Walsh GL, Komaki R, et al: Ann Intern Med 129:100–104, 1998.	
Single agent	
Cisplatin	100 mg/m^2 IV on day 1
Appropriate IV prehydration, posthydration along with mannitol and electrolytes	
Repeat cycle every 3 weeks.	
Adapted from Bonomi PD, Finkelstein D, Aisner S, et al: Am J Clin Oncol 16:342–345, 1993.	
Ifosfamide	1.5 g/m^2 infused continuously on days 1-5
Mesna	Continuous infusion as appropriate
Repeat cycle every 3 weeks.	
Adapted from Highley MS, Underhill CR, Parnis FX, et al: J Clin Oncol 17:2737–2744, 1999.	

Table prepared by Ishmael Jaiyesimi, DO

Induction chemotherapy consists of cyclophosphamide (500 mg/m^2 IV on day 1), doxorubicin (20 $mg/m^2/d$, continuous infusion, on days 1–3), cisplatin (30 $mg/m^2/d$ IV on days 1–3), and prednisone (100 mg/d PO on days 1–5), repeated every 3–4 weeks for 3 courses. Twenty-two evaluable patients were consecutively treated from 1990 to 2000 in a prospective phase II study at M. D. Anderson Cancer Center. After induction chemotherapy, 17 of 22 patients (77%) had major responses, including 3 complete responses.

Twenty-one patients underwent surgical resection. All patients received postoperative radiation therapy and consolidation chemotherapy. With a median follow-up of 50.3 months, overall survival rates at 5 years and 7 years were 95% and 79%, respectively. The rate of disease progression-free survival was 77% at 5 and 7 years. The multidisciplinary approaches to unresectable thymoma appear to be promising.

SUGGESTED READING

ON SMALL-CELL LUNG CANCER

Auperin A, Arriagada R, Pignon J-P, et al: Prophylactic cranial irradiation for patients with small-cell lung cancer in complete remission. Prophylactic Cranial Irradiation Overview Collaborative Group. N Engl J Med 341:476–484, 1999.

De Ruysscher D, Pijls-Johannesma M, Bentzen SM, et al: Time between the first day of chemotherapy and the last day of chest radiation is the most important predictor of survival in limited-disease small-cell lung cancer. J Clin Oncol 24:1057-1063, 2006.

Fried DB, Morris DE, Poole C, et al: Systematic review evaluating the timing of thoracic radiation therapy in combined modality therapy for limited-stage small-cell lung cancer. J Clin Oncol 22:4837-4845, 2004.

Glisson BS: Recurrent small cell lung cancer: Update. Semin Oncol 30:72-78, 2003.

Hanna N, Bunn PA Jr, Langer C, et al: Randomized phase III trial comparing irinotecan/cisplatin with etoposide/cisplatin in patients with previously untreated extensive-stage small-cell lung cancer. J Clin Oncol 24:2038-2043, 2006.

Janne PA, Freidlin B, Saxman S, et al: Twenty-five years of clinical research for patients with limited-stage small cell lung carcinoma in North America. Cancer 95:1528-1538, 2002.

Movsas B, Moughan J, Komaki R, et al: Radiotherapy (RT) Patterns of Care Study (PCS) in lung carcinoma. J Clin Oncol 24:4553–4559, 2003.

Neill HB, Herndon JE, Miller AA, et al: Randomized phase III intergroup trial of etoposide and cisplatin with or without paclitaxel and granulocyte colony-stimulating factor in patients with extensive stage small-cell lung cancer. Cancer and Leukemia Group B Trial 9732. J Clin Oncol 23:3752–3759, 2005.

Turrisi A, Kim K, Blum R, et al: Twice-daily compared with once-daily thoracic radiotherapy in limited small-cell lung cancer treated concurrently with cisplatin and etoposide. N Engl J Med 340:265–271, 1999.

Videtic GM, Stitt LW, Dar AR, et al: Continued cigarette smoking by patients receiving concurrent chemoradiotherapy for limited-stage small-cell lung cancer is associated with decreased survival. J Clin Oncol 21:1544-1549, 2003.

ON MESOTHELIOMA

Hazarika M, White RM Jr, Booth BP, et al: Pemetrexed in malignant pleural mesothelioma. Clin Cancer Res 11:982–992, 2005.

ON THYMOMA

Kim ES, Putnam JB, Komaki R, et al: A phase II study of a multidisciplinary approach with induction chemotherapy, followed by surgical resection, radiation therapy, and consolidation chemotherapy for unresectable malignant thymomas: Final report. Lung Cancer 44:369–379, 2004.

CHAPTER 8

Breast cancer overview

Risk factors, screening, genetic testing, and prevention

Lori Jardines, MD, Bruce G. Haffty, MD, Paul Fisher, MD,
Jeffrey Weitzel, MD, and Melanie Royce, MD, PhD

Breast cancer is the most common malignancy in women, accounting for 31% of all female cancers. Breast cancer also is responsible for 15% of cancer deaths in women, making it the number-two cause of cancer death. An estimated 178,480 new invasive breast cancer cases diagnosed in women in the United States in the year 2007, and 40,460 women will die of this cancer. There are approximately 2 million breast cancer survivors in the United States.

This chapter provides an overview of breast cancer, with discussions of epidemiology, etiology and risk factors, genetic cancer risk assessment, signs and symptoms, screening and diagnosis, prevention (including lifestyle changes and chemoprevention), staging, and prognosis. The three chapters to follow focus on the management of stages 0 and I, stage II, and stages III and IV breast cancer.

Epidemiology

Gender Breast cancer is relatively uncommon in men; the female-to-male ratio is approximately 100:1. It accounts for < 1% of all cancer cases in men, and an estimated 450 men will die of the disease in 2007. The incidence of breast cancer in men has remained relatively stable over the past decades, except in Africa, where for unclear reasons the incidence is rising. *BRCA* mutations are associated with an increased risk for breast cancer in men.

The most common presentation in men is asymmetric gynecomastia, often related to a single effect of drug therapy (such as from digoxin) or liver failure. All palpable masses in men should be carefully examined. Based upon the findings on physical examination, mammography and breast ultrasonography should be considered. Fine-needle aspiration (FNA) or core biopsy can be used to distinguish between gynecomastia and breast cancer. Core biopsy may be performed if the FNA is nondiagnostic.

Age The risk of developing breast cancer increases with age. The disease is uncommon in women younger than 40 years of age; only about 0.8% of breast cancers occur in women < 30 years old and approximately 6.5% develop in women between 30 and 40 years old.

TABLE 1: Survival of women with breast cancer, according to stage, without chemotherapy

Stage	Survival rate at 8 years (%)
I	90
II	70
III	40
IV	10

Race Caucasian women have a higher overall rate of breast cancer than African-American women; however, this difference is not apparent until age 50 and is marked only after menopause. The incidence of breast cancer in American Asian and Hispanic women is approximately half that in American Caucasian women. Breast cancer risk is extremely low in Native-American women.

Geography There is at least a fivefold variation in the incidence of breast cancer among different countries, although this difference appears to be narrowing. The incidence of breast cancer is significantly lower in Japan, Thailand, Nigeria, and India than in Denmark, the Netherlands, New Zealand, Switzerland, the United Kingdom, and the United States. Women living in North America have the highest rate of breast cancer in the world. It has been suggested that these trends in breast cancer incidence may be related, in some way, to dietary influences, particularly dietary fat consumption (see section on "Etiology and risk factors").

Socioeconomic status The incidence of breast cancer is higher in women of higher socioeconomic background. This relationship is most likely related to lifestyle differences, such as age at first birth.

Disease site The left breast is involved slightly more frequently than the right, and the most common locations of the disease are the upper outer quadrant and retroareolar region. The risk of contralateral breast cancer in women with *BRCA* mutations is approximately 40% at 10 years after the initial diagnosis of breast cancer. This risk is higher in *BRCA1* than *BRCA2* mutation carriers and those first diagnosed at age < 50.

Risk for breast cancer may be reduced in women who take tamoxifen. It may also be reduced in women who undergo bilateral salpingo-oophorectomy (BSO), especially when this procedure is performed in women younger than age 50. The protective effect of BSO is pronounced among women who develop breast cancer premenopausally.

Survival Survival rates for patients with nonmetastatic breast cancer have improved in recent years (Table 1). These improvements may be secondary to advances in adjuvant chemotherapy and radiation therapy. The contribution of screening mammography to breast cancer–specific survival is variable, favoring a reduction in breast cancer mortality of up to 25% in some series. Its impact on overall survival is less certain.

Etiology and risk factors

Numerous risk factors have been associated with the development of breast cancer, including genetic, environmental, hormonal, and nutritional influences. Despite all of the available data on breast cancer risk factors, 75% of women with this cancer have no risk factors.

Genetic factors Hereditary forms of breast cancer constitute only 5%–7% of breast cancer cases overall. However, the magnitude of the probability that a woman will develop cancer if she inherits a highly penetrant cancer gene mutation justifies the intense interest in predictive testing. Commercial testing is available for several genes (*BRCA1, BRCA2,* and *p53)* associated with a high risk for breast cancer development.

Elevated risk for breast cancer is also associated with mutations in the *PTEN* gene in Cowden's syndrome (described later), and a modest increased risk (relative risk of 3.9–6.4) may be seen in women who are heterozygous for a mutation in the *ATM* gene, which is associated with the recessive disease ataxia-telangiectasia in the homozygous state. A moderately increased risk for breast cancer (2-fold for women and 10-fold for men) was recently associated with a variant (1100 delC) in the cell-cycle checkpoint kinase gene, CHEK2, among families without *BRCA* gene mutations.

BRCA1 gene The *BRCA1* gene is located on chromosome 17. This gene is extremely large and complex, and more than 1,000 different mutations have been discovered, distributed along the entire gene. *BRCA1* mutations are inherited in an autosomal-dominant fashion and are associated with an increased risk for breast, ovarian, and, to a lesser degree, prostate cancers. A *BRCA1* mutation carrier has a lifetime risk of developing breast cancer on the order of 56%–85% and a 15%–45% lifetime risk of developing ovarian cancer.

BRCA2 gene The *BRCA2* gene was localized to chromosome 13. *BRCA2* is approximately twice as large as *BRCA1* and similarly complex.

Alterations in *BRCA2* have been associated with an increased incidence of breast cancer in both women (similar to *BRCA1*) and men (6% lifetime risk). Increased risk for ovarian cancer, pancreatic cancer, prostate cancer, and melanoma has also been reported. Together, *BRCA1* and *BRCA2* account for most hereditary breast and ovarian cancer families and approximately half of hereditary breast cancer families.

The incidence of *BRCA* gene mutations in the general breast cancer population is unknown, since most of the data have come from studies of high-risk populations. In one population-based study of women with breast cancer, only 9.4% of women < 35 years of age at the time of diagnosis and 12.0% of women < 45 years old who also had a first-degree relative with breast cancer had germline *BRCA1* or *BRCA2* mutations. However, a 40-year-old woman of Ashkenazi Jewish ancestry who has breast cancer has a 20%–30% probability of bearing one of three founder *BRCA* gene mutations, based on data from high-risk clinics, testing vendors, and Israeli series.

Li-Fraumeni syndrome This rare syndrome is characterized by premenopausal breast cancer in combination with childhood sarcoma, brain tumors, leukemia, and adrenocortical carcinoma. Tumors frequently occur in childhood and early adulthood and often present as multiple primaries in the same individual. Germline mutations in the *p53* gene on chromosome 17p have been documented in persons with this syndrome. Inheritance is autosomal dominant, with a penetrance of at least 50% by age 50.

Cowden's syndrome is inherited as an autosomal-dominant trait and is notable for a distinctive skin lesion (trichilemmoma) and mucocutaneous lesions. Patients with this uncommon syndrome have a high incidence of GI polyps and thyroid disorders; lifetime estimates for breast cancer among women with this syndrome range from 25%–50%. Germline mutations in the *PTEN* gene, located on chromosome 10q23, are responsible for this syndrome.

Family history The overall relative risk of breast cancer in a woman with a positive family history in a first-degree relative (mother, daughter, or sister) is 1.7. Premenopausal onset of the disease in a first-degree relative is associated with a threefold increase in breast cancer risk, whereas postmenopausal diagnosis increases the relative risk by only 1.5. When the first-degree relative has bilateral disease, there is a fivefold increase in risk. The relative risk for a woman whose first-degree relative developed bilateral breast cancer prior to menopause is nearly 9.

Proliferative breast disease The diagnosis of certain conditions after breast biopsy is also associated with an increased risk for the subsequent development of invasive breast cancer. They include moderate or florid ductal hyperplasia and sclerosing adenosis, which pose only a slightly increased risk of breast cancer (1.5–2.0 times); atypical ductal or lobular hyperplasia, which moderately increases risk (4–5 times); and lobular carcinoma in situ (LCIS), which markedly increases risk (8–11 times; see more detailed discussion of LCIS in chapter 9). Patients who have a family history of breast cancer along with a personal history of atypical epithelial hyperplasia have an 8-fold increase in breast cancer risk when compared with patients with a positive family history alone and an 11-fold increase in breast cancer risk when compared with patients who do not have atypical hyperplasia and have a negative family history.

Personal cancer history A personal history of breast cancer is a significant risk factor for the subsequent development of a second, new breast cancer. This risk has been estimated to be as high as 1% per year from the time of diagnosis of an initial sporadic breast cancer. Women with *BRCA*-associated cancer have a 3%–5% per year risk of contralateral breast cancer (cumulative lifetime risk of up to 64% in high-risk cohorts). Women with a history of endometrial, ovarian, or colon cancer also have a higher likelihood of developing breast cancer than those with no history of these malignancies.

Menstrual and reproductive factors Early onset of menarche (< 12 years old) has been associated with a modest increase in breast cancer risk (twofold or less). Women who undergo menopause before age 30 have a twofold reduction in breast cancer risk when compared with women who undergo menopause after age 55. A first full-term pregnancy before age 30 appears to have a protective effect against breast cancer, whereas a late first full-term pregnancy or nulliparity may be associated with a higher risk. There is also a suggestion that lactation protects against breast cancer development.

Radiation exposure An increased rate of breast cancer has been observed in survivors of the atomic bomb explosions in Japan, with a peak latency period of 15–20 years. More recently, it has been noted that patients with Hodgkin's lymphoma who are treated with mantle irradiation, particularly women who are younger than age 20 at the time of radiation therapy, have an increased incidence of breast cancer.

Exogenous hormone use Epidemiologic data provide strong evidence for an association between plasma estrogens and breast cancer risk.

The 1996, large meta-analysis of the relationship between oral contraceptive use and breast cancer risk showed that a history of recent oral contraceptive use was a better predictor of breast cancer risk than duration of use. (Meta-analysis consisted of 54 earlier studies including 53,297 women with breast cancer and 100,239 women without breast cancer.) The increase in risk for current users was modest (24% for ever users vs never users). These data were based primarily on older high-dose and moderate-dose oral contraceptive pills and not the recently introduced low-dose pills. Therefore, it is likely that the small increase in breast cancer risk associated with the early formulations of oral contraceptives will diminish with the new low-dose pills.

In regard to hormone replacement therapy (HRT) or postmenopausal hormone use, results from the Women's Health Initiative (WHI) showed that the overall risks of estrogen plus progestin outweigh the benefits. This large randomized clinical trial sponsored by the National Institutes of Health (NIH) included more than 16,000 healthy women. Results from the WHI trial were published in 2002 after an average 5.6 years of follow-up and included a 26% increase in risk of invasive breast cancer among women taking estrogen plus progestin, compared with women taking placebo. In addition, in women taking these hormones, there were increased risks of heart disease, stroke, and blood clots.

The NIH stopped the estrogen-alone arm of the WHI trial in March 2004. No increase in breast cancer risk was observed in the estrogen-alone arm during the study period (7 years of follow-up). The NIH concluded that estrogen alone does not appear to increase or decrease a woman's risk of heart disease, although it does appear to increase her risk of stroke and decrease her risk of hip fracture.

Alcohol Moderate alcohol intake (two or more drinks per day) appears to modestly increase breast cancer risk.

High-fat diet Diets that are high in fat have been associated with an increased risk for breast cancer. Women who have diets high in animal fat from red meat or high-fat dairy foods have an increased risk of developing breast cancer. Whether the increase in breast cancer risk is associated with the fat content or an unknown carcinogen in these foods is unclear.

TABLE 2: Features indicating an increased likelihood of a *BRCA* mutation

Early-onset breast cancer
Ovarian cancer (with or without a family history of breast or ovarian cancer)
Breast and ovarian cancers in the same woman
Bilateral breast cancer
Ashkenazi Jewish heritage
Male breast cancer

Obesity Alterations in endogenous estrogen levels secondary to obesity may enhance breast cancer risk. Obesity appears to be a factor primarily in postmenopausal women.

Genetic cancer risk assessment

Genetic testing clearly has the potential to benefit carefully selected and counseled families. Education and adequately trained health care professionals are key elements in the successful integration of genetic cancer risk assessment into clinical practice.

The genetic risk assessment process begins with an assessment of perceived risk and the impact of cancer on the patient and family. This information forms the framework for counseling.

Comprehensive personal and family histories Detailed information regarding personal, reproductive, and hormonal risk factors is noted. Family history, including age at disease onset, types of cancer, and current age or age at death, is obtained for all family members going back at least three generations.

Documentation of cancer cases is crucial to accurate risk estimation. Pathology reports, medical record notes, and death certificates may all be used in determining the exact diagnosis.

Pedigree construction and evaluation The family pedigree is then constructed and analyzed to determine whether a pattern of cancer in the family is consistent with genetic disease. Sometimes, small family structure or lack of information about the family limits assessment of a hereditary trait; other times, clues such as ancestry or early age at diagnosis influence risk assessment and the usefulness of genetic testing.

Individual risk assessment Several models are used to estimate the likelihood that a detectable *BRCA1* or *BRCA2* mutation is responsible for the disease in the family. The BRCAPRO computer program is a cancer risk assessment tool that uses a family history of breast or ovarian cancer in first- and second-degree relatives to calculate the probabilities that either a *BRCA1* or

TABLE 3: Risk management options for *BRCA* mutation carriers[a]

Recommended for breast cancer detection

- Monthly self-examination of the breast beginning in late teen years
- Beginning at age 25 (or at least 10 years before the earliest onset cancer in the kindred):
  - Clinician breast examination every 6 months
  - Annual mammography
  - Consider annual breast MRI if there is significant mammographic density
  - Discussed as options:
    - Bilateral risk reduction mastectomy (total or skin-sparing)
    - Participation in clinical trials for chemoprevention

Recommended for ovarian cancer detection or prevention

- Risk reduction salpingo-oophorectomy recommended upon completion of childbearing
- Pelvic examination and Pap smear annually
- Serum CA-125 every 6 months
- Transvaginal ultrasonography every 6 months

[a] Also offered to women at increased risk because of a positive family history of hereditary breast and ovarian cancers but for whom genotypic information is not available.

BRCA2 mutation is responsible for the disease. It includes a Bayesian calculation (of conditional probability) to account for age-specific penetrance differences. If genetic testing is not performed or results are uninformative, the empiric breast cancer risk is estimated by the phenotype as well as the Claus model (derived from the Cancer and Hormone Study, which uses age at onset of breast cancer among first- and second-degree relatives). Personal and family characteristics that are associated with an increased likelihood of a *BRCA1* or *BRCA2* mutation are summarized in Table 2.

Education about the principles of genetics and hereditary cancer patterns is provided. Information on the application of genetic testing (appropriateness, limitations, advantages, and disadvantages) is also given.

Genetic counseling and testing Informed consent is obtained before genetic testing is performed. For individuals who decide to undergo testing, a post-test counseling session is scheduled to disclose and explain the results in person.

Customized screening and prevention recommendations Regardless of whether or not a woman undergoes genetic testing, a customized management plan is delineated, with the goal of prevention or early detection of malignancy, within the context of her personal preferences and degree of risk (Table 3).

Laboratory methods

Several techniques/strategies for detecting mutations in cancer genes have been adopted by different researchers and commercial vendors. Current technology misses 8%–10% of pathologic alterations in *BRCA1* and *BRCA2* (generally large rearrangements).

Directed assays are available for specific founder or ancestral mutations that are common in a given population. Among Ashkenazi Jews, 1 in 40 individuals bears one of three founder mutations (185delAG and 5382insC in *BRCA1* and 6174delT in *BRCA2)*; these mutations account for 25% of early-onset breast cancer in this population. Moreover, 95% of Ashkenazi Jews with a *BRCA* gene mutation will have one of the three founder mutations.

The lifetime risk of breast cancer was 82% among founder mutation carriers in a large cohort of Jewish families identified via a New York breast cancer study. The lifetime risk of ovarian cancer was 54% for *BRCA1* and 23% for *BRCA2*, similar to the risk in multiplex families from the Breast Cancer Linkage Consortium (BCLC). However, a population-based study indicated a lifetime breast cancer risk of 40%–73%.

Limitations All of the approaches to detecting mutations have limitations. In general, discovery of an inactivating or "deleterious" mutation of either *BRCA1* or *BRCA2* indicates a high probability that a person will develop breast and/or ovarian cancer.

One of the greatest challenges is the interpretation of missense mutations. These mutations are more likely to be significant if located in an evolutionarily conserved or functionally critical region of the protein. In the absence of a clear disease association, it is often difficult to exclude the possibility that a given missense alteration simply represents a rare polymorphism. A testing service may designate such changes as "genetic variants of uncertain significance."

Testing strategies

In general, testing should be initiated with the youngest affected individual in a given family. Even if one is convinced that a family has hereditary breast and ovarian cancers based on clinical criteria, there is only a 50% chance that an offspring or sibling of an affected patient will have inherited the deleterious allele. Therefore, only a positive test result (detection of a known or likely deleterious mutation) is truly informative.

Until the "familial mutation" is known, a negative test result could mean either that the unaffected person being tested did not inherit the cancer susceptibility mutation or that the person inherited the disease-associated gene, but the mutation was not detectable by the methods used.

In many cases, no affected family members are available for testing. In that case, one may proceed with genetic testing of an unaffected person, but only after she has been thoroughly counseled regarding its risks, benefits, and limitations.

Unless there is a suggestive family history, cancer susceptibility testing is not considered appropriate for screening unaffected individuals in the general population. However, it may be reasonable to test unaffected persons who are members of an ethnic group in which specific ancestral mutations are prevalent and whose family structure is limited (ie, the family is small, with few female relatives or no information due to premature death from noncancerous causes).

A recent study of 491 BRCA carriers with stage I or II breast cancer indicated that the risk of ovarian cancer was 12.7% at 10 years for BRCA1 (6.8% for BRCA2), and ovarian cancer was the cause of death in 25% of the stage I breast cancer patients *(Metcalfe K, Lynch HT, Ghadirian P, et al: Gynecol Oncol 96:222-226, 2005).*

Impact of genetic cancer risk status on management

Data from the BCLC suggest that the cumulative risk of developing a second primary breast cancer is approximately 65% by age 70 among *BRCA* gene mutation carriers who have already had breast cancer. A large, retrospective cohort study of BRCA carriers with a history of limited-stage breast cancer indicated up to a 40% risk of contralateral breast cancer at 10 years.

Thus, knowledge of the genetic status of a woman affected with breast cancer might influence the initial surgical approach (eg, bilateral mastectomy might be recommended for a mutation carrier instead of a more conservative procedure). Moreover, since ovarian cancer risk may be markedly increased in women with *BRCA1* mutations (and to a lesser degree with *BRCA2* mutations), additional measures, such as surveillance for presymptomatic detection of early-stage tumors or consideration of oophorectomy, may be warranted. According to data from *BRCA* carriers who underwent risk reduction salpingo-oophorectomy (RRSO), breast cancer risk may also be decreased by the reduction in ovarian hormone exposure.

Retrospective data suggest that bilateral mastectomy in women who are at high risk for the disease based upon family history significantly reduces the risk for developing breast cancer by approximately 90%. Women who opt for risk reduction mastectomy should be offered reconstruction. Skin-sparing mastectomy may enhance the cosmetic results of reconstruction and should be discussed with the patient's surgeon. This procedure entails removing the breast tissue (including the nipple-areolar complex).

Potential benefits and risks of genetic testing

The ability to identify individuals at highest risk for cancer holds the promise of improved prevention and early detection of cancers. Patients who are *not* at high risk can be spared anxiety and the need for increased surveillance. Recent studies suggest a better emotional state among at-risk relatives who undergo testing than among those who choose not to know their status. The patient's perception of risk is often much higher than risk estimated by current models.

The efficacy of bilateral risk reduction mastectomy (RRM) has been confirmed in a large prospective study of 483 women with *BRCA* mutations. With a mean follow-up of 6.4 years, RRM reduced the risk of breast cancer by 90% (95% in women who also underwent risk reduction salpingo-oophorectomy; *Rebbeck TR, Friebel T, Lynch HT, et al: J Clin Oncol 22:1055-1062, 2004).*

Potential risks Potential medical, psychological, and socioeconomic risks must be addressed in the context of obtaining informed consent for genetic testing.

Concerns about insurance Fear about adverse effects of testing on insurability remains the premier concern among patients. Close behind that is concern about the cost of analyzing large complex genes ($2,975 for full sequencing of *BRCA1* and *BRCA2).*

Legal and privacy issues The legal and privacy issues surrounding genetic testing are as complex as the testing technologies. Although several state laws regarding the privacy of medical information, genetic testing, and insurance and employment discrimination have been passed, they vary widely.

The 1996 Health Insurance Portability and Accountability Act (US public law 104-191) stipulates that genetic information may not be treated as a preexisting condition in the absence of a diagnosis of the condition related to such information. It further prohibits group medical plans from basing rules for eligibility or costs for coverage on genetic information. However, the law does not address genetic privacy issues and does not cover individual policies. Many states have laws addressing genetic discrimination, but gaps remain.

ASCO recommendations for genetic testing

Updated guidelines from the American Society of Clinical Oncology (ASCO) recommend that cancer predisposition testing be offered only in the following situations: (1) a person has a strong family history of cancer or early onset of disease; (2) the test can be adequately interpreted; and (3) the results will influence the medical management of the patient or family member. The National Comprehensive Cancer Network (NCCN) published practice guidelines for genetics/familial high-risk cancer screening, and up-to-date versions are available at www.nccn.org.

Signs and symptoms

Mammographic findings Increasing numbers of breast malignancies are being discovered in asymptomatic patients through the use of screening mammography. Mammographic features suggestive of malignancy include asymmetry, microcalcifications, a mass, or an architectural distortion.

When these features are identified on a screening mammogram (see Figures 1–5), they should, in most cases, be further evaluated with a diagnostic mammogram (and, in some cases, with a breast ultrasonographic image or in highly selected cases with MRI [Figure 6]) prior to determining the need for a tissue diagnosis. Often, pseudolesions, such as those caused by summation artifact, dust on the mammographic cassettes, and dermal calcifications, are correctly identified in this manner. All mammographic lesions (and the examinations themselves) must be unambiguously categorized according to one of the six Breast Imaging Reporting Data System (BI-RAD) classifications developed by the American College of Radiology (ACR, Table 4).

Breast lump When signs or symptoms are present, the most common presenting complaint is a lump within the breast. The incidence of this complaint can range from 65%–76%, depending on the study. Inflammatory breast cancer is particularly aggressive, although relatively uncommon, accounting for about 5% of all breast cancers. On breast palpation, there often is no definite mass, but the breast appears to be engorged with erythema, skin edema (peau d'orange), and skin ridging. Ultrasonography may help to distinguish mastitis or abscess from inflammatory breast cancer. Antibiotics, which are prescribed for presumed mastitis, are not helpful for women with inflammatory carcinoma.

Paget's disease has been associated with intraductal carcinoma involving the terminal ducts of the breasts and may have an associated invasive component. It presents as an eczematoid change in the nipple, a breast mass, or bloody nipple discharge. Cytology may be helpful in establishing the diagnosis; however, negative cytologic results should not preclude a biopsy.

Other local symptoms Breast pain is the presenting symptom in ~5% of patients, breast enlargement in 1%, skin or nipple retraction in ~5%, nipple discharge in ~2%, and nipple crusting or erosion in 1%.

Screening and diagnosis

Screening

Breast self-examination The role of breast self-examination is controversial. The American Cancer Society (ACS) recommends that beginning in their 20s, women should be instructed in the technique and informed about both the benefits and limitations of this screening tool. Other groups have suggested that routine breast self-examination may lead to more false-positive results and therefore more benign biopsies. One meta-analysis of 12 studies involving a total of 8,118 patients with breast cancer correlated the performance of breast self-examination with tumor size and regional lymph node status. Women who performed breast self-examination were more likely to have smaller tumors and less likely to have axillary node metastases than those who did not.

A major problem with breast self-examination as a screening technique is that it is rarely performed well. Only 2%–3% of women do an ideal examination a year after instruction has been provided.

Clinical breast examination The ACS recommends that women begin clinical breast examination at the age of 20 and have an examination every 3 years between ages 20 and 39, and annually beginning at age 40. Beginning at age 40, the clinical breast examination should be timed to occur near or prior to screening mammography. If the clinician detects an abnormality, the patient should then undergo diagnostic imaging rather than screening. Clinical breast examination should be performed and a complete breast history obtained when a woman presents for routine health care. The clinical examination should include inspection and palpation of the breast and regional lymph nodes. Between 14% and 21% of breast cancers are detected by clinical breast examination.

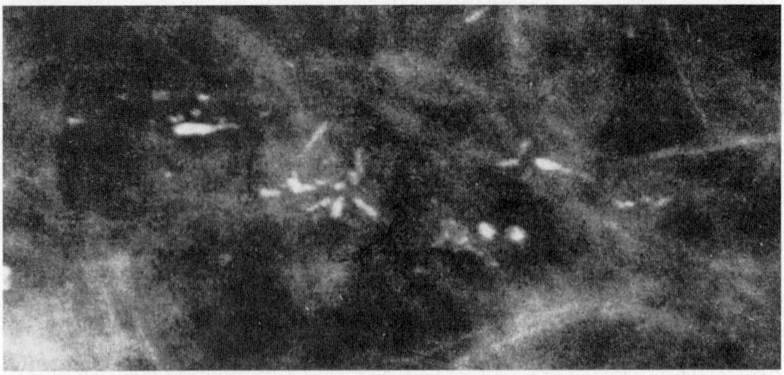

FIGURE 1: Malignant calcifications (comedocarcinoma) in a classic linear dot and dash configuration (BI-RAD 5 lesion). BI-RAD = Breast Imaging Reporting Data System.

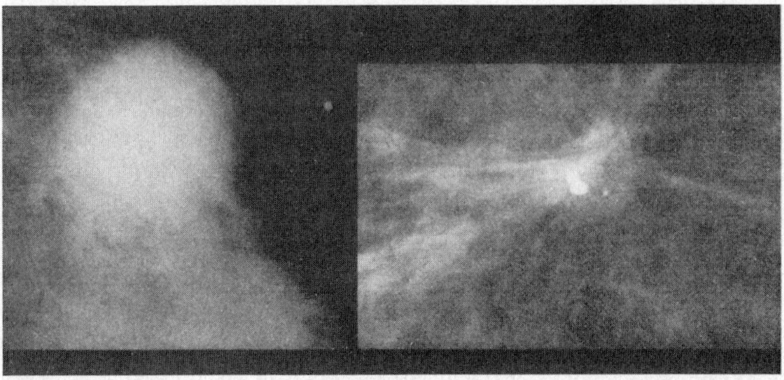

FIGURE 2: Left panel: A dense mass with partially unsharp margins (BI-RAD 4 lesion), which proved to be a fibroadenoma. Right panel: A small, spiculated mass (BI-RAD 5 lesion), which has engulfed a coarse, benign calcification. This lesion proved to be an invasive ductal carcinoma, not otherwise specified (NOS). BI-RAD = Breast Imaging Reporting Data System.

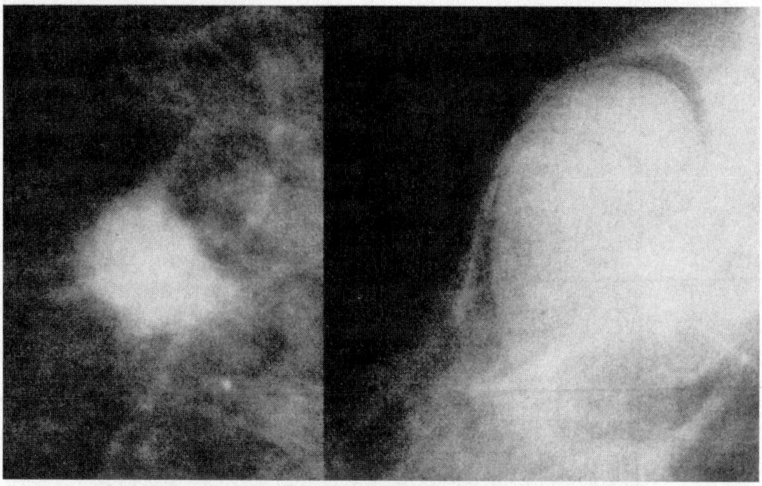

FIGURE 3: Left panel: This focal mass with truly nonsharp margins (BI-RAD 4 lesion) was diagnosed as a tubular carcinoma on stereotactic core biopsy. Right panel: A well-circumscribed lesion containing fat (BI-RAD 2 lesion), which is pathognomonic for a breast hamartoma (fibroadenolipoma). BI-RAD = Breast Imaging Reporting Data System.

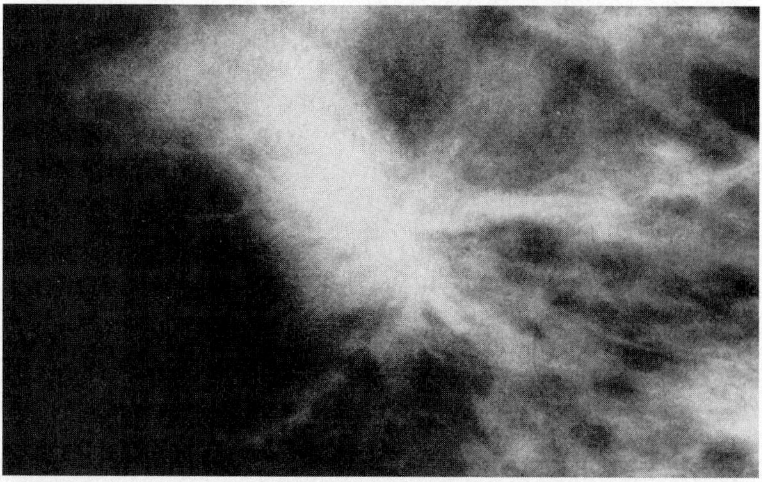

FIGURE 4: Focal architectural distortion may be difficult to see, but, if confirmed, it has the highest positive predictive value for breast carcinoma. This BI-RAD 4 lesion proved to be an invasive lobular carcinoma, which often has a subtle mammographic appearance. BI-RAD = Breast Imaging Reporting Data System.

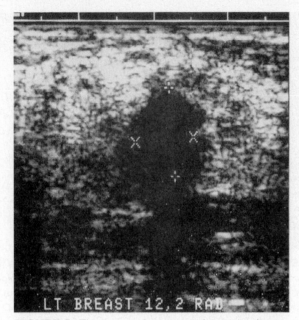

FIGURE 5: This breast ultrasonographic image demonstrates a hypoechoic, solid mass, which exhibits posterior shadowing and is taller than wide. This BI-RAD 4 lesion proved to be an invasive ductal carcinoma, not otherwise specified (NOS). BI-RAD = Breast Imaging Reporting Data System.

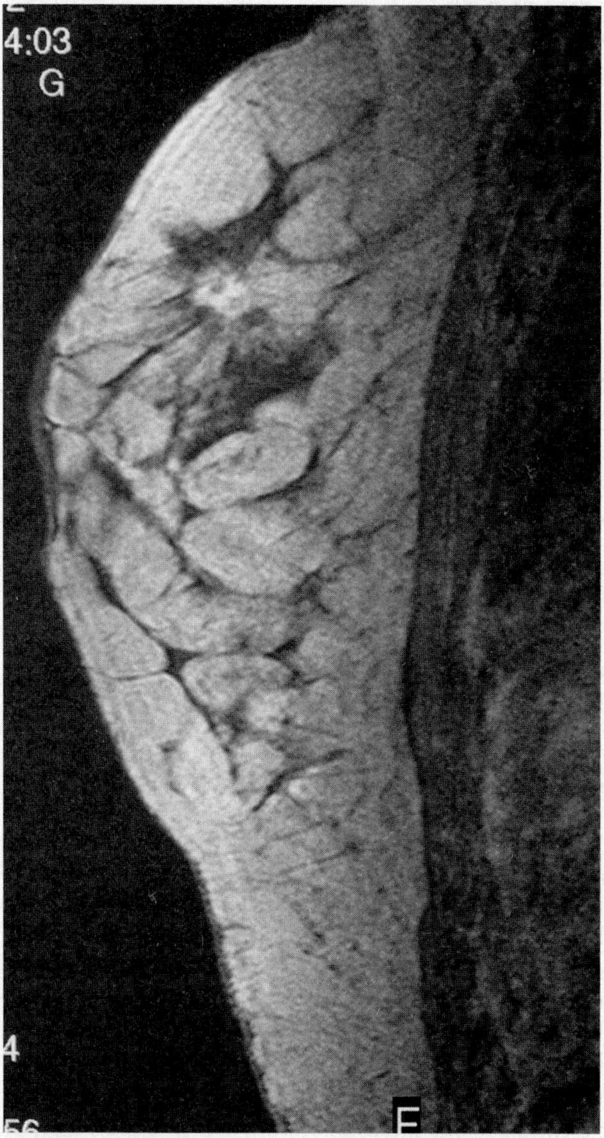

FIGURE 6: A 42-year-old woman presents with axillary adenopathy, which was positive on fine-needle aspiration. Results of a clinical breast exam, mammography, and ultrasonography were normal. A 7-mm enhancing cancer is clearly seen on this MRI of the breast.

TABLE 4: BI-RAD classification of mammographic lesions

BI-RAD class	Description	Probability of malignancy (%)	Follow-up
0	Needs additional evaluation	1	Diagnostic mammogram, ultrasonographic image
1	Normal mammogram	0	Yearly screening
2	Benign lesion	0	Yearly screening
3	Probably benign lesion	< 2	Short interval follow-up
4[a]	Suspicious for malignancy	20	Biopsy
5	Highly suspicious for malignancy	90	Biopsy
6	Biopsy-proven malignancy	100	Treatment

BI-RAD = Breast Imaging Reporting Data System

[a] The American College Radiology recommends that each site be dividied into three subcategories: 4A, low suspicion; 4B, intermediate suspicion; and 4C, moderate concern but not classic for malignancy.

Mammography Despite conflicting coverage in the lay press, the benefit of screening mammography is well established by the findings of an evidence-based clinical trial. The ACS, the ACR, and the American Medical Association have updated their guidelines since 1997 and recommend annual mammography beginning at age 40. The National Cancer Institute (NCI) also updated its guidelines in 1997, recommending that women undergo screening mammography every 1–2 years beginning in their 40s. The US Preventive Services Task Force updated its guidelines in 2002 and now recommends mammography every 1–2 years, alone or with clinical breast examination, for women aged 40 and older.

Screening mammography is performed in the asymptomatic patient to detect an occult breast cancer. This contrasts with diagnostic mammography, which is performed in a patient with a breast abnormality (palpable mass, bloody nipple discharge, or some other clinical finding) to further identify the etiology of the problem.

Physical examination and mammography are complementary. Mammography has a sensitivity of 85%–90% and, thus, would miss 10%–15% of clinically evident tumors while detecting the majority of cases an average of 2 years prior to any perceptible clinical signs or symptoms.

Screening recommendations for average-risk patients No upper age limit has been suggested, and the previous recommendation for a “baseline” mammogram between the ages of 35 and 40 has been withdrawn. Thus, both the ACS and the NCCN recommend annual mammography starting at age 40 for women at average risk of breast cancer.

Screening recommendations for high-risk patients Based on epidemiologic evidence that premenopausal familial breast cancer often presents at similar ages among affected family members, many breast imaging centers recommend that yearly screening for such high-risk individuals begin 5–10 years prior to the youngest age at which a first-degree relative was diagnosed with breast cancer. For example, according to this algorithm, a woman whose mother developed breast cancer at age 45 could begin yearly screening at age 35, in addition to biannual clinical breast examinations. Screening for women at genetic risk may begin at age 25. These commonly used screening algorithms are not based on formal studies but have arisen based on the natural history of the disease. They are, however, in keeping with the recommendations of the NCCN guidelines.

Digital mammography was approved by the US Food and Drug Administration (FDA) in 2000 and is rapidly being adopted by leading breast cancer centers worldwide. Initial trials indicate a comparable sensitivity to film-based mammography, with the benefit of a reduced risk of women called back from screening for additional work-up. The FDA also approved computer-aided detection systems for mammography beginning in 2001. Mammograms are scanned by a computer and possible lesions are marked for further review by a radiologist. A number of studies have shown a reduced risk of "missed cancers" when computer-aided diagnosis is thus employed.

Screening ultrasonography Sensitivity of mammography is diminished when the breast tissue is dense. There have been recent reports in the literature concerning the role of screening breast ultrasonography in women with dense breasts on mammography and normal mammography and clinical breast examination. The results from a multicenter trial of leading breast imagers (ACRIN) may soon become available. Currently, there is no support in the literature for screening ultrasonography, with only anecdotal evidence of adequate sensitivity and specificity. Furthermore, ultrasonography and MRI are used as adjunct studies and should not replace mammography. However, breast MRI appears to be an effective screening tool for high-risk women, particularly those with *BRCA1* and *BRCA2* mutations.

Breast MRI is a sensitive tool for detecting occult breast cancer foci. Due to its limited specificity and high cost, MRI is not likely to become a screening tool for avergage-risk women. However, the role of breast MRI for detecting breast cancers in high-risk women (ie, *BRCA* gene mutation carriers) continues to evolve.

Two major studies recently demonstrated the increased sensitivity of MRI for detecting cancers in women with inherited susceptibility to breast cancer compared with clinical breast examination, mammography, or ultrasonography. The sensitivity of breast MRI is > 75%, in contrast to mammography and ultrasonography, which is approximately 30% each. The combined sensitivity of MRI plus mammography is about 95%, suggesting that it may be a viable strategy for screening young women at high-risk for breast cancer.

Evaluation of a cystic mass

FNA When a dominant breast mass is present and the history and physical examination suggest that it is a cyst, the mass can simply be aspirated with a fine needle. Aspiration of a simple benign breast cyst should yield nonbloody fluid and result in complete resolution of the lesion.

Ultrasonography can also be used to determine whether a lesion is solid or cystic and whether a cyst is simple or complex. A complex cyst does not meet the strict criteria of a simple cyst. For example, a complex cyst may demonstrate low level echoes within the cyst fluid or a thickened cyst wall. These features may also be caused by cyst aspiration (presumably due to postaspiration bleeding); for this reason, many clinicians perform ultrasonography prior to or at the time of FNA.

Biopsy A biopsy is indicated if the cyst fluid is bloody, the lesion does not resolve completely after aspiration, or the cyst recurs after repeated aspirations. Cytologic examination of the fluid is not routinely indicated, as the yield for positive cytology is so low. Cystic carcinoma accounts for < 1% of all breast cancers. However, an intraluminal solid mass is a worrisome sign suggesting (intra) cystic carcinoma and should be biopsied.

Evaluation of a solid mass

A solid, palpable mass can be evaluated in a variety of ways. The decision to observe a patient with a solid breast mass that appears to be benign should be made only after careful clinical and radiologic examinations. Either FNA for cytology or percutaneous core biopsy should also be performed.

Mammography is used to assess the radiologic characteristics of the mass and is important for the evaluation of the remainder of the ipsilateral breast as well as the contralateral breast.

FNA is a simple, easy-to-perform method for obtaining material for cytologic examination. The overall incidence of false-positive results ranges from 0%–2.5% (0.7% when performed by experienced technicians), and the incidence of false-negative results varies from 3%–27% (3%–9% in experienced hands). Reasons for false-negative readings include less-than-optimal technique in preparing the cytologic material, a missed lesion on aspiration, tumor necrosis, and incorrect cytologic interpretation. FNA is limited in its ability to distinguish invasive from noninvasive cancers.

Biopsy In the past, an excisional biopsy of a small breast mass or incisional biopsy of a larger breast mass was performed to establish a histologic diagnosis of breast cancer. In recent years, excisional biopsy is being performed less often, except for a presumably benign lesion. For a suspected malignancy, core biopsy is the preferred diagnostic tool. With a core biopsy, the surgeon can plan for the cancer surgery, allowing for definitive surgical management in a single procedure. Core biopsy is also more advantageous than an FNA because architectural as well as cellular characteristics can be evaluated.

Image-guided core biopsies

When a palpable mass is extremely deep within the breast or a mass is relatively small, an ultrasonography-guided core biopsy can be performed to increase the diagnostic yield. When the procedure is performed with a large core needle (8 to 11 gauge) and vaccum assistance, a mass up to approximately 2–3 cm can be excised.

Ductal lavage

Ductal lavage is currently being developed and analyzed as a minimally invasive tool to identify cellular atypia within breast ducts in women who are already at high risk for developing breast cancer. Nipple aspiration is performed, and ducts that produce fluid should undergo lavage. The ductal orifice is cannulated and infused with 2–6 mL of saline. The ductal effluent is collected and evaluated by cytology. A careful record is maintained of each duct that has been lavaged by means of a nipple grid and photography.

The results of the cytologic evaluation may then be used to guide women in their decision-making process with respect to interventions to reduce their risk for breast cancer. For high-risk women who undergo ductal lavage and the cytology is benign, repeat lavage cn be performed in 1–3 years, although the optimal time for repeat lavage is not currently known. When mild atypia is identified by ductal lavage, the location of the duct should be carefully recorded using a nipple grid and photography to ensure the accurate localization of the duct. A repeat lavage can then be performed in 6–12 months. Women who have benign cytology and mild atypia on ductal lavage should also consider tamoxifen or participation in a chemoprevention trial.

Severe atypia is seen in approximately 6% of women who undergo ductal lavage. Patients with severe atypia on ductal lavage should undergo a thorough evaluation, including a repeat lavage, to confirm this diagnosis and exclude malignancy. The evaluation could also include repeated mammography with ductography, breast MRI, and/or ductoscopy. If no suspicious lesions are found, patients should be carefully followed. Fewer than 1% of patients have had malignant cells identified on ductal lavage.

Lavage of the duct producing the malignant cells should be repeated to confirm the diagnosis. If the diagnosis is confirmed, patients should then undergo the same evaluation as patients with marked atypia. Any suspicious lesion should be biopsied. Patients without suspicious lesions can be offered duct excision after the ductal system has been injected with dye or after close follow-up. These patients should also consider tamoxifen.

Evaluation of nonpalpable mammographic abnormalities

Excisional biopsy Prior to 1991, almost all nonpalpable mammographic lesions were excised using surgical excision. This technique has become less prevalent with the availability of image-guided percutaneous biopsy techniques.

Stereotactic and ultrasonography-guided core biopsies have revolutionized the management of nonpalpable breast lesions, and currently the majority

The Continuing Outcomes Relevant to Evista (CORE) trial, a 4-year follow-up to the Multiple Outcomes of Raloxifene (MORE) trial that examined the effect of long-term therapy with raloxifene (Evista) in postmenopausal women with breast cancer, found that daily intake of the agent reduced the risk of invasive breast cancer by 59%. Compared with placebo, the incidence of invasive estrogen-receptor–positive breast cancer was also reduced in the raloxifene arm ($P < .001$). Women who took raloxifene were more likely to develop blood clots in their legs or lungs, but the increased risk was not statistically significant. However, long-term use of raloxifene did not increase the risk of uterine cancer, as does long-term use of tamoxifen (*Martino S, Cauley JA, Barrett-Connor E, et al: J Natl Cancer Inst 96:1751-1761, 2004*).

of biopsies can be performed percutaneously, which is quicker, less invasive, and less expensive than excisional biopsy. Tissue acquisition is performed with automated core needles or directional vacuum-assisted biopsy probes. Guidance for percutaneous biopsy is usually provided by stereotaxis, ultrasonography, and, more recently, MRI.

Numerous studies comparing the sensitivity and specificity of stereotactic biopsy vs surgical biopsy have consistently found the two procedures to be statistically equivalent. The long-term false-negative rate for stereotactic biopsy is 1.4%, which equals best published results with surgical biopsy.

Up to 80% of patients with nonpalpable mammographic lesions are candidates for stereotactic core biopsy. Lesions near the chest wall or immediately behind the nipple often cannot be reached on the stereotactic table. Diffuse lesions, such as scattered calcifications or a large asymmetric density, are subject to undersampling with the percutaneous approaches. Some patients are unable to lie prone on the stereotactic table for the duration of the examination. Finally, stereotactic units and trained personnel are not universally available.

Ultrasonography-guided core biopsies are another accurate percutaneous technique, useful for lesions best imaged by ultrasonography. Since the biopsy gun is handheld and guided in real time by the ultrasound imager, there is more variability in performance, depending on the experience and skill of the practitioner. The overall reported accuracy rate of ultrasonography-guided biopsy is comparable to rates achieved with stereotactic and surgical biopsies.

Ultrasonography-guided or stereotactic FNA is another biopsy option. Although somewhat less invasive than core biopsy, FNA provides only cytologic (not histologic) pathology results. This technique can result in both false-positive and false-negative results, whereas a false-positive result has not been reported to date for core breast biopsies. FNA is most successful in centers that have an experienced cytopathologist, who, ideally, is available on site to review smears for adequacy during FNA procedures.

Breast MRI is currently used to search for an occult primary tumor in the setting of known metastasis, evaluate the extent of disease in a biopsy-proven breast carcinoma (useful if breast conservation is being considered), and assess lesions in implant-augmented breasts. It also is useful for screening high-risk women with dense breasts on mammography and nondiagnostic ultransonography or evaluating a borderline lesion when it is obscured by dense tissue. Breast MRI has a high sensitivity, and recent clinical developments have improved its specificity. Breast MRI examinations have recently been facilitated by the development of computer-aided detection (CAD) software, which can help to streamline the interpretation of these images and produce a more uniform result.

Breast surgeons are increasingly utilizing breast MRI for surgical planning. In a study reported by Bedrosian et al (a retrospective review of 267 patients who had preoperative MRI prior to undergoing definitive surgery), preoperative breast MRI changed the planned surgical approach in 26% of cases, including 16.5% of cases of breast conservation switched to mastectomy. Imaging centers across the United States have a varying degree of expertise in performing, interpreting, and providing a standard reporting nomenclature for breast MRI. The ACR is currently developing an accreditation program in breast MRI to address this issue.

> Kauff et al reported their findings of a multicenter prospective analysis of risk-reducing salpingo-oophorectomy (RRSO) to prevent BRCA-associated breast and ovarian cancers. During a median follow-up of 40 months, RRSO was associated with a 52% reduction in breast cancer risk and a 91% reduction in ovarian cancer risk, with the greatest risk reduction occurring in women with the *BRCA2* gene mutation. A total of 886 female *BRCA1* or *BRCA2* mutation carriers older than age 30 were enrolled from 1 of 11 study centers between 1994 and 2004. Women were treated with either ovarian surveillance (n = 325) or RRSO (n = 561). The investigators believe their results confirm that RRSO is highly protective against *BRCA*-associated breast and ovarian cancers. This protection may differ between carriers of *BRCA1* and *BRCA2* mutations (*Kauff ND, Domchek SM, Friebel TM, et al: J Clin Oncol [abstract] 24:49s, 2006*).

Ultrasonography Stavros et al have described ultrasonographic features of solid masses that suggest benign or malignant disease, such as sharp margins (benign) and taller-than-wide lesions (malignant). Although these features are useful for clinical decision-making, their utility in increasing the specificity of the breast lesion work-up has not been verified.

Sestamibi nuclear medicine scanning can help differentiate benign from malignant mammographic asymmetries and may play a role in evaluating palpable masses. Due to its limited spatial resolution and scatter, this technique is not reliable for lesions 1 cm or smaller.

Prevention

LIFESTYLE CHANGES ASSOCIATED WITH BREAST CANCER RISK REDUCTION

There is increasing evidence that lifestyle changes may alter an individual's breast cancer risk.

Physical activity has been associated with a reduction in breast cancer risk. The benefit was greatest in younger, premenopausal women. The activity can be related to leisure or work-time activities.

It has been suggested that women who exercise 3.5–4.0 times per week have a reduced incidence of breast cancer, compared with women who do not exercise. Exercise's protective effect may be associated with a reduction in the frequency of ovulatory cycles and circulating estrogen and progesterone levels.

Alcohol consumption Numerous studies on the effects of alcohol consumption on breast cancer risk and the results of a cohort study addressing this issue have been published. When compared with nondrinkers, women who consumed 2.3–4.5 bottles of beer per day, 2.5–5.6 glasses of wine per day, or 2–4 shots of liquor per day had a 41% higher risk of developing invasive breast cancer. Some reports indicate that the consumption of a moderate amount of alcohol (red wine) may decrease the risk of breast cancer, although these results are not conclusive. The biologic basis for the association between alcohol consumption and an increased risk of breast cancer is unclear. It has been proposed that there is a positive correlation between alcohol and estrogen levels.

> Low-fat intake has been hypothesized to reduce the risk for breast cancer. To assess the effects of undertaking a low-fat dietary pattern on breast cancer incidence, a randomized, controlled, primary prevention trial of 48,835 postmenopausal women, aged 50 to 79 years, without prior breast cancer, was conducted at 40 US clinical centers from 1993 to 2005. Women were randomly assigned to the dietary modification intervention group (n = 19,541) or the comparison group (n = 29,294). The intervention was designed to promote dietary change of reducing total fat to 20% and increasing daily consumption of vegetables and fruit to at least 5 servings and grains to at least 6 servings. Comparison group participants were not asked to make dietary changes. Overall, a low-fat dietary pattern did not result in a statistically significant reduction in invasive breast cancer risk over an 8.1-year average follow-up period. The number of women who developed invasive breast cancer (annualized incidence rate) was 655 (0.42%) in the intervention group and 1072 (0.45%) in the comparison group (hazard ratio, 0.91; 95% CI, 0.83-1.01). Secondary analyses suggests that among adherent women having a high-fat diet at baseline, a greater risk reduction might be achieved and that dietary effect varied by hormone receptor characteristics of the tumor *(Prentice RL, Caan B, Chlebowski RT, et al: JAMA 295(6):629-642, 2006).*

Alterations in diet and tobacco use A reduced incidence of breast cancer has been observed in countries where the diet is typically low in fat. However, no reduction in breast cancer risk has been observed in the United States when women followed low-fat diets. An association between red meat consumption or tobacco use and breast cancer risk has not been demonstrated.

Lactation Although it has been suggested that lactation may protect against breast cancer, it is unclear whether lactation reduces breast cancer risk. A recent study failed to demonstrate any breast cancer risk reduction in women who breast-fed and showed no dose-response effect in women who breast-fed for longer periods.

CHEMOPREVENTION

Breast Cancer Prevention Trial

The NIH and NCI have publicized the results of the National Surgical Adjuvant Breast and Bowel Project (NSABP) Breast Cancer Prevention Trial (BCPT). Women who had a risk of developing breast cancer equivalent to that of women 60 years of age qualified as participants in this double-blind, randomized

TABLE 5: Examples of eligible risk profiles used in the Breast Cancer Prevention Trial

Age (yr)	Risk profile
35	Two affected first-degree relatives plus personal history of biopsy
40	Two affected first-degree relatives plus no live births
45	Two affected first-degree relatives *or* one affected first-degree relative plus personal history of biopsy

trial. (For representative eligibility profiles, see Table 5.) A total of 13,388 women were randomized to receive tamoxifen or placebo.

Benefits of therapy The summary results indicate that tamoxifen prevented about half of both invasive and noninvasive breast cancers in all age groups. In addition to this reduction in invasive and noninvasive breast cancers. A secondary benefit of tamoxifen appeared to be a reduction in the incidence of hip fracture (Table 6). At present, no survival advantage has been shown for participants in this trial.

TABLE 6: Number of events among Breast Cancer Prevention Trial participants

Type of event	Placebo	Tamoxifen	Total
Invasive breast cancer	154 (5)[a]	85 (3)[a]	239 (8)[a]
Noninvasive breast cancer	59	31	90
Hip fracture	20	9	29
Colles' fracture	12	7	19
Spinal fracture	39	31	70
Endometrial cancer	14	33	47
All other invasive cancers	88	85	173
Fatal stroke	3	4	7
Nonfatal stroke	21	30	51
Transient ischemic attack	21	18	39
Fatal pulmonary embolism	0	2	2
Nonfatal pulmonary embolism	6	15	21
Deep vein thrombosis requiring hospitalization	3	3	6
Deep vein thrombosis not requiring hospitalization	16	27	43
Total	**456**	**380**	**836**

[a] Numbers in parentheses indicate the number of deaths due to breast cancer.

TABLE 7: TNM staging system for breast cancer

Primary tumor (T)

Tx	Primary tumor cannot be assessed
T0	No evidence of primary tumor
Tis	(DCIS) Carcinoma in situ
Tis	(LCIS) Carcinoma in situ
Tis	Paget's disease of the nipple with no tumor
T1	Tumor ≤ 2 cm in greatest dimension
T1mic	Microinvasion ≤ 0.1 cm in greatest dimension
T1a	Tumor > 0.1 but not > 0.5 cm in greatest dimension
T1b	Tumor > 0.5 cm but not >1 cm in greatest dimension
T1c	Tumor > 1 cm but not > 2 cm in greatest dimension
T2	Tumor > 2 cm but not > 5 cm in greatest dimension
T3	Tumor > 5 cm in greatest dimension
T4	Tumor of any size, with direct extension to (a) the chest wall or (b) skin only, as described below
T4a	Extension to the chest wall, not including the pectoralis muscle
T4b	Edema (including peau d'orange) or ulceration of the skin of the breast or satellite skin nodules confined to the same breast
T4c	Both T4a and T4b
T4d	Inflammatory carcinoma

Note: Paget's disease associated with a tumor is classified according to the size of the tumor.

Regional lymph nodes (N)

Nx	Regional lymph nodes cannot be assessed (eg, previously removed)
N0	No regional lymph node metastasis
N1	Metastasis in movable ipsilateral axillary lymph node(s); pathologic involvement of one to three axillary lymph nodes
N2	Metastasis in ipsilateral axillary lymph node(s) fixed or matted, or in clinically apparent[a] ipsilateral internal mammary nodes in the *absence* of clinically evident axillary lymph node metastasis; pathologic involvement of four to nine axillary lymph nodes
N2a	Metastasis in ipsilateral axillary lymph nodes fixed to one another (matted) or to other structures
N2b	Metastasis only in clinically apparent[a] ipsilateral internal mammary nodes and in the *absence* of clinically evident axillary lymph node metastasis
N3	Metastasis in ipsilateral infraclavicular lymph node(s) with or without axillary lymph node involvement, or in clinically apparent[a] ipsilateral internal mammary lymph node(s) and in the presence of clinically evident axillary lymph node metastasis; or metastasis in ipsilateral supraclavicular lymph node(s) with or without axillary or internal mammary lymph node involvement; pathologic involvement of 10 or more axillary lymph nodes
N3a	Metastasis in ipsilateral infraclavicular lymph node(s) and axillary lymph node(s)
N3b	Metastasis in ipsilateral internal mammary lymph node(s) and axillary lymph node(s)
N3c	Metastasis in ipsilateral supraclavicular lymph node(s)

[a] "Clinically apparent" is defined as detected by imaging studies (excluding lymphoscintigraphy) or by clinical examination or grossly visible pathologically.

Pathologic classification (pN)	
pNX	Regional lymph nodes cannot be assessed (eg, previously removed)
pN0	No regional lymph node metastasis
pN0(I–)	No regional lymph node metastasis histologically; negative IHC
pN0(I+)	No regional lymph node metastasis histologically; positive IHC; no IHC cluster > 0.2 mm
pN0(mol–)	No regional lymph node metastasis histologically; negative molecular findings (RT-PCR)
pN0(mol+)	No regional lymph node metastasis histologically; positive molecular findings (RT-PCR)
pN1	Metastasis in 1 to 3 axillary lymph nodes, and/or internal mammary nodes with microscopic disease detected by SLN dissection but not clinically apparent
pN1mi	Micrometastasis (>0.2 mm but ≤2.0 mm)
pN1a	Metastasis in 1 to 3 axillary lymph nodes
pN1b	Metastasis in internal mammary nodes with microscopic disease detected by SLN dissection but not clinically apparent
pN1c	Metastasis in 1 to 3 axillary lymph nodes and in internal mammary lymph nodes with microscopic disease detected by SLN dissection but not clinically apparent
pN2	Metastasis in 4 to 9 axillary lymph nodes, or in clinically apparent internal mammary lymph nodes in the absence of axillary lymph node metastasis to ipsilateral axillary lymph node(s) fixed to each other or other structures
pN2a	Metastasis in 4 to 9 axillary lymph nodes (at least 1 tumor deposit >2.0 mm)
pN2b	Metastasis in clinically apparent internal mammary lymph nodes in the absence of axillary lymph node metastasis
pN3	Metastasis in ≥10 axillary lymph nodes, or in infraclavicular lymph nodes, or in clinically apparent ipsilateral mammary lymph nodes(s) in the presence of 1 or more positive axillary lymph node(s); or, in >3 axillary lymph nodes with clinically negative microscopic metastasis in internal mammary lymph nodes; or in ipsilateral supraclavicular lymph nodes
pN3a	Metastasis in ≥10 axillary lymph nodes (at least 1 tumor deposit >2.0 mm); or, metastasis to the infraclavicular lymph nodes
pN3b	Metastasis in clinically apparent ipsilateral internal mammary lymph nodes in the presence of ≥1 positive axillary lymph node(s); or, in >3 axillary lymph nodes and in internal mammary lymph nodes with microscopic disease detected by sentinel lymph node dissection but not clinically apparent
pN3c	Metastasis in ipsilateral supraclavicular lymph nodes
Distant metastasis (M)	
Mx	Distant metastasis cannot be assessed
M0	No distant metastasis
M1	Distant metastasis

continued on following page

DCIS = ductal carcinoma in situ; IHC = immunohistochemistry; LCIS = lobular carcinoma in situ; RT-PCR = reverse transcriptase polymerase chain reaction; SLN = sentinel lymph node

TABLE 7: TNM staging system for breast cancer *(continued)*

Stage grouping			
Stage 0	Tis	N0	M0
Stage I	T1[b]	N0	M0
Stage IIA	T0	N1	M0
	T1[b]	N1	M0
	T2	N0	M0
Stage IIB	T2	N1	M0
	T3	N0	M0
Stage IIIA	T0	N2	M0
	T1[b]	N2	M0
	T2	N2	M0
	T3	N1-2	M0
Stage IIIB	T4	N0	M0
	T4	N1	M0
	T4	N2	M0
Stage IIIC	Any T	N3	M0
Stage IV	Any T	Any N	M1

[b] T1 includes T1mic

From: Greene FL, Page DL, Fleming ID, et al (eds): AJCC Cancer Staging Manual, 6th ed. New York, Springer-Verlag, 2002.

Side effects Tamoxifen-treated women younger than age 50 had no apparent increase in side effects. However, women older than age 50 experienced serious side effects, including vascular events and endometrial cancer. Particularly worrisome was the increased incidence of endometrial cancer in the tamoxifen-treated patients (Table 6). In addition, a significant increase in pulmonary embolism and deep vein thrombosis was noted, especially in women older than age 50 (Table 6).

Current recommendations

Based on results of the BCPT, the FDA has approved tamoxifen for use in women at high risk (1.66% chance of getting breast cancer in the next 5 years, based on the Gail model) of breast cancer.

The NCI and NSABP are in the process of developing risk profiles based on age, number of affected first-degree relatives with breast cancer, number of prior breast biopsies, presence or absence of atypical hyperplasia or LCIS, age at menarche, and age at first live birth. These risk profiles may help guide women in making the decision as to whether or not to take tamoxifen.

An ASCO working group published an assessment of tamoxifen use in the setting of breast cancer risk reduction. All women older than 35 years of age with a Gail model risk of > 1.66% (or the risk equivalent to that of women 60 years of age) should be considered candidates for this treatment strategy. Comorbid conditions, such as a history of deep vein thrombosis, must be a part of the consent process and treatment decision.

Although the BCPT results establish tamoxifen as the standard of care for the primary chemoprevention of breast cancer in high-risk women, concern over the side effects of tamoxifen has prompted a continuing search for an agent that displays a more desirable efficacy/toxicity profile. Raloxifene (Evista), approved for the prevention of osteoporosis in postmenopausal women, displays antiestrogenic properties in the breast and endometrium and estrogenic effects in the bone, making it an attractive candidate for comparison with tamoxifen.

The Study of Tamoxifen and Raloxifene (STAR or NSABP P-2) began in July 1999 at almost 400 centers in North America. A total of19,747 postmenopausal women, or women ≥ 35 years old at increased risk of breast cancer by Gail criteria, were randomized to receive either tamoxifen (20 mg/d) or raloxifene (60 mg/d) for 5 years. Study endpoints included invasive and noninvasive breast cancers, cardiovascular disease, endometrial cancer, bone fractures, and vascular events. This trial completed accrual in November 2004, and results should be forthcoming.

Initial findings from the STAR trial suggest that both tamoxifen and raloxifene (Evista) are equally effective in reducing the risk of developing invasive breast cancer in postmenopausal women at increased risk of developing the disease. On the other hand, it appears that raloxifene was less effective than tamoxifen in preventing noninvasive breast cancer. Although trends indicated that raloxifene may be associated with fewer adverse events, in most cases, there was not a statistical difference between the two groups, except regarding cataracts and cataract surgery, in which there was a clear significant advantage to raloxifene (*Wickerham DL, Costantino JP, Vogel V, et al: J Clin Oncol [abstract] 24:2s, 2006*). Moreover, preliminary STAR data on patient-reported outcomes (PROs) revealed that there were no significant differences between the drugs in PROs for physical and mental health or depression. Although the severity of symptoms was generally low in this sample, the pattern differed; women on raloxifene reported more musculoskeletal problems and weight gain, whereas women on tamoxifen reported more vasomotor and gynecologic difficulties (*Ganz PA, Land SR, Wickerham DL, et al: J Clin Oncol [abstract] 24:18s, 2006*).

Staging and prognosis

Staging system The most widely used system to stage breast cancer is the American Joint Committee on Cancer (AJCC) classification, which is based on tumor size, the status of regional lymph nodes, and the presence of distant metastasis (Table 7).

Clinical staging is performed initially and is determined after the physical examination and appropriate radiologic studies have been performed.

Pathologic staging Pathologic stage is determined following surgery for operable breast cancer. Pathologic tumor size may differ from clinical tumor size. In addition, axillary nodal metastases that were not clinically evident may be detected after pathologic examination. With the advent of powerful molecular techniques, isolated tumor cells (ITC) can be identified in histologically negative nodes. In the current AJCC staging, pathologic staging of nodes for detection of ITCs were included to obtain more information and hopefully gain insight into the biologic significance of these ITCs.

Prognostic factors Numerous prognostic factors for breast cancer have been identified.

Lymph node status Axillary nodal metastasis is the most important prognostic factor. Axillary nodal involvement and survival were evaluated in patients with breast cancer. Survival was examined relative to the number of nodes involved and the location of nodes that contained metastatic deposits. For any given number of positive nodes, survival was independent of the *level* of involvement but was directly related to the *number* of involved nodes.

Overall, patients who have node-negative disease have a 10-year survival rate of 70% and a 5-year recurrence rate of 19%. As the number of positive nodes increases, so does the likelihood of relapse. Patients with > 10 positive lymph nodes have a recurrence rate of 72%–82%. The majority of patients who develop recurrence after initial curative treatment of early-stage breast cancer will have distant metastases.

Hormone-receptor status In general, hormone receptor–positive tumors have a more indolent course than do hormone receptor–negative tumors. However, the hormone-receptor status of a tumor is a stronger predictive than prognostic factor; that is, hormone receptor–negative tumors are unlikely to respond to endocrine therapy in contrast to hormone receptor–positive tumors.

Other factors that have been utilized to predict outcome are histologic grade, lymphovascular permeation, S-phase fraction, and ploidy.

More recently, molecular prognostic factors have been evaluated to determine their utility in predicting outcome. They include the growth factor receptors (epidermal growth factor receptor and c-*erb*B-2/*neu*), tumor-suppressor genes (*p53*), proteolytic enzymes that may be associated with invasion of disease and metastasis (cathepsin D), and metastasis-suppressor genes (*nm23*).

Of these molecular markers, HER2/*neu* or c-erbB-1/*neu* is probably the most widely studied in breast cancer to date. HER2/*neu* amplification is often associated with a more aggressive behavior and thus poorer outcome for patients with HER2/*neu*-positive tumors. Fortunately, targeted therapy with trastuzumab (Herceptin) has changed the course of treatment, providing longer survival when used in combination with chemotherapy for patients with metastatic disease.

SUGGESTED READING

ON RISK FACTORS AND GENETIC CANCER RISK ASSESSMENT

American Society of Clinical Oncology policy statement update: Genetic testing for cancer susceptibility. J Clin Oncol 21:2397–2406, 2003.

Daly M, National Comprehensive Cancer Network: Genetic/familial high-risk assessment: Breast and ovarian. Clinical Practice Guidelines in Oncology v.1.2005.

Metcalfe K, Lynch HT, Ghadirian P, et al: Contralateral breast cancer in *BRCA1* and *BRCA2* mutation carriers. J Clin Oncol 22:2328–2335, 2004.

Metcalfe KA, Lynch HT, Ghadirian P, et al: The risk of ovarian cancer after breast cancer in BRCA1 and BRCA2 carriers. Gynecol Oncol 96:222–226, 2005.

Weitzel JN, Lagos V, Blazer KR, et al: Prevalence of BRCA mutations and founder effect in high-risk Hispanic families. Cancer Epidemiol Biomarkers Prev 14:1666–1671, 2005.

ON PREVENTION

Anderson GL, Judd HL, Kaunitz AM, et al: Effects of estrogen plus progestin on gynecologic cancers and associated diagnostic procedures. The Women's Health Initiative Randomized Trial. JAMA 290:1739–1748, 2003.

Rebbeck TR, Friebel T, Lynch HT, et al: Bilateral prophylactic mastectomy reduces breast cancer risk in *BRCA1* and *BRCA2* mutation carriers: The PROSE Study Group. J Clin Oncol 22:1055–1062, 2004.

ON SCREENING AND DIAGNOSIS

Bedrosian I, Mick R, Orel SG, et al: Changes in the surgical management of patients with breast cancer based on preoperative magnetic resonance imaging. Cancer 98:468–473, 2003.

Kriege M, Biekelmans CTM, Boetes C, et al: Efficacy of MRI and mammography for breast cancer screening in women with a familial or genetic predisposition. N Engl J Med 351:427–437, 2004.

Schnall MD, Blume J, Bluemke DA, et al: MRI detection of distinct incidental cancer in women with primary breast cancer studied in IBMC 6883. J Surg Oncol 92:32–38, 2005.s

Warner E, Plewes DB, Hill KA, et al: Surveillance of *BRCA1* and *BRCA2* mutation carriers with magnetic resonance imaging, ultrasound, mammography, and clinical breast examination. JAMA 292:1317–1325, 2004.

SUGGESTED READING

ON RISK FACTORS AND GENETIC CANCER RISK ASSESSMENT

CHAPTER 9

Stages 0 and I breast cancer

Lori Jardines, MD, Bruce G. Haffty, MD, and Melanie Royce, MD, PhD

This chapter focuses on the diagnosis and management of early-stage breast cancer, ie, stages 0 and I disease. This is an important area, since more noninvasive and small breast cancers are being diagnosed due to the increasing use of screening mammography. Treatment of these malignancies will continue to evolve as the results of clinical trials lead to further refinements in therapy.

STAGE 0 BREAST CANCER

Stage 0 breast cancer includes noninvasive breast cancer—lobular carcinoma in situ (LCIS) and ductal carcinoma in situ (DCIS)—as well as Paget's disease of the nipple when there is no associated invasive disease.

LOBULAR CARCINOMA IN SITU

LCIS is nonpalpable, produces no consistent mammographic changes, and is often an incidental finding after breast biopsy performed for another reason.

The biologic behavior of LCIS continues to be an issue of debate. Most clinicians agree that it is a marker for increased risk for all types of breast cancer (both noninvasive and invasive).

Epidemiology and etiology

The incidence of LCIS has doubled over the past 25 years and is now 2.8 per 100,000 women. In the past, the peak incidence of LCIS was in women in their 40s. Over the past 3 decades, the peak incidence has increased to the 50s. The incidence of LCIS decreases in women who are in their 60s–80s. It has been suggested that the increase in the age of peak incidence of LCIS is related to the use of hormone replacement therapy (HRT). It is also possible that the use of HRT prevents the usual regression of LCIS normally seen at the time of menopause.

Signs and symptoms

LCIS is nonpalpable and has no consistent features on breast imaging. Most often, LCIS is found in association with a completely separate mammographic abnormality or palpable mass.

Risk of invasive cancer

Approximately 20%–25% of women with LCIS will develop invasive cancer within 15 years after the diagnosis of LCIS. More often, the invasive cancer is ductal in origin, and both breasts are at risk. At this point, there are no reliable molecular markers to determine which patients with LCIS will progress to invasive cancer.

Just as the incidence of LCIS has increased, there has also been an associated increase in the incidence of cases of infiltrating lobular carcinoma in postmenopausal women. The increase in invasive lobular carcinoma peaks in women in their 70s.

Pathology

LCIS appears to arise from the terminal duct-lobular apparatus, and the disease tends to be multifocal, multicentric, and bilateral. Subsequently, other types of LCIS have also been described and include pleomorphic LCIS. This entity tends to be associated with infiltrating lobular carcinoma, and the cytologic features are similar to those of intermediate- or high-grade DCIS. Pleomorphic LCIS may be more aggressive, with a higher likelihood of progression to invasion than classic LCIS.

Treatment options

The management of LCIS is continuing to evolve since the disease appears to be heterogeneous. Presently, treatment options include close follow-up, participation in a chemoprevention trial, tamoxifen, or bilateral prophylactic total mastectomy with or without reconstruction. At present, the decision for a given treatment will depend upon the patient's individual risk profile for DCIS or invasive breast cancer after careful counseling. In the future, treatment decisions may be based upon an analysis of a series of molecular markers, which can separate those patients with a low risk for invasion from those who are at high risk for disease progression.

DUCTAL CARCINOMA IN SITU

DCIS is being encountered more frequently with the expanded use of screening mammography. In some institutions, DCIS accounts for 25%–50% of all breast cancers.

Epidemiology

DCIS, like invasive ductal carcinoma, occurs more frequently in women, although it accounts for approximately 5% of all male breast cancers. The average age at diagnosis of DCIS is 54–56 years, which is approximately a decade later than the age at presentation for LCIS.

Signs and symptoms

The clinical signs and symptoms of DCIS include a mass, breast pain, or bloody nipple discharge. On mammography, the disease most often appears as microcalcifications. Because these microcalcifications are nonpalpable and are not always associated with a mass, DCIS is often discovered with mammography alone. Approximately 5% of patients who present with pathologic nipple discharge will have underlying breast cancer, and many of them will have DCIS alone.

Risk of invasive cancer

The risk of developing an invasive carcinoma following a biopsy-proven diagnosis of DCIS is between 25% and 50%. Virtually all invasive cancers that follow DCIS are ductal and ipsilateral and generally present in the same quadrant within 10 years of the diagnosis of DCIS. For these reasons, DCIS is considered a more ominous lesion than LCIS (which is considered a marker for risk) and appears to be a more direct precursor of invasive cancer.

Pathology

A variety of histologic patterns are seen with DCIS, including solid, cribriform, and papillary. Some researchers have divided DCIS into two subgroups: comedo and noncomedo types. As compared with the noncomedo subtypes, the comedo variant has a higher proliferative rate, overexpression of HER2/*neu*, and a higher incidence of local recurrence and microinvasion. DCIS is less likely to be bilateral and has approximately a 30% incidence of multicentricity.

Treatment of noninvasive breast carcinoma

DUCTAL CARCINOMA IN SITU

Breast-conserving surgery

Breast-conservation surgery, followed by radiation therapy to the intact breast, is now considered the standard treatment of DCIS. Since the incidence of positive lymph nodes after axillary lymph node dissection for DCIS is ~ 1%–2%, axillary dissection is not indicated in most instances.

The most important factor in determining local control within the breast is margin status. A surgical margin of 1 mm has been associated with a 43% chance of having residual disease at the time of reexcision. When a surgical margin of 10 mm can be obtained, there is an extremely low rate of recurrence (4%). A 10-mm surgical margin may not be practical, however, when trying to provide a good cosmetic outcome. When breast-conserving therapy is used alone (without irradiation), a margin of at least 10 mm is required, and the tumor should be small (< 1 cm) and a noncomedo type. Although a wide margin is always desirable, narrower margins are acceptable for DCIS when radiation therapy is used after lumpectomy.

Sentinel node biopsy

The sentinel lymph node is the first node in the draining lymphatic basin that receives primary lymph flow. The technique of sampling the first draining lymph node was initially described in the management of patients with melanoma to determine who would benefit from regional lymph node dissection and was performed using a vital blue dye. This same technique has been used in patients with breast cancer, and sentinel lymph node biopsy represents a minimally invasive way to determine whether the axilla is involved with disease. If the sentinel lymph node is negative, the patient may be spared lymph node dissection. The precise methods for identifying the sentinel lymph node (filtered vs unfiltered Tc-99m sulfur colloid and/or blue dye) and assessing the node (hematoxylin and eosin staining vs immunohistochemistry [IHC] vs polymerase chain reaction [PCR]) are being studied.

When blue dye is used, it can be injected into the breast parenchyma at the primary tumor or subareolar site. The radioactive tracer can be injected subdermally or intraparenchymally at the site of the primary tumor or in the subareolar location. The site and technique of injection will be based upon individual patient factors, including the type and location of the previous breast biopsy.

When lymphatic mapping and sentinel lymph node biopsy are performed, a blue vital dye and/or a radioactive tracer (generally technetium-labeled sulfur colloid) can be used. When a radiotracer is used, lymphoscintigraphy can also be performed to aid in locating the sentinel node. When a sentinel node biopsy is performed using blue dye, the axillary surgery should be performed carefully to avoid disrupting the blue-stained afferent lymphatic channels. When a radioisotope is used, a hand-held gamma counter is used to locate the sentinel node.

Axillary lymph node dissection is not routinely recommended for patients with DCIS. Recently, however, investigators have used sentinel lymph node biopsy to determine whether individuals with DCIS may harbor occult nodal metastases. Current studies have identified metastatic disease to the axillary nodes in up to 12% of patients who have undergone sentinel lymph node biopsy. Despite this relatively high percentage of positive sentinel nodes, recurrence in the nodal basins is rare (about 2%). Based on this and recent work, there is no indication for routine sentinel lymph node biopsy in patients with DCIS.

Factors associated with an increased risk of axillary metastasis with a diagnosis of DCIS are extensive DCIS requiring mastectomy, suspicion of microinvasion, DCIS associated with a palpable mass, and evidence of lymphovascular permeation or invasion seen on review of the slides. These factors likely are associated with a preoperatively nondiagnosed invasive component. However, for patients diagnosed with DCIS who are scheduled for mastectomy, sentinel lymph node sampling, prior to mastectomy, is a reasonable practice. In the event that an occult invasive cancer within the mastectomy is found, a negative sentinel node would be reassuring and perhaps would make it possible to avoid follow-up axillary dissection.

Adjuvant radiation therapy

Retrospective series of patients with DCIS, as well as subsets of patients with early invasive cancer, have been treated with conservative surgery alone, omitting radiation therapy to the intact breast. In addition, several prospective, randomized trials have attempted to address this issue of omission of breast irradiation for both invasive cancer and DCIS. It is clear from all of these series that omission of breast irradiation results in a significantly higher ipsilateral breast tumor recurrence rate but has not, as yet, had an impact on overall survival.

Two large prospective randomized trials have demonstrated a significant reduction in local relapse with the use of postlumpectomy irradiation in treatment of DCIS. In the National Surgical Adjuvant Breast and Bowel Project (NSABP) B-17, the local recurrence rate at 8 years was reduced from 27% to 12% with postlumpectomy irradiation.

Similar results have been reported by a European cooperative group study of 1,010 women with DCIS randomly assigned to receive either 50 Gy of radiotherapy to the whole breast over 5 weeks or no further treatment. With a median follow-up of 4.25 years, the 4-year local relapse-free rate was 91% in the radiotherapy arm vs 84% in the observation arm. Hazard ratios with postexcision radiotherapy were 0.62 for all local relapses, 0.65 for DCIS recurrences, and 0.60 for noninvasive recurrences.

Both trials showed that radiotherapy reduces the risk of both noninvasive and invasive recurrences. Identification of a subgroup of patients who did not benefit from postlumpectomy irradiation has not as yet been clearly defined.

The Van Nuys Prognostic Index (VNPI), based on tumor size, grade, presence of necrosis, and width of the excision margin, is an algorithm commonly used to predict local recurrence after breast-conserving surgery for DCIS. In some series, VNPI lacked discriminatory power for guiding further patient management. In studies performed by this group, it appears that the width of the excision margin is the most important predictor of local recurrence after breast-conserving surgery for DCIS.

One study demonstrated acceptable local control in patients with DCIS treated by excision alone, provided that wide negative margins were obtained. In this retrospective series of 469 patients, radiation therapy did not lower the local recurrence rate in patients with wide ($\geq$ 10 mm) negative margins but did produce a significant benefit in patients with close ($\leq$ 1 mm) margins. The authors concluded that radiation therapy is unlikely to benefit patients with wide negative margins and small tumors. These findings need to be confirmed in prospective, randomized trials.

Although there may be some patients for whom wide excision alone is appropriate therapy, the available literature has not consistently identified the specific subgroup of patients. Clearly, the omission of radiation therapy in subsets of patients remains a controversial issue worthy of further investigation. It is hoped that ongoing randomized studies will help to resolve some of the conflicts generated by selective, retrospective studies.

Two trials have addressed the need for postlumpectomy radiation therapy (RT) in older women with breast cancer. Both studies randomized patients, following lumpectomy and adjuvant hormonal therapy, to receive RT or observation. Both studies confirmed statistically significant improvements in local control with RT, and local relapse rates were acceptable in carefully selected patients. The authors concluded that selected elderly patients may be treated with hormonal therapy alone (without RT) following breast-conserving therapy (*Hughes KS, Schnaper LA, Berry D, et al: N Engl J Med 351:971-977, 2004; Fyles AW, McCready DR, Manchul LA, et al: N Engl J Med 351:963-970, 2004*).

Adjuvant tamoxifen therapy

Adjuvant therapy is not routinely employed for patients with DCIS. However, the use of tamoxifen for the prevention of secondary breast cancers in women at high risk for breast cancer, which includes women previously diagnosed with DCIS, has led some clinicians to consider the use of tamoxifen in women diagnosed with DCIS. In NSABP B-24, 1,804 women with DCIS treated with lumpectomy and irradiation were randomly assigned to receive placebo or tamoxifen. At a median follow-up of 74 months, women in the tamoxifen group had fewer breast cancer events than those in the placebo group (8.2% vs 13.4%; $P = .0009$). Tamoxifen decreased the incidence of both ipsilateral and contralateral events. The risk of ipsilateral invasive cancers was reduced by tamoxifen, regardless of the presence or absence of comedo-necrosis or margin involvement.

In a recent analysis of NSABP B-24, it was found that the benefit from tamoxifen is derived exclusively by patients with hormone receptor-positive disease. Based on these results, tamoxifen may be considered as adjuvant therapy for patients with hormone receptor-positive DCIS. The role of tamoxifen or other estrogen receptor modulators is likely to evolve rapidly over the next decade, and additional data on the use of hormonal agents as adjuvant therapy for DCIS are eagerly awaited.

STAGE I BREAST CANCER

Stage I breast cancer ranges from microinvasive tumors (≤ 0.1 cm) to tumors ≤ 2 cm without evidence of spread to the regional lymph nodes.

Pathology of invasive breast cancer

Ductal carcinoma Most cases of invasive carcinomas of the breast are ductal in origin. Of the different histologic subtypes of ductal carcinoma that have been described, tubular, medullary, mucinous (colloid), and papillary subtypes have been associated with a favorable outcome.

Lobular carcinoma Approximately 5%–10% of invasive breast cancers are lobular in origin. This histology has been associated with synchronous and metachronous contralateral primary tumors in as many as 30% of cases.

TABLE 1: Contraindications to breast conservation

Absolute contraindications	Relative contraindications
Multicentric disease[a]	Tumor size vs breast size
Diffuse malignant microcalcifications	Tumor location
Pregnancy	Collagen vascular disease (excluding rheumatoid arthritis)
Persistently positive surgical margins	
Previous breast or mantle irradiation	

[a] If a satisfactory cosmetic outcome is anticipated, multicentric disease is considered to be a relative contraindication.

Treatment of stage I breast cancer

SURGICAL AND RADIATION TREATMENTS

Multiple studies have demonstrated that patients with stage I breast cancer who are treated with either breast-conservation therapy (lumpectomy and radiation therapy) or modified radical mastectomy have similar disease-free and overall survival rates.

Breast-conservation therapy

Extent of local surgery The optimal extent of local surgery has yet to be determined and, in the literature, has ranged from excisional biopsy to quadrantectomy. A consensus statement on breast-conserving therapy issued by the National Cancer Institute (NCI) recommended that the breast cancer be completely excised with negative surgical margins.

The extent of axillary surgery also continues to evolve. In recent years, patients with early-stage breast cancer who have clinically node-negative disease have the option to undergo sentinel lymph node biopsy rather than axillary node dissection. The present standard of care for patients with a positive sentinel node is complete nodal dissection. A study is under way to determine whether patients with a positive sentinel node require further axillary surgery.

Patient selection Specific guidelines must be followed when selecting patients for breast conservation. Patients may be considered unacceptable candidates for conservative surgery and radiation therapy either because the risk of breast recurrence following the conservative approach is significant enough to warrant mastectomy or the likelihood of an unacceptable cosmetic result is high. Some patients who are candidates for breast conservation can undergo breast MRI to identify sites of additional disease within the breast that may preclude breast-conserving treatment, although this is not a standard for evaluation. Contraindications to breast-conserving surgery are listed in Table 1.

Risk factors for ipsilateral recurrence For patients undergoing conservative surgery followed by radiation therapy to the intact breast, the risk of ipsilateral breast tumor recurrence has been reported to range from 0.5% to 2.0% per year, with long-term failure rates varying from 7% to 20%. Risk factors for ipsilateral breast tumor recurrence include, but are not limited to, young age (< 35–40 years), an extensive intraductal component, major lymphocytic stromal reaction, peritumoral invasion, presence of tumor necrosis, and positive resection margins. After a wide excision has been performed, the specimen should be oriented and inked; the pathologist may then ink each margin a different color. If a positive surgical margin is present, the color-coded system will guide the reexcision to obtain negative surgical margins with the removal of the least amount of breast tissue possible.

Earlier studies demonstrated that an extensive intraductal component was a risk factor for local relapse. However, in subsequent reports, when negative surgical margins are achieved, patients with an extensive intraductal component can be safely treated with breast conservation. Although it is desirable to achieve negative surgical margins, the available data do not preclude the use of conservative treatment, provided that adequate radiation doses (> 6,000 cGy) to the tumor bed are employed. The role of the remaining risk factors previously cited in predicting recurrence is unclear, and patients should not be denied breast conservation because of their presence.

Cosmetic considerations include primary tumor size and location, overall breast size, total body weight, and a history of preexisting collagen vascular disease.

Tumor size and breast size are important in determining whether the patient will have an acceptable cosmetic outcome after surgical resection. Patients with large tumors with respect to breast size may consider neoadjuvant chemotherapy to reduce the size of the primary tumor and allow breast preservation. (See chapter 11 for discussion of neoadjuvant chemotherapy.)

Obese women with large, pendulous breasts may experience marked fibrosis and retraction of the irradiated breast, making a good to excellent cosmetic outcome less likely. Techniques of brachytherapy may prove beneficial for these women. Women in this situation can undergo bilateral reduction mammoplasty after the wide excision of the primary tumor site has been completed. The partial mastectomy specimen should be evaluated by the pathologist to ensure adequate resection margins. Radio-opaque clips can be left to mark and identify the primary tumor site for the radiation oncologist. The follow-up mammograms will be more difficult to interpret due to scarring and radiotherapy effect.

Patients with collagen vascular disease may develop more severe reactions following radiation therapy. Although initial anecdotal reports demonstrated higher complication rates in patients with collagen vascular disease, a case-controlled study of patients with early-stage breast cancer showed higher complication rates only in those patients with scleroderma. Other case-controlled studies have also failed to demonstrate significantly higher complication rates in patients with collagen vascular disease undergoing radiation therapy. It appears that most patients without active significant collagen vascular diseases may be candidates for breast-conserving surgery and irradiation, although this approach remains controversial.

In some instances, it is necessary to excise skin to obtain a negative surgical margin. This does not necessarily preclude the patient from undergoing breast-conserving therapy and does not mean the patient should have a poor cosmetic outcome. When skin must be removed to obtain a negative surgical margin, complex skin closures, such as V-Y advancement flaps or Z-plasties, can be utilized to enhance cosmesis.

Patients with centrally located tumors Traditionally, patients who have centrally located tumors requiring excision of the nipple-areolar complex have not been offered the option of breast conservation. However, the cosmetic result achieved after local tumor excision that includes the nipple-areolar complex may not differ significantly from that obtained following mastectomy and reconstruction.

Furthermore, conservatively treated patients with subareolar lesions do not necessarily need to have the nipple-areolar complex sacrificed, as long as negative surgical margins can be achieved. However, if the complex is not removed, the remaining breast tissue and overlying skin remain sensate. Recent studies also indicate that the incidence of local recurrence is not increased when primary tumors in this location are treated conservatively.

Genetically predisposed breast cancer patients For women harboring germline mutations in *BRCA1* or *BRCA2*, there are limited data regarding long-term outcome. Studies, to date, have shown acceptable local control rates in the short term and increased but acceptable rates of acute, subacute, and chronic normal tissue reactions with lumpectomy followed by radiation therapy. Women with germline *BRCA1* and *BRCA2* mutations, however, are at high risk for second primary tumors in the contralateral breast.

A study from Yale University demonstrated high rates of second primary tumors in the ipsilateral breast. This study suggests that if breast-conserving therapy is chosen, some prophylactic measures, such as selective estrogen receptor modulators or oophorectomy, might be considered to reduce the risk of second primary tumors in the ipsilateral or contralateral breast. Other studies also indicate a trend toward higher rates of late local relapses in *BRCA* carriers. Further studies are clearly warranted to assess the long-term risks and benefits of breast-conserving strategies in women harboring mutations in *BRCA1* and *BRCA2*.

Role of axillary lymph node dissection The role of axillary lymph node dissection in the management of breast cancer has been questioned, particularly when a patient with a clinically negative axilla is undergoing breast-conservation therapy. In most instances, the breast surgery is performed with the patient under local anesthesia and sedation on an outpatient basis. When axillary lymph node dissection is added, the surgery is performed with the patient under general anesthesia.

It has also been suggested that if the status of the nodes will not alter therapy, the dissection is unnecessary and the axilla can be treated with irradiation. On the other hand, if axillary lymph node staging is not performed, the patient will not be accurately staged and important prognostic information will be unavailable.

Patients who may not be candidates for sentinel node biopsy are women who are pregnant or breast-feeding and women who have had prior irradiation. A prior excisional biopsy does not preclude the use of lymphatic mapping and sentinel node biopsy. It has recently been suggested that sentinel node biopsy accurately evaluates the axilla, even in patients with tumors > 5 cm and those who have been treated with neoadjuvant chemotherapy.

Once the sentinel node(s) have been identified, they can be sent to pathology for frozen section or touch-prep analysis.

Sensitivity and specificity In breast cancer, lymphatic mapping has been performed using a vital blue dye and/or lymphoscintigraphy. Studies have suggested that the success rate for identifying the sentinel node can be increased when these techniques are used in combination. The ability to identify the sentinel node can reach as high as 97% when blue dye and Tc-99m sulfur colloid are used together. When blue dye is used alone, the success rate is 83%, and when Tc-99m sulfur colloid is used alone, the success rate is 94%.

Results from a multi-institution practice have demonstrated that sentinel lymph node biopsy using dual-agent injection provides optimal sensitivity. In the study, 806 patients were enrolled by 99 surgeons for sentinel lymph node biopsy by single-agent (blue dye alone or radioactive colloid alone) or dual-agent injection at the discretion of the surgeons. All patients underwent complete level I/II dissection following the sentinel procedure. There were no significant differences in the identification of a sentinel node among patients who underwent single- compared with dual-agent injection. However, the false-negative rate was 11.8% for single-agent vs 5.8% for dual-agent injections ($P = .05$).

The sensitivity and specificity of sentinel lymph node biopsy are high, and the likelihood of a false-negative result is extremely low. False-negative rates vary among series, ranging from 0% to 11%. In one series, in 18% of the cases where the frozen-section evaluation of the node was negative, the final pathologic evaluation revealed metastatic disease, and the patient ultimately required lymph node dissection. This potential result can be distressing to patients; however, they should be informed of this possibility at the time of the procedure.

Patients whose sentinel node biopsy is normal do not require a complete node dissection, since the risk of an axillary recurrence is extremely low. Many institutions are using IHC in the evaluation of the sentinel node. When there is no evidence of metastatic disease by routine hematoxylin and eosin staining and the node is IHC–, the node is considered pN0 (i–). When there are isolated tumor cells seen but no cluster is greater than 0.2 mm, the node is staged as pN0 (i+) and the patient does not require a complete node dissection. If the focus of metastatic disease in the node is greater than 0.2 mm but less than 2 mm, the node is staged as pN1mi. In this instance, consideration should be given to performing a complete axillary node dissection or axillary radiation therapy, unless the patient is participating in a clinical trial. The likelihood that nonsentinel lymph nodes will also contain metastatic disease increases as the size of the primary tumor increases.

Radiation therapy after breast-conserving surgery

Based on the results of a number of retrospective single-institution experiences, as well as several prospective randomized clinical trials, breast-conserving surgery followed by radiation therapy to the intact breast is now considered a standard treatment for the majority of patients with stage I or II invasive breast cancer.

Radiation dose and protocol Radiation therapy after breast-conservation surgery should employ careful treatment planning techniques that minimize treatment of the underlying heart and lungs. To achieve the optimal cosmetic result, efforts should be made to obtain a homogeneous dose distribution throughout the breast. Doses of 180–200 cGy/d to the intact breast, to a total dose of 4,500–5,000 cGy, are considered standard.

Additional irradiation to the tumor bed is often administered. Although the necessity of a boost to the tumor bed has been questioned, at least two randomized clinical trials have demonstrated a small but statistically significant reduction in ipsilateral breast tumor relapses with the use of a radiation boost to the tumor bed following whole-breast irradiation of 50 Gy. In one of these trials, involving more than 5,000 women randomized to receive either a 16-Gy boost to the tumor bed or not, a 3% absolute reduction in local relapse was seen with the use of the radiation boost (4.3% vs 7.3%; $P < .0001$). This effect was particularly evident in patients younger than age 50. The boost is directed at the original tumor bed with either electron-beam irradiation or an interstitial implant, to bring the total dose to 50–66 Gy.

Regional nodal irradiation For patients who undergo axillary dissection and are found to have negative nodes, regional nodal irradiation is no longer routinely employed. For patients with positive nodes, radiation therapy to the supraclavicular fossa and/or internal mammary chain may be considered on an individualized basis (see chapter 10).

Partial breast irradiation There have been several reports demonstrating promising re-

In a recent meta-analysis evaluating radiation therapy following breast-conserving surgery, a search of the literature identified 15 trials with a pooled total of 9,422 patients available for analysis, who were randomized following breast-conserving therapy to undergo radiation therapy or observation. The relative risk of ipsilateral breast tumor recurrence after surgery was 3.00 (95% CI = 2.65 to 3.40). Mortality data were available for 13 trials, with a pooled total of 8,206 patients. The relative risk of mortality was 1.086 (95% CI = 1.003 to 1.175), corresponding to an estimated 8.6% relative excess mortality if radiotherapy was omitted. The authors concluded that omission of radiotherapy is associated with a large increase in risk of ipsilateral breast tumor recurrence and a small increase in the risk of mortality (*Vinh-Hung V, Verschraegen CL: J Natl Cancer Inst 21:115-121, 2004*).

sults with the use of partial breast irradiation, a potentially more convenient option for patients than the extended course of postoperartive radiotherapy.

Additional options are now available to shorten the radiotherapy treatment time to 1–5 days (accelerated) and to focus an increased dose of radiation on just the breast tissue around the excision cavity (partial breast). Current accelerated partial breast irradiation (APBI) approaches include interstitial brachytherapy, intracavitary (balloon) brachytherapy, and accelerated external beam (three-dimensional conformal) radiotherapy. Intraoperative radiotherapy is even shorter, with the entire treatment given as a single dose delivered immediately after surgery. Each approach has benefits and limitations.

Ongoing randomized trials will shape how APBI is utilized in routine clinical practice. Some of the more important outcomes from these trials will be local toxicity, local and regional recurrence, and overall survival. If APBI is ultimately demonstrated to be as safe and effective as whole-breast radiotherapy, breast conservation may become an even more appealing choice, and the overall impact of treatment may be further reduced for certain women with newly diagnosed breast cancer.

Mastectomy options

Patients who are not candidates for breast conservation or who are not interested in breast conservation are offered mastectomy. For patients who desire immediate reconstruction at the time of mastectomy, a skin-sparing approach is recommended, provided it is oncologically safe. In most instances, the mastectomy can be performed through a circumareolar incision, where the nipple-areolar complex (NAC) is excised in continuity with the breast tissue. If a biopsy has been performed, this skin should also be excised with the mastectomy specimen. There have been reports in the literature in which the NAC has been spared during the course of a skin-sparing mastectomy. This concept awaits further study and is not considered standard of care.

MEDICAL TREATMENT

Medical management of local disease depends on clinical and pathologic staging. Systemic therapy is indicated only for invasive (infiltrating) breast cancers.

In the past, systemic therapy was not offered to patients with stage I disease (tumors up to 2.0 cm). However, adjuvant chemotherapy and hormonal therapy have been shown to improve disease-free and overall survival in selected patients with node-negative disease.

The sequence of systemic therapy and radiation therapy for patients treated with breast-conserving therapy has been the subject of considerable debate. Although concurrent CMF (cyclophosphamide, methotrexate, fluorouracil [5-FU]) and radiation therapy have been used with accetable toxicity, the concurrent use of chemoradiation therapy has fallen out of favor due to reports of enhanced toxicities. Delaying chemotherapy for 6–8 weeks of radiation therapy does not appear to negatively impact systemic disease or survival. Recent studies do not demonstrate a compromise in local control if radiation is delayed until chemotherapy is complete. Currently, the majority of patients receiving chemotherapy and radiation therapy are treated with chemotherapy prior to radiation therapy (see sidebar).

For patients receiving tamoxifen or other hormonal agents, there had been considerable controversy regarding whether the hormonal agents should be administered during or after radiation therapy. Theoretically, tamoxifen may place cells in a resting state, making them less radiosensitive. Three retrospective studies, conducted independently but recently published together, all reached a similar conclusion: The timing of therapy had no impact on local relapse rates (see sidebar).

> The Harvard sequencing trial of 244 patients, which randomized patients treated with conservative surgery and irradiation to receive chemotherapy or radiotherapy first, was recently updated. With a median follow-up of 135 months, there was no significant difference between the chemotherapy-first and radiotherapy-first groups with respect to time to any event, metastasis, or death (*Bellon JR, Come SE, Gelman RS, et al: J Clin Oncol 23:1934-1940, 2005*).

Treatment regimens

Multiagent therapy with CMF, CMF and prednisone (CMFP), sequential methotrexate and 5-FU (MF), and Adriamycin (doxorubicin) and cyclophosphamide (AC) has been used in patients with node-negative disease (Table 2). Hormonal therapy with tamoxifen (20 mg PO every day for 5 years) has been shown to be of value in women ≥ 50 years of age with estrogen- and/or progesterone-receptor–positive tumors. (See chapter 10 for further discussion about tamoxifen and the ATAC trial [Arimidex and Tamoxifen Alone or in Combination] as well as for adjuvant chemotherapy regimens for node-positive breast cancer [Table 1].)

Taxanes (ie, paclitaxel and docetaxel [Taxotere]) are now routinely used in the adjuvant therapy for node-positive breast cancer. The role of taxanes in node-negative disease is still evolving.

Node-negative tumors < 1.0 cm The reduction in the odds of recurrence and death with adjuvant therapy is similar in estrogen-receptor–negative and [node]-negative patients. Therefore, patients who have the lowest risk of recurrence are least likely to benefit from systemic treatment when the attendant risks of treatment are considered. None of the reported trials in node-negative breast cancer included women with tumors < 1.0 cm, and because of the low risk of recurrence (≤ 10%) in this group, systemic adjuvant therapy is not used routinely. Recent results from the NSABP in this group of patients are provocative in suggesting a potential benefit from systemic therapy.

> Three retrospective studies evaluated the sequencing of tamoxifen and radiation therapy in conservatively managed patients and reached a similar conclusion. Whether tamoxifen was administered concurrently with radiation therapy or sequentially after radiation therapy, there was no difference in local control (*Ahn PH, Vu HT, Lannin D, et al: J Clin Oncol 23:17-23, 2005; Harris EE, Christensen VJ, Hwang WT, et al: J Clin Oncol 23:11-16, 2005; Pierce LJ, Hutchins LF, Green SR, et al: J Clin Oncol 23:24-29, 2005*).

TABLE 2: Adjuvant chemotherapy regimens for node-negative breast cancer

Regimen	Dose and frequency
MF	
Methotrexate	100 mg/m^2 IV on days 1 and 8
5-FU	600 mg/m^2 IV on days 1 and 8 (1 h after methotrexate)
Folinic acid	10 mg/m^2 PO q6h × 6 doses (24 h after methotrexate)
Repeat every 4 weeks for 12 cycles.	
CMF (Bonadonna regimen)	
Cyclophosphamide	600 mg/m^2 IV on day 1
Methotrexate	40 mg/m^2 IV on day 1
5-FU	600 mg/m^2 IV on day 1
Repeat every 3 weeks for 9 cycles.	
or	
Cyclophosphamide	100 mg/m^2 IV on days 1-14
Methotrexate	40 mg/m^2 IV on days 1 and 8
5-FU	600 mg/m^2 IV on days 1 and 8
Repeat every 28 days for 6 cycles.	
CMFP	
Cyclophosphamide	100 mg/m^2 PO on days 1-14
Methotrexate	40 mg/m^2 IV on days 1 and 8
5-FU	600 mg/m^2 IV on days 1 and 8
Prednisone	40 mg/m^2 PO on days 1 and 14
Repeat every 4 weeks for 6 cycles.	
FAC	
5-FU	500 mg/m^2 IV on days 1 and 4 or 8
Adriamycin (doxorubicin)	50 mg/m^2 IV by continuous 72-h infusion on days 1-3 (or 50 mg/m^2 on day 1)
Cyclophosphamide	500 mg/m^2 IV on day 1
Repeat at 21-day intervals if hematologic recovery occurs for 6 cycles.	
CAF	
Cyclophosphamide	600 mg/m^2 IV on day 1
Adriamycin (doxorubicin)	60 mg/m^2 IV on day 1
5-FU	600 mg/m^2 IV on day 1
Repeat every 21-28 days.	
FEC	
5-FU	500 mg/m^2 IV on day 1
Epirubicin	100 mg/m^2 IV on day 1
Cyclophosphamide	500 mg/m^2 IV on day 1
Repeat every 21 days.	
AC	
Adriamycin (doxorubicin)	60 mg/m^2 IV on day 1
Cyclophosphamide	600 mg/m^2 IV on day 1
Repeat every 21-28 days depending on hematologic recovery for 4 cycles.	

In this validation study, the likelihood of distant recurrence in tamoxifen-treated patients with node-negative, estrogen receptor-positive breast cancer was tested using a reverse transcriptase (RT)-PCR assay of 21 prospectively selected genes (16 cancer-related genes and 5 reference genes) in paraffin-embedded tumor tissue. The levels of expression of the 21 genes were used in a prospectively defined algorithm to calculate a recurrence score and to determine a risk group for each patient.

The proportions of patients categorized as having a low, intermediate, or high risk by the RT-PCR assay were 51%, 22%, and 27%, respectively. The Kaplan-Meier estimates of the rates of distant recurrence at 10 years in the low-, intermediate-, and high-risk groups were 6.8%, 14.3%, and 30.5%, respectively. The rate in the low-risk group was significantly lower than that in the high-risk group ($P < .001$). In a multivariate Cox model, the recurrence score provided significant predictive power that was independent of age and tumor size ($P < .001$). The recurrence score was also predictive of overall survival ($P < .001$) and could be used as a continuous function to predict distant recurrence in individual patients.

A randomized trial to determine whether reducing dietary fat intake was effective in influencing relapse-free survival in postmenopausal women with primary breast cancer was conducted in 2,437 women with early-stage resected breast cancer. Patients, 48–79 years old, were randomized in a 40:60 ratio to dietary intervention (group 1) or control groups (group 2). The dietary intervention included eight biweekly individual counseling sessions with trained nutritionists. Dietary fat intake reduction was greater in the dietary group than in the control group. After a median follow-up of 60 months, there were 277 reported relapse events. Breast cancer recurrence was 12.4% in group 1 versus 9.8% in group 2, or a 24% reduction in the risk of recurrence for the women on the low-fat diet. The largest risk reduction (42%) was seen among women on the low-fat diet whose tumors were ER-negative (*Chlebowski RT, Blackburn GL, Elashoff RE, et al. Proc Am Soc Clin Oncol [abstract] 23:10, 2005*).

Node-negative tumors ≥ 1.0 cm The selection of a specific treatment program and the characteristics that predict risk of recurrence and death in women with node-negative breast cancer require further delineation and clarification in clinical trials. At present, women with tumors ≥ 1.0 cm who have poor histologic or nuclear differentiation, negative estrogen receptors, a high S-phase percentage, or high Ki-67 can be considered appropriate candidates for adjuvant systemic therapy.

An update of the NSABP B-20 trial indicated a significant advantage in the estrogen-receptor–positive, node-negative population when chemotherapy with CMF or sequential MF is added to tamoxifen in the adjuvant setting. Patients receiving CMF plus tamoxifen appeared to derive the greatest benefit. Benefits with respect to both disease-free and overall survival have been reported for patients given chemotherapy and tamoxifen.

Chemotherapy and ovarian function suppression are both effective adjuvant therapies for patients with early-stage breast cancer. The efficacy of their sequential combination was investigated by the International Breast Cancer Study Group (IBCSG) Trial VIII. This study randomized more than 1,000 pre- and perimenopausal women with lymph node-negative breast cancer to receive either goserelin (Zoladex) for 24 months (n = 346), 6 courses of "classic" CMF chemotherapy (n = 360), or 6 courses of classic CMF followed by 18 months of goserelin (CMF then goserelin; n = 357). The primary outcome was disease-free survival.

In this study, patients with estrogen-receptor–negative tumors achieved better 5-year disease-free survival rates if they received CMF (84% and 88% for CMF and CMF then goserelin, respectively) than if they received goserelin alone (73%). However, for patients with estrogen-receptor–positive disease, chemotherapy alone and goserelin alone provided similar outcomes (81% 5-year disease-free survival rates for both treatment groups), whereas sequential therapy provided a statistically nonsignificant improvement compared with either modality alone.

Follow-up of long-term survivors

There is no consensus among oncologists as to the optimal follow-up routine for long-term breast cancer survivors. Based on guidelines from the National Comprehensive Cancer Network (NCCN), patients with stage 0 breast cancer should undergo a medical history and physical examination every 6 months for 5 years and then annually thereafter; mammography should be performed every year. Patients with stage I breast cancer should undergo a medical history and physical examination every 4 to 6 months for 5 years and then annually thereafter. In stage I patients, mammography should be performed every 6 months in the ipsilateral breast after radiation therapy following breast-conservation surgery and then annually thereafter, including the contralateral breast; if mastectomy was performed, mammography should be performed annually in the contralateral breast. Women receiving tamoxifen should undergo pelvic examination every 12 months if the uterus is present. All other follow-up evaluations are dictated by the development of symptoms.

SUGGESTED READING

Fisher B, Dignam J, Tan-Chiu E, et al: Prognosis and treatment of patients with breast tumors of 1 cm or less and negative axillary lymph nodes. J Natl Cancer Inst 93:112–120, 2001.

Fyles AW, McCready DR, Manchul LA, et al: Tamoxifen with or without breast irradiation in women 50 years of age or older with early breast cancer. N Engl J Med 351:963–970, 2004.

Gibson GR, Lesnikoski B-A, Yoo J, et al: A comparison of ink-directed and traditional whole cavity reexcision for breast lumpectomy specimens with positive margins. Ann Surg Oncol 8:693–704, 2001.

Giuliano AE, Haigh PI, Brennan MB, et al: Prospective observational study of sentinel lymphadenectomy without further axillary dissection in patients with sentinel node-negative breast cancer. J Clin Oncol 18:2553–2559, 2000.

Haffty B, Ward B, Pathare P, et al: Reappraisal of the role of axillary lymph node dissection in the conservative treatment of breast cancer. J Clin Oncol 15:691–700, 1997.

Haigh PI, Hansen NM, Qi K, et al: Biopsy method and excision volume do not affect success rate of subsequent sentinel node dissection in breast cancer. Ann Surg Oncol 7:21–27, 2000.

Hughes KS, Schnaper LA, Berry D, et al: Cancer and Leukemia Group B; Radiation Therapy Oncology Group; Eastern Cooperative Oncology Group: Lumpectomy plus tamoxifen with or without irradiation in women 70 years of age or older with early breast cancer. N Engl J Med 351:971–977, 2004.

Julien J-P for the EORTC Breast Cancer Cooperative Group: Radiotherapy in breast conserving treatment for ductal carcinoma in situ: First results of the European Organization for Research and Treatment of Cancer (EORTC) randomised phase III trial. Lancet 355:528–533, 2000.

Kerlikowske K, Molinaro A, Cha I, et al: Characteristics associated with recurrence among women with ductal carcinoma in situ treated by lumpectomy. J Natl Cancer Inst 95:1692–1702, 2003.

King TA, Fey JV, Van Zee KJ, et al: A prospective analysis of the effect of blue-dye volume on sentinel lymph node mapping success and incidence of allergic reaction in patients with breast cancer. Ann Surg Oncol 11:535–541, 2004.

Klauber-DeMore N, Tan LK, Liberman L, et al: Sentinel lymph node biopsy: Is it indicated in patients with high-risk ductal carcinoma in situ and ductal carcinoma in situ with microinvasion? Ann Surg Oncol 7:636–642, 2000.

McMasters KM, Tuttle TM, Carlson DJ, et al: Sentinel lymph node biopsy for breast cancer: A suitable alternative to routine axillary dissection in multi-institution practice when optimal technique is used. J Clin Oncol 18:2560–2566, 2000.

Paik S, Shak S, Tang G, et al: A multigene assay to predict recurrence of tamoxifen-treated, node-negative breast cancer. N Engl J Med 351:2817–2826, 2004.

Pierce LJ, Strawderman M, Narod SA, et al: Effect of radiotherapy following breast-conserving treatment in women with breast cancer and germline *BRCA1/2* mutations. J Clin Oncol 18:3360–3369, 2000.

Sakorafas GH, Tsiotou AG: Ductal carcinoma in situ (DCIS) of the breast: Evolving perspectives. Cancer Treat Rev 26:103–125, 2000.

Vinh-Hung V, Verschraegen C: Breast-conserving surgery with or without radiotherapy: Pooled-analysis for risks of ipsilateral breast tumor recurrence and mortality. J Natl Cancer Inst 96:115–121, 2004.

Voogd AC, Nielsen M, Peterse JL, et al: Differences in risk factors for local and distant recurrence after breast-conserving therapy or mastectomy for stage I and II breast cancer: Pooled results of two large European randomized trials. J Clin Oncol 19:1688–1697, 2001.

CHAPTER 10

Stage II breast cancer

Lori Jardines, MD, Bruce G. Haffty, MD, and Melanie Royce, MD, PhD

This chapter focuses on the treatment of stage II breast cancer, which encompasses primary tumors > 2 cm in greatest dimension that involve ipsilateral axillary lymph nodes as well as tumors up to 5 cm without nodal involvement.

Stage II breast cancer is further subdivided into stages IIA and IIB. Patients classified as having stage IIA breast cancer include those with T0-1, N1, and T2, N0 disease. Stage IIB breast cancer includes patients with T2, N1, and T3, N0 disease. Therefore, this patient population is more heterogeneous than the populations with stage 0 and stage I disease. The pretreatment evaluation and type of treatment offered to patients with stage II breast cancer are based on tumor size, nodal status, and estrogen-receptor status.

Treatment

SURGICAL AND RADIATION TREATMENT

Multiple studies have demonstrated that patients with stage II breast cancer who are treated with either breast-conservation therapy (lumpectomy and radiation therapy) or modified radical mastectomy have similar disease-free and overall survival rates.

Breast-conservation therapy

The optimal extent of local surgery has yet to be determined and, in the literature, has ranged from excisional biopsy to quadrantectomy. A consensus statement issued by the National Cancer Institute (NCI) recommended that the breast cancer be completely excised with negative surgical margins and that a level I–II axillary lymph node dissection be performed. Patients should subsequently be treated with adjuvant breast irradiation.

Patients with tumors > 4–5 cm may not be optimal candidates for breast conservation due to the risk of significant residual tumor burden and the potential for a poor cosmetic result following lumpectomy (or partial mastectomy). Neoadjuvant chemotherapy, typically used for locally advanced breast cancer, is increasingly used in earlier stage, operable breast cancers to reduce the size of the primary tumor and allow conservative treatment.

In a recent study of more than 300 patients treated with neoadjuvant chemotherapy at the M. D. Anderson Cancer Center, promising results were reported. At a median follow-up of 60 months, the 5-year actuarial rates of intrabreast tumor recurrence-free and locoregional recurrence-free survival were 95% and

91%, respectively. The authors concluded that breast-conservation therapy after neoadjuvant chemotherapy results in acceptably low rates of recurrence-free survival in appropriately selected patients, even those with T3 or T4 disease. Advanced nodal involvement at diagnosis, residual tumor larger than 2 cm, multifocal residual disease, and lymphovascular space invasion predict higher rates of recurrence.

In some patients, preoperative chemotherapy results in sufficient reduction in tumor response that breast-conserving therapy becomes possible. The NSABP B-18 trial showed that preoperative doxorubicin-based chemotherapy decreases tumor size by > 50% in approximately 90% of operable breast cancers, resulting in a greater frequency of lumpectomy.

In a subsequent trial, NSABP B-27, women with invasive breast cancer were randomized to receive 4 cycles of preoperative AC chemotherapy followed by surgery or 4 cycles of preoperative AC (Adriamycin [doxorubicin] and cyclophosphamide) followed by 4 cycles of docetaxel (Taxotere) followed by surgery, or 4 cycles of preoperative AC chemotherapy followed by surgery followed by 4 cycles of postoperative docetaxel. A higher rate of complete pathologic response was seen at surgery in patients treated with AC followed by docetaxel vs AC alone. There were no significant differences in disease-free and overall survival between the treatment groups. However, those who had a complete pathologic response in the breast had significant improvement in disease-free (hazard ratio [HR], 0.45; $P < .0001$) and overall survival (HR, 0.33; $P < .0001$) compared with those with residual disease after preoperative chemotherapy. Since preoperative chemotherapy does not have a negative impact on survival, the preoperative approach is a reasonable option and has gained favor among many patients.

Preoperative chemotherapy had an ability to convert patients requiring mastectomy to candidates for breast-conserving surgery. However, there was an increase in local recurrence in the "converted" group compared with those deemed eligibile initially for breast-conserving surgery.

The timing of sentinel node biopsy in patients undergoing preoperative chemotherapy is controversial. Preoperative chemotherapy can sterilize the axillary nodes and lead to errors in determination of nodal involvement. Formal studies are required to determine whether sentinel node biopsy can be safely performed after the patient has completed neoadjuvant chemotherapy.

Radiation therapy after breast-conserving surgery

For patients with stages I and II breast cancer, radiation therapy following lumpectomy remains an acceptable standard of care. Randomized trials as well as single-institution experiences have consistently demonstrated a significant reduction in local relapse rates for radiotherapy following breast-conserving surgery. Furthermore, small but significant differences in distant metastasis and disease-free survival have been observed in randomized trials comparing lumpectomy alone with lumpectomy and radiation therapy for patients with invasive breast cancer.

Based on the results of a number of retrospective single-institution experiences, as well as several prospective randomized clinical trials, breast-conserving surgery followed by radiation therapy to the intact breast is now considered standard treatment for the majority of patients with stage II invasive breast cancer.

Radiation dose and protocol Radiation dose to the intact breast follows the same guidelines as are used in patients with stages 0 and I disease, described in chapter 9.

Regional nodal irradiation For patients who undergo axillary lymph node dissection and are found to have negative lymph nodes, regional nodal irradiation is no longer employed routinely. For patients with positive lymph nodes, radiation therapy to the supraclavicular fossa and/or internal mammary chain may be considered on an individualized basis.

Regional nodal irradiation should be administered using careful treatment planning techniques to minimize the dose delivered to the underlying heart and lungs. Prophylactic nodal irradiation to doses of 4,500–5,000 cGy results in a high rate of regional nodal control and may improve disease-free survival in subsets of patients.

Given the widespread use of systemic therapy for patients with both node-negative and node-positive disease, the role of axillary dissection has recently come into question. In patients with clinically negative axillae who do not undergo axillary dissection, radiation therapy to the supraclavicular and axillary regions at the time of breast irradiation results in a high rate (> 95%) of regional nodal control with minimal morbidity.

Radiation therapy after mastectomy

Available data suggest that in patients with positive postmastectomy margins, primary tumors > 5 cm, or involvement of four or more lymph nodes at the time of mastectomy, the risk of locoregional failure remains significantly high enough to consider postmastectomy radiation therapy.

Several prospective randomized trials have evaluated the role of postmastectomy radiotherapy in addition to chemotherapy. Most of these trials have been limited to patients with pathologic stage II disease or patients with T3 or T4 primary lesions. All of these trials have shown an improvement in locoregional control with the addition of adjuvant irradiation, and several recent trials have demonstrated a disease-free and overall survival advantage in selected patients. Clinical practice guidelines developed by the American Society of Clinical Oncology (ASCO) support the routine use of postmastectomy radiation therapy for women with stage III or T3 disease or who have four or more involved axillary lymph nodes.

Most ongoing trials evaluating dose-intensive chemotherapy, with or without bone marrow or stem-cell transplantation, routinely include postmastectomy radiation therapy to the chest wall and/or regional lymph nodes to minimize locoregional recurrence.

For the first time, the type of taxane (paclitaxel vs docetaxel) and the schedule of therapy (every 3 weeks vs weekly) were compared in the adjuvant therapy of operable breast cancer. The E1199 trial included a total of 4,988 patients with lymph node-positive or high-risk (tumor ≥ 2 cm) node-negative breast cancer. After a median follow-up of 46.5 months, there were no significant differences in the hazard ratios (HR) comparing taxane (0.985; $P = 0.83$) or schedule (1.043; $P = 0.54$) for disease-free survival (DFS). There was a trend toward improved DFS associated with weekly paclitaxel (HR 1.20; 95%; $P = 0.06$) and fewer grade 3/4 toxicities (24% vs 4%; *Sparano JA, Wang M, Martino S, et al: San Antonio Breast Cancer Symposium, San Antonio, Texas [abstract], December 8-11, 2005*).

Current recommendations There is no clearly defined role for postmastectomy irradiation in patients with small (T1 or T2) primary tumors and negative nodes.

For patients with four or more positive lymph nodes, with or without a large primary tumor, postmastectomy radiation therapy should be considered to lower the rate of local relapse and improve disease-free survival. For patients with T1 or T2 tumors and one to three positive nodes, postmastectomy radiation therapy may have a benefit with respect to disease-free and overall survival. However, controversies and uncertainties regarding this issue remain, and individualized decision-making, based on the patient's overall condition and specific risk factors, is reasonable.

Minimizing pulmonary and cardiac toxicities Early trials employing postmastectomy radiation therapy showed that the modest improvement in breast cancer mortality was offset by an excess risk of cardiovascular deaths, presumably due to the radiation treatment techniques used, which resulted in delivery of relatively high radiation doses to the heart. Recent trials employing more modern radiation therapy techniques have *not* demonstrated an excess of cardiac morbidity and, hence, have shown a slight improvement in overall survival due to a decrease in breast cancer deaths. Thus, in any patient being considered for postmastectomy radiation therapy, efforts should be made to treat the areas at risk while minimizing the dose to the underlying heart and lungs.

Radiation dose and protocol The available literature suggests that doses of 4,500–5,000 cGy should be sufficient to control subclinical microscopic disease in the postmastectomy setting. Electron-beam boosts to areas of positive margins and/or gross residual disease, to doses of ~6,000 cGy, may be considered.

In patients who have undergone axillary lymph node dissection, even in those with multiple positive nodes, treatment of the axilla does not appear to be necessary in the absence of gross residual disease. Treatment of the supraclavicular and/or internal mammary chain should employ techniques and field arrangements that minimize overlap between adjacent fields and decrease the dose to underlying cardiac and pulmonary structures.

MEDICAL TREATMENT

Medical management of local disease depends on clinical and pathologic staging. Systemic therapy is indicated only for invasive (infiltrating) breast cancers.

A discussion of the sequencing of chemotherapy and irradiation and hormonal therapy with irradiation is provided in chapter 9.

Treatment regimens

Systemic adjuvant therapy has been shown to decrease the risk of recurrence and in some cases also the risk of death. Systemic therapy may be divided into chemotherapy and endocrine (hormonal) therapy. Chemotherapy often involves use of combination regimens, given for 4 to 8 cycles. Chemotherapy is most often delivered after primary surgery for breast cancer and before radiation therapy for those who are candidates for irradiation.

> Nonanthracyline-containing regimens with activity in breast cancer, such as docetaxel and cyclophosphamide (TC), are promising alternatives to doxorubicin. Mature results of a study comparing doxorubicin and cyclophosphamide (AC) vs TC in 1,016 patients who had complete surgical excision of the primary tumor have been presented. At 5 years, the disease-free survival was significantly better ($P = .027$) for TC (86%; 95% confidence interval [CI], 84%–88%) than for AC (81%; 95% CI, 79%–83%). Overall survival between the treatments was not statistically significant (89% vs 88%, $P = .188$). In general, TC appeared to be a more tolerable regimen *(Jones SE, Savin MA, Holmes FA, et al. San Antonio Breast Cancer Symposium, San Antonio, Texas [abstract], December 8-11, 2005)*.

Chemotherapy Multiagent therapy with cyclophosphamide, methotrexate, and fluorouracil (5-FU, CMF regimen); cyclophosphamide, methotrexate, 5-FU, and prednisone (CMFP); AC; and sequential methotrexate and 5-FU (MF) has been used in patients with node-negative disease (see Table 2 in Chapter 9).

For node-positive disease, systemic chemotherapy has changed over the past few years. Anthracycline-containing regimens are being used with greater frequency and have been shown to be of greater benefit than nonanthracycline-containing regimens (eg, CMF). Epirubicin (Ellence) was approved by the US Food and Drug Administration (FDA) for use in combination with cyclophosphamide and 5-FU (CEF regimen) for the adjuvant treatment of patients with node-positive breast cancer following resection of the primary tumor.

In a pivotal trial conducted by the NCI of Canada, premenopausal women with node-positive breast cancer were randomly allocated to receive either CEF or CMF, administered monthly for 6 months. With a median follow-up of 59 months, the 5-year relapse-free survival rates were 53% and 63% ($P = .009$), and 5-year survival rates were 70% and 77% for CEF and CMF, respectively ($P = .03$).

Several trials have also shown the benefit of incorporating taxanes (paclitaxel and docetaxel) in the adjuvant treatment of node-positive breast cancer, and they are now routinely used in this setting. Taxanes can either be given in combination with an anthracycline or sequentially, either before or after an anthracycline.

The Breast Cancer International Research Group (BCIRG) compared Taxotere (docetaxel), Adriamycin (doxorubicin), and cylophosphamide (TAC regimen) with 5-FU, Adriamycin, and cyclophosphamide (FAC regimen) in 1,480 women with node-positive breast cancer (BCIRG 001/TAX 316). At a median follow-up of 55 months, the estimated 5-year disease-free survival rate was 75% for patients treated with TAC vs 68% for those treated with FAC. This represents a statistically significant reduction in the risk of relapse of 28% ($P = .001$). Furthermore, treatment with TAC resulted in a statistically significant reduction in

Goldstein et al presented the results of E2197 at the 2005 ASCO meeting. In this clinical trial, 2,885 patients with node-positive or high-risk node-negative breast cancer were randomized to receive 4 cycles of AT (Adriamycin 60 mg/m^2; Taxotere, 60 mg/m^2 IV q3wk) or AC (Adriamycin, 60 mg/m^2; cyclophosphamide, 600 mg/m^2 IV q3wk). Patients with ER+ and/or PR+ disease also received tamoxifen (20 mg daily) for 5 years. The primary endpoint of the trial was disease-free survival. At median follow-up of 53 months, there was no difference between the two treatment groups, with a 4-year disease-free survival of 87% for both. Furthermore, overall survival was not statistically different (hazard ratio, 1.09; 95% confidence interval, 0.85–1.40; *P* = .49). A considerably higher incidence of neutropenia was observed in the AT arm than in the AC arm (19% vs 16%, respectively). Overall, both regimens produced outcomes that were better than expected. *(Goldstein LJ, O'Neill A, Sparano J, et al: J Clin Oncol [abstract] 23(suppl):7s, 2005).*

the risk of death (30%; *P* = .008). Although there was more febrile neutropenia with TAC, it was ameliorated with growth factor support.

In another study by the Cancer and Leukemia Group B (CALGB 9344), 3,121 women with operable, node-positive breast cancer were randomly assigned to receive 3 doses of doxorubicin with a standard dose of cyclophosphamide followed by either no further therapy or 4 cycles of paclitaxel (175 mg/m^2). This study did not show any substantial benefit from dose escalation of doxorubicin. However, the addition of 4 cycles of paclitaxel improved the disease-free and overall survival. At 5 years, the disease-free survival was 65% and 70%, and overall survival was 77% and 80% after AC vs AC plus paclitaxel, respectively. An unplanned subset analysis showed that the majority of the benefit was seen in those with estrogen receptor-negative tumors. Tamoxifen was given to 94% of patients with hormone receptor-positive tumors. Toxicity was modest with the addition of 4 cycles of paclitaxel.

In a similar study by the National Surgical Adjuvant Breast and Bowel Project (NSABP B-28), the addition of paclitaxel (225 mg/m^2) did not initially result in improvement of either disease-free or overall survival. However, with longer follow-up (median 67 months), improvement in disease-free survival in favor of AC followed by paclitaxel has emerged.

Dose-dense treatment CALGB 9741 tested two novel concepts: dose density and sequential therapy. A total of 2,005 women with operable, node-positive breast cancer were randomly assigned to receive one of the following regimens: (1) sequential Adriamycin (A) × 4 (doses) followed by Taxol (T) × 4 followed by cyclophosphamide (C) × 4, with doses every 3 weeks; (2) sequential A × 4 followed by T × 4 followed by C × 4, every 2 weeks with filgrastim (Neupogen); (3) concurrent AC × 4 followed by T × 4, every 3 weeks; or (4) concurrent AC × 4 followed by T × 4, every 2 weeks with filgrastim. At a median follow-up of 36 months, there was an improvement in disease-free (risk ratio = 0.74; *P*=.010) and overall survival (risk ratio = 0.69; *P*=.013) in favor of dose density. Four-year disease free survival was 82% for the dose-dense regimens and 75% for the others. There was no difference in disease-free or overall survival between the concurrent (dose-dense) and sequential schedules.

The dosages, schedules, and frequencies of chemotherapy regimens used for node-positive breast cancer are detailed in Table 1. Other regimens also used in node-negative (Chapter 9) and/or metastatic disease (Chapter 11) are listed in their respective chapters.

Recommendations All patients with stage II breast cancer should be considered for systemic adjuvant therapy. Adjuvant chemotherapy in node-positive breast cancer improves disease-free and overall survival by 24% and 15%, respectively. Risk reductions for multiagent chemotherapy are proportionately the same in patients with node-negative and node-positive disease.

Chemotherapy for women 50 years of age and older is similar to that for younger women. However, multiagent chemotherapy affords the greatest benefit in women younger than age 50 with respect to reductions in the risk of recurrence and death from breast cancer. For instance, CMF or AC chemotherapy improves disease-free survival in women aged 50 to 69 by 18%, vs 33% for women younger than age 50. Limited data are available from randomized trials regarding women aged 70 and older. However, in the absence of comorbidity, such as heart, renal, or liver disease, systemic adjuvant therapy can be offered to women ≥ 70 years old.

Endocrine (hormonal) therapy

The Early Breast Cancer Trialists' Collaborative Group (EBCTCG) overview analyses demonstrated a significant advantage with the addition of tamoxifen (20 mg/d oral) for 5 years to the adjuvant therapy regimen of women with estrogen receptor-positive breast cancer regardless of age. Treatment with tamoxifen reduced the risk of death by 14% in women younger than age 50 and by 27% in those 50 years of age and older. Long-term follow-up from the NSABP conclusively demonstrates that there is no benefit to continuing tamoxifen therapy beyond 5 years.

Premenopausal women

Approximately 60% of premenopausal women with primary breast cancer have estrogen receptor-positive tumors. For this group of patients, the benefit of adjuvant endocrine therapy, either tamoxifen or ovarian ablation, was established in the EBCTCG overview. Endocrine therapy has comparable efficacy to that of chemotherapy. For premenopausal women, however, the long-term morbidity associated with permanent ovarian suppression may be significant. Ovarian suppression with luteinizing hormone-releasing hormone (LHRH) analogs offers an alternative to permanent ovarian ablation, which is potentially reversible on cessation of therapy.

The Zoladex Early Breast Cancer Research Association (ZEBRA) trial is a randomized trial directly comparing goserelin (Zoladex) monotherapy with CMF in premenopausal women 50 years of age and younger with node-positive, stage II breast cancer. The primary efficacy population included 1,614 patients: 797 randomized to receive goserelin and 817, CMF. Estrogen-receptor status was known for 92.5% of patients; 80% had estrogen receptor-positive tumors.

TABLE 1: Adjuvant chemotherapy regimens in node-positive breast cancer

Regimen	Dose and frequency
TAC	
Taxotere (docetaxel)	75 mg/m^2 IV on day 1
Adriamycin (doxorubicin)	50 mg/m^2 IV on day 1
Cyclophosphamide	500 mg/m^2 IV on day 1
Repeat every 21 days for 6 cycles.	
Martin M, Pienkowski T, Mackey J, et al: Eur J Cancer 2(suppl):70, 2004.	
AC → T (conventional regimen)	
Adriamycin (doxorubicin)	60 mg/m^2 IV on day 1
Cyclophosphamide	600 mg/m^2 IV on day 1 × 4 cycles
followed by	
Taxol (paclitaxel)	175 mg/m^2 IV by 3-h infusion every 3 weeks × 4 cycles
Dose-dense (concurrent regimen)	
Adriamycin	60 mg/m^2 IV on day 1 every 2 weeks
Cyclophosphamide	600 mg/m^2 IV on day 1 every 2 weeks × 4 cycles
followed by	
Paclitaxel	175 mg/m^2 IV by 3-h infusion every 2 weeks × 4 cycles
Dose-dense (sequential regimen)	
Adriamycin	60 mg/m^2 IV on day 1 every 2 weeks × 4 cycles
followed by	
Paclitaxel × 4 cycles	175 mg/m^2 IV by 3-h infusion every 2 weeks
followed by	
Cyclophosphamide	600 mg/m^2 IV on day 1 every 2 weeks × 4 cycles
Citron M, Berry DA, Cirrincione C, et al: J Clin Oncol 21:1431–1439, 2003.	
A-CMF	
Adriamycin (doxorubicin)	75 mg/m^2 IV on day 1
Repeat every 3 weeks for 4 courses.	
Cyclophosphamide	600 mg/m^2 IV on day 1
Methotrexate	40 mg/m^2 IV on days 1 and 8
5-FU	600 mg/m^2 on day 1
Repeat every 3 weeks for eight courses.	
Buzzoni R, Bonadonna G, Valagussa P, et al: J Clin Oncol 9:2134–2140, 1991.	

At a median follow-up of 6 years, the estrogen receptor-positive patients treated with goserelin fared comparably to those who received CMF in terms of disease-free survival (HR = 1.01; P= .94) and overall survival (HR = 0.99; P= .92). Not surprisingly, CMF was superior to goserelin in patients with estrogen

Regimen	Dose and frequency
AC → T + trastuzumab	
Adriamycin (doxorubicin)	60 mg/m^2 IV on day 1
Cyclophosphamide	600 mg/m^2 IV over 30 minutes on day 1
Repeat every 21 days for 4 cycles.	
followed by	
Taxol (paclitaxel)	175 mg/m^2 IV by 3-h infusion on day 1
Repeat every 21 days for 4 cycles.	
NOTE: All patients should receive dexamethasone (20 mg orally) 12 and 6 hours before paclitaxel, diphenhydramine (50 mg IV), and ranitidine (50 mg IV) 30 to 60 minutes before paclitaxel.	
Or	
Taxol (paclitaxel)	80 mg/m^2 IV over 1 hour weekly for 12 doses
NOTE: All patients should receive dexamethasone (20 mg orally) 12 and 6 hours before the first dose of paclitaxel. If no hypersensitivity reaction occurs, convert to dexamethasone (10 mg IV), completed 30 minutes before each subsequent paclitaxel administration (dexamethasone may be tapered during the 12 weeks of paclitaxel).	
along with	
Trastuzumab	4 mg/kg IV, loading dose over 90 minutes on day of the first paclitaxel cycle (On the weeks paclitaxel is given, trastuzumab will be given after paclitaxel.)
	2 mg/kg IV, maintenance dose over 30 minutes every week for 51 weeks starting on day 8

Romond E, et al: J Clin Oncol [abstract] 23(suppl): plenary session, 2005.

receptor-negative tumors. The onset of amenorrhea occurred sooner with goserelin; by 6 months, more than 95% of patients on goserelin were amenorrheic, vs 59% for CMF recipients. Reversibility of amenorrhea was also greater for goserelin; 1 year after cessation of goserelin treatment, 23% remained amenorrheic, vs 77% for CMF recipients.

Several studies have compared adjuvant chemotherapy with combined endocrine therapies in premenopausal women, consisting of tamoxifen for 5 years and an LHRH agonist for 2 to 3 years. Overall, combination endocrine treatment yielded better results than chemotherapy alone. Whether a strategy of combined endocrine therapy is better than tamoxifen alone, either with or without chemotherapy, in premenopausal patients with hormone receptor-positive tumors is the subject of several ongoing clinical trials.

In the Suppression of Ovarian Function Trial (SOFT), following adjuvant chemotherapy, tamoxifen alone is being compared with tamoxifen plus ovarian function suppression/ablation vs ovarian function suppression plus an aromatase inhibitor (exemestane [Aromasin]). The role of ovarian suppression and aromatase inhibitors in this setting is being further investigated by the complementary Tamoxifen and Exemestane Trial (TEXT) comparing ovarian suppression with the LHRH analog triptorelin (Trelstar) plus tamoxifen vs triptorelin plus exemestane.

The ATAC Trialists' Group has presented its 5-year results on the effect of anastrozole (Arimidex) on bone mineral density (BMD). Breast cancer patients treated with anastrozole had significant bone loss, with lumbar BMD declining by about 2% per year during the first 2 years of treatment and then by nearly 1% annually in years 3–5. No patient with normal BMD at baseline, however, developed osteoporosis. Regular monitoring of BMD and strategies of bone protection are likely to be required in patients receiving anastrozole in the presence of preexisting osteopenia (*Coleman RE, on behalf of the ATAC Trialists' Group: J Clin Oncol [abstract] 24:5s, 2006*).

Currently, almost all premenopausal women with lymph node-positive, hormone receptor-positive breast cancer receive chemotherapy. Whether combined endocrine therapies alone may be sufficient to achieve excellent outcomes without chemotherapy is a question being investigated in the Premenopausal Endocrine Responsive Chemotherapy (PERCHE) trial. This trial is comparing ovarian function suppression with an LHRH agonist plus chemotherapy followed by tamoxifen or exemestane vs ovarian function suppression and tamoxifen or exemestane without chemotherapy for premenopausal patients with hormone receptor-positive tumors.

Postmenopausal women

For many years, tamoxifen has been the standard adjuvant endocrine therapy for postmenopausal women with hormone receptor-positive tumors. However, demonstrable benefits of aromatase inhibitors, as from several large, randomized clinical trials, have led to increasing use of these agents in the adjuvant treatment of postmenopausal women with hormone receptor-positive tumors.

The Arimidex, Tamoxifen, Alone or in Combination (ATAC) trial was the first large randomized trial demonstrating the superiority of an aromatase inhibitor over tamoxifen in the adjuvant treatment of postmenopausal women with hormone receptor-positive breast cancer. After the initial ATAC analyses, the combination arm was closed because of low efficacy. The ATAC trial was recently updated, with a median follow-up of 68 months.

In this updated analysis, only 8% of patients remain on trial treatment. Compared with tamoxifen, anastrozole (Arimidex) led to significant improvements in disease-free survival (HR = 0.87; $P = .01$), time to disease recurrence (HR = 0.79; $P = .0005$), and time to distant recurrence (HR = 0.86; $P = .04$). Additionally, substantial reduction in the incidence of contralateral breast cancer was observed with anastrozole compared with tamoxifen (42% reduction; $P = .01$). No differences have yet emerged in overall survival.

The safety profile of anastrozole remains unchanged from the previous analyses. No new safety concerns have emerged with additional months of follow-up. In general, toxicities were less common with anastrozole than with tamoxifen, with significantly fewer cases of hot flashes, vaginal bleeding/discharge, endometrial cancer, and thromboembolic events in the anastrozole-treated patients. Arthralgias occurred more frequently with anastrozole. Fracture rates were also higher with anastrozole (HR = 1.44; $P < .0001$); however, the low incidence of hip fractures was similar in the two groups.

Recently presented results from the BIG (Breast International Group) 1-98 trial also demonstrated the benefit of up-front use of Letrozole (Femara) compared with tamoxifen for 5 years as adjuvant endocrine therapy for postmenopausal women with hormone receptor-positive breast cancer. The study was later modified to include a crossover for both agents, and the results from crossover treatment arms were censored at 2 years in this analysis. In the core analysis, 8,010 patients were included; median follow-up was 25.8 months with more than 1,200 patients followed for at least 5 years.

> The first mature analysis of the Intergroup Exemestane Study suggests that switching to exemestane (Aromasin) after 2–3 years of tamoxifen significantly improves disease-free and overall survival compared with remaining on tamoxifen. A total of 4,724 postmenopausal women with estrogen receptor-positive early breast cancer have now been followed for a median of nearly 5 years. Women who switched to exemestane were less likely to have thromboembolic or serious gynecologic events than women who continued on tamoxifen but were more likely to experience a bone fracture (*Coombes RC, Paridaens R, Jassem J, et al: J Clin Oncol [abstract] 24:9s, 2006*).

Letrozole significantly prolonged disease free survival, with a 19% decrease in risk of recurrence ($P = .003$), compared with tamoxifen and significantly decreased the risk of distant metastasis by 27% ($P = .0012$). There was a trend toward better overall survival with letrozole (HR = 0.86), but it was not statistically significant. Unlike the ATAC trial, similar benefits in disease-free survival were observed in the estrogen receptor+/progesterone receptor+ and estrogen receptor+/progesterone receptor– subgroups. The safety profile was similar to that seen in prior studies of aromatase inhibitors, except for the higher incidence of hypercholesterolemia and grade 3–5 cardiac events noted for letrozole, which merits closer scrutiny.

Other randomized trials have investigated the use of an aromatase inhibitor after tamoxifen. Two sequential strategies after tamoxifen were studied: (1) a switch to an aromatase inhibitor after 2 or 3 years of tamoxifen, to complete a 5-year course of endocrine therapy or (2) a switch to an aromatase inhibitor after 5 years of tamoxifen, to complete 10 years of endocrine therapy, also called extended adjuvant therapy. With either strategy, the use of an aromatase inhibitor after tamoxifen provided significant reduction in events (recurrence, contralateral breast cancer, or death).

In the Intergroup Exemestane Study (IES), 4,742 patients who had received 2 to 3 years of tamoxifen were randomized to receive either additional tamoxifen or a switch to exemestane, to complete a 5-year course of endocrine therapy. After a median follow-up of 30.6 months, there was a significant reduction in risk, with an HR of 0.68 ($P < .001$) in favor of exemestane. Disease-free survival 3 years after randomization was 91.5% in the exemestane group and 86.8% in the tamoxifen group; this represents a 32% reduction in risk, or an absolute benefit in disease-free survival of 4.7%. Distant disease-free survival was also better in the exemestane group (HR = 0.66; $P = .0004$). Contralateral breast cancer occurred in 9 and 20 patients in the exemestane and tamoxifen groups, respectively ($P = .04$). Overall survival was not significantly different in the two groups.

Severe toxic effects of exemestane were rare, and toxicity profiles were similar

In the ABCSG Trial 6a, postmenopausal women who had received tamoxifen in combination with aminoglutethimide (Cytadren) or tamoxifen alone for 5 years were rerandomized to either anastrozole (Arimidex) or placebo for 3 years. Over 800 patients were included in the analysis, with a median follow-up of 5 years. Significantly fewer patients receiving anastrozole had relapsed compared with placebo (hazard ratio = 0.64; 95% confidence interval, 0.4–0.99; *P* = .047), although no statistically significant difference in overall survival has yet emerged (*Jakesz R, Samonigg H, Greil R, et al: J Clin Oncol [abstract] 23(suppl):10s, 2005*).

to those previously reported for aromatase inhibitors. Exemestane was associated with a higher incidence of arthralgia and diarrhea, and there was an increased trend for osteoporosis and visual disturbances. Fractures were more frequent in the exemestane group, although no significant statistical difference was noted between the two groups. Gynecologic symptoms, vaginal bleeding, and muscle cramps were more common with tamoxifen, and thromboembolic events were significantly more frequent with tamoxifen.

Three other randomized trials showed a benefit to switching to anastrozole after 2 to 3 years of tamoxifen treatment vs continued tamoxifen for a total of 5 years. The ITA (Italian Tamoxifen Arimidex) trial, with 448 patients enrolled and a median follow-up of 36 months, showed significant benefits in event-free (HR = 0.35; 95% confidence interval [CI], 0.20–0.63; *P*= .0002) and recurrence-free survival (HR = 0.35; 95% CI, 0.18–0.68; *P*= .001) in the women switched to anastrozole. There were 19 total events in the tamoxifen group (n = 225) and 10 in the anastrozole group (n = 223). The 3-year difference in recurrence-free survival was 5.8% (95% CI, 5.2–6.4%). Significantly longer locoregional recurrence-free survival (HR = 0.15; 95% CI, 0.03–0.65; *P*= .003) was noted for the anastrozole group. The difference in distant recurrence-free survival approached statistical significance (HR = 0.49; 95% CI, 0.22–1.05; P = .06).

A combined analysis of the ABCSG (Austrian Breast and Colorectal Cancer Study Group) Trial 8 and ARNO 95 Trial, with 3,224 patients and a median follow-up of 28 months, investigated a similar strategy. It showed that sequential endocrine therapy with tamoxifen for 2 years followed by anastrozole for 3 years was superior to 5 years of tamoxifen in terms of event-free (HR = 0.6; 95% CI, 0.44–0.81; *P* = .0009) and distant recurrence-free survival (HR = 0.61; 95% CI, 0.42–0.87; *P* = 0.0067). No statistically significant difference in overall survival has emerged at this point (*P*= .16).

In the MA-17 trial, 5,187 postmenopausal women who had taken tamoxifen for 5 years were randomly assigned to receive either letrozole or placebo for an additional 5 years. After the first interim analysis, the independent data and safety monitoring committee recommended termination of the trial since letrozole therapy after the completion of standard tamoxifen treatment significantly improved disease-free survival. With a median follow-up of approximately 27 months, the 4-year disease-free survival rates for letrozole and placebo were 93% and 87%, respectively (*P*< .001). No significant difference was noted in overall survival. However, in an updated analysis, an advantage in distant disease-free and overall survival was reported in the subset of women with node-positive disease. Toxicities associated with letrozole were similar to those seen with aromatase inhibitors in other trials.

Recent guidelines from the American Society of Clinical Oncology (ASCO) and the National Comprehensive Cancer Network (NCCN) highlight the appropriate use of aromatase inhibitors in postmenopausal women with hormone receptor-positive breast cancer. Aromatase inhibitors have a significant role in reduction of recurrence in early-stage breast cancer and should be included as part of the adjuvant endocrine therapy for postmenopausal women with hormone receptor-positive disease. Using an aromatase inhibitor as up-front therapy or switching at some point after 2 to 3 years of tamoxifen is an acceptable strategy. Since the risk of breast cancer recurrence after completion of adjuvant endocrine therapy remains substantial, extended therapy with an aromatase inhibitor is another viable strategy for patients who are completing 5 years of tamoxifen.

Several questions on the optimal use of aromatase inhibitors remain, and we must await completion of ongoing trials and/or development of new trials for answers. For instance, neither the optimal timing nor the duration of aromatase inhibitor therapy has been established, and the role of biomarkers (such as HER2/*neu* status) in selecting optimal endocrine therapy remains controversial. Furthermore, long-term effects of aromatase therapy, including osteoporosis, have not yet been well characterized.

HER2-positive tumors

Recent results suggest that patients with HER2/*neu*-expressing breast cancers associated with axillary lymph node metastasis benefit significantly from intensive, doxorubicin-containing adjuvant chemotherapy. Furthermore, studies demonstrating significant benefit to the addition of trastuzumab (Herceptin) to chemotherapy in metastatic breast cancer have prompted several groups to study this agent in the adjuvant setting. Some of these studies have completed accrual, and early results are astoundingly positive.

Three major trials of trastuzumab in the adjuvant setting were presented at 2005 meeting of ASCO. NSABP (National Surgical Adjuvant Breast and Bowel Project) B-31 and NCCTG (North Central Cancer Treatment Group) 9831 were jointly analyzed to include a total of 3,351 HER2-positive patients, with a median follow-up of 2.4 years. Both trials included two similar treatment arms: adjuvant chemotherapy with AC followed by paclitaxel with or without weekly trastuzumab for 1 year. Although there were differences between the two studies, including a third treatment arm in N9831 sequencing trastuzumab after paclitaxel that was not included in the joint analysis, the common question addressed was the effect of adding trastuzumab to AC followed by paclitaxel.

Both disease-free (hazard ratio = 0.48; $P = 3 \times 10^{-12}$) and distant disease-free (hazard ratio = 0.47; $P = 8 \times 10^{-10}$) survival were so highly statistically significant for trastuzumab, such results were unlikely to be due to chance alone. Furthermore, there appears to be an early survival benefit to the addition of trastuzumab (hazard ratio = 0.67; $P = .015$; disease-free survival: 87% vs 75%; overall sur-

The BCIRG 006 study evaluated the benefit of adjuvant trastuzumab (H) in 3,222 patients with HER2-positive breast cancer. Unique to this study was a nonanthracycline-containing regimen, which was expected to minimize the cardiotoxicity seen with trastuzumab following anthracycline-based chemotherapy. There were three treatment arms: 1) doxorubicin and cyclophosphamide (AC) followed by docetaxel (T); 2) AC→TH; or 3) TCH. At a median follow-up of 23 months, disease-free survival in the two trastuzumab-containing arms were statistically significant. There was a statistically significant higher incidence of cardiac events in the AC→TH arm but not in the TCH arm when compared with AC→T. There was also a statistically significant higher incidence of asymptomatic declines in left ventricular ejection fraction with AC→TH in comparison to AC→T. Longer follow-up is needed to confirm whether the efficacy of a nonanthracycline-based adjuvant trastuzumab regimen will be comparable to an anthracycline-based regimen (*Slamon D, Eiermann W, Robert N, et al. San Antonio Breast Cancer Symposium, San Antonio, Texas [abstract], December 8-11, 2005*).

overall survival: 94% vs 92%) despite the short follow-up. There was a small, but increased, risk of congestive heart failure with the use of Trastuzumab in these studies (approximately 3.8%). Since the dramatic results are changing the way breast cancer is treated and many clinicians are likely to use trastuzumab for similar groups of patients, the same monitoring used in these trials can be adopted in clinical practice to minimize cardiac toxicity.

The international HERA trial had a different design and assessed HER2-positive patients who received a variety of chemotherapeutic regimens, randomized to either observation vs 1 or 2 years of every-3-week trastuzumab. Results were reported by Piccart-Gebhart for only the 1 year of trastuzumab vs observation arm, which included 5,090 patients, with 1-year medial follow-up. Similar to the previously mentioned joint analysis, reduction in recurrences and improvement in progression-free survival were noted for women who received trastuzumab. The hazard ratios were approximately 0.5 ($P < .001$) for both recurrence-free and distant disease-free survival in favor of trastuzumab. No statistically significant differences in overall survival have been noted in this early analysis.

There are unresolved questions about the adjuvant use of trastuzumab, including sequential vs concurrent use with chemotherapy, the optimal duration, and whether anthracyclines can be omitted. Furthermore, the long-term safety of trastuzumab in this setting remains to be determined.

High-dose chemotherapy Because of the higher rate of recurrence in patients with stage IIB breast cancer, high-dose chemotherapy can also be considered as part of a clinical trial. See chapter 11 for a discussion of the current status of this approach.

Toxic effects of medical therapy

Chemotherapy The most frequent acute toxicities are nausea/vomiting, alopecia, and hematologic side effects, such as leukopenia and thrombocytopenia. Neutropenia, with its attendant risk of infection, is a potentially life-threatening complication that requires prompt medical attention and broad-spectrum antibiotics until hematologic recovery occurs.

TABLE 2: Follow-up recommendations for asymptomatic long-term breast cancer survivors as per NCCN guidelines

Intervention*	Year 1	Year 2	Years 3–5	Year 6+
History and physical exam	Every 4 mo	Every 4 mo	Every 6 mo	Annually
Mammography	Annually (or 6 mo after post BCS irradiation)	Annually	Annually	Annually
Chest x-ray	Annually?	NRR	NRR	NRR
Pelvic exam[a]	Annually	Annually	Annually	Annually
Bone density[b]	Every 1 to 2 yr	Every 1 to 2 yr	Every 1 to 2 yr	

NCCN = National Comprehensive Cancer Network; NRR = not routinely recommended; BCS = breast-conserving surgery

[a] For patients with an intact uterus on tamoxifen

[b] For patients at risk for osteoporosis

* Bone scan, liver function tests, and tumor markers are not routinely recommended and are performed only if clinically indicated.

Other toxicities may include amenorrhea, cystitis, stomatitis, myocardial failure, and nail/skin changes. Amenorrhea is drug- and dose-related and is often permanent in women older than age 40. Recent evidence demonstrates that chemotherapy-induced ovarian failure in the adjuvant chemotherapy setting is associated with a high risk of rapid bone demineralization in the first 6–12 months after treatment. Thus, premenopausal women undergoing adjuvant chemotherapy must be closely evaluated to prevent the development of early osteoporosis. Cardiac failure, although rare, is potentially life-threatening and may be irreversible.

Endocrine therapy Toxicities with tamoxifen or aromatase inhibitors include hot flashes, menstrual irregularities, vaginal discharge, and weight gain. Thrombophlebitis and endometrial hyperplasia are more common with tamoxifen. Arthralgias, osteoporosis, and fractures are more common with aromatase inhibitors, although the incidence of hip fractures is low.

Follow-up of long-term survivors

There is no consensus among oncologists as to the appropriate and optimal follow-up routine for long-term breast cancer survivors. Recommendations for follow-up testing vary. The vast majority of relapses, both locoregional and distant, occur within the first 3 years. Surveillance is most intensive in the initial 5 years; thereafter, the frequency of follow-up visits and testing is reduced (Table 2).

History and physical examination Surveillance methods include a detailed history and physical examination at each office visit. They are performed every 4–6 months for 5 years after completion of initial therapy, then annually thereafter. Patients at higher risk of recurrence or complications of treatment may require surveillance at shorter intervals. Patients who have been treated by mastectomy can be seen in the office annually after they have been disease-free for 5 years. Patients who were treated with breast-conserving surgery and radiotherapy can be followed at 6-month intervals until they have been disease-free for 6–8 years and then annually.

Approximately 71% of breast cancer recurrences are detected by the patients themselves, and they will report a change in their symptoms when questioned carefully. In patients who are asymptomatic, physical examination will detect a recurrence in another 15%. Therefore, a patient's complaint on history or a new finding on physical examination will lead to the detection of 86% of all recurrences.

Mammography should be performed annually in all patients who have been treated for breast cancer. For patients who have undergone breast-conserving surgery, the first follow-up mammogram should be performed approximately 6 months after completion of radiation therapy. The risk of developing contralateral breast cancer is approximately 0.5%–1.0% per year. In addition, approximately one-third of ipsilateral breast tumor recurrences in patients who have been treated by conservation surgery and radiotherapy are detected by mammography alone. As the time interval between the initial therapy and follow-up mammography increases, so does the likelihood that local breast recurrence will develop elsewhere in the breast rather than at the site of the initial primary lesion.

Chest x-ray Routine chest radiographs detect between 2.3% and 19.5% of recurrences in asymptomatic patients and may be indicated on an annual basis.

Liver function tests detect recurrences in relatively few asymptomatic patients, and their routine use has been questioned. However, these tests are relatively inexpensive, and it may not be unreasonable to obtain them annually.

Tumor markers There is no evidence that tumor markers, such as carcinoembryonic assay (CEA), CA-15-3, and CA-57-29, provide an advantage in survival or palliation of recurrent disease in asymptomatic patients. Therefore, the use of tumor markers to follow long-term breast cancer survivors is not recommended.

Bone scans Postoperative bone scans are also not recommended in asymptomatic patients. In the NSABP B-09 trial, in which bone scans were regularly performed, occult disease was identified in only 0.4% of patients.

Liver and brain imaging Imaging studies of the liver and brain are not indicated in asymptomatic patients. PET scans are not routinely recommended. Their utility is primarily as an adjunct study, often to establish the extent of metastatic disease.

Pelvic examinations Women with intact uteri who are taking tamoxifen should have yearly pelvic examinations because of their risk of tamoxifen-associated endometrial carcinoma, especially among postmenopausal women. The vast majority of women with tamoxifen-associated uterine carcinoma have early vaginal spotting, and any vaginal spotting should prompt rapid evaluation. However, since neither endometrial biopsy nor ultrasonography has demonstrated utility as a screening test in any population of women, routine use of these tests in asymptomatic women is not recommended.

Bone density Premenopausal women who become permanently amenorrheic from adjuvant chemotherapy and postmenopausal women who are treated with an aromatase inhibitor are at increased risk for bone fracture from osteopenia/osteoporosis. These patients should undergo monitoring of bone health every 1 to 2 years.

SUGGESTED READING

Boccardo F, Rubagotti A, Puntoni M, et al: Switching to anastozole versus continued tamoxifen treatment of early breast cancer: Preliminary results of the Italian Tamoxifen Anastrozole Trial. J Clin Oncol 23:5138–5147, 2005.

Chen AM, Meric-Bernstam F, Hunt KK, et al: Breast conservation after neoadjuvant chemotherapy: The M. D. Anderson Cancer Center experience. J Clin Oncol 22:2303–2312, 2004.

Citron ML, Berry DA, Cirrincione C, et al: Randomized trial of dose-dense versus conventionally scheduled and sequential versus concurrent combination chemotherapy as postoperative adjuvant treatment of node-positive primary breast cancer: First report of Intergroup trial C9741/Cancer and Leukemia B trial 9741. J Clin Oncol 21:1431–1439, 2003.

Coombes RC, Hall E, Gibson LJ, et al: A randomized trial of exemestane after 2 to 3 years of tamoxifen therapy in postmenopausal women with primary breast cancer. N Engl J Med 350:1081–1092, 2004.

Goss PE, Ingle JN, Martino S, et al: A randomized trial of letrozole in postmenopausal women after 5 years of tamoxifen therapy for early-stage breast cancer. N Engl J Med 349:1793–1802, 2003.

Henderson IC, Berry DA, Demetri GD, et al: Improved outcomes from adding sequential paclitaxel but not from escalating doxorubicin dose in an adjuvant chemotherapy regimen for patients with node-positive primary breast cancer. J Clin Oncol 21:976–983, 2003.

Jakesz R, Kaufmann M, Gnant M, et al: Benefits of switching postmenopausal women with hormone-sensitive early breast cancer to anastrozole after 2 years of adjuvant tamoxifen: Combined results from 3,123 women enrolled in the ABCSG Trial 8 and the ARNO 95 Trial (abstract). Breast Cancer Res Treat 88(suppl 2):S7, 2004.

Jonat W, Kaufmann M, Sauerbrei W, et al: Goserelin versus cyclophosphamide, methotrexate, and fluorouracil as adjuvant therapy in premenopausal patients with node-positive breast cancer: The Zoladex Early Breast Cancer Research Association Study. J Clin Oncol 20:4628–4635, 2002.

Mamounas EP, Bryant J, Lembersky BC, et al: Paclitaxel (T) following doxorubicin/cyclophosphamide (AC) as adjuvant chemotherapy for node-positive breast cancer: Results from NSABP B-28 (abstract). Proc Am Soc Clin Oncol 22:4, 2003.

Martin M, Pienkowski T, Mackey J, et al; Breast Cancer International Research Group 001 Investigators: Adjuvant docetaxel for node-positive breast cancer. N Engl J Med 352:2302–2313, 2005.

Piccart-Gebhart MJ, Procter M, Leyland-Jones B, et al; Herceptin Adjuvant (HERA) Trial Study Team: Trastuzumab after adjuvant chemotherapy in HER2-positive breast cancer. N Engl J Med 353:1659–1672, 2005.

Pierce LJ, Hutchins LF, Green SR, et al: Sequencing of tamoxifen and radiotherapy after breast-conserving surgery in early-stage breast cancer. J Clin Oncol 23:24–29, 2005.

Romond EH, Perez EA, Bryant J, et al: Trastuzumab plus adjuvant chemotherapy for operable HER2-positive breast cancer. N Engl J Med 353:1673–1684, 2005.

Thurlimann BJ, Keshaviah A, Mouridsen H, et al: Randomized double-blind phase III study to evaluate letrozole (L) vs tamofixen (T) as adjuvant endocrine therapy for postmenopausal women with receptor-positive breast cancer (abstract). J Clin Oncol 23(suppl):6s, 2005.

Winer EP, Hudis C, Burstein HJ, et al: American Society of Clinical Oncology technology assessment on the use of aromatase inhibitors as adjuvant therapy for postmenopausal women with hormone receptor-positive breast cancer: Status report. J Clin Oncol 23:619–629, 2005.

CHAPTER 11

Stages III and IV breast cancer

Lori Jardines, MD, Bruce G. Haffty, MD, Melanie Royce, MD, PhD, and Ishmael Jaiyesimi, DO

This chapter addresses the diagnosis and management of locally advanced, locally recurrent, and metastatic breast cancer, ie, stages III and IV disease.

Approximately 20%–25% of patients present with locally advanced breast cancer. Inflammatory breast cancer is a particularly aggressive form of breast cancer that falls under the heading of locally advanced disease and accounts for 1%–3% of all breast cancers.

Locoregional recurrence of breast cancer remains a major clinical oncologic problem. Rates of locoregional recurrence may vary from < 10% to > 50%, depending on initial disease stage and treatment.

Metastatic disease is found at presentation in 5%–10% of patients with breast cancer. The most common sites of distant metastasis are the lungs, liver, and bone.

The optimal therapy for stage III breast cancer continues to evolve. Recently, the use of neoadjuvant chemotherapy has been effective in downstaging locally advanced breast cancer prior to surgical intervention. The optimal neoadjuvant chemotherapeutic regimens continue to evolve, and studies are being performed to evaluate new agents and delivery methods.

Diagnosis

Locally advanced disease

Patients with locally advanced breast cancer do not have distant metastatic disease and are in this group based on tumor size and/or nodal status. Such patients often present with a large breast mass or axillary nodal disease, which is easily palpable on physical examination. In some instances, the breast is diffusely infiltrated with disease, and no dominant mass is evident.

Patients with inflammatory breast cancer often present with erythema and edema of the skin of the breast (peau d'orange) and may not have a discrete mass within the breast. These patients often are treated with antibiotics unsuccessfully for presumed mastitis.

Mammography is beneficial in determining the local extent of disease in the ipsilateral breast, as well as in studying the contralateral breast.

Fine-needle aspiration (FNA) or biopsy The diagnosis of breast cancer can be confirmed by either FNA cytology or core biopsy. Core biopsy is preferred to perform the wide variety of marker analyses.

Search for metastasis The presence of distant metastatic disease should be ruled out by physical examination, chest radiography, CT of the liver, bone scan, and CT of the chest. ^{18}Fluorodeoxyglucose-positron emission tomography (FDG-PET) has moderate accuracy for detecting axillary metastasis. It is highly predictive for nodal tumor involvement when multiple intense foci of tracer uptake are identified but fails to detect small nodal metastasis. The addition of FDG-PET to the standard workup of patients with locally advanced breast cancer may lead to the detection of unexpected distant metastases. Abnormal PET findings should be confirmed to prevent patients from being denied appropriate treatment.

Locoregional recurrence

Biopsy or FNA Locoregional recurrence of breast cancer can be diagnosed by surgical biopsy or FNA cytology. Whichever modality is appropriate, material should be sent for hormone-receptor studies, since there is only an 80% concordance in hormone-receptor status between the primary tumor and recurrent disease. When the suspected recurrent disease is not extensive, the biopsy procedure of choice is a negative margin excisional biopsy. For an extensive recurrence, an incisional biopsy can be used.

Search for distant metastasis Prior to beginning a treatment regimen for a patient with locoregional recurrence, an evaluation for distant metastasis should be instituted, since the findings may alter the treatment plan.

Distant metastasis from the breasts

Metastatic breast cancer may be manifested by bone pain, shortness of breath secondary to a pleural effusion, parenchymal or pulmonary nodules, or neurologic deficits secondary to spinal cord compression or brain metastases. In some instances, metastatic disease is identified after abnormalities are found on routine laboratory or radiologic studies.

Assessment of disease extent by radiography, CT, and radionuclide scanning is important. Organ functional impairment may be determined by blood tests (liver/renal/hematologic) or may require cardiac and pulmonary function testing. Biopsy may be required to confirm the diagnosis of metastasis; this is especially important when only a single distant lesion is identified.

Metastasis to the breasts

The most common source of metastatic disease to the breasts is a contralateral breast primary. Metastasis from a nonbreast primary is rare, representing < 1.5% of all breast malignancies. Some malignancies that could metastasize to the breast include non-Hodgkin lymphoma, leukemias, melanoma, lung cancer (particularly small-cell lung cancer), gynecologic cancers, soft-tissue sarcomas, and GI adenocarcinomas. Metastasis to the breasts from a nonbreast primary is more common in younger women. The average age at diagnosis ranges from the late 30s to 40s. Treatment depends on the status and location of the primary site.

Mammographic findings Mammography in patients with metastatic disease to the breasts most commonly reveals a single lesion or multiple masses with distinct or semidiscrete borders. Less common mammographic findings include skin thickening or axillary adenopathy.

FNA or biopsy FNA cytology has been extremely useful in establishing the diagnosis when the metastatic disease has cytologic features that are not consistent with a breast primary. When cytology is not helpful, core biopsy or even open biopsy may be necessary to distinguish primary breast cancer from metastatic disease.

Treatment

TREATMENT OF LOCALLY ADVANCED DISEASE

The optimal treatment for patients with locally advanced breast cancer has yet to be defined, due to the heterogeneity of this group. There are approximately 40 different substage possibilities with the different combinations of tumor size and nodal status. Between 66% and 90% of patients with stage III breast cancer will have positive lymph nodes at the time of dissection, and approximately 50% of patients will have four or more positive nodes.

Patients with locally advanced breast cancer have disease-free survival rates ranging from 0% to 60%, depending on the tumor characteristics and nodal status. In general, the most frequent type of treatment failure is due to distant metastases, and the majority of them appear within 2 years of diagnosis.

With the increased utilization of multimodality therapy, including chemotherapy, radiation therapy, and surgery, survival for this patient population has improved significantly.

Neoadjuvant systemic therapy

Neoadjuvant therapy with cytotoxic drugs permits in vivo chemosensitivity testing, can downstage locally advanced disease and render it operable, and may allow breast-conservation surgery to be performed. Preoperative chemotherapy requires a coordinated multidisciplinary approach to plan for surgical and radiation therapy. A multimodality treatment approach can provide improved control of locoregional and systemic disease. When neoadjuvant therapy is used, accurate pathologic staging is not possible.

Active regimens Preoperative chemotherapy regimens reported to result in high response rates (partial and complete responses) include CAF (cyclophosphamide, doxorubicin [Adriamycin], and fluorouracil [5-FU]), FAC (5-FU, Adriamycin, and cyclophosphamide), CMF (cyclophosphamide, methotrexate, and 5-FU), and CMFVP (cyclophosphamide, methotrexate, 5-FU, vincristine, and prednisone). Combination chemotherapy with an anthracycline-

TABLE 1: Doses and schedules of chemotherapy agents commonly used in patients with metastatic breast cancer

Drug/combination	Dose and schedule
FAC	
5-FU	500 mg/m^2 IV on days 1 and 8
Adriamycin	50 mg/m^2 IV on day 1
Cyclophosphamide	500 mg/m^2 IV on day 1
Repeat cycle every 3-4 weeks.	
TAC	
Taxotere	75 mg/m^2 IV on day 1
Adriamycin	50 mg/m^2 IV on day 1
Cyclophosphamide	500 mg/m^2 IV on day 1
Repeat cycle every 21 days.	
FEC	
5-FU	500 mg/m^2 IV on day 1
Epirubicin	100 mg/m^2 IV on day 1
Cyclophosphamide	500 mg/m^2 IV on day 1
Repeat cycle every 21 days.	
Note: An absolute granulocyte count < 1,500/μL and/or platelet count <100,000/μL on day 21 will cause a treatment delay of at least 1 week. Treatment wil be terminated if hematology recovery takes more than 3 weeks.	
Paclitaxel	175 mg/m^2 by 3-h IV infusion every 3 weeks or 80-100 mg/m^2/week
Docetaxel	60-100 mg/m^2 by 1-h IV infusion every 3 weeks or 40 mg/m^2/week
Repeat if hematologic recovery has occurred (ie, absolute granulocyte count ≥ 1,500/μL and platelet count ≥ 100,000/μL).	
Capecitabine	2,000 to 2,500 mg/m^2 PO bid (divided dose, AM and PM) for 14 days, followed by 1-week rest
Repeat cycle every 21 days.	
Capecitabine + docetaxel	
Capecitabine	1,000 to 1,250 mg/m^2 orally twice daily on days 1 to 14, followed by 1-week rest
Docetaxel	75 to 100 mg/m^2 IV infusion over 1 hour
Repeat cycle every 3 weeks.	
Vinorelbine + trastuzumab	
Vinorelbine	25 mg/m^2 IV on day 1 every week
Trastuzumab	4 mg/kg IV loading dose, then 2 mg/kg IV every week

[a]See pages 1061 and 1072 for information on capecitabine + lapatinib.

based regimen—FAC or AC—is used most often. Recently published data suggest that the AT regimen of Adriamycin and docetaxel (Taxotere) given concomitantly may produce equivalently high response rates. Combination agents for metastastic breast cancer also include paclitaxel plus trastuzumab (Herceptin) with carboplatin (Paraplatin), gemcitabine (Gemzar) and paclitaxel, and

Drug/combination	Dose and schedule
Docetaxel or paclitaxel + carboplatin + trastuzumab (every-3-week dosing)	
Docetaxel	75 mg/m^2 IV on day 1 every 21 days
	or
Paclitaxel	175 mg/m^2 IV on day 1 every 21 days
	plus
Carboplatin	AUC of 5 to 6 on day 1 every 21 days
	plus
Trastuzumab	4 mg/kg IV loading dose on day 1, followed by 2 mg/kg weekly
Note: Patients must be premedicated with dexamethasone prior to docetaxel.	
Trastuzumab	4 mg/kg IV loading dose, then 2 mg/kg weekly 8 mg/kg IV loading dose, then 6 mg/kg every 3 weeks
Paclitaxel or docetaxel + carboplatin + trastuzumab (weekly dosing)	
Paclitaxel	80 mg/m^2 IV on day 1 every week
	or
Docetaxel	35 mg/m^2 IV on day 1 every week
	plus
Carboplatin	AUC 2 IV on day 1 every week
	plus
Trastuzumab	4 mg/kg IV loading dose, then 2 mg/kg every week
Gemcitabine + paclitaxel	
Gemcitabine	1,250 mg/m^2 IV on days 1 and 8 (as a 30-minute infusion) every 21 days
Paclitaxel	175 mg/m^2 IV on day 1 (over 3 hours) every 21 days
Note: Standard paclitaxel premedications should be given.	
Pegylated doxorubicin	
Doxil	30 to 50 mg/m^2 IV on day 1 every 21 to 28 days
Nab-paclitaxel (nanoparticle albumin-bound paclitaxel)	
Abraxane	260 mg/m^2 IV on day 1 every 3 weeks

AUC = area under the curve

capecitabine (Xeloda) and docetaxel (Table 1). Although not yet definitive, recent data indicate that enhancing dose density may increase the pathologic complete response rate for women with locally advanced disease. The doses of these combination chemotherapy regimens are given in Table 1, chapter 10.

There seems to be no difference in survival in women with locally advanced disease who receive chemotherapy before or after surgery. Neoadjuvant chemotherapy results in complete response rates ranging from 20%–53% and partial response rates (≥ 50% reduction in bidimensionally measurable disease) ranging from 37%–50%, with total response rates ranging from 80%–90%. Patients with large lesions are more likely to have partial responses. Pathologic complete responses (pCRs) do occur and are more likely to be seen in patients with smaller tumors. A pCR in the primary tumor is often predictive of a complete axillary lymph node response. Patients with locally advanced breast cancer who have a pCR in the breast and axillary nodes have a significantly improved disease-free survival rate compared with those who have less than a pCR. However, a pCR does not entirely eliminate the risk for recurrence.

Patients should be followed carefully while receiving neoadjuvant systemic therapy to determine treatment response. In addition to clinical examination, it may also be helpful to document photographically the response of ulcerated, erythematous, indurated skin lesions. Physical examination, mammography, and breast ultrasonography are best for assessing primary tumor response, whereas physical examination and ultrasonography are used to evaluate regional nodal involvement.

The role of MRI in evaluating response to preoperative chemotherapy is still evolving. Dynamic contrast-enhanced MRI performed at baseline, during chemotherapy, and before surgery has yielded more than 90% diagnostic accuracy in identifying tumors achieving a pCR and can potentially provide functional parameters that may help to optimize neoadjuvant chemotherapy strategies. However, despite its high sensitivity, a large number of patients still may have either false-negative or false-positive results on MRI scanning.

Multimodality approach

A multimodality treatment plan for locally advanced breast cancer (stage IIIA and IIIB, M1 supraclavicular nodes) is shown schematically in Figure 1. This approach has been shown to result in a 5-year survival rate of 84% in patients with stage IIIA disease and a 44% rate in those with stage IIIB disease. The most striking benefit has been seen in patients with inflammatory breast cancer, with 5-year survival rates of 35%–50% reported for a multimodality treatment approach including primary chemotherapy followed by surgery and radiation therapy and additional adjuvant systemic therapy. The same chemotherapy drugs, doses, and schedules used for single-modality therapy are employed in the multimodality approach.

Surgery Traditionally, the surgical procedure of choice for patients with locally advanced breast cancer has been mastectomy. In recently published studies, some patients with locally advanced breast cancer who responded to treatment with neoadjuvant chemotherapy became candidates for breast-conservation therapy and were treated with limited breast surgery and adjuvant breast irradiation. Patients who have been downstaged using neoadjuvant chemotherapy should be evaluated carefully before proceeding with conservative treatment. It may be helpful to mark the site of the primary tumor with the placement of a clip during the course of percutaneous biopsy prior to beginning adjuvant therapy. There can sometimes be a complete clinical and/or radiographic response after neoadjuvant chemotherapy or hormonal therapy, and this may facilitate a wide local incision.

The role of sentinel node biopsy in the treatment of breast cancer after neoadjuvant chemotherapy has yet to be defined. Studies have shown that pathologically positive axillary lymph nodes can be sterilized when neoadjuvant chemotherapy is utilized. There are other biologic concerns with sentinel node

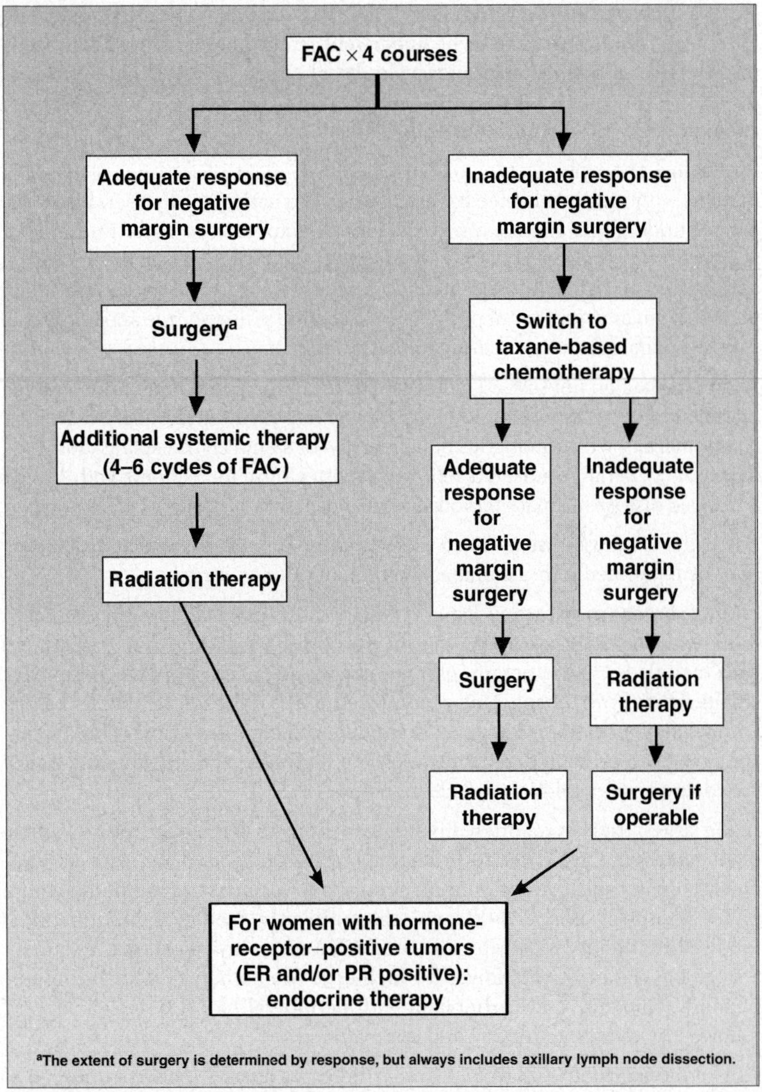

FIGURE 1: Multimodality approach to locally advanced breast cancer

biopsy after neoadjuvant chemotherapy. The lymphatics may undergo fibrosis or may become obstructed by cellular debris, making the mapping procedure unreliable, with false-negative rates of up to 25%. The rate of conversion from positive to negative nodes can be enhanced when 4 cycles of a doxorubicin-based regimen are followed by 4 cycles of docetaxel. Sentinel node biopsy will only be accurate then if all the metastatic deposits within the axilla respond in a similar fashion to chemotherapy. Preliminary data from the National Surgical

Adjuvant Breast and Bowel Project (NSABP) B-27 trial demonstrated an 11% false-negative rate in women who underwent sentinel node biopsy after receiving 4 cycles of doxorubicin and cyclophosphamide followed by 4 cycles of docetaxel. However, patients with clinically positive nodes prior to neoadjuvant chemotherapy should have full node dissection.

Radiation therapy remains an integral component of the management of patients with locally advanced breast cancer. For patients with operable breast cancer undergoing mastectomy, radiation therapy to the chest wall and/or regional lymph nodes (to a total dose of 5,000–6,000 cGy) is usually employed, as discussed in chapter 10. Recent randomized trials suggest that postmastectomy patients with any number of positive nodes derive a disease-free and/or overall survival benefit from postmastectomy irradiation.

Available data do not suggest a problem in delaying radiation therapy until the completion of systemic chemotherapy. Even in patients undergoing high-dose chemotherapy with autologous bone marrow or stem-cell transplantation, irradiation is generally indicated following mastectomy for patients with locally advanced disease (primary tumors ≥ 5 cm and/or ≥ four positive axillary nodes).

For patients whose disease is considered to be inoperable, radiation therapy may be integrated into the management plan prior to surgery.

High-dose chemotherapy Patients with locally advanced breast cancer and those with multiple positive nodes may be candidates for protocol treatment with high-dose chemotherapy plus autologous stem-cell support. Preliminary results from three prospective, randomized trials of high-dose chemotherapy with autologous stem-cell support in women with high-risk primary breast cancer have been presented. All three trials are summarized in Table 2, and two of the trials are discussed in more detail below.

In the largest trial yet reported, investigators from all of the bone marrow transplant centers in the Netherlands randomly assigned 885 women with stages II and III breast cancer with 4 or more tumor-positive nodes to a standard therapy arm of 5 courses of FEC (5-FU, epirubicin [Ellence], and cyclophosphamide) followed by radiation therapy and tamoxifen or an investigational treatment arm of 4 cycles of FEC followed by high-dose chemotherapy with cyclophosphamide, thiotepa, and carboplatin with peripheral blood stem-cell support followed by radiation therapy and tamoxifen.

After a median follow-up of 57 months, there was a trend toward improved 5-year relapse-free survival rates in the high-dose group, but it was not statistically significant (hazard ratio [HR] = 0.83; *P* = .09). In the subgroup of patients with 10 or more positive nodes, however, the relapse-free survival rate reached statistical significance (HR = 0.71; *P* = .05). There was also a suggestion that the benefit seen in the high-dose group may be confined to patients with HER2/*neu*-negative tumors.

The second-largest trial evaluating high-dose chemotherapy was conducted by the Cancer and Leukemia Group B (CALGB) in patients with stage II or III breast cancer involving 10 or more axillary lymph nodes. This trial examined the value of consolidation high-dose therapy with cyclophosphamide, cisplatin,

TABLE 2: Randomized studies of high-dose chemotherapy in primary breast cancer

Investigators	Number of patients	Follow-up (median)	Survival benefit?	*P* value
Rodenhuis et al	885	36 mo	Yes	$P < .05$
Peters et al	783	36 mo	No	NS
Scandinavian Breast Cancer Study Group	525	20 mo	No	NS

NS = not significant

and carmustine (BiCNU) with autologous stem-cell support following adjuvant therapy with cyclophosphamide, doxorubicin, and 5-FU. Preliminary results of this study, with 783 participants, showed a reduction in relapse frequency of over 30% in patients receiving high-dose chemotherapy; a 3-year survival rate of 68% was observed in patients treated with high-dose chemotherapy, vs a 64% rate in those who received intermediate-dose consolidation therapy with the same drugs. However, follow-up is not yet long enough to define the ultimate benefit of this approach. Moreover, toxicity to date has been significantly higher and the relapse rate significantly lower in the high-dose group.

Nonrandomized studies of high-dose chemotherapy plus autologous stem-cell support have shown a disease-free survival of ~70%, as compared with historic data showing a 30% 5-year disease-free survival rate with conventional-dose chemotherapy.

To date, the results of available clinical trials have not all shown improved disease-free and overall survival in patients treated with dose-intensive regimens. However, trial design, power, and strategy have all been questioned. Outside the context of a clinical trial, high-dose chemotherapy cannot be recommended for patients with primary or metastatic breast cancer.

TREATMENT OF LOCOREGIONAL RECURRENCE AFTER EARLY INVASIVE CANCER OR DCIS

When a patient develops a local failure after breast-conservation treatment for early invasive cancer or ductal carcinoma in situ (DCIS), it is generally in the region of the initial primary tumor. The risk of ipsilateral breast tumor recurrence after conservative treatment in patients with early invasive cancer ranges from 0.5%–2.0% per year, with long-term local failure rates plateauing at about 15%–20%. Local failure rates after wide excision alone for DCIS vary from 10%–63%, as compared with rates between 7% and 21% after wide excision plus radiation therapy. Most patients whose disease recurs after conservative treatment for DCIS can be treated with salvage mastectomy. In one study, 14% of patients who developed local recurrence had synchronous distant metastatic disease.

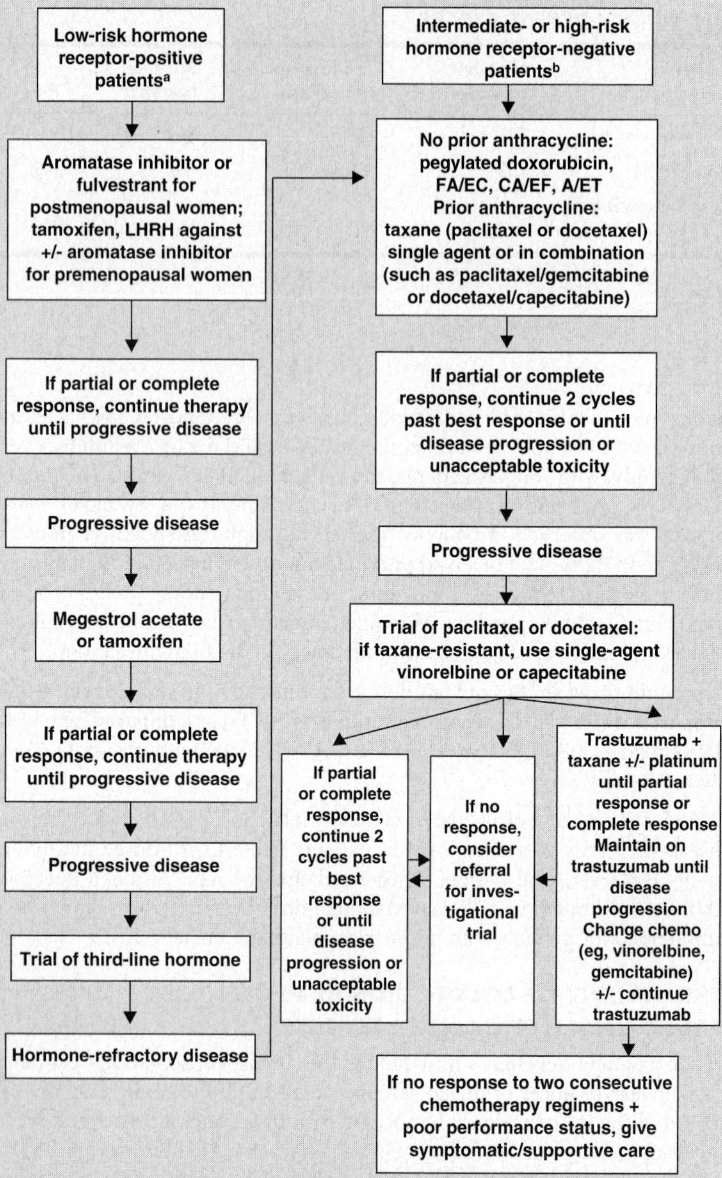

Low-risk hormone receptor-positive patients[a]
Aromatase inhibitor or fulvestrant for postmenopausal women; tamoxifen, LHRH against +/- aromatase inhibitor for premenopausal women
If partial or complete response, continue therapy until progressive disease
Progressive disease
Megestrol acetate or tamoxifen
If partial or complete response, continue therapy until progressive disease
Progressive disease
Trial of third-line hormone
Hormone-refractory disease
Intermediate- or high-risk hormone receptor-negative patients[b]
No prior anthracycline: pegylated doxorubicin, FA/EC, CA/EF, A/ET
Prior anthracycline: taxane (paclitaxel or docetaxel) single agent or in combination (such as paclitaxel/gemcitabine or docetaxel/capecitabine)
If partial or complete response, continue 2 cycles past best response or until disease progression or unacceptable toxicity
Progressive disease
Trial of paclitaxel or docetaxel: if taxane-resistant, use single-agent vinorelbine or capecitabine
If partial or complete response, continue 2 cycles past best response or until disease progression or unacceptable toxicity
If no response, consider referral for inves-tigational trial
Trastuzumab + taxane +/- platinum until partial response or complete response Maintain on trastuzumab until disease progression Change chemo (eg, vinorelbine, gemcitabine) +/- continue trastuzumab
If no response to two consecutive chemotherapy regimens + poor performance status, give symptomatic/supportive care

[a]Low-risk patients include those with a long disease-free interval, tumors that are positive for hormone receptors (estrogen and progesterone), or bone-only disease, as well as those without extensive visceral involvement

[b]Intermediate- or high-risk patients include those with rapidly progressive disease, visceral involvement, hormone-refractory disease, or tumors that are negative for hormone receptors

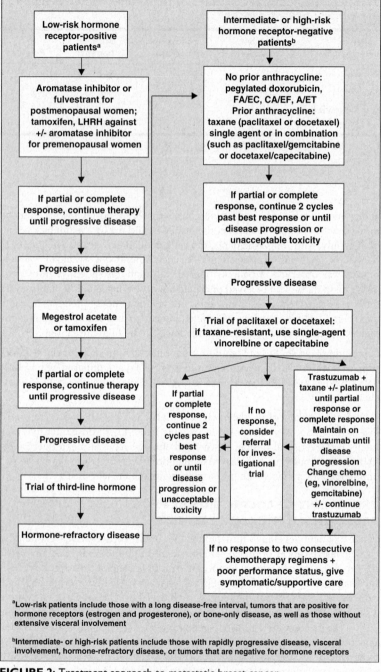

FIGURE 2: Treatment approach to metastatic breast cancer

The optimal treatment of a local or regional recurrence after mastectomy has yet to be defined. Locoregional recurrences are associated with initial nodal status and primary tumor size. Appropriate treatment may result in long-term control of locoregional disease. In many instances, these patients develop simultaneous distant metastasis, or distant disease develops some time after the locoregional recurrence manifests itself.

Recurrence of invasive cancer after breast conservation

Recurrence after wide excision and breast irradiation For patients with early invasive cancer who have undergone conservative surgery followed by irradiation and whose cancer recurs in the ipsilateral breast, salvage mastectomy is the most common treatment modality. The same is true for ipsilateral recurrence (of invasive or in situ disease) after conservative treatment for DCIS, when there is no evidence of distant metastatic disease.

Some studies with limited follow-up have reported acceptable results with repeated wide local excision for ipsilateral breast tumor relapses following conservative surgery and radiation therapy. Selection criteria for this approach are unclear, however, and use of this salvage procedure remains controversial. Although the use of limited-field reirradiation has been reported, selection criteria for this management option and long-term follow-up data are lacking.

Recurrence after wide excision alone In patients initially treated with wide local excision alone who sustain an ipsilateral breast tumor recurrence, small series with limited follow-up suggest that wide local excision followed by radiation therapy to the intact breast at the time of local recurrence may be a reasonable treatment alternative. In this situation, standard radiation doses would be employed.

Recurrent disease in the chest wall after mastectomy

In general, patients who develop minimal recurrent disease in the chest wall after a long disease-free interval may be treated by excision alone, although this approach is controversial and may not be ideal. Locoregional control obtained by radiation therapy alone is related to the volume of residual disease and may not be durable. When possible, disease recurring in the chest wall or axillary nodes should be resected and radiation therapy should be delivered to aid in local control.

Radiation treatment techniques are generally similar to those employed for patients treated with standard postmastectomy irradiation and consist of photon- and/or electron-beam arrangements directed at the chest wall and adjacent lymph node regions. Treatment planning should strive for homogeneous dose distributions to the target areas while minimizing the dose to the underlying cardiac and pulmonary structures.

Radiation dose and protocol Conventional fractionation of 180–200 cGy/d to the area of locoregional recurrence and immediately adjacent areas at risk, to a total dose of 4,500–5,000 cGy, is indicated. A boost to the area of recurrence or gross residual disease, to a dose of approximately 6,000 cGy, results in acceptable long-term locoregional control.

> A double-blind, placebo-controlled study of exemestane (Aromasin) demonstrated that it had a modest effect on bone loss in women with early-stage postmenopausal breast cancer who had already undergone surgery and irradiation. The investigators evaluated its effects on bone loss in 147 women with bone mineral density (BMD) levels that fell within 2 SDs of the mean level for women aged 65. Patients were randomized to receive exemestane orally for 2 years or placebo. Exemestane was well tolerated, and no patient who had a normal BMD level at baseline developed osteoporosis. Of the 19 patients with osteopenia at baseline, 6 in the exemestane arm and 5 in the placebo arm developed osteoporosis in the spine, and 3 in the exemestane arm and 5 in the placebo arm developed osteoporosis in the femoral neck. Nine patients had bone fractures. The authors concluded that exemestane had no effect on the spine and little effect on the femoral neck (*Lonning PE, Geisler J, Krag LE, et al: J Clin Oncol 23:5126-5137, 2005*).

Radical chest wall resection A select group of patients with local chest wall recurrence secondary to breast cancer may be candidates for a radical chest wall resection, which may include resection of skin, soft tissue, and bone. Flap coverage or prosthetic chest wall reconstruction is required. Appropriate candidates would include patients who do not have distant metastases and who have persistent or recurrent chest wall disease after chest wall irradiation and patients who present with a chest wall recurrence after a long disease-free interval.

ADJUVANT SYSTEMIC THERAPY FOR LOCOREGIONAL RECURRENCE

Ipsilateral breast tumor recurrence

Limited data support the use of adjuvant systemic therapy at the time of ipsilateral breast tumor recurrence. Retrospective studies have suggested a 20%–50% risk of systemic metastases in patients who sustain an ipsilateral breast tumor recurrence. A study conducted at Yale University found that ipsilateral breast tumor recurrence was a significant predictor of distant metastases, particularly among women who relapsed within 4 years of the original diagnosis; these women had a rate of distant metastasis of approximately 50%. Similar findings were noted by the NSABP investigators.

These data suggest that women whose tumors recur in the ipsilateral breast within the first few years following the original diagnosis may be considered for adjuvant systemic therapy. Given the lack of prospective, randomized data, specific treatment recommendations for these women remain highly individualized.

Regional nodal recurrence and postmastectomy recurrence of disease in the chest wall

Although there are limited data addressing the use of adjuvant systemic therapy at the time of locoregional relapse following mastectomy, given the high rate of systemic metastasis in this population, these patients may be considered for adjuvant systemic therapy. A randomized trial demonstrated a disease-free survival benefit with the use of adjuvant tamoxifen following radiation therapy at the time of postmastectomy recurrence of disease in the chest wall in patients with estrogen-receptor–positive tumors. The 5-year disease-free survival rate was increased from 36% to 59%, and the median disease-free survival was prolonged by > 4.5 years.

Patients with estrogen-receptor–negative tumors and aggressive locoregional recurrences may also be considered for systemic cytotoxic chemotherapy, given their relatively poor prognosis and the high rate of metastasis.

To determine whether weekly infusion of paclitaxel improves response rates vs the standard 3-hour infusion, 577 patients with metastatic breast cancer who had received one or two prior regimens were randomized to receive standard (175 mg/m²) or weekly (80 mg/m²) paclitaxel. Weekly paclitaxel was shown to be superior with respect to response rate (40% vs 28%; *P* = .017), time to disease progression (9 vs 5 mo; *P* = .0008), and overall survival (24 vs 16 mo). When trastuzumab (Herceptin) became standard therapy for HER2-positive tumors, all patients with HER2-positive disease received trastuzumab, whereas patients with HER2-negative disease were randomized to receive either addition of trastuzumab or not. The addition of trastuzumab did not improve any of these end points. Weekly paclitaxel caused more grade 3 sensory/motor neuropathy and less grade ≥ 3 granulocytopenia. The authors concluded that weekly is superior to standard paclitaxel in the management of metastatic breast cancer (*Seidman AD, Broadwater G, Carney W, et al: J Clin Oncol [abstract] 23[suppl]:18s, 2005*).

MEDICAL TREATMENT OF METASTATIC BREAST CANCER

Patients with metastatic cancer can be divided into two groups: those with stage IV disease at presentation and those who develop metastases after primary treatment. The management of stage IV disease depends on the site and extent of metastases, comorbid conditions, and clinical tumor characteristics.

Patients with delayed metastatic disease can be divided into two groups, ie, so-called low risk and intermediate or high risk, based on the biologic aggressiveness of the disease. As shown schematically in Figure 2, the management approach to these two groups differs.

Low-risk patients

The low-risk group includes patients who develop metastatic disease after a long disease-free interval (ie, a long disease-free interval from primary breast cancer diagnosis to presentation with metastasis), those whose tumors are positive for hormone receptors (estrogen and progesterone), those with bone-only disease, and those without extensive visceral organ involvement.

Hormone therapy Low-risk patients, whose tumor is hormone receptor-positive (ie, estrogen receptor-positive and/or progesterone receptor-positive), may be treated with a trial of hormone therapy.

First-line hormonal therapy consists of an aromatase inhibitor, with careful serial assessment of clinical and disease responses.

Hormone therapy may be associated with a "flare" response, a temporary worsening of signs and symptoms of disease within the first few weeks of treatment. This response generally means clinical benefit will follow.

If the tumor initially responds to first-line hormone therapy and then progresses, a second hormonal manipulation is warranted. Various hormonal agents are available (Table 3). They may be used sequentially and may provide disease

TABLE 3: Doses and schedules of hormonal agents commonly used in patients with metastatic breast cancer

Agent	Dose and schedule
Postmenopausal	
Tamoxifen	20 mg PO every day
or	
Toremifene	60 mg PO every day
Anastrozole	1 mg PO every day
or	
Letrozole	2.5 mg PO every day
or	
Exemestane	25 mg PO every day
Fulvestrant	250 mg IM every month
Megestrol	40 mg PO 4 times a day
Fluoxymesterone	10 mg PO 3 times a day
Aminoglutethimide	250 mg PO 4 times a day
Premenopausal	
Tamoxifen	20 mg PO every day
Luteinizing hormone-releasing hormone analogues	
Leuprolide	7.5 mg IM depot every 28 days 22.5 mg IM every 3 months 30 mg IM every 4 months
Goserelin	3.6 mg SC depot every 28 days 10.8 mg SC every 3 months
Megestrol	40 mg PO 4 times a day
Fluoxymesterone	10 mg PO 3 times a day

palliation for prolonged periods in some patients.

Second-line hormonal agents The choice of second-line endocrine therapy depends on the front-line endocrine agent used. Typically, if tamoxifen was used, the second-line agent includes an aromatase inhibitor or fulvestrant (Faslodex) for postmenopausal women. For premenopausal women, the choice may be megestrol or induction of menopause with an LHRH (luteinizing hormone-releasing hormone) agonist with or without an aromatase inhibitor. If aromatase inhibitors were used as front-line agents for postmenopausal women, second-line options can be to change to another class of aromatase inhibitor, fulvestrant, or tamoxifen.

The most commonly used second-line hormonal agents had been progestational drugs, such as megestrol. Recent randomized trials have indicated that the aromatase inhibitors, such as anastrozole (Arimidex), letrozole (Femara), fulvestrant, and exemestane (Aromasin), are equally effective for palliation of metastatic disease, have less toxicity, and may provide a survival advantage compared with megestrol. Therefore, they are the drugs of choice for second-line therapy following tamoxifen administration. Tamoxifen may also be considered as second-line therapy for patients initially treated with an aromatase inhibitor.

Hormonal therapy continues until evidence of disease progression or drug-related toxicity precludes further therapy with the same agent. If a partial or complete response to the first hormonal treatment is documented at the time of disease progression, a second hormonal agent may provide further palliation of symptoms and avoid the initiation of systemic chemotherapy. However, subsequent hormonal responses tend to be of shorter duration, and, ultimately, the disease will become refractory to hormonal treatment.

> When added to capecitabine (Xeloda), the dual tyrosine kinase inhibitor lapatinib provided significant benefit to patients with metastatic breast cancer and HER2-positive tumors previously treated with trastuzumab (Herceptin). The combination of lapatinib (Tykerb) and capecitabine nearly doubled the time to disease progression compared with capecitabine alone (8.5 vs 4.5 months). Enrollment in the study was halted based on the superior efficacy and acceptable tolerability of the combination regimen. *(Geyer CE, Cameron D, Chan S, et al: J Clin Oncol [abstract] 24:special session, 2006).* Lapatinib was approved by FDA in March 2007 in combination with capecitabine for metastatic breast cancer.

Cytotoxic agents Hormone-refractory disease can be treated with systemic cytotoxic therapy. FAC, paclitaxel, TAC (Taxotere [docetaxel], Adriamycin [doxorubicin], cyclophosphamide), or docetaxel may be used in this situation. (For a more detailed discussion of these agents, see section on "Intermediate- or high-risk patients." For doses, see Table 1.)

A prospective, multicenter study assessed the role of circulating tumor cells in predicting survival in 177 metastatic breast cancer patients before the start of a new treatment. Patients with levels of circulating tumor cells ≥ 5/7.5 mL of whole blood had a shorter median progression-free survival (2.7 vs 7.0 months; $P < .001$) and shorter overall survival (10.1 vs > 18 months; $P < .001$) than those with < 5/7.5 mL circulating tumor cells. Of all the variables in the statistical model, the levels of circulating tumor cells at baseline and at the first follow-up visit were the most significant predictors of progression-free and overall survival in this group of patients.

Intermediate- or high-risk patients

Intermediate- or high-risk patients include those with rapidly progressive disease or visceral involvement, as well as those with disease shown to be refractory to hormonal manipulation by a prior therapeutic trial.

Anthracycline-containing combinations, such as FAC (see Table 1), are preferred for these patients. However, newer combinations of doxorubicin and a taxane are gaining favor for use in patients who have not received > 450 mg/m^2 of an anthracycline and whose relapse has occurred more than 12 months after the completion of adjuvant therapy.

Single agents Many single cytotoxic drugs have shown some activity in metastatic breast cancer (Table 1). They include vinblastine, mitomycin (Mutamycin), thiotepa, capecitabine, vinorelbine, and gemcitabine.

One study explored the relationship between circulating HER2 extracellular domain (ECD) and tissue HER2 status and examined its predictive value in a cohort of metastatic breast cancer patients treated with weekly trastuzumab (Herceptin) and paclitaxel. Retrospective analysis of patients treated on a previous trial evaluated the associations between pretreatment serum HER2 ECD and tissue HER2 status and the change in serum HER2 ECD after 12 weeks of therapy and response. Stored serum samples were available for 55 of 95 patients (58%). Statistically significant association were found between HER2 status and baseline serum HER2 ECD level. Patients whose ECD normalized after 12 weeks of therapy had a higher response proportion thatn did those with persistently high ECD levels (68% vs 15%; *P* = .005). A relative decline of more than 55% from baseline HER2 ECD predicted response to trastuzumab-based therapy (*Fornier MN, Seidman AD, Schwartz MK, et al: Ann Oncol 16:234-239, 2005*).

Paclitaxel One of the most active agents is paclitaxel. It has demonstrated antitumor activity in patients with anthracycline-resistant disease, as well as in those who have received three or more prior chemotherapy regimens for metastatic disease.

High-dose paclitaxel (250 mg/m^2 over 3 hours) has not been shown to be superior to 175 mg/m^2 over 3 hours. The higher dose regimen is associated with greater hematologic and neurologic toxicities.

Docetaxel, approved by the US Food and Drug Administration (FDA) for anthracycline-resistant locally advanced or metastatic breast cancer, has demonstrated overall response rates of 41% in patients with doxorubicin-resistant disease. It has been shown to be superior to mitomycin/vinblastine in patients whose disease progressed after an anthracycline-based chemotherapy regimen.

The recommended starting dose of docetaxel—100 mg/m^2 as a 1-hour IV infusion—requires premedication with dexamethasone to avoid fluid retention and the capillary leak syndrome. The usual regimen of dexamethasone is 8 mg twice daily for a total of 3 days, beginning 24 hours prior to the administration of docetaxel.

Although 100 mg/m^2 is the dose of docetaxel approved by the FDA, many recent trials have demonstrated a high rate of grade 4 hematologic toxicity at this dose level; a dose of 60–70 mg/m^2 may achieve equivalent therapeutic benefit with improved safety. As with paclitaxel, the docetaxel dosage must be modified in patients who have hepatic impairment, manifested by elevated transaminase or alkaline phosphatase levels.

Capecitabine, an orally active fluorinated pyrimidine carbonate, has been shown to have a substantial antitumor effect in patients whose disease has recurred or progressed after prior anthracycline or taxane therapy. Prolonged survival, limited toxicity, and response in visceral as well as soft-tissue disease add to the benefit of capecitabine. Toxicities include diarrhea, stomatitis, and hand-foot syndrome.

New approaches Multiple new approaches to treating metastatic breast cancer are being explored. Weekly schedules of docetaxel and paclitaxel have been reported to produce high response rates and lower toxicity than 3-week schedules. Combinations of doxorubicin with paclitaxel or docetaxel have also shown substantial antitumor activity, as have combinations of capecitabine and docetaxel, carboplatin and paclitaxel, and gemcitabine and cisplatin. These newer combinations need to be compared with standard AC or FAC (CAF) regimens in phase III trials. Recent studies also suggest that sequential weekly chemotherapy may be as effective as more intensive combinations with respect to overall survival in patients with metastatic breast cancer.

Bevacizumab (Avastin) is the first antiangiogenic agent to demonstrate benefit in women with breast cancer. The phase III ECOG 2100 trial, which randomized patients to receive either standard doses of weekly paclitaxel or the same chemotherapy with bevacizumab as front-line treatment for metastatic disease, was presented at the 2005 ASCO meeting. The overall response rate was significantly better with the combination (28.2% vs 14.2%; $P < .0001$). Noteworthy were the significant increases in progression-free and overall survival for patients treated with the combination, although the survival data are still immature. Toxicities associated with the bevacizumab combination included hypertension, proteinuria, and neuropathy. There was also a trend toward an increase in thrombosis and bleeding, but it was not statistically significant *(Miller KD, Wang M, Gralow J, et al: Breast Cancer Res Treat [abstract] 94[suppl 1]:56, 2005).*

Monoclonal antibody therapy

Trastuzumab, a humanized monoclonal antibody to the HER2/*neu* protein, has been approved for use as a single agent in second- and third-line therapy for metastatic breast cancer and in combination with paclitaxel as first-line therapy in this setting. A randomized trial consisting of 469 women showed that the combination of trastuzumab with chemotherapy yielded a 45% overall response rate, as compared with a 29% rate with chemotherapy alone—a 55% increase. The addition of trastuzumab had the greatest impact on response when combined with paclitaxel. Among the study group as a whole, 79% of women treated with trastuzumab chemotherapy were alive at 1 year, as compared with 68% of those given chemotherapy alone.

An update of these data has shown a superior median overall survival with chemotherapy plus trastuzumab compared with chemotherapy alone (25.4 vs 20.9 months). The survival advantage was seen with both AC plus trastuzumab and paclitaxel plus the monoclonal antibody.

In another single-arm trial involving 222 women who had not responded to prior chemotherapy, trastuzumab shrunk tumors by 50% in 14% of women, with a median duration of response of 9 months. Overall, trastuzumab was well tolerated in both trials. Due to an increased risk of cardiac dysfunction observed in women treated with trastuzumab plus an anthracycline, trastuzumab should not be used in combination with this drug class.

It is important to point out that trastuzumab also produces cardiac toxicity when administered by itself, particularly in patients who have had extensive prior exposure to an anthracycline. Finally, essentially all of the clinical benefit of trastuzumab (alone or in combination) is confined to patients whose breast cancer expresses high (3+) levels of the HER2/*neu* oncoprotein.

In one randomized trial, patients with one to three newly diagnosed brain metastases (breast as well as other sites) were randomly allocated to receive either whole brain radiation therapy (WBRT, 164 patients) or WBRT followed by a stereotactic radiosurgery boost (167 patients). Univariate analysis showed that there was a survival advantage in the WBRT and surgery group for patients with a single brain metastasis (median survival 6.5 vs 4.9 months; *P* = .0393). Patients in the stereotactic surgery group were more likely to have a stable or improved Karnofsky performance status score at 6 months' follow-up than were patients allocated to WBRT alone (43% vs 27%, respectively; *P* = .03; *Andrews DW, Scottt CB, Sperduto PW, et al: Lancet 363:1665-1672, 2004*).

High-dose chemotherapy

Patients who present with or subsequently develop distant metastasis may be candidates for high-dose intensive chemotherapy programs with autologous stem-cell support. Multiple feasibility and phase II studies of this approach have been undertaken. The majority of programs include the use of multiple alkylating agents. The role of high-dose chemotherapy in metastatic disease remains controversial, and analysis and observation of ongoing clinical trials continue to be important.

The results from multiple centers indicate an overall 5-year disease-free survival rate of 25% in patients with metastatic disease treated with high-dose chemotherapy. However, it must be remembered that these results were obtained in a select patient population—generally individuals < 60 years of age with good performance status; chemotherapy-sensitive disease; and normal cardiac, pulmonary, renal, and hepatic function. The use of intensive supportive outpatient care, such as colony-stimulating factors and antibiotics, has significantly reduced the morbidity and mortality associated with the high-dose chemotherapy approach.

In recently presented randomized trials of high-dose chemotherapy in patients with metastatic breast cancer (Table 4), it appears that most of the benefit occurs in women with low-bulk disease, especially those in complete clinical remission. A meta-analysis with longer follow-up also demonstrated a benefit for the addition of high-dose therapy to standard, anthracycline-containing chemotherapy for advanced disease in the setting of patients in complete clinical remission. This therapeutic modality remains investigational for patients with stage IV disease, however; women referred for high-dose therapy should be enrolled in a clinical trial.

Adjunctive bisphosphonate therapy

Multiple published reports have now confirmed the benefit of bisphosphonates as an adjunct to treatment of patients with bone metastasis. Use of these agents results in a significant reduction in skeleton-related events, including pathologic fracture, bone pain, and the need for radiation therapy to bone. Pamidronate and zoledronic acid (Zometa), both in IV formulations, are available in the United States. Oral bisphosphonates used for this indication, such ibandronate (Boniva) and clodronate, are not in the US market.

Patients with breast carcinoma who had all types of bone metastases (osteolytic, mixed, or osteoblastic) were randomized to receive treatment with either 4 or 8

TABLE 4: Randomized studies of high-dose chemotherapy in metastatic breast cancer

Investigators	Number of patients	Median follow-up (yr)	Survival rate (%) High-dose treatment	Survival rate (%) Standard treatment	P value
Stadtmauer et al	553	3	32.0	38.0	NS
Lotz et al	61	5	29.8	18.5	NS

NS = not significant

mg of zoledronic acid as a 15-minute infusion or 90 mg of pamidronate as a 2-hour infusion every 3–4 weeks for 12 months. The proportion of patients who had a skeleton-related event (defined as a pathologic fracture, spinal cord compression, radiotherapy, or surgery to bone) was comparable between treatment groups (approximately 45%). However, among patients who had breast carcinoma with at least one osteolytic lesion, treatment with 4 mg of zoledronic acid was more effective than 90 mg of pamidronate in reducing skeletal complications.

The most commonly reported adverse events for both zoledronic acid and pamidronate were bone pain, nausea, fatigue, emesis, and fever. The 4-mg dose of zoledronic acid results in elevated serum creatinine levels in about 7.7% of patients, vs 6.0% with pamidronate. A larger proportion of patients had elevated serum creatinine levels with 8-mg of zoledronic acid; therefore, this dose is not recommended. Symptomatic hypocalcemia, although relatively rare, requires frequent monitoring of calcium and phosphate levels during treatment.

ROLE OF RADIATION THERAPY IN METASTATIC DISEASE

Irradiation remains an integral component of the management of metastatic breast carcinoma. Although bone metastases are the most commonly treated metastatic sites in patients with breast cancer, brain metastases, spinal cord compression, choroidal metastases, endobronchial lung metastases, and metastatic lesions in other visceral sites can be effectively palliated with irradiation.

Radiation dose and schedule Depending on the disease site and volume of the radiation field, fractionation schedules ranging from 20 Gy in 5 fractions to 30 Gy in 10 fractions are used most commonly. In some situations, more protracted courses using lower daily doses may be indicated.

Bone metastasis For patients with widespread bone metastasis, hemibody irradiation (6–7 Gy in one fraction to the upper body or 8 Gy to the lower body) has been shown to be effective. Strontium-89 chloride (Metastron) and other systemic radionuclides also provide effective palliation for widespread bone disease.

Consolidation after high-dose chemotherapy Since patients with metastatic disease treated with high-dose chemotherapy and autologous bone marrow or stem-cell transplantation often develop progressive disease in previously involved sites, studies have suggested the use of "consolidative radiation therapy" for patients undergoing high-dose chemotherapy. Although this approach appears to be well tolerated and preliminary data are encouraging, whether it will affect survival remains to be determined.

ROLE OF SURGERY IN METASTATIC DISEASE

There are selected indications for surgical intervention in patients with metastatic breast cancer, and the role of surgery at this point is generally palliative. Most commonly, palliative surgery is offered to patients with brain metastases, spinal cord compression, fractures, or symptomatic pleural or pericardial effusions not controlled by other means. It is also used for GI complications stemming from metastatic deposits. The curative benefit of surgery in the treatment of metastatic disease to the lungs or liver is not proven, but, in highly selected cases, surgery may be beneficial.

Spinal cord compression Patients with spinal cord compression who have progressive symptoms during irradiation, disease recurrence after irradiation, or spinal instability or who require diagnosis are candidates for surgery.

Solitary brain metastasis Patients with a long disease-free interval and solitary brain metastasis may be candidates for resection. Evidence suggests an improved disease-free survival, overall survival, and quality of life in this subset of patients when treated with surgery combined with postoperative cranial irradiation, as compared with radiation therapy alone.

Gamma- and cyber-knife radiosurgery is increasingly used to manage brain metastases. In some instances, these modalities have been used in patients who have multiple metastatic brain lesions or in patients who had previously received conventional treatment modalities for brain metastases, including whole-brain irradiation. No radiation-induced dementia and a remarkably low incidence of local failure were reported with these treatments. Although in the past, local control of brain metastasis was an issue, these treatment modalities are shifting the question of survival to that of systemic control.

Chest wall resection It is extremely rare for a patient with distant metastatic disease to be a candidate for chest wall resection; however, patients with symptomatic recurrence of disease in the chest wall who have limited distant disease and a life expectancy of > 12 months may be appropriate candidates.

Solitary liver metastatic disease Although rarely indicated, patients with single metastases or a prolonged disease-free or disease-stable interval may be candidates for resection.

Follow-up of long-term survivors

For recommendations on the type and timing of follow-up evaluations, see chapter 10.

SUGGESTED READING

Berry DA, Broadwater G, Klein JP, et al: High-dose versus standard chemotherapy in metastatic breast cancer: Comparison of Cancer and Leukemia Group B Trials with data from the Autologous Blood and Marrow Transplant Registry. J Clin Oncol 20:743–750, 2002.

Cristofanilli M, Budd GT, Ellis MJ, et al: Circulating tumor cells, disease progression, and survival in metastatic breast cancer. N Engl J Med 351:781–791, 2004.

Green MC, Buzdar AU, Smith T, et al: Weekly paclitaxel improves pathologic complete remission in operable breast cancer when compared with paclitaxel once every 3 weeks. J Clin Oncol 23:5983–5992, 2005.

Howell A, Robertson JF, Quaresma AJ, et al: Fulvestrant, formerly ICI 182,780, is as effective as anastrozole in postmenopausal women with advanced breast cancer progressing after prior endocrine treatment. J Clin Oncol 20:3396–3403, 2002.

Kuerer HM, Hunt K: The rationale for integration of lymphatic mapping and sentinel node biopsy in the management of breast cancer after neoadjuvant chemotherapy. Semin Breast Dis 5:80–87, 2002.

Loesch D, Robert N, Asmar L, et al: Phase II multicenter trial of a weekly paclitaxel and carboplatin regimen in patients with advanced breast cancer. J Clin Oncol 20:3857–3864, 2002.

Martincich L, Montemurro F, De Rosa G, et al: Monitoring response to primary chemotherapy in breast cancer using dynamic contrast-enhanced magnetic resonance imaging. Breast Cancer Res Treat 83:67–76, 2004.

O'Shaughnessy J, Miles D, Vukelja S, et al: Superior survival with capecitabine plus docetaxel combination therapy in anthracycline-pretreated patients with advanced breast cancer: Phase III trial results. J Clin Oncol 20:2812–2823, 2002.

Robertson JF, Osborne CK, Howell A, et al: Fulvestrant versus anastrozole for the treatment of advanced breast carcinoma in postmenopausal women: A prospective combined analysis of two multicenter trials. Cancer 98:229–238, 2003.

Rodenhuis S, Bontenbal M, Beex LV, et al: High-dose chemotherapy with hematopoietic stem-cell rescue for high-risk breast cancer. N Engl J Med 349:7–16, 2003.

Rosen LS, Gordon DH, Dugan W Jr, et al: Zoledronic acid is superior to pamidronate for the treatment of bone metastases in breast carcinoma patients with at least one osteolytic lesion. Cancer 100:36–43, 2004.

Sledge GW, Neuberg D, Bernardo P, et al: Phase III trial of doxorubicin, paclitaxel, and the combination of doxorubicin and paclitaxel as front-line chemotherapy for metastatic breast cancer: An intergroup trial (E1193). J Clin Oncol 21:588–592, 2003.

van der Hoeven JJ, Krak NC, Hoekstra OS, et al: 18F-2-fluoro-2-deoxy-d-glucose positron emission tomography in staging of locally advanced breast cancer. J Clin Oncol 22:1253–1259, 2004.

Wahl RL, Siegel BA, Coleman RE, et al: Prospective multicenter study of axillary nodal staging by positron emission tomography in breast cancer: A report of the staging breast cancer with PET study group. J Clin Oncol 22:277–285, 2004.

CHAPTER 12

Esophageal cancer

I. Benjamin Paz, MD, Jimmy J. Hwang, MD, and Rajesh V. Iyer, MD

Although still relatively uncommon in Western countries, esophageal cancer is fatal in the vast majority of cases. In the United States, an estimated 15,560 new cases will be diagnosed in the year 2007, and 13,940 deaths will result from the disease. This high percentage of deaths rivals that of pancreatic cancer and is more than four times that of rectal cancer.

The esophagus extends from the cricopharyngeal sphincter to the gastroesophageal (GE) junction and is commonly divided into the cervical, upper to mid-thoracic, and thoracic portions. This can be important, as histology and optimal treatment approaches may vary considerably based on the site of the cancer. It may not be possible to determine the site of origin if the cancer involves the GE junction itself.

Epidemiology

Gender Esophageal cancer is seven times more common and slightly more lethal in men than in women.

Age Adenocarcinoma of the esophagus (now more common in the United States than the squamous cell type) has a median age at diagnosis of 69 years. The incidence of squamous cell cancer of the esophagus increases with age as well and peaks in the seventh decade of life.

Race The incidence of squamous cell esophageal cancer is three times higher in blacks than in whites, whereas adenocarcinomas are more common in white men.

Geography Evidence for an association between environment and diet and esophageal cancer comes from the profound differences in incidence observed in different parts of the world. Esophageal cancer occurs at a rate 20–30 times higher in China than in the United States. An esophageal "cancer belt" extends from northeast China to the Middle East.

Survival Although the overall outlook for patients diagnosed with esophageal cancer has improved in the past 30 years, most patients still present with advanced disease, and their survival remains poor. One-third to one-half of patients treated with either chemoradiation therapy or chemoradiation therapy plus surgery are alive at 2 years, without recurrence of esophageal cancer.

Disease site The rate of cancer of the distal esophagus is about equal to that of the more proximal two-thirds. In general, squamous cell carcinoma is found in the body of the esophagus, whereas adenocarcinoma predominates in lesions closer to the GE junction.

Etiology and risk factors

Cigarettes and alcohol Squamous cell carcinomas of the esophagus have been associated with cigarette smoking and/or excessive alcohol intake. Furthermore, cigarette smoking and alcohol appear to act synergistically, producing high relative risks in heavy users of tobacco and alcohol. Esophageal adenocarcinoma is increased twofold in smokers.

Diet High-fat, low-protein, and low-calorie diets have been shown to increase the risk of esophageal cancer. Exposure to nitrosamines has been proposed as a factor in the development of both squamous cell carcinoma and adenocarcinoma of the esophagus.

Barrett's esophagus and other factors Gastroesophageal reflux disease (GERD) and Barrett's esophagus (adenomatous metaplasia of the distal esophagus) have been linked to adenocarcinoma of the esophagus. Tylosis, Plummer-Vinson syndrome, history of head and neck cancer, and achalasia have also been associated with a higher-than-normal risk of developing squamous cell cancer of the esophagus.

Signs and symptoms

Because symptoms do not alert the patient until the disease is advanced, few esophageal cancers are diagnosed at an early stage.

Dysphagia The most common presenting complaint is dysphagia, which generally is not noted until the esophageal lumen is narrowed to one-half to one-third of normal, due to its elasticity.

Weight loss is common and has a significant role in prognosis (> 10% of total body weight as poor prognosis).

Cough that is induced by swallowing is suggestive of local extension into the trachea with resultant tracheoesophageal fistula.

Odynophagia and pain Pain with swallowing (odynophagia) is an ominous sign. Patients who describe pain radiating to the back may well have extraesophageal spread. Supraclavicular or cervical nodal metastases may be appreciated on examination.

Hoarseness may be a sign of recurrent laryngeal nerve involvement due to extraesophageal spread.

Metastatic disease may present as malignant pleural effusion or ascites. Bone metastasis can be identified by pain involving the affected site or by associated hypercalcemia. The most common metastatic sites are retroperitoneal or celiac lymph nodes.

The American College of Surgeons conducted a study utilizing its national cancer database to assess the presentation, stage distribution, and treatment of patients diagnosed with esophageal cancer between 1994 and 1997 (n = 5,044). The most common presenting symptoms were dysphagia (74.0%), weight loss (57.3%), reflux (20.5%), odynophagia (16.6%), and dyspnea (12.1%). The American College of Surgeons Database finds 50% of patients present with tumors in the lower third of the esophagus; 42% have adenocarcinoma histology, and 52% have squamous histology. Barrett's esophagus was found in 39% of those patients with adenocarcinoma. Patients undergoing initial surgical resection had the following stage distribution: stage I (13.3%), II (34.7%), III (35.7%), and IV (12.3%).

Diagnosis

In Western countries, the diagnosis of esophageal cancer is generally made by endoscopic biopsy of the esophagus. In the Far East, cytologic evaluation is frequently utilized.

Endoscopic ultrasonography (EUS) is extremely accurate (> 90%) in establishing the depth of tumor invasion (T stage) but less accurate (70%–80%) in determining nodal involvement (N stage) unless combined with fine-needle aspiration (FNA) of the involved nodes (93% accuracy) when nodes greater than 5 mm are biopsied. The addition of FNA increases the sensitivity from 63% to 93% and the specificity from 81% to 100%. EUS is not reliable in determining the extent of response to neoadjuvant treatment.

Endoscopy and barium x-rays Endoscopy allows for direct visualization of abnormalities and directed biopsies. Barium x-rays are less invasive and provide a good assessment of the extent of esophageal disease.

Bronchoscopy should be performed to detect tracheal invasion in all cases of esophageal cancer except adenocarcinoma of the distal third of the esophagus.

CT scan Once a diagnosis has been established and careful physical examination and routine blood tests have been performed, a CT scan of the chest, abdomen, and pelvis should be obtained to help assess tumor extent, nodal involvement, and metastatic disease.

PET A prospective trial designed to evaluate the utility of PET vs CT and EUS was performed by obtaining these studies in 48 consecutive patients prior to esophagectomy. PET achieved a 57% sensitivity, 97% specificity, and 86% accuracy compared with CT, which was 99% sensitive, 18% specific, and 78% accurate. In terms of nodal staging, PET was correct in 83% of cases, as compared with 60% of cases for CT and 58% for EUS ($P = .006$). This analysis suggests the improved accuracy of PET in the staging work-up of patients with esophageal cancer.

Numerous studies report the accuracy of PET scanning in determining the presence of metastatic disease, with sensitivity approaching 90% and specificity over 90%.

As PET becomes more widely available, its use will probably become an important part of the preoperative evaluation of these patients. In a prospective trial of 39 patients with esophageal cancer, PET detected additional sites of metastatic disease at the initial evaluation when compared with conventional imaging. After induction therapy, PET did not add to the estimation of locoregional resectability and did not detect new distant metastases. However, this study suggested that changes in [^{18}fluorodeoxyglucose] FDG-PET following induction therapy may predict disease-free and overall survival after induction therapy and resection in patients with esophageal cancer. A large prospective national trial will evaluate the use of PET in the treatment of esophageal cancer.

Bone scan A bone scan should be obtained if the patient has bone pain or an elevated alkaline phosphatase level.

Thoracoscopy/laparoscopy Investigators have recently begun to examine the role of surgical staging prior to definitive therapy. These procedures are designed to allow pathologic review of regional lymph nodes and the accurate assessment of extraesophageal tumor spread by direct visualization. A recently completed multi-institution trial (Cancer and Leukemia Group B [CALGB] 9380) found these procedures to be feasible in over 70% of patients; they resulted in the upstaging of patients in 38% of cases reviewed. Further investigations need to be completed to determine the appropriate use of these tools in treatment algorithms for patients with esophageal cancer.

Warning Staging studies should be performed in a sequential manner. Invasive, lower yield, and less accurate studies and procedures should only be undertaken if management would change on the basis of specific findings.

Screening and surveillance

HIGH-RISK PATIENTS

Adenocarcinoma The role of screening patients with GERD and surveillance of patients with Barrett's esophagus by upper GI endoscopy remains under investigation. In 833 patients studied by endoscopy, there was a 13% incidence of intestinal metaplasia (Barrett's esophagus). Dysplasia or cancer was seen in 31% of patients with long-segment Barrett's esophagus, in 10% of short-segment Barrett's esophagus, and in 6% of GE-junction intestinal metaplasia.

Squamous cell carcinoma Mass screening in the high-risk areas of China and Japan is considered appropriate.

Pathology

Adenocarcinoma The incidence of esophageal adenocarcinoma involving the GE junction has risen 4%–10% per year since 1976 in the United States and Europe. As a result, adenocarcinoma is now the predominant histologic subtype of esophageal cancer. The distal one-third of the esophagus is the site of origin of most adenocarcinomas.

Squamous cell carcinomas occur most often in the proximal two-thirds of the esophagus. Squamous cell carcinoma is still the most prevalent histologic subtype worldwide.

TABLE 1: 1983 and 2002 AJCC TNM staging systems for esophageal cancer

1983 Classification (clinical)		2002 Classification (pathologic)
Primary tumor (T)		
Tis	Carcinoma in situ	Same
T1	Tumor involves ≤ 5 cm of esophageal length, produces no obstruction, and has no circumferential involvement	Tumor invades lamina propria or submucosa
T2	Tumor involves > 5 cm of esophageal length, causes obstruction, or involves the circumference of the esophagus	Tumor invades muscularis propria
T3	Extraesophageal spread	Tumor invades adventitia
T4	Not applicable	Tumor invades adjacent structures
Regional lymph nodes (N)		
Nx	Regional nodes cannot be assessed	Same
N0	No nodal metastases	No regional nodal metastases
N1	Unilateral, mobile, regional nodal metastases (if clinically evaluable)	Regional nodal metastases
N2	Bilateral, mobile, regional nodal metastases (if clinically evaluable)	Not applicable
N3	Fixed nodes	Not applicable
Distant metastases (M)		
M0	No distant metastases	Same
M1	Distant metastases	Distant metastases
		Tumors of lower thoracic esophagus: M1a Metastases in celiac lymph nodes M1b Other distant metastases
		Tumors of mid-thoracic esophagus: M1a Not applicable M1b Nonregional lymph nodes and/or other distant metastases
		Tumors of upper thoracic esophagus: M1a Metastases in cervical nodes M1b Other distant metastases

Stage grouping	1983 T	1983 N	1983 M	2002 T	2002 N	2002 M
Stage I	T1	N0 or NX	M0	T1	N0	M0
Stage II	T2	N0 or NX	M0			
Stage IIA				T2-3	N0	M0
Stage IIB				T1-2	N1	M0
Stage III	T3	Any N	M0	T3 T4	N1 Any N	M0 M0
Stage IV	Any T	Any N	M1	Any T	Any N	M1
Stage IVA				Any T	Any N	M1a
Stage IVB				Any T	Any N	M1b

TABLE 2: Treatment options and survival by stage in esophageal cancer

Stage[a]		Standard treatment	5-Year survival rate (%)
Stage 0	(Tis N0 M0)	Surgery	> 90
Stage I	(T1 N0 M0)	Surgery	> 70
Stage IIA	(T2-3 N0 M0)	Surgery, chemoradiation therapy, or combination	15-30
Stage IIB	(T1-2 N1 M0)	Surgery, chemoradiation therapy, or combination	10-30
Stage III	(T3 N1 M0 or T4 Any N M0)	Chemoradiation therapy Palliative resection of T3a tumors	< 10
Stage IV	(Any T Any N M1)	Radiation therapy ± intraluminal intubation and dilation ± chemotherapy	Rare

[a] According to the AJCC TNM system definitions (see Table 1)

Note: Surgical results are based on the pathologic staging system, whereas patients treated with combined-modality therapy or neoadjuvant chemoradiation therapy are clinically staged.

Other tumor types Other, less frequently seen histologic subtypes include mucoepidermoid carcinoma, small-cell carcinoma, sarcoma, adenoid cystic leiomyosarcoma, and primary lymphoma of the esophagus. Occasionally, metastatic disease from another site may present as a mass in the esophagus or a mass pressing on the esophagus.

Metastatic spread The most common sites of metastatic disease are the regional lymph nodes, lungs, liver, bone, adrenal glands, and diaphragm. Adenocarcinoma can also metastasize to the brain.

Staging and prognosis

Based on data demonstrating that the depth of penetration has important prognostic significance, the American Joint Committee on Cancer (AJCC) TNM staging system for esophageal cancer was changed from a clinical one (1983) to a pathologic one in 2002. Both the clinical and pathologic staging systems are shown in Table 1, as patients may be cured without an operation. Although pathologic information obtained from an esophagectomy specimen is of prognostic importance, postoperative therapy to improve prognosis has not been rigorously tested. Moreover, recurrence rates for stage I (30%) and stage II (70%) cancers suggest early systemic spread undetected by current noninvasive staging.

Pathologic information obtained from an esophagectomy specimen is of significant prognostic importance. Immunohistochemical analysis of the initial biopsy specimen may also have prognostic relevance. Clinical staging has been shown to be of prognostic importance, particularly in patients managed with primary radiotherapy or chemoradiation therapy.

Histology and grade Neither histology nor grade has been shown to be of prognostic importance in esophageal carcinoma.

Other prognostic factors Patient age, performance status, and degree of weight loss are of prognostic importance. The prognostic implications of tumor-suppressor genes and oncogenes are an area of active investigation.

Treatment

Treatment options for the various disease stages are given in Table 2, along with 5-year survival rates.

TREATMENT OF LOCALIZED DISEASE

Only 40%–60% of patients with esophageal cancer present with clinically localized disease. The National Comprehensive Cancer Network (NCCN) guidelines state that patients with clinically localized disease may be treated with resection or chemotherapy plus irradiation (Tables 3 and 4). The overall 5-year survival rates for either surgery alone or combined chemotherapy and irradiation appear equivalent.

Chemoradiation therapy as primary management of localized or locoregionally confined esophageal cancer has been shown to be superior to irradiation alone. A series of randomized trials have demonstrated that adjuvant postoperative chemoradiation therapy does not offer a survival advantage to patients with esophageal cancer. Adequate patient selection, tumor staging, and treatment standardization will be required before the optimal therapeutic modalities in these patients will be determined.

Surgery

Preoperative medical evaluation helps determine the patient's risk of developing postoperative complications and mortality. In addition to the staging and nutritional status, it should include an evaluation of the pulmonary, cardiac, renal, and hepatic functions.

Extent of surgical resection The extent of resection depends on the location of the primary tumor, histology of the tumor, and nature of the procedure (palliative vs curative). Retrospective study has reported that superficial mucosal lesions may be treated via endoscopic mucosal resection, but those patients with submucosal invasion require esophagectomy. For tumors of the intrathoracic esophagus (squamous cell carcinomas) and tumors with extensive Barrett's esophagus (adenocarcinomas), it is necessary to perform a total esophagectomy with cervical anastomosis to achieve a complete resection. For distal lesions of the abdominal esophagus (adenocarcinomas) and cardia, it is often possible to perform an intrathoracic esophageal anastomosis above the azygos vein, although many surgeons would prefer to perform a total esophagectomy.

TABLE 3: Chemotherapy regimens for esophageal carcinoma

Drug/combination	Dose and schedule
Cisplatin/fluorouracil/radiation therapy	
Cisplatin	75 mg/m^2 IV on day 1 of weeks 1, 5, 8, and 11
Fluorouracil	1 g/m^2/d IV infused continuously on days 1-4 of weeks 1, 5, 8, and 11
Radiation therapy	200 cGy/d 5 days per week (total regional treatment, 3,000 cGy), followed by a 2,000-cGy boost field (total, 5,000 cGy) in 5 weeks

Give chemotherapy concurrently with radiation therapy.

Adapted from Herskovic A, Martz K, al-Sarraf M, et al: N Engl J Med 326:1593–1598, 1992.

Table prepared by Ishmael Jaiyesimi, DO

The resected esophagus may be replaced with tubularized stomach in patients with tumors of the intrathoracic esophagus or with a colon interposition in patients with tumors involving the proximal stomach, since such involvement makes this organ unsuitable for esophageal reconstruction. The esophageal replacement is usually brought up through the posterior mediastinum, although the retrosternal route is often used in palliative procedures.

Patient selection The indications for esophagectomy in esophageal cancer vary from center to center within the United States.

Clearly, patients with distant metastases, evidence of nodal metastases in more than one nodal basin, or tumor extension outside the esophagus (airway, mediastinum, vocal cord paralysis) are candidates for palliative therapy. Patients with disease limited to the esophagus and no evidence of nodal metastases (stages I and IIA) may be treated with esophagectomy, although these patients can also be considered for definitive treatment with chemoradiation therapy.

Method of resection Considerable controversy also exists among surgeons regarding the method of resection. To date, two randomized studies have compared transhiatal esophagectomy (without thoracotomy) with the Ivor-Lewis (transthoracic) esophagectomy (with thoracotomy). These studies failed to show differences between the two procedures with regard to operative morbidity and mortality. In a recent randomized trial of 220 patients treated either with a transthoracic or transhiatal esophageal resection, there was a trend toward an improvement in 5-year survival. A meta-analysis failed to show differences in 5-year survival rates. Over the past 5 years, successful attempts have been made to use minimally invasive approaches to esophageal cancer with thoracoscopy and laparoscopy. Although those studies have shown a decrease in morbidity and the minimally invasive approach appears to be oncologically sound from the point of view of resection margins, the number of nodes resected is still not comparable to that of the standard transthoracic approach.

The need for pyloric drainage (pyloroplasty) following esophagectomy is another area of debate. A meta-analysis of nine randomized trials that included

TABLE 4: Chemotherapy regimens for gastric esophageal cancer

Dose/combination	Dose and schedule
Adjuvant fluorouracil/leucovorin/radiation therapy for gastric and gastroesophageal junction adenocarcinoma	
Fluorouracil	425 mg/m^2 IV on days 1-5
Leucovorin	20 mg/m^2 IV on days 1-5 immediately before fluorouracil for 1 cycle then 3-4 weeks later
Followed by	
Radiation therapy	4,500 cGy (180 cGy a day) given concurrently with
Fluorouracil	400 mg/m^2 IV on days 1-4 and on the last 3 days of radiation therapy
Leucovorin	20 mg/m^2 IV on days 1-4 and on the last 3 days of radiation therapy
One month after completion of radiation therapy:	
Fluorouracil	425 mg/m^2 IV on days 1-5
Leucovorin	20 mg/m^2 IV on days 1-5 immediately before fluorouracil
Repeat cycle every 28 days for 2 cycles.	

Adapted from Macdonald JS, Smalley S, Benedetti J, et al: Proc Am Soc Clin Oncol 19:1, 2000.

Table prepared by Ishmael Jaiyesimi, DO

553 patients showed a trend favoring pyloric drainage in improving gastric emptying and nutritional status, whereas bile reflux was better in the nondrainage group. The gastric emptying time evaluated by scintigraphy was twice as long in the nondrainage group as in the pyloric drainage groups.

Lymphadenectomy Considerable controversy exists regarding the need for radical lymphadenectomy in esophageal disease. Much of the controversy is due to the fact that different diseases are being compared.

Japanese series include mostly patients with squamous cell carcinomas of the intrathoracic esophagus, with 80% of the tumors located in the proximal and middle sections of the esophagus. Americans report combined series, with at least 40%–50% of patients with adenocarcinomas of the distal esophagus. Skinner and DeMeester favor en bloc esophagectomy with radical (mediastinal and abdominal) lymphadenectomy, based on 5-year survival rates of 40%–50% in patients with stage II disease, as compared with rates of 14%–22% in historic controls.

In a retrospective study, Akiyama found a 28% incidence of cervical node metastases in patients with squamous cell carcinomas located in the middle and distal portions of the esophagus, as opposed to 46% in those with tumors of the proximal third. Overall survival at 5 years was significantly better in patients who underwent extended lymphadenectomy (three fields) than in those who had conventional lymphadenectomy (two fields); this finding was true in patients with negative nodes (84% and 55%, respectively) and in those with positive nodes (43% and 28%, respectively). Extended lymphadenectomy afforded no survival advantage in patients with tumors in the distal third of the esophagus.

In a study of 1,000 patients with esophagogastric junction adenocarcinomas, the tumors were classified according to the location of the center of the tumor mass in adenocarcinomas of the distal esophagus, cardia, and subcardia. The tumors located in the cardia and subcardia regions spread primarily to the paragastric and left gastric vessel nodes and did not benefit from extended esophagectomy. Kato et al have studied the use of sentinel node mapping to improve the sensitivity of lymphadenectomy.

Preoperative chemotherapy

The frequency of metastatic disease as the cause of death in patients with esophageal cancer has resulted in exploration of the early application of systemic therapy for esophageal cancer. The first of the two large studies was intergroup study 113. A total of 440 patients were treated with surgical resection alone or preceded by 3 cycles of cisplatin and 5-FU. Objective responses were reported in only 19% of patients receiving chemotherapy. No difference in resectability, operative mortality, median survival (14.9 months with chemotherapy vs 16.1 months with surgery alone), or 2-year survival (35% vs 37%) was reported.

However, the Medical Research Council evaluated 802 patients with resectable esophageal cancer in a similar study. Patients randomized to receive chemotherapy were administered two cycles of cisplatin (80 mg/m^2) and fluorouracil (5-FU; 1 g/m^2/d as a continuous infusion for 4 days). Microscopically complete resection was performed more frequently in patients receiving chemotherapy, with no difference found in postoperative complications or mortality. Moreover, patients receiving neoadjuvant chemotherapy had significantly longer median survivals (16.8 months vs 13.3 months) and 2-year survivals (43% vs 34%) than patients treated with surgery alone. The reasons for the differences in the outcomes are unclear but may be related to the chemotherapy regimen and schedule employed in the intergroup study, patient population, or study design. As a result, the role of neoadjuvant chemotherapy remains in question but is promising, especially with the potentially more efficacious newer generation of chemotherapy agents.

Polee et al have evaluated a biweekly combination of cisplatin and paclitaxel in this setting in a phase II study, with promising results. Objective responses occurred in 59% of 49 patients. No patients had progressive disease. Although 71% of patients had severe neutropenia, it was often asymptomatic. Forty-seven patients underwent resection subsequently. Complete pathologic responses occurred in 14% of patients. The median survival of patients in this study was 20 months, but it was 32 months in patients who had disease responsive to chemotherapy. The 3-year survival rate was 32%.

Given the uncertainty about the efficacy of preoperative chemotherapy and chemoradiation therapy, some investigators have administered preoperative chemotherapy, followed by chemoradiation therapy, then surgery. The true utility of this approach will need to be defined by randomized studies, but clearly, it is feasible, without a significant increase in toxicity or operative morbidity. Interestingly, these reports have also demonstrated that most patients had significant improvement or resolution of dysphagia with the induction chemotherapy alone.

Adjuvant/postoperative chemotherapy

As the most common source of treatment failure in patients with esophageal cancer who have undergone surgical resection, postoperative chemotherapy has also undergone limited investigation. The Eastern Cooperative Oncology Group (ECOG) conducted a phase II study of 4 cycles of cisplatin (75 mg/m^2) and paclitaxel (175 mg/m^2 over 3 hours) every 3 weeks. Fifty-five eligible patients were treated. Therapy was well tolerated, with grade 3 or 4 neutropenia in 5% of patients, nausea/vomiting in 12% of patients, and neuropathy in 8% of patients. The 2-year survival rate was 60%, which exceeded the investigators' expectations. However, the predominant pattern of failure was distant, with the first site of disease recurrence being distant metastases alone in 76% of patients. Although this combination was not recommended for further investigation as adjuvant therapy, the promising results should encourage further evaluation of this type of treatment.

Radiotherapy

Although radiotherapy alone is inferior to chemoradiation therapy in the management of locoregionally confined esophageal cancer, it may offer palliation to patients with advanced local disease too frail for chemotherapy.

Preoperative radiotherapy has been shown to be of little value in converting unresectable cancers into resectable ones or in improving survival. However, it decreases the incidence of locoregional recurrence.

Postoperative radiotherapy (usually to 50 or 60 Gy) can decrease locoregional failure following curative resection but has no effect on survival.

Brachytherapy Intraluminal isotope radiotherapy (intracavitary brachytherapy) allows high doses of radiation to be delivered to a small volume of tissue. Retrospective studies suggest that a brachytherapy boost may result in improved rates of local control and survival over external-beam radiotherapy alone. This technique can be associated with a high rate of morbidity if not used carefully.

A multi-institution prospective trial was conducted by the Radiation Therapy Oncology Group (RTOG) to determine the feasibility and toxicity of chemotherapy, external-beam irradiation, and esophageal brachytherapy in potentially curable patients with esophageal cancer. Nearly 70% of patients were able to complete external-beam irradiation, brachytherapy, and at least 2 cycles of 5-FU/cisplatin. The median survival was 11 months, and the 1-year survival was 49%.

> The latest Patterns of Care study, comprising patients from 1996–1999, found a lower risk of death for those patients treated with chemoradiotherapy followed by surgery vs those treated with chemoradiotherapy alone (hazard ratio, 0.32; $P < .0001$). This finding requires further study by randomized trials (*Suntharalingam M, Moughan J, Coia LR, et al: J Clin Oncol 23:2325-2331, 2005*).

Tepper et al have presented the results of CALGB 9781, a prospective, randomized Intergroup trial of trimodality therapy vs surgery alone for stages I–III esophageal cancer (*Tepper JE, Krasna M, Niedzwiecki D, et al: J Clin Oncol [abstract] 24:181s, 2006*). Although 500 patients were targeted for enrollment, only 56 patients were accured. The preoperative treatment regimen was cisplatin/fluorouracil/radiotherapy followed by surgery vs surgery alone. Although mortality was similar, there were more hematologic (54%) and esophagitis (40%) toxicities with the preoperative arm. Intent-to-treat analysis showed improved median survival for the preoperative arm (4.5 vs 1.8 yrs) and better 5-year overall survival (39% vs 16%). This study further supports the other previously published studies supporting preoperative chemoradiotherapy over surgery alone. In a retrospective, single-institution review, Rizk et al found no increase in mortality for preoperative chemoradiotherapy vs surgery alone (*Rizk NP, Bains M, Flores R, et al: J Clin Oncol [abstract] 24:184s, 2006*).

Because of the 12% incidence of fistula formation, the investigators urged caution in the routine application of brachytherapy as part of a definitive treatment plan.

Chemoradiation therapy

Preoperative chemoradiation therapy Initial trials of preoperative chemoradiation therapy reported unacceptably high operative mortality (~26%). Subsequent trials reported operative mortality of 4%–11%, median survival as long as 29 months, and 5-year survival rates as high as 34%. In general, 25%–30% of patients have no residual tumor in the resected specimen, and this group tends to have a higher survival rate than those who have a residual tumor discovered by the pathologist.

The superiority of preoperative chemoradiation therapy over surgery alone in esophageal adenocarcinoma has been investigated in several prospective trials. The first trial included 113 patients with adenocarcinoma of the esophagus. These patients were randomized to receive either preoperative chemoradiation therapy (two courses of 5-FU and cisplatin given concurrently with 40 Gy of radiotherapy in 15 fractions) or surgery alone. Median survival was statistically superior in the combined-modality arm than in the surgery-alone arm (16 vs 11 months). Rates of 3-year survival again statistically favored the combined-modality arm (32% vs 6%). Although toxicity was not severe, the short survival in the surgery control arm has minimized the impact of these results in the United States.

Another trial performed at the University of Michigan enrolled 100 patients and randomized them to undergo surgery alone or preoperative chemoradiation therapy (cisplatin, 20 mg/m^2/d), 5-FU (300 mg^2/d), and vinblastine (1 mg/m^2/d) and radiotherapy (45 Gy/1.5 Gy bid). With a median follow-up of 8.2 years, the 3-year survival was 16% (surgery alone) vs 30% (induction chemoradiation therapy). This difference did not reach statistical significance, as the study was designed to detect a relatively large increase in median survival from 1 to 2.2 years.

An Australian study of 257 patients by Burmeister et al also found no overall survival or progression-free survival for those patients randomized to receive preoperative chemoradiation therapy vs surgery alone.

A meta-analysis of randomized trials comparing neoadjuvant chemoradiation therapy followed by surgery with surgery alone found that neoadjuvant concurrent chemoradiation therapy improved 3-year survival (odds ratio, 0.66) compared with surgery alone, with a nonsignificant trend toward increased mortality with neoadjuvant treatment.

Newer chemotherapy agents are active and may improve outcome over these older trials. A phase II trial of 129 patients employed paclitaxel/carboplatin [Paraplatin]/5-FU with 45 Gy of radiation therapy followed by esophagectomy. A pathologic complete response was seen in 38% of patients, with a median survival of 22 months and a 3-year survival of 41%.

Another phase II trial from the University of Michigan administered paclitaxel/cisplatin with 45 Gy of radiation therapy twice daily (1.5 Gy bid). In this study, 19% of patients exhibited a pathologic complete response, with a 24-month median survival and a 3-year survival of 34%. A phase II trial from Memorial Sloan-Kettering Cancer Center combined cisplatin and irinotecan (Camptosar) with 50.4 Gy of radiation therapy followed by surgery. Twenty-five percent of patients had a pathologic complete response. Ongoing studies by the RTOG are employing these newer chemotherapy agents.

Primary chemoradiation therapy Patients with locally advanced esophageal cancer (T1-4 N0-1 M0) may be cured with definitive chemoradiation therapy. Randomized trials have demonstrated a survival advantage for chemoradiation therapy over radiotherapy alone in the treatment of esophageal cancer. In an RTOG randomized trial involving 129 patients with esophageal cancer, irradiation (50 Gy) with concurrent cisplatin and 5-FU provided a significant survival advantage (27% vs 0% at 5 years) and improved local control over radiation therapy alone (64 Gy). Median survival also was significantly better in the combined-therapy arm than in the irradiation arm (14.1 vs 9.3 months).

A recently completed randomized intergroup trial was designed to investigate the role of high-dose irradiation in conjunction with systemic therapy. This study compared doses of 50.4 Gy with 64.8 Gy. Both treatment arms of the study administered concurrent 5-FU and cisplatin. This trial was stopped after an interim analysis revealed no statistically significant difference in survival between the two groups. The authors concluded that higher dose radiation therapy did not offer any survival benefit compared with the 50.4-Gy dose.

Patient selection Patients with disease involving the mid to proximal esophagus are excellent candidates for definitive chemoradiation therapy because resection in this area can be associated with greater morbidity than resection of more distal tumors.

Most of the trials demonstrating the efficacy of chemoradiation therapy have had a high proportion of patients with squamous cell cancers. Chemoradiation therapy has thus become standard treatment of locoregionally confined squamous cell cancer of the esophagus. It is essential that chemotherapy be given concurrently with irradiation when this approach is chosen as primary treatment for esophageal cancer. A typical regimen is 50–60 Gy over 5–6 weeks, with cisplatin (75 mg/m^2) and 5-FU (1 g/m^2/24 h for 4 days) on weeks 1, 5, 8, and 11.

The literature also supports offering patients with adenocarcinoma primary surgery, preoperative chemoradiation therapy, or primary chemoradiation therapy with surgical salvage if necessary. Entering these patients on protocols will allow us to further define standard treatment.

Sequential preoperative chemotherapy and radiation therapy Only modest benefits have been found with preoperative chemoradiation therapy to date, with systemic failure continuing to be an important problem. Thus, sequential therapy with chemotherapy followed by chemoradiation therapy has been explored.

Ajani et al reported a series of 43 patients who received 12 weeks of cisplatin and irinotecan followed by weekly paclitaxel with infusional 5-FU and concurrent radiation therapy (4,500 cGy) and then esophagectomy. Therapy was well tolerated, with no deaths from chemotherapy or chemoradiation therapy, and an operative mortality rate of 5%. Cisplatin and irinotecan induced responses in 37% of patients, and 91% of patients underwent complete resection. Pathologic complete responses occurred in 26% of patients, and some tumor shrinkage was noted in 63% of patients. With a median follow-up of more than 30 months, the median disease progression-free survival was 10.2 months, the median survival was 22.1 months, and the 2-year survival was 42%. The patients who had a pathologic response to therapy had significantly better outcomes than the rest of the study population. However, systemic recurrences remained a prominent cause of failure, with five patients experiencing recurrence first in the brain and an additional five patients, in the liver.

Esophagectomy following induction chemotherapy and chemoradiation Controversy exists regarding the need for esophagectomy following chemoradiation therapy. Although previously described studies randomized patients to receive surgery with or without preoperative chemoradiation therapy, Stahl et al randomized patients to receive chemoradiation therapy with or without surgery. Also, all 172 patients in the study underwent initial induction chemotherapy (bolus 5-FU, leucovorin, etoposide, and cisplatin for 3 cycles). Those randomized to receive preoperative chemoradiation therapy received cisplatin/etoposide with 40 Gy of radiation, followed by surgery 3 to 4 weeks later. Those randomized to receive definitive chemoradiation therapy received cisplatin/etoposide with 65 Gy of radiation.

After a 6-year median follow-up, the local progression-free survival favored the group undergoing surgery (64% vs 41%). However, the treatment-related mortality was higher in those patients undergoing surgery (13% vs 4%), and so overall survival was statistically equivalent (at 3 years, 31% vs 24%). Since induction chemotherapy was used in all patients, these results should not be extrapolated to indicate the value of esophagectomy following chemoradiotherapy alone.

The incidence of residual disease in patients who have a complete clinical response to chemoradiation therapy is 40%-50%, and those patients who have a pathologic complete response to chemoradiation therapy have the best survival rates with surgery.

Treatment in elderly patients Since more patients are being diagnosed with esophageal cancer at older ages, research is ongoing as how to best treat elderly patients. Retrospective studies from Nallapareddy et al have have found chemoradiaton therapy is tolerable in elderly patients, whereas Rice et al have found a trimodality approach of chemoradiation therapy followed by surgery is also tolerable in the elderly. Close monitoring for toxicities such as dehydration, nutritional concerns, anemia, and postoperative arrhythmia was recommended in these two studies.

TREATMENT OF ADVANCED DISEASE

The goal of esophageal cancer treatment is generally palliative for patients with bulky or extensive retroperitoneal lymph nodes or distant metastatic disease. Therapeutic approaches should temper treatment-related morbidity with the overall dismal outlook.

Local treatment In patients with a good performance status, the combination of 5-FU/mitomycin (Mutamycin), or 5-FU/cisplatin, and radiotherapy (50 Gy) results in a median survival of 7–9 months. This regimen usually renders patients free of dysphagia until death.

Photodynamic therapy (PDT) Porfimer sodium (Photofrin) and an argon-pumped dye laser can provide effective palliation of dysphagia in patients with esophageal cancer. A prospective, randomized multicenter trial comparing PDT with neodymium/yttrium-aluminum-garnet (Nd:YAG) laser therapy in 236 patients with advanced esophageal cancer found that improvement of dysphagia was equivalent with the two treatments.

A recent review of 119 patients treated with endoluminal palliation reported a significant improvement in dysphagia scores and an increased ability to relieve stenosis caused by tumor when PDT was used in conjunction with laser therapy and irradiation.

Other approaches include external-beam radiotherapy with or without intracavitary brachytherapy boost, simple dilatation, placement of stents, and laser recannulization of the esophageal lumen.

Palliative resection for esophageal cancer is rarely warranted, although it does provide relief from dysphagia in some patients.

Chemotherapy Recently published phase I and II studies have demonstrated moderate response rates to taxanes in esophageal cancer. Taxanes in combination with platinum compounds and fluoropyrimidines are being tested in regimens with irradiation.

Although chemotherapy alone may produce an occasional long-term remission, there is no standard regimen for patients with metastatic cancer. Patients with advanced disease should be encouraged to participate in well-designed trials exploring novel agents and chemotherapy combinations.

CHEMOTHERAPY IN ADVANCED ESOPHAGEAL CANCER

In Britain, the ECF regimen, a combination of epirubicin (Ellence, 50 mg/m^2) and cisplatin (60 mg/m^2), both repeated every 21 days, with continuous infusion of 5-FU (200 mg/m^2/d), is considered to be a standard regimen for advanced esophagogastric cancers. Although the regimen has been fairly well tolerated, infusional 5-FU has rendered the combination unpopular in other countries. Several phase III studies have been performed and consistently demonstrated objective responses in about 40% of patients, with a median survival of 9 months and 1-year survival of 36%–40%. The main severe toxicities of this regimen are neutropenia, in about one-third of patients (32%–36%), lethargy (18%), and nausea and vomiting (11%–17%).

Attempts to improve the efficacy of this regimen, which is logistically difficult to administer, are ongoing. Given the accepted role of capecitabine (Xeloda), a 5-FU prodrug, in colorectal and breast cancers, as well as oxaliplatin, a study evaluating the potential roles of these drugs is being performed. Sumpter et al have reported the preliminary data from large, multicenter phase II study (REAL-2; see sidebar). A regimen with intravenous chemotherapy on one day combined with oral capecitabine, rather than infusional 5-FU, would gain much greater acceptance than ECF if the efficacy and toxicity of the regimens were similar.

With the advent of many new chemotherapeutic agents (the taxoids, paclitaxel and docetaxel [Taxotere], irinotecan, and gemcitabine [Gemzar]) with varying mechanisms of activity, further studies have been conducted, and each of these drugs has demonstrated activity, with responses achieved in approximately 15%–30% of patients.

However, the primary route of investigation for these new agents has been in combination with cisplatin and/or 5-FU. The results available to date suggest promising activity, with response rates often around 50% in phase II studies. Irinotecan (65 mg/m^2) and cisplatin (30 mg/m^2) administered weekly for 4 weeks every 6 weeks have also been active, with responses in 20 of 35 patients (57%) and an impressive median survival of 14.6 months.

Following the example of the combination of irinotecan and 5-FU/leucovorin in colon cancer, the investigators have explored a modification of that schedule, with therapy administered for 2 weeks, with cycles repeated every 3 weeks. This simple modification has been investigated in 27 patients and was well tolerated, with severe neutropenia in 18% of

In REAL-2, patients with locally advanced or unresectable esophageal or gastric cancers received epirubicin (Ellence) and oxaliplatin (Eloxatin; 130 mg/m^2 every 3 weeks) or cisplatin and infusional 5-FU or capecitabine (Xeloda; 625 mg/m^2 twice daily, continuously). The results of the full study, which has enrolled 1,000 patients, are expected in 2006, although the interim toxicity analyses of the first 204 patients have been published. The response rates in the four different combinations were similar. The combination of epirubicin, oxaliplatin, and capecitabine may have been slightly superior to ECF (48% vs 31%). In particular, the use of capecitabine did not produce significantly different "fluoropyrimidine toxicities," such as stomatitis, diarrhea, and hand-foot syndrome (*Sumpter K, Harper-Wynne C, Cunningham D, et al: Br J Cancer 92:1976-1983, 2005*).

TABLE 5: Combination chemotherapy

Agents	Response rate (%)	Survival
Cisplatin/fluorouracil	19-40	Median = 7 months, 1 year = 27%
Cisplatin/paclitaxel	37-43	Median = 6-9 months
Cisplatin/gemcitabine	38-47	Median = 7-10 months
Cisplatin/irinotecan	57	Median = 14.6 months
Cisplatin/vinorelbine	33	Median = 6.8 months
Cisplatin/etoposide	45-48	Median = 8-10 months, 1 year = 26%-41%
Epirubicin/cisplatin/ fluorouracil	40-42	Median = 9 months, 1 year = 36%-40%
Cisplatin/fluorouracil/ paclitaxel	48	Median = 10.8 months, 1 year = 38%
Carboplatin/paclitaxel	45-50	Median = 9-11 months, 1 year = 43%-46%

patients and severe diarrhea in 11% of patients.

Paclitaxel (180 mg/m^2 over 3 hours) and cisplatin (60 mg/m^2 over 3 hours) administered every 14 days have been extensively evaluated in Europe and were reported to produce objective responses in 43% of 51 patients, including two complete responses, and 43% of patients were alive 1 year after initiation of therapy (Table 5).

Because of the toxic and logistic difficulties of using cisplatin, carboplatin has become a popular chemotherapeutic drug. Several studies of carboplatin with paclitaxel in esophageal cancer have been undertaken. El-Rayes et al administered carboplatin (area under the curve of 5) with paclitaxel (200 mg/m^2 over 3 hours) every 3 weeks in 33 chemotherapy-naive patients. Objective responses were reported in 45% of patients, with a median survival of 9 months and 1-year and 2-year survival rates of 43% and 17%.

Polee et al explored a weekly schedule of these drugs in a phase I study. With therapy administered for 3 consecutive weeks, followed by a 1-week break, a dose of carboplatin (area under the curve of 4) with paclitaxel (100 mg/m^2) was recommended for further investigation. Responses were noted in half of the 40 patients, with a median survival of 11 months and 1-year survival of 46%. Both of these combinations were well tolerated, with the primary toxicity of myelosuppression.

Lorenzen et al treated 24 patients with esophageal and esophagogastric carcinomas and measurable disease with docetaxel (75 mg/m^2 IV) and capecitabine (1,000 mg/m^2 orally twice daily from days 1–14), with cycles repeated every 3 weeks. Only seven of the patients had adenocarcinomas, and eight had received prior chemotherapy. This combination had interesting antitumor activity, with objective responses in 11 patients (46%), including 56% of previously untreated patients, 2 of 8 patients who had received prior chemotherapy. Although patient numbers were small, there was no clear difference in response rates by histology. The therapy was reported to be fairly well tolerated overall, although dose reductions were necessary in 41% of patients. The main grade 3 and 4 toxicities were neutropenia (42% of patients, including two patients with neutropenic fever), diarrhea and neuropathy (13% of patients each), and hand-foot syndrome in 29% of patients.

The antimetabolite gemcitabine has also been evaluated in combination with cisplatin in esophageal cancer. A Southwest Oncology Group Study reported by Urba combined 1,000 mg/m^2 of gemcitabine on days 1, 8, and 15 with 100 mg/m^2 of cisplatin on day 15 in 64 patients. Approximately one-quarter of these patients had received prior chemotherapy. Therapy was well tolerated, with severe neutropenia occurring in 31% of patients. The median survival of patients treated on this study was 7.3 months, and the 1-year survival rate was 20%. However, the heterogeneity of the patient population makes the efficacy of the therapy somewhat difficult to assess.

Kroep et al tested a somewhat different schedule of these drugs, based on preclinical data suggesting that cytotoxicity is higher when cisplatin is administered 24 hours before gemcitabine. Thus, cisplatin (50 mg/m^2) was given on days 1 and 8, and gemcitabine (800 mg/m^2 over 30 minutes), on days 2, 9, and 16, with cycles repeated every 28 days. Objective responses were noted in 39% of 36 patients, with stable disease in 17 patients, and a median survival of 9.8 months. Aside from myelosuppression, this combination was also well tolerated.

Oxaliplatin may also have a role in the treatment of esophageal cancer, both as a radiosensitizer and an agent in advanced disease. Mauer and colleagues reported the results of treatment with oxaliplatin, 5-FU, and leucovorin according to the FOLFOX4 schedule (oxaliplatin, 85 mg/m^2 on day 1; leucovorin, 500 mg/m^2 over 2 hours on days 1 and 2; and 5-FU, 400 mg/m^2 bolus, then 600 mg/m^2 over 22 hours on days 1 and 2, repeated every 14 days). Of 35 patients who were treated, objective responses were noted in 40%. The median survival rate was 7.1 months, 1-year survival rate was 31%, and 2-year survival of 11%. The median progression-free survival was 4.6 months. Although differences in patient populations were noted, these results are similar to those of other reported combinations

The primary toxicity of these regimens is severe neutropenia, occurring in about 40%–70% of patients. Severe diarrhea, nausea, and vomiting occur in ~10%–15% of patients in many studies. Fatigue and asthenia also were significant side effects with both therapies.

With improving toxicity profiles and modest improvements in therapeutic outcomes, second-line therapy for advanced esophageal cancer is also increasingly being explored. Muro et al treated 28 Japanese patients with squamous cell carcinoma of the esophagus with docetaxel (70 mg/m^2) every 3 weeks; these patients had previously received cisplatin and 5-FU. As expected, severe neutropenia was the dominant toxicity (88%, including nine episodes of febrile neutropenia), with severe anorexia, fatigue, and anemia also reported. Objective responses were noted in 16% of these patients.

In addition, Lordick et al determined that irinotecan (55 mg/m^2) and docetaxel (25 mg/m^2) given on days 1, 8, and 15, with cycles repeated every 28 days, were tolerable, with severe asthenia in 21% of 24 patients and severe diarrhea in 13%. However, only three partial responses (13%) and eight patients with stable disease were noted, with a resultant median survival of 26 weeks. Although these studies suggest the feasibility of second-line cytotoxic chemotherapy in esophageal cancer, the significant toxicity and limited objective response rate warrant its use only with caution and preferably on a clinical study.

Novel agents are also being actively investigated, with great hope for the future. The combination of paclitaxel with the cyclin-dependent kinase inhibitor flavopiridol has demonstrated promising activity in patients with esophageal cancer. A phase I study of this combination reported one complete, one partial, and one minor response in seven patients treated.

Oral tyrosine kinase inhibitors of the epidermal growth factor receptor have also been investigated in esophageal cancer. Gefitinib (Iressa), at a daily dose of 500 mg, was evaluated by Ferry et al as second-line therapy in esophageal adenocarcinomas, with partial responses in 12% of 26 patients, with an additional 12 patients having stable disease. A similar patient population was studied by Van Groeningen et al with similar results: partial responses in 3 of 34 patients (8%) and stable disease in 6 patients. Toxicities were expected (rash, diarrhea, vomiting, and transaminase level elevation. In another study, however, Radovich et al found only 1 response in 23 patients treated with erlotinib (Tarceva,150 mg daily). As with lung cancer, the optimal population for therapy with these targeted therapies remains to be elucidated.

In addition to flavopiridol and the epidermal growth factor receptor antagonists, it is anticipated that other targeted therapies, such as vascular endothelial growth factor antagonists, will be evaluated in this disease. Such avenues of exploration, in addition to early diagnosis and therapy for early-stage disease, are the most likely path toward significant improvements in the therapy for esophageal cancer.

SUGGESTED READING

Ajani JA, Walsh G, Komaki R, et al: Preoperative induction of CPT-111 and cisplatin chemotherapy followed by chemoradiotherapy in patients with locoregional carcinoma of the esophagus or gastroesophageal junction. Cancer 100:2347–2354, 2004.

Armanios M, Xu R, Forastiere AA, et al; Eastern Cooperative Oncology Group: Adjuvant chemotherapy for resected adenocarcinoma of the esophagus, gastro-esophageal junction, and cardia: Phase II trial (E8296) of the Eastern Cooperative Oncology Group. J Clin Oncol 22:4495–4499, 2004.

Burmeister BH, Smithers BM, Gebski V, et al; Trans-Tasman Radiation Oncology Group; Australasian Gastro-Intestinal Trials Group: Surgery alone versus chemoradiotherapy followed by surgery for resectable cancer of the oesophagus: A randomised, controlled phase II trial. Lancet Oncol 6:659–668, 2005.

Downey RJ, Akhurst T, Ilson D, et al: Whole body 18FDG-PET and the response of esophageal cancer to induction therapy: Results of a prospective trial. J Clin Oncol 21:428–432, 2003.

Ferry DR, Anderson M, Beddows K, et al: Phase II trial of gefitinib (ZD1839) in advanced adenocarcinoma of the oesophagus incorporating biopsy before and after gefitinib (abstract). J Clin Oncol 22(suppl):14s, 2004.

Gerson LB, Triadafilopoulos G: Screening for esophageal adenocarcinomas: An evidence-based approach. Am J Med 113:499–505, 2002.

Hulscher JB, van Sandick JW, de Boer AG, et al: Extended transthoracic resection compared with limited transhiatal resection for adenocarcinoma of the esophagus. N Engl J Med 347:1662–1669, 2002.

Kaklamanos IG, Walker GR, Ferry K, et al: Neoadjuvant treatment for resectable cancer of the esophagus and the gastroesophageal junction: A meta-analysis of randomized clinical trials. Ann Surg Oncol 10:754–761, 2003.

Kinkel K, Lu Y, Both M, et al: Detection of hepatic metastases from cancers of the gastrointestinal tract by using noninvasive imaging methods (US, CT, MR imaging, PET): A meta-analysis. Radiology 224:748–756, 2002.

Kroep JR, Pinedo HM, Giaccone G, et al: Phase II study of cisplatin preceding gemcitabine in patients with advanced oesophageal cancer. Ann Oncol 15:230–235, 2004.

Lorenzen S, Duyster J, Lersch C, et al: Capecitabine plus docetaxel every 3 weeks in first- and second-line metastastic oesophageal cancer: Final results of a phase II trial. Br J Cancer 92:2129–2133, 2005.

Mauer AM, Kraut EH, Krauss SA, et al: Phase II trial of oxaliplatin, leucovorin, and fluorouracil in patients with advanced carcincoma of the esophagus. Ann Oncol 16:1320–1325, 2005.

Medical Research Council Esophageal Cancer Working Group: Surgical resection with or without preoperative chemotherapy in esophageal cancer: A randomized controlled trial. Lancet 359:1727–1733, 2002.

Meluch AA, Greco FA, Gray JR, et al: Preoperative therapy with concurrent paclitaxel/carboplatin/infusional 5-FU and radiation therapy in locoregional esophageal cancer: Final results of a Minnie Pearl Cancer Research Network phase II trial. Cancer J 9:251–260, 2003.

Muro K, Hamaguchi T, Ohtsu A, et al: A phase II study of single-agent docetaxel in patients with metastatic esophageal cancer. Ann Oncol 15:955–959, 2004.

Nguyen NT, Roberts P, Follette DM, et al: Thoracoscopic and laparoscopic esophagectomy for benign and malignant disease: Lessons learned from 46 consecutive procedures. J Am Coll Surg 197:902–913, 2003.

Radovich D, Kelsen D, Shah M, et al: OSI-774 in advanced esophageal cancer: A phase II study (abstract). J Clin Oncol 22(suppl):14s, 2004.

Santharalingam M, Moughan J, Coia LR, et al: Outcome results of the 1996–1999 patterns of care survey of the national practice for patients receiving radiation therapy for carcinoma of the esophagus. J Clin Oncol 23:2325–2331, 2005.

Stahl M, Stuschke M, Lehmann N, et al: Chemoradiation with and without surgery in patients with locally advanced squamous cell carcinoma of the esophagus. J Clin Oncol 23:2310–2317, 2005.

Sumpter KA, Harper-Wynne C, Cunningham D, et al: Report of two protocol planned interim analyses in a randomised, multicentre phase III study comparing capecitabine with fluorouracil and oxaliplatin with cisplatin in patients with advanced oesophagogastric cancer receiving ECF. Br J Cancer 92:1976–1983, 2005.

Urschel JD, Blewett CJ, Young JE, et al: Pyloric drainage (pyloroplasty) or no drainage in gastric reconstruction after esophagectomy: A meta-analysis of randomized controlled trials. Dig Surg 19:160–164, 2002.

Urschel JD, Vasan H: A meta-analysis of randomized controlled trials that compared neoadjuvant chemoradiation and surgery to surgery alone for resectable esophageal cancer. Am J Surg 185:538–543, 2003.

Van Groeningen C, Richel D, Giaccone G, et al: Gefitinib phase II study in second-line treatment of advanced esophageal cancer (abstract). J Clin Oncol 22(suppl):14s, 2004)

Visbal AL, Allen MS, Miller DL, et al: Ivor Lewis esophagogastrectomy for esophageal cancer. Ann Thorac Surg 71:1803–1808, 2001.

Walsh TN, Noonan N, Hollywood D, et al: A comparison of multinodal therapy and surgery for esophageal adenocarcinoma. N Engl J Med 335:462–467, 1996.

CHAPTER 13

Gastric cancer

Charles D. Blanke, MD, Lawrence R. Coia, MD, and
Roderich E. Schwarz, MD, PhD

Gastric cancer is more common than esophageal cancer in Western countries but is less fatal. More than 28,000 new cases of gastric cancer will be diagnosed in the United States in the year 2006, with 12,500 deaths attributable to cancer of the stomach (11,430) and small intestine (1,070) combined. Worldwide, gastric cancer represents approximately 930,000 new cases and accounts for more than 700,000 deaths. The incidence and mortality of gastric cancer have been declining in most developed countries, including the United States; the age-adjusted risk (world estimate) fell 5% from 1985-1990.

Gastric cancer is defined as any malignant tumor arising from the region extending between the gastroesophageal (GE) junction and the pylorus. It may not be possible to determine the site of origin if the cancer involves the GE junction itself, a situation that has become more common in recent years.

Epidemiology

Gender Gastric cancer occurs more frequently in men, with a male-to-female ratio of 2.3:1.0; mortality is approximately doubled in men.

Age The incidence of gastric cancer increases with age. In the United States, most cases occur between the ages of 65 and 74 years, with a median age of 70 for males and 74 for females.

Race Gastric cancer occurs 2.2 times more frequently in American blacks than whites; in black males, it tends to occur at a younger age (68 years).

Geography Evidence of an association between environment and diet and gastric cancer comes from the profound differences in incidence seen in various parts of the world. Almost 40% of cases occur in China, where it is the most common cancer, but age-adjusted incidence rates are highest in Korea.

Survival Most patients still present with advanced disease, and their survival remains poor. From 1989 to 1995, only 20% of patients with gastric cancer presented with localized disease. The relative 5-year survival rate for gastric cancer of all stages is 22%.

Incidence Significant increases in age-adjusted incidence rates for tumors arising in the gastric cardia have been seen in males. Rates for other gastric adenocarcinomas either have not significantly changed (black males) or have declined (white males). Overall, rates of gastric adenocarcinoma rose for white females between 1974 and 1994.

GASTRIC

Etiology, risk factors, and prevention

Diet and environment Studies of immigrants have demonstrated that high-risk populations (eg, Koreans) have a dramatic decrease in the risk of gastric carcinoma when they migrate to the West and change their dietary habits. Low consumption of vegetables and fruits and high intake of salts, nitrates, and smoked or pickled foods have been associated with an increased risk of gastric carcinoma. Conversely, the increasing availability of refrigerated foods has contributed to the decline in incidence rates. Recent laboratory data from Japan suggest that oolong tea may contain a substance that can kill stomach cancer cells.

Occupational exposure in coal mining and processing of nickel, rubber, and timber has been reported to increase the risk of gastric carcinoma. Cigarette smoking may also increase the risk.

Intestinal metaplasia, a premalignant lesion, is common in locations where gastric cancer is common and is seen in 80% of resected gastric specimens in Japan.

Individuals with blood group A may have a greater risk of gastric carcinoma than individuals with other blood groups. The risk appears to be for the infiltrative type of gastric carcinoma (rather than the exophytic type).

Gastric resection Although reports have suggested that patients undergoing gastric resection for benign disease (usually peptic ulcer disease) are at increased risk of subsequently developing gastric cancer, this association has not been definitely proven. Gastric resection may result in increased gastric pH and subsequent intestinal metaplasia in affected patients.

Pernicious anemia Although it has been widely reported that pernicious anemia is associated with the subsequent development of gastric carcinoma, this relationship also has been questioned.

Genetic abnormalities The genetic abnormalities associated with gastric cancer are still poorly understood. Abnormalities of the tumor-suppressor gene TP53 (alias *p53*) are found in over 60% of gastric cancer patients and the adenomatous polyposis coli *(APC)* gene, in over 50%. The significance of these findings is not clear at present.

Overexpression, amplification, and/or mutations of oncogenes c-Ki-*ras*, HER-2/*neu (aka* c-*erb*-b2), and c-*myc* most likely play a role in the development of some gastric neoplasms. A high S-phase fraction has been associated with an increased risk of relapse as well.

Germline E-cadherin gene mutations strongly predispose patients to diffuse-type gastric cancer. Prophylactic gastrectomy has been described as a preventive and therapeutic option.

Family history Family members of a patient with gastric cancer have a twofold to threefold higher risk of stomach cancer than the general population.

Prevention Recent studies strongly implicate cyclo-oxygenase 2 (COX-2) in the development of many human cancers, including gastric cancer. Potential mechanisms of oncogenesis include stimulation of tumor angiogenesis, inhibition of apoptosis, immune suppression, and enhancement of invasive potential. Furthermore, COX-2 inhibitors have been shown to decrease the size of gastric adenomas in mice. This information strongly suggests that COX-2 inhibitors may play a role in the prevention, and even treatment, of GI tumors. However, trials with COX-2 inhibitors in other advanced GI malignancies, such as colon cancer, have not been positive, so patients should not be treated with these agents outside the setting of a clinical trial.

Helicobacter pylori infection is associated with gastric lymphomas and adenocarcinomas. The overall risk of developing malignancy in the presence of infection is low; however, more than 40%-50% of gastric cancers are linked with *H pylori*. The bacterium has been designated a class I carcinogen. Antibiotics alone can cure localized, node-negative MALT (mucosa-associated lymphoid tissue) lymphomas in about 50% of patients. With regard to gastric adenocarcinoma, *H pylori* infection is associated with a 2.8-fold increase in the relative risk of the disease compared with uninfected controls. Data from Japan and China suggest that *H pylori* infection can lead to chronic atrophic gastritis. This condition appears to be a major risk factor for gastric cancer. Eradication of *H pylori* should thus decrease the incidence of gastric cancer by preventing it.

Signs and symptoms

Most gastric cancers are diagnosed at an advanced stage. Presenting signs and symptoms are often nonspecific and typically include pain, weight loss, vomiting, and anorexia.

Hematemesis is present in 10%-15% of patients.

Physical findings Peritoneal implants to the pelvis may be palpable on rectal examination (Blumer's shelf). Extension of disease to the liver may be appreciated as hepatomegaly on physical examination. Nodal metastases can be found in the supraclavicular fossa (Virchow's node), axilla, or umbilical region. Ascites can accompany advanced intraperitoneal spread of disease.

Screening and diagnosis

Routine screening for gastric cancer is generally not performed in Western countries because the disease is so uncommon. However, screening appears more effective in high-incidence areas. Mass screening, as has been practiced in Japan since the 1960s, has probably contributed to the 2.5-fold improvement in long-term survival compared with Western countries, though differences in biology may also play a role.

Endoscopy and barium x-rays The diagnosis of gastric cancer in a patient presenting with any constellation of the symptoms previously described revolves around the use of upper endoscopy or double-contrast barium x-rays. The advantage of endoscopy is that it allows for direct visualization of abnormalities and directed biopsies. Barium x-rays do not facilitate biopsies but are less invasive and may provide information regarding motility.

CT scan Once a diagnosis has been established and careful physical examination and routine blood tests have been performed, a CT scan of the chest, abdomen, and pelvis should be obtained to help assess tumor extent, nodal involvement, and metastatic disease. CT may demonstrate an intraluminal mass arising from the gastric wall or focal or diffuse gastric wall thickening. It is not useful in determining the depth of tumor penetration unless the carcinoma has extended through the entire gastric wall. Direct extension of the gastric tumor to the liver, spleen, or pancreas can be visualized on CT, as can metastatic involvement of celiac, retrocrural, retroperitoneal, and porta hepatis nodes. Ascites, intraperitoneal seeding, and distant metastases (liver, lungs, bone) can also be detected.

Endoscopic ultrasonography (EUS) is a staging technique that complements information gained by CT. Specifically, depth of tumor invasion, including invasion of nearby organs, can be assessed more accurately by EUS than by CT. Furthermore, perigastric regional nodes are more accurately evaluated by EUS, whereas regional nodes farther from the primary tumor are more accurately evaluated by CT. Specific ultrasonographic features may aid in the diagnosis and staging of patients with gastric lymphomas.

Capsule video endoscopy A capsule containing a tiny camera is swallowed by the patient. Two pictures per second are taken. Once clinical studies demonstrated that the procedure was safe and effective, the US Food and Drug Administration (FDA) cleared this device for clinical use in 2001. The capsule can be especially helpful in imaging the small intestine.

Laparoscopy Laparoscopy is particularly suited to detect small-volume visceral and peritoneal metastases missed on CT scan. It should be performed prior to curative-intent locoregional therapy or preoperative chemoradiation therapy.

Bone scan A bone scan should be obtained if the patient has bony pain or an elevated alkaline phosphatase level.

PET scan PET scanning may be used to show distant and metastatic disease and may also be helpful in assessing response to neoadjuvant therapy. In the latter setting, PET response correlates with better survival.

Pathology

Adenocarcinoma is the predominant form of gastric cancer, accounting for approximately 95% of cases. Histologically, adenocarcinomas are classified as intestinal or diffuse; mixed types occur but are rare. Intestinal-type cancers are characterized by cohesive cells that form glandlike structures and are often preceded by intestinal metaplasia. Diffuse-type cancers are composed of infiltrating gastric mucous cells that infrequently form masses or ulcers.

Primary lymphoma of the stomach is increasing in frequency and, occasionally, may be difficult to distinguish from adenocarcinoma.

Stromal tumors GI stromal tumors (GISTs) are mesenchymal tumors of the GI tract, most commonly arising from the stomach. These tumors share an ancestor with, or arise from, the interstitial cells of Cajal (the pacemaker cells of the gut). GISTs commonly express KIT (CD117), but this is not required for diagnosis. Most GISTs have mutations in either the C-KIT or PDGFR (platelet-derived growth factor receptor) genes.

Other histologic types Infrequently, other histologic types are found in the stomach, such as squamous cell carcinomas, small-cell carcinomas, and carcinoid tumors. Metastatic spread of disease from primaries in other organs (eg, breast cancer and malignant melanoma) is also seen occasionally.

Metastatic spread Gastric carcinomas spread by direct extension (lesser and greater omentum, liver and diaphragm, spleen, pancreas, transverse colon); regional and distant nodal metastases; hematogenous metastases (liver, lungs, bone, brain); and peritoneal metastases. Multicentricity characterizes up to 20% of gastric cancers.

Staging and prognosis

At present, epithelial gastric cancers are most commonly staged by the TNM system. Stromal tumors, lymphomas, carcinoids, and sarcomas are not covered by these TNM criteria. The most recent update of this staging system (Table 1) allows for a more precise nodal classification based on the number of lymph nodes involved.

A more detailed Japanese staging system has been shown to have prognostic importance in gastric cancer. However, these results have not yet been duplicated in the United States, and this system is not widely used around the world. Resected GISTs are placed into strata categorizing risk of recurrence (very low, low, intermediate, high). The strata are determined by tumor size and mitotic rate.

Prognostic factors Aneuploidy may predict a poor prognosis in patients with adenocarcinoma of the distal stomach. High plasma levels of vascular endothelial growth factor (VEGF) and the presence of carcinoembryonic antigen (CEA) in peritoneal washings predict poor survival in surgically resected patients. As with colorectal cancer, intratumoral levels of dihydropyrimidine dehydrogenase (DPD) may be prognostic of gastric cancer; low levels appear to predict better response to fluorouracil (5-FU)–based chemotherapy and longer survival. The prognostic implications of tumor-suppressor genes and oncogenes are an area of active investigation. Patients with cancers of the diffuse type fare worse than those with intestinal-type lesions.

TABLE 1: TNM staging system for gastric cancer

Primary tumor (T)	
Tx	Primary tumor cannot be assessed
T0	No evidence of primary tumor
Tis	Carcinoma in situ: intraepithelial tumor without invasion of the lamina propria
T1	Tumor invades lamina propria or submucosa
T2	Tumor invades muscularis propria or subserosa[a]
T2a	Tumor invades muscularis propria
T2b	Tumor invades subserosa
T3	Tumor penetrates the serosa (visceral peritoneum) without invasion of adjacent structures[b,c]
T4	Tumor invades adjacent structures[b,c]
Regional lymph nodes (N)	
Nx	Regional lymph node(s) cannot be assessed
N0	No regional lymph node metastasis
N1	Metastasis in 1-6 regional lymph nodes
N2	Metastasis in 7-15 regional lymph nodes
N3	Metastasis in > 15 regional lymph nodes
Distant metastasis (M)	
Mx	Distant metastasis cannot be assessed
M0	No distant metastasis
M1	Distant metastasis
Stage grouping	
See Table 2	

From Greene FL, Page DL, Fleming ID, et al (eds): AJCC Cancer Staging Manual, 6th ed. New York, Springer-Verlag, 2002.

a *Note:* A tumor may penetrate the muscularis propria with extension into the gastrocolic or gastrohepatic ligaments, or into the greater or lesser omentum, without perforation of the visceral peritoneum covering these structures. In this case, the tumor is classified as T2. If there is perforation of the visceral peritoneum covering the gastric ligaments or the omentum, the tumor should be classified as T3.

b *Note:* The adjacent structures of the stomach include the spleen, transverse colon, liver, diaphragm, pancreas, abdominal wall, adrenal gland, kidneys, small intestine, and retroperitoneum.

c *Note:* Intramural extension of disease to the duodenum or esophagus is classified by the depth of greatest invasion in any of these sites, including the stomach.

Treatment

PRIMARY TREATMENT OF LOCALIZED DISEASE

Management of gastric cancer relies primarily on surgical resection of the involved stomach, with reconstruction to preserve intestinal continuity, as resection provides the only chance for cure. Radiotherapy and chemotherapy have been tested as adjuncts to surgery and in patients with unresectable tumors.

Preoperative chemoradiation therapy is an active area of current investigation.

> Proper pathologic staging of resected gastric cancer remains inadequate in the United States. Instead of the recommended minimum of 15 lymph nodes (LNs) examined, 8 of the 9 regions in the SEER registry had a median of 6 to 9 LNs identified. Fewer LNs examined correlated with lower overall survival (*Coburn NG, Swallow C, Quan ML, et al: J Clin Oncol [abstract] 23:309s, 2005*). Higher numbers of LNs resected and examined (up to 40 and more) are linked to superior survival, regardless of stage or even advanced nodal involvement (*Schwarz RE, Smith DD: ASCO GI 2005 [abstract #6]:85, 2005; Smith DD, Schwarz RR, Schwarz RE: J Clin Oncol 23:7114-7124, 2005*).

Surgery

The objectives of operative treatment for potentially curable gastric cancers are confirmation of resectability, performance of a complete resection, facilitation of appropriate pathologic staging, and reestablishment of GI continuity and function.

Confirmation of resectability Laparoscopy has emerged as an excellent tool to assess the extent of disease and resectability before the surgeon performs an open laparotomy. Laparoscopy adds to the accuracy of preoperative imaging primarily in cases of peritoneal spread or small liver metastases. As a result, morbidity, hospital stay, and costs have been reduced significantly in patients with unresectable lesions. In addition, peritoneal washings can be obtained.

The initial experience with laparoscopic ultrasonography has shown that its value lies in identifying lesions with a high risk of recurrence (T2b or >, N+), for which a preoperative chemotherapy protocol may be available.

Extent of resection The extent of gastric resection depends on the site and extent of the primary cancer. Subtotal gastrectomy is preferred over total gastrectomy, since it leads to comparable survival but lower morbidity. A 5-cm margin of normal stomach appears to be sufficient in proximal and distal resections. For lesions of the GE junction or the proximal third of the stomach, proximal subtotal gastrectomy can be performed. If total gastrectomy is necessary, transection of the distal esophagus and proximal duodenum is required, and omentectomy is performed. In Japan, there is a growing experience with more limited resections of early-stage gastric cancer. This trend includes endoscopic mucosal resection (EMR) of nonulcerated T1 N0 lesions and pylorus-preserving gastrectomy. Laparoscopic resections are also being performed more frequently.

Extent of lymphadenectomy The extent of lymph node resection, including the number removed at the time of gastrectomy, continues to be controversial. Preferably, lymphadenectomy includes the lymphatic chains along the celiac, left gastric, splenic, and hepatic arteries, which allows for more precise lymph node staging. The exact level designation of lymph nodes varies with the site and intragastric location of the primary tumor. Based on the TNM staging criteria, 15 or more lymph nodes should be obtained and examined for an accurate N classification. Removal of lymph nodes immediately adjacent to the stomach (paracardial, paragastric at the lesser or greater curvature, parapyloric) has been termed D1 dissection. A more extensive D2 dissection would also remove retroperitoneal "second echelon" lymph nodes along the celiac trunk, left gastric artery, hepatic artery, splenic artery, and splenic hilus.

The international multicenter MAGIC (Medical Research Council Adjuvant Gastric Infusional Chemotherapy) trial showed that a chemotherapy regimen of ECF (epirubicin, cisplatin, and fluorouracil) given before and after surgery can provide a significant survival benefit in patients with potentially curable gastric cancer. Patients enrolled in the trial had resectable adenocarcinoma of the stomach, esophagogastric junction, or lower esophagus. They were randomized to either perioperative ECF and surgery (n = 250), or to surgery alone (n = 253). Resected tumors were significantly smaller and less advanced among patients who received perioperative chemotherapy. With a median follow-up of 4 years, compared with patients who received surgery alone, patients treated with perioperative therapy plus surgery had a higher likelihood of overall survival (hazard ratio [HR] for death, 0.75; 95% confidence interval [CI] 0.60 to 0.93, *P* = .009; 5-year survival rate 36% vs 23%) and of progression-free survival (HR for progression, 0.66; 95% CI 0.53 to 0.81, *P* < .001) (*Cunningham D, Allum WH, Stenning SP, et al: N Engl J Med 355:11-20, 2006*).

Improved long-term survival rates for Japanese patients had been attributed to the extended lymphadenectomies routinely performed in this country. Because the improvement in survival after gastrectomy during recent decades was usually associated with the performance of extended lymph node dissections (D2 dissections or greater), this practice appeared to be sensible if performed with acceptable complication rates. Retrospective data had shown that D2 lymphadenectomy is safe and does not increase morbidity.

On the other hand, two European randomized trials showed no significant differences in overall long-term survival between D1 and D2 dissection groups. Both studies found higher postoperative morbidity and mortality in the D2 (extended) group, largely due to a higher rate of splenectomy and/or partial pancreatectomy performed with those dissections. When a subset of patients with N2 disease were studied in long-term follow-up in the Dutch randomized trial, a survival advantage was shown with D2 dissection. Extended lymphadenectomy should primarily be performed in specialized centers by experienced surgeons, and splenectomy and pancreatectomy should be avoided; for adequate staging, at least 15 lymph nodes should be removed and analyzed.

Reconstruction methods After distal gastrectomy, Billroth I gastroduodenostomy or, more commonly, Billroth II gastrojejunostomy is an appropriate method for reconstruction. Reflux esophagitis is a common problem when the gastric reservoir is too small. After total or subtotal gastrectomy, a Roux-en-Y esophagojejunostomy is commonly performed.

Resection of extragastric organs may be required to control T4 disease. Such a resection can be associated with long-term survival. Splenectomy should be avoided unless it is indicated by direct tumor extension, because it significantly increases the rate of complications.

NEOADJUVANT THERAPY

Prompted by the promising results and acceptable toxicity of preoperative (neoadjuvant) chemoradiation therapy in other parts of the GI tract (eg, esophagus, rectum), there is growing interest in neoadjuvant therapy for gastric cancer. Neoadjuvant treatment may be performed in an attempt to convert an

TABLE 2: Treatment and survival by stage in patients with gastric carcinoma

Stage			Treatment	5-Year overall survival rate[a] (%)
Stage 0 (in situ)			Surgery	> 90%
Tis	N0	M0		
Stage IA			Surgery	60%-80%
T1	N0	M0		
Stage IB			Surgery ± CRT	50%-60%
T1	N1	M0		
T2a/b	N0	M0		
Stage II			Surgery + CRT	30%-50%
T1	N2	M0		
T2a/b	N1	M0		
T3	N0	M0		
Stage IIIA			Surgery + CRT	~20% (distal tumors)
T2a/b	N2	M0		
T3	N1	M0		
T4	N0	M0		
Stage IIIB			Same as for stage IIIA Consider preoperative CRT	~10%
T3	N2	M0		
Stage IV			Palliative chemotherapy, radiation therapy, and/or surgery, neoadjuvant CRT	< 5%
T4	N1-2	M0		
Any T	N3	M0		
Any T	Any N	M1		

Sources of data: American College of Surgeons Commission on Cancer and American Cancer Society

[a] Some American centers are reporting superior 5-year survival rates to those presented here. Confirmation of these results on a national level may be forthcoming.

CRT = chemoradiation therapy

initially unresectable cancer to resectable status, or it may be used in advanced but resectable disease. In a study by Ajani et al, preoperative induction chemotherapy followed by chemoradiation therapy resulted in an RO resection rate of 70% and a pathologic complete response rate of 30%, with a median survival of 34 months.

Most promising to date are the results from a still unpublished European trial using pre- and postoperative ECF (epirubicin [Ellence], cisplatin, and 5-FU). Cunningham and associates randomized patients to receive preoperative and postoperative chemotherapy vs surgery alone. The 5-year survival rate for those offered systemic ECF therapy in addition to surgery was 36%, vs 23% for those who only underwent surgery. Chemotherapy also enhanced resectability. It remains to be seen whether these positive results, achieved with relatively uncommon (in the United States) chemotherapy and without irradiation, will lead to the adoption of this regimen in the United States.

ADJUVANT THERAPY

The 5-year survival rate after "curative resection" for gastric cancer is only between 30% and 40% (Table 2). Treatment failure stems from a combination of local or regional recurrence and distant metastases. Investigators have studied adjuvant therapy in the hope of improving treatment results. A North American Intergroup trial randomizing resected patients (stages IB-IV[M0]) to receive chemoradiation therapy or observation showed significant improvement in median disease-free (median 19 vs 30 months) and overall (26 vs 35 months) survival with adjuvant therapy, and the use of postoperative chemoradiation therapy, usually with continuous infusion of 5-FU, is the standard of care in the United States.

Radiotherapy

Radiotherapy can decrease the rate of locoregional failure but has not been shown to improve survival as a single postoperative modality. Postoperative radiotherapy may be appropriate in patients who are not candidates for chemotherapy.

Chemotherapy

Chemotherapy alone as a surgical adjunct does not have a defined role in the United States. Randomized trials of chemotherapy plus surgery vs resection alone have showed no definite survival advantage, with the possible exception of patients with widespread nodal involvement who may do better with chemotherapy. Interestingly, a recent meta-analysis included both Western and Asian studies; it showed a significant survival benefit with the use of chemotherapy in the Asian trials, but there was no benefit in the Western studies, possibly due to differences in biology or drug metabolism. No specific regimen could be recommended.

Chemoradiation therapy

Patients with T3-T4 any N M0 tumors are at highest risk of locoregional recurrence after potentially curative surgery (surgery in which all macroscopic tumor has been resected with no evidence of metastatic disease) for gastric cancer. Even patients with node-negative disease (T3 N0) have a gastric cancer-related mortality of about 50% within 5 years. Mortality is significantly worse in patients with node-positive disease or in those with incomplete (R1, R2) resection.

In the North American Intergroup trial mentioned in the section on "Adjuvant therapy," patients were randomized to receive chemoradiation therapy or observation following resection of stages IB-IV (M0) adenocarcinoma of the stomach. Chemoradiation therapy following resection of these high-risk patients significantly improved both disease-free and overall survival. Because of the apparent benefit of reducing locoregional recurrences, but not distant recurrences, it is possible that more routine use of D2 lymphadenectomy may modify this recommendation in the future.

D2 lymphadenectomy was performed in only 10% of the patients in this trial. Subgroup analysis revealed that outcome did not differ based upon the type of lymphadenectomy ($P = .80$). Still, since only a small percentage of patients underwent the recommended D2 dissection, further research is necessary before firm conclusions can be made in this area.

Despite this trial, significant controversy regarding the need for adjuvant treatment persists and is perhaps growing. Many studies support the contention that aggressive, formal D2 resection may obviate the need for adjuvant treatment in many cases. Other studies and subgroup analyses support the recommendations for adjuvant treatment as concluded in the North American trial. These conflicting results, as well as distinct differences in results between Eastern and Western nations, suggest that this issue may take many years to resolve. In the interim, it is appropriate to recommend adjuvant chemoradiotherapy in the vast majority of cases in North America.

Unresectable tumors

Patients with unresectable gastric cancers and no evidence of metastatic disease can be expected to survive approximately 6 months without any treatment.

Palliative resection Palliative resection, bypass, and/or stenting may be appropriate for some patients with obstructive lesions. Palliative resection may also be suitable for patients with bleeding gastric cancers that are not resectable for cure. Generally, resection appears to offer better palliative results than bypass.

Radiotherapy Radiation therapy alone can provide palliation in patients with bleeding or obstruction who are not operative candidates. Radiotherapy may convert unresectable cancers to resectable tumors.

Chemoradiation therapy Patients with locally advanced disease may be appropriately treated with chemoradiation therapy. This approach can provide relatively long-lasting palliation and may render some unresectable cancers resectable. Older studies have shown that postoperative chemoradiation therapy can reduce relapse rates and prolong survival in patients with incompletely resected stomach cancer.

MEDICAL TREATMENT OF ADVANCED GASTRIC CANCER

When possible, all newly diagnosed patients with disseminated gastric cancer should be considered candidates for clinical trials, and those with good performance status should be offered systemic therapy. Even though cure is not expected with chemotherapy, such treatment may provide palliation in selected patients and sometimes durable remissions. At least four randomized chemotherapy trials have suggested improvement in survival and probably quality of life vs best supportive care alone.

TABLE 3: Chemotherapy regimen for gastric cancer

Drug/combination	Dose and schedule
ECF	
Epirubicin	50 mg/m^2 IV on day 1
Cisplatin	60 mg/m^2 IV on day 1
Repeat the cycle every 3 weeks to a maximum of 8 cycles.	
5-FU	200 mg/m^2/d as a continuous IV infusion for up to 6 months

Webb A, Cunningham D, Scarffe HJ, et al: J Clin Oncol 15:261–267, 1997.

Table prepared by Ishmael Jaiyesimi, DO

Single-agent therapy

Several agents have established activity in gastric cancer: 5-FU, platinums (cisplatin, oxaliplatin [Eloxatin], and carboplatin [Paraplatin]), mitomycin (Mutamycin), etoposide, some anthracyclines (doxorubicin and epirubicin), taxanes (paclitaxel and docetaxel [Taxotere]), irinotecan (Camptosar), antimetabolites (pemetrexed [Alimta], methotrexate, trimetrexate (Neutrexin), and oral fluoropyrimidines (uracil and tegafur [UFT], S-1, capecitabine [Xeloda]). 5-FU and cisplatin have been used most commonly. The responses seen with single-agent chemotherapy have been traditionally partial and mostly short-lived, with little, if any, impact on overall survival.

Shah and colleagues combined bevacizumab (Avastin) and irinotecan (Camptosar) and cisplatin in patients with previously untreated metastatic gastric and gastroesophageal junction adenocarcinomas. The combination was well tolerated. Of 20 patients, 2 developed thromboembolic events, and 1 had a gastric perforation. Of 16 patients with an intact primary tumor, 1experienced a gastric perforation. Of 10 patients with measurable disease completing 2 or more cycles, 5 partial responses and 4 minor responses (15%-29% reduction) were seen. Although still preliminary, the early evidence of potential activity was encouraging. The toxicity profile of this regimen clearly warrants further scrutiny *(Shah MA, Ilson D, Saltz L, et al: Proc Comb GI Symp [abstract] 2:95, 2005).*

Novel agents recently tested in patients with advanced gastric cancer include the epidermal growth factor receptor inhibitor erlotinib (Tarceva) and bevacizumab (Avastin), a VEGF inhibitor. Unfortunately, a phase II trial of erlotinib showed no responses among patients with advanced gastric cancer. Bevacizumab has looked promising when given with chemotherapy (see sidebar).

Combination chemotherapy

Response rates are consistently higher when combination chemotherapy regimens are used in gastric cancer. Combination therapy has been generally preferred over single agents (Table 3).

In the 1980s, the combination of 5-FU, doxorubicin, and mitomycin (FAM) was considered the standard regimen in the treatment of advanced gastric cancer. However, the North

Central Cancer Treatment Group (NCCTG) randomly compared this regimen with 5-FU plus doxorubicin and single-agent 5-FU and found no difference in survival among the patients treated with the three regimens.

Several different regimens, including FAMTX (5-FU, doxorubicin, and methotrexate) and ELF (etoposide, leucovorin, and 5-FU), have been tested. Most regimens show markedly better response rates and longer survival in early trials than in phase III studies. No combination has been confirmed as superior. However, ECF approaches standard of care in Canada and in some parts of Europe. This regimen has proved superior to FAMTX in terms of objective response rate and survival and superior to the mitomycin, cisplatin, 5-FU (MCF) regimen in terms of toxicity. A combination of docetaxel, cisplatin, and 5-FU was shown to offer superior survival rates vs cisplatin and 5-FU; however, grade 3/4 toxic events occurred in 81% of patients treated with triple therapy. The search for the optimal combination regimen continues, with the promising newer agents being introduced in combination regimens.

Newer agents with somewhat similar mechanisms of action to those of classic drugs have been tried in patients with advanced gastric cancer. An early report of a phase III trial including epirubicin and comparing capecitabine with 5-FU and oxaliplatin with cisplatin showed no early decrease in efficacy but possibly more febrile neutropenia. Additional analysis is necesssary.

Gastric cancer patients should be encouraged to participate in well-designed clinical trials. Outside experimental regimens, the recommended therapy for patients with good performance status is a 5-FU– or cisplatin–based regimen.

Chemotherapy in the elderly

The benefits of chemotherapy for the general population with metastatic gastric cancer are well established. Until recently, however, there were few trials examining systemic treatment in the elderly.

Trumper and associates examined the results of 1,080 patients entered onto three randomized trials of chemotherapy and compared the outcomes between patients aged 70 and older and those younger than age 70. There were no significant differences in grades 3/4 hematologic or nonhematologic toxicities. Additionally, no significant differences were identified in response rates between the age groups. Multivariate analysis controlling for performance status, locally advanced disease status, and treatment showed no significant differences in overall or failure-free survival by age. The authors concluded that patients with gastric cancer aged 70 and older obtain the same benefit as younger patients from palliative chemotherapy with respect to symptomatic and standard responses and survival without increased toxicities.

SUGGESTED READING

Ajani JA, Mansfield PF, Janjan N, et al: Multi-institutional trial of preoperative chemoradiotherapy in patients with potentially resectable gastric cancer. J Clin Oncol 22:2774–2780, 2004.

Bennett JJ, Gonen M, D'Angelica M, et al: Is detection of asymptomatic recurrence after curative resection associated with improved survival in patients with gastric cancer? J Am Coll Surg 201:503–510, 2005.

Blay JY, Bonvalot S, Casali P, et al: Consensus meeting for the management of gastrointestinal stromal tumors: Report of the GIST Consensus Conference of 20-21 March 2004 under the auspices of ESMO. Ann Oncol 16:566–578, 2005.

Cunningham D, Jost LM, Purkalne G, et al: ESMO Guidelines Task Force. ESMO Minimum Clinical Recommendations for diagnosis, treatment and follow-up of gastric cancer. Ann Oncol 16(suppl 1):i22–i23, 2005.

Demetri GD, von Mehren M, Blanke CD, et al: Efficacy and safety of imatinib mesylate in advanced gastrointestinal stromal tumors. N Engl J Med 347:472–480, 2002.

Hartgrink HH, van de Velde CJ, Putter H, et al: Extended lymph node dissection for gastric cancer: Who may benefit? Final results of the randomized Dutch gastric cancer group trial. J Clin Oncol 22:2069–2077, 2004.

Miner TJ, Jaques DP, Karpeh MS, et al: Defining palliative surgery in patients receiving noncurative resections for gastric cancer. J Am Coll Surg 198:1013–1021, 2004.

Ott K, Fink U, Becker K, et al: Prediction of response to preoperative chemotherapy in gastric carcinoma by metabolic imaging: Results of a prospective trial. J Clin Oncol 21:4604–4610, 2003.

Smith DD, Schwarz RR, Schwarz RE: Impact of total lymph node count on staging and survival after gastrectomy for gastric cancer: Data from a large US-population database. J Clin Oncol 23:7114–7124, 2005.

Sumpter K, Harper-Wynne C, Cunningham D, et al: Report of two protocol planned interim analyses in a randomised multicentre phase III study comparing capecitabine with fluorouracil and oxaliplatin with cisplatin in patients with advanced oesophagogastric cancer receiving ECF. Br J Cancer 92:1976–1983, 2005.

CHAPTER 14

Pancreatic, neuroendocrine GI, and adrenal cancers

Al B. Benson III, MD, Robert J. Myerson, MD, PhD, and John Hoffman, MD

PANCREATIC

PANCREATIC CANCER

Pancreatic cancer is the fifth leading cause of cancer death in the United States. In the year 2007, an estimated 37,170 new cases are expected to be diagnosed and 33,370 deaths are expected to occur.

Incidence and epidemiology

Gender The incidence of pancreatic cancer is slightly higher in males than in females. These gender differences are most prominent among younger individuals.

Age The peak incidence of pancreatic carcinoma occurs in the seventh decade of life. Two-thirds of new cases occur in people > 65 years old.

Race The incidence of pancreatic cancer is higher in the black population, with an excess risk of 40%-50% over that in whites. Perhaps more importantly, black males probably have the highest risk of pancreatic cancer worldwide.

Survival Cancer of the pancreas is a highly lethal disease historically, with few reports of 5-year survivors. However, more recent series have shown a decrease in both operative mortality and overall morbidity. There has also been a significant increase in 5-year survival after curative resection (21%–25%). Factors that appear to be important in predicting long-term survival after resection include clear surgical margins, negative lymph nodes, and reduced perioperative mortality.

Adenocarcinoma of the pancreas, the most common histologic type, has a median survival of 9–12 months and an overall 5-year survival rate of 3% for all stages. At the time of diagnosis, over 50% of patients with pancreatic adenocarcinoma have clinically apparent metastatic disease. Among patients whose disease is considered to be resectable, 50% will die of recurrent tumor within 2 years.

Etiology and risk factors

The specific risk factors for pancreatic cancer are not as striking as those for other GI malignancies, such as esophageal and gastric carcinomas. There does, however, appear to be a significant relationship between pancreatic cancer and environmental carcinogens.

Cigarette smoking Cigarette smoke is one of the carcinogens directly linked to the causation of pancreatic malignancies. Heavy cigarette smokers have at least a twofold greater risk of developing pancreatic carcinoma than nonsmokers. In Japan, cigarette smoking carries an even greater risk, which can be as much as 10-fold in men smoking one to two packs of cigarettes daily.

N-nitroso compounds, found particularly in processed meat products, reliably induce pancreatic cancer in a variety of laboratory animals. No study has directly linked dietary carcinogens to pancreatic cancers in humans.

PANCREATIC

Caffeine The contribution of caffeine consumption to the development of pancreatic carcinoma is controversial. A case-controlled study showed a correlation between caffeine consumption and pancreatic cancer. However, other studies have been unable to confirm this relationship.

Alcohol A clear-cut relationship between alcohol use and pancreatic carcinoma has not been shown.

Diabetes does not seem to be a risk factor for pancreatic cancer. However, 10% of all patients with pancreatic carcinoma present with new-onset diabetes.

Genetic factors Cancer of the pancreas is a genetic disease. To date, more than 80% of resected pancreatic cancers have been found to harbor activating point mutations in K-*ras*. In addition, the tumor-suppressor genes *p16, p53,* and *DPC4* are all frequently inactivated in this cancer.

Familial pancreatic carcinoma has been associated with the following genetic syndromes: hereditary pancreatitis, ataxia-telangiectasia, hereditary nonpolyposis colorectal cancer (HNPCC), familial atypical mole melanoma (FAMM) syndrome, Peutz-Jeghers syndrome, and familial breast cancer. Families with *p16* germline mutations may be at higher risk of developing pancreatic cancer than those without these mutations.

Signs and symptoms

The initial clinical features of pancreatic carcinoma include anorexia, weight loss, abdominal discomfort or pain, and new-onset diabetes mellitus or thrombophlebitis. The vague nature of these complaints may delay diagnosis for several months.

Pain Specific symptoms usually relate to localized invasion of peripancreatic structures. The most common symptom is back pain, which stems from tumor invasion of the splanchnic plexus and retroperitoneum or pancreatitis. This pain is described as severe, gnawing, and radiating to the middle of the back. Pain can also be epigastric or in the right upper quadrant if bile duct obstruction is present.

Jaundice In a majority of cases, patients with pancreatic cancer present with epigastric or back pain and/or jaundice. Painless or sometimes painful jaundice occurs with early lesions near the intrapancreatic bile duct.

GI symptoms Tumor invasion of the duodenum or gastric outlet may give rise to nausea or vomiting as a presenting symptom. This symptom is rare early in the course of the disease. Changes in bowel habits related to pancreatic insufficiency may also be present, along with associated steatorrhea.

Glucose intolerance Recent onset of glucose intolerance in an elderly patient associated with GI symptoms should alert physicians to the possibility of pancreatic carcinoma.

A palpable gallbladder occurring in the absence of cholecystitis or cholangitis suggests malignant obstruction of the common bile duct until proven otherwise. This so-called Courvoisier's sign is present in about 25% of all patients with pancreatic cancer.

Other physical findings include Trousseau's syndrome (migratory superficial phlebitis), ascites, Virchow's node (left supraclavicular lymph node), or a periumbilical mass (Sister Mary Joseph's node).

Screening and diagnosis

Early diagnosis of pancreatic carcinoma is difficult but essential if surgical resection and cure are to be improved. Defining early lesions at a resectable stage remains a diagnostic challenge. To date, leading medical organizations have not recommended routine screening of asymptomatic individuals for pancreatic cancer.

Serum markers The use of serologic tumor markers for pancreatic carcinoma, such as CA19-9, was originally thought to be appropriate as a screening tool. However, since the prevalence of pancreatic carcinoma in the general population is extremely low (0.01%), many false-positive screening results are generated. Also, the sensitivity of CA19-9 is not high (20%) in stage I cancers. Nevertheless, CA19-9 may be a useful marker for diagnosing patients at high risk with the appropriate symptoms, such as smokers, recent-onset diabetics, those with familial pancreatic cancer, or those with unexplained weight loss or diarrhea. This marker also is useful in following disease and in assessing the adequacy of resection or therapy.

No currently available serum marker is sufficiently accurate to be considered reliable for screening asymptomatic patients.

Laparoscopy is useful for staging patients with pancreatic carcinoma and for formulating treatment plans. Approximately 10%–15% of patients thought to have resectable disease are found to have distant metastases at laparoscopy. The false-negative rate of laparoscopy is < 10%. The strongest indications for laparoscopy are locally advanced disease and tumors of the body and tail of the pancreas.

Peritoneal cytology also is being explored for the diagnosis of pancreatic carcinoma. Cytology is positive in 5%-10% of patients who are thought to have localized disease. There are anecdotal cases of long-term survival after resection where positive cytology of peritoneal washings was noted. However, the clinical/prognostic value of this test is not yet known.

Imaging techniques

Imaging for pancreatic carcinoma is best performed with conventional ultrasonography and CT.

Ultrasonography The limit of sonographic resolution for early pancreatic carcinoma is a diameter of 1.0–1.5 cm. A mass located in the pancreatic head will produce dilatation of the common bile duct and pancreatic duct. The actual sensitivity of ultrasonography in the diagnosis of pancreatic carcinoma is ~ 70%.

CT provides better definition of the tumor and surrounding structures than does ultrasonography and is operator-independent. CT correctly predicts unresectable tumors in 85% of patients and resectable tumors in 70% of patients. Findings of tumor unresectability on CT scanning include distant lymphadenopathy, encasement or occlusion of the superior mesenteric artery (SMA) or celiac artery, occlusion of the portal vein or superior mesenteric vein (SMV), and distant metastases. Spiral CT increases the accuracy of detecting pancreatic carcinoma in general and vessel encasement in particular. This technique permits rapid data acquisition and computer-generated three-dimensional (3D) images of the mesenteric arterial and venous tributaries in any plane. Spiral CT is quicker and less expensive and uses less contrast medium than angiography.

PET The use of positron emission tomography with ^{18}fluorodeoxyglucose (FDG-PET) in the evaluation of patients with pancreatic cancer is expanding. A recent study of 126 patients with focal, malignant, or benign pancreatic lesions showed high sensitivity of FDG-PET for detection of small pancreatic neoplasms. Lack of focal glucose uptake excludes pancreatic neoplasms (sensitivity 85.4%, specificity 60.9%).

MRI At present, MRI is not as accurate as CT in diagnosing and staging pancreatic carcinoma. MRI may be as useful as CT in staging and can provide magnetic resonance angiography and magnetic resonance cholangiopancreatography (MRC) images if needed. As yet, MRC is not a standard test for the diagnosis of pancreatic carcinoma, but it may become helpful in the future.

Endoscopic ultrasonography (EUS) is a newer modality for the diagnosis of pancreatic carcinoma, with an overall diagnostic accuracy rate of approximately 85%–90%. For the assessment of regional lymph node metastases, the accuracy of EUS is 50%–70%. This technique is also important in the evaluation of portal vein/SMV involvement by tumor. In addition, EUS-guided fine-needle cytology of periampullary tumors may yield new information with respect to the diagnosis of pancreatic cancer and may be less risky in spreading cells by needle tracking than by percutaneous biopsies.

In a comparison of EUS and spiral CT, both techniques showed comparable efficacy in detecting tumor involvement of lymph nodes and the SMVs and portal veins. However, EUS is less helpful in the evaluation of the SMA.

Endoscopic retrograde cholangiopancreatography (ERCP) may someday be supplanted as a diagnostic tool by EUS, although, at present, ERCP is used in many clinics. Also, if a patient presents with jaundice and the CT scan reveals dilatation of the common bile duct without an obvious mass, ERCP may be complementary to spiral CT. ERCP findings of pancreatic cancer include an abrupt or tapered cutoff of either or both the main pancreatic and common bile ducts.

Pathology

Adenocarcinoma arising from the exocrine gland ductal system is the most common type of pancreatic cancer, accounting for 95% of all cases. Two-thirds of these cancers originate in the pancreatic head, and the remainder arise in the body or tail. Most ductal carcinomas are mucin-producing tumors and usually are associated with a dense desmoplastic reaction.

Although most pancreatic adenocarcinomas arise from the ductal epithelium, pancreatic acinar carcinomas and cancers arising from mucinous cystic neoplasms are also found.

Multicentricity, which is usually microscopic, is not unusual.

Metastatic spread Perineural invasion occurs in the majority of patients with pancreatic carcinoma. In addition, pancreatitis distal to and surrounding the tumor is usually present. Most patients present with lymph node metastases in the region of the pancreaticoduodenal drainage basins. The subpyloric and inferior pancreatic head, SMA, and para-aortic lymph node groups also may be involved.

Staging and prognosis

Pancreatic adenocarcinoma is staged according to local spread of disease, nodal status, and distant metastatic involvement using the American Joint Committee on Cancer (AJCC) TNM system (Table 1). The T staging of the primary tumor includes an analysis of direct extension of disease to the duodenum, bile duct, or peripancreatic tissues. A T4 advanced cancer may extend directly to the SMA or celiac axis, meaning that the cancer is unresectable.

Independent prognostic factors Lymph node metastases and tumor size and differentiation have independent prognostic value in patients with pancreatic carcinoma. Significantly improved survival is seen in patients with smaller lesions, lymph node-negative tumors, and tumors in which the surgical margins are not involved.

Lymph node and margin status Prior to the age of adjuvant therapy, lymph node status was the most dominant prognostic factor (Figure 1). It is now rivaled by surgical margin status in series where surgical margins have been meticulously examined.

TABLE 1: TNM staging of pancreatic tumors

Primary tumor (T)	
Tx	Primary tumor cannot be assessed
T0	No evidence of a primary tumor
Tis	Carcinoma in situ
T1	Tumor limited to the pancreas, ≤ 2 cm in diameter
T2	Tumor limited to the pancreas, > 2 cm in diameter
T3	Tumor extends beyond the pancreas but without involvement of the celiac axis or the superior mesenteric artery
T4	Tumor involves the celiac axis or the superior mesenteric artery (unresectable primary tumor)
Regional lymph nodes (N)	
N0	No involved regional lymph nodes
N1	Any involved regional lymph nodes
Distant metastases (M)	
Mx	Presence of distant metastases cannot be assessed
M0	No distant metastases
M1	Distant metastases

Stage grouping			
Stage 0	Tis	N0	M0
Stage IA	T1	N0	M0
Stage IB	T2	N0	M0
Stage IIA	T3	N0	M0
Stage IIB	T1-3	N1	M0
Stage III	T4	Any N	M0
Stage IV	Any T	Any N	M1

From Fleming ID, Cooper JS, Henson DE, et al (eds): AJCC Cancer Staging Manual, 6th ed. New York, Springer-Verlag, 2002.

Treatment

SURGICAL TREATMENT OF RESECTABLE DISEASE

The rate of resection for curative intent ranges from 10% to > 75%, with the higher percentage resulting from both a more aggressive approach and better preoperative staging for resectability. Also, there is growing evidence that patients with potentially resectable pancreatic cancer have a shorter hospital stay, reduced surgical mortality, and an overall better outcome if the surgery is performed at "high-volume" medical centers staffed by experienced surgeons (approximately 16 operable cases per year).

Extended resections may include portal or superior mesenteric vessels, colon, adrenal, or stomach. If resection of adjacent organs or tissues results in the conversion of a positive to a negative resection margin, it is of great potential benefit to the patient.

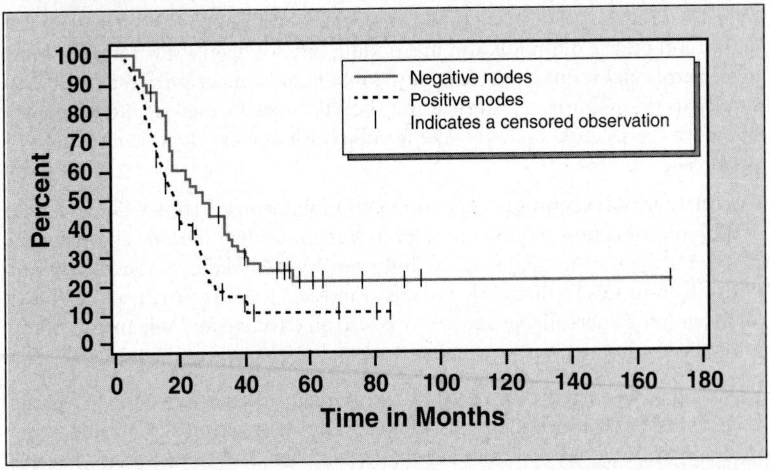

FIGURE 1: Actuarial survival as a function of regional lymph node status in patients with pancreatic cancer.

Determination of resectability

The initial approach to surgery for pancreatic carcinoma includes a determination of resectability. This determination should be first made preoperatively with high-quality CT or MRI and perhaps EUS. Operative determination of resectability includes careful examination of the liver, porta hepatis, and portal and superior mesenteric vessels. The head of the pancreas and uncinate process are mobilized by an extensive Kocher maneuver to evaluate the head of the pancreas. The SMA is palpated, and its relationship to the tumor is assessed. The hepatic artery and celiac trunk are examined to make certain there is no vascular encasement.

Criteria for unresectability include distant metastases and involvement of the SMA and celiac axis.

Operative intervention

Intraoperative biopsy Most patients with resectable periampullary tumors can successfully undergo pancreaticoduodenectomy without an intraoperative biopsy. A time-consuming frozen section interpretation may not be informative, and histologic confirmation may be impossible with small lesions associated with peritumoral pancreatitis. Most large series of pancreaticoduodenectomy for carcinoma include resections of benign pathology based on clinical judgment. A negative fine-needle cytology should not deter an experienced surgeon from proceeding with resection. However, medicolegal considerations may prompt a biopsy.

Whipple vs pylorus-preserving procedure If the tumor is deemed to be resectable, a standard pancreaticoduodenectomy (Whipple procedure) or pylorus-preserving Whipple procedure (PPW) is performed. The PPW theoretically eliminates the nutritional problems caused by a reduced gastric reservoir and gastric dumping, but this finding has not been shown to alter long-term nutritional status. If there is any doubt about cancer proximity or blood supply to the pylorus, an antrectomy should be performed. If the tumor approaches the pylorus or involves the subpyloric nodes, classic antrectomy is preferred.

Reconstruction technique The most common reconstruction technique after a Whipple resection requires a single retrocolic jejunal loop to complete the pancreaticojejunostomy, which is followed by a cholangiojejunostomy and gastrojejunostomy. A duct-mucosal anastomosis is preferred to the pancreaticojejunostomy. Pancreaticogastrostomy is also an effective and safe means of creating the anastomosis.

Postoperative complications Operative mortality of pancreaticoduodenectomy is currently < 6% in major surgical centers. The leading causes of postoperative mortality include postoperative sepsis, hemorrhage, and cardiovascular events. Most of the septic complications arise from pancreaticojejunostomy leaks.

In many series, early delayed gastric emptying is the leading cause of morbidity for pylorus-preserving procedures. The number-two cause of morbidity, seen in 5%–15% of all patients, is a leak or fistula from the pancreatic anastomosis. Today, most fistulas close spontaneously with the addition of somatostatin analog treatment and adequate drainage. Pancreatic fistulas heal with conservative measures in more than 95% of patients.

An analysis of 200 patients who underwent resection of pancreatic adenocarcinoma in the era prior to adjuvant therapy found that the most important factors influencing long-term survival were the diameter of the primary tumor, status of the resected lymph nodes, and status of the resected margins. Patients with tumors < 3 cm in diameter had significantly longer median survival and 5-year survival rates (21 months and 28%, respectively) than those with tumors ≥ 3 cm (11.5 months and 15%). Patients with no lymph node involvement had a 5-year survival rate of 36%, as compared with < 5% for those with positive nodes. Patients who underwent resections with negative margins had a 5-year survival rate of 26%, vs 8% for those with positive margins. The type of resection (pylorus-preserving vs standard Whipple procedure) did not influence survival.

SURGICAL PALLIATION

Surgical palliation is also considered in patients undergoing exploration with curative intent. Jaundice, gastric obstruction, and pain may be alleviated by surgical palliation.

Biliary tract obstruction Either a choledochojejunostomy or cholecystojejunostomy can be used to bypass the biliary obstruction. Recurrent jaundice and cholangitis are less likely to develop when the common duct is used for decompression.

Duodenal obstruction Although duodenal obstruction is rare as a presenting symptom, duodenal involvement may occur eventually in 25% of patients. Some authors believe that prophylactic bypasses are safe and should be performed in all patients. One phase III trial supports prophylactic bypass, but the subject remains controversial.

Pain relief Severe back pain may be an incapacitating symptom. Pain relief may be achieved by chemoablation of the celiac plexus or by alcohol injection, which may be performed intraoperatively or percutaneously. An intraoperative injection of 25 mL of ethanol (95%) on both sides of the celiac axis will ablate tumor pain. (For further discussion of these techniques, see chapter 37 on "Pain Management.")

NEOADJUVANT AND ADJUVANT THERAPIES

Radiation therapy

Even with apparently adequate surgical resection, pancreatic cancer has a high risk of locoregional recurrence. Moreover, most lesions are unresectable, even when there is no apparent distant metastatic disease. Thus, there is a theoretical rationale for the adjunctive use of radiation therapy, either before or after surgery, in almost all patients. Preoperative (neoadjuvant) radiation therapy may help render locally advanced lesions resectable with negative margins (R0 resection). Postoperative (adjuvant) radiation therapy may help eliminate suspected residual microscopic disease in the tumor bed and/or regional lymphatics. Alternative radiation techniques, including intensity-modulated radiotherapy (IMRT) and 3D conformal radiation therapy, are being explored.

With an effective chemotherapeutic agent, there is greater potential for adequate locoregional cytotoxicity—as well as control of subclinical distant disease—than could be obtained with limited doses of adjuvant radiation therapy alone.

Preoperative chemoradiation therapy Several single-institution studies have evaluated the role of preoperative irradiation in conjunction with fluorouracil (5-FU)- and gemcitabine (Gemzar)-based chemotherapy. In these studies, 60%–80% of the lesions were completely resected 1.0–1.5 months after the completion of chemoradiotherapy. Median survival has ranged from 16 to 36 months, but no phase III trials have been conducted to evaluate preoperative therapy vs postoperative sequencing.

Preoperative radiation therapy, to 4,500-5,000 cGy, in conjunction with chemotherapy should be considered for patients with pancreatic adenocarcinoma who are medically fit but who have marginally resectable disease. There are research initiatives to further address the role of neoadjuvant

A Radiation Therapy Oncology Group (RTOG)/Southwest Oncology Group (SWOG)/ Eastern Cooperative Oncology Group (ECOG) intergroup trial, the largest of its kind, compared infusional 5-FU with gemcitabine (Gemzar), both agents given before and after chemoradiation therapy, in patients with resected pancreatic cancer. Radiation therapy was administered without a treatment break and was given with continuous-infusion 5-FU in both arms. The study accrued 442 patients and demonstrated a survival advantage for patients with pancreatic head adenocarcinoma who received gemcitabine vs those treated with 5-FU (median overall survival 20.6 vs 16.9 months, P = .033). *(Regine WF, Winter KW, Abrams R, et al: J Clin Oncol [abstract] 18S:180s, 2006).*

chemotherapy. For example, phase II studies explore high-dose gemcitabine and high-dose gemcitabine and cisplatin with short-term radiation therapy to locally advanced cancer.

Postoperative chemoradiation therapy A small Gastrointestinal Tumor Study Group (GITSG) trial demonstrated a significant prolongation of survival (median survival increase, from 11 to 20 months) among patients with pancreatic adenocarcinoma who received irradiation plus bolus 5-FU chemotherapy after curative resection, as compared with those given no adjuvant treatment. An improvement in the long-term cure rate was also observed among those given chemoradiation therapy.

The European Organization for Research and Treatment of Cancer (EORTC) completed a trial of 218 patients similar to that of the GITSG trial but without maintenance chemotherapy. Reported data suggest no significant difference between split-course radiation therapy with bolus 5-FU and observation only after curative resection (two-tailed *P* value = .099); however, there was a trend toward benefit in median survival favoring those who received treatment. The European trial is difficult to interpret because 20% of patients randomized to receive postoperative treatment were not treated, and the study was inadequately powered for survival.

The GITSG study utilized 4,000 cGy of radiation delivered in a split-course fashion—with a planned 2-week break midway through the treatment. However, single-institution studies indicate that 4,500–5,000 cGy can be safely delivered in 5.0–5.5 weeks without a treatment break.

Careful attention to field size is important. The GITSG trial allowed portals as large as 20 × 20 cm. However, ports that are approximately 12 × 12 cm are usually sufficient to cover the tumor bed with a 2- to 3-cm margin. The use of multiple beams and high-energy photons is also important.

A total of 541 patients were enrolled in a trial conducted by the European Study Group for Pancreatic Cancer (ESPAC). This study evaluated the benefits of adjuvant therapy. The design was complex, attempting to assess several options. It included no further therapy after surgery, chemoradiation therapy (bolus 5-FU with split-course radiotherapy), chemotherapy (5-FU with leucovorin), and chemoradiation therapy followed by chemotherapy.

Interpretation of the results is confounded by the fact that some institutions opted for a full 2 × 2 randomization (all four options), whereas others allowed only two options (no further therapy vs chemotherapy or no further therapy vs chemoradiation therapy). Patients receiving these two options could also have therapy other than that prescribed in the randomization. Furthermore, no data were collected regarding time to disease recurrence or whether treatment was given after recurrence. Curiously, the median survival of those in the control group was more than 17 months, much longer than those of the control groups from the GITSG and EORTC trials.

Only the 5-FU with leucovorin arm would be considered a state-of-the-art approach, and it was demonstrated to improve survival significantly (*P* = .0005). This finding would suggest a strong benefit to postoperative chemotherapy. If radiation therapy is included, it would probably best be given after 1 to 2 months of full-dose chemotherapy. Most practitioners would recommend continuous-course radiation therapy rather than split-course treatment.

The ESPAC is now conducting a postoperative trial comparing gemcitabine and 5-FU. In the United States, the findings of several phase II trials of postoperative regimens as well as a phase III trial will be available soon. In addition, the GI Intergroup is considering a randomized phase II trial to explore new combinations incorporating the monoclonal antibodies bevacizumab (Avastin) and cetuximab (Erbitux), each given with gemcitabine; irradiation will be given with oral capecitabine (Xeloda).

A recent German randomized phase III trial including 368 patients with resected pancreatic cancer compared postoperative gemcitabine (Gemzar) given for 6 months versus observation. Disease-free survival was significantly superior for patients receiving postoperative gemcitabine (median survival 14.2 months versus 7.48 months; $P = .001$). This survival benefit was seen for both patients with node-negative and node-positive disease and for those who had undergone either an R0 or R1 resection. *(Neuhaus P, Dettle H, Post S, et al: J Clin Oncol [abstract] 23[suppl]:311s, 2005).*

Locally advanced but potentially resectable lesions

These lesions comprise 10%–15% of cases presenting to physicians. Data from Phase II preoperative chemoradiotherapy trials indicate that trimodality therapy is crucial for margin-free resection and long-term survival. A meta-analysis from the ESPAC1 trial showed that chemotherapy alone is ineffective for patients having had an R1 (residual microscopic disease at a margin) resection, thus adding further support to both chemotherapy and radiation therapy for these borderline resectable patients. ACOSOG (American College of Surgeons Oncology Group) will be mounting a trial with preoperative capecitabine, bevacizumab, and radiation therapy for these patients within the next year.

TREATMENT OF UNRESECTABLE DISEASE

Irradiation can prolong and/or improve quality of life in some patients with unresectable adenocarcinoma of the pancreas. It is better combined with chemotherapy. Long-term survival is, unfortunately, highly unusual.

Chemoradiation therapy The addition of chemotherapy to radiation therapy has been shown to improve the survival of patients with unresectable pancreatic adenocarcinoma, with moderate doses of radiation only slightly less effective than higher doses. In a GITSG trial of unresectable disease, moderate-dose radiation (4,000 cGy) with 5-FU chemotherapy significantly improved survival, as compared with higher doses of radiation (6,000 cGy) and no chemotherapy (median survival, 9.6 vs 5.2 months). The GITSG has also compared chemotherapy plus irradiation with chemotherapy alone and demonstrated a significant improvement with combined-modality therapy (median survival, 42 vs 32 weeks).

Based on these data, except in a protocol setting, the palliative management of a patient with unresectable pancreatic adenocarcinoma who has significant local symptoms should probably consist of moderate doses of radiation (4,000–

5,000 cGy) in conjunction with 5-FU–based chemotherapy. As in adjuvant treatment, carefully shaped portals approximately 12 × 12 cm should be used.

Approaches under investigation At present, numerous trials are exploring a variety of chemoradiation therapy approaches, including single-agent or combination therapy with oral or infusional 5-FU, paclitaxel, cisplatin, gemcitabine, docetaxel (Taxotere), and oxaliplatin (Eloxatin). Trials with combined gemcitabine and irradiation are of particular interest due to the activity of this drug in pancreatic cancer and the fact that it is a potent radiosensitizer. The benefit of irradiation for patients with locally advanced disease, however, remains a research question because of toxicity concerns and the relatively brief survival rates. Therefore, an Eastern Cooperative Oncology Group (ECOG) trial is evaluating gemcitabine alone vs gemcitabine and irradiation for this group of patients.

If gemcitabine is given either before or after a course of radiation therapy, full doses of 1,000 mg/m^2 are possible. If irradiation and gemcitabine are given concurrently, doses of either modality must be sharply reduced. A current phase II trial is combining "full-dose" gemcitabine (1,000 mg/m^2) with radiation therapy directed at the primary tumor alone (36 Gy). In addition, a Radiation Therapy Oncology Group (RTOG) randomized trial evaluated radiation therapy (50.4 Gy) and weekly gemcitabine and paclitaxel with or without the farnesyl transferase inhibitor R115777 for locally advanced pancreatic cancer. In that trial, the gemcitabine dose was 75 mg/m^2/wk and the paclitaxel dose was 40 mg/m^2/wk. Radiation was conventionally fractionated to a dose of 50.4 Gy. Both these trials are now completed and being analyzed.

The dose of gemcitabine that can be given concurrently with irradiation depends on the volume and dose of radiation. If full doses of gemcitabine (1,000 mg/m^2/wk) are given concurrently with irradiation, the dose of radiation must be markedly reduced to avoid unacceptable GI toxicity.

TREATMENT OF METASTATIC ADENOCARCINOMA

Pancreatic adenocarcinoma is still one of the most frustrating, resistant solid neoplasms to treat, and therapy for metastatic disease remains palliative. Few agents have demonstrated activity of > 10%. Moreover, most of the reported series have been small, and not all encouraging results have been duplicated.

Chemotherapy

As metastatic pancreatic carcinoma is incurable, the anticipated risks of chemotherapy, which are often substantial, must be balanced against the gains that may be achieved; unfortunately, they are few. Patients who are debilitated due to their underlying or comorbid disease should not be offered chemotherapy, as their likelihood of deriving any benefit is exceedingly slim. However, patients who desire therapy and who, while symptomatic, still have a good performance status may be offered "standard" chemotherapy (Table 2) or, if possible, should be encouraged to participate in a clinical trial.

5-FU Historically, single-agent 5-FU has been associated with a response rate of 25% in pancreatic cancer. FAM (5-FU, Adriamycin [doxorubicin], and

TABLE 2: Chemotherapy regimens for pancreatic cancer

Drug/combination	Dose and schedule
Fluorouracil/radiation therapy (GITSG regimen)	
Fluorouracil	500 mg/m^2/d IV bolus for 3 consecutive days once every 4 weeks during radiation therapy
Radiation therapy	Two courses of 2,000 cGy each, separated by 2 weeks (total dose, 4,000 cGy)
Gastrointestinal Tumor Study Group: Cancer 59:2006–2010, 1987.	
Infusional 5-FU with radiation therapy	
Concurrent radiation therapy and chemotherapy phase:	
Fluorouracil	150-250 mg/m^2/d, 24 hours/d during radiation therapy
Radiation therapy	Median dose of 4,500 cGy/25 fractions (range 4,000 cGy/20 fractions to 5,040 cGy/28 fractions)
Fisher B, Perera F, Kocha W, et al: Int J Radiat Oncol Biol Phys 45:291–295, 1999.	
Single-agent regimen	
Gemcitabine	1,000 mg/m^2 IV infused over 30 minutes once a week for 7 weeks, followed by a 1-week rest period
Subsequent cycles once a week for 3 consecutive weeks of every 4 weeks	
Burris HA, Moore MJ, Andersen J, et al: J Clin Oncol 15:2403–2413, 1997.	
Erlotinib plus gemcitabine	
Erlotinib	100 mg oral daily
Gemcitabine	1,000 mg/m^2 IV infused over 30 minutes once a week for 7 weeks, followed by a 1-week rest period
Subsequent cycles once a week for 3 consecutive weeks of every 4 weeks	
Moore MJ, Goldstein D, Hamm J, et al: J Clin Oncol 23(suppl):1s, 2005. Abstract 1.	

Table prepared by Ishmael Jaiyesimi, DO

mitomycin [Mutamycin]) and 5-FU plus doxorubicin offer no advantage over 5-FU alone. 5-FU plus leucovorin appears to be ineffective.

Gemcitabine is indicated for the treatment of locally advanced or metastatic pancreatic adenocarcinoma. Gemcitabine was compared with 5-FU in a group of 126 previously untreated patients and showed a small, but statistically significant, improvement in response rate. Median survival in the gemcitabine group was 5.7 months, with 18% of patients alive at 12 months, as compared with a median survival of 4.4 months in the group receiving 5-FU, with 2% of patients alive at 12 months. Perhaps more important, clinical benefit response (a composite measurement of pain, performance status, and weight) occurred in 23.8% of the gemcitabine-treated group, as compared with 4.8% of the 5-FU–treated group. Due to its palliative potential, gemcitabine has become the standard of care for patients with unresectable pancreatic adenocarcinoma.

A recent randomized, phase II trial of dose-intense gemcitabine administered by standard infusion vs a fixed-dose rate (10 mg/m^2/min) suggested an im-

> Three Intergroup metastatic pancreatic trials recently completed accrual. ECOG completed a trial of gemcitabine (Gemzar) vs fixed-rate infusion gemcitabine vs fixed-rate gemcitabine plus oxaliplatin (Eloxatin), accruing 832 patients. At a median follow-up of 12.2 months, neither of the two investigational regimens was significantly better than standard gemcitabine (both only had approximately one month longer median survival). *(Poplin E, Levy DE, Berlin J, et al: J Clin Oncol [abstract] 18S:180s, 2006)*. The CALGB compared bevacizumab (Avastin) plus gemcitabine with gemcitabine alone, showing no difference between the regimens (unpublished). The SWOG trial evaluates gemcitabine with or without cetuximab (Erbitux) and results are pending.

proved 1-year survival with the fixed-dose rate.

Combination therapy There have been a number of recent attempts to improve the therapeutic outcome for patients with metastatic pancreatic cancer by comparing promising combinations of agents in randomized clinical trials. Unfortunately, the results have been disappointing. The ECOG compared gemcitabine with or without 5-FU, demonstrating a median survival of 5.4 months for gemcitabine vs 6.7 months for the combination; however, this difference was not statistically significant. Another trial explored the addition of irinotecan (Camptosar) to gemcitabine. There was no survival benefit when this regimen was compared with gemcitabine alone, although the combination did increase the tumor response rate (16.1% vs 4.4%, $P < .001$).

Combination trials were presented during the 2004 meeting of ASCO (American Society of Clinical Oncology). A European study of the topoisomerase inhibitor exatecan (DX-89511) vs gemcitabine included 339 patients, showing no significant difference in survival. Furthermore, pain, quality of life, and time to tumor progression were worse in the exatecan arm. Another trial evaluated exatecan and gemcitabine vs gemcitabine alone in 349 patients. Efficacy parameters were similar for both arms of the trial.

> The National Cancer Institute of Canada has presented a randomized phase III study comparing gemcitabine (Gemzar) with or without erlotinib (Tarceva) in 530 patients with metastatic pancreatic cancer. The combination produced improvement in both overall (6.37 versus 5.91 months; hazard ratio: 0.81; $P = .025$) and progression-free survival (hazard ratio: 0.76; $P = .003$). As with other epidermal growth factor receptor-targeted agents, skin rash was associated with response. Diarrhea was increased with the combination *(Moore MJ, Goldstein D, Hamm J, et al: J Clin Oncol [abstract] 23[suppl]:1s, 2005)*.

A phase III study of 565 patients compared gemcitabine with the combination of gemcitabine plus the multitargeted antifolate pemetrexed (Alimta) and demonstrated a significant response benefit with the combination (14.8% vs 7.1%, $P = .004$). However, overall and disease progression-free survival were comparable. There was increased hematologic toxicity with the combination.

A fourth trial evaluated standard-dose gemcitabine vs a fixed-rate infusion of gemcitabine plus oxaliplatin. The trial accrued 326 patients and showed a superior response rate for the combination (26.8% vs 11.3%) and superior disease progression-free survival (5.8 vs 3.7 months). Although these results were not statistically significant, a trend toward increased survival was shown with the gemcitabine/oxaliplatin combination. Furthermore, during the 2003 meeting of ASCO, a trial exploring the combination of cisplatin plus gemcitabine showed no survival advantage for the combination.

A recent European randomized trial for patients with advanced pancreatic cancer compared capecitabine/gemcitabine vs gemcitabine accruing 533 patients showing a survival benefit for patients receiving capecitabine/gemcitabine (overall survival 7.4 vs 6 months, P = .026, response: 14% vs 7%, P = .008). *(Cunningham D, Chau I, Stocken D, et al, ECCO Abstract PS11, 2005).*

Agents with marginal activity include mitomycin, doxorubicin, ifosfamide (Ifex), streptozocin (Zanosar), and docetaxel. To date, monoclonal antibody therapy and hormonal manipulation have been ineffective. A phase II study of the anti–epidermal growth factor receptor (EGFR)–antibody cetuximab combined with gemcitabine has shown a 12% partial response rate and 39% stable disease in advanced pancreatic cancer. Side effects included rash/folliculitis and fatigue. A phase III trial of the combination is accruing patients.

The ECOG is also exploring EGFR-directed therapy in pancreatic cancer with a new randomized phase II trial comparing docetaxel and irinotecan with or without cetuximab. The trial will correlate EGFR expression with outcome after therapy. Other "targeted" therapies are under investigation.

Novel approaches A progressively better understanding of the molecular biology of pancreatic cancer has revealed numerous new therapeutic targets. Areas of active current research include attempts to replace tumor-suppressor genes (ie, *p53*) and to inhibit K-*ras* protein function.

Many patients seek "complementary" or "alternative" treatment strategies. The NCI (National Cancer Institute) has activated a phase III study of gemcitabine vs intensive pancreatic proteolytic enzyme therapy with ancillary nutritional support for patients with pancreatic cancer based on phase II data.

PANCREATIC ENDOCRINE TUMORS

Pancreatic endocrine tumors (PETs) cover a spectrum of neoplasms. Many, although not all, originate from the pancreatic islets of Langerhans.

Approximately 20% of patients with Zollinger-Ellison syndrome develop the syndrome in the setting of the MEN-1 (multiple endocrine neoplasia type 1) syndrome. MEN-1 is inherited as an autosomal-dominant trait and is characterized by tumors of multiple endocrine organs, including the pituitary, pancreas, and parathyroid. The gene for MEN-1, which has been localized to the long arm of chromosome 11, was recently identified and named *MENIN*.

PETs are not rare. Autopsy studies have documented an incidence as high as 1.5%. Most of these lesions are clinically silent.

The normal islet contains α, β, γ cells and enterochromaffin cells, which primarily secrete glucagon, insulin, somatostatin, and serotonin, respectively. All of these hormones may be secreted in excess by PETs. Other hormones that may be secreted by these tumors include vasoactive intestinal peptide (VIP), gastrin, pancreatic polypeptide (PP), and calcitonin. The aggressiveness of a PET in terms of its metastatic potential appears to be due to the cell of origin.

Types of tumors

Insulinomas are β-cell tumors of the pancreatic islets that produce insulin. Four-fifths of insulinomas occur as a solitary lesion, and < 10% of these tumors demonstrate malignant potential (in terms of invasiveness or the development of metastases). In patients with the multiple endocrine neoplasia type 1 (MEN-1) syndrome, insulinomas are multicentric (10% of patients). In addition, a small group of insulinomas are associated with diffuse islet-cell hyperplasia or nesidioblastosis.

Gastrinomas are gastrin-secreting tumors associated with the Zollinger-Ellison syndrome (ZES). These tumors can be either sporadic or familial. Sporadic gastrinomas do not have associated endocrinopathies, whereas hereditary gastrinomas occur in patients with MEN-1 syndrome. Patients with the sporadic form of ZES may have single or multiple gastrinomas. This finding contrasts with patients with hereditary MEN-1 PETs, who generally have a more diffuse tumor process within the pancreas.

It is known that 80%–90% of gastrinomas are located within the "gastrinoma triangle," defined as the junction of (1) the cystic and common duct, (2) the second and third portions of the duodenum, and (3) the neck and body of the pancreas. Although tumors most characteristically are located within the pancreas, a significant percentage of patients with ZES demonstrate primary tumors of the duodenal wall. Extrapancreatic and extraintestinal locations occur in approximately 10% of patients.

More than 90% of gastrinomas are malignant. The spectrum of clinical disease progression includes localized tumors, regional lymph node metastases, and widespread metastatic disease.

Other types Approximately three-quarters of VIPomas and approximately half of all glucagonomas and somatostatinomas are malignant.

'Nonfunctional' tumors Although many PETs cause considerable morbidity due to the inappropriately elevated levels of the hormones that they secrete, even "nonfunctional" PETs, ie, those without an associated demonstrable hormone-related syndrome (such as PPomas, neurotensinomas, and nonsecretory PETs), may be aggressive. Nonfunctional tumors account for up to 30% of all PETs. Two-thirds of these nonfunctional tumors will demonstrate metastatic lesions at some point during the patient's lifetime.

Signs and symptoms

The symptom complex that is observed depends on which hormone or hormones are secreted in excess.

Insulinomas are associated with symptoms of recurrent hypoglycemia. Diagnosis of these tumors is made by the demonstration of inappropriately elevated levels of insulin, proinsulin, and C peptide at the time of hypoglycemia and an elevated insulin-glucose ratio (> 0.3).

Gastrinomas Symptoms of gastrinoma-ZES are due to the effect of elevated levels of circulating gastrin. Ulceration of the upper GI tract is seen in > 90% of patients. Diarrhea is the second most common symptom. Approximately 25% of gastrinomas occur in the context of MEN-1 and are associated with parathyroid hyperplasia and hypercalcemia.

The diagnosis of ZES is established by the demonstration of hypergastrinemia (fasting serum gastrin concentration > 1,000 pg/mL) and gastric acid hypersecretion in a patient with ulcerative disease.

VIPomas An excess of VIP causes a profuse, watery diarrhea, hypokalemia, hypophosphatemia, and hypochlorhydria (WDHA syndrome).

Glucagonomas are associated with a rash (described as a necrotizing migratory erythema), glossitis, cheilosis, constipation and ileus, venous thrombosis, and hyperglycemia. Not all of these manifestations are secondary to elevated glucagon levels alone. The etiology of these signs and symptoms remains unknown, but some patients respond to supplemental zinc and amino acid infusions.

Somatostatinomas, which are rare, are associated with elevated blood glucose levels, achlorhydria, cholelithiasis, and diarrhea.

Tumor localization

Insulinomas Ultrasonography, CT, MRI, and selective arteriography with portal vein sampling have been utilized for the preoperative localization of insulinomas. The sensitivity of these preoperative imaging tests ranges from approximately 30% to 60%. This is because 40% of insulinomas are ≤ 1 cm and two-thirds of these tumors are < 1.5 cm.

Because the success of preoperative localization tests is disappointing and 90% of these tumors will be found and successfully resected by an experienced endocrine surgeon, there is a general trend toward performing fewer tests. Some centers utilize preoperative ultrasonography if the patient has not undergone prior pancreatic surgery. Other centers still routinely employ portal vein catheterization and angiography. Most centers with EUS availability use the modality as a standard diagnostic tool for these tumors.

More recently, intraoperative sonography has been shown to aid the surgeon. In one series, 84% of tumors not localized preoperatively were correctly located by surgical exploration and intraoperative sonography. Many lesions not discovered by surgical palpation may be found by this technique. At present, there is much less reliance on blind distal resection than was previously advocated. Obviously, the technique of intraoperative ultrasonography may not be as helpful in the MEN-1 syndrome, in which multiple small insulinomas may be found.

Gastrinomas CT, ultrasonography, selective abdominal angiography, selective venous sampling of gastrin, intraoperative ultrasonography, EUS, and intraoperative endoscopy have all been reported to be useful in localizing gastrinomas. More recently, somatostatin receptor scintigraphy (SRS) has become a valuable tool for PET localization; several studies have suggested greater sensitivity and specificity with SRS than with other diagnostic tests.

Treatment

Surgery for insulinomas

For larger insulinomas in the body or tail of the pancreas, a distal pancreatectomy may be preferable to enucleation. For tumors in the head of the pancreas, enucleation of the tumor is usually possible. Patients with MEN-1 or islet-cell hyperplasia may benefit from an 80% distal pancreatectomy. If the insulinoma is not found at surgery, a blind pancreatectomy is not warranted. Further imaging and venous sampling studies may reveal the exact location of the tumor.

A surgical cure results in normal values on subsequent provocative testing, during which blood insulin and glucose concentrations are measured simultaneously. Some insulinoma recurrences actually represent persistent disease after incomplete tumor excisions or overlooked secondary multiple tumors.

Surgery for gastrinoma-ZES

The ideal treatment of gastrinoma-ZES is surgical excision of the gastrinoma. However, this approach is possible in only 20% of patients, most of whom have a sporadic tumor. With the development of effective antisecretory agents and preoperative localization with octreotide scanning, the majority of patients demonstrating widespread metastatic disease can be identified and spared surgical exploration. In addition, some series report that patients with nonmetastatic sporadic gastrinoma may have a higher incidence of extrapancreatic sites than was previously thought. One series has reported that two-thirds of gastrinomas are extrapancreatic.

Patients with sporadic gastrinoma All patients with sporadic gastrinoma should undergo localization studies and be considered for exploratory laparotomy, with the goal of potential cure of ZES. Recent evidence suggests that resection of primary gastrinoma decreases the incidence of liver metastases and ZES. Overall, surgery produces complete remission in approximately 60% of patients with sporadic ZES, and subsequent survival is excellent.

Patients with ZES and MEN-1 Some experts believe that surgery should not be used in the management of patients with MEN-1 and ZES. Instead, they recommend treatment with antisecretory medications. This approach is somewhat controversial, as some authors believe that all patients without demonstrated liver metastases should undergo surgery to remove duodenal and pancreatic gastrinomas.

Moreover, since many patients with ZES and MEN-1 die of metastatic gastrinoma at a young age, a surgical approach may be warranted. Surgery should be performed only if imaging studies localize the tumor. Although radical surgery may not provide a cure, removal of large tumors may decrease metastatic potential and increase survival.

Surgical procedure During surgery, the entire pancreas should be mobilized and scanned ultrasonographically to permit a thorough examination of the pancreatic head, duodenum, stomach, mesentery, liver, and splenic hilum. Intraoperative endoscopy with transillumination of the bowel wall may also be useful in identifying duodenal lesions. In general, enucleation is the treatment of choice, except for lesions within the duodenal wall, which may require pancreaticoduodenectomy. If no tumor is found, blind distal pancreatectomy should be avoided, since 90% of gastrinomas are located within the gastrinoma triangle. (This triangle is formed by the angles at the junction between the cystic and common bile ducts, the junction between the second and third parts of the duodenum, and the junction between the head and neck of the pancreas.)

Surgical resection of liver metastases is controversial. However, several authors have demonstrated meaningful survival in patients with small, isolated lesions. The use of ablative procedures, with open, laparoscopic, or percutaneous techniques, can reduce the neurohormonal tumor burden.

Radiation therapy for PETs

Adjuvant therapy The role of adjuvant radiation therapy for PETs of the pancreas is unclear. Because of the rarity of these lesions and their often indolent behavior, the role of this therapy will probably never be demonstrated. However, postoperative irradiation can be considered for patients with positive nodes or microscopically close margins. Concurrent chemotherapy with such agents as 5-FU and/or streptozocin also can be considered. Radiation doses are the same as are used in adjuvant treatment of pancreatic cancer.

Palliative therapy Anecdotal reports indicate that pancreatic PETs may respond to palliative doses of irradiation. Long-term control of unresectable disease has been reported.

Chemotherapy for PETs

PETs are more sensitive to chemotherapy than are carcinoid tumors.

Single agents Agents that have demonstrated antitumor activity include recombinant human interferon alfa-2a and alfa-2b (Roferon-A, Intron A, respectively), 5-FU, doxorubicin, dacarbazine, and streptozocin.

Combination regimens Combination chemotherapy is often more effective than monotherapy. For example, in an ECOG study, the combination of 5-FU and streptozocin demonstrated a higher response rate than streptozocin alone (63% vs 36%) in PETs, as well as a better complete response rate (33% vs 12%) and median survival duration (26.0 vs 16.5 months). Therapy with doxorubicin plus streptozocin was superior to therapy with both 5-FU plus streptozocin and single-agent chlorozotocin in terms of response and survival and is the combination most widely used in the United States. Etoposide combined with cisplatin is active in poorly differentiated neuroendocrine malignancies but is marginally effective in well-differentiated lesions.

TREATMENT OF SYMPTOMS

Octreotide

Octreotide (Sandostatin) is often successful in palliating symptoms in patients with PETs, although this success depends somewhat on the cell type. For example, insulinomas are marginally responsive to octreotide, whereas gastrinomas and VIPomas often respond. However, compared with carcinoid tumors, the median duration of response of PETs to octreotide is significantly shorter (~ 10 weeks).

Recent Surveillance, Epidemiology, and End Results (SEER) data between 1973 and 1999 suggest increasing median survival of patients with metastatic carinoid tumors since the era of sandostatin treatment.

As discussed more fully in the section on carcinoid tumors below, a promising experimental approach for patients whose tumors express somatostatin receptors is the use of octreotide conjugated to a therapeutic radioisotope.

Other agents

Omeprazole (Prilosec), an inhibitor of the function of the parietal cell hydrogen pump, is more effective than H_2-receptor antagonists in blocking gastric acid production and is useful in the symptomatic management of gastrinomas.

Other agents available for symptomatic treatment of insulinomas include diazoxide (Hyperstat), an insulin-release inhibitor, and, more recently, glucagon, by continuous infusion through a portable pump. Both of these agents are used in conjunction with frequent high-carbohydrate meals.

Patients with the glucagonoma syndrome are treated symptomatically with insulin, high-protein meals, supplemental zinc, amino acid infusions, and anticoagulants.

Hepatic arterial embolization

Hepatic arterial embolization, with or without chemotherapy (chemoembolization), is an alternative palliative therapy for patients with either carcinoid tumors or a PET who have predominant liver metastases or who are symptomatic. Embolization is best reserved for patients with < 75% tumor involvement of the liver, bilirubin level < 2 mg/dL, and an ECOG performance status of ≤ 2.

CARCINOID TUMORS OF THE GI TRACT

Carcinoid tumors typically arise from components derived from the primitive gut, lungs, and, rarely, the gonads. Approximately 85% of all carcinoids originate from the gut, predominantly the appendix, followed by the small bowel and rectum.

These tumors have the propensity to cause considerable morbidity by virtue of creating a syndrome of hormonal excess. For example, although the majority of carcinoids are hormonally inert, these neoplasms may produce excessive amounts of serotonin (from dietary tryptophan), prostaglandins, kinins (secondary to kallikrein release), and a variety of other hormones, which may account for the "carcinoid syndrome." Recent SEER data suggest an increase in the incidence of carcinoid tumors between 1973 and 1990.

Signs and symptoms

Flushing The most common sign of the carcinoid syndrome is flushing, which is often triggered by alcohol, catecholamines, or emotional stress. It ranges in severity from a minor annoyance to profound vasodilatation with near syncope and hypotension.

Diarrhea is also common and is due to GI hypermotility. It usually occurs after meals and is rarely voluminous, bulky, or foul-smelling.

Abdominal cramps Diarrhea may be associated with crampy pain, although other etiologies for the pain must be considered, including bowel obstruction due to tumor or mesenteric fibrosis.

Bronchospasm Patients may also develop bronchospasm, which may be mediated by histamine. This problem is often associated with (although less common than) flushing.

Valvular heart disease A late finding is right-sided valvular heart disease, although left-sided lesions may be noted occasionally. The fibrous deposits may lead to tricuspid insufficiency and/or pulmonary stenosis. Valve replacement is rarely necessary, however.

Symptom triad If there is sufficient shunting of dietary tryptophan from niacin to serotonin synthesis, patients may develop diarrhea, dermatitis, and dementia, although this symptom triad is rare if patients maintain adequate intake of a balanced diet.

Diagnosis

Diagnostic studies include CT/MRI of the abdomen and a 24-hour urine test for 5-hydroxyindoleacetic acid (5-HIAA). Some radiologists prefer to obtain a triple-phase CT scan of the liver to detect these highly vascular liver metastases.

Octreotide scanning Indium-111 octreotide scintigraphy (OctreoScan) has been shown to have a higher sensitivity for detecting pancreatic tumors and is superior to CT or MRI for detecting metastatic disease, particularly extrahepatic disease. One study suggests that indium-111 octreotide scintigraphy can reduce costs by avoiding unnecessary surgeries. Also, a positive scan may predict which patients may benefit from treatment with somatostatin analogs (eg, octreotide). Initial studies with a new peptide tracer, indium-111 DOTA-lanreotide, suggest high tumor uptake and a more favorable dosimetry than is seen with indium-111 DTPA-D-Phel-octreotide.

Prognosis

Site and size of tumor The site of tumor origin is potentially prognostic, as most appendiceal carcinoids (75%) are < 1 cm when found and are usually cured by resection. Similarly, rectal carcinoids are usually small and completely resectable for cure.

In contrast, small bowel carcinoids tend to present at a more advanced stage, and approximately one-third have multicentric primary lesions. However, if the disease is completely resectable, patients have a 20-year survival rate of 80%; patients with unresectable intra-abdominal or hepatic metastases have median survival durations of 5 and 3 years, respectively.

Treatment

The management of carcinoid tumors focuses not only on treating bulky disease, in common with other solid malignancies, but also on treating the complications of hormonal excess.

TREATMENT OF BULKY DISEASE

Surgery

Appendiceal carcinoids For tumors that are found incidentally in the appendix and that are probably between 1 and 2 cm, appendectomy is the treatment of choice. For tumors > 2 cm, a right hemicolectomy and lymph node dissection are appropriate.

Small intestines and rectal carcinoids should be resected with a wedge lymphadenectomy to evaluate nodal disease. Duodenal lesions should be locally excised if small (< 2 cm), with radical resection reserved for larger tumors.

Tumor debulking Liver resection or ablation of liver metastases with cryotherapy or radiofrequency techniques is useful in patients with limited extrahepatic disease and/or asymptomatic carcinoid syndrome. Tumor debulking can protect liver functional reserve and improve quality of life.

Liver transplantation may be of benefit in selected patients without extrahepatic disease whose cancer progresses after other therapeutic interventions.

Radiation therapy

Carcinoid tumors are responsive to radiation therapy and frequently are well palliated with this modality. Overall, treatment with higher radiation doses (29–52 Gy) has been associated with higher response rates (40%–50%) than treatment with lower doses (10%).

Chemotherapy

Since carcinoid tumors tend to be resistant to most chemotherapeutic agents, there are no standard regimens for the treatment of unresectable tumors.

Single agents Agents that have reported activity include 5-FU, doxorubicin, and recombinant human interferon alfa-2a and alfa-2b. However, the response rate with these agents is in the range of 10%–20%, the response duration is < 6 months, and complete remission is rare.

Combination regimens Combination chemotherapy regimens represent little improvement over single-agent therapy, with response rates ranging from 25% to 35%, response durations < 9 months, and rare complete remissions.

TREATMENT OF SYMPTOMS

Somatostatin analogs

Octreotide The most active agent is the somatostatin analog octreotide. Even though native somatostatin is effective in controlling many symptoms, due to its short half-life (< 2 minutes), this agent would have to be administered via continuous infusion to be clinically useful. However, octreotide may be administered subcutaneously every 8–12 hours, facilitating outpatient therapy. The initial dose of octreotide is 100–600 μg/d in two to four divided doses, although the effective dose varies between patients and must be titrated to the individual patient's symptoms.

Octreotide not only is useful in managing the chronic problems of the carcinoid syndrome but also is effective in treating carcinoid crisis (volume-resistant hypotension), which may be precipitated by surgery or effective antitumor treatment.

Octreotide is well tolerated, although chronic treatment may be associated with cholelithiasis, increased fecal fat excretion, fluid retention, nausea, and glucose intolerance. Occasional objective antitumor responses have been observed in patients who have received octreotide; the median duration of symptomatic improvement is 1 year. One report evaluating the cost-effectiveness of octreotide suggested that it may double survival time. Other somatostatin analogs, including lanreotide and vapreotide, are under investigation.

SMS 201-995 pa LAR is a long-acting somatostatin analog that allows for monthly dosing, avoiding the need for three daily injections. This new agent improves quality of life while apparently maintaining the same activity seen with daily octreotide. The usual monthly dose is 20 or 30 mg.

Patients who demonstrate disease resistance with somatostatin analog treatment alone may benefit from combination therapy with interferon-α and this somatostatin analog.

Radiolabeled somatostatin analogs A promising experimental treatment approach involves the use of octreotide or other somatostatin analogs conjugated to radioisotopes (eg, indium-111 or yttrium-90) in patients whose tumors express somatostatin receptors (eg, those with a positive OctreoScan result). This approach allows targeted in situ radiotherapy by taking advantage of internalization of the radioligand into the cell to produce DNA damage and cell death, with little effect on normal tissue. Initial reports have shown favorable results with this technique.

Other agents

Other agents that have been used for symptomatic management include H_1- and H_2-receptor antagonists, methoxamine (Vasoxyl), cyproheptadine, and diphenoxylate with atropine. The symptom complex of diarrhea, dermatitis, and dementia may be prevented or treated with supplemental niacin.

Hepatic arterial embolization

Hepatic arterial embolization with such agents as Ivalon or Gelfoam, with or without chemotherapy (chemoembolization), is an option for patients with either a carcinoid tumor or an islet-cell carcinoma who have predominant liver metastases or who are symptomatic. These lesions often are hypervascular, and, thus, peripheral hepatic embolization may provide symptomatic relief in some patients. It is unclear whether this therapy has any effect on patient survival.

ADRENOCORTICAL CARCINOMA

Adrenocortical carcinoma is a rare, highly malignant neoplasm that accounts for about 0.2% of cancer deaths. Long-term survival is dismal overall; the survival rate is 23% at 5 years and 10% at 10 years.

Etiology

The etiology of adrenocortical cancer is unknown, but some cases have occurred in families with a hereditary cancer syndrome.

Signs and symptoms

Approximately half of adrenocortical neoplasms produce hormonal and metabolic syndromes of hormone hypersecretion (such as Cushing's syndrome, virilizing or feminizing syndromes, and hyperaldosteronism). In children, Cushing's syndrome is rare but is often due to adrenal carcinoma. Mixed syndromes, such as Cushing's syndrome and virilization, strongly suggest adrenal carcinoma. The combination of hirsutism, acne, amenorrhea, and rapidly progressing Cushing's syndrome in a young female is a typical presentation. In men, estrogen-secreting tumors are associated with gynecomastia, breast tenderness, testicular atrophy, impotence, and decreased libido.

Often the diagnosis of adrenocortical carcinoma is not evident until the discovery of metastases or until the primary tumor becomes large enough to produce abdominal symptoms. Smaller tumors may be discovered incidentally, when unrelated abdominal complaints are investigated radiographically.

Treatment

Surgery

Complete surgical resection is the treatment of choice in patients with localized disease, as it offers the best chance of extending the disease-free interval and survival.

Medical therapy

Mitotane (Lysodren) is one of only a few effective agents; it exerts a specific cytolytic effect on adrenocortical cells and has been used to treat unresectable or metastatic adrenocortical carcinoma. Only 15%–30% of patients experience objective tumor regression, with a median duration of about 7 months. Mitotane is given at a dose of 4–8 g/d as tolerated, although the dose is variable.

Chemotherapy Doxorubicin has been of benefit in a limited number of patients, and combination chemotherapy is under investigation.

Suramin (Metaret), a sulfonated drug that is cytotoxic to human adrenocortical carcinoma cell lines, has been evaluated but has not proven useful in inoperable adrenocortical cancer. Innovative chemotherapy programs are clearly needed for this disease.

Controlling hormone hypersecretion Hormone hypersecretion can be controlled medically in most cases. Agents that are effective in reducing steroid production and in palliating associated clinical syndromes include the antifungal drug ketoconazole (Nizoral), 800 mg/d; aminoglutethimide (Cytadren), 1–2 g/d; and metyrapone (Metopirone), 1–4 g/d or higher as needed to control cortisol levels. These agents may be used alone or with mitotane.

PHEOCHROMOCYTOMA

Pheochromocytomas are catecholamine-secreting tumors that arise from chromaffin cells in the adrenal medulla or extra-adrenal sympathetic ganglia. These tumors constitute a surgically correctable cause of hypertension in 0.1%–1.0% of hypertensive persons.

Only about 10% of pheochromocytomas are considered to be malignant. The vast majority (90%) of pheochromocytomas are found in the adrenal medulla, and 97% are located below the diaphragm. Approximately 10% each of pheochromocytomas are bilateral, malignant, multifocal, extra-adrenal, found in children, or associated with a familial syndrome.

Pheochromocytomas in patients with familial syndromes, such as MEN-2 and von Hippel-Lindau syndrome (VHL), are less likely to be malignant than other adrenal lesions. In contrast, pheochromocytomas in patients with a family history of malignant pheochromocytoma are more apt to be malignant.

Epidemiology and etiology

Pheochromocytomas occur in all age groups, but the incidence peaks in the third to fifth decades of life. Most pheochromocytomas (90%) are sporadic. Approximately 10% of cases are inherited as an autosomal-dominant trait, either independently or as a part of the MEN-2 syndrome; bilateral tumors are more common in this setting.

Both MEN-2A and MEN-2B include medullary thyroid carcinoma and pheochromocytoma. MEN-2A includes hyperparathyroidism, whereas MEN-2B includes ganglioneuromas and marfanoid habitus. In MEN-2 families, pheochromocytoma occurs in 5.5%–100% (mean, 40%), depending on the kindred studied. Bilateral medullary hyperplasia is almost always present. Pheochromocytomas are bilateral in 70% of cases and usually multicentric, but they are rarely extra-adrenal or malignant.

Signs and symptoms

Patients can present with various symptoms, ranging from mild labile hypertension to hypertensive crisis, myocardial infarction, or cerebral vascular accident, all of which can result in sudden death. The classic pattern of paroxysmal hypertension occurs in 30%-50% of cases; sustained hypertension may also occur and resembles essential hypertension. A characteristic presentation includes "spells" of paroxysmal headaches, pallor or flushing, tremors, apprehension, palpitations, hypertension, and diaphoresis.

Diagnosis

The diagnosis of pheochromocytoma relies on an appropriate history and documentation of excessive catecholamine production.

Catecholamine measurements Measurement of 24-hour urinary catecholamines and their metabolites, vanillylmandelic acid and metanephrine, is commonly used; the metanephrine level is considered to be the most specific single test. Serum catecholamine measurements are more susceptible to false elevations due to stress-related physiologic fluctuations. The evaluation of serum catecholamines after clonidine suppression, however, provides a useful diagnostic tool that is more convenient than urine collection. Dynamic provocative tests are rarely indicated.

Radiologic studies Almost all pheochromocytomas are localized in the abdomen, mostly in the adrenal medulla; other locations include the posterior mediastinum or any distribution of the sympathetic ganglia. After the diagnosis is established biochemically, radiologic methods may be needed for preoperative localization of the lesion; CT and MRI are most widely used. Iodine methyliodobenzyl guanidine (MIBG) and SRS provide a "functional" image; they are most helpful in the detection of occult contralateral or extra-adrenal lesions.

Differentiating benign from malignant tumors The histologic differentiation between benign and malignant lesions is extremely difficult and often impossible to make; this distinction may require the development of lymph node, hepatic, bone, or other distant metastases. Recurrent symptoms of pheochromocytoma, often emerging many years after the original diagnosis, are suggestive of malignancy. Biochemical confirmation of recurrent catecholamine hypersecretion and localization of metastatic lesion(s) with iodine-131–MIBG scan constitute diagnostic proof.

Treatment

PREOPERATIVE MEDICAL MANAGEMENT

Phenoxybenzamine (Dibenzyline), an oral, long-acting, noncompetitive α-adrenoceptor blocker, is a widely used, very helpful first drug; it is given at a dose of 10–40 mg/d. Propranolol, a β-blocker (20–80 mg/d), is usually added after a few days to prevent tachycardia or arrhythmia. The use of β-blockers alone is hazardous because they may precipitate a paradoxical rise in blood pressure. The tyrosine hydroxylase inhibitor metyrosine (Demser) may be added in patients whose blood pressure is not well controlled with the combination of an α- and a β-blocker.

SURGERY

The principles of pheochromocytoma resection are complete tumor resection, avoidance of tumor seeding, and minimal tumor manipulation. Adrenalectomy can be performed by means of an open anterior transabdominal, open posterior retroperitoneal, laparoscopic lateral transabdominal, or laparoscopic posterior retroperitoneal approach. In the past, an open anterior approach was the standard because it allowed for complete exploration and inspection for potential tumor foci. However, with the improved accuracy of preoperative imaging and increased experience with laparoscopic procedures, there is little need for exploration in areas in which a tumor has not been identified.

Except in tumors < 6 cm, the laparoscopic approach to pheochromocytoma is probably the technique of choice. In the absence of obvious local tumor invasion or metastatic disease, a laparoscopic procedure is acceptable to many experienced endocrine surgeons.

The most critical intraoperative aspect of surgery is control of blood pressure immediately after removal of the tumor, when all agonistic effects are abolished and the effects of α- and β-blockers are still present. Close cooperation with the anesthesiologist to expand fluid volume and prepare the appropriate infusions of agonists to support vascular stability is critical.

TREATMENT OF METASTATIC MALIGNANT PHEOCHROMOCYTOMA

The treatment of choice for metastatic malignant pheochromocytoma remains problematic.

Medical and radiation therapy

Medical therapy with α- or β-blockers, as well as metyrosine, is almost always required to maintain hemodynamic stability. Chemotherapy utilizing streptozocin-based regimens or the combination of cyclophosphamide, vincristine, and dacarbazine has yielded promising responses. Treatment with iodine-131–MIBG or (in Europe) with radiolabeled somatostatin has met with only limited success. In most cases, uncontrolled catecholamine hypersecretion eventually escapes biochemical blockade, and fatal hypertensive crisis ensues.

Surgery

In those cases in which limited and resectable lesions can be identified, surgery can effect complete and lasting remission of the disease.

SUGGESTED READING

ON PANCREATIC CANCER

Choti MA: Adjuvant therapy for pancreatic cancer–The debate continues. N Engl J Med 350:1249–1251, 2004.

Chua YJ, Cunningham D: Adjuvant treatment for resectable pancreatic cancer. J Clin Oncol 23:4532–4537, 2005.

Goggins M: Molecular markers of early pancreatic cancer. J Clin Oncol 23:4524–4531, 2005.

Louvet C, Labianca R, Hammel P, et al; GERCOR;GISCAD: Gemcitabine in combination with oxaliplatin compared with gemcitabine alone in locally advanced or metastatic pancreatic cancer: Results of a GERCOR and GISCAD phase III trial. J Clin Oncol 23:3509–3516, 2005.

Milano MT, Chmura SJ, Garofalo MC, et al: Intensity-modulated radiotherapy in treatment of pancreatic and bile duct malignancies: Toxicity and clinical outcome. Int J Radiat Oncol Biol Phys 1:445–453, 2004.

Neoptolemos JP, Stocken DD, Friess H, et al; European Study Group for Pancreatic Cancer: A randomized trial of chemoradiotherapy and chemotherapy after resection of pancreatic cancer. N Engl J Med 350:1200–1210, 2004. Erratum in: N Engl J Med 351:726, 2004.

Rocha Lima CM, Green MR, Rotche R, et al: Irinotecan plus gemcitabine results in no survival advantage compared with gemcitabine monotherapy in patients with locally advanced or metastatic pancreatic cancer despite increased tumor response rate. J Clin Oncol 15:3776–3783, 2004.

Stocken DD, Buchler MW, Dervenis C, et al: Meta-analysis of randomised adjuvant therapy trials for pancreatic cancer. Br J Cancer 92:1372–1381, 2005.

Tempero M, Plunkett W, Ruiz Van Haperen V, et al: Randomized phase II comparison of dose-intense gemcitabine: Thirty-minute infusion and fixed dose rate infusion in patients with pancreatic adenocarcinoma. J Clin Oncol 15:3402–3408, 2003.

Willett CG, Czito BG, Bendell JJ, et al: Locally advanced pancreatic cancer. J Clin Oncol 23:4538–4544, 2005.

Wong GY, Schroeder DR, Carns PE, et al: Effect of neurolytic celiac plexus block on pain relief, quality of life, and survival in patients with unresectable pancreatic cancer: A randomized controlled trial. JAMA 3:1092–1099, 2004.

Yeo CJ: The Johns Hopkins experience with pancreaticoduodenectomy with or without extended retroperitoneal lymphadenectomy for periampullary carcinoma. J Gastrointest Surg 4:231–232, 2000.

ON NEUROENDOCRINE GI TUMORS

Bajetta E, Procopio G, Ferrari L, et al: Update on the treatment of neuroendocrine tumors. Expert Rev Anticancer Ther 3:631–642, 2003.

Brentjens R, Saltz L: Islet cell tumors of the pancreas: The medical oncologist's perspective. Surg Clin North Am 81:527–542, 2001.

Faiss S, Pape UF, Bohmig M, et al: Prospective, randomized, multicenter trial on the antiproliferative effect of lanreotide, interferon alfa, and their combination for therapy of metastatic neuroendocrine gastroenteropancreatic tumors. The International Lanreotide and Interferon Alfa Study Group. J Clin Oncol 15:2689–2696, 2003.

Fazio N, Oberg K: Prospective, randomized, multicenter trial on the antiproliferative effect of lanreotide, interferon alfa, and their combination for therapy of metastatic neuroendocrine gastroenteropancreatic tumors. J Clin Oncol 22:573–574, 2004.

Kvols LK, Krenning EP, Pauwels S, et al: Phase I study of 90Y-SMT487 (Octreother) in patients with somatostatin receptor (SS-R) positive neuroendocrine (NE) tumors (abstract). Proc Am Soc Clin Oncol 19:207, 2000.

Kwekkeboom DJ, Teunissen JJ, Bakker WH, et al: Radiolabeled somatostatin analog [177Lu-DOTA0,Tyr3]octreotate in patients with endocrine gastroenteropancreatic tumors. J Clin Oncol 23:2754–2762, 2005.

Moertel CG, Lefkopoulo M, Lipsitz S, et al: Streptozocin-doxorubicin, streptozocin-fluorouracil, or chlorozotocin in the treatment of advanced islet-cell carcinoma. N Engl J Med 326:519–523, 1992.

Norton JA, Alexander HR, Fraker DL, et al: Comparison of surgical results in patients with advanced and limited disease with multiple endocrine neoplasia type 1 and Zollinger-Ellison syndrome. Ann Surg 234:495–506, 2001.

Oberg K, Kvols L, Caplin M, et al: Consensus report on the use of somatostatin analogs for the management of neuroendocrine tumors of the gastroenteropancreatic system. Ann Oncol 15:966–973, 2004.

O'Toole D, Maire F, Ruszniewski P: Ablative therapies for liver metastases of digestive endocrine tumours. Endocr Relat Cancer 10:463–468, 2003.

Ruszniewski P, Malka D: Hepatic arterial chemoembolization in the management of advanced digestive endocrine tumors. Digestion 62(suppl 1):79–83, 2003.

Sarmiento JM, Que FG: Hepatic surgery for metastases from neuroendocrine tumors. Surg Oncol Clin N Am 12:231–242, 2003.

Virgolini I, Patri P, Novotny C, et al: Comparative somatostatin receptor scintigraphy using in-111-DOTA-lanreotide and in-111-DOTA-Tyr3-octreotide versus F-18-FDG-PET for evaluation of somatostatin receptor-mediated radionuclide therapy. Ann Oncol 12(suppl 2):S41–S45, 2001.

Waldherr C, Pless M, Maecke HR, et al: The clinical value of [90Y-DOTA]-D-Phel-Tyr3-octreotide (90Y-DOTATOC) in the treatment of neuroendocrine tumours: A clinical phase II study. Ann Oncol 12:941–945, 2001.

ON ADRENAL NEOPLASMS

Jossart GH, Burpee SE, Gagner M: Surgery of the adrenal glands. Endocrinol Metab Clin North Am 29:57–68, 2000.

Kendrick ML, Lloyd R, Erickson L, et al: Adrenocortical carcinoma: Surgical progress or status quo? Arch Surg 136:543–549, 2001.

Sosa JA, Udelsman R: Imaging of the adrenal gland. Surg Oncol Clin N Am 8:109–127, 1999.

Vassilopoulou-Sellin R, Schultz PN: Adrenocortical carcinoma: Clinical outcome at the end of the 20th century. Cancer 92:1113–1121, 2001.

Wajchenberg BL, Albergaria Pereira MA, Medonca BB, et al: Adrenocortical carcinoma: Clinical and laboratory observations. Cancer 88:711–736, 2000.

ON CARCINOIDS

Anthony LB, Kang T, Shyr T: Malignant carcinoid syndrome: Survival in the octreotide era. J Clin Oncol 23(suppl):328s, 2005. Abstract 4084.

Goede AC, Winslet MC: Surgery for carcinoid tumours of the lower gastrointestinal tract. Colorectal Dis 5:123–128, 2003.

Kolby L, Persson G, Franzen S, et al: Randomized clinical trial of the effect of interferon alpha on survival in patients with disseminated midgut carcinoid tumours. Br J Surg 90:687–693, 2003.

Krenning EP, de Jong M: Therapeutic use of radiolabelled peptides. Ann Oncol 11(suppl 3):267–271, 2000.

Modlin IM, Lye KD, Kidd M: A 5-decade analysis of 13,715 carcinoid tumors. Cancer 97:934–959, 2003.

Moller JE, Connolly HM, Rubin J, et al: Factors associated with progression of carcinoid heart disease. N Engl J Med 348:1005–1015, 2003.

Oberg K: Carcinoid tumors: Molecular genetics, tumor biology, and update of diagnosis and treatment. Curr Opin Oncol 14:38–45, 2002.

Schell SR, Camp ER, Caridi JG, et al: Hepatic artery embolization for control of symptoms, octreotide requirements, and tumor progression in metastatic carcinoid tumors. J Gastrointest Surg 6:664–670, 2002.

Talamonti MS, Stuart KE, Yao JC: Neuroendocrine tumors of the gastrointestinal tract: How aggressive should we be? ASCO 2004 Educational Book, pp 206–218.

van der Horst-Schrivers AN, Wymenga AN, de Vries EG: Carcinoid heart disease. N Engl J Med 348:2359–2361, 2003.

ON PHEOCHROMOCYTOMAS

Baghai M, Thompson GB, Young WF Jr, et al: Pheochromocytomas and paragangliomas in von Hippel-Lindau disease: A role for laparoscopic and cortical-sparing surgery. Arch Surg 137:682–689, 2002.

Goldstein RE, O'Neill JA Jr, Holcomb GW III, et al: Clinical experience over 48 years with pheochromocytoma. Ann Surg 229:755–764, 1999.

Lenders JW, Eisenhofer G, Mannelli M, et al: Phaeochromocytoma. Lancet 366:665–675, 2005.

Rose B, Matthay KK, Price D, et al: High-dose 131I-metaiodobenzylguanidine therapy for 12 patients with malignant pheochromocytoma. Cancer 98:239–248, 2003.

Safford SD, Coleman RE, Gockerman JP, et al: Iodine-131 metaiodobenzylguanidine is an effective treatment for malignant pheochromocytoma and paraganglioma. Surgery 134:956–962, 2003; discussion 962–963.

Vaughan ED Jr: Diseases of the adrenal gland. Med Clin North Am 88:443–466, 2004.

Zendron L, Fehrenbach J, Taverna C, et al: Pitfalls in the diagnosis of phaeochromocytoma. Br Med J 13:629–630, 2004.

CHAPTER 15

Liver, gallbladder, and biliary tract cancers

Lawrence D. Wagman, MD, John M. Robertson, MD, and Bert O'Neil, MD

HEPATOCELLULAR CANCER

Hepatocellular carcinoma is one of the most common malignancies in the world, with approximately 1 million new cases recorded annually.

Epidemiology

Gender Hepatocellular carcinoma is the most common tumor in males worldwide, with a male-to-female ratio of 5:1 in Asia and 2:1 in the United States.

Geography Tumor incidence varies significantly, depending on geographic location. In the United States, hepatocellular carcinoma represents < 2% of all tumors, whereas in the Far East and sub-Saharan Africa, this neoplasm occurs at an incidence of 150 per 100,000 population and comprises almost 50% of all diagnosed tumors. A study analyzing SEER (Surveillance, Epidemiology, and End Results) data has shown that the incidence of hepatocellular carcinoma is rising in both white and black populations in the United States, with a current incidence of about 3.4 cases per 100,000 in whites and 5.6 per 100,000 in blacks. Modeling of the spread of hepatitis C virus (HCV) suggests that this number may continue to increase dramatically.

Age The incidence of hepatocellular cancer increases with age. The mean age at diagnosis is 53 years in Asia and 67 years in the United States.

Race The incidence of hepatocellular tumors is higher in Asian immigrants and blacks than in whites.

Survival In patients who undergo curative resection, the 5-year survival rate is approximately 20%. Recurrence is common, with metastases arising in the remaining liver, lungs, bone, kidneys, and heart. Most patients present with unresectable disease. Patients with unimpaired liver function who can undergo resection may experience significantly longer survival than those whose disease is not resected.

A large 5-year randomized study performed in China has confirmed that treatment of chronic hepatitis B infection with the antiviral lamivudine not only decreases the risk of progression to cirrhosis of the liver but also decreases the rate of progression to hepatocellular cancer. Treated patients had a 3.9% risk of hepatocellular cancer over 5 years, compared with 7.4% for those in the placebo group (hazard ratio: 0.49; *P* = 0.047; *Liaw YF, Sung J, Chow WC, et al: N Engl J Med 351:1521-1531, 2004*).

Etiology and risk factors

Hepatitis B The close geographic relationship between hepatitis B incidence and hepatocellular carcinoma rates is well recognized. In endemic areas of hepatitis B, approximately 90% of all patients with hepatocellular carcinoma are positive for hepatitis B surface antigen (HBsAg). The presence of the hepatitis B "e" antigen has been found to increase risk ninefold. The most compelling epidemiologic evidence of a causal relationship between hepatitis B infection and hepatocellular carcinoma is the observation of a significant decline in the incidence of childhood hepatocellular carcinoma after the introduction of a national immunization program in Taiwan. The hepatitis B "x" gene, which can interact with *p53*, has been a focus of study on the pathogenesis of hepatocellular carcinoma.

Hepatitis C has also been implicated in hepatocellular carcinoma development. The molecular mechanisms of HCV infection and carcinogenesis are poorly understood. Unlike patients with hepatitis B infection, patients with hepatocellular carcinoma infected with hepatitis C usually have cirrhotic livers at diagnosis; this finding suggests an extended period of infection (or hepatic damage) before malignancy develops.

Alcohol Patients with alcoholic cirrhosis are at risk for hepatocellular carcinoma, but the addition of HCV infection increases that risk dramatically.

Other possible etiologies include aflatoxin, hemochromatosis, hepatic venous obstruction, thorotrast (a contrast agent no longer used for radiologic procedures), androgens, estrogens, and α_1-antitrypsin deficiency.

Signs and symptoms

Nonspecific symptoms Patients usually present with abdominal pain and other vague symptoms, including malaise, fever, chills, anorexia, weight loss, and jaundice.

Physical findings An abdominal mass is noted on physical examination in one-third of patients. Less common findings include splenomegaly, ascites, abdominal tenderness, muscle wasting, and spider nevi. Up to 10% of patients may present with an acute abdomen due to a ruptured tumor.

Screening and diagnosis

Presently, no organization recommends routine screening of average-risk, asymptomatic adults for liver, gallbladder, and biliary tract cancers.

α-Fetoprotein is produced by 70% of hepatocellular carcinomas. The normal range for this serum marker is 0–20 ng/mL, and a level > 200 ng/mL is essentially diagnostic for hepatocellular cancer in the absence of chronic, active hepatitis B infection. In the presence of active hepatitis B infection, the diagnostic cutoff is considered to be at least 1,000 ng/mL. In the setting of hepatitis C infection, the cutoff for diagnosis of hepatocellular carcinoma has not been well studied. In hepatitis C, values > 200 ng/mL appear to be highly predictive of hepatocellular carcinoma. False-positive results may be due to acute or chronic hepatitis, germ-cell tumors, or pregnancy. In its guidelines for diagnosis of hepatic masses suspicious for hepatocellular carcinomas, the NCCN does not recommend biopsy for patients with an α-fetoprotein level > 400 ng/mL, except in the presence of hepatitis B surface antigen positivity. In that situation, a cutoff value of 4,000 ng/mL is recommended for biopsy.

Hepatitis B and C Given the association between hepatitis B and C and hepatocellular cancer, blood should be sent for hepatitis B and C antigen and antibody determinations.

Imaging The initial diagnostic test in the symptomatic patient may be ultrasonography, as it is noninvasive and can detect lesions as small as 1 cm. Ultrasound findings should be followed up with more specific imaging.

Triple-phase, high-resolution CT and contrast-enhanced MRI are the primary imaging modalities used to diagnose and stage hepatocellular carcinoma. Recent reports have documented a high number of false-positive results with CT angioportography (CTAP) and CT hepatic angiography (CTHA). CT scan predicts resectability in only 40%–50% of cases and does not accurately determine the functional extent of cirrhosis. Major difficulties arise when the liver parenchyma is not homogeneous and the lesions are smaller than 1 cm.

Laparoscopy is useful for the evaluation of small tumors, the extent of cirrhosis, peritoneal seeding, and the volume of noninvolved liver and therefore may be used prior to open laparotomy for resection. Laparoscopic or intraoperative ultrasonography should be used to confirm preoperative imaging tests. The laparoscopic results may change surgical management in up to one-third of selected patients.

High-risk patients should be screened for hepatocellular carcinoma using ultrasonography and serum α-fetoprotein levels. At present, however, there is no standard screening interval, and screening has not been shown to affect survival. Data suggest that, for screened patients, there is an increase in the proportion of cancers that are resectable. A study comparing 6-month and 12-month survival intervals in a cohort of HIV-infected patients with hemophilia showed no substantial benefit to more frequent screening.

Pathology

Three morphologic patterns of hepatocellular carcinoma have been described: nodular, diffuse, and massive. Diffuse and massive types account for > 90% of cases. The nodular type usually has multiple lesions in both lobes.

TABLE 1: TNM staging of liver and intrahepatic bile duct tumors

Primary tumor (T)	
Tx	Primary tumor cannot be assessed
T0	No evidence of primary tumor
T1	Solitary tumor without vascular invasion
T2	Solitary tumor with vascular invasion or multiple tumors (none > 5 cm)
T3	Multiple tumors > 5 cm or tumor involving a major branch of the portal or hepatic vein(s)
T4	Tumor(s) with direct invasion of adjacent organs other than the gallbladder or perforation of the visceral peritoneum
Regional lymph nodes (N)	
Nx	Regional lymph nodes cannot be assessed
N0	No regional lymph node metastasis
N1	Regional lymph node metastasis
Distant metastasis (M)	
Mx	Distant metastasis cannot be assessed
M0	No distant metastasis
M1	Distant metastasis

Stage grouping			
Stage I	T1	N0	M0
Stage II	T2	N0	M0
Stage IIIA	T3	N0	M0
Stage IIIB	T4	N0	M0
Stage IIIC	Any T	N1	M0
Stage IV	Any T	Any N	M1

From Greene FL, Page DL, Fleming ID, et al (eds): AJCC Cancer Staging Manual, 6th ed. New York, Springer-Verlag, 2002.

Histologic arrangements Several histologic arrangements have been identified: trabecular, compact, pseudoglandular or acinar, clear cell, and a fibrolamellar variant, which is associated with a relatively favorable prognosis.

Staging and prognosis

The staging system for hepatocellular cancer is based on the number and size of lesions and the presence or absence of vascular invasion (Table 1). The Okuda staging system accounts for the degree of liver dysfunction and may better predict prognosis than the TNM stage. However, the Okuda staging system does not adequately predict resectability. Because of the limited value of standard staging, the most important factors determining survival are technical resectability of lesions and degree of dysfunction of the normal liver. Groups in Italy and China have created prognostic indices that may prove useful for making treatment decisions.

Of the 5%–30% of patients who can undergo resection, factors associated with improved survival include curative resection, small tumor size, well-differentiated tumors, and normal performance status. Cirrhosis, nodal metastases, and an elevated prothrombin time are indicative of a poor prognosis, as are male sex, age > 50 years, poor performance status, duration of symptoms < 3 months, tumor rupture, aneuploidy, high DNA synthesis rate, hypocalcemia, vascular invasion, and a high serum α-fetoprotein level.

Treatment

SURGERY

Surgery is the form of treatment that offers the greatest potential for cure, even though only a small minority of patients will actually be cured. Unfortunately, many patients whose disease is thought to be resectable are clinically understaged preoperatively.

Only stage I or II tumors have a significant likelihood of being resectable for cure. However, a large tumor may still be potentially resectable for cure. Moreover, contiguous involvement of large vessels (including the portal vein and inferior vena cava) or bile ducts does not automatically mitigate against a resection, especially in patients with a fibrolamellar histology, although such resections are considerably more difficult.

Bilobar disease may be addressed with formal resection, tumor ablation techniques (eg, cryoablation, radiofrequency ablation, and ethanol injection ablation), or a combination of the two modalities.

Contraindications to resection include imminent clinical hepatic failure (jaundice in the absence of biliary obstruction), hypoalbuminemia, ascites, renal insufficiency, hypoglycemia, prolongation of the prothrombin and partial thromboplastin times, main portal vein involvement, extrahepatic metastatic disease, or other comorbid diseases that would preclude surgery of any kind.

Noncirrhotic vs cirrhotic patients Resection should be performed in all noncirrhotic patients when feasible. Resection of hepatocellular carcinoma in the presence of cirrhosis is more controversial due to its increased morbidity in this setting. Cirrhosis has been a major deterrent to resection in western nations. Resectability rates vary from 0%–43% for cirrhotic patients, whereas up to 60% of patients without cirrhosis undergo resection. Use of the modified Child-Pugh classification of liver reserve may guide the surgeon in preoperative assessment of liver function status and may aid in the selection of operable patients.

When resection is performed in the presence of cirrhosis, Child class A patients fare better than Child class B or C patients. Survival rates at 5 years following resection range from 4% to 36%, with noncirrhotic patients living longer than cirrhotic patients.

Transplantation Owing to the risk of hepatic failure following resection in cirrhotic patients, transplantation has become an option for patients with hepatocellular cancer and cirrhosis. In a study of 181 patients with hepatocellular carcinoma, Starzl and Iwatsuki found similar overall 5-year survival rates in patients treated with transplantation vs resection (36% vs 33%). Survival rates were similar in the two groups when tumors were compared for TNM stage. However, survival was significantly improved in patients with concomitant cirrhosis if they were treated with transplantation. Tumor recurrence rates for stages II and III tumors were significantly lower after transplantation than after resection, but no differences were seen for stage IV tumors.

Patients with cirrhosis and single tumors < 5 cm or multiple tumors (up to 3 with none > 3 cm) can be considered for transplantation. Larger tumors may be treated with resection when feasible. Chemoembolization followed by transplantation may be considered in selected patients. The use of transplantation is significantly limited by the scarcity and lack of immediate availability of donor organs. Recently, changes in the organ allocation system have decreased waiting times for patients with documented hepatocellular cancer.

ADJUVANT AND PALLIATIVE THERAPIES

Given the high risk of recurrence after resection, the multifocal nature of hepatocellular carcinoma, and its association with chronic liver disease, nonresectional therapies can play an important role in management. A number of prognostic factors have been identified for patients with unresectable hepatocellular carcinoma. These factors, taken alone, can have a great effect on survival rates, making cross-treatment comparisons more difficult because considerable selection bias may be present in any nonrandomized trial.

Radiation therapy

Adjuvant treatment Intrahepatic recurrence has been observed in up to two-thirds of patients treated with partial hepatectomy for hepatocellular carcinoma. Such a recurrence may represent growth at the resected edge, metastatic disease, or a new primary tumor. There is no evidence, however, that adjuvant radiation therapy can reduce this risk.

Unresectable disease Whole-liver radiation therapy can provide palliation in patients with unresectable tumors but is limited to a total dose of ≤ 30 Gy due to the risk of radiation-induced liver disease. Whole-liver irradiation has been combined with chemotherapy and transcatheter arterial chemoembolization, with objective response rates of approximately 40%–50% and median survival rates of about 18 months. Patients with tumor regrowth after chemoembolization may respond to radiotherapy.

A phase II study of proton beam radiation therapy for hepatocellular carcinoma found a complete response rate of 80% in 30 people with solitary nonmetastatic tumors measuring ≤ 10 cm in maximum dimension. The progression-free survival rate was 96%, with an actuarial overall survival rate of 66% at 2 years. Eight patients developed proton-induced hepatic insufficiency at 1 to 4 months after treatment, with four deaths in this group (*Kawashima M, Furuse J, Nishio T, et al: J Clin Oncol 23:1839-1846, 2005*).

Radiation therapy has also been delivered using yttrium-90 microspheres infused via the hepatic artery. This approach has encouraging response rates and a low toxicity profile and may be complementary with other forms of therapy.

Three-dimensional conformal radiation therapy treatment planning can allow patients with nondiffuse disease to be safely irradiated to doses well above the whole-liver tolerance dose, with doses up to 90 Gy given safely to selected patients.

Multiple institutions have reported response rates as high as 90% with acceptable toxicity when conformal radiation therapy was combined with transcatheter arterial chemoembolization (TACE). Good response and local control rates have also been reported for proton, carbon ion, and stereotactic radiotherapy.

The controversy about the survival benefits of TACE (transcatheter arterial chemoembolization) continues with a large French randomized study in which 138 patients received tamoxifen (20 mg daily) or tamoxifen along with TACE using epirubicin (Ellence) as the chemotherapy agent. TACE was repeated every 2 months until disease progression or stabilization and could be repeated at tumor progression for patients who had responded and then progressed. The majority of patients in both groups had Child's A cirrhosis. Overall survival was no different for the two groups, although there was a trend toward improvement in median survival (12 vs 16 months) favoring TACE in patients with Okuda I disease. Forty percent of patients treated experienced liver failure. Based on these results, a less intensive schedule of embolization should be considered. Further study is necessary to clarify the survival benefits of TACE, which still cannot be considered standard therapy (*Doffoel M, Vetter D, Bouche O, et al: J Clin Oncol [abstract] 23[suppl]309s, 2005*).

Hepatic TACE

Normal hepatocytes receive most of their blood supply from the portal vein, whereas tumors create new blood vessels from branches of the hepatic arterial system. This target is exploited by embolization of the hepatic artery with any number of substances, resulting in radiographic response rates in about 50% of patients and evidence of tumor liquefaction in over two-thirds of patients. Embolization is accomplished by advancing a catheter within the tumor-feeding branch of the hepatic artery. Materials injected have included Gelfoam powder, polyvinyl alcohol, iodized oil (Lipiodol), collagen, and autologous blood clot. Chemoembolization should be reserved for symptomatic tumors, reducing tumor size for resection or ablation, or as a bridge while awaiting transplant.

The effect of TACE on survival remains controversial, with randomized studies returning mixed results. A randomized, controlled trial in Spain was stopped early due to a survival benefit, but the number of analyses of data performed represents a potential problem for interpreting these data.

Intratumoral ethanol injection

The direct injection of 95% ethanol into a neoplastic lesion causes cellular dehydration and coagulation necrosis. Intratumoral ethanol ablation is employed via a percutaneous route under ultrasonographic guidance. Percutaneous intratumoral ethanol injection is best suited for use in patients with few lesions, each < 5 cm, although larger lesions may be injected multiple times.

Although intratumoral ethanol injection appears to be an effective palliative modality in certain patients, its effect on patient survival is unclear.

CRYOTHERAPY AND RADIOFREQUENCY ABLATION

Similar to ethanol ablation, cryotherapy and radiofrequency ablation (RFA) techniques are suitable for treatment of localized disease. Cryotherapy has been used intraoperatively to ablate small solitary tumors outside a planned resection (ie, in patients with bilobar disease). Cryotherapy must be performed using laparotomy, which limits its use in the palliative setting. RFA can be performed either via laparotomy or percutaneously and has limitations similar to those of ethanol ablation. As with ethanol ablation, there are no data about a survival advantage with these therapies, which may prove to be most useful for temporary tumor control in patients awaiting liver transplants. A randomized trial comparing RFA with ethanol injection found a significant benefit to RFA for local recurrence-free survival (96% vs 62% at 2 years) but not for overall survival (98% vs 88%).

A cautionary note regarding percutaneous RFA has been raised by publication of a report from Barcelona, citing 4 of 32 patients in a series who developed needle-track tumor seeding relating to subcapsular tumor location and poorly differentiated tumors.

Chemotherapy

Systemically administered chemotherapy has, for the most part, been disappointing in patients with hepatocellular carcinoma. This fact relates to both low rates of response to available agents and to difficulty with toxicity for modestly active agents because of liver dysfunction. Agents with partial response rates near or above 10% include doxorubicin, fluorouracil (5-FU), and cisplatin. Two newer agents, oxaliplatin (Eloxatin) and gemcitabine (Gemzar), which do not require liver metabolism or excretion, have garnered some interest. Both agents appear to be more active when partnered with a second agent, but results from phase II combination studies are mixed.

Intra-arterial chemotherapy (HAI) Use of HAI, principally floxuridine (fluorodeoxyuridine [FUDR]), has good biologic rationale but is hampered by high rates of biliary complications and the requirement for surgical pump placement in patients who are generally poor surgical candidates. A meta-analysis concluded that HAI after curative liver resection improved survival significantly at both 2 (23% benefit) and 3 (28% benefit) years.

Biologic therapy Interferon-alpha (IFN-α) has been shown to have potential beneficial effects in prevention of hepatocellular carcinoma; however, recent randomized studies have failed to show a benefit in patients with preexisting cirrhosis and advanced cancers. Adjuvant interferon, however, was associated with a reduction in recurrence in two small randomized trials. This finding needs to be confirmed in a much larger trial. Moderate-to-high doses of interferon are poorly tolerated by patients with frankly cirrhotic livers.

Between 2002 and 2003, 272 European patients with hepatocellular cancer were randomized to receive octreotide (Sandostatin LAR; 30 mg monthly) or placebo. Patients were stratified by center and the Cancer of the Liver Italian Program (CLIP) score; patients with a CLIP score > 3 were excluded. At a planned interim analysis, median overall survival was 6.5 months for octreotide and 7.3 months for placebo. The independent data monitoring committee recommended discontinuation of enrollment based on the low likelihood of finding a difference in favor of octreotide.

An exciting and innovative therapy for hepatocellular cancer (HCC) has been reported. Based on the observation that HCC lacks the enzyme capable of synthesizing the nonessential amino acid arginine, an arginine-depleting therapy was tested in patients with HCC. The treatment (arginine deaminase conjugated to pegylated polyethylene glycol) has few side effects, and in patients treated at a dose that completely suppressed serum arginine levels, the response rate was astounding (9 of 19 patients). Formal phase III testing of this compound is under way *(Izzo F, Marra P, Beneduce G, et al: J Clin Oncol 22:1815-1822, 2004).*

Retinoid therapy In one randomized Japanese trial, polyprenoic acid has been shown to significantly decrease the rate of recurrence of hepatocellular carcinoma after curative resection. A survival advantage was also demonstrated with long-term follow-up. Unfortunately, this compound has been unavailable for further study.

Hormone therapy A small trial reported a survival benefit at 1 year for patients treated with medroxyprogesterone. This result needs to be validated. In one randomized study, people with variant estrogen receptors had a significant improvement in median survival from 7 to 18 months when megestrol was given.

Biochemotherapy Recent results of combination biochemotherapy in a study of 154 patients by Leung et al have been encouraging. Using a combination of cisplatin, interferon-α-2a (Roferon-A), doxorubicin, and 5-FU for 4 days out of 28 days, they have shown a response rate of around 20%. Moreover, 10% of patients whose tumors were initially thought to be unresectable subsequently underwent complete resection. Eight of these patients had documented pathologic complete remissions. A recently published phase III study of PIAF (cisplatin [Platinol]/interferon-α-2b/doxorubicin [Adriamycin]/5-FU) vs single-agent doxorubicin has confirmed a higher response rate for PIAF, but survival was not significantly better than with doxorubicin. Of note, all patients in this series had hepatitis B-associated hepatocellu-

Testing of modern targeted therapies in hepatocellular cancer (HCC) has begun. A group led by Philip at Karmanos Cancer Institute has reported results of a phase II trial of the epidermal growth factor receptor (EGFR)-targeting agent erlotinib (Tarceva) in HCC and biliary tumors. Erlotinib was administered orally, 150 mg daily, to 35 patients with HCC. As of this report, 20 patients were evaluable, with an end point of disease progression-free survival at 6 months. Seven patients met the end point, and 3 of 20 patients had partial radiographic response, signaling interesting activity *(Philip PA, Mahoney M, Thomas J, et al: J Clin Oncol 23:2332-2338, 2005).*

Based on promising response rates and occasional complete pathologic response rates, the PIAF (cisplatin [Platinol]/ interferon-alpha-2b/doxorubicin [Adriamycin]/fluorouracil) regimen was tested against single-agent doxorubicin in a multicenter study performed in China. Not surprisingly, the phase III response rate with PIAF was lower than that in a phase II study, at 20.4% The response rate to doxorubicin was 10%. Despite this difference, there was no improvement in overall survival for the patients receiving the combination therapy. Combination therapy outside a clinical trial should be used with caution, given the comorbidities of patients with hepatocellular cancer *(Yeo W, Mok TS, Zee B, et al: J Natl Cancer Inst 97:1532-1538, 2005).*

lar carcinoma. Patt et al have studied a less-toxic regimen of continuous 5-FU with interferon-α-2b, demonstrating a median survival of 15.5 months.

Targeted therapies

Novel agents are now being studied in hepatocellular carcinoma (see boxed items), and some show promise for improving the outlook for this difficult disease.

BILIARY TRACT CANCERS

Gallbladder carcinoma is diagnosed approximately 5,000 times a year in the United States, making it the most common biliary tract tumor and the fifth most common GI tract cancer. Approximately 4,500 cases of bile duct tumors occur each year in the United States.

Epidemiology

GALLBLADDER CANCER

Gender Women are more commonly afflicted with gallbladder cancer than are men, with a female-to-male ratio of 1.7:1.

Age The median age at presentation of gallbladder cancer is 73 years.

Race An incidence five to six times that of the general population is seen in southwestern Native Americans, Hispanics, and Alaskans.

BILE DUCT CANCER

Gender Bile duct tumors are found in an equal number of men and women.

Age Extrahepatic bile duct tumors occur primarily in older individuals; the median age at diagnosis is 70 years.

Etiology and risk factors

GALLBLADDER CANCER

The risk of developing gallbladder cancer is higher in patients with cholelithiasis or calcified gallbladders and in typhoid carriers.

BILE DUCT CANCER

Ulcerative colitis is a clear risk factor for bile duct tumors. Patients with ulcerative colitis have an incidence of bile duct cancer that is 9-21 times higher than that of the general population. This risk does not decline after total colectomy for ulcerative colitis.

Other risk factors Primary sclerosing cholangitis, congenital anomalies of the pancreaticobiliary tree, and parasitic infections are also associated with bile duct tumors. No association of bile duct cancer with calculi, infection, or chronic obstruction has been found.

Signs and symptoms

GALLBLADDER CANCER

Early disease In the early stages, gallbladder cancer is usually asymptomatic.

Late disease Later, symptoms similar to those of benign gallbladder disease arise; they include right upper quadrant pain, nausea, vomiting, fatty food intolerance, anorexia, jaundice, and weight loss. This nonspecificity of symptoms delays presentation for medical attention and contributes to the low curability of gallbladder cancer.

Physical findings may include tenderness, an abdominal mass, hepatomegaly, jaundice, fever, and ascites.

BILE DUCT CANCER

Jaundice is the most frequent symptom found in patients with high bile duct tumors; it is present in up to 98% of such patients.

Nonspecific signs and symptoms Patients who do not present with jaundice have vague complaints, including abdominal pain, weight loss, pruritus, fever, and an abdominal mass.

Diagnosis

GALLBLADDER CANCER

Gallbladder carcinomas are often diagnosed at an advanced stage, such that by the time symptoms have developed, most tumors are unresectable.

Laboratory values in patients with gallbladder carcinoma are nonspecific but may include anemia, leukocytosis, and an elevated bilirubin level.

Ultrasonography is useful for defining a thickened gallbladder wall and may show tumor extension into the liver.

CT is more helpful than ultrasonography in assessing adenopathy and spread of disease into the liver, porta hepatis, or adjacent structures. MRI may be used to evaluate intrahepatic spread.

Endoscopic retrograde cholangiopancreatography (ERCP) or transhepatic cholangiography (THC) may be useful in the presence of jaundice to determine the location of biliary obstruction and involvement of the liver.

TABLE 2: TNM staging of gallbladder cancer

Primary tumor (T)	
Tx	Primary tumor cannot be assessed
T0	No evidence of primary tumor
Tis	Carcinoma in situ
T1	Tumor invades the lamina propria or muscle layer
T1a	Tumor invades the lamina propria
T1b	Tumor invades the muscle layer
T2	Tumor invades perimuscular connective tissue; no extension beyond the serosa or into the liver
T3	Tumor perforates the serosa (visceral peritoneum) and/or directly invades the liver and/or one other adjacent organ or structure, such as the stomach, duodenum, colon, pancreas, omentum, or extrahepatic bile ducts
T4	Tumor invades the main portal vein or hepatic artery or invades two or more extrahepatic organs or structures
Regional lymph nodes (N)	
Nx	Regional lymph nodes cannot be assessed
N0	No regional lymph node metastasis
N1	Regional lymph node metastasis
Distant metastasis (M)	
Mx	Distant metastasis cannot be assessed
M0	No distant metastasis
M1	Distant metastasis

Stage grouping			
Stage 0	Tis	N0	M0
Stage IA	T1	N0	M0
Stage IB	T2	N0	M0
Stage IIA	T3	N0	M0
Stage IIB	T1	N1	M0
	T2	N1	M0
	T3	N1	M0
Stage III	T4	Any N	M0
Stage IV	Any T	Any N	M1

From Greene FL, Page DL, Fleming ID, et al (eds): AJCC Cancer Staging Manual, 6th ed. New York, Springer-Verlag, 2002.

BILE DUCT CANCER

Cholangiocarcinoma may present earlier than gallbladder cancer by virtue of the development of biliary obstruction with jaundice, which may be painless. Tissue confirmation of suspected bile duct cancer can be difficult. The goals of the diagnostic evaluation include the determination of the level and extent of obstruction, the extent of local invasion of disease, and the identification of metastases.

Many patients with cholangiocarcinoma are thought to have metastatic

TABLE 3: Staging of bile duct tumors

Primary tumor (T)			
Tx	Primary tumor cannot be assessed		
T0	No evidence of primary tumor		
T1	Tumor confined to the bile duct histologically		
T2	Tumor invades beyond the wall of the bile duct		
T3	Tumor invades the liver, gallbladder, pancreas, and/or ipsilateral branches of the portal vein (right or left) or hepatic artery (right or left)		
T4	Tumor invades any of the following sites: main portal vein or its branches bilaterally; common hepatic artery; or other adjacent structures, such as the colon, stomach, duodenum, or abdominal wall		
Regional lymph nodes (N)			
Nx	Regional lymph nodes cannot be assessed		
N0	No regional lymph node metastasis		
N1	Regional lymph node metastasis		
Distant metastasis (M)			
Mx	Distant metastasis cannot be assessed		
M0	No distant metastasis		
M1	Distant metastasis		
Stage grouping			
Stage 0	Tis	N0	M0
Stage IA	T1	N0	M0
Stage IB	T2	N0	M0
Stage IIA	T3	N0	M0
Stage IIB	T1	N1	M0
	T2	N1	M0
	T3	N1	M0
Stage III	T4	Any N	M0
Stage IV	Any T	Any N	M1

From Greene FL, Page DL, Fleming ID, et al (eds): AJCC Cancer Staging Manual, 6th ed. New York, Springer-Verlag, 2002.

adenocarcinoma of an unknown primary, although occasionally the metastatic lesion may produce biliary dilatation without the primary lesion itself being radiographically visualized.

Ultrasonography It is generally accepted that ultrasonography should be the first imaging procedure in the evaluation of the jaundiced patient.

CT is a complementary test to ultrasonography, but both tests are accurate for staging in only 50% of patients and for determining resectability in < 45% of patients.

Cholangiography is essential to determine the location and nature of the obstruction. Percutaneous THC is used for proximal lesions, and ERCP is used for distal lesions. Magnetic resonance cholangiopancreatography (MRCP) may replace invasive studies in the near future. Histologic confirmation of tumor can be made in 45%–85% of patients with the use of exfoliative or brush cytology during cholangiography.

Pathology

GALLBLADDER CANCER

Histologic types Over 85% of gallbladder neoplasms are adenocarcinomas and the remaining 15% are squamous cell or mixed tumors.

Route of spread The initial route of spread of gallbladder cancer is locoregional rather than distant. For patients undergoing resection for presumed high-risk gallbladder masses or preoperatively defined disease limited to the gallbladder, 25% of patients will have lymphatic involvement and 70% will have direct extension of disease into the liver defined at operation.

BILE DUCT CANCER

Adenocarcinoma Morphologically, more than 90% of bile duct tumors are adenocarcinomas. Three macroscopic appearances have been identified: The papillary and nodular types occur more frequently in the distal bile duct, whereas the sclerosing type is found in the proximal bile duct. Patients with papillary lesions have the best prognosis.

Other histologic types Unusual malignant diseases of the biliary tract include adenosquamous carcinoma, leiomyosarcoma, and mucoepidermoid carcinoma.

Route of spread Most bile duct tumors grow slowly, spreading frequently by local extension and rarely by the hematogenous route. Nodal metastases are found in up to one-third of patients.

Staging and prognosis

GALLBLADDER CANCER

Gallbladder cancer is staged primarily at the time of surgery, and staging is determined by lymphatic involvement and extension of disease into adjacent structures (Table 2).

Stage Survival of gallbladder carcinoma is directly related to disease stage. The 5-year survival rate is 83% for tumors that are confined to the gallbladder mucosa; this rate decreases to 33% if the tumor extends through the gallbladder. For patients who have involvement of the lymph nodes or metastatic disease, 5-year survival rates range from 0%–15%.

Type of therapy Median survival is also improved in patients who have undergone curative resection, as compared with those who have had palliative procedures or no surgery (17 months vs 6 and 3 months, respectively).

BILE DUCT CANCER

Over 70% of patients with cholangiocarcinoma present with local extension, lymph node involvement, or distant spread of disease. The AJCC (American Joint Committee on Cancer) staging system for extrahepatic tumors is shown in Table 3.

Stage Survival for these patients is poor and is directly related to disease stage. Median survival is 12–20 months for patients with disease limited to the bile ducts and ≤ 8 months when the disease has spread.

Tumor location Survival is also related to tumor location, with patients with distal lesions doing better than those with mid or proximal tumors.

Success of therapy Curative resection and negative margins result in improved survival.

Treatment

In the absence of polyps identified ultrasonographically and confirmed by CT during the work-up of suspected cholelithiasas, relatively few patients with gallbladder cancer are diagnosed prior to surgery. Only 1%–2% of cholecystectomy specimens are found to contain malignancy.

SURGERY FOR GALLBLADDER CANCER

Surgical management of gallbladder carcinoma is based on the local extension of the tumor.

Early-stage disease Tumors that invade the mucosa, those that do not penetrate the muscularis, and those that penetrate full thickness but do not abut the liver or muscularis require cholecystectomy alone. Laparoscopic cholecystectomy may be adequate for T1 tumors. If there is direct extension of disease to or through the serosa, the resection should include the gallbladder bed (segments IVb and V) and a porta hepatis lymphadenectomy. Disease that involves the gallbladder node is particularly curable and should be resected. Nodal disease beyond the pericholedochal nodes defines the surgically incurable patient.

SURGERY FOR BILE DUCT CANCER

The rate of resectability is 15%–20% for high bile duct tumors and up to 70% for distal lesions.

Assessing resectability Higher resolution CT or MRI with biliary reconstruction may be supplemented with hepatic arteriography, portal venography, or duplex imaging preoperatively to assess resectability.

Preoperative treatments Three randomized trials have shown no benefit to preoperative decompression of the biliary tree in patients with obstructive jaundice. Some authors advocate the preoperative placement of biliary stents to facilitate dissection of the hilus. This procedure should be performed immediately prior to resection to reduce the risk of cholangitis and maintain the duct at its maximally dilated size.

Proximal tumors Local excision is often possible for proximal lesions. Hepatic resection is indicated for high bile duct tumors with quadrate lobe invasion or unilateral intrahepatic ductal or vascular involvement. Resection is not indicated in situations in which a clear surgical margin cannot be obtained.

Both 5-FU and gemcitabine have modest activity in biliary malignancies. A group in Toronto recently published results of combination therapy with capecitabine (Xeloda) and gemcitabine (Gemzar). The mix of cholangiocarcinoma and gallbladder cancer in the 45 patients studied was nearly 50:50. The overall response rate was 31%, and the median survival was a promising 14 months. This regimen is a reasonable alternative to gemcitabine and cisplatin for biliary tract neoplasms (*Knox JJ, Hedley D, Oza A, et al: J Clin Oncol 23:2332-2338, 2005*).

Mid-ductal and distal tumors Mid-ductal lesions can often be removed by resection of the bile duct with associated portal lymphadenectomy. Distal or mid-ductal lesions that cannot be locally excised should be removed by pancreaticoduodenectomy.

Reconstruction techniques Biliary-enteric continuity is usually reconstructed with a Roux-en-Y anastomosis to the hilum for high lesions and in a standard drainage pattern following pancreaticoduodenectomy.

Liver transplantation has been attempted for unresectable tumors, but early recurrence and poor survival have prevented the widespread application of this approach.

Surgical bypass For patients found to have unresectable disease at surgical exploration, operative biliary bypass may be performed using a variety of techniques. Bypass results in excellent palliation and obviates the need for further intervention.

ADJUVANT RADIATION THERAPY FOR BILIARY TRACT CANCER

A review of the patterns of initial disease recurrence after resection of gallbladder cancer (80 patients, in whom disease recurred in 53) and hilar cholangiocarcinoma (76 patients, in whom disease recurred in 52) found a distinct difference with regard to total locoregional failure vs total distant failure. Hilar cholangiocarcinomas were much more likely to include locoregional failure alone or as a component (65% of all failures), compared with gallbladder cancer (28% of all failures). Distant failure was found alone or as a component in 72% of all recurrences of gallbladder cancer but only in 36% of hilar cholangiocarcinomas.

A recent report compared a group of patients with unresectable hilar cholangiocarcinoma prospectively treated with radiation therapy, bolus fluorouracil, or capecitabine (Xeloda) and liver transplantation with patients with resectable hilar cholangiocarcinoma treated with resection only during the same period at the same institution. Survival rates were superior for all 71 neoadjuvantly treated patients with unresectable disease (58% at 5 years) and for the 38 patients who ultimately underwent transplantation (82% at 5 years), suggesting that further evaluation of this approach is reasonable; however, the separate contributions of the neoadjuvant therapy and liver transplantation could not be evaluated (*Rea DJ, Heimbach JK, Rosen CB, et al: Ann Surg 242:451-461, 2005*).

Despite these observations, there are no good prospective data to define the role of adjuvant radiation or chemoradiation treatment. For bile duct tumors, a review of 192 patients found that a benefit from adjuvant chemoradiation therapy was more evident in distal tumors than in intrahepatic or perihilar tumors. Another retrospective review, however, found that on multivariate analysis, only lymph node status was prognostically significant.

ADJUVANT CHEMOTHERAPY

A recently published randomized trial performed in Japan showed that treatment with 5-FU and mitomycin (Mutamycin) produced a survival benefit in patients with resected gallbladder cancers. These data came from a planned subset of a larger trial in which 112 patients with gallbladder cancer were randomized. At 5 years, 26% of chemotherapy-treated patients were alive, compared with 14% of those treated with surgery and observation alone. These data warrant consideration of chemotherapy for these patients, but definitive conclusions would require a larger randomized trial.

> A trial of capecitabine (Xeloda) and oxaliplatin (Eloxatin) was performed in patients with cholangiocarcinoma at M. D. Anderson Cancer Center. In this population (28 patients), half of whom were previously treated, the response rate was 17.8%. Survival data were not available at the time this abstract was presented at the 2005 ASCO meeting (*Glover KY, Thomas MB, Brown TD, et al: J Clin Oncol [abstract] 23:338s, 2005*).

TREATMENT OF UNRESECTABLE DISEASE

Like pancreatic adenocarcinoma, unresectable biliary tract carcinoma has a poor prognosis.

Stenting

Many patients with unresectable disease, particularly those with pain, nausea, or pruritus, will benefit from nonsurgical percutaneous or endoscopic stenting.

Radiation therapy

There are few data on radiation therapy for unresectable gallbladder cancer, other than reports of intraoperative radiation therapy. External-beam radiation therapy would be anticipated to provide a palliative benefit.

There is considerable experience using brachytherapy alone or combined with external-beam radiation therapy for unresectable bile duct tumors. Median survival ranges from 10–24 months, and 5-year survival rates are approximately 10% with these approaches. Cholangitis, however, may occur more frequently in people treated with brachytherapy. A randomized trial of stenting alone vs with photodynamic therapy (PDT) found a significantly longer median survival and improved quality of life in the PDT group. Although it is unlikely that all of the tumor was treated with PDT, this study did show the importance of local control and its association with quality of life. Radiation therapy may also ultimately play a role in the promotion of viral replication for gene therapy.

Chemotherapy

Because biliary tract malignancies are uncommon cancers, the number of clinical trials and the number of patients in those trials are limited. Generally speaking, responses to chemotherapy are infrequent and brief. However, newer drugs and drug combinations are better tolerated and stand to improve on past results.

5-FU has historically been the most active single agent, with single-agent response rates in the 10%–20% range.

Capecitabine (Xeloda), a prodrug of 5-FU (see chapter 16), produced responses in 4 of 8 gallbladder cancers but in only 1 of 18 cholangiocarcinomas in a phase II study presented by Hassan et al from M. D. Anderson Cancer Center.

Gemcitabine Multiple studies have documented gemcitabine as an active agent, particularly in gallbladder cancer. Cisplatin and gemcitabine may be a synergistic doublet, with reported response rates for gallbladder cancer in the range of 30%–50%.

Other agents with reported activity in biliary tract malignancies include oxaliplatin, cisplatin, docetaxel (Taxotere), mitomycin, doxorubicin, and the nitrosoureas. Combination regimens do not clearly improve on the results of single-agent chemotherapy and as such remain investigational.

Hepatic arterial chemotherapy There is limited experience with hepatic arterial chemotherapy for biliary tract neoplasms, but there are case reports of responses to floxuridine in the literature.

Treatment recommendations In the absence of a clinical trial, patients should be offered gemcitabine or 5-FU (or capecitabine), with or without leucovorin. Other agents, such as doxorubicin or cisplatin, may be added, but, as noted, there is no unequivocal evidence that combination chemotherapy produces any substantial benefits in improving quality of life or survival.

SUGGESTED READING

ON HEPATOCELLULAR CARCINOMA

Gupta S, Bent S, Kohlwes J: Test characteristics of alpha-fetoprotein for detecting hepatocellular carcinoma in patients with hepatitis C: A systematic review and critical analysis. Ann Intern Med 1394:46–50, 2003.

Kawashima M, Furuse J, Nishio T, et al: Phase II study of radiotherapy employing proton beam for hepatocellular caricinoma. J Clin Oncol 23:1839–1846, 2005.

Lencioni RA, Allgaier H-P, Cioni D, et al: Small hepatocellular carcinoma in cirrhosis: Randomized comparison of radio-frequency thermal ablation versus percutaneous ethanol injection. Radiology 228:235–240, 2003.

Llovet J, Bruix J: Systematic review of randomized trials for unresectable hepatocellular carcinoma: Chemoembolization improves survival. Hepatology 37:429–442, 2003.

Mathurin P, Raynard B, Dharancy S, et al: Meta-analysis: Evaluation of adjuvant therapy after curative liver resection for hepatocellular carcinoma. Aliment Pharmacol Ther 17:1247–1261, 2003.

Mok TS, Yeo W, Yu S, et al: An intensive surveillance program detected a high incidence of hepatocellular carcinoma among hepatitis B virus carriers with abnormal alpha-fetoprotein levels or abdominal ultrasonography results. J Clin Oncol 23:8041–8047, 2005.

Yao FY, Bass NM, Ascher NL, et al: Liver transplantation for hepatocellular carcinoma: Lessons from the first year under the Model of End-Stage Liver Disease (MELD) organ allocation policy. Liver Transpl 10:621–630, 2004.

Yeo W, Mok TS, Zee B, et al: A randomized phase III study of doxorubicin versus cisplatin/interferon alpha-2b/doxorubicin/fluorouracil (PIAF) combination chemotherapy for unresectable heaptocellular carcinoma. J Natl Cancer Inst 97:1532–1538, 2005.

ON GALLBLADDER TUMORS

Doval DC, Sekhon JS, Gupta SK, et al: A phase II study of gemcitabine and cisplatin in chemotherapy-naive, unresectable gall bladder cancer. Br J Cancer 90:1516–1520, 2004.

Jarnagin WR, Ruo L, Little SA, et al: Patterns of initial disease recurrence after resection of gallbladder carcinoma and hilar cholangiocarcinoma: Implications of adjuvant therapeutic strategies. Cancer 98:1689–1700, 2003.

Patt YZ, Hassan MM, Aguayo A, et al: Oral capecitabine for the treatment of hepatocellular carcinoma, cholangiocarcinoma, and gallbladder carcinoma. Cancer 101:578–586, 2004.

Takada T, Amano H, Yasuda H, et al: Is postoperative adjuvant chemotherapy useful for gallbladder carcinoma? A phase III multicenter prospective randomized controlled trial in patients with resected pancreaticobiliary carcinoma. Cancer 95:1685–1695, 2002.

ON BILE DUCT TUMORS

Alberts SR, Al-Khatib H, Mahoney MR, et al: Gemcitabine, 5-fluorouracil, and leucovorin in advanced biliary tract and gallbladder carcinoma: A North Central Cancer Treatment Group phase II trial. Cancer 103:111–118, 2005.

Knox JJ, Hedley D, Oza A, et al: Combining gemcitabine and capecitabine in patients with advanced biliary cancer: A phase II trial. J Clin Oncol 23:2332–2338, 2005.

Ortner ME, Caca K, Berr F, et al: Successful photodynamic therapy for nonresectable cholangiocarcinoma: A randomized prospective study. Gastroenterology 125:1355–1363, 2003.

Rea DJ, Heimbach JK, Rosen CB, et al: Liver transplantation with neoadjuvant chemoradiation is more effective than resection for hilar cholangiocarcinoma. Ann Surg 242:451–461, 2005.

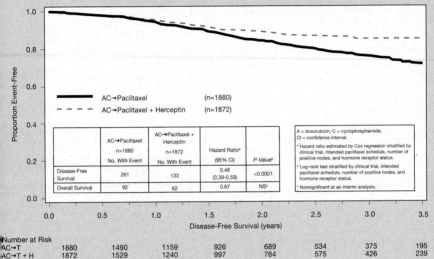

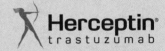

Herceptin®
trastuzumab

HERCEPTIN® [Trastuzumab] BRIEF SUMMARY
Please see full prescribing information including DOSAGE AND ADMINISTRATION.

WARNINGS:
Cardiomyopathy
Herceptin administration can result in left ventricular dysfunction and congestive heart failure (CHF). Left ventricular function should be evaluated in all patients prior to and during treatment with Herceptin.

The incidence and severity of left ventricular cardiac dysfunction/CHF was highest in patients who received Herceptin concurrently with anthracycline-containing chemotherapy regimens. Discontinue Herceptin treatment in patients receiving adjuvant therapy for breast cancer and strongly consider discontinuation of Herceptin in patients with metastatic breast cancer who develop a clinically significant decrease in left ventricular function. (See **WARNINGS: Cardiomyopathy**, See **DOSAGE AND ADMINISTRATION: Dose Modifications**)

Infusion Reactions
Pulmonary Toxicity
Herceptin administration can result in serious infusion reactions and pulmonary toxicity. Rarely, these have been fatal. In most cases, symptoms occurred during or within 24 hours of administration of Herceptin. Herceptin infusion should be interrupted for patients experiencing dyspnea or clinically significant hypotension. Patients should be monitored until signs and symptoms completely resolve. Discontinuation of Herceptin should be strongly considered for infusion reactions manifesting as anaphylaxis, angioedema, pneumonitis, or acute respiratory distress syndrome. (See **WARNINGS**.)

INDICATIONS AND USAGE
Herceptin (Trastuzumab), as part of a treatment regimen containing doxorubicin, cyclophosphamide, and paclitaxel, is indicated for the adjuvant treatment of patients with HER2-overexpressing, node-positive breast cancer. (See **CLINICAL STUDIES** and **DOSAGE AND ADMINISTRATION**)

Herceptin as a single agent is indicated for the treatment of patients with metastatic breast cancer whose tumors overexpress the HER2 protein and who have received one or more chemotherapy regimens for their metastatic disease.

Herceptin in combination with paclitaxel is indicated for treatment of patients with metastatic breast cancer whose tumors overexpress the HER2 protein and who have not received chemotherapy for their metastatic disease. (See **PRECAUTIONS: HER2 Testing** and **CLINICAL STUDIES: HER2 Detection**).

CONTRAINDICATIONS
None.

WARNINGS
Cardiomyopathy
Herceptin can cause left ventricular cardiac dysfunction. Cardiac dysfunction in patients receiving Herceptin therapy can be serious with disabling cardiac failure, death, and mural thrombosis leading to stroke (see **BOXED WARNINGS: Cardiomyopathy**).

Among women receiving adjuvant therapy for breast cancer in Study 1, 16% (136/844) of patients discontinued Herceptin therapy due to clinical evidence of myocardial dysfunction or significant decline in LVEF (see **DOSAGE AND ADMINISTRATION: Dose Modifications**). There was one death due to cardiomyopathy among patients receiving Herceptin. If Herceptin therapy is discontinued for left ventricular cardiac dysfunction, patients should be closely monitored for evidence of clinical deterioration and further decline in left ventricular function.

Among 32 patients receiving adjuvant chemotherapy (Studies 1 and 2) with clinical cardiac events as determined by ACREC, one patient died of cardiomyopathy and all other patients were receiving cardiac medication at last follow-up. Approximately half of the surviving patients had recovery to a normal LVEF (defined as ≥50%) on continuing medical management at the time of last follow-up. The safety of continuation or resumption of Herceptin in patients with Herceptin-induced left ventricular cardiac dysfunction has not been studied.

In the adjuvant setting, among patients who completed AC chemotherapy and received at least one dose of paclitaxel, 2% [32/1677] of patients in the Herceptin arm and 0.4% [7/1600] of patients in the control arm experienced clinically symptomatic, laboratory-confirmed cardiomyopathy as determined by an external review committee (ACREC).

Among patients with metastatic breast cancer, the incidence of CHF was 11% versus 1% in patients receiving paclitaxel with or without Herceptin and 28% versus 7% in patients receiving AC chemotherapy with or without Herceptin, respectively. The incidence of CHF in patients with metastatic breast cancer receiving Herceptin monotherapy was 7%.

An exploratory analysis for risk factors for symptomatic cardiomyopathy was conducted in patients receiving adjuvant treatment for breast cancer.

The analysis is limited by the number and type of variables collected and how they were defined. Declining LVEF to below the lower limit of normal after completion of AC chemotherapy or during Herceptin treatment, a reported history of prior or concurrent use of anti-hypertensive medications, and increasing age were associated with an increased risk of Herceptin-induced symptomatic cardiomyopathy. Similar limited analyses in patients receiving chemotherapy for metastatic breast cancer identified prior cardiotoxic therapy (e.g., anthracycline or radiation therapy to the chest) and increasing age as potentially associated with an increased risk of Herceptin-induced CHF.

Candidates for treatment with Herceptin should undergo a thorough baseline cardiac assessment, including history, physical examination, and an assessment of LVEF by echocardiogram or MUGA scan. Patients receiving Herceptin should undergo frequent monitoring for deteriorating left ventricular function. The following recommended schedule is consistent with that used in Studies 1 and 2: at baseline prior to AC chemotherapy, immediately prior to initiation of Herceptin, 3 months after initiation of Herceptin with paclitaxel, 3 months after initiation of Herceptin monotherapy, and 3 months after completion of Herceptin monotherapy. More frequent monitoring should be employed in patients with preexisting cardiac dysfunction. Monitoring will not identify all patients who will develop cardiac dysfunction.

Infusion Reactions
In clinical trials, infusion reactions consisted of a symptom complex characterized by fever and chills, and on occasion included nausea, vomiting, pain (in some cases at tumor sites), headache, dizziness, dyspnea, hypotension, rash, and asthenia. These reactions were usually mild to moderate in severity (see **ADVERSE REACTIONS: Infusion Reactions**).

However, in postmarketing reports, serious and fatal infusion reactions were reported infrequently. Severe reactions which include bronchospasm, hypoxia, and severe hypotension, were usually reported during or immediately following the initial infusion. However, the onset and clinical course were variable including progressive worsening, initial improvement followed by clinical deterioration, or delayed post-infusion events with rapid clinical deterioration. For fatal events, death occurred within hours to days following a serious infusion reaction.

Herceptin infusion should be interrupted in all patients experiencing dyspnea or clinically significant hypotension and medical therapy administered, which may include epinephrine, corticosteroids, diphenhydramine, bronchodilators, and oxygen. Patients should be evaluated and carefully monitored until complete resolution of signs and symptoms. Permanent discontinuation should be strongly considered in all patients with severe infusion reactions.

There are no data regarding the most appropriate method of identification of patients who may safely be retreated with Herceptin after experiencing a severe infusion reaction. Herceptin has been readministered to some patients who fully recovered from the previous severe reaction. Prior to readministration of Herceptin, the majority of these patients were prophylactically treated with pre-medications including antihistamines and/or corticosteroids. While some of these patients tolerated retreatment, others had severe reactions again despite the use of prophylactic pre-medications.

Exacerbation of Chemotherapy-Induced Neutropenia
In randomized, controlled clinical trials in women with metastatic breast cancer designed to assess the impact of the addition of Herceptin on chemotherapy, the per-patient incidences of moderate to severe neutropenia and of febrile neutropenia were higher in patients receiving Herceptin in combination with myelosuppressive chemotherapy as compared to those who received chemotherapy alone. Deaths due to sepsis in patients with severe neutropenia have been reported in patients receiving Herceptin and myelosuppressive chemotherapy, although in controlled clinical trials, the incidence of septic death was not significantly increased. (See **ADVERSE REACTIONS: Neutropenia** and **Infection**).

Pulmonary Toxicity
Herceptin use can result in serious and fatal pulmonary toxicity. Pulmonary toxicity includes dyspnea, pneumonitis, pulmonary infiltrates, pleural effusions, non-cardiogenic pulmonary edema, pulmonary insufficiency and hypoxia, acute respiratory distress syndrome, and pulmonary fibrosis. Such events can occur as sequelae of infusion reactions (see **WARNINGS: Infusion Reactions**). Patients with symptomatic intrinsic lung disease or with extensive tumor involvement of the lungs, resulting in dyspnea at rest, appear to have more severe toxicity.

PRECAUTIONS
HER2 Testing
Detection of HER2 protein overexpression is necessary for selection of patients appropriate for Herceptin therapy because these are the only patients studied and for whom benefit has been shown (see **INDICATIONS AND USAGE**). Patients enrolled in metastatic breast cancer clinical studies were required to have immunohistochemical evidence of HER2 protein overexpression. In trials of adjuvant therapy, patients were required to have evidence of HER2 protein overexpression and/or HER2 gene

amplification. Assessment for HER2 overexpression and of HER2 gene amplification should be performed by laboratories with demonstrated proficiency in the specific technology being utilized. Improper assay performance, including use of suboptimally fixed tissue, failure to utilize specified reagents, deviation from specific assay instructions, and failure to include appropriate controls for assay validation, can lead to unreliable results. Refer to the HercepTest®, the PathVysion®, or any other FDA-approved test kit package inserts for full instructions on assay performance (see **CLINICAL STUDIES: HER2 Detection: HER2 Protein Overexpression Detection Methods** and **HER2 Gene Amplification Detection Methods**).

Drug Interactions

There have been no formal drug interaction studies performed with Herceptin in humans. Administration of paclitaxel in combination with Herceptin resulted in a two-fold decrease in Herceptin clearance in a non-human primate study and in a 1.5-fold increase in Herceptin serum levels in clinical studies (see **CLINICAL PHARMACOLOGY: Pharmacokinetics**).

Carcinogenesis, Mutagenesis, Impairment of Fertility

Carcinogenesis

Herceptin has not been tested for its carcinogenic potential.

Mutagenesis

No evidence of mutagenic activity was observed in Ames tests using six different test strains of bacteria, with and without metabolic activation, at concentrations of up to 5000 µg/mL Trastuzumab. Human peripheral blood lymphocytes treated *in vitro* at concentrations of up to 5000 µg/plate Trastuzumab, with and without metabolic activation, revealed no evidence of mutagenic potential. In an *in vivo* mutagenic assay (the micronucleus assay), no evidence of chromosomal damage to mouse bone marrow cells was observed following bolus intravenous doses of up to 118 mg/kg Trastuzumab.

Impairment of Fertility

A fertility study has been conducted in female cynomolgus monkeys at doses up to 25 times the weekly human maintenance dose of 2 mg/kg Herceptin and has revealed no evidence of impaired fertility.

Pregnancy Category B

There are no adequate and well-controlled studies in pregnant women. Because animal reproduction studies are not always predictive of human response, Herceptin should be used during pregnancy only if the potential benefit to the mother justifies the potential risk to the fetus.

In the postmarketing setting, oligohydramnios has been reported in women who received Herceptin during pregnancy, either in combination with chemotherapy or as a single agent. Given the limited number of reported cases, the high background rate of occurrence of oligohydramnios, the lack of clear temporal relationships between drug use and clinical findings, and the lack of supportive findings in animal studies, an association between Herceptin and oligohydramnios has not been established.

Reproduction studies have been conducted in cynomolgus monkeys at doses up to 25 times the weekly human maintenance dose of 2 mg/kg Herceptin and have revealed no evidence of impaired fertility or harm to the fetus. However, HER2 protein expression is high in many embryonic tissues including cardiac and neural tissues; in mutant mice lacking HER2, embryos died in early gestation (1). Placental transfer of Herceptin during the early (Days 20–50 of gestation) and late (Days 120–150 of gestation) fetal development period was observed in monkeys.

Nursing Mothers

A study conducted in lactating cynomolgus monkeys at doses 25 times the weekly human maintenance dose of 2 mg/kg Herceptin demonstrated that Trastuzumab is secreted in the milk. The presence of Trastuzumab in the serum of infant monkeys was not associated with any adverse effects on their growth or development from birth to 3 months of age. It is not known whether Herceptin is secreted in human milk. Because human IgG is secreted in human milk, and the potential for absorption and harm to the infant is unknown, women should be advised to discontinue nursing during Herceptin therapy and for 6 months after the last dose of Herceptin.

Pediatric Use

The safety and effectiveness of Herceptin in pediatric patients have not been established.

Geriatric Use

Herceptin has been administered to 257 patients who were 65 years of age or over (124 in the adjuvant treatment and 133 in metastatic breast cancer treatment settings). The risk of cardiac dysfunction was increased in geriatric patients as compared to younger patients in both those receiving treatment for metastatic disease or adjuvant therapy. Aside from cardiac dysfunction, limitations in data collection and differences in study design of the 2 studies of Herceptin in adjuvant treatment of breast cancer preclude a determination of whether the toxicity profile of Herceptin in older patients is different from younger patients. The reported clinical experience is not adequate to determine whether the efficacy improvements (ORR, TTP, OS, DFS) of Herceptin treatment in older patients is different from that observed in patients <65 years of age for metastatic disease and adjuvant treatment.

HERCEPTIN® [Trastuzumab] BRIEF SUMMARY

ADVERSE REACTIONS

Because clinical trials are conducted under widely varying conditions, adverse reaction rates observed in the clinical trials of a drug cannot be directly compared with rates in the clinical trials of another drug and may not reflect the rates observed in practice. The adverse reaction information from clinical trials does, however, provide a basis for identifying the adverse events that appear to be related to drug use and for approximating rates.

The most serious toxicities of Herceptin are:

- Cardiomyopathy
- Pulmonary toxicity (respiratory failure, pneumonitis, pulmonary infiltrates)
- Infusion reactions
- Febrile neutropenia/exacerbation of chemotherapy-induced neutropenia

Please refer to the **BOXED WARNINGS** and/or **WARNINGS** sections for detailed descriptions of these serious adverse reactions.

The most common adverse reactions in patients receiving Herceptin are fever, nausea, vomiting, infusion reactions, diarrhea, infections, increased cough, headache, fatigue, dyspnea, rash, neutropenia, anemia, and myalgia. Adverse reactions requiring interruption or discontinuation of Herceptin treatment include severe infusion reactions, CHF, and significant decline in left ventricular cardiac function. (See **DOSAGE AND ADMINISTRATION: Dose Modifications**)

Where specific percentages are noted, these data are based on clinical studies of Herceptin alone or in combination with chemotherapy in women with metastatic breast cancer or in combination with and following chemotherapy in women receiving adjuvant treatment for breast cancer.

Additional adverse reactions have been identified during post-marketing use of Herceptin in the metastatic breast cancer population. Because these reactions are reported voluntarily from a population of uncertain size, it is not always possible to reliably estimate their frequency or establish a causal relationship to Herceptin exposure. Decisions to include these reactions in labeling are typically based on one or more of the following factors: (1) seriousness of the reaction, (2) frequency of reporting, or (3) strength of causal connection to Herceptin.

Cardiomyopathy

See **BOXED WARNINGS: Cardiomyopathy** and **WARNINGS: Cardiomyopathy**.

Herceptin can cause left ventricular myocardial dysfunction, characterized by signs and symptoms of congestive heart failure and a decline in LVEF. Cardiac dysfunction due to Herceptin therapy can be serious with disabling cardiac failure, death, and mural thrombosis leading to stroke (see **BOXED WARNINGS: Cardiomyopathy**). Herceptin can also cause asymptomatic decline in LVEF.

Serial measurement of cardiac function (LVEF) was obtained only in clinical trials in the adjuvant treatment of breast cancer. There were 6% of patients who were unable to receive Herceptin following completion of AC chemotherapy due to cardiac dysfunction (LVEF <50% or ≥15 point decline in LVEF from baseline to end of AC). Following initiation of Herceptin therapy, the incidence of new-onset dose-limiting myocardial dysfunction was higher among patients receiving Herceptin and paclitaxel as compared to those receiving paclitaxel alone (see Table 5).

Table 5

Per Patient Incidence* of New Onset Myocardial Dysfunction (LVEF Decline Below 50%) by Time Period Following the Initiation of Paclitaxel +/- Herceptin

Timepoint following initiation of chemotherapy	**AC→T**	**AC→TH**
Paclitaxel +/- Herceptin Treatment (Month 3–6)	5.0 % (66/1330)	11.6 % (171/1469)
During Herceptin Monotherapy / Observation (Month 6–9)	4.1 % (46/1125)	8.8 % (96/1090)

*Incidence is proportion of patients with LVEF <50% during the time period in patients with a normal LVEF at the start of that time period.

Among patients receiving adjuvant therapy for breast cancer (Studies 1 and 2), investigator-identified cases of cardiac adverse events underwent a secondary review by subcommittees each of which used different criteria for classification of a cardiac event. The per-patient incidence of clinical cardiac adverse events, as determined either by a central study committee or by an external safety committee (ACREC) that was blinded to treatment assignment, was increased among those receiving Herceptin. The results are presented in Table 6.

Table 6
Incidence of Clinical Cardiac Events in Adjuvant Breast Cancer

	Study 1		Study 2	
	AC→T (n = 876)	AC→T + H (n = 920)	AC→T (n = 724)	AC→T + H (n = 757)
ACREC	6 0.68%	19 2.07%	1 0.14%	13 1.72%
Study-specific subcommittee	10 1.14%	31 3.37%	0 0.00%	20 2.64%

Approximately half of the clinical cardiac events among patients in the Herceptin arm were identified by the end of paclitaxel therapy (month 6) and approximately 90% were identified by one year following completion of paclitaxel (month 15).

The incidence of treatment emergent congestive heart failure among patients in the metastatic breast cancer trials was classified for severity using the New York Heart Association classification system (I–IV, where IV is the most severe level of cardiac failure) (see Table 7).

Table 7
Incidence and Severity of Cardiac Dysfunction in Metastatic Breast Cancer

	Herceptin[a] Alone n = 213	Herceptin + Paclitaxel[b] n = 91	Paclitaxel[b] n = 95	Herceptin + Anthracycline + Cyclo-phosphamide[b] n = 143	Anthracycline + Cyclo-phosphamide[b] n = 135
Any Cardiac Dysfunction	7%	11%	1%	28%	7%
Class III–IV	5%	4%	1%	19%	3%

[a]Open-label, single-agent Phase II study (94% received prior anthracyclines).
[b]Randomized Phase III study comparing chemotherapy plus Herceptin to chemotherapy alone, where chemotherapy is either anthracycline/cyclophosphamide or paclitaxel.

In the metastatic breast cancer trials the probability of cardiac dysfunction was highest in patients who received Herceptin concurrently with anthracyclines.

Infusion Reactions

During the first infusion with Herceptin, a symptom complex most commonly consisting of chills and/or fever was observed in approximately 40% of patients in clinical trials. The symptoms were usually mild to moderate in severity and were treated with acetaminophen, diphenhydramine, and meperidine (with or without reduction in the rate of Herceptin infusion); permanent discontinuation of Herceptin for infusional toxicity was required in <1% of patients. Other signs and/or symptoms may include nausea, vomiting, pain (in some cases at tumor sites), rigors, headache, dizziness, dyspnea, hypotension, elevated blood pressure, rash, and asthenia. Infusional toxicity occurred in 21% and 35% of patients, and was severe in 1.4% and 9% of patients, on second or subsequent Herceptin infusions administered as monotherapy or in combination with chemotherapy, respectively. (See **BOXED WARNINGS: Infusion Reactions** and **WARNINGS: Infusion Reactions**).

Anemia

In randomized controlled clinical trials, the overall incidence of anemia (30% vs. 21% [Study 3]), of selected NCI CTC Grade 2–5 anemia (12.5% vs. 6.6% [Study 1]), and of anemia requiring transfusions (0.1% vs. 0 patients [Study 2]) were increased in patients receiving Herceptin and chemotherapy compared with those receiving chemotherapy alone.

Neutropenia

In randomized controlled clinical trials in the adjuvant setting, the incidence of selected NCI CTC Grade 4–5 neutropenia (2% vs. 0.7% [Study 2]) and of selected Grade 2–5 neutropenia (7.1% vs. 4.5% [Study 1]) were increased in patients receiving Herceptin and chemotherapy compared with those receiving chemotherapy alone. In a randomized, controlled trial in patients with metastatic breast cancer, the incidences of NCI-CTC Grade 3/4 neutropenia (32% vs. 22%) and of febrile neutropenia (23% vs. 17%) were also increased in patients randomized to Herceptin in combination with myelosuppressive chemotherapy as compared to chemotherapy alone (see **ADVERSE REACTIONS: Infection**).

Following the administration of Herceptin as a single agent (Study 4), the incidences of NCI-CTC Grade 3 leukopenia, thrombocytopenia, and anemia were all <1%. No Grade 4 hematologic toxicities were observed.

Infection

The overall incidences of infection (46% vs. 30% [Study 3]), of selected NCI-CTC Grade 2–5 infection/febrile neutropenia (22% vs. 14% [Study 1]) and of selected Grade 3–5 infection/febrile neutropenia (3.3% vs. 1.4%) [Study 2]), were higher in patients receiving Herceptin and chemotherapy compared with those receiving chemotherapy alone. The most common site of infections in the adjuvant setting involved the upper respiratory tract, skin, and urinary tract.

HERCEPTIN® [Trastuzumab] BRIEF SUMMARY

In a randomized, controlled trial in treatment of metastatic breast cancer, the reported incidence of febrile neutropenia was higher (23% vs. 17%) in patients receiving Herceptin in combination with myelosuppressive chemotherapy as compared to chemotherapy alone (see **WARNINGS: Exacerbation of Chemotherapy-Induced Neutropenia**).

Pulmonary Toxicity

Among women receiving adjuvant therapy for breast cancer, the incidence of selected NCI-CTC Grade 2–5 pulmonary toxicity (14% vs. 5% [Study 1]) and of selected NCI-CTC Grade 3–5 pulmonary toxicity and spontaneously reported Grade 2 dyspnea (3.4 % vs. 1% [Study 2]) was higher in patients receiving Herceptin and chemotherapy compared with chemotherapy alone. The most common pulmonary toxicity was dyspnea (NCI-CTC Grade 2–5: 12% vs. 4% [Study 1]; NCI-CTC Grade 2–5: 2.5% vs. 0.1% [Study 2]). Pneumonitis/pulmonary infiltrates occurred in 0.7% of patients receiving Herceptin compared with 0.3% of those receiving chemotherapy alone. Fatal respiratory failure occurred in 3 patients receiving Herceptin, one as a component of multi-organ system failure, as compared to 1 patient receiving chemotherapy alone.

Among women receiving Herceptin for treatment of metastatic breast cancer, the incidence of pulmonary toxicity was also increased. Pulmonary adverse events have been reported in the post-marketing experience as part of the symptom complex of infusion reactions (see **BOXED WARNINGS: Infusion Reactions; Pulmonary Toxicity** and **WARNINGS: Infusion Reactions**). Pulmonary events include bronchospasm, hypoxia, dyspnea, pulmonary infiltrates, pleural effusions, non-cardiogenic pulmonary edema, and acute respiratory distress syndrome. For a detailed description, see **WARNINGS**.

Thrombosis/Embolism

In three randomized, controlled clinical trials, the incidence of thrombotic adverse events was higher in patients receiving Herceptin and chemotherapy compared to chemotherapy alone in two studies (3.0 vs. 1.3% [Study 1] and 2.1% vs. 0% [Study 3]).

Diarrhea

Of patients treated with Herceptin as a single agent, 25% experienced diarrhea. An increased incidence of diarrhea, primarily mild to moderate in severity, was observed in patients receiving Herceptin in combination with chemotherapy for treatment of metastatic breast cancer. Among women receiving adjuvant therapy for breast cancer, the incidence of treatment-related NCI-CTC Grade 2 and all Grade 3–5 diarrhea (6.2% vs. 4.8% [Study 1]) and of treatment-related NCI-CTC Grade 3–5 diarrhea (1.6% vs. 0% [Study 2]) were higher in patients receiving Herceptin and chemotherapy compared with chemotherapy alone.

Glomerulopathy

In the postmarketing setting, rare cases of nephrotic syndrome with pathologic evidence of glomerulopathy have been reported. The time to onset ranged from 4 months to approximately 18 months from initiation of Herceptin therapy. Pathologic findings included membranous glomerulonephritis, focal glomerulosclerosis, and fibrillary glomerulonephritis. Complications included volume overload and congestive heart failure.

Immunogenicity

Among 903 women with metastatic breast cancer, human anti-human antibody (HAHA) to Trastuzumab was detected in one patient using an enzyme-linked immunosorbent assay (ELISA). This patient did not experience an allergic reaction. Samples for assessment of HAHA were not collected in studies of adjuvant breast cancer.

The data reflect the percentage of patients whose test results were considered positive for antibodies to Herceptin in ELISA assay, and are highly dependent on the sensitivity and specificity of the assay. Additionally, the observed incidence of antibody positivity in an assay may be influenced by several factors including sample handling, timing of sample collection, concomitant medications, and underlying disease. For these reasons, comparison of the incidence of antibodies to Herceptin with the incidence of antibodies to other products may be misleading.

Adjuvant Breast Cancer

Safety data for Herceptin in the adjuvant breast cancer setting are based on two randomized, controlled clinical trials [Study 1 and Study 2] in which 1635 women received at least one dose of Herceptin in combination with paclitaxel adjuvant therapy for breast cancer and 1571 women in the control arms who received at least one dose of paclitaxel chemotherapy and for whom any follow-up safety data were recorded.

Because the initial treatment was similar in both study arms (4 cycles of AC chemotherapy), comparisons of adverse events are limited to the post-AC period. Data collection was limited in both studies.

The data in Table 8 were obtained from 1772 patients enrolled in Study 1. Among these patients, the median age was 49 years (range 22 to 78 years); 83% of patients were White, 8% were Black, 4% were Hispanic, and 4% were Asian/Pacific Islander. The data in Study 2 were obtained from 1434 patients enrolled, of which 732 received Herceptin. The median age was 49 years (range 24 to 80 years); 86% of patients were White, 6% were Black, 3% were Hispanic, and 4% were Asian/Pacific Islander. Herceptin was administered at a loading dose of 4 mg/kg followed by 2 mg/kg weekly, for a maximum of 52 weeks.

Table 8

Study 1: Selected Non-Cardiac Adverse Events with Higher Incidence (≥2%) in the Herceptin + Chemotherapy Arm*

NCI-CTC (v.2.0) Toxicity Term	AC→Paclitaxel + Herceptin (n=903)		AC→Paclitaxel (n=869)	
	Grade 2–5	Gr. 3–5	Grade 2–5	Gr. 3–5
Arthralgia	31%	6%	28%	6%
Fatigue	28%	2%	22%	3%
Infection	22%	6%	14%	4%
Hot Flashes	17%	0%	15%	0.2%
Anemia	13%	1%	7%	1%
Dyspnea	12%	2%	4%	1%
Rash/ desquamation	11%	1%	7%	1%
Neutropenia	7%	4%	5%	3%
Headache	6%	1%	4%	1%
Insomnia	3.7%	0.4%	1.5%	0%

* Only Grade 3–5 adverse events, treatment-related Grade 2 events, and Grade 2–5 dyspnea were collected during and for up to 3 months following protocol-specified treatment.

In Study 2, data collection was limited to the following investigator-attributed treatment-related adverse reactions: NCI-CTC Grade 4 and 5 hematologic toxicities, Grade 3–5 non-hematologic toxicities, selected Grade 2–5 toxicities associated with taxanes (myalgia, arthralgias, nail changes, motor neuropathy, sensory neuropathy) and Grade 1–5 cardiac toxicities occurring during chemotherapy and/or Herceptin treatment. The following non-cardiac adverse reactions of Grade 2–5 toxicities occurred at an incidence of at least 2% greater among patients randomized to Herceptin plus chemotherapy as compared to chemotherapy alone: arthralgia (11% vs. 8.4%), myalgia (10% vs. 8%), nail changes (9% vs. 7%), and dyspnea (2.5% vs. 0.1%). The majority of these events were grade 2 in severity.

Metastatic Breast Cancer

Where specific percentages are noted these data are based on clinical studies of Herceptin alone or in combination with chemotherapy for the treatment of metastatic breast cancer. Data in Table 9 are based on the experience for Herceptin in a randomized controlled trial in which 464 patients were treated with chemotherapy alone (n = 230), Herceptin in combination with chemotherapy (n = 234), and four open-label studies of Herceptin as a single agent which enrolled 352 patients. Data regarding serious adverse events are based on experience in 958 patients (including some with other cancer diagnoses) enrolled in clinical trials of Herceptin conducted prior to marketing.

Among the 464 patients treated in Study 3, the median age was 52 years (range: 25–77 years). Eighty-nine percent were White, 5% Black, 1% Asian and 5% other racial/ethnic groups. All patients received 4 mg/kg initial dose of Herceptin followed by 2 mg/kg weekly. The percentages of patients who received Herceptin treatment for ≥6 months and ≥12 months were 58% and 9%, respectively.

Among the 352 patients treated in single agent studies (213 patients from Study 4), the median age was 50 years (range 28–86 years), 100% had breast cancer, 86% were White, 3% were Black, 3% were Asian, and 8% in other racial/ethnic groups. Most of patients received 4 mg/kg initial dose of Herceptin followed by 2 mg/kg weekly. The percentages of patients who received Herceptin treatment for ≥6 months and ≥12 months were 31% and 16%, respectively.

HERCEPTIN® [Trastuzumab] BRIEF SUMMARY

Table 9

Per-Patient Incidence of Adverse Events Occurring in ≥5% of Patients in Uncontrolled Studies or at Increased Incidence in the Herceptin Arm (Study 3)
(Percent of Patients)

	Single Agent n = 352	Herceptin + Paclitaxel n = 91	Paclitaxel Alone n = 95	Herceptin + AC n = 143	AC Alone n = 135
Body as a Whole					
Pain	47	61	62	57	42
Asthenia	42	62	57	54	55
Fever	36	49	23	56	34
Chills	32	41	4	35	11
Headache	26	36	28	44	31
Abdominal pain	22	34	22	23	18
Back pain	22	34	30	27	15
Infection	20	47	27	47	31
Flu syndrome	10	12	5	12	6
Accidental injury	6	13	3	9	4
Allergic reaction	3	8	2	4	2
Cardiovascular					
Tachycardia	5	12	4	10	5
Congestive heart failure	7	11	1	28	7
Digestive					
Nausea	33	51	9	76	77
Diarrhea	25	45	29	45	26
Vomiting	23	37	28	53	49
Nausea and vomiting	8	14	11	18	9
Anorexia	14	24	16	31	26
Heme & Lymphatic					
Anemia	4	14	9	36	26
Leukopenia	3	24	17	52	34
Metabolic					
Peripheral edema	10	22	20	20	17
Edema	8	10	8	11	5
Musculoskeletal					
Bone pain	7	24	18	7	7
Arthralgia	6	37	21	8	9
Nervous					
Insomnia	14	25	13	29	15
Dizziness	13	22	24	24	18
Paresthesia	9	48	39	17	11
Depression	6	12	13	20	12
Peripheral neuritis	2	23	16	2	2
Neuropathy	1	13	5	4	4
Respiratory					
Cough increased	26	41	22	43	29
Dyspnea	22	27	26	42	25
Rhinitis	14	22	5	22	16
Pharyngitis	12	22	14	30	18
Sinusitis	9	21	7	13	6
Skin					
Rash	18	38	18	27	17
Herpes simplex	2	12	3	7	9
Acne	2	11	3	3	<1
Urogenital					
Urinary tract infection	5	18	14	13	7

OVERDOSAGE

There is no experience with overdosage in human clinical trials. Single doses higher than 500 mg have not been tested.

HOW SUPPLIED

Herceptin (Trastuzumab) is supplied as a lyophilized, sterile powder nominally containing 440 mg Trastuzumab per vial under vacuum.

Each carton contains one vial of 440 mg Herceptin® (Trastuzumab) and one vial containing 20 mL of Bacteriostatic Water for Injection, USP, 1.1% benzyl alcohol. NDC 50242-134-68.

REFERENCE

1. Lee KS, Simon H, Chen H, Bates B, Hung MC, Hauser C. Requirement for neuroregulin receptor, erbB2, in neural and cardiac development. *Nature* 1995;378:394–396.

Herceptin®
[Trastuzumab]

Genentech
BIONCOLOGY

Manufactured by:
Genentech, Inc.
1 DNA Way
South San Francisco, CA 94080-4990

4839800
Initial US Approval September 1998
Revision Date November, 2006

CHAPTER 16

Colon, rectal, and anal cancers

Joshua D. I. Ellenhorn, MD, Carey A. Cullinane, MD,
Lawrence R. Coia, MD, and Steven R. Alberts, MD

COLORECTAL CANCER

Despite the existence of excellent screening and preventive strategies, colorectal carcinoma (CRC) remains a major public health problem in Western countries. The American Cancer Society (ACS) estimated that in 2006, 148,610 people were diagnosed with CRC, and 55,170 died of the disease. CRC is the third most common type of cancer in both sexes (after prostate and lung cancers in men and lung and breast cancers in women) and the second most common cause of cancer death in the United States.

About 72% of new CRCs arise in the colon, and the remaining 28% arise in the rectum. Rectal cancer is defined as cancer arising below the peritoneal reflection, up to approximately 12–15 cm from the anal verge.

The lifetime risk of being diagnosed with CRC in the United States is estimated to be 5.9% for men and 5.5% for women. Despite these daunting statistics, the incidence rates of CRC have been declining in both men and women since 1998, likely reflecting early detection efforts with removal of precancerous polyps.

Epidemiology

Gender Overall the incidence of CRC and mortality rates are higher in men than in women; tumors of the colon are slightly more frequent in women than in men (1.2:1), whereas rectal carcinomas are more common in men than in women (1.7:1).

Age The vast majority, 91%, of all new CRC cases occur in individuals older than age 50. In the United States, the median age at presentation is 72 years.

Race The incidence and mortality rates of CRC are highest among African-American men and women compared with white men and women (15% higher and 40% higher, respectively). The incidence rates among Asian Americans, Hispanics/Latinos, and American Indians/Alaskan natives are lower than those among whites.

Geography The incidence of CRC is higher in industrialized regions (the United States, Canada, the Scandinavian countries, northern and western Europe, New

TABLE 1: Five-year relative survival rates in colorectal cancer[a] by stage at diagnosis (1995–2000)

Time of detection	5-year survival rate (%)
All stages	
In early, localized stage	64
After spread to adjacent organs or lymph nodes	67
After spread to distant sites	10
Unstaged	35

[a] Source: Cancer Facts & Figures—2005. Atlanta: American Cancer Society; 2005. Surveillance, Epidemiology, and End Results (SEER) Program.

Zealand, Australia) and lower in Asia, Africa (among blacks), and South America (except Argentina and Uruguay).

Survival Five-year survival rates (Table 1) for patients with CRC have improved in recent years. This fact may be due to wider surgical resections, modern anesthetic techniques, and improved supportive care. In addition, better pathologic examination of resected specimens, preoperative staging, and abdominal exploration reveal clinically occult disease and allow treatment to be delivered more accurately. Survival also has improved through the use of adjuvant chemotherapy for colon cancer and adjuvant chemoradiation therapy for rectal cancer.

Etiology and risk factors

The specific causes of CRC are unknown, but environmental, nutritional, genetic, and familial factors, as well as preexisting diseases, have been found to be associated with this cancer. A summary of selected risk factors for CRC is shown in Table 2.

Environment Asians, Africans, and South Americans who emigrate from low-risk areas assume the colon cancer risk for their adopted country, suggesting the importance of environmental factors in CRC. Smoking and alcohol intake (four or more drinks per week) increase the risk of CRC.

Diet Diets rich in fat and cholesterol have been linked to an increased risk of colorectal tumors. Dietary fat causes endogenous production of secondary bile acids and neutral steroids and increases bacterial degradation and excretion of these acids and steroids, thereby promoting colonic carcinogenesis. Historically, diets rich in cereal fiber or bran and yellow and green vegetables are said to have protective effects, although recent studies have failed to prove a risk reduction with increasing dietary fiber intake. A protective role also has been ascribed to calcium salts and calcium-rich foods, because they decrease colon-cell turnover and reduce the cancer-promoting effects of bile acid and fatty acids.

TABLE 2: Selected risk factors for colorectal cancer

Risk factor	Relative risk
Family and medical histories	
Family history (first-degree relative)	1.8
Inflammatory bowel disease (diagnosed ≥ 10 years)	1.5
Modifiable factors that increase risk	
Obesity (body mass index ≥ 30)	1.5–2.0
Red meat (≥ 7 servings/week vs 1 serving/month)	1.5
Cigarette use (current vs never)	1.5
Alcohol (≥ 4 drinks/week vs none)	1.4
Modifiable factors that decrease risk	
Physical activity (more than 3 hours/week vs none)	0.6
Vegetable and fruit consumption (≥ 5 vs < 3 servings/day)	0.7

Source: Colorectal Cancer Facts & Figures–2005. Atlanta: American Cancer Society; 2005.

Physical activity Several studies have reported a lower risk of CRC in individuals who participate in regular physical activity. High levels of physical activity may decrease the risk by as much as 50%. Being overweight or obese has been consistently associated with a higher risk of CRC.

Inflammatory bowel disease Patients with inflammatory bowel disease (ulcerative colitis, Crohn's disease) have a higher incidence of CRC. The risk of CRC in patients with ulcerative colitis is associated with the duration of active disease, extent of colitis, development of mucosal dysplasia, and duration of symptoms.

The risk of CRC increases exponentially with the duration of colitis, from approximately 3% in the first decade to 20% in the second decade to > 30% in the third decade. CRC risk also is increased in patients with Crohn's disease, although to a lesser extent.

Adenomatous polyps Colorectal tumors develop more often in patients with adenomatous polyps than in those without polyps. There is approximately a 5% probability that carcinoma will be present in an adenoma; the risk correlates with the histology and size of the polyp. The potential for malignant transformation is higher for villous and tubulovillous adenomas than for tubular adenomas. Adenomatous polyps < 1 cm have a slightly greater than 1% chance of being malignant, in comparison with adenomas > 2 cm, which have up to a 40% likelihood of malignant transformation.

Cancer history Patients with a history of CRC are at increased risk of a second primary colon cancer or other malignancy. The risk of a second CRC is higher if the first diagnosis was made prior to age 60.

Prior surgery Following ureterosigmoidostomy, an increased incidence of colon cancer at or near the suture line has been reported. Cholecystectomy also has

A study designed to determine the usefulness of immunohistochemical analysis for the diagnosis of mismatch repair (MMR) gene defective colorectal tumors in 172 cases of colorectal cancer detected microsatellite instability (MSI) in 13 (1.6%) tumors. All showed loss of protein expression of hMLH1 (11 of 13) or hMSH2 (2 of 13; $P <$ .000). Patients with MMR-defective tumors more frequently had poorly differentiated tumors (5 of 13 [38%] vs 18 of 159 [11%]; $P = .02$) located in the ascending colon (8 of 13 [62%] vs 30 of 159 [19%]; $P = .0001$) and a personal history of other neoplasms (4 of 13 [31%] vs 18 of 159 [11%]; $P =$ .05). There were no differences in age, family history of cancer, or TNM stage (*Jover R, Paya A, Alenda C, et al: Am J Clin Pathol 122:389-394,2004*).

been associated with colon cancer in some studies but not in others.

Family history and genetic factors Individuals with a first-degree relative with the disease have an increased risk of developing CRC. Those with two or more relatives with the disease make up about 20% of all people with CRC. The risk of developing CRC is significantly increased in several forms of inherited susceptibility (Table 3). About 5%–10% of all patients with CRC have an inherited susceptibility to the disease. The risks of developing CRC in the subgroups of familial or hereditary CRC vary from 15% in relatives of patients with CRC diagnosed before 45 years of age, through 20% for family members with two first-degree relatives with CRC, to approximately 70%–95% in patients with familial adenomatous polyposis and hereditary nonpolyposis CRC (HNPCC).

Familial adenomatous polyposis (FAP) is inherited as an autosomal-dominant trait with variable penetrance. Patients characteristically develop pancolonic and rectal adenomatous polyps. Approximately 50% of patients with FAP will develop adenomas by 15 years of age and 95% by age 35. Left untreated, 100% of patients with FAP will develop CRC, with an average age at diagnosis ranging from 34 to 43 years. Total colectomy, usually performed on patients in their mid-to-late teens, is the preventive treatment of choice in this group of patients. The familial adenomatous polyposis coli *(APC)* gene has been localized to chromosome 5q21. Currently, it is possible to detect mutations in the *APC* gene in up to 82% of families with FAP. Mutations in the *APC* gene combined with mutational activation of proto-oncogenes, especially K-*ras*, occur sequentially in the neoplastic transformation of bowel epithelium in patients with FAP. Use of cyclo-oxygenase-2 (COX-2) inhibitors such as celecoxib (Celebrex) has been shown to reduce the number of polyps in patients with FAP.

HNPCC is transmitted as an autosomal-dominant trait. It is associated with germline mutations in one of five DNA mismatch repair genes (*MSH2, MLH1, PMS1, PMS2,* and *MSH6)*. The incidence of a mutated mismatch repair gene is approximately 1 in 1,000 people. The Amsterdam criteria were proposed in 1991 as a way to help identify patients at risk of HNPCC. In 1999, they were revised (Amsterdam II) to recognize extracolonic manifestations as part of the family history. The criteria include the following factors:

- three or more relatives with a histologically verified HNPCC-associated cancer (colorectal, endometrial, small bowel, ureter, or renal pelvis), one of whom is a first-degree relative of the other two (FAP should be excluded)

TABLE 3: Hereditary polyposis syndromes

Adenomatous polyposis

Familial adenomatous polyposis (FAP)

Characterized by hundreds or thousands of sessile or pedunculated polyps throughout the large intestine; histologic examination reveals microscopic adenomas; average age at onset of polyps, 25 years; at onset of symptoms, 33 years; at diagnosis, 36 years; at diagnosis of colon cancer, 42 years; extracolonic features include mandibular osteomas, upper GI polyps, and congenital hypertrophy of the retinal pigment epithelium.

An attenuated form of FAP that is clinically characterized by the presence of tens or hundreds of polyps exists

Gardner's syndrome

Same colonic manifestations as FAP; extracolonic features more evident and varied, including osteomas of the skull, mandible, and long bones; desmoid tumors; dental abnormalities; neoplasms of the thyroid, adrenal glands, biliary tree, and liver; upper GI polyps; and congenital hypertrophy of the retinal pigment epithelium; fibromatosis of the mesentery is a potentially fatal complication (occurring in 8%–13% of patients)

Turcot's syndrome

This rare syndrome is characterized by malignant colon and brain tumors. Two different types of Turcot's have been identified: one characterized by an adenomatous polyposis coli (APC) mutation resulting in colon cancer and malignant glioblastoma; the second characterized by a mismatch repair gene mutation resulting in colon cancer and astrocytoma

Hamartomatous polyposis

Peutz-Jeghers syndrome

In infancy and childhood, melanin deposits manifest as greenish-black to brown mucocutaneous pigmentation (which may fade at puberty) around the nose, lips, buccal mucosa, hands, and feet; polyps (most frequent in the small intestines; also found in the stomach and colon) are unique hamartomas with branching bands of smooth muscle surrounded by glandular epithelium; may produce acute and chronic GI bleeding, intestinal obstruction, or intussusception; 50% of patients develop cancer (median age at diagnosis, 50 years); ovarian cysts and unique ovarian sex-cord tumors reported (5%–12% of female patients)

Juvenile polyposis

Three forms: familial juvenile polyposis coli (polyps limited to the colon), familial juvenile polyposis of the stomach, and generalized juvenile polyposis (polyps distributed throughout the GI tract); polyps are hamartomas covered by normal glandular epithelium, found mostly in the rectum in children and sometimes in adults; may produce GI bleeding, obstruction, or intussusception; mixed juvenile/adenomatous polyps or synchronous adenomatous polyps may lead to cancer, but gastric cancer has not been reported in patients with familial juvenile polyposis of the stomach

Cowden's disease (multiple hamartoma syndrome)

Multiple hamartomatous tumors of ectodermal, mesodermal, and endodermal origin; mucocutaneous lesions are prominent and distinctive; also reported: breast lesions ranging from fibrocystic disease to cancer (50% of patients), thyroid abnormalities (10%–15%), cutaneous lipomas, ovarian cysts, uterine leiomyomas, skeletal and developmental anomalies, and GI polyps; no associated risk of cancer in GI polyps; probably does not warrant clinical surveillance

Poynter and colleagues investigated the association between HMG-CoA reductase inhibitors (statins) and colorectal cancer in a population-based case-controlled study of incident colorectal cancer. In analyses including 1,953 patients with colorectal cancer and 2,015 controls, the use of statins for at least 5 years was associated with a significantly reduced relative risk of colorectal cancer. The use of statins was associated with a 50% reduction in colorectal cancer risk (*Poynter JN, Gruber SB, Higgins PDR, et al: N Engl J Med 352:2184-2192, 2005*).

- CRC involving at least two generations.
- one or more CRC diagnosed before the age of 50.

The Bethesda criteria were developed based upon an analysis of high-risk patients who did not meet the Amsterdam criteria but still demonstrated germline mutations in either the *MSH2* or *MLH1* gene. These criteria are much less restrictive than the Amsterdam criteria and serve to help identify those individual patients at risk of HNPCC who might benefit from further evaluation. They include the following:

- individuals with cancer in families who meet the Amsterdam criteria
- individuals with two HNPCC-related cancers, including synchronous and metachronous CRCs or associated extracolonic cancers; endometrial, ovarian, gastric, hepatobiliary, small bowel, or transitional cell carcinoma of the renal pelvis or ureter
- individuals with CRC and a first-degree relative with CRC and/or HNPCC-related extracolonic cancer and/or a colorectal adenoma; one of the cancers diagnosed at age younger than 45 years; and the adenoma diagnosed at age younger than 40 years
- individuals with CRC or endometrial cancer diagnosed at age < 45 years
- individuals with right-sided CRC with an undifferentiated pattern (solid/cribriform) on histology diagnosed at age < 45 years
- individuals with signet ring-cell–type CRC diagnosed at age < 45 years
- individuals with colorectal adenomas diagnosed at age < 40 years.

Mutations in the DNA mismatch repair genes *MLH1* or *MSH2* can be found in approximately 40% of individuals who meet these criteria. Genetic evaluation for HNPCC should be considered in families that meet the Amsterdam criteria, in affected individuals who meet the Bethesda criteria, and in first-degree relatives of those individuals with known mutations. For situations in which HNPCC is suspected but the first three Bethesda criteria are not met, microsatellite instability (MSI) testing may be considered. Over 90% of HNPCCs will demonstrate MSI, compared with 15%–20% of sporadic CRC, and thus a normal result in the absence of compelling clinical criteria usually excludes the diagnosis of HNPCC. Alternatively, *MSH6* may be involved in a substantial proportion of patients in whom HNPCC is suspected and should be considered in those with tumors that are low in MSI.

TABLE 4: American Cancer Society guidelines on screening and surveillance for the early detection of colorectal adenomas and cancer—Average risk

Test	Interval (beginning at age 50)	Comment
FOBT or FIT and flexible sigmoidoscopy	FOBT annually and flexible sigmoidoscopy every 5 years	Flexible sigmoidoscopy together with FOBT is preferred over FOBT or flexible sigmoidoscopy alone. All positive test results should be followed up with colonoscopy.[a]
Flexible sigmoidoscopy	Every 5 years	All positive test results should be followed up with colonoscopy.[a]
FOBT	Annually	The recommended take-home multiple sample method should be used. All positive test results should be followed up with colonoscopy.[a,b]
Colonoscopy	Every 10 years	Colonoscopy provides an opportunity to visualize, sample, and/or remove significant lesions.
Double-contrast barium enema	Every 5 years	All positive test results should be followed up with colonoscopy.

[a] If colonoscopy is unavailable, not feasible, or not desired by the patient, double-contrast barium enema (DCBE) alone or the combination of flexible sigmoidoscopy and DCBE is an acceptable alternative. Adding flexible sigmoidoscopy to DCBE may provide a more comprehensive diagnostic evaluation than DCBE alone in finding significant lesions. A supplementary DCBE may be needed if a colonoscopic exam fails to reach the cecum, and a supplementary colonoscopy may be needed if a DCBE identifies a possible lesion or does not adequately visualize the entire colorectum.

[b] There is no justification for repeating FOBT in response to an initial positive finding.

FOBT = fecal occult blood test; FIT = fecal immunochemical test

Adapted with permission from Smith RA, von Eschenbach AC, Wender R, et al: CA Cancer J Clin 53:27–43, 2003.

Chemoprevention

Chemoprevention aims to block the action of carcinogens on cells before the development of cancer.

Antioxidants and calcium Controlled trials of vitamins C and E and calcium have produced mixed results. Clinical trials have shown that calcium supplementation modestly decreases the risk of colorectal adenomas.

Nonsteroidal anti-inflammatory drugs inhibit colorectal carcinogenesis, possibly by reducing endogenous prostaglandin production through COX inhibition. Sulindac (Clinoril) has induced regression of large bowel polyps in patients with FAP. Controlled studies have shown a reduction in the incidence of colorectal polyps with regular, long-term use of aspirin.

TABLE 5: American Cancer Society guidelines on screening and surveillance for the early detection of colorectal adenomas and cancer—Increased or high risk

Risk category	Age to begin	Practice
Increased risk		
A single, small (< 1 cm) adenoma	3-6 years after initial polypectomy	Colonoscopy[a]
If the exam is normal, the patient can thereafter be screened as per average-risk guidelines.		
A large (> 1 cm) adenoma, multiple adenomas, or adenomas with high-grade dysplasia or villous change	Within 3 years after the initial polypectomy	Colonoscopy[a]
If the exam is normal, repeat examination in 3 years; if the exam is normal then, the patient can thereafter be screened as per average-risk guidelines.		
Personal history of curative-intent resection of colorectal cancer	Within 1 year after cancer resection	Colonoscopy[a]
If the exam is normal, repeat examination in 3 years; if the exam is normal then, repeat examination every 5 years.		
Either colorectal cancer or adenomatous polyps in any first-degree relative before age 60 or in two or more first-degree relatives at any age (if not a hereditary syndrome)	Age 40, or 5-10 years before the youngest case in the immediate family	Colonoscopy[a]
Every 5-10 years. Colorectal cancer in relatives more distant than first-degree relatives does not increase risk substantially above the average-risk group.		
High risk		
Family history of familial adenomatous polyposis (FAP)	12 years	Early surveillance with endoscopy and counseling to consider genetic testing
If the genetic test result is positive, colectomy may be indicated. These patients are best referred to a center with experience in the management of FAP.		
Family history of hereditary nonpolyposis colorectal cancer (HNPCC)	Age 21	Colonoscopy and counseling to consider genetic testing
If the genetic test result is positive or the patient has not undergone genetic testing, every 1-2 years until age 40, then annually. These patients are best referred to a center with experience in the management of HNPCC.		
Inflammatory bowel disease, chronic ulcerative colitis, Crohn's disease	Cancer risk begins to be significant 8 years after the onset of pancolitis or 12-15 years after the onset of left-sided colitis	Colonoscopy with biopsies for dysplasia
Every 1-2 years. These patients are best referred to a center with experience in the surveillance and management of inflammatory bowel disease.		

[a] If colonoscopy is unavailable, not feasible, or not desired by the patient, double-contrast barium enema (DCBE) alone or the combination of flexible sigmoidoscopy and DCBE is an acceptable alternative. Adding flexible sigmoidoscopy to DCBE may provide a more comprehensive diagnostic evaluation than DCBE alone in finding significant lesions. A supplementary DCBE may be needed if a colonoscopic exam fails to reach the cecum, and a supplementary colonoscopy may be needed if a DCBE identifies a possible lesion or does not adequately visualize the entire colorectum.

Adapted with permission from Smith RA, von Eschenbach AC, Wender R, et al: CA Cancer J Clin 53:27–43, 2003.

Postmenopausal hormones Women who use postmenopausal hormones appear to have a lower rate of CRC than do those who do not.

Signs and symptoms

Early stage During the early stages of CRC, patients may be asymptomatic or complain of vague abdominal pain and flatulence, which may be attributed to gallbladder or peptic ulcer disease. Minor changes in bowel movements, with or without rectal bleeding, are also seen; they are frequently ignored and/or attributed to hemorrhoids or other benign disorders.

Left side of the colon Cancers occurring in the left side of the colon generally cause constipation alternating with diarrhea; abdominal pain; and obstructive symptoms, such as nausea and vomiting.

Right side of the colon Right-sided colon lesions produce vague, abdominal aching, unlike the colicky pain seen with obstructive left-sided lesions. Anemia resulting from chronic blood loss, weakness, weight loss, and/or an abdominal mass may also accompany carcinoma of the right side of the colon.

Rectum Patients with cancer of the rectum may present with a change in bowel movements; rectal fullness, urgency, or bleeding; and tenesmus.

Pelvic pain is seen at later stages of the disease and usually indicates local extension of the tumor to the pelvic nerves.

Screening and diagnosis

Screening

Fecal occult blood testing (FOBT) or fecal immunochemical test (FIT) guaiac-based fecal occult blood tests are, in themselves, inexpensive but have been associated with many false-positive and false-negative results. Almost all colonic polyps and > 50% of all CRCs go undetected because they are not bleeding at the time of the test. The newer FOBTs, including a guaiac-based product called Hemoccult SENSA and immunochemical tests for hemoglobin (HemeSelect), appear to have better sensitivity than the older tests without sacrificing specificity.

Three large randomized controlled clinical trials have demonstrated decreased CRC mortality associated with detection of earlier-stage cancer and adenomas by FOBT. Recently, results from a large trial also showed a decreased incidence of CRC associated with FOBT, largely because of increased use of polypectomy resulting from diagnostic endoscopy following positive tests.

Digital rectal examination is simple to perform and can detect lesions up to 7 cm from the anal verge.

Sigmoidoscopy Flexible proctosigmoidoscopy is safe and more comfortable than examination using a rigid proctoscope. Almost 50% of all colorectal neoplasms are within the reach of a 60-cm sigmoidoscope. Even though flexible sigmoidoscopy visualizes only the distal portion of the colorectum, the identification of adenomas can lead to colonoscopy. When we add the percentage of colorectal neoplasms in the distal 60 cm of the colorectum to the percentage of patients with distal polyps leading to complete colonoscopy, 80% of those individuals with a significant neoplasm anywhere in the colorectum can be identified.

Colonoscopy (optical) provides information on the mucosa of the entire colon, and its sensitivity in detecting tumors is extremely high. Most physicians consider colonoscopy to be the best screening modality for CRC. Colonoscopy can be used to obtain biopsy specimens of adenomas and carcinomas and permits the excision of adenomatous polyps. For this reason, colonoscopy is the only screening modality ever shown to reduce the incidence of cancer in screened individuals. Colonoscopy is the best follow-up strategy for evaluating patients with positive guaiac-based FOBTs and the best screening modality for high-risk patients.

Limitations of colonoscopy include its inability to detect some polyps and small lesions because of blind corners and mucosal folds and the fact that sometimes the cecum cannot be reached. A supplementary double-contrast barium enema may be needed if a colonoscopic exam fails to reach the cecum.

Colonoscopy (CT virtual) Some recent studies have suggested that CT virtual colonoscopy may have sensitivity and specificity for detecting neoplastic polyps that approach those of optical colonoscopy. Unfortunately, other studies have demonstrated clear superiority of optical colonoscopy. Until additional confirmatory studies are available, virtual CT colonoscopy should not replace routine optical colonoscopic screening.

Barium enemas can accurately detect CRC; however, the false-negative rate associated with double-contrast barium enemas ranges from 2% to 61% because of misinterpretation, poor preparation, and difficulties in detecting smaller lesions. A supplementary colonoscopy may be needed if a double-contrast barium enema does not adequately visualize the entire colon or to obtain histopathology or perform polypectomy in the event of abnormal findings.

Recommendations for average-risk individuals Adults at average risk should begin colorectal cancer screening at age 50. The ACS guidelines on screening and surveillance for the early detection of colorectal adenomatous polyps and cancer provide several options for screening average-risk individuals (Table 4).

For those individuals who elect FOBT/FIT alone, or in combination with flexible sigmoidoscopy, a single test of a stool sample in the clinical setting (as, for instance, is often performed with the stool sample collected on the fingertip during a digital rectal examination) is not an adequate substitute for a full set of samples using the take-home card system. Because combining flexible sigmoidoscopy with FOBT/FIT can substantially increase the benefits of either test alone, the ACS regards annual FOBT/FIT accompanied by flexible sigmoidoscopy every 5 years as a better choice than either FOBT/FIT or flexible sigmoidoscopy alone.

The choice of colonoscopy or double-contrast barium enema for screening may depend on factors such as personal preference, cost, and the local availability of trained clinicians to perform a high-quality examination. For those who elect either colonoscopy or double-contrast barium enema for screening, there is no need for annual FOBT/FIT. Digital rectal examination should be performed at the time of the sigmoidoscopy or colonoscopy.

Recommendations for screening increased-risk and high-risk individuals
Risk of CRC is even higher among individuals with hereditary syndromes or a history of inflammatory bowel disease of significant duration.

Those individuals who have been diagnosed as having adenomatous polyps or a personal history of curative-intent resection of CRC should undergo a colonoscopy to remove all polyps from the colorectum, after which a colonoscopic exam should be repeated at an interval to be determined on the basis of the size, multiplicity, and histologic appearance of the adenoma(s) (Table 5). If colonoscopy is not available, or not feasible, flexible sigmoidoscopy followed by double-contrast barium enema may be used for surveillance.

A family history of either CRC or colorectal adenomas increases the risk of developing CRC. Risk is higher for individuals with a family history involving first-degree relatives, those family members with younger age of onset, and those with multiple affected family members. Individuals with a single first-degree relative diagnosed with CRC or an adenomatous polyp after age 60, or with affected relatives who are more distant than first-degree relatives, can be considered to be at "average risk." In general, colonoscopy is recommended 5–10 years prior to the earliest diagnosis in the family or age 40, whichever is earlier. Subsequent colonoscopy should be repeated at intervals to be determined on the basis of the initial examination. If a colonoscopy is not available or feasible, flexible sigmoidoscopy followed by a double-contrast barium enema can be used.

Individuals at elevated risk due to the known or likely presence of FAP or HNPCC should begin surveillance at an early age with endoscopic examination (Table 5). There is ample evidence to support endoscopic surveillance as a method of early detection. A program of biennial colonoscopy starting at age 20 to 25 years is recommended for HNPCC carriers. For those with FAP, it is recommended that regular sigmoidoscopy start at the age of 12 years and continue at 2-year intervals. DNA testing of at-risk individuals provides the opportunity to identify those who should undergo intensive surveillance and those who are at average risk.

Individuals with a history of extensive inflammatory bowel disease affecting the colon should begin colonoscopic surveillance with biopsy for dysplasia every 1–2 years after 8 years of symptoms. Prophylactic colectomy should be considered in the presence of persistent dysplasia.

TABLE 6: TNM staging of colorectal cancer

TNM stage	Primary tumor[a]	Lymph node metastasis[b]	Distant metastasis[c]	Modified Astler-Coller
Stage 0	Tis	N0	M0	–
Stage I	T1	N0	M0	A
	T2	N0	M0	B1
Stage IIA	T3	N0	M0	B2
IIB	T4	N0	M0	B3
Stage IIIA	T1-2	N1	M0	C1[d]
IIIB	T3-4	N1	M0	C2-3[d]
IIIC	Any T	N2	M0	C1-3[d]
Stage IV	Any T	Any N	M1	D

[a] Tis = carcinoma in situ; T1 = tumor invades submucosa; T2 = tumor invades muscularis propria; T3 = tumor invades through the muscularis propria into the subserosa or into nonperitoneal pericolic or perirectal tissues; T4 = tumor perforates the visceral peritoneum or directly invades other organs or structures

[b] N0 = no regional lymph node metastasis; N1 = metastases in one to three pericolic or perirectal lymph nodes; N2 = metastases in four or more pericolic or perirectal lymph nodes

[c] M0 = no distant metastasis; M1 = distant metastasis

[d] C1 = T2 N1, T2 N2 C2 = T3 N1, T3 N2 C3 = T4 N1, T4 N2

From Greene FL, Page DL, Fleming ID, et al (eds): AJCC Cancer Staging Manual, 6th Ed. New York, Springer-Verlag, 2002.

Diagnosis

Initial work-up An initial diagnostic work-up for patients suspected of having colorectal tumors should include:

- digital rectal examination and FOBT
- colonoscopy
- biopsy of any detected lesions.

Adequate staging prior to surgical intervention requires:

- chest x-ray
- CT scan of the abdomen and pelvis
- CBC with platelet count
- liver and renal function tests
- urinalysis
- measurement of carcinoembryonic antigen (CEA) level.

FDG-PET scanning FDG ([18]fluorodeoxyglucose)-PET scanning has emerged as a highly sensitive study for the evaluation of patients who may be candidates for resection of isolated metastases from CRC. Although not usually recommended in the evaluation of primary disease, this modality can aid in the staging of recurrence.

Pathology

Adenocarcinomas constitute 90%–95% of all large bowel neoplasms. These tumors consist of cuboidal or columnar epithelium with multiple degrees of differentiation and variable amounts of mucin.

Mucinous adenocarcinoma is a histologic variant characterized by huge amounts of extracellular mucus in the tumor and the tendency to spread within the peritoneum. Approximately 10% of colorectal adenocarcinomas are mucinous. It is more commonly seen in younger patients.

Signet-ring–cell carcinoma is an uncommon variant, comprising 1% of colorectal adenocarcinomas. These tumors contain large quantities of intracellular mucinous elements (causing the cytoplasm to displace the nucleus) and tend to involve the submucosa, making their detection difficult with conventional imaging techniques.

Other tumor types Squamous cell carcinomas, small-cell carcinomas, carcinoid tumors, and adenosquamous and undifferentiated carcinomas also have been found in the colon and rectum. Nonepithelial tumors, such as sarcomas and lymphomas, are exceedingly rare.

Metastatic spread CRC has a tendency toward local invasion by circumferential growth and for lymphatic, hematogenous, transperitoneal, and perineural spread. Longitudinal spread is usually not extensive, with microscopic spread averaging only 1–2 cm from gross disease, but radial spread is common and depends on anatomic location.

The most common site of extralymphatic involvement is the liver, with the lungs the most frequently affected extra-abdominal organ. Other sites of hematogenous spread include the bones, kidneys, adrenal glands, and brain.

Staging and prognosis

The TNM staging classification, which is based on the depth of tumor invasion in the intestinal wall, the number of regional lymph nodes involved, and the presence or absence of distant metastases, has largely replaced the older Dukes' classification scheme (Table 6).

Pathologic stage is the single most important prognostic factor following surgical resection of colorectal tumors. The prognosis for early stages (I and II) is favorable overall, in contrast to the prognosis for advanced stages (III and IV). However, there appears to be a superior survival for patients with stage III disease whose disease is confined to the bowel wall (ie, $\leq$ T2, N+).

Histologic grade may be correlated with survival. Five-year survival rates of 56%–100%, 33%–80%, and 11%–58% have been reported for grades 1, 2, and 3 colorectal tumors, respectively.

Other prognostic factors (such as age at diagnosis, presurgical CEA level, gender, presence and duration of symptoms, site of disease, histologic features, obstruction or perforation, perineural invasion, venous or lymphatic invasion, ploidy status, and S-phase fraction) have not consistently been correlated with overall disease recurrence and survival. Furthermore, the size of the primary lesion has had no influence on survival. Elevated expression of thymidylate synthase and allelic loss of chromosome 18 have been correlated with a poor prognosis.

Treatment

PRIMARY TREATMENT OF LOCALIZED DISEASE

Management of colorectal carcinoma relies primarily on resection of the bowel with the adjacent draining lymph nodes. The need for adjuvant systemic or local chemotherapy or immunotherapy, with or without concurrent irradiation, depends on tumor location (colon vs rectum) and stage of disease.

Surgery

Colon The primary therapy for adenocarcinoma of the colon is surgical extirpation of the bowel segment containing the tumor, the adjacent mesentery, and draining lymph nodes. It is recommended that at least 12 lymph nodes be available for examination by a pathologist to confirm the accuracy of a node-negative diagnosis. Surgical resection can be performed by open or laparoscopic approach. The type of resection depends on the anatomic location of the tumor. Right, left, or transverse colectomy is the surgical treatment of choice in patients with right, left, or transverse colonic tumors, respectively. Tumors in the sigmoid colon may be treated with wide sigmoid resection. The length of colon resected depends largely on the requirement for wide mesenteric nodal clearance.

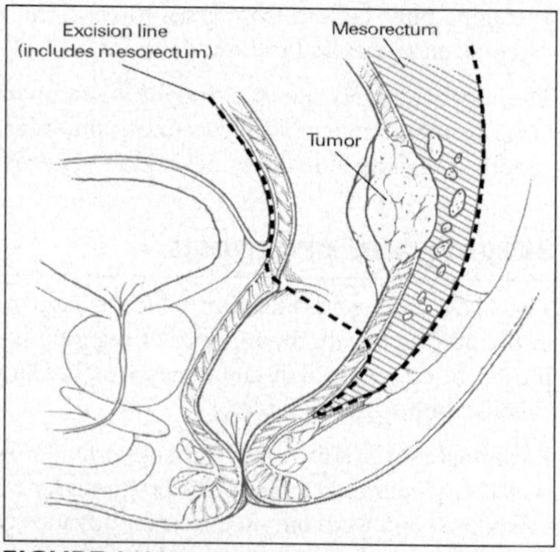

FIGURE 1: Mesorectal excision
Adapted with permission from N Engl J Med 345:690–692, 2001.

Rectum For rectal carcinoma, the distal surgical margin should be at least 2 cm, although some investigators have suggested that a smaller but still negative margin may be adequate.

The resection should include the node-bearing mesorectum surrounding the rectum. This procedure, which is termed total mesorectal excision (TME), is accomplished using a sharp dissection technique (see Figure 1). The use of TME has been associated with a significant reduction in local recurrence rates for patients with rectal cancer.

Posteriorly, the mesorectal dissection is carried out along the presacral fascia. Anteriorly, the dissection follows the posterior vaginal wall in females or Denonvilliers' fascia in males, either of which may be resected in the presence of an anterior wall rectal cancer. Reported rates of local recurrence following TME for rectal cancer have generally been < 10%, compared with rates of recurrence up to 30% prior to the advent of TME. Selective use of radiation therapy can improve upon the results of TME alone.

> A large, single-institution, retrospective review compared the long-term results of transanal excision of T1 rectal cancers in 151 patients with those of radical surgery in 168 patients. At 5 years, the overall occurrence rate for transanal excision was 23% and only 6% for radical surgery. Multivariate analysis revealed that the type of operation performed was the only factor predictive of outcome. Although limited by its retrospective nature, this study suggests that transanal excision may not yield an equivalent outcome to radical surgery in patients with these early rectal cancers (*Bentrem DJ, Okabe S, Wong WD, et al: Ann Surg 242:472-479, 2005*).

Sphincter-sparing approaches Technologies (eg, circular stapling devices) and the application of surgical techniques, such as coloanal anastomosis and creation of intestinal pouches, are employed to maintain anal sphincter function for tumors in the lower one-third of the rectum. If the tumor is located proximally between 6 and 15 cm from the anal verge, a low anterior resection with end-to-end anastomosis may be performed.

Abdominoperineal resection, removing the anus and sphincter muscle with permanent colostomy, may be necessary if the tumor is located in the distal rectum and other characteristics of the tumor (eg, bulky size, proximity to the sphincter musculature) preclude an oncologically adequate sphincter-sparing approach. An alternative procedure for tumors 2–5 cm from the anal verge is to resect the entire rectum, sparing the anoderm and anal sphincter musculature, and to perform a coloanal anastomosis. Either procedure can be performed with autonomic nerve preservation, minimizing bladder and sexual function morbidity.

Local excision alone may be indicated for selected patients who have small (< 3–4 cm), T1, well to moderately differentiated rectal cancers without histologic evidence of lymphovascular involvement, provided that a full-thickness negative margin can be achieved. In most series, transanal excision for these good histology T1 lesions results in excellent long-term control. However, some studies with long-term follow-up demonstrated significant local recurrence rates, even with T1 lesions. For T2 or T3 tumors, the standard therapy remains a transabdominal resection because of the risk of mesorectal nodal spread. Preoperative transrectal ultrasonography is useful in defining lesions that can be resected by local excision alone. A trial sponsored by the CALGB (Cancer and Leukemia Group B) demonstrated reasonable results for patients

Two prospective randomized trials involving laparoscopic colorectal resection have been published. A multicenter group in the United States randomized 872 patients with right, left, or sigmoid colon cancers to receive laparoscopic vs open colectomy. At 3 years of follow-up, there were no differences in recurrence rates or survival *(The Clinical Outcomes of Surgical Therapy Study Group: N Engl J Med 350:2050-2059, 2004)*. A similar study randomized 403 patients with rectosigmoid carcinoma to receive laparoscopic vs open colectomy. At 5 years of follow-up, there were no differences in recurrence rates or survival *(Leung KL, Kwok SP, Lam SC, et al: Lancet 363:1187-1192, 2004)*. Although the operative time for laparoscopy was longer, both studies demonstrated a reduction in postoperative hospitalization and narcotic use.

with T2 rectal cancer undergoing negative margin local excision followed by fluorouracil (5-FU) and external-beam radiation therapy. The locoregional recurrence rate at 6 years was only 14%. Good results with local excision alone following chemoradiotherapy for rectal cancer have been reported. The role of local excision alone in this clinical scenario awaits confirmatory studies.

Laparoscopic colonic resection The use of laparoscopic colonic and rectal resection is becoming an oncologically acceptable method of treating cancers of the colon and rectum. The potential advantages include a shorter hospital stay, reduced postoperative ileus, decreased time away from work, fewer adhesive complications, and a lower risk of hernia formation. The potential disadvantages compared with open transabdominal resection include longer operative time, higher operative costs, and technical considerations related to operative skill.

Patterns of failure

The natural history and patterns of failure following "curative" resection are different for colon and rectal carcinomas. Locoregional failure as the only or major site of recurrence is common in rectal cancer, whereas colon cancer tends to recur in the peritoneum, liver, and other distant sites, with a lower rate of local failure. As a result, local therapy, such as irradiation, may play a significant role in the treatment of rectal tumors but is not used routinely for colon cancers.

ADJUVANT THERAPY FOR COLON CANCER

Compared with 5-FU and leucovorin, capecitabine (Xeloda) provides an equivalent or superior benefit in the adjuvant treatment of resected stage III colon cancer. Patients in the capecitabine arm also experienced fewer severe toxicities, including less stomatitis and neutropenic fever/sepsis *(Cassidy J, Scheithauer W, McKendrick H, et al: Proc Am Soc Clin Oncol [abstract] 23:247S, 2004)*.

Approximately 75% of all patients with colorectal carcinoma will present at a stage when all gross carcinoma can be surgically resected. Nevertheless, despite the high resectability rate, almost half of all patients with colorectal adenocarcinoma die of metastatic disease, primarily because of residual disease that is not apparent at the time of surgery. These individuals are candidates for adjuvant local or systemic therapies.

TABLE 7: Adjuvant chemotherapy regimens for colorectal adenocarcinoma (nonmetastatic)

Drug/combination	Dose and schedule
Adjuvant low-dose leucovorin/fluorouracil	
Leucovorin	20 mg/m^2 IV bolus on days 1-5 immediately before fluorouracil
Fluorouracil	425 mg/m^2/d IV bolus on days 1-5
Repeat cycle at 4 weeks, 8 weeks, and then every 5 weeks for 6 cycles.	
Poon MA, O'Connell MJ, Moertel CG, et al: J Clin Oncol 7:1407–1418, 1989.	
Adjuvant high-dose leucovorin/fluorouracil	
Leucovorin	500 mg/m^2 IV infused over 2 hours every week for 6 weeks
Fluorouracil	500 mg/m^2 IV infused over 1 hour after the start of leucovorin every week for 6 weeks
Repeat cycle every 8 weeks for 6 cycles.	
Wolmark N, Rockette H, Fisher B, et al: J Clin Oncol 11:1879–1887, 1993.	
FLOX	
Fluorouracil	500 mg/m^2 IV bolus weekly for 6 weeks
Leucovorin	500 mg/m^2 IV weekly for 6 weeks each 8-week cycle x 3
Oxaliplatin	85 mg/m^2 IV administered on weeks 1,3, and 5 of each 8-week cycle x 3
Wolmark N, Wieand S, Kuebler JP, et al: J Clin Oncol 23(suppl):246s, 2005. Abstract.	
Capecitabine	
Capecitabine	1,250 mg/m^2 twice daily on days 1–14 every 3 weeks for 24 weeks
Twelves C, Wong A, Nowacki MP, et al: N Engl J Med 352:2696–2704, 2005.	
Oxaliplatin/fluorouracil/leucovorin (FOLFOX4)	
Oxaliplatin	85 mg/m^2 IV piggbyback over 2 hours on day 1only
Leucovorin	200 mg/m^2/d over 2 hours on day 1 given simultaneously with oxaliplatin
Fluorouracil	400 mg/m^2 IV bolus over 2 to 4 minutes
Fluorouracil	600 mg/m^2 continuous infusion over 22 hours on days 1 and 2 every 14 days for 12 cycles
Andre T, Boni C, Mounedji-Boudiaf L, et al: N Engl J Med 350:2343–2351, 2004.	

Systemic chemotherapy

Systemic combined chemotherapy is the principal adjuvant therapy for colon cancer (Table 7). When determining the benefit of adjuvant therapy for stage II disease, several factors should be taken into consideration, including the number of lymph nodes analyzed after surgery, the prognostic features (T4 lesion, perforation, peritumoral lymphovascular invasion, poorly differentiated histol-

> A randomized trial (NSABP C-07) compared a noninfusional 5-FU, oxaliplatin, and leucovorin regimen (FLOX; see Table 7) with that same regimen without oxaliplatin in resected stage II and III colon cancer. FLOX resulted in a statistically significant improvement in 3-year disease-free survival (76.5% vs 71.6%; $P < .004$; *Wolmark H, Wieand HS, Kuebler JP, et al: Proc Am Soc Clin Oncol [abstract] 23:246s, 2005*).

ogy), anticipated life expectancy, and comorbid conditions.

5-FU, synthesized by Heidelberger in 1957, remains an important agent in the treatment of advanced colon carcinoma. 5-FU may be administered as a bolus injection either weekly or daily for 5 days, every 4–5 weeks. With these regimens, response rates have been approximately 10%–15%. The development of permanent venous access devices and portable infusion pumps has permitted the continuous infusion of 5-FU on an outpatient basis. Commonly used continuous infusion regimens of 5-FU are 750–1,000 mg/m²/d for 5 days. Protracted infusions have administered 5-FU at 200–400 mg/m²/d for up to 12 weeks.

The pattern of 5-FU toxicity differs depending on whether it is administered as a bolus or continuous infusion than by other methods. Bolus administration has pronounced myelotoxic effects, whereas the dose-limiting toxic effects of continuous infusion 5-FU are mucositis and diarrhea. Palmar-plantar erythrodysesthesia (hand-foot syndrome) has been reported with protracted infusions.

Overall, the incidence of side effects is significantly lower when 5-FU is delivered by continuous infusion. A meta-analysis of more than 1,200 patients treated with either continuous infusion or bolus regimens of 5-FU demonstrated superior response rates and a small survival advantage for the continuous infusion regimens.

Infusional 5-FU is now an important component of therapy when combined with either irinotecan or oxaliplatin.

Biochemical modulation of 5-FU Interest in the biochemical modulation of 5-FU by leucovorin is based on preclinical studies demonstrating that leucovorin raises the level of N_5,N_{10}-methylenetetrahydrofolate and, thus, forms a stable tertiary complex of thymidylate synthase (TS), the folate coenzyme, and 5-FU (in the form of 5-fluorodeoxyuridine). The use of 5-FU with leucovorin results in higher response rates than 5-FU alone and may prolong survival.

Although there is no agreement as to the optimal dose of leucovorin, two dosing schedules have been approved by the FDA:

- "low-dose" leucovorin regimen, consisting of leucovorin, 20 mg/m²/d, immediately followed by 5-FU, 425 mg/m²/d
- "high-dose" leucovorin regimen, consisting of leucovorin, 200 mg/m²/d, immediately followed by 5-FU, 370 mg/m²/d

With both schedules, leucovorin and 5-FU are administered by rapid IV injections daily for 5 consecutive days. Courses of both schedules are repeated at 4 weeks, 8 weeks, and every 5 weeks thereafter. There is no survival difference between these two regimens.

5-FU plus leucovorin Studies have demonstrated the benefits of 5-FU plus leucovorin (folinic acid) in the adjuvant treatment of colon carcinomas. Acceptable adjuvant regimens of 5-FU plus leucovorin for colon cancer include:

- a "low-dose" leucovorin (Mayo Clinic) regimen, consisting of leucovorin (20 mg/m^2) immediately followed by 5-FU (425 mg/m^2), both given by rapid IV injections daily for 5 consecutive days, with courses repeated every 4 weeks for 6 months
- a "high-dose" weekly leucovorin regimen, consisting of 5-FU (500 mg/m^2) by rapid IV injection given at 1 hour during a 2-hour infusion of leucovorin (500 mg/m^2) weekly for 6 weeks, with courses repeated every 8 weeks for 6 cycles. More recently, completed randomized trials by the National Surgical Adjuvant Breast and Bowel Project (NSABP) have used 3 rather than 6 cycles of therapy

An analysis of survival data from patients with stage II or III disease treated in four consecutive NSABP adjuvant chemotherapy trials showed similar relative reductions in disease recurrence and mortality as well as similar improvements in overall survival in patients with stage II and III disease.

5-FU, oxaliplatin (Eloxatin), and leucovorin (FOLFOX) Oxaliplatin has been approved by the FDA for adjuvant therapy for resected stage III CRC. In a phase III trial for resected stages II and III colon cancer from Europe (MOSAIC), the use of FOLFOX compared with the same infusional regimen without oxaliplatin led to a higher 3-year disease-free survival rate (78% vs 73%) in those receiving FOLFOX.

Monoclonal antibody 17-1A (edrecolomab) A randomized study of 17-1A antibody in patients with stage III colon cancer showed it to be inferior to 5-FU and leucovorin. Its addition to 5-FU and leucovorin did not improve disease-free or overall survival. A trial of the antibody in stage II colon cancer recently completed accrual. No results are yet available from this trial.

Irinotecan (CPT-11, Camptosar) Two phase III trials of FOLFIRI (5-FU/irinotecan/leucovorin) compared with the same infusional regimen without irinotecan in either patients with resected stages II and III colon cancer (PETACC3) or high-risk stage III (ACCORD-2) did not show a benefit to the use of irinotecan in the adjuvant setting. Given the results of these two studies, the use of irinotecan currently is not considered a primary option for patients with resected stage II or III colon cancer.

Capecitabine (Xeloda) is an oral fluorinated pyrimidine recently approved by the FDA for adjuvant therapy for patients with stage III colon cancer who have undergone complete resection of the primary tumor when treatment with fluoropyrimidine therapy alone is preferred. Capecitabine was not inferior to bolus 5-FU and low-dose leucovorin for disease-free survival, with a hazard ratio in the capecitabine group of 0.87 (95% confidence interval: 0.75 to 1.00). Capecitabine is an alternative for patients who are unlikely to tolerate 5-FU, leucovorin, and oxaliplatin.

For patients with stage III (T1-4, N1-2, M0) carcinoma, 6 months of 5-FU/leucovorin and capecitabine or 5-FU/leucovorin and oxaliplatin should be consid-

TABLE 8: Five-year overall survival in Patterns of Care Study (PCS) vs the National Cancer Data Base (NCDB), Gastrointestinal Tumor Study Group (GITSG), and Mayo/North Central Cancer Treatment Group (Mayo/NCCTG) studies

Study	5-year survival	
Bimodality vs trimodality	**S + RT**	**S + RT + CT**
Stage II		
PCS	61%	81%
NCDB	55%	62%
Stage III		
PCS	33%	65%
NCDB	39%	42%
Postop CRT vs postop RT	**Postop RT**	**Postop CRT**
GITSG (7175)	52%	59%
Mayo/NCCTG (7945)	48%	57%
PCS	50%	69%

S = surgery; RT = radiation therapy; CT = chemotherapy; CRT = concurrent radiation therapy and chemotherapy

Adapted from Coia LR, Gunderson LL, Haller D, et al: Cancer 86:1952–1958, 1999.

ered. Patients with stage IV disease who are candidates for surgery should be considered for neoadjuvant chemotherapy (FOLFIRI or FOLFOX with bevacizumab [Avastin]) followed by synchronous or staged colectomy and hepatic resection.

Radiation therapy

Postoperative irradiation to the tumor bed should be considered in patients with T3 node-positive and T4 (B3 or C3) tumors located in retroperitoneal portions of the colon because more than 30% of these patients develop a local recurrence. Retrospective studies suggest improved local control with irradiation, particularly in patients with positive resection margins. If available, intraoperative radiotherapy may be considered for patients with T4 or recurrent cancers as an additional boost.

ADJUVANT THERAPY FOR RECTAL CANCER

Local recurrence alone or in combination with distant metastases occurs in up to 50% of patients with rectal carcinoma. Nodal metastases and deep bowel wall penetration are significant risk factors for locoregional failure.

In the absence of nodal metastases, the rate of local recurrence may be as low as 5%–10% for stage I rectal cancer and 15%–30% for stage II tumors. In stage III disease, the incidence of pelvic failure increases to 50% or more. The use of TME significantly reduces this risk of local recurrence; however, local recurrence remains a concern in patients with stages II and III disease.

Local recurrence in the pelvis is complicated by involvement of contiguous organs, soft and bony tissue, and deep nodal disease. Presenting symptoms vary from vague pelvic fullness to sciatica related to mass effect in the fixed space of the bony pelvis and invasion of the sciatic nerve.

Because local recurrence in the absence of metastatic disease is more common in rectal cancer than in colon cancer, aggressive resections, such as pelvic exenteration (anterior and posterior), sacral resection, and wide soft-tissue and pelvic floor resection, have been employed to treat these recurrences. Modern techniques of pelvic floor reconstruction, creation of continent urinary diversion, and vaginal reconstruction may be required for functional recovery.

The recent findings of the NSABP R-02 trial indicated postoperative adjuvant chemotherapy resulted in similar survival rates to those of postoperative chemoradiation therapy but was associated with a significantly higher rate of locoregional failure.

Pre- or postoperative radiation therapy

Radiation therapy has been used to reduce the locoregional recurrence rate of rectal tumors. Preoperative radiation therapy has been demonstrated to reduce local tumor recurrence, even in patients undergoing TME surgery. However, with the exception of one recent study, preoperative therapy has not affected overall survival in patients with stage II or III rectal cancer. An improvement in local control also has been observed with postoperative irradiation, but again with no benefit with regard to disease-free or overall survival. Preoperative radiation therapy reduced local recurrence rates when combined with total mesorectal resection (8% vs 2%; $P < .001$) in a Dutch phase III trial. In a French study of 762 patients, preoperative chemoradiation therapy compared with preoperative radiotherapy reduced local failure rates in patients with T3–T4 rectal cancers from 16.5% to 8%.

Chemoradiation therapy

Postoperative chemoradiation therapy Clinical trials of surgical adjuvant treatment indicate that postoperative radiation therapy with concurrent chemotherapy (chemoradiation therapy) is superior to postoperative radiation therapy alone or surgery alone. Postoperative chemoradiation therapy is a standard of care for patients with stage II or III rectal cancer based largely on the findings of the North Central Cancer Treatment Group (NCCTG) and Gastrointestinal Tumor Study Group (GITSG) trials. A summary of the 5-year survival results of the Patterns of Care Study (PCS) of the American College of Radiology and the results of the National Cancer Data Base (NCDB), both of which are representative of American national averages, is shown in Table 8.

The most effective combination of drugs, optimal mode of administration, and sequence of irradiation and chemotherapy still need to be determined. Radiation doses of 45–55 Gy are recommended in combination with 5-FU–based chemotherapy. Postoperative bolus 5-FU administration with irradiation is inferior to protracted venous infusion, resulting in lower 3-year rates of both overall survival (68% vs 76%) and disease-free survival (56% vs 67%).

TABLE 9: Chemotherapy for advanced or metastatic disease

Drug/combination	Dose and schedule
Oxaliplatin/fluorouracil/leucovorin (FOLFOX6)	
Leucovorin	400 mg/m^2 IV infused over 2 hours on day 1
Oxaliplatin	85 mg/m^2 IV infused over 2 hours on day 1
Fluorouracil	400 mg/m^2 IV bolus on day 1 then 1,200 mg/m^2/d for 2 days (total 2,400 mg/m^2 over 46-48 hours) continuous infusion
Cycle repeated every 2 weeks.	
Maindrault-Goebel F, Louvet C, Andre T, et al: Eur J Cancer 35:1338–1342, 1999.	
Capecitabine/oxaliplatin (CAPOX)	
Oxaliplatin	130 mg/m^2 IV infused on day 1 only followed by
Capecitabine	1,000 mg/m^2 IV orally twice daily in the evening on day 1 to the morning of day 15
Cycle repeated every 3 weeks.	
Cassidy J, Tabernero J, Twelves C, et al: J Clin Oncol 22:2084-2091, 2004.	
Fluorouracil as an irradiation enhancer—bolus	
Leucovorin	20 mg/m^2 IV bolus on days 1-5, 29-33 immediately before fluorouracil
Fluorouracil	325 mg/m^2/d IV bolus on days 1-5, 29-33
Hyams DM, Mamounas EP, Petrelli N, et al: Dis Colon Rectum 40:131–139, 1997.	
Fluorouracil as an irradiation enhancer—continuous infusion	
Fluorouracil	225 mg/m^2/d IV continuous infusion during irradiation
O'Connell MJ, Martenson JA, Wieand HS, et al: N Engl J Med 331:502–507, 1994.	

An adjuvant treatment combining chemotherapy and pelvic irradiation in patients with stage II or III disease used the following regimen: 5-FU, 500 mg/m^2/d administered as a rapid IV infusion on days 1–5 and 450 mg/m^2/d on days 134–138 and days 169–173. Patients received a protracted IV infusion of 5-FU, 225 mg/m^2/d, by portable ambulatory infusion pump during the entire period of pelvic irradiation. Pelvic radiation therapy began on day 64 with a multiple-field technique to the tumor bed and nodal groups. A total of 4,500 cGy in 180-cGy fractions was administered over a 5-week period. Patients received a minimal boost dose of 540 cGy to the entire tumor bed, adjacent nodes, and 2 cm of adjacent tissue. A second boost dose of 360 cGy was allowed in selected patients with excellent displacement of the small bowel.

Neoadjuvant therapy For rectal cancers approaching the anal sphincter, preoperative (neoadjuvant) irradiation or the combination of chemotherapy and irradiation will significantly reduce the size of the majority of tumors. This approach allows for sphincter-preserving surgery in many patients. In addition, the long-term morbidity of radiation therapy for rectal cancer may be reduced if it is administered prior to surgery. The use of preoperative chemo-

Irinotecan/fluorouracil/leucovorin (FOLFIRI)

Leucovorin	400 mg/m^2 IV infused over 2 hours prior to 5-FU on days 1 and 2
Irinotecan	180 mg/m^2 IV infused over 90 minutes on day 1
Fluorouracil	400 mg/m^2 IV bolus on day 1, then 600 mg/m^2 IV over 22 hours continuous infusion on days 1 and 2

Repeat cycle every 2 weeks.

Andre T, Louvet C, Maindrault-Goebel F, et al: Eur J Cancer 35:1343–1347, 1999.

Fluorouracil and leucovorin plus bevacizumab

Leucovorin	500 mg/m^2 IV infused over 2 hours once a week for 6 weeks, then a 2-week rest period
Fluorouracil	500 mg/m^2 IV bolus slow push 1 hour after leucovorin infusion once a week for 6 weeks, then a 2-week rest period
Bevacizumab	5 mg/kg IV continuous infusion over 90 minutes every 2 weeks

Kabbinavar F, Hurwitz H, Fehrenbacher I, et al: J Clin Oncol 21:60–65, 2003.

therapy and radiation therapy is particularly important for patients presenting with locally advanced, unresectable rectal cancer, as the disease of the majority will be rendered resectable following neoadjuvant therapy. One additional role of neoadjuvant therapy may be in facilitating transanal excision of T2 and T3 rectal cancers in poor surgical risk patients. A number of investigators have reported good results with transanal excision of T2 and T3 tumors following a complete response to neoadjuvant therapy. However, this approach cannot be considered the current standard of care.

Preoperative vs postoperative chemoradiation therapy Preoperative chemoradiation therapy may be preferred to postoperative adjuvant treatment, particularly in patients with T3 or T4 lesions. Such treatment may enhance resectability and may be associated with a lower frequency of complications compared with postoperative treatment. In a report of a randomized trial conducted by the German Rectal Cancer Study, Sauer et al found that compared with postoperative chemoradiotherapy, preoperative chemoradiotherapy significantly decreased local failure (7% vs 11%; $P = .02$) and sphincter preservation in low-lying tumors (39% vs 19%; $P < .004$). In addition, the incidence of chronic anastomotic recurrence was also lowest in the preoperative chemoradiotherapy group (2.7% vs 8.5%; $P = .001$).

TREATMENT OF ADVANCED AND METASTATIC COLON CANCER

Surgery

Local recurrences from colon cancers usually occur at the site of anastomosis, in the resection bed, or in the contiguous and retroperitoneal (para-aortic, paracaval) lymph nodes. Anastomotic recurrences heralded by symptoms are the most curable, followed by local soft-tissue recurrences. Regional and retro-

The OPTIMOX2 trial showed that a chemotherapy-free interval, after 6 cycles of FOLFOX7, led to an 8-week decrease in progression-free survival versus continuing 5-FU and leucovorin during this interval. It is unclear whether this finding impacts overall survival (*Maindrault-Goebel F, Lledo G, Chibaudel B, et al: J Clin Oncol [abstract] 24:147s, 2006*). Research continues on the benefits of "stop-and-go" chemotherapy for metastatic colorectal cancer.

peritoneal lymph node recurrences portend a poor prognosis and systemic disease.

Metastasectomy Metastases to the liver and lungs account for most cases of non-nodal systemic disease in CRC. Resection of metastases, or metastasectomy, has gained recognition as a viable treatment. Resection of liver metastases results in cure rates of 5%–60%, depending on the number of metastases and stage of disease. Resection of solitary metastases in patients with stage I or II disease results in a 5-year survival rate of ~40%.

Adjuvant therapy after resection of hepatic metastases has been assessed in several randomized trials. Intra-arterial administration of floxuridine, using a hepatic artery catheter, alternating with systemic 5-FU and leucovorin, improves overall survival and reduces the risk of recurrence within the liver.

Chemotherapy The development of chemotherapy for advanced CRC has become a very active field (Table 9). After decades of 5-FU–based treatment, and of little clinical gains, the arrival of new, effective agents has significantly changed the way this cancer is treated. Although 5-FU remains the backbone of most regimens, the new agents irinotecan and oxaliplatin are rapidly becoming an important part of front-line treatment of this disease in the United States and abroad. The rapid development of newer agents, such as the molecular-targeted agents, holds the promise that progress will continue in chemotherapy for CRC.

5-FU, leucovorin, and oxaliplatin Oxaliplatin combined with infusional 5-FU and leucovorin was approved by the FDA in 2004 as first-line therapy. Oxaliplatin has demonstrated activity in patients with pretreated, 5-FU–resistant CRC when used alone (10% response rate) or in combination with 5-FU (45% response rate). In patients with untreated metastatic colon cancer, response rates of 27% have been reported with oxaliplatin alone, and rates as high as 57% have been noted when the drug is combined with 5-FU. Patients receiving oxaliplatin, infusional 5-FU, and leucovorin have achieved overall survivals of > 20 months in several reported trials. However, many of these patients have received second- and even third-line therapies at the time of disease progression. Oxaliplatin's toxicity profile includes nausea/vomiting and cumulative, reversible peripheral neuropathy. Patients may also develop a reversible, cold-induced, acute pharyngolaryngeal neuropathy.

A multicenter, randomized phase III study (ASCO 2002, 2003) showed improved outcome with regard to response rate, time to disease progression, and overall survival for patients receiving first-line therapy for metastatic CRC with oxaliplatin, infusional 5-FU, and leucovorin, compared with IFL. At the time of the 2003 presentation, the time to disease progression for the oxaliplatin combination was 8.7 months, compared with 6.9 months for the irinotecan combination. The oxaliplatin regimen also had a significantly better overall survival (19.5 vs 14.8 months) and response rate (45% vs 31%).

The BICC-C trial compared three different ways of giving irinotecan (FOLFIRI, mIFL, CapeIri). Bevacizumab was added in extension to this trial to the FOLFIRI and mIFL arms. FOLFIRI was better tolerated and produced a longer overall survival than did the other regimens. mIFL, with or without bevacizumab, produced significant toxicity and a high 60-day mortality compared with FOLFIRI (*Fuchs C, Marshall J, Mitchell E, et al: J Clin Oncol [abstract] 24:147s, 2006*). mIFL should no longer be considered for use in standard patient care.

Irinotecan has significant clinical activity in patients with metastatic CRC whose disease has recurred or spread after standard chemotherapy. Its FDA approval was based on two phase III trials showing that irinotecan (350 mg/m^2 once every 3 weeks) significantly increased survival, compared with best supportive care and infusional 5-FU, respectively, in patients with recurrent or progressive cancer following first-line 5-FU therapy. Irinotecan increased the median survival by 27% and 41%, respectively, in the two trials.

Irinotecan is active in patients whose disease progressed while receiving 5-FU. Reproducible 15%–20% response rates in this patient population led to the approval of irinotecan for use in patients with 5-FU–refractory disease. The dosage schedules most commonly used are 125 mg/m^2 weekly for 4 weeks, followed by a 2-week rest period (United States), and 350 mg/m^2 every 3 weeks (Europe).

The primary toxicities of irinotecan are diarrhea and neutropenia. Intensive loperamide is important in the management of the former complication. An initial 4-mg loading dose is given at the first sign of diarrhea, followed by 2-mg doses every 2 hours until diarrhea abates for at least a 12-hour period.

5-FU, leucovorin, and irinotecan (FOLFIRI) Several randomized trials have shown improved response rates and overall survival when irinotecan is added to an infusional regimen of 5-FU and leucovorin. However, more severe toxicity (grade 3/4, primarily diarrhea and neutropenia) occurs with the addition of irinotecan. The infusional regimen, however, appears to be better tolerated than a similar bolus regimen (IFL). Although there has not been a direct comparison of these regimens, the bolus regimen may cause severe and life-threatening diarrhea and neutropenia shortly after the initiation of therapy.

In a phase III trial comparing the sequence of FOLFIRI followed by FOLFOX or the reverse sequence for patients with metastatic colorectal cancer, no difference in median survival was seen. Grade 3 or 4 mucositis, nausea, and vomiting occurred more frequently with FOLFIRI, whereas grade 3 or 4 neutropenia and neurosensory toxicity were more frequent with FOLFOX. Response rates were similar between the two groups. However, there did appear to be a higher proportion of patients with liver metastases responding to FOLFOX than FOLFIRI. The results of this clinical trial and others stress the importance of using all available agents in the treatment of metastatic colorectal cancer, and the sequence of their use appears to be less important.

Capecitabine In a phase III trial of previously untreated patients with metastatic colon cancer, capecitabine produced higher response rates than 5-FU and leucovorin. Overall survival and time to disease progression were similar (noninferior) to those with 5-FU and leucovorin. The recommended dose of capecitabine is 2,500 mg/m^2 each day, given as a twice-daily dose, for 14 days followed by a 1-week rest period. The side effects of capecitabine tend to be similar to those seen with prolonged infusion of 5-FU, with hand-foot syndrome being the most common.

Molecular-targeted agents A variety of monoclonal antibodies and small molecules are being evaluated in clinical trials and preclinical studies. Three of these agents (cetuximab [Erbitux], bevacizumab, and panitumumab [Vectibix]) have been FDA approved for use.

Cetuximab is a human/mouse chimeric antibody directed against the epithelial growth factor receptor (EGFR). In a randomized trial of patients with CRC refractory to irinotecan, patients were randomized to receive either cetuximab and irinotecan or cetuximab alone. The addition of cetuximab to irinotecan led to a significantly higher response rate compared with cetuximab alone. The median survival for those receiving cetuximab and irinotecan was also longer. Based on the results of this study, cetuximab has been approved by the FDA for use in patients whose disease is refractory to irinotecan with tumors expressing EGFR.

Bevacizumab is a humanized monoclonal antibody that binds circulating vascular endothelial growth factor (VEGF). When given with either 5-FU and leucovorin or IFL as first-line therapy in patients with metastatic CRC, bevacizumab led to improved outcome. The addition of bevacizumab to 5-FU and leucovorin resulted in significant improvement in disease progression-free survival. Even better results were seen with IFL. The addition of bevacizumab to IFL resulted in significant improvement in overall survival and response rate. These studies led to FDA approval of bevacizumab. It is indicated for use in first-line therapy for metastatic CRC when combined with 5-FU–based chemotherapy, such as FOLFOX.

Panitumumab is a monoclonal antibody that targets the epidermal growth factor receptor (EGFR). In a pivotal phase III trial, 463 patients with metastatic colorectal cancer who had failed previous standard therapy were randomized between panitumumab (6 mg/kg q2wk) plus best supportive care (BSC) vs BSC alone. Patients in the panitumumab arm achieved a significantly improved time to disease progression (96 d vs 60 d, $P = .000000001$) and objective response rate (8% vs 0%). On the basis of the results of this trial, the FDA approved panitumumba for the treatment of patients with colorectal cancer that has metastasized following standard chemotherapy.

Intrahepatic floxuridine administration Renewed interest in regional delivery of floxuridine into the liver has followed the introduction of effective implantable infusion pumps. These pumps allow chemotherapeutic agents to be delivered in higher concentration directly into the hepatic artery.

Randomized trials have shown a considerably higher therapeutic response rate with intrahepatic administration (IA) of floxuridine than with systemic therapy.

A meta-analysis of studies comparing IV vs IA fluorinated pyrimidines in patients with unresectable, liver-confined, metastatic disease has indicated a small advantage for IA therapy.

Intrahepatic chemotherapy is costly and associated with gastroduodenal mucosal ulceration, hepatitis, and sclerosing cholangitis. The addition of dexamethasone to floxuridine infusions appears to decrease biliary sclerosis.

TREATMENT OF ADVANCED RECTAL CANCER

Radiation therapy

Radiation therapy is moderately effective in palliating the symptoms of advanced rectal cancer. Pain is decreased in 80% of irradiated patients, although only 20% report complete relief. Bleeding can be controlled in more than 70% of patients. Obstruction cannot be reliably relieved by irradiation, and diverting colostomy is recommended. Only 15% of patients with recurrent rectal cancers achieve local disease control with irradiation, and median survival is < 2 years.

Chemoradiation therapy may be useful to convert fixed unresectable lesions into resectable lesions. These regimens have generally used protracted infusions of 5-FU (200–250 mg/m^2/d) delivered via a portable infusion pump during pelvic radiation therapy (450 cGy over 5 weeks).

Intraoperative radiotherapy (localized irradiation given to the tumor or tumor bed at the time of resection) is under active investigation in advanced and locoregionally recurrent rectal cancer.

Laser photoablation

Laser photoablation is occasionally employed for temporary relief of obstructive rectal cancer in patients who are not surgical candidates because of the presence of distant metastases, surgical comorbidity, or extensive intra-abdominal disease.

Follow-up of long-term survivors

Patients who have completed therapy for CRC require monitoring for potential treatment-related complications, recurrent disease, and new metachronous cancers. Specific follow-up recommendations for these patients are controversial. Guidelines for post-treatment surveillance/monitoring adopted by the National Comprehensive Cancer Network (NCCN), a consortium of 19 American cancer centers, are shown in Table 10.

ANAL CANAL CARCINOMA

Epidemiology, etiology, and risk factors

In the United States, about 3,990 new cases of anal canal carcinoma are diagnosed each year. Overall, it is slightly more common in women than men.

TABLE 10: NCCN recommendations for post-treatment surveillance/monitoring*

- History and physical examination every 3 months for 2 years, then every 6 months for a total of 5 years
- CEA level evaluation every 3 months for 2 years, then every 6 months or years 2-5 for T2 or greater lesions
- Colonoscopy in 1 year, repeat in 1 year if results are abnormal or at least every 2-3 years if results are negative for polyps. If no preoperative colonoscopy has been performed due to an obstructing lesion, colonoscopy in 3-6 months
- Abdominal/pelvic CT scan in addition to chest x-ray or chest CT for patients with resected stage IV disease only: Every 6 months for 2 years, then every 6-12 months for a total of 5 years

* http://www.nccn.org

CEA = carcinoembryonic antigen; NCCN = National Comprehensive Cancer Network

More than 80% of anal canal tumors occur in individuals > 60 years of age. Recent epidemiologic studies suggest that receptive anal intercourse is strongly related to anal cancer.

The incidence rate of anal cancer for single men is reported to be six times that for married men. In people < 35 years old, anal carcinoma is more common in men than women. A history of genital warts has been observed, suggesting that papillomavirus may be an etiologic factor.

Signs and symptoms

The diagnosis of anal canal carcinoma is usually delayed because the symptoms (bleeding, pain, and sensation of mass) are so often attributed to benign anorectal disorders, such as hemorrhoids or anal fissures.

Diagnosis

Evaluation should include a careful rectal examination, endoscopic examination with description of lesion size, and assessment of whether there is invasion of disease into adjacent organs (vagina, urethra, or bladder). Reexamination under general anesthesia may be necessary. A diagnostic incisional biopsy is required.

Pelvic CT is suggested to evaluate pelvic nodes. Although distant metastases are uncommon at diagnosis, a chest x-ray and liver function tests are recommended. Suspicious inguinal nodes discovered on physical examination must be assessed pathologically. The incidence of inguinal nodal metastases at diagnosis varies from 13% to 25%. The presence of perirectal, inguinal, and pelvic lymph node involvement correlates with tumor size and is unusual for tumors < 2 cm in diameter. Formal groin dissection is not advised; needle aspiration should be performed, with limited surgical biopsy if results of aspiration are inconclusive.

Pathology

Squamous cell carcinomas Most anal canal malignancies are squamous cell carcinomas. They have been classified as cloacogenic carcinomas, basaloid carcinomas, transitional cell carcinomas, or mucoepidermoid carcinomas. However, there is little difference in the natural history of these various types.

Unusual tumors arising in the anal canal include small-cell carcinomas, anal melanomas, and adenocarcinomas.

Small-cell carcinomas of the anal canal are aggressive neoplasms similar in natural history to bronchogenic small-cell carcinomas. If such a histology is identified, the clinician should be alerted to the possibility of early distant metastases, and treatment should include chemotherapeutic regimens used in bronchogenic small-cell carcinomas.

Anal melanomas Although advanced anal melanomas generally are associated with a dismal survival, prognosis may be related to the depth of disease penetration. Early anal melanomas < 2.0 mm in depth can be cured with wide excision. More advanced disease can be treated with local excision and external-beam irradiation with excellent local control. Abdominoperineal resection is indicated only rarely in the management of anal melanoma, because lesions large enough to require radical surgery are almost always associated with distant spread of disease.

Adenocarcinomas are uncommon cancers associated with a poor prognosis. Treatment should be aggressive and based on a multimodality approach. The rarity of this tumor precludes the development of specific clinical trials.

Staging

Size of the primary tumor is the most important clinical predictor of survival for patients with anal carcinomas. Both the International Union Against Cancer (UICC) and the American Joint Committee on Cancer (AJCC) have agreed on a unified staging system (Table 11). The TNM classification distinguishes between anal canal carcinoma and anal margin tumors, since the latter exhibit biologic behavior similar to that of other skin cancers and are staged as skin cancers.

Treatment

Surgery

In selected individuals with small superficial T1 tumors, local excision has achieved adequate local control and survival. However, most studies of local excision have been retrospective, with small numbers of patients. Prior to the advent of primary radiotherapy and combined-modality treatment (see later in this chapter), abdominoperineal resection was considered to be the conventional treatment for patients with invasive anal canal cancer. Unfortunately, even with radical surgical procedures, local recurrences are frequent. Currently, radical extirpative surgery is indicated only after the failure of combined-modality treatment.

TABLE 11: TNM classification of anal canal tumors

Primary tumor (T)	
Tx	Primary tumor cannot be assessed
T0	No evidence of primary tumor
Tis	Carcinoma in situ
T1	Tumor ≤ 2 cm in greatest dimension
T2	Tumor > 2 cm but not > 5 cm in greatest dimension
T3	Tumor > 5 cm in greatest dimension
T4	Tumor of any size that invades adjacent organs (eg, vagina, bladder, urethra, bladder)[a]
Regional lymph nodes (N)	
Nx	Regional lymph nodes cannot be assessed
N0	No regional lymph node metastasis
N1	Metastasis in perirectal lymph node(s)
N2	Metastasis in unilateral internal iliac and/or inguinal lymph node(s)
N3	Metastasis in perirectal and inguinal lymph nodes and/or bilateral internal iliac and/or inguinal lymph nodes
Distant metastasis (M)	
Mx	Distant metastasis cannot be assessed
M0	No distant metastasis
M1	Distant metastasis
Grade (G)	
Gx	Grade of differentiation cannot be assessed
G1	Well differentiated
G2	Moderately differentiated
G3	Poorly differentiated
G4	Undifferentiated

Stage groupings

Stage 0	Tis	N0	M0
Stage I	T1	N0	M0
Stage II	T2	N0	M0
	T3	N0	M0
Stage IIIA	T1-3	N1	M0
	T4	N0	M0
Stage IIIB	T4	N1	M0
	Any T	N2-3	M0
Stage IV	Any T	Any N	M1

[a] Direct invasion of the rectal wall, perirectal skin, subcutaneous tissue, or the sphincter muscle(s) is not classified as T4.

From Greene FL, Page DL, Fleming ID, et al (eds): AJCC Cancer Staging Manual, 6th Ed. New York, Springer-Verlag, 2002.

TABLE 12: Chemotherapy regimens for anal canal cancer

Drug/combination	Dose and schedule
Fluorouracil/mitomycin/radiation therapy	
Fluorouracil	1 $g/m^2/d$ IV infused continuously on days 1-4 and 29-32
Mitomycin	15 mg/m^2 IV on day 1
Irradiation	200 cGy/d for 5 days per week (total dose, 3,000 cGy)
Give chemotherapy concurrently with irradiation; start both modalities on the same day.	
Leichman L, Nigro ND, Vaitkevicius VK, et al: Am J Med 78:211–215, 1985.	
Fluorouracil/cisplatin/radiation therapy	
Fluorouracil	1 $g/m^2/d$ IV infused continuously for 4 days
Cisplatin	25 $mg/m^2/d$ IV on days 2-5 following standard hydration
Irradiation	200 cGy/d for 5 days per week (total dose, 3,000 cGy)
Give chemotherapy concurrently with irradiation, except in elderly or frail patients.	
Wagner JP, Mahe MA, Romestaing P, et al: Int J Radiat Oncol Biol Phys 29:17–23, 1994.	

Table prepared by Ishmael Jaiyesimi, DO

Radiation therapy

Trials of primary external-beam radiotherapy in patients with anal canal carcinomas have used doses varying between 4,500 and 7,550 cGy. Local control rates of 60%–90%, with 5-year survival rates of 32%–90%, are similar to the results of surgical series when the trials are controlled for tumor size.

Interstitial radiation therapy alone has been used primarily in Europe for early-stage lesions. A relatively high radiation dose is delivered to a small volume. This modality carries a high potential for radiation necrosis and fails to incorporate treatment of the inguinal nodes.

Combined-modality treatment

Chemotherapy given concurrently with irradiation is the preferred therapy for most patients with anal canal cancer (Table 12). Investigators from Wayne State University pioneered the use of simultaneous pelvic irradiation and chemotherapy in the treatment of patients with anal canal carcinomas. They demonstrated that the majority of such patients could be treated with this combination, obviating the need for an abdominoperineal resection. The original study design used 3,000 cGy over 3 weeks with 5-FU (1,000 $mg/m^2/d$) as a continuous infusion on days 1–4 and then repeated on days 29–32. Mitomycin (Mutamycin), 15 mg/m^2, was administered as an IV bolus on day 1. A total of 4 to 6 weeks after the completion of therapy, patients had a deep muscle biopsy of the anal canal scar.

An updated analysis of this experience demonstrated that 38 of 45 patients (84%) were rendered disease free after chemotherapy and irradiation. Individuals who had positive results on biopsy underwent an abdominoperineal resection.

Because of the success of this experience, other investigators have attempted to implement infusional 5-FU and mitomycin with irradiation as definitive therapy. Most studies have used similar schedules of 5-FU and mitomycin but have used higher doses of pelvic irradiation (4,500–5,700 cGy). Five-year survival rates > 70% have been reported.

A randomized trial from the Radiation Therapy Oncology Group (RTOG) showed that the use of mitomycin with irradiation and 5-FU increased complete tumor regression and improved colostomy-free survival over irradiation and 5-FU alone. At 4 years, the colostomy-free survival rate was higher in the mitomycin arm than in the 5-FU–alone arm (71% vs 59%), as was the disease-free survival rate (73% vs 51%). Current studies are examining the role of cisplatinum versus mitomycin along with radiation therapy and 5-FU.

Several investigators have compared the results of irradiation alone vs irradiation plus chemotherapy. Cummings et al found that with identical irradiation doses and techniques, the local control rate for cancers > 2 cm rose from 49% with radiation therapy alone to 85% when 5-FU and mitomycin were combined with irradiation. Papillon and Montbarbon found an increase in the rate of local control with a combined-modality approach compared with pelvic irradiation alone (81% vs 66%). Two recent randomized studies have shown improved local control with chemoradiation therapy over irradiation.

A complete response to combined chemotherapy and radiation therapy is expected in 80%–90% of patients with anal cancer. It is important to evaluate the response of therapy with a careful examination of the anal canal after treatment. Anal canal cancers can continue to regress for up to 3 or more months after completion of treatment. For this reason, it is recommended that a biopsy be performed no sooner than 3 months after the completion of treatment, unless there is evidence of progression or other evidence to suggest early recurrence. If pathologic evidence of recurrence is diagnosed, abdominoperineal resection is expected to yield long-term disease control and survival in 40%–60% of patients.

Chemotherapy

Reports of other chemotherapeutic agents in anal cancer have been relatively anecdotal, with limited phase II studies. Because of the activity of cisplatin in other squamous cell carcinomas, this agent has been employed as a single agent or combined with infusional 5-FU in advanced disease.

SUGGESTED READING

ON COLORECTAL CARCINOMA

Andre T, Boni C, Mounedji-Boudiaf L, et al: Oxaliplatin, fluorouracil, and leucovorin as adjuvant treatment for colon cancer. N Engl J Med 350:2343–2351, 2004.

Benson AB III, Goldberg RM: Optimal use of the combination of irinotecan and 5-fluorouracil. Semin Oncol 30(3 suppl 6):68–77, 2003.

Bentrem DJ, Okabe S, Wong WD, et al: T1 adenocarcinoma of the rectum: Transanal excision or radical surgery? Ann Surg 242:472–477, 2005.

Cunningham D, Humblet Y, Siena S, et al: Cetuximab monotherapy and cetuximab plus irinotecan in irinotecan-refractory metastatic colorectal cancer. N Engl J Med 351:337–345, 2005.

Clinical Outcomes of Surgical Therapy Study Group: A comparison of laparoscopically assisted and open colectomy for colon cancer. N Engl J Med 350:2050–2059, 2004.

Goldberg RM, Sargent DJ, Morton RF, et al: A randomized controlled trial of fluorouracil plus leucovorin, irinotecan, and oxaliplatin combinations in patients with previously untreated metastatic colorectal cancer. J Clin Oncol 22:23–30, 2004.

Kapiteijn E, Marijnen CA, Nagtegaal ID, et al; Dutch Colorectal Cancer Group: Preoperative radiotherapy combined with total mesorectal excision for resectable rectal cancer. N Engl J Med 345:638–646, 2001.

Leung KL, Kwok SP, Lam SC, et al: Laparoscopic resection of rectosigmoid carcinoma: Prospective randomised trial. Lancet 363:1187–1192, 2004.

Le Voyer TE, Sigurdson ER, Hanlon AL, et al: Colon cancer survival is associated with increasing number of lymph nodes analyzed: A secondary survey of intergroup trial INT-0089. J Clin Oncol 21:2912–2919, 2003.

Poynter JN, Gruber SB, Higgins PD, et al: Statins and the risk of colorectal cancer. N Engl J Med 352:2184–2192, 2005.

Sauer R, Becker H, Hohenberger W, et al; German Rectal Cancer Study Group: Preoperative versus postoperative chemoradiotherapy for rectal cancer. N Engl J Med 351:1731–1740, 2004.

Swanson RS, Compton CC, Stewart AK, et al: The prognosis of T3N0 colon cancer is dependent on the number of lymph nodes examined. Ann Surg Oncol 10:65–71, 2003.

Tournigand C, Andre T, Achille E, et al: FOLFIRI followed by FOLFOX6 or the reverse sequence in advanced colorectal cancer: A randomized GERCOR study. J Clin Oncol 22:229–237, 2004.

Twelves C, Wong A, Nowacki MP, et al: Capecitabine as adjuvant treatment for stage III colon cancer. N Engl J Med 352:2696–2704, 2005.

ON ANAL CANAL CARCINOMA

Ghouti L, Houvenaeghel G, Moutardier V, et al: Salvage abdominoperineal resection after failure of conservative treatment in anal epidermoid cancer. Dis Colon Rectum 48:16–22, 2005.

CHAPTER 17

Prostate cancer

Judd W. Moul, MD, FACS, Brent K. Hollenbeck, MD, Kathleen W. Beekman, MD, Joseph Lattanzi, MD, and Maha Hussain, MD

Prostate cancer is the most common cancer in American men. Despite the fact that this cancer will be diagnosed in an estimated 218,890 American men in the year 2007 and will lead to the death of approximately 27,050 men, there is no universally agreed-upon strategic plan for its diagnosis and management.

Epidemiology

Age The risk of developing prostate cancer begins to increase at age 50 years in white men who have no family history of the disease and at age 40 years in black men and those who have a first-degree relative (father, brother) with prostate cancer. Risk increases with age, but, unlike other cancers, prostate cancer has no "peak" age or modal distribution. There has been a downward "age migration" in the PSA (prostate-specific antigen) era such that the median age at diagnosis is now approximately 60 years old.

Race The highest incidence of prostate cancer in the world is found in American black men, who have approximately a 9.8% lifetime risk of developing this cancer. This rate is slightly higher than the 8% lifetime risk for American white men. Black men have an incidence of prostate cancer that is 1.6 times that of white men.

The Japanese and mainland Chinese populations have the lowest rates of prostate cancer. Interestingly, although Japanese immigrants to the United States have a higher incidence of prostate cancer than Japanese people living in Japan, their rate is still about half that of American whites.

Socioeconomic status appears to be unrelated to the risk of prostate cancer, and the explanation for racial variability is unknown. However, an interplay of diet, hormonal factors, and genetics likely acounts for the variability.

Geography The incidence of prostate cancer is highest in Scandinavian countries (22 cases per 100,000 population) and lowest in Asia (5 per 100,000). Risk may be inversely related to ultraviolet light exposure, as the incidence increases the farther one lives from the equator. However, recent studies show extremely high rates in populations of African heritage, such as Jamaicans.

> Preclinical data support the hypothesis that nonsteroidal anti-inflammatory drugs (NSAIDs) may interfere with prostate carcinogenesis. The American Cancer Society examined a large cohort of over 70,000 men who completed a mailed self-administered questionnaire, including information on demographic, medical, and lifestyle factors. Follow-up questionnaires were sent to update exposure information and to ascertain newly diagnosed cancers. There was no protection from prostate cancer with current NSAID use. However, long-time users (30 or more pills per month for 5 or more years) had a significantly decreased risk of prostate cancer (*Jacobs EJ, Rodriguez C, Mondul AM, et al: J Natl Cancer Inst 97:975-980, 2005*).

Etiology and risk factors

Family history Men who have a first-degree relative with prostate cancer have approximately a twofold increased risk of developing prostate cancer during their lifetime. An individual who has two first-degree relatives with prostate cancer has a ninefold increase in lifetime risk.

True hereditary prostate cancer occurs in a small number of men and tends to develop at an early age (< 55 years old).

Dietary fat Studies have suggested that dietary fat may increase the risk of prostate cancer. However, no definitive proof of its role has yet been found.

Vasectomy Several large epidemiologic studies suggest that vasectomy may increase the relative risk of prostate cancer by as much as 1.85. However, these same studies do not report an increased risk of dying from prostate cancer associated with vasectomy but do indicate a statistically increased risk of dying from lung cancer. These findings argue against an association between vasectomy and prostate cancer. Currently, this association is unproven and does not constitute grounds for fundamental changes in the use of vasectomy.

Sexual activity/sexually transmitted disease A large prospective study of more than 29,000 men demonstrated an association between high ejaculatory frequency (more than 21 ejaculations/month) and a decreased risk of prostate cancer, with a lifetime relative risk of 0.67. However, there may be several confounding factors associated with high sexual activity, such as differences in prostate cancer screening or lifestyle. There was no associated increased risk for men in the lowest ejaculatory frequency category.

Prevention Active research on chemoprevention of prostate cancer is ongoing. The only prospective randomized trial to demonstrate an effect was the Prostate Cancer Prevention Trial (PCPT), which showed a 24.8% reduction in the risk of prostate cancer among men randomized to receive finasteride (Proscar) daily versus those men on the placebo arm. Finasteride as a chemopreventive agent has not been universally accepted, however, because patients in the treatment arm were possibly more likely to exhibit higher-grade prostate cancer. Recent follow-up studies of the PCPT suggest that finasteride probably does not induce high-grade disease, and the observation may be a detection artifact. Other agents under study include vitamin E and selenium, both of which have been associated with a decreased risk of prostate cancer. A large prospective randomized trial to evaluate the effects of these agents in healthy men is currently under way.

Signs and symptoms

Early-stage disease Men with organ-confined prostate cancer often are completely asymptomatic. Men with a large component of benign prostatic hyperplasia often present with bladder outlet obstruction unrelated to prostate cancer.

Locally advanced disease Bladder outlet obstruction is the most common sign of locally advanced prostate cancer. A few men with locally advanced disease present with hematuria, urinary tract infections, and irritative voiding symptoms secondary to bladder outlet obstruction.

Advanced disease Rarely, men with bulky lymph node metastasis may present with bilateral lower-extremity edema. Men with bony metastasis often present with bone pain and, uncommonly, with lower-extremity weakness or paralysis from spinal cord compression.

> The optimal threshold PSA level to recommend prostate biopsy continues to be controversial. In the latest data from the Prostate Cancer Prevention Trial, Thompson et al studied 8,575 men in the placebo arm, all of whom started the trial with a PSA level of 3.0 ng/mL or less. PSA cutoff values of 1.1, 2.1, 3.1, and 4.1 ng/mL yielded sensitivities of 83.4%, 52.6%, 32.2%, and 20.5% and specificities of 38.9%, 72.5%, 86.7%, and 93.8%, respectively. The authors concluded that there is no one cutpoint with simultaneous high sensitivity and specificity and that there is a continuous risk of prostate cancer with rising PSA (*Thompson IM, Ankerst DP, Chi C, et al: JAMA 294:66-70, 2005*).

Screening and diagnosis

Prostate cancer screening with PSA and digital rectal examination (DRE) has resulted in not only an increase in prostate cancer detection but also a stage shift. More cancers are now being detected at earlier stages, when they are potentially curable. Prior to screening efforts, most prostate cancers were detected when they produced local symptoms or distant metastases, at which point treatment for cure often was impossible.

Digital rectal examination Prostate biopsy prompted by abnormal findings on DRE, such as nodularity or induration of the prostate, leads to a diagnosis of prostate cancer in only 15%–25% of cases. This rate compares with a prostate cancer prevalence of < 5% among men of similar age without an abnormal DRE. Although neither accurate nor sensitive for prostate cancer detection, abnormal DRE is associated with a fivefold increased risk of cancer present at the time of screening.

PSA is a serine protease produced by the prostatic epithelium and secreted in the seminal fluid in large quantities. The level of PSA in serum is increased by inflammation of the prostate, urinary retention, prostatic infection, benign prostatic hyperplasia, prostate cancer, and prostatic manipulation. The optimal threshold to recommend prostatic biopsy has come under increasing scrutiny. The overall sensitivity for PSA levels is approximately 70%, but it is not as specific and does not allow for differentiation between indolent and aggressive disease. For example, by using a threshold of 4.1 ng/mL, the majority of cancers in men < age 60 would potentially be missed. However, a PSA

D'Amico et al studied 1,095 men with localized prostate cancer to determine what factors predicted for death following radical prostatectomy. All men had clinical stage disease of up to T2, and the median PSA level was 4.3 ng/mL. Men were followed for a median of 5.3 years. On multivariate analysis, the most important factors associated with death from prostate cancer were PSA velocity > 2.0 ng/mL/yr, the absolute PSA value, a Gleason score of 8-10, and clinical stage T2. There were only 27 deaths from prostate cancer in this study. However, the data suggest that PSA velocity is an important prognostic factor for men with localized prostate cancer. Whether PSA velocity is a useful predictor in screening is currently under study (*D'Amico AV, Chen MH, Roehl KA, et. al: N Engl J Med 351:125-135, 2004*).

cutoff of 4.1 ng/mL only has a positive predictive value of approximately 30%, meaning two out of three men would undergo biopsy for benign disease.

A more worthwhile approach for PSA screening may be to use the rate of rise in PSA (PSA velocity) in combination with the absolute PSA value. This approach has been shown to be useful recently in the form of age-adjusted PSA velocity, but accepted guidelines are still controversial.

Another commonly employed test for patients with a PSA level < 10 ng/mL is the percent-free PSA level. There is an inverse relationship between the percent-free PSA level and the risk of a cancer diagnosis. Most urologists utilize a cutoff of 10% to prompt a recommendation for biopsy. In men who have never had a prostate biopsy but who have a total PSA level > 4.0, a percent-free PSA less than 25% may suggest a 50%–60% probability of prostate cancer. In men who have had a prior negative biopsy but who have a persistently elevated PSA level > 4.0, a percent-free PSA < 10% should prompt a repeat biopsy.

Current screening recommendations The American Cancer Society and the American Urological Association (AUA) recommend that the PSA test and the DRE should be offered annually beginning at age 50 to men who have a life expectancy of at least 10 years. In high-risk men (African Americans and those with a first-degree relative diagnosed with prostate cancer), screening should be offered at an earlier age (40–45 years old). Prior to testing, physicians should discuss with their patients the potential benefits of early prostate cancer detection and its implications in the need for subsequent treatment so that patients can make an informed decision about undergoing screening.

There are currently two ongoing major prostate cancer screening trials: The Prostate, Lung, Colorectal, and Ovarian (PLCO) trial in the United States funded by the National Cancer Institute and the European Organization for Research and Treatment of Cancer (EORTC) trial. The National Comprehensive Cancer Network (NCCN) has recently published aggressive screening guidelines on its website (www.nccn.org). These new controversial guidelines call for baseline PSA levels at a younger age (generally age 40) and suggest that any young man with a PSA level > 0.7 ng/mL (median in men aged 40–49) be tested annually.

Biopsy When indicated, prostate biopsy usually is performed as an office procedure by transrectal ultrasonographic guidance using an automated 18-gauge biopsy gun. The procedure is performed with, at most, local anesthesia and carries a risk of significant infection of only 1 in 200 cases. Additional side effects of hematuria and hematochezia are common for 2–3 days following the biopsy. Hematospermia may last for up to 4–6 weeks. Since about the year 2000, prostate biopsy includes laterally directed extended core protocols employing 8–12 biopsy cores per procedure. Multiple studies have demonstrated that the addition of the lateral cores improves the accuracy of biopsy.

> A cohort of 223 men with clinically localized disease was followed expectantly in Sweden (mean follow-up of 21 years). Substantial declines in disease progression-free, metastasis-free, and prostate-specific survivals were demonstrated at 15 to 20 years' follow-up. Between the two time intervals (0 to 15 years vs 15 to 20 years), the prostate cancer mortality rates increased from 15/1,000/year to 44/1,000/yr ($P = .01$), suggesting that treatment should be principally directed at patients with a life expectancy > 15 years *(Johansson JE, Andren O, Andersson SO, et al: JAMA 291:2713-2719, 2004).*

If the biopsy result is negative, these men are typically followed conservatively with serial PSA levels and DRE repeated annually. Repeat biopsy is performed only when PSA levels rise at abnormal rates (> 0.8 ng/mL/yr) or if DRE findings show new nodularity or induration. Men in whom high-grade prostatic intraepithelial neoplasia is found on biopsy usually should undergo repeat biopsy, since one-third to one-half will be found to have prostate cancer.

Recently, a new test, the UPM-3 urine test, has become more widely available. This test, performed on voided urine after an "attentive" DRE, is based on reverse transcriptase-polymerase chain reaction assay for a PSA product (DD3). It is becoming useful, not as a primary screening test, but to dictate the need for repeat prostate biopsy in men with persistently elevated PSA levels.

Pathology

Adenocarcinomas make up the vast majority of prostate carcinomas. A total of 70% of prostate adenocarcinomas occur in the peripheral zone, 20% in the transitional zone, and approximately 10% in the central zone.

Other tumor types are relatively rare and include ductal adenocarcinoma, which occurs in the major ducts and often projects into the urethra; and mucinous adenocarcinoma, which secretes abundant mucin and does not arise from the major ducts. Transitional carcinoma of the prostate occurs within the ducts and, to a lesser extent, in the prostatic acini. Typically, primary transitional carcinomas are aggressive cancers that have a poor prognosis. Similarly, neuroendocrine (small-cell) tumors are rare and aggressive, have a poor prognosis, and typically require aggressive surgical management.

Histologic grade The grading system developed by Gleason from data accumulated by the Veterans Administration Cooperative Urologic Research Group appears to provide the best prognostic information in addition to clinical stage and is the predominant grading system in widespread use.

TABLE 1: TNM staging system of prostate cancer

Localized disease	
T1a	Tumor incidental histologic finding in ≤ 5% of resected tissue; not palpable
T1b	Tumor incidental histologic finding in > 5% of resected tissue
T1c	Tumor identified by needle biopsy (eg, because of elevated PSA level)
T2a	Tumor involves one-half of one lobe or less
T2b	Tumor involves more than one-half of one lobe but not both lobes
T2c	Tumor involves both lobes
Local extension	
T3a	Extracapsular extension (unilateral or bilateral)
T3b	Tumor invades seminal vesicle(s)
T4	Bladder invasion, fixed to pelvic side wall, or invasion of adjacent structures
Metastatic disease	
N1	Positive regional lymph nodes
M1	Distant metastasis

Adapted from Greene FI, Page DL, Fleming ID, et al (eds): AJCC Cancer Staging Manual, 6th ed. New York, Springer-Verlag, 2002.

Metastatic spread Adenocarcinoma of the prostate may spread locally through direct extension into periprostatic fat or via the ejaculatory ducts into seminal vesicles; lymphatically to regional lymph nodes, including the hypogastric and obturator lymph nodes; and hematogenously to bone. The most common sites of bony metastases are the lumbosacral spine (probably related to venous drainage of the prostate through Baston's plexus) and the axial skeleton, but any bone, including the skull and ribs, can be involved. Rare sites of metastatic spread include the liver and lungs.

Prevention

Until 2004, there was no intervention known to prevent prostate cancer. The primary objective of the Prostate Cancer Prevention Trial was to describe the prevalence of histologically proven prostate cancer among men randomized to receive daily finasteride (a 5-alpha-reductase inhibitor that decreases prostate size and serum/prostate dihydrotestosterone levels) or placebo. The authors described a 24.8% reduction in the prevalence of prostate cancer among men taking finasteride, suggesting that it either prevents or delays the appearance of prostate cancer. The caveat of their findings, however, was that these cancers that developed in the treatment arm were of a higher grade.

TABLE 2: D'Amico et al risk stratification for clinically localized prostate cancer

Low risk	Diagnostic PSA < 10.0 ng/mL *and* highest biopsy Gleason score ≤ 6 *and* clinical stage T1c or T2a
Intermediate risk	Diagnostic PSA > 10 but < 20 ng/mL *or* highest biopsy Gleason score = 7 *or* clinical stage T2b
High risk	Diagnostic PSA > 20 ng/mL *or* highest biopsy Gleason score ≤ 8 *or* cinical stage T2c/T3

PSA = prostate-specific antigen

Prognosis and natural history

Staging systems The most widely used and universally accepted staging system for prostate cancer is the TNM system (Table 1). In the TNM system, T1 and T2 tumors are confined to the gland, whereas T3 and T4 tumors have local extension.

Risk-adapted staging The development of the "Partin Tables" in 1993 ushered in a new era of combining clinical stage, Gleason score, and PSA level to predict pathologic stage after radical prostatectomy. More recently, this has led to the D'Amico et al risk groupings for newly diagnosed men with clinically localized disease (Table 2). Patients are divided into three risk groups (low, intermediate, or high) of occult micrometastases and relapse after initial local therapy. Although not perfect, this system is currently in widespread use and allows a framework for multimodal and multidisciplinary treatment strategies based on risk grouping.

Prognosis The optimal management of patients with prostate cancer varies widely and is highly dependent upon a patient's age, overall health, and tumor risk assessment. The natural history of the disease process can be heterogeneous, ranging from an incidental finding unlikely to result in cancer-specific mortality, to very aggressive, resulting in early widespread metastatic disease and death. Therefore, treating physicians should carefully consider the value of curative therapy with potential toxicity in the context of a patient's comorbidities and life expectancy.

Among patients with clinically localized prostate cancer treated conservatively (observation or hormonal therapy alone), those with a low Gleason score (2–4) have a small risk of dying of their cancer within 15 years (4%–7%). However, those with poorly differentiated tumors (Gleason score 8–10) have a greater risk of dying of prostate cancer than of any other cause, even when the cancer is diagnosed in the eighth decade of life. Indeed, a man diagnosed before the age of 60 with a clinically localized, Gleason score 8–10 prostate

TABLE 3: Risk of dying of clinically localized prostate cancer without definitive locoregional therapy

	Age			
Gleason score	55-59	60-64	65-69	70-74
2-4	4%	5%	6%	7%
5	6%	8%	10%	11%
6	18%	23%	27%	30%
7	70%	62%	53%	42%
8-10	87%	81%	72%	60%

Adapted from Albertsen PC, Hanley JA, Fine J: JAMA 293:2095–2101, 2005.

cancer has an 87% risk of dying of the disease within 15 years if untreated (Table 3).

D'Amico et al combined a number of national datasets to report 10-year cancer-specific mortality rates for men undergoing radical prostatectomy or external-beam radiotherapy (EBRT) by this risk grouping and age at diagnosis. These 10-year mortality graphs are useful to counsel contemporary-era men contemplating surgery or radiation therapy. Given recent advances in the treatment of metastatic disease, identifying men at high risk for metastatic disease following local therapy is important, as these agents are incorporated earlier in the disease course.

Treatment of localized prostate cancer

There are several treatment options for localized prostate cancer, including radical prostatectomy, EBRT, and brachytherapy (interstitial radiation/seeds). Multiple treatment series with each modality have documented the validity of the risk-stratification model based on clinical palpation stage, Gleason score, and serum PSA level. More recently, it has been suggested that biopsy quantification may also be an important factor. Specifically, counting the number of involved needle biopsy cores or the percentage of each core involved by cancer may be prognostic. Low-risk patients experience a favorable 85%–90% freedom from recurrence, compared with approximately 75% and 35%–50% for the intermediate- and high-risk patients, respectively. Although no randomized studies have been performed, contemporary

Long-term (median, 6.2 years) follow-up of quality of life (QOL) following localized prostate cancer therapies (prostatectomy, external-beam radiation therapy [EBRT], and brachytherapy) has demonstrated that QOL continues to evolve for patients treated with either interstitial therapy or EBRT. Specifically, irritative urinary and bowel symptoms seemed to abate among those treated with brachytherapy, whereas incontinence worsened among men treated with either brachytherapy or EBRT. This finding underscores the need for long-term follow-up when measuring QOL after localized prostate cancer therapies (*Miller DC, Sanda MG, Dunn RL, et al: J Clin Oncol 23:2772-2780, 2005*).

series, which stratify patients by the risk model, demonstrate remarkably similar outcomes independent of the treatment modality. For this reason, treatment recommendations should be individualized based on patient preference, life expectancy, and discussion of potential toxicities.

Evidence among 1,095 men with localized prostate cancer suggests that those with a higher preoperative PSA velocity (> 2 ng/mL in this study) were at greater risk of death from prostate cancer after radical prostatectomy than those with more indolent PSA velocities, highlighting the role of such an indicator in predicting the aggressiveness of the disease *(D'Amico AV, Chen MH, Roehl KA, et al: N Engl J Med 351:125-135, 2004)*. A subsequent study confirmed that the adverse implications of a higher PSA velocity (> 2 ng/cc/yr) were generalizable to men treated with radiation therapy. Pretreatment PSA dynamics should be studied in more detail and considered in patient education and treatment decisions for multimodality therapy *(D'Amico AV, Renshaw AA, Sussman B, et al: JAMA 294:440-447, 2005)*.

TREATMENT OF CLINICALLY LOCALIZED DISEASE (T1, T2)

Radical prostatectomy

Radical prostatectomy can be performed retropubically through a lower midline incision—an approach that may include pelvic lymph node dissection. Alternatively, some urologists prefer the perineal approach. With the latter approach, a separate incision is required if lymph node removal is desired. Compared with patients managed with watchful waiting, those treated with radical prostatectomy have a lower risk of distant metastases and improved disease-specific survival, although no benefit in overall survival has yet been demonstrated.

Although the morbidity of radical prostatectomy was a major concern in the past, improvements were made during the 1980s. The hazards of anesthesia, risk of blood loss, and hospital stay have all been minimized. Nationwide, Medicare data suggest that surgical outcomes are significantly better at those centers performing > 40 prostatectomies per year than at other hospitals with a lower surgical volume.

Transfusion is usually unnecessary, and treatment-related mortality is < 0.05% at leading prostate cancer centers. The average hospital stay of a man undergoing radical prostatectomy is now approximately 1 to 3 days at leading referral centers in the United States; several institutions routinely discharge patients within 24 hours. Although urinary incontinence is common in the first few months after prostatectomy, most men recover urinary control; at some leading centers, 90%–98% of men report few or no long-term urinary problems.

Nerve-sparing radical prostatectomy is appropriate for men with small-volume disease. It offers those men with good potency prior to

The first trial to empirically demonstrate better survival after treatment (compared with no treatment or androgen ablation) for localized prostate cancer was reported by Bill-Axelson and colleagues. The authors found a 44%, 40%, and 67% decrease in the risk of prostate cancer mortality, distant metastases, and local disease progression among men randomized to receive radical prostatectomy compared with those managed expectantly. This finding represents the only localized prostate cancer treatment modality backed by empirical evidence favoring treatment *(Bill-Axelson A, Holmberg L, Ruutu M, et al: N Engl J Med 352:1977-1984, 2005)*.

> Stephenson et al reported the outcome of 501 patients treated with salvage radiotherapy for increasing PSA levels after radical prostatectomy at five US academic institutions. Although preradiotherapy PSA values had risen to a median of 0.72 ng/mL, 45% of patients had undetectable PSA values 4 years after radiotherapy. Patients lacking adverse risk factors (a Gleason score of 8 or higher, preradiotherapy PSA level > 2.0 ng/mL, negative surgical margins, PSA doubling time < 10 months, and seminal vesicle invasion) achieved a 77% rate of undetectable PSA levels at 4 years, and salvage rates were significantly lower when adverse features were present. These data suggest that earlier salvage therapy is optimal while PSA values are still as low as possible (*Stephenson AJ, Shariat SF, Zelefsky MJ, et al: JAMA 291:1325-1332, 2004*).

surgery the probability of recovering that function following the operation. By permitting better visualization of Santorini's dorsal venous plexus, the apical prostate, the urethra, and the striated urethral sphincter, the nerve-sparing technique also reduces blood loss and improves recovery of urinary continence. In appropriately selected individuals, a nerve-sparing procedure confers no greater risk of prostate cancer recurrence after considering other relevant clinical information (PSA, Gleason score, margin status, seminal vesicle involvement, and the presence of extraprostatic spread).

Referral centers have reported that 50%–90% of patients who are fully potent prior to surgery recover erections following a nerve-sparing procedure, but the quality (rigidity and duration) of these recovered erections may be compromised compared with preoperative erections. Erection recovery rates can be higher than 80% in patients < 60 years of age and lower in older men. Potency may return anywhere from 2–24 months following surgery. Regardless of potency, sensation of the penis is not changed after this procedure, and men still experience orgasm. Nerve-sparing radical prostatectomy has not compromised cancer control outcomes in well-selected men with early-stage disease. Also, a recent study has suggested that early postoperative use of sildenafil (Viagra) may facilitate the return of natural erections more quickly. Generally speaking, recovery of erectile function after radical prostatectomy is mediated by age (the younger, the better), pretreatment erectile function (the stronger, the better), and a nerve-sparing approach (bilateral is better than unilateral, which is better than none, which is better than wide dissection).

Laparoscopic radical prostatectomy

Laparoscopic prostatectomy was initially described by Schuessler in 1997 but was abandoned because of its technical difficulty and long operative time with little apparent benefit over the conventional technique. A resurgence in the technique was prompted by improved instrumentation and refinements in the procedure itself, although the laparoscopically naive urologist must endure a substantial learning curve (with attendant perioperative morbidity) prior to meeting the outcome standards set by the open technique.

The robotic-assisted prostatectomy was developed to overcome some of the difficulties of the standard laparoscopic prostatectomy (eg, intracorporeal suturing). The robotic technique allows for three-dimensional (3D) visualization of the operative field and provides for a significantly wider range of movements intracorporeally than do standard laparoscopic instruments. This advance has prompted the assimilation of the technique into the armamentarium of many urologists.

Current evidence suggests that in experienced hands, the laparoscopic and robotic techniques have similar oncologic efficacy to that of the open procedure. However, the length of follow-up (usually < 12 months) in these studies is limited, suggesting that a measure of caution be taken when interpreting the results. Furthermore, recent studies suggest the learning curve is prolonged, with 200–250 cases necessary before results can be compared with those of experienced surgeons. Long-term effects of these modalities on sexual and urinary health (as measured by a psychometrically valid survey) have not been reported, and such data are critical in the context of the prostatectomy patient when evaluating technical results. Though it is a promising advance in the treatment of prostate cancer, published data suggest further research in this area is warranted.

> The first published report to examine the use of hormonal therapy (HT) for prostate-specific antigen (PSA)-only or biochemical recurrence after radical prostatectomy was authored by Moul et al. Using the Center for Prostate Disease Research (CPDR) multicenter database, the authors studied 1,352 men who had PSA recurrence postoperatively, comparing 355 men who received HT with 997 who were observed. For men with high-risk disease, including a PSA doubling time of < 12 months or a Gleason score of 8 or higher, early HT before the PSA level reached 10 ng/mL was an independent predictor of delayed clinical metastases. Although this is the first study to show a benefit to early HT in this setting, the study was not randomized, and longer follow-up is needed (*Moul J, Wu H, Sun L, et al: J Urol 171:1141-1147, 2004*).

Despite the perception that laparoscopic robotic prostatectomy is "minimally invasive," it actually is an intraperitoneal operation, whereas the open retropubic prostatectomy is a pure retroperitoneal approach. Whether this poses any short- or long-term risk remains unknown.

Pelvic lymph node dissection Studies now indicate that regional pelvic lymph node dissection may not be necessary for patients with stage T1c disease if the total Gleason score is < 7 and the PSA level is < 10.0 ng/mL, ie, low-risk individuals. Selected intermediate-risk men may also not require this staging procedure, but in high-risk men, it is still considered imperative.

Neoadjuvant hormonal therapy

Approximately 15%–35% of men who undergo radical prostatectomy for clinical stage T2 prostate cancer will be found to have pathologic T3 disease following surgery. This finding led some investigators to evaluate the efficacy of neoadjuvant androgen deprivation therapy in prospective clinical trials. Early data from these trials suggested that neoadjuvant hormonal therapy led to a reduction in positive surgical margins. However, these findings need to be considered in a technical context: Androgen deprivation therapy causes artifactual changes in prostate morphology that cause difficulties for the pathologic identification of prostate cancer foci.

Indeed, more recent data from prospective studies have shown no benefit of neoadjuvant therapy with regard to disease progression-free survival. At present, therefore, it appears that neoadjuvant hormonal therapy does not improve the curative potential of radical prostatectomy but instead is associated with morphologic alterations that complicate the prognostic utility of standard pathology. Consequently, neoadjuvant hormonal therapy should be reserved for evaluation as an experimental modality in the context of clinical trials.

Adjuvant therapy post prostatectomy

The potential indications for adjuvant therapy following radical prostatectomy in patients with clinical T1 or T2 malignancy include pathologic evidence of T3 disease, positive nodes, a rising PSA level, and positive surgical margins, among others. Possible adjuvant treatments include radiation therapy and androgen deprivation either alone or in combination. Best available evidence suggests that early salvage radiotherapy (eg, postprostatectomy PSA level < 1.0 ng/mL) affords the best results in terms of subsequent biochemical recurrence.

Radiation therapy Men with positive margins or pathologic T3 disease following radical prostatectomy are potential candidates for adjuvant EBRT. Some controversy exists as to the efficacy of early postoperative therapy versus intervention once a biochemical failure has been documented.

Valicenti et al demonstrated that the 5-year PSA control rate with immediate postoperative radiation therapy for patients with pathologic T3 disease was 89%, compared with 55% for a matched-pair analysis of surgery alone. Additionally, they demonstrated a favorable dose response in patients receiving EBRT doses above 64.8 Gy.

More recently, Bolla et al reported the results of a randomized, controlled study of observation vs EBRT in 500 patients with pathologic T3 disease following radical prostatectomy. Although to date there are no data demonstrating an overall survival difference, with a median follow-up of 5 years, the progression-free survival was significantly improved with treatment (74% vs 53%).

Less controversy exists regarding the role of salvage radiation therapy for PSA recurrence. Approximately 60%–70% of patients with favorable disease after surgical failure (PSA level < 2.0 ng/mL, a slow PSA doubling time, and a long interval to failure after surgery) will experience durable disease-free survival after adjuvant radiotherapy, presumably due to a smaller tumor burden and a lower likelihood of occult metastatic disease.

Stephenson et al evaluated a large number of patients with persistent or increasing PSA levels after surgery from five American academic institutions. Forty-five percent of patients were free of disease at 4 years. Patients with no adverse risk features achieved a 4-year progression-free probability of 77%. Patients who experience PSA failure after radical prostatectomy should be restaged with pelvic CT, bone scan, and DRE. Patients with no evidence of metastatic disease should be evaluated for adjuvant radiotherapy.

Hormonal therapy Significant controversy exists within the academic community as to the timing of initiating androgen deprivation following radical prostatectomy. Clinical trials have documented a benefit only for those patients with nodal involvement.

Treatment recommendations for postprostatectomy recurrence

Following radical prostatectomy, it is expected that serial PSA levels will become undetectable. Any detectable PSA level (> 0.2 ng/mL) following surgery indicates possible recurrent disease and the need for restaging and possible salvage therapies, including radiation or hormonal therapy, experimental protocols, or observation. However, some patients can develop low levels of detectable PSA after prostatectomy without cancer recurrence, presumably due to small foci of benign prostate tissue in situ. Although there is concern for recurrence when the PSA level is > 0.2 ng/mL, most clinicians will wait until a PSA threshold > 0.4 ng/mL is reached to assume that the rise in PSA level represents real recurrence.

Definitive radiation therapy

EBRT EBRT utilizes high-energy photons to destroy cancer cells by damaging cellular DNA. Traditional EBRT utilized bony landmarks and standard beam arrangements to deliver dose to the pelvic region. Technologic advances in treatment planning, driven by improved computing power and the incorporation of individualized patient anatomy, have led to dramatic improvements in treatment delivery. (For a more complete discussion of radiation therapy techniques, see chapter 1.)

3D conformal EBRT creates 3D representations of target structures (ie, the prostate) and designs highly tailored treatment portals utilizing various angles to create a volume of high radiation dose that conforms to the target shape. The anatomic information used to define the target is generally derived from CT images obtained while the patient is placed in an immobilization device in the precise treatment position. With the selective delivery of dose to the target and avoidance of the surrounding normal tissue, the therapeutic ratio is improved. This approach has permitted the use of doses far higher than tolerable with traditional therapy, with fewer bowel and bladder complications.

Treatment volumes in patients with low-risk disease are designed to encompass the prostate plus a margin for daily variations. Patients with a high risk for periprostatic extension and/or regional lymph node metastasis receive initial pelvic treatment of 45–50 Gy, followed by a coned-down boost to the prostate.

RTOG (Radiation Therapy Oncology Group) 9413 was designed to test the addition of whole pelvic radiation and the timing of androgen deprivation in the treatment of high-risk patients (lymph node-positive potential > 15% or locally advanced [Gleason score ≥ 6 and > cT2c] cancers). At a median follow-up of 59.5 months, Roach et al noted an improved 4-year disease progression-free survival (60%) among those receiving whole pelvic radiotherapy in conjunction with neoadjuvant androgen deprivation, compared with other treatment arms (44%–50%).

EBRT dose The previous standard radiation dose with conventional therapy was 70 Gy given over 7 weeks; however, much recent work has suggested a positive dose response, particularly in the intermediate- and high-risk patient

Emerging evidence supports the use of high-dose (79.2 Gy) over conventional (70.2 Gy) conformal radiotherapy. Among patients with localized prostate cancer, men randomized to receive high-dose therapy were 49% less likely to experience biochemical failure than those treated with conventional-dose radiotherapy (*Zietman AL, DeSilvio ML, Slater JD, et al: JAMA 294:1233-1239, 2005*).

populations. Multiple single-institution experiences have demonstrated that 3D conformal EBRT techniques with doses of 75 Gy and higher can be delivered with minimal toxicities.

A randomized trial from the M. D. Anderson Cancer Center compared 70 Gy given conventionally with 78 Gy delivered with a conformal boost. It showed an advantage in freedom from failure for the higher dose arm in patients with a PSA level > 10 ng/mL. Kupelian et al presented pooled data for nearly 5,000 patients from 9 institutions over a narrow time range (1994–1995) to remove treatment technique, stage migration, and lead-time bias. They demonstrated favorable biochemical control outcomes for doses higher than 72 Gy in all risk groups.

The RTOG has completed a dose-escalation trial to assess toxicity with 3D conformal EBRT. In this multi-institutional trial, 78 Gy (prescribed as a minimum to the tumor volume in 2-Gy fractions) was well tolerated, with only 3% of patients experiencing significant (grade 3+) acute gastrointestinal/genitourinary (GI/GU) morbidity and a 6% rate of significant late toxicity. A comparison trial is being conducted by the RTOG (P0126); it will accrue 1,520 cases and provide information regarding any beneficial effect on mortality with higher radiation doses. Although no standard exists, doses ≥ 75 Gy with 3D conformal EBRT techniques appear to be well tolerated and improve biochemical response rates.

Intensity-modulated radiation therapy (IMRT) is becoming a widely used treatment for prostate cancer. This refinement of conformal therapy employs high nonuniform beam intensity profiles and dynamic multileaf collimation to create even more conformal dose distributions. Further improving the therapeutic index compared with 3D conformal EBRT, IMRT is associated with reduced toxicity, permitting further dose escalations previously unattainable.

Albertson et al updated their study of the Connecticut Tumor Registry examining 20-year outcomes of conservative management of clinically localized prostate cancer. For low-risk men with Gleason 2-4 disease, the risk of death from prostate cancer remains low, between 15 and 20 years of follow-up. The authors concluded that aggressive treatment is not supported by their data for low-risk men with low-grade disease, even with long follow-up (*Albertsen PC, Hanley JA, Fine J: JAMA 293:2095-2101, 2005*).

IMRT was pioneered in several major centers, and Memorial Sloan-Kettering Cancer Center has reported a series of 772 patients treated with doses between 81 and 86.4 Gy. With a median follow-up of 24 months, the side-effect profile was improved, despite these higher doses, with less than 1% of patients experiencing late grade 3+ GI/GU toxicity. The early PSA relapse-free survival rates for favorable, intermediate, and unfavorable risk groups were 92%, 86%, and 81%, respectively. Although IMRT is quickly becoming the standard of care at most institutions, some caution should be exercised. The precision of dose delivery and the complexity of treatment planning demand a strong commitment by both physicians and physics personnel to ensure high-quality IMRT.

Androgen ablation with EBRT Two potential benefits of the use of transient androgen ablation prior to EBRT have been identified. First, there may be some synergy between the apoptotic response induced by androgen deprivation and radiotherapy that may increase local control.

Second, androgen deprivation results in an average 20% decrease in prostate volume. This volume reduction not only may reduce the number of target cells, and thereby improve tumor control, but also may shrink the prostate and, thus, diminish the volume of rectum and bladder irradiated during conformal therapy. Complete androgen blockade can be achieved with luteinizing hormone-releasing hormone (LHRH) agonists plus an oral antiandrogen.

The survival benefits of androgen suppression therapy (AST) for patients with intermediate-risk disease have been uncertain. A recent single-institution prospective trial by D'Amico et al randomized patients with a PSA level > 10 ng/mL, a Gleason score ≥ 7, or radiographic evidence of extraprostatic disease to receive EBRT (70 Gy) alone or the same EBRT with 6 months of AST. After a median follow-up of 4.5 years, patients treated with combined EBRT and AST were found to have improved disease progression-free, prostate cancer-specific, and overall survival ($P = .04$). Although hormone therapy for 3 years has been shown to be beneficial in locally advanced cases, this trial in men with more localized disease showed a benefit to shorter duration of hormone therapy. However, it is not known whether high-dose radiotherapy will obviate the need for AST in this group of patients.

Interstitial radiotherapy In the 1970s, the use of permanently placed radioactive iodine implants produced initial results as good as those obtained with other available radiotherapy techniques and posed a small risk of impotence and other morbidity when compared with conventional EBRT and radical prostatectomy. However, ultimate control rates were unacceptable. The technique used (freehand placement of seeds during laparotomy) was found to distribute the radioactive seeds unevenly throughout the gland, and, thus, cold regions may have contributed to the relatively poor outcome.

The advent of improved imaging and seed placement techniques coupled with better patient selection has resulted in vast improvements in cancer control. The perception of fewer side effects in a single outpatient treatment has also contributed to a recent surge in this treatment modality. Transrectal ultrasonography is now utilized to guide seed placement from a transperineal approach, which has corrected the problem of poor seed placement in experienced hands. Two radioactive seed isotopes have been used: iodine (I-125), with a half-life of 60 days, and palladium (Pd-103), with a shorter half-life (17 days) and subsequent higher dose rate. The advantage of the brachytherapy technique is that substantial dose can be delivered to the prostate with minimal effect on the surrounding tissue.

Although concentrating dose with brachytherapy represents a potential advantage over EBRT, it also highlights the need for appropriate patient selection. Significant dose falloff 2–3 mm beyond placement of the seeds within the gland limits the application of seed monotherapy in patients with potential periprostatic or regional disease extension. Large studies from several leading institutions have now matured and confirm the long-term effectiveness and safety of this approach in low-risk populations. Favorable results have also been reported in selected intermediate-risk patients. Typical monotherapy doses of 145 Gy for I-131 and 125 Gy for Pd-103 are utilized. To date, the data do not support the use of either isotope over the other.

In addition to disease risk factors, certain patient selection factors are important in considering implants. A large prostate size (> 60 cc) may make the procedure more challenging, both from the perspective of increased prostate gland swelling due to the increased number of needles and the difficulty of the pubic bone obstructing needle placement. Patients with outlet obstruction symptoms (American Urological Society score > 15) have an increased risk of requiring catheterization following implantation. Patients who have undergone prior transurethral resection of prostate (TURP) have been reported to have an increased risk of incontinence; recognizing this risk and placing seeds farther from the defect may help to minimize this risk. Therefore, with proper counseling, patients with small TURP defects may still be considered implant candidates.

For patients with intermediate- or high-risk disease, implants may be combined with EBRT. There is sound logic in combining high-dose therapy to the prostate with an implant and moderate doses of EBRT to the regional tissues to sterilize micrometastatic disease. In this situation, an implant (110 Gy of I-131 or 100 Gy of Pd-104) usually either precedes or follows 20–45 Gy delivered to the pelvis. Some reports have suggested an increase in rectal toxicity with this approach; however, this is likely due to the poor quality of the implant. At least one study from a leading implant center suggested no significant increase in severe early or late GI/GU morbidity with combination therapy. The value of supplemental EBRT needs to be evaluated in comparison to full-dose EBRT in terms of long-term morbidity and cancer control.

High-dose–rate (HDR) devices Besides permanent implants, which deliver low-dose–rate (LDR) radiotherapy, brachytherapy for prostate cancer has been delivered using temporary high-dose–rate devices, usually in patients with locally advanced disease. In this technique, a high dose (minimum, approximately 5 Gy) is delivered to the prostate over ≤ 1 hour by remotely inserting a highly radioactive source into catheters placed into the prostate under ultrasonographic guidance while the patient is under anesthesia. Several treatments are given on separate occasions, and EBRT is used for approximately 5 weeks as well.

More reports are accumulating on the application of HDR brachytherapy to prostate cancer. Various dose-fractionation combinations of HDR with or without combined pelvic EBRT have been employed, with a dose-response relationship apparent in biochemical control. Although the follow-up is short and no prospective randomized trials evaluating this approach have yet been published, it appears that HDR prostate brachytherapy in combination with pelvic EBRT may be effective. The long-term consequences for normal tissue of delivering large doses per fraction using this technique are unclear.

MEDICATIONS AND DEVICES TO MANAGE IMPOTENCE AFTER PROSTATECTOMY, EBRT, OR BRACHYTHERAPY

Treatment for postprostatectomy impotence includes the phosphodiesterase inhibitors sildenafil, vardenafil (Levitra), and tadalafil (Cialis); prostaglandin E_1, administered as a urethral suppository (Muse); intercavernosal injection (Caverject, Edex); or vacuum-pump erection aids that are useful for improving erections in men who have poor erectile function after prostatectomy, radiation therapy, or brachytherapy. These therapies are effective in 15%–40% of men with postprostatectomy impotence and in 50%–75% of men with postradiotherapy erectile dysfunction. Insertion of a penile prosthesis is typically offered to patients only after unsuccessful trials with the previously mentioned, less invasive interventions.

DETECTION AND TREATMENT OF RECURRENCE

Significance and definition of a rising PSA level post irradiation

The use of PSA levels following definitive therapy (either radiotherapy or radical prostatectomy) can detect early recurrences that may be amenable to salvage treatment. A rising PSA profile following radiotherapy is unequivocal evidence of the presence of a residual prostatic neoplasm. However, the definition of a rising PSA level after radiation therapy varies in the literature. A 1996 consensus conference recommended that PSA failure be considered to have occurred after three consecutive PSA level rises, with the rate of failure defined as halfway between the first rise and the previous PSA level.

Moreover, patients with a rising PSA level after irradiation may be a heterogeneous group, including patients with truly localized failure as well as those with metastatic disease. Also, certain patients will have a slowly rising PSA level after irradiation and may not require additional treatment. In patients who do not receive androgen ablation, the 5-year actuarial risk of distant metastasis from the time that the PSA level begins to rise is ~50%. A rapidly emerging key concept in rising PSA levels is PSA velocity, or more specifically PSA doubling time. Multiple recent studies have found that a PSA doubling time < 10–12 months predicts early clinical relapse if biochemical recurrence is untreated.

Treatment recommendations for recurrence postirradiation

In general, men who have clear evidence of a rising PSA level 2 years after definitive radiotherapy for localized prostate cancer should be advised about the options of hormonal therapy (see section on "Treatment of locally advanced disease [T3, T4]"), salvage surgery, salvage cryotherapy, observation, or experimental therapy.

If patients have minimal comorbidity, good life expectancy, and only local evidence of disease recurrence, salvage surgery is an option but should be preceded by a bone scan, CT scan, cystoscopy, and extensive counseling because urinary

> Freedland et al have updated the Johns Hopkins PSA recurrence after radical prostatectomy series originally reported by Pound et al in 1999. In 379 men with biochemical (PSA only) recurrence, median survival had not been reached after 16 years of follow-up after this recurrence. Patients were risk-stratified for cancer-specific mortality based on PSA doubling time, pathologic Gleason score, and time from surgery to biochemical recurrence, and nomogram tables were constructed (*Freedland SJ, Humphreys EB, Mangold LA, et al: JAMA 294:433-439, 2005*).

difficulties after salvage prostatectomy are substantial and highly prevalent.

TREATMENT OF LOCALLY ADVANCED DISEASE (T3, T4)

The treatment of patients with locally advanced prostate cancer is centered on a multimodality and multidisciplinary approach, including radiation therapy (EBRT with or without HDR interstitial therapy), androgen ablation plus EBRT, or radical prostatectomy with or without androgen deprivation.

EBRT with and without HDR interstitial therapy For patients with locally extensive prostate cancer, local failure remains a potential problem after EBRT. This problem has prompted investigations into alternative means to intensify therapy.

One strategy has been to deliver large fractions of radiotherapy using HDR interstitial techniques in combination with EBRT. The large interstitial fractions, which may be on the order of 5 Gy, deliver a high dose to the prostate but spare normal tissues, due to the rapid dose falloff outside the implanted volume. Early experience with this strategy is encouraging, but long-term data on outcome, particularly in patients with locally extensive disease, and on morbidity are awaited.

Patients with locally advanced prostate cancer probably are not good candidates for permanent prostate implants. Patients with stage T3-T4 tumors are at high risk of gross extraprostatic involvement, and this localized therapy may not offer adequate dosimetric coverage of extraprostatic disease.

> RTOG 92-02 was designed to test the utility of long-term (24 months) androgen blockade compared with short-term (4 months) deprivation among men with locally advanced prostate cancer (T2c-T4). Among all randomized subjects, there was no overall survival benefit among those treated with long-term blockade. A secondary analysis demonstrated that a subset of men with a Gleason score of 8-10 experienced a survival benefit with long-term deprivation (81% vs 71% survival at 5 years, $P = .04$; *Hanks GE, Pajak TF, Porter A, et al: J Clin Oncol 21:3972-3978, 2004*).

As mentioned in the previous section, there may be a synergistic effect between hormonal therapy given in conjunction with radiation therapy. In addition to enhancing apoptosis and producing local cytoreduction, the use of early androgen deprivation may possibly delay or even prevent the development of metastatic disease.

The current body of evidence from two large randomized trials (RTOG 85-10 and EORTC) suggests that immediate long-term androgen deprivation in conjunction with EBRT improves outcomes among men with locally advanced or high-risk (Gleason score ≥ 8) prostate cancer compared with radiation therapy alone. An analysis of RTOG 85-31 by Horwitz et al, which employed early indefinite androgen deprivation, demonstrated that patients with locally advanced disease (T3N0) had improved cause-specific failure and distant metastatic failure compared with EBRT alone. Furthermore, a comparison to RTOG 86-10, which studied similar patients treated with only 4 months of hormonal therapy, favored the long-term approach. The EORTC trial randomized 415 patients and demonstrated a 15% overall survival benefit to 3 years of combined therapy versus radiation therapy alone.

Radical prostatectomy with or without adjuvant therapy

Surgical monotherapy can be considered a reasonable option for patients with locally advanced prostate cancer. Stage T3 disease can be successfully treated with low morbidity and significant reductions in risk of local recurrence, with clinical overstaging (up to 26%) reported by Yamada et al. Well- and moderately differentiated cancers have cancer-specific survival rates of 76% at 10 years, comparable to those of other treatment modalities.

The Mayo Clinic has one of the largest radical prostatectomy series for T3 disease, consisting of more than 1,000 patients. In this population, of whom 34% received adjuvant therapy, 15-year cancer-specific survival and local recurrence rates were 77% and 21%, respectively. Ninety-eight men who were found to have nodal metastases following radical prostatectomy and pelvic lymphadenectomy were randomized to receive immediate androgen deprivation or be followed until clinical disease progression. At a median follow-up of 7 years, 18 of 51 men in the observation group had died, compared with only 4 of 47 in the treatment group ($P = .02$).

Treatment of node-positive disease

Whether any local treatment adds to the overall survival duration in patients with known nodal involvement is debatable. Until recently, the standard of care had been to perform frozen-section pathologic analysis on pelvic lymph nodes at the time of radical prostatectomy, prior to removal of the prostate. If this analysis revealed micrometastases, radical prostatectomy was thought to be contraindicated. Although retrospective in nature, recent data from several American centers, including one large study from the Mayo Clinic, have reported a survival benefit in men who undergo radical prostatectomy despite the presence of micrometastases to regional pelvic lymph nodes. These men tend to do better and survive longer when started on early hormonal therapy, either with orchiectomy or an LHRH agonist.

Radiation therapy There are also compelling data that long-term survival is achievable in these patients with combination radiation and hormonal therapy. Data from the M. D. Anderson Cancer Center indicate a benefit to pelvic/prostate radiation therapy plus immediate hormonal manipulation compared with hormones alone. A subset analysis of patients with node-positive disease from RTOG 85-31 revealed immediate hormonal therapy plus radiation therapy resulted in 5- and 9-year cause-specific survival rates of 84% and 76%, respectively. Therefore, aggressive locoregional therapy appears to be effective in this cohort of unfavorable patients.

TABLE 4: Hormonal approaches to the treatment of advanced prostate cancer

Method	Mechanism of action	Side effects
Surgical castration	Removal of testicular androgens	Hot flashes (50%), psychological effects
Diethylstilbestrol (DES)	Inhibition of gonadotropin secretion	Gynecomastia, cardiovascular risks at high doses
LHRH analogs (goserelin, leuprolide)	Inhibition of gonadotropin secretion	Hot flashes (50%), less gynecomastia than with DES, fatigue
Antiandrogens (bicalutamide, flutamide, nilutamide)	Blockade of binding of dihydrotestosterone to its receptor	Abnormal liver function studies, diarrhea (10%)

LHRH = luteinizing hormone-releasing hormone

TREATMENT OF ADVANCED SYSTEMIC DISEASE

Defining advanced disease

Metastatic prostate cancer The most common sites of metastatic disease are the bone and pelvic and abdominal lymph nodes. Other, less common sites include the liver and lungs. Complications of metastatic prostate cancer include pain, fatigue, skeletal fractures, spinal cord compression, urinary outlet obstruction, and failure to thrive. First-line hormonal therapy for men with metastatic prostate cancer delays these complications.

Rising PSA level A large series of more than 2,000 patients treated with radical prostatectomy at Johns Hopkins University demonstrated that approximately 17% of cases recurred, with only 5.8% being local disease. In the remaining patients, disease recurred initially with either a rise in PSA level alone (9.7%) or evidence of clinical metastases (1.7%).

Outcomes for men with only a rising PSA level can vary greatly. Time to PSA recurrence (< vs > 2 years), PSA doubling time (< vs > 9 months), and Gleason score (8-10 vs 5-7) are among the important factors for predicting the development of metastatic disease and survival. The major developments for hormonal therapy in advanced prostate cancer were achieved prior to routine PSA testing and were often complicated by problematic study design. There are no prospective data that confirm a benefit to early hormonal therapy for men with a rising PSA alone. However, for patients with a rising PSA level who are at high risk for the development of metastases, some physicians agree that early hormonal therapy is likely to benefit this group of patients as well as those with radiologic evidence of metastatic disease.

First-line therapies for advanced disease

The standard first-line treatment of advanced prostate cancer, regardless of whether local treatment has been applied, is to ablate the action of androgens by medical or surgical means. For the majority of patients, androgen ablation can result in a decline in PSA level, palliation of disease-related symptoms, and regression of metastatic disease on imaging.

Petrylak and colleagues from the Southwest Oncology Group (SWOG) reported on 770 men with hormone-refractory prostate cancer (HRPC) randomized to receive mitoxantrone (Novantrone) plus prednisone vs docetaxel (Taxotere) plus estramustine (Emcyt) plus dexamethasone. The docetaxel arm had improved survival by a median of 2 months, showing for the first time that a chemotherapy drug could extend survival in HRPC. A second trial by Eisenberger et al showed a similar survival benefit of docetaxel with prednisone given on an every-3-week schedule (*Petrylak D, Tangen C, Hussain M, et al: N Engl J Med 351:1513-1520, 2004*).

Bilateral orchiectomy The advantages of orchiectomy over other means of castration include an immediate decline in testosterone levels and ease of compliance for patients. Given these advantages, however, many men still opt for medical castration, with the potential advantage of intermittent hormonal therapy. In addition, the psychological impact of orchiectomy can be significant. Nonetheless, bilateral orchiectomy may be appropriate for a select group of patients.

LHRH analogs LHRH agonists, such as leuprolide and goserelin (Zoladex), interfere with the normal pulsatile secretion of LH from the pituitary gland, resulting in an eventual decline in serum testosterone levels. The effect is reversible with cessation of therapy. Because LH is initially increased with LHRH agonists, testosterone levels may actually increase initially as well. This finding can result in a transient rise in PSA levels and potential growth of metastatic sites. Because of this initial "flare response" with LHRH agonists, consideration should be given to the administration of an antiandrogen prior to the LHRH, especially in patients who are at risk for complications from the disease (such as spinal cord compression, worsening pain, or urinary outlet obstruction; Table 4).

A pure LHRH antagonist (abarelix [Plenaxis]) has been approved by the FDA. Its main advantage is the lack of an LHRH surge or flare, and it is indicated in men with impending spinal cord compression or other now uncommon clinical scenarios where a flare could be harmful. However, this drug must be administered every 2 weeks in the first month and monthly thereafter. Also, it can rarely be associated with an anaphylactic reaction.

Antiandrogens Antiandrogens function to block the binding of dihydrotestosterone (DHT) to the androgen receptor, blocking the translocation of the DHT-androgen receptor complex into the nuclei of cells. There are two general classes: steroidal and nonsteroidal. Steroidal antiandrogens include cyproterone and megestrol. The most commonly used antiandrogens include the nonsteroidal agents flutamide, bicalutamide (Casodex), and nilutamide (Nilandron). These agents differ slightly in their affinity for the androgen receptor and their side-effect profiles.

Typically, antiandrogens are used in combination with surgical or medical castration. Some trials comparing antiandrogens alone with LHRH analogs have shown similar efficacy, but more recent trials suggest that monotherapy with antiandrogens may be inferior in terms of time to disease progression and possibly survival. For example, a randomized trial of monotherapy with high-dose bicalutamide (150 mg daily) compared with flutamide plus goserelin demonstrated that patients treated with bicalutamide monotherapy had fewer side effects, such as loss of libido or erectile dysfunction, and trended toward improved quality of life. However, in patients with radiographic evidence of metastases, bicalutamide monotherapy was associated with a small 6-week decrease in survival (hazard ratio, 1.3). Despite this finding, for men who are intolerant to the side effects of LHRH analogs, monotherapy with antiandrogens can be considered after careful discussion with patients.

Antiandrogen monotherapy with flutamide or bicalutamide is also sometimes used to treat PSA recurrence. Used alone or in combination with a 5-alpha reductase inhibitor (finasteride or dutasteride), this approach is associated with fewer side effects than traditional androgen suppression therapy, but the approches have not been approved by the US FDA. A significant downside is nipple tenderness or gynecomastia, but this "peripheral blockade" approach may preserve potency and libido.

Combined androgen blockade Combined androgen blockade (CAB) refers to the elimination of testicular androgens in combination with blockade of adrenal androgens, generally with an LHRH analog and an antiandrogen agent. The use of CAB is somewhat controversial. Several randomized trials comparing LHRH antagonists alone versus CAB have demonstrated a survival benefit with CAB. However, in one of the largest trials conducted by the United States Intergroup, more than 1,300 men were randomized to undergo orchiectomy versus orchiectomy plus flutamide. There was no significant advantage to CAB in terms of time to disease progression or overall survival. Some investigators believe that bicalutamide, a more potent agent, may be associated with greater survival when used as part of CAB.

Many investigators believe that the advantages observed in trials that include an LHRH antagonist exist because of the "flare phenomenon," which occurs with LHRH antagonists alone and may be lost with a short period of treatment with antiandrogens during the expected flare period. The American Society of Clinical Oncology does not recommend the routine use of CAB over monotherapy with an LHRH antagonist or orchiectomy.

Diethylstilbestrol (DES) Estrogen administration, in the form of DES, also produces chemical castration. DES inhibits prostate growth, primarily through the inhibition of the hypothalamic-pituitary-gonadal axis, which blocks testicular synthesis of testosterone and thus lowers plasma testosterone levels. Since doses higher than 3 mg/d cause significant cardiovascular mortality, DES has fallen out of favor as a first-line therapy to induce castration.

Ketoconazole (Nizoral) Ketoconazole is an antifungal agent that can inhibit adrenal and testicular steroid synthesis at higher doses, leading to a decline in adrenal and testicular androgens. It has the benefit of a rapid decline in test-

TABLE 5: The incidence of complications from advanced prostate cancer with immediate vs deferred androgen deprivation

Complication	Immediate	Deferred
Pathologic fracture	2.3%	4.5%
Spinal cord compression	2.0%	5.0%
Ureteric obstruction	7.0%	11.8%
Extraskeletal metastases	7.9%	11.8%

osterone, which can be useful for patients who present emergently with a complication of newly diagnosed advanced disease. Ketoconazole is started at a dose of 200 mg three times daily and increased to a total dose of 400 mg three times daily. Ketoconazole is associated with significant side effects (such as fatigue, nausea, and vomiting), however, and must be given with supplemental hydrocortisone to avoid symptoms of adrenal insufficiency. Because of the side effects, its use is more common in the second-line setting, where responses can be expected in 20%–40% of patients following progression with CAB.

Early vs late treatment Whether to treat patients early with hormonal therapy or wait until patients become symptomatic has been tested in a large European trial conducted by the Medical Research Council. Men were randomized to receive immediate hormonal therapy (orchiectomy or an LHRH analog) versus delayed therapy which was initiated with symptomatic progression. Men who were treated with early therapy were less likely to experience urinary obstructive symptoms requiring intervention, pathologic fractures, and cord compression than those treated in the delayed arm (Table 5). The survival benefit was less clear, however, because many of the men in the delayed arm died before they received any hormonal therapy. This study was also complicated by the initiation of PSA monitoring during the study period. Many patients and physicians currently are not comfortable delaying therapy until the onset of symptoms while the PSA level is rising; this fact limits the applicability of its findings in the modern era.

Other smaller trials have examined this issue as well. A Cochrane Database review was conducted in 2002; it demonstrated an increase in progression-free survival and a small, but significant, improvement in survival with early hormonal therapy.

Treatment recommendations Just as for localized disease, initial treatment for advanced prostate cancer must be individualized. A patient who presents with a rising PSA level only after local treatment and a slow PSA doubling time, a prolonged time to PSA recurrence, and a low initial Gleason score may not require immediate therapy, especially if there are other more significant comorbidities. However, a patient with multiple metastatic sites will need immediate treatment, generally with orchiectomy or CAB initially followed by monotherapy with an LHRH analog, to prevent the sequelae of metastatic disease, such as fracture, spinal cord compression, and ureteral obstruction. Ketoconazole may be considered as the initial systemic therapy for patients presenting with cord compression as the first presentation of prostate cancer. Given the overall limitations of hormone therapy, all appropriate patients should be offered access to clinical trials.

For patients with a rising PSA level who are at high risk for the development of metastases, a discussion regarding the potential advantages to early treatment and an explanation of the lack of randomized prospective data are warranted. Some investigators favor early treatment for these patients based on the data from the Medical Research Council trial and the Cochrane Database review, understanding that this information is extrapolated from data obtained prior to PSA testing and from patients with clinical and radiographic metastases.

Second-line hormonal therapies

Outcomes with initial androgen ablation can vary from responses that last from months to years; they also vary as a function of the Gleason grade, pretreatment PSA velocity, and extent of disease at the time of initiating treatment. Once PSA levels begin to rise with androgen ablation, the disease is often referred to as "hormone refractory." This term is actually a misnomer, because preclinical data suggest that tumors may become hypersensitive to androgens, resulting in worsened disease if androgen ablation is removed entirely. Moreover, many patients have disease that remains sensitive to further hormonal manipulations, such as second-line antiandrogens, steroids, or ketoconazole.

An example of this sensitivity to hormonal manipulation is exemplified in the antiandrogen withdrawal response. Up to one-third of patients with a rising PSA level while receiving treatment with an antiandrogen will have a decline in PSA level and or clinical regression with antiandrogen withdrawal. The mechanism of this response has not been fully elucidated but supports the hypothesis that the androgen receptor remains important in progressive disease.

Although second-line hormonal therapy has demonstrated benefit in terms of PSA levels and response, there are no data to demonstrate a survival advantage with second-line hormonal therapy. Its role has further come into question, with data that support the use of docetaxel (Taxotere) chemotherapy for men with metastatic androgen-independent prostate cancer to improve survival. It is unknown whether the survival benefit with docetaxel is limited after multiple hormonal therapies.

For patients with a rising PSA level only, timing of chemotherapy is even less clear. The Eastern Cooperative Oncology Group attempted a trial comparing ketoconazole/hydrocortisone with docetaxel in patients with a rising PSA level but no evidence of metastatic disease after hormonal therapy, but the trial was closed early due to lack of accrual. Until prospective data are available, physicians will need to counsel patients carefully on the different options and timing of those options available at the time of progression, including second-line hormonal manipulation, chemotherapy, and especially clinical trials.

TABLE 6: Chemotherapy regimens for prostate cancer

Drug/combination	Dose and schedule
Mitoxantrone/prednisone	
Mitoxantrone	12 mg/m^2 IV on day 1
Prednisone	5 mg PO bid
Repeat cycle every 21 days.	
Tannock IF, Osoba D, Stockler MR, et al: J Clin Oncol 14:1756–1764, 1996.	
Docetaxel/estramustine	
Docetaxel	60 mg/m^2 on day 2 every 21 days
Estramustine	280 mg orally on days 1 to 5 every 21 days
Dexamethasone	60 mg orally given as a premedication before docetaxel
Petrylak DP, Tangen CM, Hussain MHA, et al: N Engl J Med 351:1513–1520, 2004.	
Docetaxel/prednisone	
Docetaxel	75 mg/m^2 IV every 3 weeks
Prednisone	5 mg orally twice daily started on day 1
Note: Standard docetaxel premedication should be given prior to the administration of docetaxel	
Tannock IF, de Wit R, Berry WR, et al: N Engl J Med 351:1502–1512, 2004.	

Table prepared by Ishmael Jaiyesimi, DO

Chemotherapy for androgen-independent disease

Docetaxel The role of chemotherapy has changed significantly over the past several years with the results of two large randomized trials demonstrating a survival benefit for men with androgen-independent metastatic prostate cancer treated with docetaxel-based chemotherapy (Table 6). Investigators from the Southwest Oncology Group randomized patients to receive mitoxantrone (Novantrone) plus prednisone versus docetaxel (60 mg/m^2) plus estramustine and dexamethasone every 3 weeks. Patients in the docetaxel arm had a significant improvement in survival by 2 months.

A second trial by Tannock et al showed a similar survival benefit of 2 months with docetaxel (75 mg/m^2) plus prednisone given every 3 weeks compared with mitoxantrone and prednisone. These trials were the first to demonstrate a survival benefit with chemotherapy in advanced prostate cancer and have sparked numerous studies involving docetaxel in combination with newer agents. Toxicities of docetaxel include myelosuppression and neuropathy, both of which can be dose-limiting.

Mitoxantrone plus prednisone Mitoxantrone (12 mg/m^2) plus prednisone has been approved for use in advanced prostate cancer based on improvement in palliation of pain and quality of life over prednisone alone despite no improvement in overall survival.

The epothilones are a new class of antimicrotubule agents active in both taxane-sensitive and taxane-resistant prostate cancer models. Two phase II trials with ixabepilone have been reported. SWOG 0111 demonstrated post-treatment confirmed PSA responses of 33%, and 72% had declines over 80%. The estimated mean progression-free survival is 6 months (95% CI, 4-8 months), and the median overall survival is 18 months (95% CI, 13-24 months; *Hussain M, Tangen CM, Lara PN, et al J Clin Oncol 23:8724-8729, 2005*). In the second study, post-treatment declines in PSA response of $\geq$ 50% were seen in 48% of men treated with ixabepilone alone and 69% of men treated with ixabepilone in combination with estramustine (Emcyt). In patients with measurable disease, partial responses were observed in 32% and 48%, respectively (*Galsky MD, Small EJ, Oh WK, et. al: J Clin Oncol 23:1439-1446, 2005*). A randomized phase II trial evaluating ixabepilone and mitoxantrone in the second-line setting post docetaxel therapy has completed accrual, and a large phase III trial is being planned.

Bisphosphonates Bone metastases from prostate cancer are associated with increased bone formation around tumor deposits, resulting in characteristic osteoblastic metastases. However, concomitant with the osteoblastic activity is a marked increase in bone resorption and osteolysis, which can be inhibited by bisphosphonates.

Studies of bisphosphonates in prostate cancer have demonstrated mixed results. A combined analysis of two multicentered randomized controlled trials comparing pamidronate with placebo in men with androgen-independent progressive prostate cancer demonstrated no benefit in terms of skeleton-related events or palliation of symptoms. A phase III trial with an oral bisphosphonate, clodronate, demonstrated no difference in either symptomatic bone metastases or prostate cancer-related deaths when compared with placebo.

A phase III trial demonstrated a reduction in skeleton-related events for men with androgen-independent metastatic prostate cancer with a more potent bisphosphonate, zoledronic acid (Zometa). However, it is important to note that this trial did not show an improvement in quality of life with zoledronic acid, nor did it demonstrate a reduction in the development of new metastases.

At this time, the recommendation for zoledronic acid in prostate cancer is limited to men with androgen-independent prostate cancer. It is important to recognize the limitations of this therapy and to understand that there is no defined role for its use in men with androgen-dependent prostate cancer. Although these men are at higher risk for osteoporosis, less potent oral bisphosphonates may be a more reasonable approach, given the long-term side effects associated with zoledronic acid (renal insufficiency and osteonecrosis of the mandible).

Newer therapies

Several new therapies for men with prostate cancer (some as single agents and some with chemotherapy) are under investigation, with promising early results. They include the endothelin receptor antagonist atrasentan, vitamin D_3 (calcitriol), the VEGF inhibitor bevacizumab (Avastin), and a new class of antimicrotubule agents (the epothilones). There are ample preclinical and early clinical data to suggest that all of these agents may have activity against prostate cancer, but no definitive trials to establish their role have yet been performed. These agents are still considered investigational. Several trials are evaluating the combinations of docetaxel and bevacizumab, docetaxel and atrasentan, and docetaxel and a vaccine.

Radiation therapy for palliating bone metastasis

Radiotherapy is effective in controlling local pain associated with skeletal prostate metastasis. In general, a treatment regimen of 30 Gy over 10 treatments results in rapid and durable local symptom control and a reduced dependence on analgesics.

For patients with more extensive bone involvement causing pain that may be difficult to address with localized EBRT, alternatives include wide-field irradiation (ie, hemibody irradiation) or systemic administration of radioactive bone-seeking isotopes that can deliver therapeutic doses to skeletal metastatic disease. Radioactive isotopes used in this fashion include strontium-89 chloride (Metastron) and samarium SM 153 lexidronam (Quadramet). A more detailed discussion of these approaches can be found in chapter 37.

SUGGESTED READING

Albertsen PC, Hanley JA, Fine J, et al: 20-year outcomes following conservative management of clinically localized prostate cancer. JAMA 293:2095–2101, 2005.

Bill-Axelson A, Holmberg L, Ruutu M, et al: Radical prostatectomy versus watchful waiting in early prostate cancer. N Engl J Med 352:1977–1984, 2005.

D'Amico AV, Chen MH, Roehl KA, et al: Preoperative PSA velocity and the risk of death from prostate cancer after radical prostatectomy. N Engl J Med 351:125–135, 2004.

D'Amico AV, Moul JW, Carroll PR, et al: Cancer-specific mortality after surgery or radiation for patients with clinically localized prostate cancer managed during the prostate-specific antigen era. J Clin Oncol 21:2163–2172, 2003.

D'Amico AV, Moul JW, Carroll PR, et al: Surrogate end point for prostate cancer-specific mortality after radical prostatectomy or radiation therapy. J Natl Cancer Inst 95:1376–1383, 2003.

D'Amico AV, Renshaw AA, Sussman B, et al: Pretreatment PSA velocity and risk of death from prostate cancer following external beam radiation therapy. JAMA 294:440–447, 2005.

Freedland SJ, Humphreys EB, Mangold LA, et al: Risk of prostate cancer-specific mortality following biochemical recurrence after radical prostatectomy. JAMA 294:433–439, 2005.

Lawton CA, Winter K, Grignon D, et al: Androgen suppression plus radiation versus radiation alone for patients with stage D1/pathologic node-positive adenocarcinoma of the prostate: Updated results based on national prospective randomized trial Radiation Therapy Oncology Group 85-31. J Clin Oncol 23:800–807, 2005.

Moul JW, Wu H, Sun L, et al: Early versus delayed hormonal therapy for prostate specific antigen only recurrence of prostate cancer after radical prostatectomy. J Urol 171:1141–1147, 2004.

Sharifi N, Gulley JL, Dahut WL: Androgen deprivation therapy for prostate cancer. JAMA 294:238–244, 2005.

Smith MR, Kabbinavar F, Saad F, et al: Natural history of rising serum prostate-specific antigen in men with castrate nonmetastatic prostate cancer. J Clin Oncol 23:2918–2925, 2005.

Stephenson AJ, Shariat SF, Zelefsky MJ, et al: Salvage radiotherapy for recurrent prostate cancer after radical prostatectomy. JAMA 291:1325–1332, 2004.

Thompson IM, Ankerst DP, Chi C, et al: Operating characteristics of prostate-specific antigen in men with an initial PSA level of 3.0 ng/ml or lower. JAMA 294:66–70, 2005.

Thompson IM, Pauler DK, Goodman PJ, et al: Prevalence of prostate cancer among men with a prostate-specific antigen level < or = 4.0 ng per milliliter. N Engl J Med 350:2239–2246, 2004.

CHAPTER 18

Testicular cancer

Patrick J. Loehrer, MD, Thomas E. Ahlering, MD,
Mark K. Buyyounouski, MD, and Douglas Skarecky, BS

TESTICULAR

Testicular cancer, although an uncommon malignancy, is the most frequently occurring cancer in young men. In the year 2007, an estimated 7,920 cases of testicular cancer will be diagnosed in the United States. For unknown reasons, the incidence of this cancer has increased since the turn of the century, from 2 cases per 100,000 population in the 1930s, to 3.7 cases per 100,000 population from 1969 to 1971, to 5.4 cases per 100,000 population from 1995–1999. The greatest rise has been observed in Puerto Rico (1973–1997: 220%). This trend seems greatest for the development of seminoma.

Most testicular tumors are of germ-cell origin. These cancers are uniquely sensitive to chemotherapy and are considered the model for the treatment of solid tumors. Perhaps the most controversial area in the management of germ-cell tumors is the proper approach to early-stage disease (ie, surveillance vs primary lymphadenectomy [for nonseminoma germ-cell tumors] or radiation therapy [for seminomas]). In advanced disease, chemotherapy plays an essential role, but novel treatment regimens are currently being evaluated through multi-institution clinical trials.

Epidemiology

Age Testicular cancer can occur at any age but is most common between the ages of 15 and 35 years. There is a secondary peak in incidence after age 60. Seminoma is the most common histology in the older population but is rare in those younger than age 10.

Race Although testicular cancer is rare in African-Americans (1.6/100,000 population), these men present with higher grade disease and have significantly worse survival at 5 and 10 years. The incidence of this cancer has increased in whites during the 20th century but has remained flat in African-Americans.

Geography Denmark has the highest incidence of testicular cancer; the Far East has the lowest.

Primary site Germ-cell tumors present most commonly in the testis (90%) and only infrequently in extragonadal sites (10%). The most common extragonadal sites (in decreasing order of frequency) are the retroperitoneum, mediastinum, and pineal gland. Many patients presumed to have a primary retroperitoneal germ-cell tumor may have an occult germ-cell tumor of the testicle. This possibility should be evaluated with testicular ultrasonography, especially when the retroperitoneal tumor is predominantly one-sided.

TABLE 1: Anticipated cure rates in patients with germ-cell tumors, according to disease stage

Stage	Incidence at presentation (%)	Cure rate (%)
I (testis alone)	40	100
II (extension to retroperitoneal lymph nodes)	40	98
III (disseminated disease)	20	80

Survival The 5-year survival rate for all patients with testicular cancer is ~95%. Cure rates are highest for early-stage disease, which is treated primarily with surgery or radiation therapy (early seminoma), and lower for advanced disease, for which chemotherapy is the primary therapy (Table 1).

Etiology and risk factors

The specific cause of germ-cell tumors is unknown, but various factors have been associated with an increased risk of this malignancy.

Prior testicular cancer Perhaps the strongest risk factor for germ-cell tumors is a history of testicular cancer. Approximately 1%–2% of patients with testicular cancer will develop a second primary in the contralateral testis over time. This represents a 500-fold increase in incidence over that in the normal male population.

Cryptorchidism Patients with cryptorchidism have a 20- to 40-fold increased risk of developing germ-cell tumors compared with their normal counterparts. Orchiopexy, even at an early age, appears to reduce the incidence of germ-cell tumor only slightly (if at all). Of note, in ~10% of patients with cryptorchidism who develop germ-cell tumors, the cancer is found in the normally descended testis. Biopsies of nonenlarged cryptorchid testes demonstrate an increased incidence of intratubal germ-cell neoplasm, a presumed precursor lesion.

Genetics Klinefelter's syndrome (47XXY) is associated with a higher incidence of germ-cell tumors, particularly primary mediastinal germ-cell tumors. For first-degree relatives of individuals affected with 47XXY, approximately a 6- to 10-fold increased risk for germ-cell tumors has been observed. In addition, patients with Down's syndrome have been reported to be at increased risk for germ-cell

The risk of contralateral testicular cancer was studied in a large population-based cohort of men diagnosed with testicular cancer before age 55 years. For 29,515 cases reported from 1973 through 2001 to the National Cancer Institute's Surveillance, Epidemiology, and End Results Program, the 15-year cumulative risk of developing a metachronous contralateral testicular cancer was 1.9%, reaffirming the practice of not performing a biopsy on the contralateral testis at initial presentation *(Fossa SD, Chen J, Schonfeld SJ, et al: J Natl Cancer Inst 97:1056-1066, 2005).*

tumors. Also thought to be at greater risk are patients with testicular feminization, true hermaphrodites, persistent müllerian syndrome, and cutaneous ichthyosis.

Family history Although familial testicular cancer has been observed, the incidence among first-degree relatives remains low. One investigator, however, reported a sixfold increased risk among male offspring of a patient with testicular cancer.

Environment Numerous industrial occupations and drug exposures have been implicated in the development of testicular cancer. Although exposure to diethylstilbestrol (DES) in utero is associated with cryptorchidism, a direct association between DES and germ-cell neoplasm is weak at best.

Reports have suggested an increased risk of testicular cancer among individuals exposed to exogenous toxins, such as Agent Orange and solvents used to clean jets. One author has suggested that based on epidemiologic evidence, ochratoxin A correlated with incidence data for testicular cancer.

Prior trauma, elevated scrotal temperature (secondary to the use of thermal underwear, jockey shorts, and electric blankets), and recurrent activities, such as horseback riding and motorcycle riding, do not appear to be related to the development of testicular cancer.

No supporting findings substantiate a viral etiology.

Fertility An increased risk of infertility exists for men with unilateral testicular cancer successfully treated with orchiectomy. For example, 40% of patients have subnormal sperm counts, and by 1 year, 25% continue to have subnormal sperm counts.

Signs and symptoms

Local disease

Scrotal mass The most common complaint of patients on presentation is a painless scrotal mass, which, on physical examination, cannot be separated from the testis. This finding distinguishes the mass from epididymitis. Not infrequently, the mass may be painful and thus may mimic epididymitis or testicular torsion.

Hydrocele Approximately 20% of patients with germ-cell tumors have an associated hydrocele.

Inguinal adenopathy Patients generally do not have inguinal adenopathy in the absence of prior scrotal violation.

Other symptoms include low back pain (from retroperitoneal adenopathy) and gynecomastia (usually bilateral). In cases of massive retroperitoneal lymphadenopathy, abdominal pain, nausea, vomiting, and constipation may be reported.

Disseminated disease

Patients with disseminated germ-cell tumors usually present with symptoms from lymphatic or hematogenous dissemination. Mediastinal adenopathy may be associated with chest pain or cough. Supraclavicular lymphadenopathy may also be present.

The cumulative 10-year risk of developing metachronous testicular cancer for patients with extragonadal germ-cell tumors is 10.3%. Patients with extragonadal tumors of the retroperitoneum and nonseminomatous cell type have a 14.3% 10-year risk for the development of metachronous testicular cancer.

Hematogenous spread to the lungs may be associated with dyspnea, cough, or hemoptysis. Infrequently, patients with extensive disease may present with signs and symptoms of CNS metastases or bone pain from osseous metastases (most common in patients with seminoma).

Metastases to the liver are not uncommon and may manifest as fullness in the upper abdomen or vague abdominal discomfort. More likely, they will be identified on CT scan in an otherwise asymptomatic patient.

Primary mediastinal germ-cell tumors

Primary mediastinal germ-cell tumors are associated with several unique syndromes, including Klinefelter's syndrome and acute megakaryocytic leukemia. In addition, mediastinal tumors have a great propensity for the development of non–germ-cell malignant histology as a major component of the tumor (eg, embryonal rhabdomyosarcoma, adenocarcinoma, and peripheral neuroectodermal tumor).

Screening and diagnosis

Screening

Self-examination Testicular self-examination is both simple to learn and safe to perform. The rarity of this disease, however, calls into question the value of routine aggressive screening procedures.

Testicular biopsy Testicular biopsy of a suspicious lesion is not recommended. Approximately 95% of patients with a mass within the testicle have a malignancy. Orchiectomy is the preferred treatment for patients with a testicular mass.

Carcinoma in situ (CIS) appears to be the precursor lesion for most testicular germ-cell tumors, except spermatocytic seminoma. Most patients harboring CIS can be expected to develop testicular cancer but with a latency period of a decade or more. The incidence of CIS in infertile men is about 0.6%. In pa-

> Virtually all adult patients with germ-cell tumors have increased copies of isochromosome 12p, usually as i(12p). This is a useful marker in patients with undifferentiated tumors who fit the clinical profile of patients with germ-cell malignancy. Kit mutations have also been observed in seminoma, especially of primary mediastinal origin. The clinical significance of this observation is unknown at present.

tients with prior testicular cancer, biopsy will reveal CIS in the contralateral testis at a rate of ~5%–6%. Men with a history of cryptorchidism and presumed extragonadal germ-cell tumor are at greater risk for CIS. Some investigators suggest routine biopsy of the contralateral testis in men with CIS.

Diagnosis

Ultrasonography can reliably identify masses within the testis. In virtually all patients, ultrasonography can distinguish a testicular from an extratesticular mass and may detect lesions that are not palpable on physical examination. Ultrasonographic findings cannot consistently differentiate benign from malignant tumors of the testis (95% of such masses are malignant). Most patients with testicular cancer, especially seminoma, have hypoechoic lesions compared to adjacent tissue. Nonseminomatous tumors, however, may have mixed signals, including hyperechoic masses, which are commonly seen with teratoma.

Serum markers Serum levels of β-subunit human chorionic gonadotropin (β-hCG) and α-fetoprotein (AFP) are elevated in ~80%–85% of patients with extensive germ-cell tumors. Patients with pure seminoma may have elevated levels of β-hCG but not AFP (a significantly elevated AFP level usually indicates the presence of nonseminomatous germ-cell elements). False-positive β-hCG levels can be seen in patients who have hypogonadism (cross-reactivity with luteinizing hormone) or who pursue the use of marijuana; AFP levels may be elevated in patients with liver dysfunction or hepatitis.

Inguinal orchiectomy When a testicular mass is discovered, the patient should undergo an orchiectomy through an inguinal incision.

Trans-scrotal incisions or biopsies should not be performed, as they ultimately lead to aberrant lymphatic drainage from the tumor.

Staging evaluation

The principal objective of the staging evaluation is to ascertain whether the patient has early-stage disease (which is amenable to local therapy, such as retroperitoneal lymphadenectomy [for nonseminoma] or radiation therapy [for seminoma]) or disseminated disease (which requires chemotherapy).

Chest x-ray A chest x-ray can determine whether or not a patient has gross supradiaphragmatic metastases, which would mandate initial chemotherapy.

Chest CT In patients with a normal chest x-ray, chest CT is recommended in both patients with seminoma and those with nonseminoma when abdominal adenopathy is found, to rule out occult metastases within the lungs or mediastinum. If such metastases are present, the patient should be treated with primary chemotherapy.

Abdominopelvic CT provides important information about the retroperitoneal lymph nodes. Usually, periaortic adenopathy is noted on the ipsilateral side of the primary tumor. Patients with primary retroperitoneal germ-cell tumors often show an enlarged retroperitoneal mass in the midline. Although hepatic metastases are infrequent, at present, CT is the most viable method of determining these metastatic lesions.

PET [18]Fluorodeoxyglucose (FDG)-PET is emerging as a significant adjunct in staging and follow-up. Seminomas are FDG-avid. In some cases, nodal and extranodal metastases not appreciated on CT scans may be noted with FDG-PET. The optimal use of FDG-PET is in patients with residual masses following systemic therapy for pure seminoma. In such cases, the scans should be performed at least 3–4 weeks beyond the last course of chemotherapy.

Other scans In the absence of symptoms or signs, a CT scan (or MRI) of the head and radionuclide bone scan are unnecessary. A lymphangiogram is rarely used today to identify microscopic nodal involvement in patients with stage I disease who choose to undergo surveillance. PET scans may be useful in patients with residual disease following chemotherapy for seminoma. If a PET scan is positive in such patients, surgical resection of the residual mass is indicated. Otherwise, the residual mass can be simply followed with periodic radiographic evaluation.

Pathology

Germ-cell tumors are classified into two broad histologic categories: seminoma and nonseminomatous germ-cell tumor (NSGCT). Patients with seminoma who have increased AFP levels or any focus of NSGCT components (including teratoma) are considered to have an NSGCT.

TABLE 2: Staging systems for testicular cancer

Royal Marsden system	TNM system	Description
I	Tx, N0, M0	Disease confined to the testis and peritesticular tissue
II	Tx, N1 or N2a,M0	Fewer than six positive lymph nodes without extension into retroperitoneal fat; no node > 2 cm (infradiaphragmatic)
A < 2 cm B 2-5 cm C > 5-10 cm D > 10 cm		
	Tx, N2b, M0	Six or more positive lymph nodes, well-encapsulated and/or retroperitoneal fat extension; any node > 2 cm
	Tx, N3, M0	Any node > 5 cm
III	Tx, Nx, M1	Supradiaphragmatic and infradiaphragmatic adenopathy (no extralymphatic metastasis)
IV		Disseminated disease (lungs, liver, bone)

Seminoma

Seminoma is the most common single histology, accounting for ~30% of all germ-cell tumors. Up to 10% of seminomas have focal syncytiotrophoblastic cells, thought to be the source of β-hCG in some cases. Elevated AFP levels connote NSGCT.

Spermatocytic seminoma, a rare subset of germ-cell tumors, often grows to large size, occurs almost exclusively in men older than age 50, and rarely, if ever, metastasizes.

Nonseminoma

Embryonal carcinoma is composed of large pleomorphic cells with different architectural patterns. This tumor may be associated with an elevation in the serum levels of β-hCG and/or AFP.

Endodermal sinus tumor (yolk sac carcinoma) is the most common testicular tumor seen in infants and young children. Like embryonal carcinoma, yolk sac tumor has a variety of architectural patterns. This tumor is associated with an elevated serum level of AFP.

Choriocarcinoma, as a pure entity, is one of the least common germ-cell tumors. These tumors have a great propensity for hematogenous spread, often skipping the retroperitoneum. Choriocarcinoma is associated with an increased serum level of β-hCG.

Teratoma is a generally benign tumor with elements from each of the germ layers (ectoderm, mesoderm, and endoderm). Teratoma is uncommonly seen as the sole histology in primary tumors, but it is frequently associated with other histologic elements, including those previously mentioned. Of patients with residual disease following chemotherapy for NSGCT, ~45% have teratoma in resected specimens.

A subset of patients with immature teratoma that contains non–germ-cell histologies (eg, sarcoma, adenocarcinoma) has been reported. In contrast to most teratomas, these tumors may grow locally and can be lethal. In addition, late recurrences of both teratoma and carcinoma have been reported in patients with teratoma. Serum markers are normal in patients with pure teratoma.

Pattern of spread

Testicular cancer spreads in a fairly predictable fashion: from the testicle to the retroperitoneal lymph nodes and later hematogenously to the lungs or other visceral sites. Only 10% of patients present with hematogenous metastases (usually in the lungs) in the absence of discernible retroperitoneal adenopathy.

Staging systems

Clinical staging systems (Royal Marsden and TNM systems) for testicular cancer are outlined in Table 2. These staging systems help define the population for appropriate primary therapy.

TABLE 3: International Germ-Cell Collaborative Group Consensus Conference criteria for good- and poor-risk testicular cancer patients treated with chemotherapy

NONSEMINOMA

Good prognosis

All of the following:

- AFP < 1,000 ng/mL, β-hCG < 5,000 IU/L, and LDH < 1.5 × upper limit of normal
- Nonmediastinal primary
- No nonpulmonary visceral metastasis

Intermediate prognosis

All of the following:

- AFP = 1,000-10,000 ng/mL, β-hCG = 5,000-50,000 IU/L, or LDH = 1.5-10 × normal
- Nonmediastinal primary site
- No nonpulmonary visceral metastasis

Poor prognosis

Any of the following:

- AFP > 10,000 ng/mL, β-hCG > 50,000 IU/L, or LDH > 10 × normal
- Mediastinal primary site
- Nonpulmonary visceral metastasis

SEMINOMA

Good prognosis

- No nonpulmonary visceral metastasis

Intermediate prognosis

- Nonpulmonary visceral metastasis

AFP = α-fetoprotein; hCG = human chorionic gonadotropin; LDH = lactic dehydrogenase

Organ-sparing surgery for testicular cancer may represent a means of preserving testicular function in highly selected patients. Patients with synchronous bilateral testicular tumors or tumors in a solitary testis may be considered for this alternative. The lesions must be < 20 mm, and there must be no evidence of metastasis. Postoperative radiotherapy for carcinoma in situ is necessary to prevent recurrence *(Yossepowitch O, Baniel J: Urology 63:421-427, 2004).*

Good- and poor-risk subgroups For patients with nonseminomas who are candidates for chemotherapy, other staging systems (such as those by Indiana University and Memorial Sloan-Kettering Cancer Center) were developed to segregate patients into good- and poor-risk categories. More recently, the International Germ-Cell Collaborative Group Consensus Conference formulated a classification that more clearly defines good- and poor-risk disease (Table 3), and it is currently being used to stratify patients in ongoing trials.

Treatment

SURGICAL TREATMENT OF STAGE I OR II DISEASE

Initial intervention for testicular cancer is radical inguinal orchiectomy. Orchiectomy may be deferred temporarily in patients with advanced-stage disease in whom the diagnosis of NSGCT can be made on clinical grounds (elevated markers). In such patients, an orchiectomy must be performed sooner or later, as there is incomplete penetration of chemotherapy into the testes.

Laparoscopic retroperitoneal lymphadenectomy was performed in 185 patients with clinical stage I-IIC disease. With a mean follow-up of 55 months, there were no deaths due to disease or surgical complications. There were no in-field recurrences, and even patients with postchemotherapy masses were successfully treated. Postoperative complications were reduced, and patients experienced less pain and returned to normal activities quicker *(Steiner H, Peschel R, Janetschek G, et al: Urology 63:550-555, 2004)*.

Further therapy hinges on the pathologic diagnosis. In general, pure seminomas (normal AFP level with or without an elevated β-hCG level) are treated with radiotherapy and/or chemotherapy, whereas most nonseminomas are treated with surgery and/or chemotherapy.

Inguinal orchiectomy

In addition to removal of the testis, the spermatic cord is dissected high into the retroperitoneum. The vas deferens is isolated from the testicular vessels and ligated separately with a permanent suture. Also, the testicular vessels are freed from the peritoneum and carefully ligated with a permanent suture.

Retroperitoneal lymphadenectomy (nonseminomas)

For patients with nonseminomatous testicular cancer and either no evidence or a small volume of disease on CT (stage I [N0] or stage II [N1, N2a, N2b] disease), retroperitoneal lymphadenectomy (RLND) is generally indicated because it (1) accurately and definitively defines the presence or absence of retroperitoneal metastases and (2) removes the retroperitoneum as a site of recurrence, thus obviating the need for surveillance with CT.

RLND can be accomplished transperitoneally or retroperitoneally through a thoracoabdominal approach. The thoracoabdominal approach is more technically difficult but eliminates the risk of postoperative small bowel obstruction and usually requires a shorter hospital stay.

Nerve-sparing surgery Regardless of the approach, urologic oncologists recommend a unilateral, nerve-sparing procedure. For right-sided tumors, the medial border of the template is the midpoint of the aorta, and for left-sided tumors, the medial border is the midpoint of the inferior vena cava (IVC). The sympathetic trunks responsible for normal bladder neck closure during ejaculation course lateral to the aorta on the left side and behind the IVC on the right side. Below the inferior mesenteric artery, both sympathetic trunks send branches to the region anterior to the aorta. The branches coalesce and then pass to the bladder neck.

Critical aspects of nerve-sparing surgery include preservation of the ipsilateral sympathetic nerve trunk and bilateral preservation of branches below the level of the inferior mesenteric artery. In our experience and that of other authors, it is possible to maintain normal ejaculatory function in virtually all patients using this technique.

TABLE 4: Chemotherapy regimens for testicular cancer

Drug/combination	Dose and schedule
BEP	
Bleomycin	30 IU IV bolus on days 2, 9, and 16
Etoposide	100 mg/m^2 IV infused over 30 minutes on days 1-5
Platinol (cisplatin)	20 mg/m^2 IV infused over 15-30 minutes on days 1-5
Repeat cycle every 21 days for 3 or 4 cycles.	
NOTE: Treat patients every 21 days on schedule, regardless of the granulocyte count. Reduce etoposide dose by 20% in patients who previously received radiotherapy or had granulocytopenia with fever/sepsis during the previous cycle. Patients receiving 4 cycles of BEP should undergo pulmonary function tests at baseline and at 9 weeks.	
Williams SD, Birch R, Einhorn LH, et al: N Engl J Med 316:1435–1440, 1987.	
EP	
Etoposide	100 mg/m^2 IV infused over 30 minutes on days 1-5
Platinol (cisplatin)	20 mg/m^2 IV infused over 15-30 minutes on days 1-5
Repeat cycle every 21 days for 4 cycles.	
NOTE: Treat patients every 21 days on schedule, regardless of the granulocyte count. Reduce etoposide dose by 20% in patients who previously received radiotherapy or had granulocytopenia with fever/sepsis during the previous cycle.	
de Wit R, Roberts JT, Wilkinson PM, et al: J Clin Oncol 19:1629–1640, 2001.	
VIP	
VePesid (etoposide)	75 mg/m^2/d IV on days 1-5
Ifosfamide	1.2 g/m^2/d IV on days 1-5
Platinol (cisplatin)	20 mg/m^2/d IV on days 1-5
Mesna	400 mg IV bolus prior to the first ifosfamide dose, then 1.2 g/m^2/d IV infused continuously on days 1-5
Repeat cycle every 21 days for 4 cycles.	
Loehrer PJ, Lauer R, Roth BJ, et al: Ann Intern Med 109:540–546, 1988.	
VeIP (salvage therapy)	
Vinblastine	0.11 mg/kg/d on days 1 and 2
Ifosfamide	1.2 g/m^2/d IV on days 1-5
Platinol (cisplatin)	20 mg/m^2/d IV on days 1-5
Mesna	400 mg/m^2 IV bolus prior to first ifosfamide dose, then 1.2 g/m^2/d IV infused continuously for 5 days
Repeat cycle every 21 days for 4 cycles.	
Loehrer PJ, Lauer R, Roth BJ, et al: Ann Intern Med 109:540–546, 1988.	
Miller KD, Loehrer PJ, Gonin R, et al: J Clin Oncol 15:1427–1431, 1997.	

Table prepared by Ishmael Jaiyesimi, DO

SURVEILLANCE (NONSEMINOMAS)

In patients with clinical stage I disease (normal serum markers and normal CT scans of the chest and abdomen), surveillance is a reasonable option. In patients with NSGCTs, the risk of recurrence is approximately 25%. Thus, close follow-up with chest x-ray, serum markers (β-hCG and AFP), and physical exam should be performed monthly during the first year, every 2 months during the second year, and every 3–4 months during the next several years. Similarly, abdominal CT scans should be performed every 2 months during the first year and every 4 months during the second year.

When followed up in this way, most patients will be detected with low-volume disease. If recurrence occurs, these cases should be curable with 3 cycles of BEP (bleomycin, 30 IU/wk × 9; etoposide, 100 mg/m^2/d ; and Platinol [cisplatin], 20 mg/m^2/d) or 4 cycles of EP (etoposide plus Platinol at the same doses; see Table 4). If patients recur with higher volume disease, up to 10% may not be cured. Thus, diligent follow-up is crucial.

RADIATION THERAPY FOR STAGE I OR II SEMINOMAS

Seminomas of the testes are exquisitely sensitive to irradiation. This characteristic, combined with their predictable lymphatic spread, makes these cancers amenable to radiotherapy. Since low radiation doses are used, acute and late side effects are few.

Stage I disease

Prophylactic radiotherapy vs surveillance vs chemotherapy Primary lymphatic drainage of the testes is to the para-aortic lymph nodes from the level of the renal vessels to the bifurcation of the aorta. Although ipsilateral pelvic nodal failures and, to a much lesser extent, inguinal failures occur following tumor resection by inguinal orchiectomy in patients with stage I disease, these sites are at a much lower risk of failure than the para-aortic region. Based on surveillance data, the overall incidence of disease failure without radiotherapy is 15%–27% (median, 20%), whereas only 2%–5% (median, 3%) of patients who are treated with radiotherapy relapse. Relapse rates with surveillance appear to be lower in patients with < 4 cm primary tumors and no evidence of rete testis involvement.

The identification of prognostic factors makes surveillance an attractive alternative to the more conventional approach of radiotherapy in selected patients. Follow-up in patients undergoing surveillance is rigorous because disease progression usually is not associated with symptoms until the tumor burden is large. Surveillance requires abdominopelvic CT scans and chest x-rays at 3- to 4-month intervals for about 3 years and then at 6-month intervals for at least an additional 2 years. Late failures beyond 5 years have been observed. Salvage rates reported in patients who relapse while undergoing surveillance are approximately 90% initially, with ultimate salvage rates after relapse of approximately 95%. Those patients who do develop recurrence usually receive 4 cycles of EP.

Single-cycle carboplatin (Paraplatin) has been studied as an alternative to adjuvant radiotherapy in a randomized trial conducted by the UK Medical Research Council/European Organization for Research on Treatment of Cancer (UKMRC/EORTC). At a median follow-up of 4 years, 3-year relapse-free survival rates were similar among the 1,477 randomized patients. However, first-echelon para-aortic nodal recurrences were more common in the chemotherapy group (74% vs 9%), raising concern regarding the efficacy of single-cycle carboplatin. Para-aortic nodal recurrences following radiotherapy are typically marginal misses at the edge of the treatment field.

Further questioning the role of single-cycle carboplatin in stage I disease, a pooled analysis of two randomized trials in advanced-stage disease demonstrated that single-agent carboplatin is inferior to cisplatin-based combination therapy. Phase II results evaluating two cycles of carboplatin (400 mg/m^2) for prophylactic treatment of stage I seminomas are more promising. However, acute toxicity (ie, the degree of lethargy and time missed from work) is unlikely to be less than that of a 2-week course of radiotherapy.

Radiation fields and doses The radiotherapy portals have traditionally included the para-aortic lymph nodes from T10–L5 and the ipsilateral hemipelvis, including the inguinal scar. However, recent studies that reduced the size of para-aortic fields and omitted hemipelvis irradiation in selected patients (eg, those who have not undergone prior orchiopexy or other pelvic, inguinal, or scrotal surgery) are encouraging. A study by Fossa and colleagues randomized 478 men with stage I seminomas to receive irradiation of the para-aortics (T11–L5) and ipsilateral hemipelvis vs irradiation of the para-aortics only. The actuarial rate of 3-year freedom from relapse was about 96% for both groups, although there were more pelvic relapses in patients given para-aortic radiation therapy only. Pelvic and/or inguinal failures occurred in < 5% of these patients. The few failures observed following radiotherapy most often occurred in the next echelon of lymph node drainage sites, such as the mediastinum or left supraclavicular fossa.

The smaller treatment volume reduces the dose to the remaining testicle and probably the risk of secondary malignancy. The ipsilateral hemipelvis is treated only when there is a history of ipsilateral inguinal surgery. Violation of the inguinal region can alter the testicular lymphatic drainage pathway to the para-aortic region. The hemiscrotum is often treated if the tumor penetrated the tunica albuginea, a trans-scrotal incision was performed, or orchiopexy was performed for cryptorchidism. However, this practice has been questioned, since the incidence of scrotal failure is low, even in the presence of these risk factors. In fact, some surgeons advocate trans-scrotal exploration to rule out benign lesions.

Side effects The acute side effects of radiotherapy are limited to nausea, vomiting, and infrequently diarrhea, all of which usually can be readily controlled with medication. Long-term complications recently reported at M. D. Anderson Cancer Center demonstrated increased mortality ratios for overall, cardiac-specific, and secondary cancer deaths for men treated with radiation therapy for seminoma between 1951 and 1999. No difference in mortality risk was noted in the first 15 years following treatment; however, over the entire period, the all-cause mortality risk was 1.59. The cardiac-specific mortality rate after 15 years was 1.61, and the secondary cancer mortality rate was 1.91.

A randomized comparison of adjuvant radiotherapy in 625 patients showed that 20 Gy in 10 treatments was as effective as 30 Gy in 15. With a median follow-up of 61 months, the absolute difference in 2-year relapse rates was 0.7%, with an estimated increase in the 2-year relapse rate associated with the lower dose of no more than 3%. When combining an additional 469 patients randomized between 20 Gy and 30 Gy as part of a subsequent trial, the estimated increase in relapse rates associated with the lower dose was further reduced, to less than 0.5% (*Jones WG, Fossa SD, Mead GM, et al: J Clin Oncol 23:1200-1208, 2005*).

Permanent infertility from scattered irradiation to the contralateral testis is uncommon, whereas prolonged aspermia for more than 1 year may occur, especially with irradiation of the hemiscrotum. Nevertheless, sperm banking is recommended for patients concerned about childbearing.

Thus, in summary, various options exist for the primary treatment of clinical stage I seminoma, including radiation therapy and observation with monitoring of serum markers and computed tomography. Primary chemotherapy has been advocated by some investigators, but risk-adapted therapy has not yet defined the optimal population.

Stage II disease

The majority of patients with infradiaphragmatic para-aortic and/or pelvic adenopathy < 5 cm are treated with radiotherapy alone. Those with larger lymph node metastases are typically treated with platinum-based chemotherapy. Among patients who are candidates for radiotherapy, it is essential that renal function be preserved in case chemotherapy is necessary for salvage treatment. Recent preliminary evidence indicates that the 5-year freedom-from-failure rates may be improved to 97% by administration of neoadjuvant carboplatin combined with reduced-field radiotherapy. Alternatively, systemic therapy alone (BEP x 3 vs EP x 4) may be used in lieu of radiation therapy.

Radiation fields The radiotherapy fields are similar to those used for stage I disease except that they are widened to include any para-aortic or pelvic adenopathy with a 2- to 3-cm margin. In the past, mediastinal and supraclavicular treatment was standard in patients with stage II disease. However, data from several series revealed only a 3% rate of mediastinal/supraclavicular relapse. In addition, late cardiac toxicity has been reported. Although treatment to supradiaphragmatic sites has largely been abandoned in these cases, one report indicates that the rate of failure in the left supraclavicular fossa is higher than was previously believed. An analysis from another group indicates the opposite, however, that supradiaphragmatic radiotherapy for stage IIA-B seminoma is unnecessary. The overall actuarial rate of freedom from disease at 5 years for patients with para-aortic adenopathy < 2 cm (IIA) is 95%, 2–5 cm (IIB) is 90%, and > 5 and < 10 cm (IIC) is 85%.

Radiation doses The involved areas are usually treated with 30–35 Gy and the uninvolved areas, with 20–25 Gy. There is no evidence of a dose-response effect above 20 Gy for uninvolved areas and above 30 Gy for involved areas.

Failures within the irradiated volume are anecdotal.

MEDICAL TREATMENT OF STAGE II NONSEMINOMAS

Over the past several years, the threshold for primary surgery in patients with stage II disease on CT scans has changed. At present, masses > 3 cm in greatest cross-sectional diameter or those with more extensive longitudinal lymphatic spread are generally handled primarily with chemotherapy. For patients with tumor sizes ≤ 3 cm, primary RLND is considered the standard approach. It should be noted that up to 25% of patients with enlarged lymph nodes on CT scans will be found to have pathologic stage I (false-positive) disease by RLND.

Adjuvant chemotherapy for nonseminomas

The risk of systemic recurrence is 5%–10% in patients with pathologic stage I nonseminomas, 15%–30% in those with completely resected stage IIA (N2a) disease, and 30%–50% in those with stage IIB (N2b) disease. Recurrence usually occurs in the lungs within the first 24 months after surgery. The risk of retroperitoneal recurrence in patients with stage I, IIA, or IIB disease is < 1% after a properly performed RLND. Following RLND, patients with complete resection of stage II disease can be considered candidates for adjuvant chemotherapy.

The decision of whether or not to prescribe adjuvant therapy following lymph node dissection is somewhat arbitrary and often depends on the patient's social circumstances and likelihood of adhering to close follow-up. A patient with completely resected carcinoma who undergoes RLND has a 70% chance of cure; thus, the majority of patients will never need chemotherapy. However, these patients must be monitored carefully with chest x-rays and serum marker determinations every month for 1 year, every 2 months for an additional year, and then every 6 months for the next 3 years. (CT scanning is not performed routinely unless clinically indicated.) The 30% of patients followed in such a manner who do develop recurrence will present with a tumor of low volume (eg, small pulmonary metastases or elevated serum markers); nearly 100% of these patients should be cured with appropriate systemic therapy.

However, some patients with resected stage II disease elect to receive adjuvant chemotherapy to minimize the risk of cancer recurrence. For such therapy, two cycles of BEP (bleomycin, 30 IU/wk × 8; etoposide, 100 mg/m^2 on days 1–5 and 29–34; and Platinol, 20 mg/m^2 on days 1–5 and 29–34) are recommended (Table 4). It should be emphasized that in a patient who agrees to close follow-up, the chance of dying of cancer should be negligible in either scenario. For patients who have persistently elevated or increasing serum markers following RLND or who have undergone incomplete lymph node dissection, three cycles of BEP are indicated.

In a study of 75 patients with stage I NSGCTs, compliance with clinical examinations was 61.5% in year 1 and 35.5% in year 2, whereas compliance with abdominal/pelvic CT was only 25.0% and 11.8% in years 1 and 2, respectively. Careful selection of highly motivated patients for surveillance is indicated.

TREATMENT OF STAGE III DISEASE

Seminomas

Chemotherapy is the treatment of choice for patients with stage III seminomas (see Table 4). The management of patients with bulky disease after chemotherapy (residual mass > 3 cm) is somewhat controversial. Investigators at Memorial Sloan-Kettering Cancer Center suggest that such patients require consolidation with radiotherapy or surgical removal of radiographically evident disease. More recent data from the Royal Marsden Hospital and the Centre Léon Bérard report a relapse rate of 10%–15% in patients with residual masses with or without postchemotherapy surgery or radiotherapy, supporting the practice of observation in patients with residual masses following chemotherapy. FDG-PET may be helpful in the decision to treat residual masses > 3 cm but should be performed 4–6 weeks after the last course of chemotherapy.

Nonseminomas

As mentioned previously, patients with nonseminomas being treated with chemotherapy can be classified as having good- or poor-risk disease (see Table 3).

Good-risk nonseminomas In patients with good-risk nonseminomas, three cycles of BEP given every 3 weeks or, alternatively, four cycles of EP at the same dosages appear to yield equivalent results. More than 90% of good-risk patients should be cured with these therapies.

Two prospective randomized trials comparing cisplatin with carboplatin in good-risk patients with disseminated germ-cell tumors have demonstrated inferior results for carboplatin-containing regimens.

Postchemotherapy resection If a patient has persistent radiographic disease with normal serum markers 4–6 weeks following chemotherapy for a NSGCT, surgical resection should be performed when possible. In patients with seminoma, a residual mass > 3 cm, and an abnormal PET scan, resection is also recommended.

Postresection chemotherapy Histologic examination of residual disease will reveal necrotic fibrous tissue in ~45% of such cases, benign teratoma in ~45%, and persistent carcinoma in ~10%–15%. If persistent carcinoma is detected in the resected specimen, two additional cycles of EP should be administered. For patients with complete resection of mature and immature teratoma or necrosis, no additional therapy is needed.

Poor-risk nonseminomas A cohort of patients with disseminated germ-cell tumors presents with advanced or poor-risk disease. "Poor risk" has been variously defined (see Table 3) but represents a patient population with a cure rate of ≤ 50% with standard cisplatin-based combination chemotherapy. Irradiation is useful in the treatment of metastatic nonseminomas to the brain.

Chemotherapy During the past few years, several trials have evaluated a variety of combination regimens in patients with poor-risk disease (Table 4). They include the use of high-dose therapy, sequential therapy, and VIP (VePesid [etoposide], ifosfamide [Ifex], and Platinol). VIP appears to be therapeutically equivalent to BEP; however, for most patients with advanced disease, BEP is the preferred regimen because it produces less myelosuppression. In patients with underlying pulmonary dysfunction, VIP is preferred.

In a study by Bhatia et al, 65 patients with recurrent testicular cancer were treated with tandem cycles of high-dose etoposide plus carboplatin followed by peripheral stem-cell transplantation as initial salvage therapy. With a median follow-up of 39 months, 37 patients (57%) remain continuously disease-free, with 3 additional patients (5%) disease-free with subsequent surgery. There was no treatment-related mortality.

A prospective intergroup trial evaluating high-dose chemotherapy and bone marrow transplantation (BMT) comparing four cycles of BEP with two cycles of BEP followed by two tandem courses of high-dose chemotherapy plus BMT in previously untreated patients with poor-risk disease was recently completed.

Postchemotherapy resection The ultimate goal of combination chemotherapy in these patients is the resolution of all radiographically visible disease and normalization of tumor markers. If residual radiographic abnormalities persist in the lungs and/or abdomen, surgical resection of residual disease is indicated.

Postchemotherapy RLND must clear the region of residual disease. In general, postchemotherapy resections are extremely difficult, and incomplete resections are unacceptable. After the retroperitoneum is cleared of persistent radiographic disease, persistent pulmonary lesions are resected. In cases with residual disease in the retroperitoneum and thorax, RLND should be performed first. If necrosis is found, the disease within the chest can be observed. If teratoma or cancer is noted, the supradiaphragmatic disease should be resected.

Complicating factors associated with postchemotherapy resection include the risk of oxygen toxicity secondary to bleomycin as well as intense fibrosis and adherence of residual disease to the aorta and other vital retroperitoneal organs. Inspired oxygen levels must remain below 35% to prevent bleomycin-related acute respiratory distress syndrome, which has a fatality rate ≥ 50%.

After successful resection, the only visible structures remaining should include the back muscles, nerves, anterior spinous ligament, aorta, IVC, renal vessels, kidneys, and ureters. Up to 20% of patients with advanced abdominal disease may require resection of a kidney or even the IVC. Operative mortality in centers with experience performing resection of these advanced-stage tumors should be < 2%.

Postresection chemotherapy As mentioned, two additional cycles of chemotherapy are indicated for patients with persistent viable carcinoma in the resected specimen. For patients with resected teratoma of nonviable necrotic tissue, no additional chemotherapy is warranted.

Salvage chemotherapy

Approximately 20%–30% of patients with disseminated germ-cell tumors do not attain complete remission with induction chemotherapy or relapse after such therapy. These patients may be candidates for salvage chemotherapy. It should be noted that occasional patients may be erroneously classified as having recurrent disease based on false-positive markers or abnormal radiographic findings. Some of these false-positive results may be due to a growing teratoma; pseudonodules from bleomycin-induced pulmonary disease; or elevated markers from other causes, such as an elevated β-hCG level from marijuana usage, cross-reactivity with luteinizing hormone, or an elevated AFP level associated with hepatitis or liver dysfunction. Another cause of persistently elevated markers is a tumor sanctuary site (eg, in the testes or brain). Assuming that false disease progression has been ruled out, several approaches to salvage therapy can be used. When possible, autologous BMT is preferred. It can achieve slightly more durable response rates than other options.

VeIP Ifosfamide is one of a few drugs (including etoposide, gemcitabine [Gemzar], and paclitaxel) that has clinical activity in patients with cisplatin-refractory disease. As second-line therapy, VeIP (vinblastine, 0.11 mg/kg on days 1 and 2, total dose=.22 mg/kg; plus ifosfamide, 1.2 g/m^2 [plus mesna (Mesnex)]; plus Platinol, 20 mg/m^2, both on days 1–5) produces durable complete remissions in ~30% of patients previously treated with BEP chemotherapy (Table 4). Toxicity is primarily hematologic, which can be minimized with the use of a colony-stimulating growth factor.

Seminoma Patients with recurrent seminoma appear to be more sensitive to salvage therapy. In a study by Miller et al, 24 patients with seminoma were treated with VeIP as second-line therapy (following relapse after cisplatin-etoposide combination therapy). Of the 24 patients, 20 patients (83%) achieved a complete response, and 13 patients (54%) are long-term survivors, including 4 of 6 with extragonadal primary sites. Thus, initial salvage therapy in these patients should be VeIP (Table 4) rather than high-dose chemotherapy with bone marrow rescue.

High-dose chemotherapy with stem-cell rescue High-dose chemotherapy with tandem courses of carboplatin and etoposide plus autologous stem-cell rescue produces durable complete remission in 5%–10% of patients whose disease is overtly refractory to cisplatin. When this approach is used in patients with recurrent, but not cisplatin-refractory, disease, improved response rates are observed; ~50% of patients with recurrence of testicular cancer (excluding extragonadal recurrence) will be cured.

Surgery Some patients with recurrent disease appear to have localized or minimally metastatic disease. In such cases, "desperation" surgery may achieve a durable complete remission. A 25% cure rate was seen in a select group of patients with elevated serum markers who underwent such surgery at Indiana University. These patients had completely resected viable carcinoma without chemotherapy following surgery.

Other agents Few drugs besides etoposide and ifosfamide have activity in patients with cisplatin-refractory disease. Oral etoposide given in a chronic schedule (50 mg/m^2/d for 21 days) has produced objective responses in ~20% of patients who were previously treated with IV etoposide. Paclitaxel has a similar response rate in minimally pretreated patients (< 6 cycles). Gemcitabine produces a response rate of ~ 15% in patients with cisplatin-refractory disease.

The Eastern Cooperative Oncology Group conducted a phase II trial of gemcitabine (1,000 mg/m^2) plus paclitaxel (110 mg/m^2) every week × 3 given every 4 weeks in patients with recurrent germ-cell tumor not thought to be curable with standard chemotherapy or surgery. Of 28 evaluable patients, 6 responded, including 3 complete responses (2 of whom are free of disease at 15+ and 25+ months).

Follow-up of long-term survivors

Delayed toxicity from systemic therapy

Delayed toxicity from systemic therapy for germ-cell tumors has been well characterized. In the absence of signs and symptoms, specific monitoring for these late effects is not generally warranted. A number of late effects have been observed.

Fertility problems and fetal malformation Fertility problems, manifested by azoospermia or oligospermia at or beyond 2 years, occur in 45%–55% of treated patients. No increased risk of fetal malformation has been observed in the offspring of men previously treated with chemotherapy for testicular cancer.

Cardiovascular disease The risk of hypertension or other cardiovascular disease may be increased in patients with testicular cancer who received chemotherapy, but this theory is controversial. The only exception is Raynaud's phenomenon, which occurs at a rate directly proportional to the number of cycles of cisplatin-based chemotherapy.

Renal and pulmonary toxicities Although renal and pulmonary dysfunction can occur acutely during therapy, long-term consequences from therapy are uncommon. A similar percentage of patients may suffer late recurrence of the primary tumor. These late recurrences typically occur over 5 years (longest 32+ years) after primary therapy, frequently present with an elevated serum level of AFP, and are particularly resistant to salvage chemotherapy. Thus, surgical resection of disease is the primary treatment strategy.

Secondary malignancies

Perhaps of greatest concern is the development of secondary malignancies.

Testicular cancer Approximately 1%–2% of patients may develop a second primary testicular cancer.

Other cancers In a large series of 40,000 men by Travis et al, the relative risk for developing secondary tumors was 1.9 for 10-year survivors of testicular cancer and remained 1.7 for 35-year survivors. The greatest elevated risk was for cancers of the pleura, pancreas, bladder, and stomach. In another large retrospective analysis of 635 patients with extragonadal germ-cell tumors treated from 1975–1996, only an increased number of hematologic and skin malignancies were observed.

The contribution of chemotherapy and/or radiation therapy to the development of these other malignancies, as opposed to a natural propensity toward their development, is unknown. However, in several series, etoposide has been shown to pose an increased risk for the development of secondary leukemia (dose-related). At higher dosages (> 2 g/m^2 cumulative), etoposide has been associated with a greater incidence of acute leukemia. Very high dosages of etoposide with stem-cell rescue do not appear to be linked to a higher risk than standard-dose chemotherapy. In one paper by Travis and colleagues, both increased dosages of radiation therapy and cisplatin were associated with an increased risk for acute leukemia. Although these risks are real, they still are low compared with the risk of death caused by testicular cancer. Nonetheless, indiscriminate use of chemotherapy for early-stage (stage I) disease should be tempered by the recognition of the long-term hazards of therapy.

Follow-up for relapse

Because the relapse rate for testicular cancer is low, patients with pathologically confirmed stage I NSGCTs require no further therapy, and follow-up can be accomplished easily with chest x-ray, tumor markers, and physical examination. Similarly, for patients who have stage II disease and receive adjuvant chemotherapy, the risk of relapse is low. For patients with either of these two clinical scenarios, follow-up tests (chest x-ray, serum markers) should be performed every 2 months for 1 year, every 4 months for the second year, every 6 months for years 3 through 5, and annually thereafter.

In patients with resected stage II, NSGCTs who do not receive adjuvant chemotherapy, the follow-up tests are the same as those listed above. However, in these patients, follow-up tests are performed every month for 1 year, every 2 months for 2 years, every 6 months for years 3 through 5, and then annually.

SUGGESTED READING

Albqami N, Janetschek G: Laparoscopic retroperitoneal lymph-node dissection in the management of clinical stage I and II testicular cancer. J Endourol 19:683–692, 2005.

Beck SD, Foster RS, Bihrle R, et al: Does the histology of nodal metastasis predict systemic relapse after retroperitoneal lymph node dissection in pathological stage B1 germ cell tumors? J Urol 174:1287–1290, 2005.

Beck SD, Foster RS, Bihrle R, et al: Impact of the number of positive lymph nodes on disease-free survival in patients with pathological stage B1 nonseminomatous germ cell tumor. J Urol 174:143–145, 2005.

Bokemeyer C, Hartmann JT, Fossa SD, et al: Extragonadal germ cell tumors: Relations to testicular neoplasia and management options. APMIS 111:49–59, 2003.

Chung PW, Warde PR, Panzarella T, et al: Appropriate radiation volume for stage IIA/B testicular seminoma. Int J Radiat Oncol Biol Phys 56:746–748, 2003.

Classen J, Schmidberger H, Meisner C, et al: Radiotherapy for stages IIA/B testicular seminoma: Final report of a prospective multicenter clinical trial. J Clin Oncol 21:1101–1106, 2003.

Classen J, Schmidberger H, Meisner C, et al: Para-aortic irradiation for stage I testicular seminoma: Results of a prospective study in 675 patients. A trial of the German testicular cancer study group (GTCSG). Br J Cancer 90:2305–2311, 2004.

Corvin S, Sturm W, Schlatter E, et al: Laparoscopic retroperitoneal lymph-node dissection with the waterjet is technically feasible and safe in testis-cancer patients. J Endourol 19:823–826, 2005.

Daugaard G, Petersen PM, Rorth M: Surveillance in stage I testicular cancer. APMIS 111:76–83, 2003.

DeSantis M, Becherer A, Bokemeyer C, et al: 2-18Fluoro-deoxy-*D*-glucose positron emission tomography is a reliable predictor for viable tumor in postchemotherapy seminoma: An update of the prospective multicentric SEMPET trial. J Clin Oncol 22:1034–1039, 2004.

Donohue JP: Evolution of retroperitoneal lymphadenectomy (RPLND) in the management of non-seminomatous testicular cancer (NSGCT). Urol Oncol 23:129–132, 2003.

Einhorn LH: Curing metastatic testicular cancer. Proc Natl Acad Sci U S A 99:4592–4595, 2002.

Fizazi K, Tjulandin S, Salvioni R, et al: Viable malignant cells after primary chemotherapy for disseminated nonseminomatous germ cell tumors: Prognostic factors and role of post surgery chemotherapy: Results from an international study group. J Clin Oncol 19:2647–2657, 2001.

Flechon A, Bompas E, Bidon P, et al: Management of post-chemotherapy residual masses in advanced seminoma. J Urol 168:1975–1979, 2002.

Fleshner N, Warde P: Controversies in the management of testicular seminoma. Semin Urol Oncol 20:227–233, 2002.

Fossa SD, Horwich A, Russell JM, et al: Optimal planning target volume for stage I testicular seminoma: A Medical Research Council Testicular Working Group. J Clin Oncol 17:1146–1154, 1999.

Hartmann JT, Nichols CR, Droz JP, et al: Prognostic variables for response and outcome in patients with extragonadal germ-cell tumors. Ann Oncol 13:1017–1028, 2002.

Hendry WF, Norman AR, Dearnaley DP, et al: Metastatic nonseminomatous germ-cell tumors of the testis. Cancer 94:1668–1676, 2002.

Hinton S, Catalano PJ, Einhorn LH, et al: Cisplatin, etoposide and either bleomycin or ifosfamide in the treatment of disseminated germ cell tumors. Cancer 97:1869–1875, 2003.

Hinton S, Catalano P, Einhorn LH, et al: Phase II study of paclitaxel plus gemcitabine in refractory germ-cell tumors (E9897): A trial of the Eastern Cooperative Oncology Group. J Clin Oncol 20:1859–1863, 2002.

Holm M, Hoei-Hansen CE, Rajpert-DeMeyts E, et al: Increased risk of carcinoma in situ in patients with testicular germ cell cancer with ultrasonic microlithiasis in the contralateral testicle. J Urol 170:1163–1167, 2003.

Houck W, Abonour R, Vance G, et al: Secondary leukemias in refractory germ cell tumor patients undergoing autologous stem-cell transplantation using high-dose etoposide. J Clin Oncol 22:2155–2158, 2004.

Huyghe E, Matsuda T, Thonneau P: Increasing incidence of testicular cancer worldwide: A review. J Urol 170:5–11, 2003.

Jones WG, Fossa SD, Mead GM, et al: Randomized trial of 30 versus 20 Gy in the adjuvant treatment of stage I testicular seminoma: A report on Medical Research Council Trial TE18, European Organisation for the Research and Treatment of Cancer Trial 30942 (ISRCTN 18525328). J Clin Oncol 23:1200–1208, 2005.

Loehrer PJ, Bosl GJ: Carboplatin for stage I seminoma and the Sword of Damocles (editorial). J Clin Oncol 23:8566–8569, 2005.

McGlynn KA, Devesa SS, Sigurdson AJ, et al: Trends in the incidence of testicular germ cell tumors in the United States. Cancer 97:63–70, 2003.

Melchior D, Mulle SC, Albers P: Extensive surgery in metastatic testicular cancer. Aktuelle Urol 34:214–222, 2003.

Oliver RT, Mason MD, Mead GM, et al: Radiotherapy versus single-dose carboplatin in adjuvant treatment of stage I seminoma: A randomised trial. Lancet 366:293–300, 2005.

Przygodzki RM, Hubbs AE, Zhao FQ, et al: Primary mediastinal seminomas: Evidence of single and multiple KIT mutations. Lab Invest 82:1369–1375, 2002.

Rick O, Bokemeyer C, Weinknecht T, et al: Residual tumor resection after high-dose chemotherapy in patients with relapsed or refractory germ cell cancer. J Clin Oncol 22:3713–3719, 2004.

Schwartz GG: Hypothesis: Does ochratoxin A cause testicular cancer? Cancer Causes Control 13:91–100, 2002.

Toner GC, Stockler MR, Boyer MJ, et al: Comparison of two standard chemotherapy regimens for good-prognosis germ-cell tumours: A randomised trial. Australian and New Zealand Germ Cell Trial Group. Lancet 357:739–745, 2001.

Travis LB, Fossa SD, Schonfeld SJ, et al: Second cancers among 40,576 testicular cancer patients: Focus on long-term survivors. J Natl Cancer Inst 97:1354–1365, 2005.

Warde P, Specht L, Horwich A, et al: Prognostic factors for relapse in stage I seminoma managed by surveillance: A pooled analysis. J Clin Oncol 20:4448–4452, 2002.

Zagars GK, Ballo MT, Lee AK, et al: Mortality after cure of testicular seminoma. J Clin Oncol 22:640–647, 2004.

CHAPTER 19

Urothelial and kidney cancers

Bruce G. Redman, DO, Mark Hurwitz, MD, Philippe E. Spiess, MD, and Louis L. Pisters, MD

UROTHELIAL CANCER

In the year 2007, an estimated 67,160 new cases of bladder cancer will be diagnosed in the United States, and approximately 13,750 patients will die of this disease.

Urothelial cancers encompass carcinomas of the bladder, ureters, and renal pelvis; these cancers occur at a ratio of 50:3:1, respectively. Cancer of the urothelium is a multifocal process. Patients with cancer of the upper urinary tract have a 30%–50% chance of developing cancer of the bladder at some time in their lives. On the other hand, patients with bladder cancer have a 2%–3% chance of developing cancer of the upper urinary tract. The incidence of renal pelvis tumors is decreasing.

Epidemiology

Gender Urothelial cancers occur more commonly in men than in women (3:1) and have a peak incidence in the seventh decade of life.

Race Cancers of the urothelial tract are also more common in whites than in blacks (2:1).

Etiology and risk factors

Cigarette smoking The major cause of urothelial cancer is cigarette smoking. A strong correlation exists between the duration and amount of cigarette smoking and cancers at all levels of the urothelial tract. This association holds for both transitional cell and squamous cell carcinomas.

Analgesic abuse Abuse of compound analgesics, especially those containing phenacetin, has been associated with an increased risk of cancers of the urothelial tract. This risk appears to be greatest for the renal pelvis, and cancer at this site is usually preceded by renal papillary necrosis. The risk associated with analgesic abuse is seen after the consumption of excessive amounts (5 kg).

Chronic urinary tract inflammation also has been associated with urothelial cancers. Upper urinary tract stones are associated with renal pelvis cancers. Chronic bladder infections can predispose patients to cancer of the bladder, usually squamous cell cancer.

Occupational exposure has been associated with an increased risk of urothelial cancers. Workers exposed to arylamines in the organic chemical, rubber, and paint and dye industries have an increased risk of urothelial cancer similar to that originally reported for aniline dye workers.

Balkan nephropathy An increased risk of cancer of the renal pelvis and ureters occurs in patients with Balkan nephropathy. This disorder is a familial nephropathy of unknown cause that results in progressive inflammation of the renal parenchyma, leading to renal failure and multifocal, superficial, low-grade cancers of the renal pelvis and ureters.

Genetic factors There are reports of families with a higher risk of transitional cell cancers of the urothelium, but the genetic basis for this familial clustering remains undefined.

Signs and symptoms

Hematuria is the most common symptom in patients presenting with urothelial tract cancer. It is most often painless, unless obstruction due to a clot or tumor and/or deeper levels of tumor invasion have already occurred.

Urinary voiding symptoms of urgency, frequency, and/or dysuria are also seen in patients with cancers of the bladder or ureters but are uncommon in patients with cancers of the renal pelvis.

Vesical irritation without hematuria can be seen, especially in patients with carcinoma in situ of the urinary bladder.

Symptoms of advanced disease Pain is usually a symptom of more advanced disease, as is edema of the lower extremities secondary to lymphatic obstruction.

Diagnosis

Initial work-up The initial evaluation of a patient suspected of having urothelial cancer consists of excretory urography, followed by cystoscopy. In patients with upper tract lesions, retrograde pyelography can better define the exact location of lesions. Definitive urethroscopic examination and biopsy can be accomplished utilizing rigid or flexible instrumentation.

At the time of cystoscopy, urine is obtained from both ureters for cytology, and brush biopsy is obtained from suspicious lesions of the ureter. Brush biopsies significantly increase the diagnostic yield over urine cytology alone. Also, at the time of cystoscopy, a bimanual examination is performed to determine whether a palpable mass is present and whether the bladder is mobile or fixed.

Evaluation of a primary bladder tumor In addition to biopsy of suspicious lesions, evaluation of a bladder primary tumor includes biopsy of selected mucosal sites to detect possible concomitant carcinoma in situ. Biopsies of the primary lesion must include bladder wall muscle to determine whether there is invasion of muscle by the overlying carcinoma.

CT For urothelial cancers of the upper tract or muscle invasive bladder cancers, a CT scan of the abdomen/pelvis is performed to detect local extension of the cancer and involvement of the abdominal lymph nodes.

Bone scan For patients with bone pain or an elevated alkaline phosphatase level, a radioisotope bone scan is performed.

A chest x-ray completes the staging evaluation.

Pathology

Transitional cell carcinomas constitute 90%–95% of urothelial tract cancers.

Squamous cell cancers account for 3%–7% of urothelial carcinomas and are more common in the renal pelvis and ureters.

Adenocarcinomas account for a small percentage (< 3%) of bladder malignancies and are predominantly located in the trigone region. Adenocarcinomas of the bladder that arise from the dome are thought to be urachal in origin.

Carcinoma in situ In approximately 30% of newly diagnosed bladder cancers, there are multiple sites of bladder involvement, most commonly with carcinoma in situ. Although carcinoma in situ can occur without macroscopic cancer, it most commonly accompanies higher disease stages.

When carcinoma in situ is associated with superficial tumors, rates of recurrence and disease progression (development of muscle invasion) are higher (50%–80%) than when no such association is present (10%). Carcinoma in situ involving the bladder diffusely without an associated superficial tumor is also considered an aggressive disease. Most patients with this type of cancer will develop invasive cancers of the bladder.

Staging and prognosis

Staging system Urothelial tract cancers are staged according to the American Joint Committee on Cancer (AJCC) TNM classification system (Table 1). Superficial bladder cancer includes papillary tumors that involve only the mucosa (Ta) or submucosa (T1) and flat carcinoma in situ (Tis). The natural history of superficial bladder cancer is unpredictable, and recurrences are common. Most tumors recur within 6–12 months and are of the same stage and grade, but 10%–15% of patients with superficial cancer will develop invasive or metastatic disease.

Prognostic factors For carcinomas confined to the bladder, ureters, or renal pelvis, the most important prognostic factors are T stage and differentiation pattern. The impact of associated carcinoma in situ on Ta and T1 lesions is

TABLE 1: TNM staging of urothelial tract cancers

Primary tumor (T)			
Tx	Primary tumor cannot be assessed		
T0	No evidence of primary tumor		
Ta	Noninvasive papillary tumor		
Tis	Carcinoma in situ: "flat tumor"		
T1	Tumor invades subepithelial connective tissue		
T2	Tumor invades muscle		
pT2a	Tumor invades superficial muscle (inner half)		
pT2b	Tumor invades deep muscle (outer half)		
T3	Tumor invades perivesical tissue		
pT3a	Microscopically		
pT3b	Macroscopically (extravesical mass)		
T4	Tumor invades any of the following: prostate, uterus, vagina, pelvic wall, abdominal wall		
T4a	Tumor invades prostate, uterus, vagina		
T4b	Tumor invades pelvic wall, abdominal wall		
Regional lymph nodes (N)			
Nx	Regional lymph nodes cannot be assessed		
N0	No regional node involvement		
N1	Metastasis in a single node, ≤ 2 cm in greatest dimension		
N2	Metastasis in a single node, > 2 cm but ≤ 5 cm in greatest dimension; or multiple lymph nodes, none > 5 cm in greatest dimension		
N3	Metastasis in a lymph node, > 5 cm in greatest dimension		
Distant metastasis (M)			
Mx	Distant metastasis cannot be assessed		
M0	No distant metastasis		
M1	Distant metastasis		
Stage grouping			
Stage 0a	Ta	N0	M0
Stage 0is	Tis	N0	M0
Stage I	T1	N0	M0
Stage II	T2a	N0	M0
	T2b	N0	M0
Stage III	T3a	N0	M0
	T3b	N0	M0
	T4a	N0	M0
Stage IV	T4b	N0	M0
	Any T	N1-N3	M0
	Any T	Any N	M1

From Greene FL, Page DL, Fleming ID, et al (eds): AJCC Cancer Staging Manual, 6th ed. New York, Springer-Verlag, 2002.

discussed previously (see section on "Pathology"). Less-differentiated Ta–T1 lesions also are associated with higher recurrence and progression rates. Patients with well-differentiated Ta lesions without carcinoma in situ have a 95% survival rate, whereas those with high-grade T1 lesions have a 10-year survival rate of 50%. The presence of lymphovascular invasion within the surgical specimen appears to be independently associated with overall survival, cause-specific survival, as well as local and distant recurrence in patients with node-negative bladder cancer at the time of cystectomy. As such, the presence of lymphovascular invasion should be included in the pathologic assessment of bladder cancer.

Muscle invasive carcinoma carries a 5-year survival rate of 20%–50%. When regional lymph nodes are involved, the 5-year survival rate is 0%–20%.

Treatment

TREATMENT OF LOCALIZED DISEASE

Surgical approaches to superficial bladder cancer

Transurethral resection Most patients with superficial bladder cancer can be treated adequately with transurethral resection (TUR). Such procedures preserve bladder function, entail minimal morbidity, and can be performed repeatedly. Survival rates > 70% at 5 years are expected. Although TUR removes existing tumors, it does not prevent the development of new lesions. Patients should be followed closely.

Laser The neodymium:yttrium-aluminum-garnet (Nd:YAG) laser has achieved good local control when used in the treatment of superficial bladder tumors. However, it has not been adopted for general use because of its limitations in obtaining material for staging and grading of tumors.

Partial cystectomy is an infrequently utilized treatment option for patients whose tumors are not accessible or amenable to TUR.

Radical cystectomy is generally not used for the treatment of superficial bladder tumors. The indications for radical cystectomy include:

- Unusually large tumors that are not amenable to complete TUR, even on repeated occasions
- Some high-grade tumors
- Multiple tumors or frequent recurrences that make TUR impractical
- Symptomatic diffuse carcinoma in situ (Tis) that proves unresponsive to intravesical therapy
- Prostatic stromal involvement.

Intravesical therapy The indications for intravesical therapy include:

- Stage T1 tumors, especially if multiple
- Multifocal papillary Ta lesions, especially grade 2 or 3

- Diffuse carcinoma in situ (Tis)
- Rapidly recurring Ta, T1, or Tis disease.

In the United States, four intravesical agents are commonly used: thiotepa, an alkylating agent; bacillus Calmette-Guérin (BCG), an immune modulator/stimulator; and mitomycin (Mutamycin) and doxorubicin, both antibiotic chemotherapeutic agents. The dose of BCG varies with the strain (50 mg [Tice] or 60 mg [Connaught]). Mitomycin doses range from 20 to 40 mg. Although all four agents reduce the tumor recurrence rate, BCG is the most effective. For the treatment of papillary Ta and T1 lesions, BCG and mitomycin have the greatest efficacy (complete response rate, approximately 50%). For the treatment of carcinoma in situ (Tis), BCG is extremely effective.

In a recent meta-analysis, comparing intravesical BCG and chemotherapy (mitomycin C, epirubicin [Ellence], doxorubicin, or sequential mitomycin/doxorubicin), intravesical BCG was shown to be superior in reducing the risk of short- and long-term treatment failure for Tis. Therefore, intravesical BCG appears to be the agent of choice for Tis.

Surgical approaches to invasive bladder cancer

Radical cystectomy Invasive bladder cancer (stage II or higher) is best treated by radical cystectomy. Candidates for radical cystectomy include:

- Patients with muscle-invasive tumor (depth of invasion is not important, merely its presence), regardless of grade
- Patients with high-grade, invasive, lamina propria tumors with evidence of lymphovascular invasion, with or without carcinoma in situ (Tis)
- Patients with diffuse carcinoma in situ or recurrent superficial cancer who do not respond to intravesical therapy.

In men, radical cystectomy includes en bloc pelvic lymph node dissection and removal of the bladder, seminal vesicles, and prostate. In women, radical cystectomy entails en bloc pelvic lymph node dissection and anterior exenteration, including both ovaries, fallopian tubes, uterus, cervix, anterior vaginal wall, bladder, and urethra.

Partial cystectomy is an infrequently utilized treatment option and should only be considered when there is a solitary lesion in the dome of the bladder and when random biopsy results from remote areas of the bladder and prostatic urethra are negative.

Urethrectomy is routinely included in the anterior exenteration performed in female patients. Urethrectomy in male patients is performed if the tumor grossly involves the prostatic urethra or if prior TUR biopsy results of the prostatic stroma are positive. Delayed urethrectomy for positive urethral cytology or biopsy is required in about 10% of male patients.

Urinary reconstruction may involve any one of the following: intestinal conduits (eg, ileal, jejunal, or colonic), continent cutaneous diversion (eg, Indiana or Kock pouch), or orthotopic reconstruction (in both male and female patients).

Surgical approaches to ureteral and renal pelvic tumors

Optimal surgical management of urothelial malignancies of the ureter and renal pelvis consists of nephroureterectomy with excision of a bladder cuff. Some tumors may respond well to local resection, and tumor specifics may allow for a more conservative intervention.

Upper ureteral and renal pelvic tumors (because of similar tumor behavior and anatomic aspects) may be considered as a group, whereas lower ureteral tumors may be considered as a separate group.

Upper ureteral and renal pelvic tumors are best treated with nephroureterectomy. Solitary, low-grade upper tract tumors may be considered for segmental excision or ureteroscopic surgery if close surveillance is feasible. Care should be exercised, however, as multicentricity is more probable and the risk of recurrence is greater than for lower ureteral lesions.

Lower ureteral lesions may be managed by nephroureterectomy, segmental resection, and neovesical reimplantation or by endoscopic resection. A 15% recurrence rate is seen after segmental resection or endoscopic excision. Careful follow-up is mandatory. Disease progression, the development of a ureteral stricture precluding periodic surveillance, and poor patient compliance are indications to abandon conservative management and perform nephroureterectomy.

ROLE OF RADIATION THERAPY

Radiation therapy for bladder cancer

Primary radiation or chemoradiation therapy Radiation therapy, either alone or in conjunction with chemotherapy, is the modality of choice for patients whose clinical condition precludes surgery, either because of extensive disease or poor overall status. Trials have shown that patients treated with irradiation and cisplatin with or without fluorouracil (5-FU) have improved local control, as compared with patients treated with irradiation alone.

Other studies suggest that TUR followed by radiation therapy combined with cisplatin or 5-FU chemotherapy, with cystectomy reserved for salvage, provides a survival equivalent to that achieved with initial radical cystectomy while allowing for bladder preservation in many patients. The extent of TUR and the absence of hydronephrosis are important prognostic factors in studies of bladder-conserving treatment. Updates from institutions in Europe and the United States on over 600 patients with long-term follow-up support the durability of outcomes previously reported.

A randomized phase III study of bladder preservation with or without neoadjuvant chemotherapy following TUR, conducted by the Radiation Treatment Oncology Group (RTOG), revealed no advantage to the use of MCV (methotrexate, cisplatin, and vinblastine) before radiation therapy and concurrent cisplatin. The favorable outcome without neoadjuvant chemotherapy may make bladder preservation a more acceptable option for a wider range of patients.

TABLE 2: Chemotherapy regimens for bladder carcinoma

Drug/combination	Dose and schedule
M-VAC	
Methotrexate	30 mg/m^2 IV on days 1, 15, and 22
Vinblastine	3 mg/m^2 IV on days 2, 15, and 22
Adriamycin (doxorubicin)	30 mg/m^2 IV on day 2
Cisplatin	70 mg/m^2 IV on day 2

NOTE: Reduce doxorubicin dose to 15 mg/m^2 in patients who have received prior pelvic irradiation. On days 15 and 22, methotrexate (30 mg/m^2) and vinblastine (3 mg/m^2) are given only if the WBC count is > 2,500 cells/mL and the platelet count is > 100,000 cells/mL.

Repeat cycles every 28-32 days even if the interim dose is withheld due to myelosuppression or mucositis.

Loehrer PJ Sr, Einhorn LH, Elson PJ, et al: J Clin Oncol 10:1066–1073, 1992.

Drug/combination	Dose and schedule
Paclitaxel/carboplatin	
Paclitaxel	200 mg/m^2 IV infused over 3 hours
Carboplatin	Dose calculated by the Calvert formula to an area under the curve (AUC) of 5 mg/mL/min IV infused over 15 minutes after paclitaxel

Repeat cycle every 21 days.

PREMEDICATIONS: Dexamethasone, 20 mg PO, 12 and 6 hours prior to paclitaxel; as well as ranitidine, 50 mg IV, and diphenhydramine, 50 mg IV, both 30-60 minutes prior to paclitaxel.

Redman B, Smith D, Flaherty L, et al: J Clin Oncol 16:1844–1848, 1998.

Drug/combination	Dose and schedule
Gemcitabine/cisplatin	
Gemcitabine	1 g/m^2 IV on days 1, 8, and 15
Cisplatin	75 mg/m^2 IV on day 1

Repeat cycle every 28 days.

Kaufman D, Stadler W, Carducci M, et al: Proc Am Soc Clin Oncol 17:320a, 1998.

Preoperative irradiation may improve survival in patients undergoing radical cystectomy. Its use is limited due to concern over complications occurring with the urinary diversions currently utilized.

Radiation dose and technique Initially, a pelvic field is treated to 4,500 cGy utilizing a four-field box technique, with 180 cGy delivered daily. The bladder tumor is then boosted to a total dose of 6,480 cGy utilizing multifield techniques, with 180 cGy delivered daily.

Radiation therapy for renal pelvic and ureteral cancers

In patients with renal pelvic and ureteral lesions who have undergone nephroureterectomy, postoperative local-field irradiation is offered if there is periureteral, perirenal, or peripelvic extension or lymph node involvement. A dose of approximately 4,500–5,040 cGy is delivered utilizing multifield techniques.

Drug/combination	Dose and schedule
PCG	
Paclitaxel	200 mg/m^2 IV infused over 3 hours on day 1
Carboplatin	Dose calculated on AUC of 5, 15-minute IV infusion on day 1
Gemcitabine	800 mg/m^2 30-minute IV on days 1 and 8

Repeat cycle every 21 days.

PREMEDICATIONS: Dexamethasone, 20 mg PO, 12 and 6 hours prior to paclitaxel; diphenhydramine, 50 mg IV, 30 minutes prior to paclitaxel; and either cimetidine, 300 mg IV, or ranitidine, 50 mg IV, 30 minutes prior to paclitaxel.

Hussain M, Vaishampayan U, Du W, et al: J Clin Oncol 19:2527–2533, 2001.

Drug/combination	Dose and schedule
Paclitaxel/cisplatin	
Paclitaxel	135 mg/m^2 IV infused over 3 hours
Cisplatin	70 mg/m^2 IV infused over 2 hours

Repeat cycle every 3 weeks until disease progression or for a maximum of 6 cycles.

PREMEDICATIONS: Dexamethasone, 20 mg PO, 12 and 6 hours prior to paclitaxel; as well as ranitidine, 50 mg IV, or cimetidine, 300 mg IV, prior to paclitaxel, and diphenhydramine, 50 mg IV, 30 minutes prior to paclitaxel.

Burch PA, Richardson RI, Cha SS, et al: Proc Am Soc Clin Oncol 18:1266a, 1999.

Drug/combination	Dose and schedule
TCG	
Taxol (paclitaxel)	80 mg/m^2 IV infused over 1 hour on days 1 and 8
Cisplatin	70 mg/m^2 on day 1
Gemcitabine	1 g/m^2 IV on days 1 and 8

Repeat cycle every 21 days.

PREMEDICATIONS: Dexamethasone, 20 mg PO, 12 and 6 hours prior to paclitaxel; as well as diphenhydramine, 50 mg IV, 30 minutes prior to paclitaxel, and either cimetidine, 300 mg IV, or ranitidine, 50 mg IV, 30 minutes prior to paclitaxel.

Vaishampayan U, Smith D, Redman B, et al: Proc Am Soc Clin Oncol 18:333a (abstract 1282), 1999.

Table prepared by Ishmael Jaiyesimi, DO

Palliative irradiation

Palliative radiation therapy is effective in controlling pain from local and metastatic disease and in providing hemostatic control. A randomized study comparing 3,500 cGy in 10 fractions vs 2,100 cGy in 3 hypofractionated treatments revealed high rates of relief of hematuria, frequency, dysuria, and nocturia with either regimen. In selected cases of bladder cancer, aggressive palliation to approximately 6,000 cGy may be warranted to provide long-term local control. Concurrent chemotherapy, such as cisplatin, should be considered.

CHEMOTHERAPY FOR ADVANCED DISEASE

Treatment of advanced metastatic urothelial cancer is palliative. Cisplatin, paclitaxel, and gemcitabine (Gemzar) have all demonstrated single-agent activity for the systemic treatment of this disease. A randomized trial showed an advantage for a regimen of M-VAC (methotrexate, vinblastine, Adriamycin [doxorubicin], and cisplatin) over cisplatin alone with regard to disease progression-free and overall survival. Combination regimens with cisplatin or carboplatin (Paraplatin), usually with paclitaxel or gemcitabine or in combination with methotrexate and vinblastine with or without doxorubicin, produce response rates of 40%–60% in patients with advanced disease, with a median survival of 12–14 months (Table 2). In another randomized trial, the combination of gemcitabine and cisplatin exhibited equivalent survival to M-VAC in metastatic bladder cancer but was clinically better tolerated. The role of combination chemotherapy in the adjuvant treatment of resected urothelial cancer remains undetermined and an area of clinical research. A randomized trial of neoadjuvant M-VAC in locally advanced resectable bladder cancer showed a trend in survival favoring M-VAC over surgery alone, but it was not statistically significant.

KIDNEY CANCER

Approximately 51,190 new cases of renal cell carcinoma will be diagnosed in the year 2007 in the United States, with an associated 12,890 deaths. There has been a steady increase in the incidence of renal cell carcinoma that is not explained by the increased use of diagnostic imaging procedures. Mortality rates have also shown a steady increase over the past 2 decades.

Epidemiology

Gender and age This malignancy is twice as common in men as in women. Most cases of renal cell carcinoma are diagnosed in the fourth to sixth decades of life, but the disease has been reported in all age groups.

Ethnicity Renal cell carcinoma is more common in persons of northern European ancestry than in those of African or Asian descent.

Etiology and risk factors

Renal cell carcinoma occurs most commonly as a sporadic form and rarely as a familial form. The exact etiology of sporadic renal cell carcinoma has not been determined. However, smoking, obesity, and renal dialysis have been associated with an increased incidence of the disease.

Genetic factors More recently, a genetic basis has been sought for this disease.

von Hippel-Lindau disease, an autosomal-dominant disease, is associated with retinal angiomas, CNS hemangioblastomas, and renal cell carcinoma.

Chromosomal abnormalities Deletions of the short arm of chromosome 3 (3p) occur commonly in renal cell carcinoma associated with von Hippel-Lindau disease. In the rare familial forms of renal cell carcinoma, translocations affecting chromosome 3p are uniformly present. Sporadic renal cell carcinoma of the nonpapillary type is also associated with 3p deletions.

Associated malignancy Two studies from large patient databases have reported a higher-than-expected incidence of both renal cell cancer and lymphoma. No explanation for this association has been found.

Signs and symptoms

Renal cell carcinoma has been associated with a wide array of signs and symptoms. The classic triad of hematuria, flank mass, and flank pain occurs in only 10% of patients and is usually associated with a poor prognosis. With the routine use of CT scanning for various diagnostic reasons, renal cell carcinoma is being diagnosed more frequently as an incidental finding.

Hematuria More than half of patients with renal cell carcinoma present with hematuria.

Other common signs/symptoms Other commonly associated signs and symptoms of renal cell carcinoma include normocytic/normochromic anemia, fever, and weight loss.

Less common signs/symptoms Less frequently occurring, but often described, signs and symptoms include polycythemia, hepatic dysfunction not associated with hepatic metastasis, and hypercalcemia. Although not a common finding at the time of diagnosis of renal cell carcinoma, hypercalcemia ultimately occurs in up to 25% of patients with metastatic disease.

Diagnosis

Contrast-enhanced CT scanning has virtually replaced excretory urography and renal ultrasonography in the evaluation of suspected renal cell carcinoma. In most cases, CT imaging can differentiate cystic from solid masses and also supplies information about lymph nodes and renal vein/inferior vena cava (IVC) involvement.

Ultrasonography is useful in evaluating questionable cystic renal lesions if CT imaging is inconclusive.

Venography and MRI When IVC involvement by tumor is suspected, either IVC venography or MRI is needed to evaluate its extent. MRI is currently the preferred imaging technique for assessing IVC involvement at most centers.

Renal arteriography is not used as frequently now as it was in the past in the evaluation of suspected renal cell carcinoma. In patients with small, indeterminate lesions, arteriography may be helpful. It is also used by the surgeon as part of the preoperative evaluation of a large renal neoplasm.

Percutaneous cyst puncture is used in the evaluation of cystic renal lesions that are thought to be potentially malignant on the basis of ultrasonography or CT imaging. Percutaneous cyst puncture permits the collection of cyst fluid for analysis, as well as the evaluation of cyst structure via instillation of contrast medium after fluid removal. Benign cyst fluid is usually clear to straw-colored and low in protein, fat, and lactic dehydrogenase (LDH) content, whereas malignant fluid is usually bloody with high protein, fat, and LDH content.

Evaluation of extra-abdominal disease sites includes a chest x-ray. In the face of a normal chest x-ray, CT imaging of the chest adds no further helpful information. A bone scan is required if a patient has symptoms suggestive of bone metastasis and/or an elevated alkaline phosphatase level.

Pathology

Renal cell carcinoma arises from the proximal renal tubular epithelium. Histologically, renal cell carcinoma can be of various cellular types: clear cell, granular cell, and sarcomatoid (spindle) variant. The majority of these tumors are mixtures of clear and granular cell types. Approximately 1%–6% of renal cell carcinomas are of the sarcomatoid variant, which is a more aggressive malignancy with a worse prognosis.

Staging and prognosis

Staging system The preferred staging system for renal cell carcinoma is the TNM classification (Table 3). The University of California has recently developed an integrated staging system termed the UCLA Integrated Staging System (UISS), which combines the 1997 TNM staging system, Fuhrman grade, and Eastern Cooperative Oncology Group (ECOG) performance status. The UISS is simple to use and is superior to TNM stage alone in differentiating patient survival following radical nephrectomy for renal cell carcinoma.

Prognostic factors The natural history of renal cell carcinoma is highly variable. However, approximately 30% of patients present with metastatic disease at diagnosis, and one-third of the remainder will develop metastasis during follow-up.

Five-year survival rates after nephrectomy for tumors confined to the renal parenchyma (T1/2) are > 80%. Renal vein involvement without nodal involvement does not affect survival. Lymph node involvement and/or extracapsular spread is associated with a 5-year survival of 10%–25%. Patients with metastatic disease have a median survival of 1 year and a 5-year survival of 0%–20%.

TABLE 3: TNM staging of renal cell carcinoma

Primary tumor (T)			
Tx	Primary tumor cannot be assessed		
T0	No evidence of primary tumor		
T1	Tumor ≤ 7 cm in greatest dimension, limited to the kidneys		
T1a	Tumor ≤ 4 cm in greatest dimension, limited to the kidneys		
T1b	Tumor > 4 cm but not > 7 cm in greatest dimension, limited to the kidneys		
T2	Tumor > 7 cm in greatest dimension, limited to the kidneys		
T3	Tumor extends into major veins or invades adrenal gland or perinephric tissues but not beyond Gerota's fascia		
T3a	Tumor directly invades adrenal gland or perirenal and/or renal sinus fat but not beyond Gerota's fascia		
T3b	Tumor grossly extends into renal vein or its segmental (muscle-containing) branches or vena cava below the diaphragm		
T3c	Tumor grossly extends into the vena cava above the diaphragm or invades the wall of the vena cava		
T4	Tumor invades beyond Gerota's fascia		
Regional lymph nodes (N)			
Nx	Regional lymph nodes cannot be assessed		
N0	No regional lymph node metastasis		
N1	Metastasis in a single regional lymph node		
N2	Metastasis in more than one regional lymph node		
Distant metastasis (M)			
Mx	Distant metastasis cannot be assessed		
M0	No distant metastasis		
M1	Distant metastasis		
Stage grouping			
Stage I	T1	N0	M0
Stage II	T2	N0	M0
Stage III	T1	N1	M0
	T2	N1	M0
	T3a	N0-N1	M0
	T3b	N0-N1	M0
	T3c	N0-N1	M0
Stage IV	T4	N0-N1	M0
	Any T	N2	M0
	Any T	Any N	M1

From Greene FL, Page DL, Fleming ID, et al (eds): AJCC Cancer Staging Manual, 6th ed. New York, Springer-Verlag, 2002.

TABLE 4: Therapeutic regimens for renal cell carcinoma

Dose and schedule
High-dose IL-2
IL-2: 600,000 or 720,000 IU/kg IV infused over 15 minutes every 8 hours until toxicity develops; or 14 consecutive doses for 5 days
After a 5- to 9-day rest period, an additional 14 doses of IL-2 are administered over a 5-day period. If patients show evidence of tumor regression or stable disease, 1-2 more courses of treatment may be given.
Fyfe G, Fisher RI, Rosenberg SA, et al: J Clin Oncol 13:688–696, 1995.
Low-dose IL-2
IL-2: 72,000 IU/kg by IV bolus every 8 hours to a maximum of 15 doses every 7-10 days for 2 cycles
NOTE: The cycles represent one course of therapy. Patients who are stable or responding after one course of therapy receive a second course. Third and fourth courses are given only if patients demonstrate further tumor regression.
Yang JC, Topalian SL, Parkinson D, et al: J Clin Oncol 12:1572–1576, 1998.
Sunitinib
50 mg PO daily for 4 weeks. Repeat every 6 weeks (4 weeks on, 2 weeks off)
Motzer RJ, Michaelson M, Redman BG, et al: J Clin Oncol 24:16–24, 2006.
Sorafenib
400 mg PO bid daily continuously until disease progression

Table prepared by Ishmael Jaiyesimi, DO

Treatment

Surgery

Radical nephrectomy is the established therapy for localized renal cell carcinoma. At surgery, the kidneys, adrenal gland, and perirenal fat (structures bound by Gerota's fascia) are removed. Also, limited regional lymph node dissection is often performed for staging purposes. Partial nephrectomy is considered in patients for whom a radical nephrectomy would result in permanent dialysis.

Since complete resection is the only known cure for renal cell carcinoma, even in locally advanced disease, surgery is considered if the involved structures can be safely removed. In the presence of metastatic disease, surgery is generally considered for palliation only. In patients with metastatic renal cell carcinoma, two randomized, controlled trials have shown a survival benefit of between 3 and 10 months with a debulking nephrectomy prior to interferon-alpha immunotherapy, as compared with immunotherapy alone. However, patients must be carefully selected prior to the nephrectomy and should have a performance status of 0 to 1 according to the World Health Organization criteria. The performance status of a patient prior to treatment is an important determinant of disease-related outcome and should be considered in making treatment decisions.

Radiation therapy for renal cell carcinoma

Primary radiation therapy Radiation therapy may be considered for palliation as the primary therapy for renal cell carcinoma in patients whose clinical condition precludes surgery, either because of extensive disease or poor overall condition. A dose of 4,500 cGy is delivered, with consideration of a boost up to 5,500 cGy.

Postoperative radiation therapy is controversial. However, it may be considered in patients with perinephric fat extension, adrenal invasion, or involved margins. A dose of 4,500 cGy is delivered, with consideration of a boost.

Palliation Radiation therapy is commonly used for palliation for metastatic and local disease.

Systemic therapy for advanced disease

Metastatic renal cell carcinoma is resistant to chemotherapeutic agents. An extensive review of currently available agents concluded that the overall response rate to chemotherapy is 6%.

Interleukin-2 The first US Food and Drug Administration (FDA)-approved treatment for metastatic renal cell carcinoma was high-dose interleukin-2 (IL-2, aldesleukin [Proleukin]; Table 4).

High-dose regimen High-dose IL-2 (720,000 IU/kg IV piggyback every 8 hours for 14 doses, repeated once after a 9-day rest) results in a 15% remission rate (7% complete responses, 8% partial responses). The majority of responses to IL-2 are durable, with a median response duration of 54 months.

The major toxicity of high-dose IL-2 is a sepsis-like syndrome, which includes a progressive decrease in systemic vascular resistance and an associated decrease in intravascular volume due to a "capillary leak." Management includes judicious use of fluids and vasopressor support to maintain blood pressure and intravascular volume and at the same time to avoid pulmonary toxicity due to noncardiogenic pulmonary edema from the capillary leak. This syndrome is totally reversible.

Other doses and schedules Because of the toxicity of high-dose IL-2, other doses and schedules have been and are being evaluated. Several trials of low-dose IL-2 (3–18 × 10^6 IU/d), either alone or combined with interferon-alpha, have reported response rates similar to those achieved with high-dose IL-2.

Multikinase inhibitors Two oral multikinase inhibitors have been recently approved by the FDA for the treatment of advanced kidney cancer.

Sorafenib (Nexavar) targets several serine/threonine and receptor tyrosine kinases. A phase III placebo-controlled trial was conducted in 769 patients with advanced renal cell carcinoma who had received prior systemic treatment. The recommended oral dose of sorafenib (400 mg twice daily) was used. The median progression-free survival was 167 days in the sorafenib group vs 84 days in the placebo group. This difference was highly significant, and results did not appear to differ between previously untreated and prior cytokine-treated patients. Toxic effects associated with sorafenib included reversible skin rashes in

> Preliminary results have been reported in two randomized phase III trials in subjects with previously untreated advanced kidney cancer. In the first trial, sunitinib was superior to interferon-alpha in terms of both median progression-free survival (47.3 vs 24.9 weeks) and overall response rate (24.8% vs 4.9%; *Motzer RJ, Hutson TE, Tomczak P, et al: J Clin Oncol [late-breaking abstract 3] 24, 2006*). In the second trial, temsirolimus (a specific inhibitor of mTOR) was superior to inerferon with respect to median overall survival (10.9 vs 7.3 months) in patients with poor-prognosis metastatic kidney cancer. Poor prognosis was defined by three of six risk factors (five Motzer criteria and more than one metastatic disease site; *Hudes G, Carducci M, Tomczak P, et al: J Clin Oncol [late-breaking abstract 4] 24, 2006*).

40% and hand-foot skin reactions in 30% of patients. Because the incidence of treatment-emergent cardiac ischemia/infarction events was higher with sorafenib (2.9% vs 0.4%), frequent blood pressure monitoring is recommended.

Sunitinib (Sutent) targets several receptor tyrosine kinases. In a single-arm, multicenter phase II trial of patients with metastatic renal cell disease, the overall response rate with sunitinib was nearly 40% (all partial responses), with a median time to disease progression of 8.7 months. Diarrhea, skin discoloration, and mucositis/stomatitis were the most common adverse events occurring more frequently with sunitinib. Decreases in left ventricular ejection fraction were noted with sunitinib, and dose reductions and/or antihypertensive or diuretic medications may be required.

Immunotherapy New immunotherapeutic approaches under investigation for the treatment of advanced renal cell cancer include the use of peripheral blood stem cell transplantations, dendritic cell-based vaccines, and monoclonal antibodies. Early reports on the use of allogeneic stem cell transplantation from HLA-matched donors to invoke a graft-vs-tumor reaction have shown encouraging preliminary results that warrant further investigation. In a recent phase III, randomized controlled trial of adjuvant autologous tumor cell vaccine in patients with renal cell carcinoma treated by radical nephrectomy, there appeared to be a benefit in 5-year progression-free survival (77.4% vs 67.8%; $P = .024$) to the well-tolerated vaccine group.

A humanized monoclonal antibody against the G250 antigen found on all clear cell, and the majority of non-clear cell, renal carcinomas is also in clinical trials.

As always, patients should be encouraged to participate in ongoing clinical trials of metastatic renal cell cancer.

SUGGESTED READING

ON UROTHELIAL CANCER

Barton Grossman H, Natale RB, Tangen CM, et al: Neoadjuvant chemotherapy plus cystectomy compared with cystectomy alone for locally advanced bladder cancer. N Engl J Med 349:859–866, 2003.

Duchesne GM, Bolger JJ, Griffiths GD, et al: A randomized trial of hypofractionated schedules of palliative radiotherapy in the management of bladder carcinoma: Results of Medical Research Council Trial BA09. Int J Radiat Oncol Biol Phys 47:379–388, 2000.

Hudson MA, Herr HW: Carcinoma in situ of the bladder. J Urol 153:564–572, 1995.

Hussain MH, Glass TR, Forman J, et al: Combination cisplatin, 5-fluorouracil, and radiation therapy for locally advanced unresectable or medically unfit bladder cancer cases: A Southwest Oncology Group study. J Urol 165:56–60, 2001.

Lotan Y, Gupta A, Shariat SF, et al: Lymphovascular invasion is independently associated with overall survival, cause-specific survival, and local and distant recurrence in patients with negative lymph nodes at radical cystectomy. J Clin Oncol 23:6533–6539, 2005.

Rodel C, Grabenbaner GG, Kuhn R, et al: Combined-modality treatment and selective organ preservation in invasive bladder cancer: Long-term results. J Clin Oncol 20:3048–3050, 2002.

Shipley WU, Kaufman DS, Zehr E, et al: Selective bladder preservation by combined modality protocol treatment: Long-term outcomes of 190 patients with invasive bladder cancer. Urology 60:62–67, 2002.

Sylvester RJ, van der Meijden AP, Witjes JA, et al: Bacillus calmette-guerin versus chemotherapy for the intravesical treatment of patients with carcinoma in situ of the bladder: A meta-analysis of the published results of randomized clinical trials. J Urol 174:86–92, 2005.

Von der Maase H, Hansen SW, Roberts JT, et al: Gemcitabine and cisplatin versus methotrexate, vinblastine, doxorubicin, and cisplatin in advanced or metastatic bladder cancer: Results of a large, randomized, multinational, multicenter, phase III study. J Clin Oncol 17:3068–3077, 2000.

ON KIDNEY CANCER

Flanigan RC, Salmon SE, Blumenstein BA, et al: Nephrectomy followed by interferon alfa-2b compared with interferon alfa-2b alone for metastatic renal cell cancer. N Engl J Med 345:1655–1659, 2001.

Jocham D, Richter A, Hoffmann L, et al: Adjuvant autologous renal tumour cell vaccine and risk of tumour progression in patients with renal-cell carcinoma after radical nephrectomy: Phase III, randomized controlled trial. Lancet 363:594–599, 2004.

Mickisch GH, Garin A, van Poppel H, et al: Radical nephrectomy plus interferon-alfa-based immunotherapy compared with interferon alone in metastatic renal-cell carcinoma: A randomized trial. Lancet 358:966–970, 2001.

Motzer RJ, Bacik J, Schwartz LH, et al: Prognostic factors for survival in previously treated patients with metastatic renal cell carcinoma. J Clin Oncol 22:454–463, 2004.

Motzer RJ, Mazumder M, Bacik J, et al: Survival and prognostic stratification of 670 patients with advanced renal cell carcinoma. J Clin Oncol 17:2530–2540, 1999.

Motzer RJ, Michaelson M, Redman BG, et al: Activity of SU11248, a multi-targeted inhibitor of vascular endothelial growth factor receptor and platelet-derived growth factor receptor, in patients with metastatic renal cell carcinoma. J Clin Oncol 24:16–24, 2006.

Parkinson DR, Sznol M: High-dose interleukin-2 in the therapy of metastatic renal cell carcinoma. Semin Oncol 22:61–66, 1995.

Rabinovitch RA, Zelefsky MJ, Gaynor JJ, et al: Patterns of failure following surgical resection of renal cell carcinoma: Implications for adjuvant local and systemic therapy. J Clin Oncol 12:206–212, 1994.

Stodlen WM, Vogelzang NJ: Low-dose interleukin-2 in the treatment of metastatic renal cell carcinoma. Semin Oncol 22:67–73, 1995.

Zisman A, Pantuck AJ, Dorey F, et al: Improved prognostication of renal cell carcinoma using an integrated staging system. J Clin Oncol 19:1649–1657, 2001.

CHAPTER 20

Cervical cancer

Dennis S. Chi, MD, Carlos A. Perez, MD, Rachelle M. Lanciano, MD, and John Kavanagh, MD

The overall incidence of invasive cervical carcinoma has declined steadily since the mid-1940s. Of the predominant gynecologic cancers, cancer of the uterine cervix is the least common, with only 11,150 new cases anticipated in the United States in 2007. Nevertheless, approximately 3,670 women die of cancer of the uterine cervix annually in the United States.

Epidemiology

Age The peak age of developing cervical cancer is 47 years. Approximately 47% of women with invasive cervical cancer are < 35 years old at diagnosis. Older women (> 65 years) account for another 10% of patients with cervical cancer. Although these older patients represent only 10% of all cases, they are more likely to die of the disease due to their more advanced stage at diagnosis.

Socioeconomic class Carcinoma of the uterine cervix primarily affects women from the lower socioeconomic class and those with poor access to routine medical care.

Geography Although invasive cervical carcinoma is relatively uncommon in the United States compared with the more common cancers in women (breast, endometrial, and ovarian cancers), it remains a significant health problem for women worldwide. In many developing countries, not only is cervical carcinoma the most frequently occurring cancer among middle-aged women, but also it is a leading cause of death. This is due, in part, to poor access to medical care and the unavailability of routine screening in many of these countries.

Etiology and risk factors

Sexual activity Invasive cervical carcinoma can be viewed as a sexually transmitted disease. If a woman is never sexually active, it is extremely unlikely that she will ever develop this cancer. Conversely, any woman who has been sexually active is at risk for invasive cervical carcinoma.

Human papillomavirus Molecular and epidemiologic evidence clearly indicates that certain types of human papillomavirus (HPV), which is sexually transmitted, are the principal causes of invasive cervical cancer and cervical intraepithelial

Gardasil, a vaccine to prevent cervical cancer, has been approved by the US FDA to be used in girls and women aged 9 to 26. The vaccine uses virus-like particles to block infection with human papillomavirus (HPV) types 16 and 18, which cause approximately 70% of cervical cancers and more than 50% of precancerous lesions of the cervix, vulva, and vagina. It is also reported to be protective against HPV types 6 and 11, which cause genital warts. Overall, more than 50,000 women have participated in the phase III trials worldwide. With follow-up ranging from 1 to 4 years, the vaccine has been reported to be 90%–100% effective in preventing infection and precancerous lesions (*Prescribing information, US FDA. Issued June 2006. No. 9682300*).

neoplasia (CIN). More than 80 HPV types have been identified, and about 40 infect the genital tract. HPV-16 and HPV-18 are the types most commonly linked with cancer, present in 70% of cervical cancers and high-grade CINs. Two vaccines are set to become available within the coming year.

Age of onset of sexual activity Population studies of women with invasive cervical carcinoma have demonstrated that early age of onset of sexual activity also plays a role in the later development of the cancer. It is postulated that during the time of menarche in early reproductive life, the transformation zone of the cervix is more susceptible to oncogenic agents, such as HPV. Women who begin sexual activity before 16 years of age or who are sexually active within 1 year of beginning menses are at particularly high risk of developing invasive cervical carcinoma.

Other risk factors include multiple sexual partners, a history of genital warts, and multiparity. Family history has been suggested as a risk factor, but the data are incomplete.

Cigarette smoking has been identified as a significant risk factor for cervical carcinoma. The mechanism may be related to diminished immune function secondary to a systemic effect of cigarette smoke and its by-products or a local effect of tobacco-specific carcinogens.

Oral contraceptives may also play a role in the development of invasive cervical carcinoma, although this theory is controversial. Given that most women who use oral contraceptives are more sexually active than women who do not, this may represent a confounding factor rather than a true independent risk factor. The exception may be adenocarcinoma of the cervix; this relatively uncommon histologic subtype may be related to previous oral contraceptive use.

Immune system alterations In recent years, alterations in the immune system have been associated with an increased risk of invasive cervical carcinoma, as exemplified by the fact that patients who are infected with the human immunodeficiency virus (HIV) have increased rates of both preinvasive and invasive cervical carcinomas. These patients also are at risk for other types of carcinoma, including Kaposi's sarcoma, lymphomas, and other squamous cell carcinomas of the head and neck and the anogenital region. (For further discussion of AIDS-related malignancies, see chapter 27.)

Data suggest that patients who are immunocompromised due to immunosuppressive medications also are at risk for both preinvasive and invasive cervical carcinomas. This association is probably due to the suppression of the normal immune response to HPV, which makes patients more susceptible to malignant transformation.

Signs and symptoms

Common symptoms A symptom of advanced cervical carcinoma is intermenstrual bleeding in a premenopausal patient. Other commonly reported symptoms include heavier menstrual flow, metrorrhagia, and/or postcoital bleeding. With effective screening, cervical cancer is generally asymptomatic.

Less common presentations Less frequently, patients with advanced cancer will present with signs of advanced disease, such as bowel obstruction and renal failure due to urinary tract obstruction. Only rarely are asymptomatic patients with a normal screening Pap smear found to have a lesion on the cervix as their only sign or symptom of cervical cancer. Foul-smelling vaginal discharge, pelvic pain, or both are occasionally observed.

Screening and diagnosis

Screening

Pap smear The paradigm for a cost-effective, easy-to-use, reliable screening test is the cervical cytology screen, or Pap smear. In every population studied, the introduction of the Pap smear has resulted in a significant reduction in the incidence of invasive cervical carcinoma, as well as a shift toward earlier stage disease at the time of diagnosis. The success of cervical cytology, as measured by the lowered incidence of cervical cancer, ironically has led to some controversy regarding the most effective application of this screening tool. With the marked reduction in the incidence of cervical carcinoma, more patients are screened and greater costs incurred to detect each additional case of cervical carcinoma.

Current screening recommendations The current recommendation of the American College of Obstetricians and Gynecologists (ACOG) is that all women who are 18 years of age or older and are sexually active be screened. If the patient has three consecutive annual cervical cytology smears that are normal, she may be safely screened at a less frequent interval of perhaps 2–3 years. There are no data to support screening patients on a less frequent basis. Any patient who has a history of cervical dysplasia should be screened at least on a yearly basis.

The current American Cancer Society (ACS) revised guidelines for cervical cancer screening follow: Cervical cancer screening should begin ~3 years after the onset of vaginal intercourse but no later than age 21. Cervical screening should be performed every year with conventional cervical cytology smears, or every 2 years using liquid-based cytology until age 30. After age 30, as an alternative to annual routine cytology, HPV DNA testing may be added to cervical cytology for screening. After this initial dual testing, women whose results are negative by both HPV DNA testing and cytology should not be rescreened before 3 years. Women whose results are negative by cytology but who are high-risk HPV DNA (type 16, 18, most commonly) positive are at a relatively low risk of having high-grade cervical neoplasia, and colposcopy should not be performed routinely in this setting. Instead, HPV DNA testing along with cervical cytology should be repeated in these women at 6 or 12 months. If test results of either modality are positive, colposcopy should then be performed.

Women who are > 70 years old with an intact cervix and who have had three or more documented, consecutive, technically satisfactory normal cervical cytology tests and no abnormal cytology tests within the 10-year period prior to age 70 may elect to cease cervical cancer screening. Women with a history of cervical cancer, in utero exposure to diethylstilbestrol (DES), and/or who are immunocompromised (including HIV+) should continue cervical cancer screening for as long as they are in reasonably good health and do not have a life-limiting chronic condition. Women > 70 years old should discuss their need for cervical cancer screening with a health care professional and make an informed decision about continuing screening based on its potential benefits, harms, and limitations.

Women who have had a supracervical hysterectomy should continue cervical cancer screening as per current guidelines. Cervical cancer screening following total hysterectomy (with removal of the cervix) for benign gynecologic disease is not indicated. Women with a history of CIN2/3 or for whom it is not possible to document the absence of CIN2/3 prior to or as the indication for hysterectomy should be screened until three documented, consecutive, technically satisfactory normal cervical cytology tests and no abnormal cytology tests (within a 10-year period) are achieved. Women with a history of in utero DES exposure and a history of cervical carcinoma should continue screening after hysterectomy for as long as they are in reasonably good health and do not have a life-limiting chronic condition.

Techniques designed to improve the sensitivity of the Pap smear have been approved by the FDA. Liquid-based cytologies such as thin prep and SurePath are commercially available techniques. Computer-based analysis of these techniques has been developed but is still under evaluation.

Diagnosis

The diagnosis of invasive cervical carcinoma can be suggested by either an abnormal Pap smear or an abnormal physical finding.

Colposcopy In the patient who has an abnormal Pap smear but normal physical findings, colposcopy is indicated. Colposcopic findings consistent with invasive cervical carcinoma include dense white epithelium covering the ectocervix, punctation, mosaicism, and especially, an atypical blood vessel pattern.

Biopsy If the colposcopic findings are suggestive of invasion, biopsies are obtained from the ectocervix and endocervix. If these biopsies demonstrate only precancerous changes but not an invasive carcinoma, the patient should undergo an excisional biopsy of the cervix. In most current clinical settings, the loop electrosurgical excision procedure (LEEP) is the most expedient method for performing an excisional biopsy. This can be easily accomplished in the office with the patient under local anesthesia and provides adequate tissue for diagnosis. Once the diagnosis of either microinvasive or invasive carcinoma has been established, the patient can be triaged accordingly.

Patient with signs/symptoms of advanced disease The patient with signs/symptoms of advanced invasive cervical carcinoma requires a cervical biopsy for diagnosis and treatment planning. In this setting, a Pap smear is superfluous and may be misleading.

Pathology

Squamous cell carcinoma The most common histology associated with invasive cervical carcinoma is squamous cell carcinoma, which accounts for approximately 80% of all carcinomas of the uterine cervix. For the most part, the decline in the annual incidence of invasive cervical carcinoma has been seen primarily among patients with this subtype.

Adenocarcinoma In the past, adenocarcinoma was relatively uncommon as a primary histology of cervical cancer. As a result of the decrease in the overall incidence of invasive squamous cell cancer and, probably, an increase in the baseline incidence of adenocarcinoma of the uterine cervix, this histology now accounts for approximately 20% of all cervical cancers.

There is controversy over whether patients with adenocarcinoma of the cervix have a worse prognosis than those with the more common squamous cell histology. The poorer prognosis associated with adenocarcinoma may be due to the relatively higher frequency of late stage at the time of diagnosis among patients with this histologic type. In several series in which patients were stratified by stage and tumor size, the outcome of cervical adenocarcinoma appeared to be similar to that of squamous lesions of the cervix.

Aggressive subtypes Among the various subtypes of adenocarcinoma, certain types are particularly aggressive and are associated with a poor prognosis. Among them are the small cell or neuroendocrine tumors, which have a poor prognosis even when diagnosed at an early stage.

Rare tumor types More rare lesions of the cervix include lymphoma, sarcoma, and melanoma. These histologic subtypes account for < 1% of all cervical cancers.

TABLE 1: AJCC and FIGO staging for carcinoma of the uterine cervix

AJC	FIGO	
Primary tumor (T)		
Tx		Primary tumor cannot be assessed
T0		No evidence of primary tumor
Tis		Carcinoma in situ
T1	I	Cervical carcinoma confined to the uterus (extension to the corpus should be disregarded)
T1a	IA	Preclinical invasive carcinoma, diagnosed by microscopy only
T1a1	IA1	Minimal microscopic stromal invasion
T1a2	IA2	Tumor with an invasive component 5 mm or less taken from the base of the epithelium and 7 mm or less in horizontal spread
T1b	IB	Clinical lesions confined to the cervix or preclinical lesions greater than stage IA
	IB1	Clinical lesions no greater than 4 cm
	IB2	Clinical lesions greater than 4 cm
T2	II	Cervical carcinoma invades beyond the uterus but not to the pelvic wall or to the lower third of the vagina
T2a	IIA	Tumor without parametrial invasion
T2b	IIB	Tumor with parametrial invasion
T3	III	Cervical carcinoma extends to the pelvic wall and/or involves the lower third of the vagina and/or causes hydronephrosis or nonfunctioning kidney
T3a	IIIA	Tumor involves the lower third of the vagina, with no exension to the pelvic wall
T3b	IIIB	Tumor extends to the pelvic wall and/or causes hydronephrosis or nonfunctioning kidney
T4[a]	IVA	Tumor invades the mucosa of the bladder or rectum and/or extends beyond the true pelvis
Regional lymph nodes[b] (N)		
Nx		Regional lymph nodes cannot be assessed
N0		No regional lymph node metastasis
N1		Regional lymph node metastasis
Distant metastasis (M)		
Mx		Presence of distant metastasis cannot be assessed
M0		No distant metastasis
M1	IVB	Distant metastasis

AJCC = American Joint Committee on Cancer; FIGO = International Federation of Gynecology and Obstetrics

[a] *Note*: The presence of bullous edema is not sufficient evidence to classify a tumor as T4.

[b] Regional lymph nodes include paracervical, parametrial, hypogastric (obturator), common, internal and external iliac, presacral, and sacral.

Modified from Greene FL, Page DL, Fleming ID, et al: AJCC Cancer Staging Manual, ed 6. N Y, Springer, 2002; Perez CA, Kavanagh BD: Uterine cervix. In: Perez CA, Brady LW, Halperin EC, eds: Principles and Practice of Radiation Oncology, ed 4, pp 1800–1915. Philadelphia, Lippincott Williams & Wilkins, 2004.

Staging and prognosis

Clinical staging: suspected early disease

When a diagnosis of invasive cervical cancer has been established histologically, an evaluation of all pelvic organs should be performed to determine whether the tumor is confined to the cervix or has extended to the adjacent vagina, parametrium, endometrial cavity, bladder, ureters, or rectum. According to the International Federation of Gynecology and Obstetrics (FIGO) guidelines for clinical staging (Table 1), diagnostic studies may include intravenous urography (IVU), cystoscopic examination of the bladder and urethra, a proctosigmoidoscopic study, a barium enema (BE), and in the case of early-stage disease, a colposcopic study of the vagina and the vaginal fornices. Colposcopic findings may be used for assigning a stage to the tumor (for instance, FIGO stage IIA), but the results must be confirmed by biopsy.

A pelvic examination must be performed as part of the staging process, and the procedure is best done with the patient completely relaxed by general anesthesia. In up to 20% of patients, the initial clinical classification of the disease has proved to be incorrect at the time of pelvic examination. Such an examination can reveal a more advanced stage of the disease than was originally found; additional biopsies (if indicated) or fractional curettage can be performed as well as colposcopy, cystoscopy, and proctosigmoidoscopy.

Clinical staging: suspected advanced disease

When studies detect ureteral obstruction, a tumor is classified as a stage IIIB lesion, regardless of the size of the primary lesion. Ureteral obstruction, either hydronephrosis or nonfunction of the kidneys, is well established as an indicator of poor prognosis, as recognized in the FIGO classification.

In women with bulky or advanced-stage tumors, the bladder mucosa also should be inspected cystoscopically for possible bullous edema, which indicates lymphatic obstruction within the bladder wall. Evidence of tumor in the bladder must be confirmed by biopsy before the lesion can be classified as stage IVA. Rectal mucosal lesions also require a biopsy via proctosigmoidoscopy, because they can be related to an inflammatory process rather than to the cervical tumor.

Surgical experience from pelvic lymphadenectomy has confirmed an error rate of 15%–25% in the clinical staging of patients with stage IB or II lesions. In 10%–30% of cases with stage II/III tumors, in addition to positive findings of occult pelvic lymph nodes, other metastases may be found in the para-aortic nodes. Unfortunately, pelvic examinations and clinical staging as defined by FIGO cannot detect such metastases.

Consequently, there is a growing body of literature showing the superiority of cross-sectional imaging (CT and MRI) over clinical staging in delineating the extent of disease in patients with cervical cancer. As stated previously, official FIGO guidelines do not incorporate the use of either CT or MRI findings into the staging of cervical cancer. However, as knowledge of prognostic factors and the value of cross-sectional imaging has accumulated, its use in treatment planning has increased without changing the official FIGO clinical staging guidelines. Similarly, although the benefits of laparoscopic extraperitoneal surgical staging have also been reported in this setting, this approach has not been incorporated into the FIGO staging system.

The value of CT scanning in the pretreatment evaluation of patients with cervical cancer is in the assessment of advanced disease (stage IIB and greater) and in the detection and biopsy of suspected lymph node metastasis. The treatment plan for patients with locally advanced disease must be modified if upper abdominal tumor masses and/or distant metastasis is discovered. The soft-tissue contrast resolution of CT scanning does not allow for consistent tumor visualization at the primary cervical site, and, therefore, neither tumor size nor early parametrial invasion can be evaluated reliably. However, T2-weighted MRI allows consistent tumor visualization and has been reported to be over 90% accurate in determining tumor size to within 5 mm of measurements of surgical specimens.

Surgical staging

Clinical staging of cervical carcinoma, although widely utilized, is not without controversy. When compared with surgical staging performed by large cooperative groups, clinical staging is frequently inaccurate in predicting locoregional spread. For many cooperative groups, including the Gynecologic Oncology Group (GOG), surgical staging may be required for patients who are entering prospective, randomized clinical protocols. However, because of the controversy of risk and benefit, the GOG considers surgical staging optional.

The most common method used to stage patients with advanced disease is extraperitoneal sampling of the pelvic and aortic lymph nodes. This approach minimizes the risk of subsequent radiation injury to the small bowel due to surgical adhesions and, in patients with advanced disease, allows for individualized treatment planning.

Work-up for advanced disease The standard work-up of a patient with advanced cervical carcinoma who is not considered a candidate for radical surgery includes an abdominopelvic CT scan with both intravenous and GI oral contrast. If there is evidence of aortic lymph node metastases, the patient should undergo fine-needle aspiration (FNA) of these enlarged lymph nodes. If FNA confirms that there is aortic lymph node metastasis, treatment should be individualized, and extended-field irradiation should be considered part of the primary treatment regimen.

If the scalene lymph nodes are negative on clinical examination and the patient is known to have positive metastatic disease to the aortic lymph nodes, consideration can be given to performing a scalene lymph node biopsy; the incidence of positive scalene nodes when aortic lymph nodes are known to be positive ranges from 0% to 17%. The rationale for biopsying the scalene nodes is that if there is disease outside the radiation therapy field, chemotherapy may be appropriate.

If the result of FNA is negative, or if the abdominopelvic CT scan does not demonstrate enlarged para-aortic lymph nodes, the patient can be considered for surgical staging.

Recent data regarding the use of PET scan in cervical cancer reveal that tumor volume can be accurately measured by PET and can separate patients into prognostic groups. In a series of 101 consecutive patients with advanced cervical cancer, 67% had positive lymph nodes on PET, which correlated with decreased survival following chemoradiation therapy.

> Grigsby et al reported on 152 patients with carcinoma of the cervix treated with irradiation and brachytherapy in some combined with weekly cisplatin for whom pre- and post-treatment FDG-PET imaging was performed. In 114 patients with a negative PET scan, the 5-year cause-specific survival was 80%, compared with 32% when persistent abnormal PET scans were noted in the irradiated volumes (20 patients), and there were no survivors in 18 patients who developed new sites of abnormal FDG uptake (*Grigsby PW, Siegel BA, Dehdashti F, et al: J Clin Oncol 22:2167-2171, 2004*).

Pros and cons of surgical staging The advantage of surgical staging is that patients with microscopic disease in the para-aortic lymph nodes can be treated with extended-field radiation therapy and, possibly, chemotherapy and potentially benefit in terms of long-term survival. The controversy regarding surgical staging stems from the fact that a small number of patients will actually benefit from the procedure; the majority of patients who undergo it will be found not to have metastatic disease and will receive the same treatment as planned prior to surgical staging; if they are found to have metastatic disease, they will be unlikely to benefit from extended-field radiation therapy. Because of this controversy, GOG considers surgical staging to be *optional* for patients with advanced-stage cervical cancer.

Laparoscopic surgery In more recent years, the introduction of minimal-access surgery has allowed surgeons to accurately stage patients via the laparoscope prior to initiation of radiation therapy. However, the safety and efficacy of laparoscopic surgical staging are areas of ongoing investigation.

Work-up for early-stage disease For patients who have early-stage disease for which surgery is contemplated, only a minimal diagnostic work-up is indicated prior to surgery. At most institutions, this would include a two-view chest x-ray. Patients who have stage IA cervical carcinoma (microinvasive carcinoma) do not require preoperative CT scanning prior to hysterectomy. For patients with a small IB carcinoma of the cervix, a CT scan of the abdomen and pelvis has a low yield and is unlikely to change the treatment plan.

Prognostic factors

Clinical stage The most important determinant of prognosis remains clinical stage, which is defined by tumor volume and extent of disease spread. The overall 5-year survival rate ranges from 95% to 100% for patients with stage IA cancer and from 75% to 90% for those with stage IB disease. Patients with stage IV disease have a ≤ 5% chance of surviving 5 years after diagnosis.

Patients with early disease For patients with early invasive carcinoma (stage IB), the size of the lesion, percentage of cervical stromal invasion, histology, tumor grade, and lymphovascular space involvement are important local factors that predict prognosis. In general, good prognostic signs are lesions that are ≤ 2 cm in diameter, superficially invasive, and well differentiated with no lymphovascular space involvement.

For patients who have undergone radical hysterectomy for early cervical carcinoma, poor prognostic factors, in addition to the local factors previously mentioned, include positive vaginal or parametrial margins and metastasis to the pelvic lymph nodes. For patients with stage IB disease and positive pelvic nodes, the 5-year survival rate drops from approximately 75%–85% to 50%.

Patients with advanced disease For patients with advanced-stage disease (stages II through IV), the primary determinants of prognosis are histology and size of the primary lesion. Survival is significantly higher for patients with small stage IIB cervical carcinomas and minimal parametrial involvement than for patients with large bulky tumors and bilateral parametrial involvement. Disease extension beyond the pelvis to the aortic nodes is associated with a significant decrease in overall survival rate. With regard to histology, a better prognosis is associated with a large-cell nonkeratinizing squamous cell cancer of the cervix, as opposed to a poorly differentiated adenocarcinoma.

Other prognostic factors Other factors that may predict outcome include the patient's general medical and nutritional status. Patients who are anemic may respond poorly to radiation therapy, as compared with those with normal hemoglobin levels. Patients with significant alterations in their immune system may not respond as well; this result is becoming increasingly apparent with regard to patients who are HIV-seropositive.

A retrospective review of 605 patients from seven institutions in Canada treated with irradiation for cervical cancer described average weekly nadir hemoglobin levels as significant prognostic factors for survival, second only in importance to tumor stage. Interestingly, Winter et al reported that hemoglobin levels during treatment were independent predictors of treatment outcome through a recent retrospective study of 494 patients from two consecutive prospective GOG trials. The pretreatment level was not a significant predictor of outcome in the multivariate regression model. Levels in the last part of treatment were the most predictive of disease recurrence and survival. However, erythropoietin should not be given outside a clinical trial, as thrombosis is a significant complication and cause/effect has not been proven.

Treatment

SURGICAL TREATMENT OF EARLY-STAGE DISEASE

The standard management of patients with early cervical carcinoma is surgical removal of the cervix. The extent of resection of surrounding tissue depends on the size of the lesion and the depth of tumor invasion.

Stage IA1 disease

> Meta-analysis shows that all conservative procedures to treat cervical intraepithelial neoplasia and microinvasive cervical cancer present similar pregnancy-related morbidities without apparent neonatal morbidities. Caution should be recommended in the treatment of young women with mild cervical abnormalities (*Kyrgiou M, Koliopoulos G, Martin-Hirsch P, et al: Lancet 367:489-498, 2006*).

Simple hysterectomy Patients who have a microinvasive squamous carcinoma of the cervix with ≤ 3 mm of tumor invasion, ≤ 7 mm of lateral extent, and no lymphovascular space involvement (stage IA1) can be treated with a simple hysterectomy. Vaginal, abdominal, and laparoscopic hysterectomies are equally effective.

Cone biopsy Although simple hysterectomy is considered the standard therapy for patients with microinvasive cervical carcinoma, there are some patients in whom preservation of future fertility is a strong consideration. A cone biopsy entails removal of the cervical transformation zone. Provided that the biopsy margins are free of dysplasia and microinvasive carcinoma, cone biopsy is probably a safe treatment for such patients who meet the criteria of having superficial invasion < 3 mm, minimal lateral extension, and no lymphovascular space involvement.

Since there is a small risk of recurrence among this population of patients treated by cone biopsy alone, they should be followed closely. Follow-up includes a Pap smear every 3 months for 2 years and then twice a year. An abnormal Pap smear is an indication for a repeat colposcopy. If such patients are successful in achieving pregnancy and have no evidence of recurrent squamous cell carcinoma, there is no need to proceed with hysterectomy at the completion of planned childbearing.

Stages IA2, IB1, and nonbulky IIA disease

Radical hysterectomy A standard treatment for patients with small cervical carcinomas (≤ 4 cm) confined to the uterine cervix or with minimal involvement of the vagina (stage IIA) is radical hysterectomy (removal of the uterus, cervix, and parametrial tissue), pelvic lymphadenectomy, and para-aortic lymph node sampling. The overall success of this treatment is similar to that of radiation therapy, and for patients with early lesions, radical hysterectomy may provide an improved quality of life. The benefits of surgical excision include rapid treatment, less time away from normal activities, and preservation of normal ovarian and vaginal function.

A recent randomized trial for patients with early-stage cervical cancer reported no difference in survival between radical hysterectomy and definitive radiation therapy. Because a significant percentage of patients following radical hysterectomy required postoperative pelvic radiotherapy, the morbidity was increased in the surgery arm. Therefore, patients selected for radical hysterectomy should have small-volume disease so adjuvant pelvic radiation therapy is unnecessary.

Currently, there are no specific contra-indications to radical hysterectomy. Several studies have demonstrated that patients ≥ 65 years old tolerate this procedure well, and age alone should not be considered a contraindication. Obesity also is not a contraindication to radical hysterectomy.

Alternatives to radical hysterectomy Reports have described laparoscopically assisted radical vaginal hysterectomy and laparoscopic abdominal radical hysterectomy as less invasive alternatives to traditional radical hysterectomy. Although these procedures are not performed in all centers, the results from centers that have the surgical expertise are promising. The use of fertility-preserving surgery by means of pelvic lymphadenectomy combined with radical vaginal trachelectomy (removal of the uterine cervix) has also been evaluated in selected women with early cervical cancer (see box). Successful pregnancies after this procedure have been reported. However, further data are needed to assess the safety and efficacy of fertility-preserving surgery. There is a lack of long-term follow-up data and survival rates between conservative and radical treatment. These techniques should be performed by fully trained surgeons. The role of laparoscopic sentinel lymph node dissection is an area of active investigation.

Complications Due to improved surgical techniques, as well as the use of prophylactic antibiotics and prophylaxis against deep vein thrombosis, the morbidity and mortality associated with radical hysterectomy have declined significantly over the past several decades. The currently accepted complication rate for radical hysterectomy includes approximately a 0.5%–1.0% incidence of urinary tract injury, a 0.5%–1.0% incidence of deep vein thrombosis, and an overall mortality of < 1.0%.

In a prospective study, the rate of recurrence, fertility, and complications was evaluated in 118 women with stages IA2 and IB1 cervical cancer who had undergone radical vaginal trachelectomy (RVT) and pelvic lymphadenectomy. Six patients received chemoradiotherapy after surgery. The average follow-up was 45 months. There were 5 recurrences and 32 complications (6 intraoperative and 26 postoperative). The 5-year pregnancy rate among women trying to conceive was 52.8%. All but two women were delivered by cesarean section, and seven babies (25%) were born prematurely. Therefore, for selected women with early-stage cervical cancer, RVT and pelvic lymphadenectomy are fertility-sparing options (*Shepherd JH, Spencer C, Herod J, et a: Br J Oncol Gynaecol 113:719-724, 2006*).

The increased awareness of the risks associated with blood transfusion is reflected in the fact that, in many cases, no transfusions are administered. The need for heterologous blood transfusion also can be decreased by encouraging autologous blood donation prior to radical hysterectomy or by using intraoperative hemodilution.

The average hospital stay for patients undergoing radical hysterectomy is between 4 and 7 days. Follow-up should include a vaginal Pap smear every 3 months for 2 years, twice a year for 3 years, and yearly thereafter.

Stages IB2 and bulky IIA disease

Numerous studies have demonstrated that patients with early-stage "bulky" lesions (> 4 cm) have a worse prognosis than those with nonbulky tumors. Therefore, patients who

One retrospective analysis compared 109 cervical cancer patients with stage IB1 (bulky disease < 4 cm) and 86 patients with stage IB2 (bulky disease > 4 cm) treated with radical hysterectomy to define predictors of nodal status and recurrence. Multivariate analysis identified only lymphovascular space involvement (LVSI) and parametrial invasion as independent predictors of positive nodes, with a median follow-up of 35 months. The significant independent predictors of disease-free survival (DFS) are LVSI and outer two-thirds depth of invasion. Neither tumor size nor nodal status was a significant predictor of DFS. So, treatment decisions based on tumor size alone should be reconsidered (*Rutledge TL, Kamelle SA, Tillmanns TD, et al: Gynecol Oncol 95:70-76, 2004*).

have undergone radical hysterectomy and pelvic lymphadenectomy for early-stage bulky cervical cancer have traditionally received postoperative adjuvant pelvic radiation therapy. However, a randomized trial from Italy demonstrated that radical hysterectomy plus radiotherapy does not improve overall or disease-free survival in patients with early-stage bulky tumors, as compared with radiation therapy alone, but does significantly increase morbidity.

Furthermore, a recent GOG trial (GOG 123) demonstrated the benefit of the addition of cisplatin chemotherapy to pelvic radiation therapy followed by extrafascial hysterectomy in this group of patients (Figure 1). Therefore, many experts believe that patients with stage IB2 and bulky IIA cervical cancer should be treated initially with chemoradiation therapy instead of radical hysterectomy. GOG attempted to compare chemoradiation therapy with radical hysterectomy followed by chemoradiation therapy for bulky stage IB2 cervical cancer, but unfortunately, the trial closed prematurely due to poor accrual.

CHEMORADIATION THERAPY FOR LOCALLY ADVANCED DISEASE

The role of curative surgery diminishes once cervical cancer has spread beyond the confines of the cervix and vaginal fornices. Intracavitary irradiation for central pelvic disease and external-beam radiation therapy for lateral parametrial and pelvic nodal disease are typically combined to encompass the known patterns of disease spread with an appropriate radiation dose while sparing the bladder and rectum from receiving full doses. The addition of intracavitary irradiation to external-beam irradiation is associated with improved pelvic control and survival over external irradiation alone, as the combination can achieve high central doses of radiation.

Radiation techniques

Intracavitary brachytherapy Radioactive isotopes, such as cesium-137, can be introduced directly into the uterine cavity and vaginal fornices with special applicators. The most commonly used applicator is the Fletcher-Suit intrauterine tandem and vaginal ovoids.

Calculating dose rates With the advent of computerized dosimetry, the dose rate to a number of points from a particular source arrangement can be calculated. Adjustments in the strength or positioning of the sources can then be made to yield a selected dose rate to one or more points.

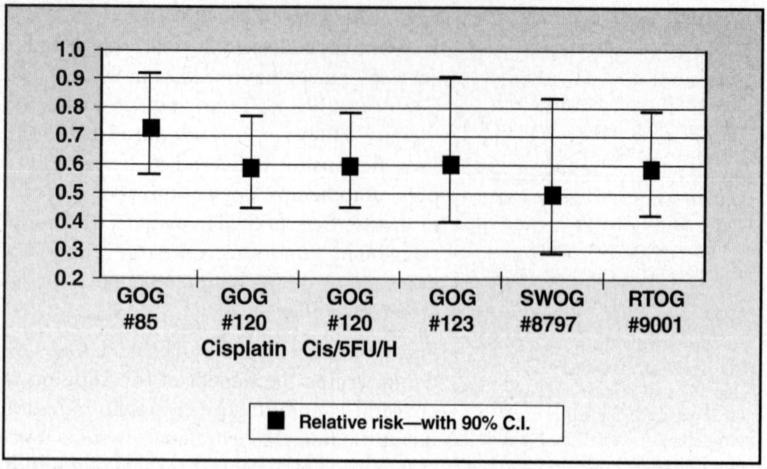

FIGURE 1: Relative risk estimate of survival from five phase III randomized, controlled clinical trials of chemoradiation therapy in women with cervical cancer. A relative risk of 1 indicates no difference in outcome between the treatment arms. A relative risk of < 1 indicates a benefit for the experimental treatment. A relative risk of 0.6, for example, indicates that the treatment has reduced the risk of death by 40%. The relative risks of survival for all five trials, with 90% confidence intervals shown, range from 0.70–0.50, indicating that the concurrent chemoradiation therapy decreased the risk of death by 30%–50% (Rose PG, Bundy BN: J Clin Oncol 20:891–893, 2002).

Quantification of acceptable implant geometry has been described by Katz and Eifel after review of 808 implants performed in 396 patients with cervical cancer treated with irradiation at M. D. Anderson Cancer Center. These guidelines set the standard for high-quality tandem and ovoid insertions.

Points of interest usually include the maximal rectal and bladder dose, as well as the dose to three standard pelvic points: A, B, and P (see Figure 2). Point A is located 2 cm cephalad from the cervical os and 2 cm lateral to the uterine canal. Anatomically, it represents the medial parametrium/lateral cervix, the approximate point at which the ureter and uterine artery cross. Point B is 5 cm lateral to the center of the pelvis at the same level as point A and approximates the region of the obturator nodes or lateral parametrium. Point P is located along the bony pelvic sidewall at its most lateral point and represents the minimal dose to the external iliac lymph nodes.

LDR vs HDR brachytherapy Standard dose rates at point A are typically 50–70 cGy/h; this level is considered low-dose-rate (LDR) brachytherapy. The applicator is placed into the uterus while the patient is under anesthesia in the operating room, and the patient must stay in the hospital for 2–3 days during the procedure. One or two implants are usually placed. Despite the fact that two insertions may allow time for regression of disease between placements, there are no data indicating that two insertions improve pelvic control or survival rates over one insertion.

Whereas LDR brachytherapy has been used successfully for decades in the treatment of carcinoma of the cervix, the use of high-dose-rate (HDR) brachytherapy has been increasing in the United States over the past decade. Dose rates are typically 200–300 cGy/min, with short treatment times allowing for stable position of the applicator.

The major benefit of HDR brachytherapy is that the procedure can be performed on an outpatient basis with less radiation exposure to personnel. The major disadvantage is biologic: large single fractions of radiation (5–10 Gy) are used with 3–10 insertions per patient, which may increase the rate of late complications.

Several series have cited comparable disease control and complication rates with HDR and LDR brachytherapy. A total of 237 patients with previously untreated invasive cervical cancer were enrolled into one randomized study to compare the clinical outcome between high-dose-rate (HDR) and low-dose-rate (LDR) intracavitary brachytherapy. The median follow-up for LDR and HDR groups was 40.2 and 37.2 months, respectively. The 3-year overall and relapse-free survival rates for all patients were 69.6% and 70.0%. There was no significant difference in the following clinical parameters between LDR and HDR groups: the 3-year overall survival rate was 70.9% and 68.4% ($P = .75$), the 3-year pelvic control rate was 89.1% and 86.4% ($P = .51$), and the 3-year relapse-free survival rate in both groups was 69.9% ($P = .35$). Considering patient convenience, the small number of medical personnel needed, and the decreased radiation exposure to health care workers, HDR intracavitary brachytherapy is an alternative to conventional LDR brachytherapy. HDR brachytherapy is an alternative to LDR brachytherapy in current GOG and Radiation Therapy Oncology Group (RTOG) advanced cervical cancer trials.

Guidelines have been published for HDR brachytherapy for cervical cancer by the American Brachytherapy Society.

External-beam pelvic radiation therapy is used in conjunction with intracavitary radiotherapy for stage IA2 disease and above when the risk of pelvic lymph node involvement is significant. The amount of external-beam irradiation delivered and the timing of its administration relative to intracavitary radiation are individualized. For example, the presence of a large exophytic cancer that distorts the cervix would initially preclude successful placement of intracavitary brachytherapy. External-beam radiotherapy would be administered first, and after significant regression of disease, it could be followed by intracavitary radiotherapy.

Various techniques have been developed to optimize external-beam irradiation, including CT simulation, conformal blocking, and, more recently, intensity-modulated radiation therapy (IMRT). These techniques reduce the volume of normal tissue having full-dose irradiation while coverage of the target is not compromised.

Several preliminary reports have been published describing highly conformal dose distributions for patients with carcinoma of the cervix in IMRT. Tumor

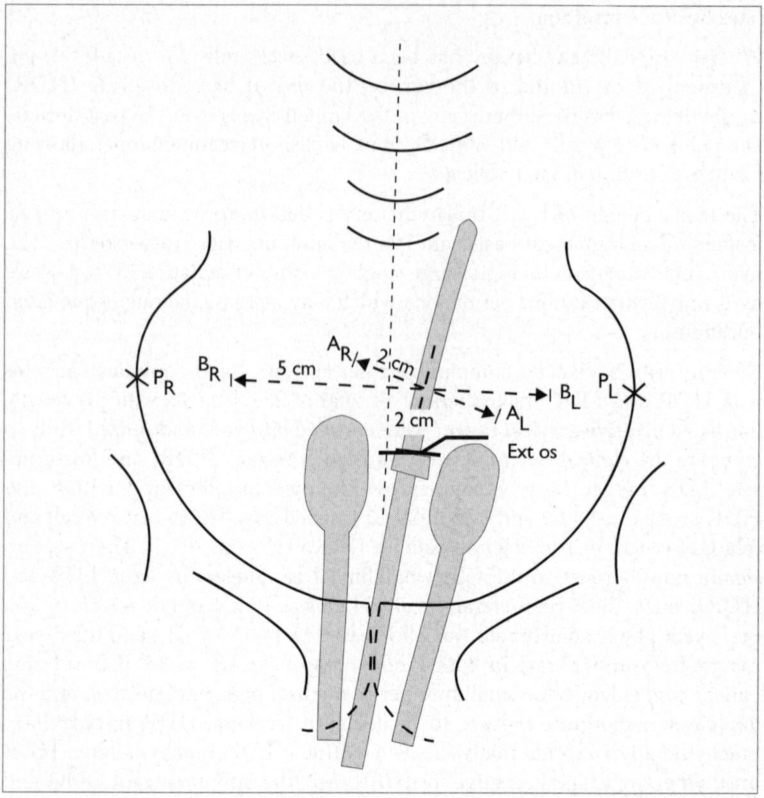

FIGURE 2: Gynecologic Oncology Group (GOG) definitions of points A, B, and P.

control has been about 80% for various stages, and no patient has developed > grade 2 GI or genitourinary toxicity.

Advanced tumors require relatively more external irradiation due to the inability of central radioisotope sources to effectively irradiate disease in the lateral parametrium. Typically, external pelvic doses of 4,000–5,000 cGy are followed by 4,000–5,000 cGy to point A with intracavitary LDR brachytherapy, for a total dose of 8,000–9,000 cGy to point A. A parametrial boost completes treatment to the lateral pelvis, for a total dose to point B or P of 6,000 cGy from external-beam irradiation and brachytherapy, depending on the extent of disease.

With HDR brachytherapy, equivalent doses are prescribed using the linear quadratic equation. The HDR/LDR dose ratio ranges from .5 to .8 depending on the number of HDR fractions.

External-beam para-aortic radiation therapy may be used in addition to external-beam pelvic irradiation when para-aortic disease is confirmed or suspected. An RTOG trial found that external-beam para-aortic irradiation con-

TABLE 2: Relationship between tumor size and outcome in patients with tumors ≥ 5 cm treated with irradiation alone[a]

Tumor size (cm)	Number of patients	Central pelvic control rate (%)	Total pelvic control rate (%)	DSS (%)
5-5.9	200	93	85	69
6-6.9	99	92	79	69
7-7.9	55	90	81	58
≥ 8	48	69	57	40

[a]Excludes patients who underwent adjuvant hysterectomy DSS = disease-specific survival

ferred a survival benefit in patients with advanced cervical cancer (stage IB > 4 cm, stage IIA, and stage IIB) over external-beam pelvic therapy alone. Although external-beam radiation therapy can successfully sterilize microscopic disease, its value in the treatment of gross para-aortic disease is limited, as the tolerance of surrounding organs (bowel, kidneys, spinal cord) precludes the delivery of sufficiently high doses to the para-aortic region.

In multivariate analysis, treatment factors associated with improved pelvic control for cervical cancer include the use of intracavitary brachytherapy, total point A dose > 8,500 cGy (stage III only), and overall treatment time < 8 weeks.

Definitive radiation therapy

CIS, stage IA disease Carcinoma in situ (CIS) and microinvasive cervical cancer (stage IA) are not associated with lymph node metastases. Therefore, intracavitary LDR brachytherapy alone, delivering approximately 5,500 cGy to point A, can control 100% of CIS and stage IA disease and is an acceptable alternative to surgery for patients who cannot undergo surgery due to their medical condition.

Stage IB disease The most important prognostic factor associated with pelvic tumor control and survival following radiation therapy for stage IB cervical cancer is tumor size. The central pelvic control rate with radiotherapy alone is excellent for tumors < 8 cm (97%), with total pelvic control and survival rates of 93% and 82%, respectively. Therefore, many experts have argued that adjuvant hysterectomy following chemoradiation therapy is unnecessary for cervical cancer < 8 cm. For bulky cervical cancers ≥ 8 cm, pelvic control and survival rates decrease to 57% and 40%, respectively, with irradiation alone, and adjuvant hysterectomy may potentially improve local control and survival rates (Table 2).

An updated RTOG trial (RTOG 90-01) for advanced cervical cancer (stage IB or IIA with tumor ≥ 5 cm or with biopsy-proven pelvic lymph node involvement and stages IIB–IVA disease) compared external-beam pelvic irra-

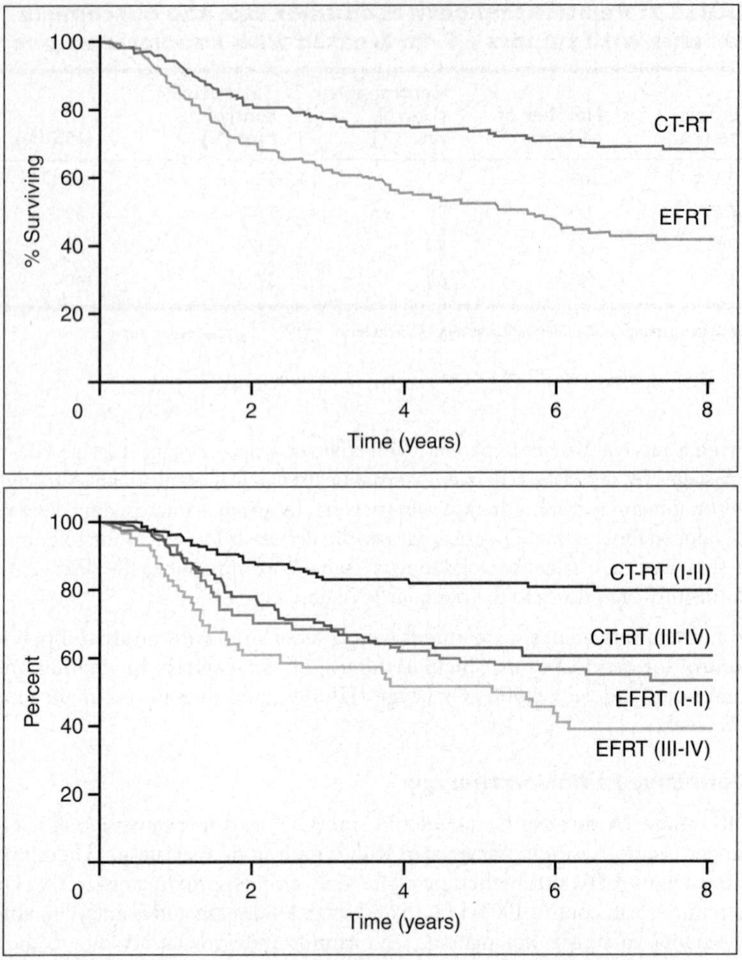

FIGURE 3: Top – Kaplan-Meier estimates of overall survival for patients who received extended-field radiotherapy (EFRT) or concurrent chemotherapy and radiotherapy (CT-RT; *P* < .0001). **Bottom** – Kaplan-Meier estimates of overall survival for patients who received EFRT or CT-RT in subgroups stratified by International Federation of Gynecology and Obstetrics stage (*P* < .0001).

Reprinted with permission from Eifel PJ, Winter K, Morris M, et al: Pelvic irradiation with concurrent chemotherapy versus pelvic and para-aortic irradiation for high-risk cervical cancer: An update of Radiation Therapy Oncology Group Trial (RTOG) 90-01. J Clin Oncol 22: 872–880, 2004. Copyright 2004, American Society of Clinical Oncology. All rights reserved.

diation plus concurrent fluorouracil (5-FU) and cisplatin with external-beam pelvic and para-aortic irradiation; in both arms, these therapies were followed by intracavitary irradiation. The addition of chemotherapy to irradiation improved 5-year survival from 55% to 79% and disease-free survival from 46% to 74% for stage IB/IIA disease by reducing the rates of both local recurrence and distant metastases. For stage III/IVA disease, chemoradiotherapy improved 5-year survival from 45% to 59% and disease-free survival from 37% to 54% (Figures 1 and 3).

GOG 123 randomized patients with stage IB bulky cervical cancer to receive either local treatment alone (external and intracavitary irradiation followed by hysterectomy) or local therapy plus weekly cisplatin. The combination of concurrent weekly cisplatin and irradiation significantly reduced the relapse rate and improved survival by 50%. The 3-year survival rate was significantly improved from 74% to 83% with the use of chemotherapy; this improvement was primarily due to a reduced risk of local recurrence (21% vs 9%).

RTOG 90-01 enrolled 390 patients with locally advanced cervical cancer. Extended-field radiotherapy (EFRT) was compared with pelvic radiotherapy and concomitant fluorouracil and cisplatin (CTRT). The median follow-up time for 228 surviving patients was 6.6 years. The overall survival rate for patients treated with CTRT was significantly greater than that for patients treated with EFRT (67% vs 41% at 8 years; $P < .001$). There was an overall reduction in the risk of disease recurrence of 51% for patients who received CTRT. The addition of fluorouracil and cisplatin to radiotherapy significantly improves the survival rate of women with locally advanced cervical cancer without increasing the rate of late treatment-related side effects (*Eifel PJ, Winter K, Morris M, et al: J Clin Oncol 22:872-880, 2004*).

On the other hand, an Australian gynecologic group randomized study with 76 patients and a Canadian randomized study with 127 patients with stage IB to IIB carcinoma of the cervix treated with chemotherapy and irradiation or irradiation alone showed no significant difference in tumor control or survival. A possible explanation for the discrepancy in the results between the five US trials and the National Cancer Institute (NCI) of Canada study has been analyzed by Lehman and Thomas.

Current treatment recommendations Concurrent radiotherapy and chemotherapy (usually cisplatin-based) with or without adjuvant hysterectomy are standard treatments for bulky IB2 cervical cancer. An alternative approach is radical hysterectomy followed by tailored postoperative chemoradiation therapy.

The use of adjuvant hysterectomy is controversial for stage IB2 cervical cancer, since dose-intense external pelvic and intracavitary irradiation plus chemotherapy may obviate the need for adjuvant surgery. The GOG trial suggests that adjuvant hysterectomy reduces the recurrence rate but does not affect survival.

The use of weekly cisplatin for 6 cycles or 5-FU and cisplatin every 3 weeks × two cycles concurrent with radiotherapy is the standard treatment approach for bulky IB2 cervical cancer.

Stages IIA–IVA disease The most important prognostic factor associated with

A total of 264 patients with recurrent or persistent stage IVB squamous cell carcinoma of the cervix were enrolled into a randomized study to compare cisplatin and cisplatin + paclitaxel (C&P). The median disease progression-free survival was 2.8 and 4.8 months, respectively, for cisplatin vs C&P ($P < .001$). The median follow-up is 2 years. There were no differences in median survival (8.8 vs 9.7 months) and in quality of life. C&P may be superior to cisplatin alone with respect to response rate and disease progression-free survival, with sustained quality of life *(Moore DH, Blessing JA, McQuellon RP, et al: J Clin Oncol 22:3113-3119, 2004).*

pelvic tumor control and survival is the bulk of pelvic disease within each stage. For stage IIB, bulky disease is variously defined as bilateral or lateral parametrial infiltration or central bulky disease > 4 cm in diameter. For stage IIIB, bulky disease is defined as bilateral sidewall involvement, lower-third vaginal involvement, or hydronephrosis.

In the previous GOG experience, in which para-aortic lymph node staging had been mandated, multivariate analysis testing revealed para-aortic lymph node involvement to be the most powerful negative prognostic factor, followed by pelvic lymph node involvement, larger tumor diameter, young age, advanced stage, and lower performance status for patients with negative para-aortic lymph nodes. Five-year survival rates for radiotherapy alone vary from 80% for stage I, 60% for stage II, and 45% for stage III disease, with corresponding pelvic control rates of 90%, 80%, and 50%, respectively.

Chemoradiation therapy A GOG phase III trial (GOG 120) compared standard pelvic external-beam irradiation/intracavitary brachytherapy plus hydroxyurea vs weekly cisplatin vs hydroxyurea, 5-FU, and cisplatin. Both the weekly cisplatin and the 5-FU–cisplatin–hydroxyurea arms produced significantly improved survival and relapse rates compared with hydroxyurea alone. Two-year disease progression-free survival rates were significantly improved from 47% to 67% and 64% with weekly cisplatin-irradiation and 5-FU–cisplatin–hydroxyurea–irradiation compared with hydroxyurea and radiotherapy (Figure 1). The improved outcome was due to the reduced rates of pelvic failure and lung metastases. Because of an improved therapeutic ratio, weekly cisplatin is the favored regimen.

GOG 165 compared standard radiation therapy plus concurrent weekly cisplatin vs concurrent protracted venous infusion 5-FU (225 mg/m^2/d over 5 weeks) as radiation sensitizers. In this study, the dose of radiation to point A (in Figure 2) had been increased by 500 cGy, and the pelvic fields were redefined to improve the dose intensity and accuracy of radiotherapy. This recently reported study confirms the efficacy of pelvic radiotherapy with weekly cisplatin. The study was closed prematurely when a planned interim analysis indicated that the 5-FU arm had a 35% higher rate of treatment failure. An editorial published with the article highlighted the future difficulties with randomized trials for this population.

Current treatment recommendations In view of the multiple randomized trials documenting a survival benefit with concurrent chemoradiotherapy, the use of concurrent weekly cisplatin or cisplatin–5-FU every 3 weeks with irradiation is standard therapy for stages IB2–IVA cervical cancer (Figure 1).

Five large randomized clinical trials demonstrated a significant survival benefit for patients treated with concurrent chemoradiotherapy, using a cisplatin-based regimen, with a 28%–50% relative reduction in the risk of death. In addition, the results of a meta-analysis of 19 randomized clinical trials of concurrent chemoradiotherapy involving 4,580 patients showed that concurrent chemoradiotherapy significantly improved overall survival (hazard ratio [HR] = 0.71; $P < .001$), as well as disease progression-free survival (HR = 0.61; $P < .0001$). In line with these results, concurrent chemoradiotherapy is currently recommended as standard therapy (Table 3).

The current phase II GOG trial for advanced cervical cancer (stages IB2–IVA) is randomizing patients to undergo pelvic radiotherapy plus cisplatin weekly or pelvic radiotherapy, cisplatin, and tirapazamine (a hypoxic cell sensitizer).

For patients without para-aortic lymph node metastases, pelvic external irradiation (4,000–5,000 cGy) should be used, followed by intracavitary LDR brachytherapy (4,000–5,000 cGy) to point A, for a total dose of 8,000–9,000 cGy to point A.

Adjuvant radiotherapy following radical hysterectomy

Node-negative disease Local failure rates approach 20% following radical hysterectomy and pelvic lymphadenectomy when pelvic lymph nodes are not involved but the primary tumor has high-risk characteristics (primary tumor > 4 cm, outer-third cervical stromal invasion, and capillary-lymphatic space invasion). A GOG trial randomized these intermediate-risk patients with node-negative disease to receive pelvic external-beam radiation therapy (5,100 cGy/30 fractions) or no further therapy following radical hysterectomy-pelvic lymphadenectomy. Postoperative irradiation produced a significant 44% reduction in recurrence; the recurrence-free rate at 2 years was 88% with irradiation vs 79% without it. Survival analysis awaits further follow-up.

Node-positive disease For patients with positive pelvic lymph nodes following radical hysterectomy-pelvic lymphadenectomy, pelvic radiotherapy reduces the pelvic failure rate from approximately 50% to 25% but does not affect survival, since distant metastases are still seen in 30% of patients. A recently reported GOG/Southwest Oncology Group (SWOG 8797) trial randomized these high-risk patients with node-positive disease (or patients with positive surgical margins) to undergo pelvic external-beam irradiation (4,930 cGy/29 fractions) vs pelvic external-beam irradiation plus concurrent 5-FU and cisplatin for 4 cycles following radical hysterectomy-pelvic lymphadenectomy. A significant improvement in disease progression-free and overall survival was seen for concurrent 5-FU–cisplatin and radiation therapy compared with radiation therapy alone (4-year survival, 81% vs 71%).

Current treatment recommendations At present, the use of adjuvant pelvic radiotherapy should be considered for patients with negative nodes who are at risk for pelvic failure and remains the standard postoperative treatment for patients with positive lymph nodes. Treatment consists of external pelvic irradiation

(45–50 Gy), with specific sites boosted with further external-beam or intracavitary irradiation as needed.

Since the combination of radical surgery and irradiation has greater morbidity than either modality alone, complete preoperative assessment is crucial to minimize the need for both.

Since concurrent chemoradiation therapy following radical hysterectomy provides a significant benefit in node-positive high-risk cervical cancer, it should be part of the postoperative treatment plan. Postoperative chemoradiation therapy following radical hysterectomy should be strongly considered for patients with negative nodes but positive margins or parametria, ≥ middle-third stromal invasion, and lymphovascular space invasion for tumors ≥ 5 cm.

SURGICAL MANAGEMENT OF RECURRENT OR METASTATIC DISEASE

Recurrent advanced disease

Pelvic exenteration For patients whose disease fails to respond to primary radiation therapy or for those with early invasive cervical carcinoma whose disease recurs after surgery or radiation therapy, pelvic exenteration offers the possibility of cure. Patients should be considered for pelvic exenteration only if they have locoregional disease that can be completely removed by this radical surgical procedure. In most cases, patients will require surgical removal of the bladder, uterus, cervix, vagina, and rectum.

Of all patients who are considered candidates for pelvic exenteration, only about half will be found to have resectable disease at the time of exploratory laparotomy. For patients who successfully undergo pelvic exenteration, 5-year survival rates range from 25% to 50%.

When the patient has central recurrence of squamous cell or adenocarcinoma of the cervix, the initial evaluation includes a complete physical examination, as well as an abdominopelvic CT or MRI scan and, usually, a chest CT scan.

Evidence of extrapelvic disease is a contraindication to pelvic exenteration. If no evidence of disease beyond the pelvis is found, the patient can be prepared for pelvic exenteration.

> A prospective study comparing the accuracy of PET scan with that of CT and/or MRI scans has been presented. Eighteen patients underwent PET scans with CT or MRI scans prior to surgical exploration for pelvic exenteration. PET scan was reported to be the most accurate method of detecting extrapelvic metastasis, with a sensitivity of 100% and a specificity of 73% (*Husain A, Akhurst T, Larson SM, et al: Gynecol Oncol [abstract] 92:417, 2004*).

Preparation for exenteration includes complete bowel preparation, a visit with the stomal therapy nurse, and counseling regarding the radical nature of the surgery and the anticipated changes in body image after the operation. In most cases, we counsel the patient that vaginal reconstruction should be performed at the time of pelvic exenteration, both for maintenance of body image and improved healing.

TABLE 3: Large randomized studies of concurrent chemoradiotherapy in cervical cancer

Author	Stage	Design	RT	CT (mg/m^2, except for HU)	No. of patients	Survival (%) CT/RT vs RT(follow-up)	*P value*
Whitney, GOG 85, 1999	IIB-IVAPAN(-) Washing cytology (-)	WP+PF × 3 vs WP+HU+PAN	IIB:40 Gy+Ra III, IVA: WP, 51Gy+Ra III, IV: 61 Gy	P:50/day 1 F:1,000/days 2-5, every 4 weeks HU:80 mg/kg/twice a week	388	55 vs 43 (8.7 years)	.018
Rose, GOG 120, 1999	IIIB-IVA PAN(-)	WP+P weekly vs WP+PF+HU vs WP+HU	IIB: 40 Gy+Ra; III, IVA: WP, 51 Gy +Ra; III, IV: 61 Gy	P:40/week for 4 weeks vs P: 50/day 1+F:1,000/days 1-4 Hu:2,000/0/week, every 4 weeks vs HU:3,000/2/week of 6 weeks	176	66 vs 67 vs 50 (3 years) 8 vs 71 (4 years)	.0040 .002
Keys GOG 123, 1999	IB ≥ 4 cm	WP + P weekly vs WP Adj TAH	WP:45 Gy + Ra	P:40/week for 6 weeks	369	83 vs 74 (3 years)	.008
Peters SWOG 8797, 2000	IA2-IIA Postsurgical pN1/pT2b/ stump(+)	WP+PF × 4 vs WP + PAN	WP:45 GyWP+PAN	P:70/day 1 + F: 1,000/days 1-4, every 3 weeks	268	81 vs 71 (4 years)	.007
Eifel RTOG 90-01,2004	IB-IVA > 5cm PAN(-)	WP+PF × 3 vs WP+PAN	WP: 45 Gy PAN:45 Gy	P:75/day 1F:1,000/days 2-5, every 3 weeks	403	67 vs 41 (8 years)	.0001

CT = chemotherapy; RT = radiotherapy; WP = whole pelvis; PAN = para-aortic lymph node; Adj = adjuvant; TAH = total abdominal hysterectomy; P = Platinol (cisplatin); F = 5-FU; Ra = radium therapy; HU = hydroxyurea

Adapted with permission from Kuzuya K: Chemotherapy for uterine cancer: Current status and perspective. Int J Clin Oncol 9:458–470, 2005.

Surgical procedure During surgery, a careful exploration is carried out to confirm that there is no evidence of unresectable disease beyond the pelvis. The pelvic sidewall spaces are opened and resectability is determined. An en bloc resection is usually performed; in some cases, especially when the recurrent tumor involves the lower vagina, a two-team approach can expedite the procedure. The actual exenterative portion of the procedure may take several hours and is usually accompanied by significant blood loss. In cases where surgical margin status may be questionable, the use of intraoperative radiation therapy is considered.

Reconstruction Following the exenterative procedure, the reconstructive portion of the procedure begins. We currently recommend to nearly all patients that they consider a continent urinary diversion. Although this step may add approximately 30–60 minutes to the surgical procedure, the improvement in quality of life is significant.

In patients who have undergone a supralevator pelvic exenteration, we frequently attempt a stapled reanastomosis of the colon. Unless there is excessive tension on the anastomosis or other problems, a diverting colostomy is not routinely indicated. About one-third of these patients suffer anastomotic breakdown in the postoperative period. At that time, a diverting colostomy can be performed. Unfortunately, Hatch et al found no benefit to the earlier use of colostomy.

Lung metastasis

For the rare patient who presents with a single isolated lung metastasis after treatment of invasive cervical carcinoma, pulmonary resection may offer the possibility of long-term disease-free survival or even cure in selected cases. For patients who have multiple lung metastases or unresectable pelvic disease, surgery offers little or no hope and produces significant morbidity and mortality.

RADIATION THERAPY FOR RECURRENT OR METASTATIC DISEASE

Local recurrence after radical hysterectomy

Local recurrence confined to the pelvis following radical hysterectomy for cervical cancer can be treated with radiotherapy with curative intent. An experience with 5-FU–based chemotherapy and concurrent pelvic external-beam irradiation resulted in a 58% complete response rate and a 45% no-evidence-of-disease rate, at a median follow-up of 57 months. The total pelvic external-beam dose was 5,280 cGy plus a boost to sites of recurrence with twice-daily 160-cGy fractions during the 5-FU infusion. Therefore, radiotherapy, with or without chemotherapy, can provide durable local control, with better results attainable for small, central recurrences, for which brachytherapy is possible.

TABLE 4: Active agents as defined by a response rate of at least 15%

Drug	No. of Patients	Responses	Response rate
Alkylating agents			
Chlorambucil	44	11	25%
Cyclophosphamide	251	38	15%
Dibromodulcitol	120	23	23%
Galactitol	36	7	19%
Ifosfamide	157	35	22%
Melphalan	20	4	20%
Heavy metal complexes			
Carboplatin	175	27	15%
Cisplatin	815	190	23%
Antibiotics			
Doxorubicin	266	45	17%
Porfiromycin	78	17	22%
Antimetabolites			
Baker's antifol	32	5	16%
5-Fluorouracil	142	29	20%
Methotrexate	96	17	18%
Plant alkaloids			
Vincristine	55	10	18%
Vindesine	21	5	24%
Vinorelbine	42	6	15%
Other agents			
Irinotecan	55	13	24%
Hexamethylmelamine	64	12	19%
ICRF-159	28	5	18%
Paclitaxel	52	9	17%
Topotecan	43	8	19%

Adapted with permission from Thigpen T: The role of chemotherapy in the management of carcinoma of the cervix. Cancer J 9:425–432, 2003.

Local recurrence after definitive radiation therapy

Local recurrence confined to the pelvis following definitive radiation therapy rarely can be cured with exenteration. In a series of patients treated with definitive radiotherapy, 21% of recurrences (80 of 376) were isolated to the pelvis. Only 29% of these localized pelvic recurrences (23 of 80) were explored for curative exenteration, and for the 43% of patients (10 of 23) deemed operable, the 5-year survival rate was 16%.

Palliation of metastatic disease

Palliative radiation therapy to sites of metastatic cervical cancer is effective. The most common sites of metastasis are distant lymph nodes, bone, and lungs. Reirradiation of the pelvis is possible in selected patients to control local symptoms, such as bleeding, but carries an increased risk of bowel complications. For previously unirradiated sites of metastatic disease, 3,000 cGy in 10 fractions provides palliation of symptoms in the majority of patients.

CHEMOTHERAPY FOR ADVANCED/RECURRENT DISEASE

Chemotherapy has traditionally been used for the palliative management of advanced or recurrent disease that can no longer be managed by surgery or radiation therapy (see Table 3). Various factors complicate the use of chemotherapy in such patients, however. Prior radiation treatment can affect the blood supply to the involved field, which may result in decreased drug delivery to the tumor site. Pelvic irradiation also reduces bone marrow reserve, thus limiting the tolerable doses of most chemotherapeutic agents. Moreover, irradiation may produce its cytotoxic effect, in part, through a mechanism similar to that of alkylating agents; thus, it is thought to be cross-resistant with some chemotherapeutic agents. A significant number of patients with advanced disease may also have impaired renal function, further limiting the use of certain chemotherapeutic regimens.

Single agents

Among the chemotherapeutic agents used for cervical cancer, cisplatin and ifosfamide (Ifex) have shown the most consistent activity as single agents (Table 4). The duration of response with any single agent is brief, ranging from 4 to 6 months, with survival ranging from 6 to 9 months.

Cisplatin has been the most extensively evaluated single agent for cervical carcinoma. A dose of 100 mg/m^2 was shown to have a higher response rate than a dose of 50 mg/m^2 (31% vs 21%), but the higher dose was associated with increased toxicity, and overall survival did not differ significantly between the two groups. A 24-hour infusion of cisplatin was tolerated better than a 2-hour infusion, with no difference in therapeutic efficacy.

Ifosfamide produces response rates ranging from 33% to 50% in various dose schedules. A dose of 1.5 g/m^2 over 30 minutes for 5 days (with mesna [Mesnex]) produced an overall response rate of 40% and a complete response rate of 20%.

Lower response rates are generally seen in patients who have had prior chemotherapy. Responses also are decreased in previously irradiated sites.

Taxanes Paclitaxel and docetaxel (Taxotere) have been reported to be active in cervical cancer. A study of paclitaxel (170 mg/m^2 over 24 hours) showed an ob-

TABLE 5: Combination chemotherapy for advanced or recurrent cervical carcinoma

Chemotherapy regimen	Number of evaluable patients	Prior radiation therapy (%)	Complete response rate (%)	Overall response rate (%)
Bleomycin/ifosfamide/cisplatin	49	86	20	69
Bleomycin/ifosfamide/carboplatin	21	49	23	60
Vinblastine/bleomycin/cisplatin	33	66	18	67
5-FU/doxorubicin/vincristine/cyclophosphamide	31	87	9	58
Paclitaxel/cisplatin[a]	130	91	–	36
Paclitaxel/carboplatin[b]	32	–	22	72
Gemcitabine/cisplatin[c]	32	69	25	63
Irinotecan/cisplatin[d]	27	–	4	37

From Lopez A, Kudelka AP, Edwards CL, et al: Carcinoma of the uterine cervix. In: Pazdur R (ed): Medical Oncology: A Comprehensive Review, 2nd ed. Melville, New York, PRR, 1996.

[a]Moore DH; [b]Mickiewicz E; [c]Mahfouf H; [d]Garin A: Proc Am Soc Clin Oncol 20: 201–207, 2001.

jective response rate of 17%, and another study of paclitaxel (250 mg/m^2 over 3 hours) demonstrated an objective response rate of 27%. Docetaxel (100 mg/m^2 over 1 hour) has yielded a response rate of 19%.

Camptothecins Irinotecan (CPT-11 [Camptosar]) and topotecan (Hycamtin), semisynthetic camptothecins, have shown activity in patients with cervical cancer, even in patients who did not respond to prior chemotherapy and prior radiation therapy. The reported objective response rates were 21% and 19%, respectively.

Combination regimens

Various combination chemotherapy regimens have been evaluated in phase II trials, and high response rates (> 50%) were noted, even in patients who had received prior radiation therapy. The results of some of these trials are summarized in Tables 5 and 6. In one study, a subset analysis showed a response rate of 72% with the combination of bleomycin, ifosfamide, and cisplatin as treatment for tumors located in previously irradiated sites. Neoadjuvant regimens of cisplatin combined with gemcitabine (Gemzar) in patients with locally advanced cervical cancer demonstrated very high activity, with a clinical response rate of 95%. Neoadjuvant ifosfamide and cisplatin, with or without paclitaxel, produced 87% and 82% response rates, respectively, among 146 evaluable patients in a randomized study.

A randomized trial was recently reported by Long et al. A total of 146 patients with advanced persistent or recurrent cervical cancer were treated with cisplatin

TABLE 6: New combination chemotherapy for cervical cancer

Author	Subjects	Design	CT regimen (mg/m^2)	No. of patients	RR (%) (95% CI)	Median survival	Remarks
Rose (GOG), 1999	CT-naive SCC	Phase II	TP: T, 135/24h + P, 75, q 3 weeks	44	46.3 (30.7–62.6)	PFI: 5.4 months OS: 10.0 months	Non-RT site vs RT site: 70% vs 23% (*P* = .008)
Piver, 1999	CT-naive SCC + adenocarcinoma	Phase II	TP: T, 135/24h + P, 75, q 4 weeks	20	45	PFS: 10.5 vs 4 months (*P* = .015) OS: 13 vs 6 months (*P* = .14)	RT field: outside vs inside Outside, better response: 60%
Papadimitriou, 1999	Stage IV/rec SCC + adenocarcinoma	Phase II	TP: T, 175/3h+P, 75, q 3 weeks with G-CSF	34	47 (30–65)	PFI: 5.5 months TTP: 5 months OS: 9 months	G3/4 neuropathy: 43%
Park, 2004	Stage IB2-IIB SCC + adenocarcinoma	Phase II NAC-surgery	TP:T, 60/3h+P, 60, q 10 days;	43	90.7		CR: 39.5%; pCR: 11.6% PR: 51.2%, downstaging: 72.1%
Mickiewicz (GOL), 2001	CT-naive	Phase II	TJ: T, 175/3h+J, AUC 5, q 3 weeks	32	71.9 (56.4–87.4)	PFI: 7 months	
Zanetta, 1999	Rec, SCC	Phase II, Salvage	TIP: T, 175/3h day 1+I, 5000, day 2+ P, 75 day 2, q 3 weeks	45	67 (51–81)	OS: Nonresponders vs responders: 6 vs 13 months	Non-RT site vs RT site: 75% vs 52%; G 3/4 myelotoxicity, 91%
D'Agostino, 2002	IB2-IVA SCC + adenocarcinoma	Phase II	TEP: T, 175+E, 100 +P, 100, q 3 weeks	42	78.5 (63.8–93.2)	PFS: 47 months	Surgical rate: 76.2%
Moore (GOG), 2004	Stage IVB/rec	Phase III, P vs TP	P:50 vs TP; T, 135/24 h+P, 50, q 3 weeks	264	19.4% vs 36.2%	PFI: 2.8 vs 4.8 months OS: 8.8 vs 9.7 months	RR: *P* = .002; PFI, < .01
Kitagawa, 2004	Rec	Phase II	T: 175/3h+J, AUC 5, q 3 weeks	28	61 (41–78)	PFS: 5.9 months	OS: NS Non-RT site RT site: 57% vs 67%

RR = relative risk; CI = confidence interval; SCC = small-cell cancer; TP = Taxol + cisplatin; PFI = progression-free interval; OS = overall survival; PFS = progression-free survival; G-CSF = granulocyte colony-stimulating factor; NAC = neoadjuvant chemotherapy; CR = complete response; pCR = pathologic complete response; TJ = Taxol + JM-8 (carboplatin); AUC = area under the curve; TIP = Taxol + ifosfamide + cisplatin; TEP = Taxol + epirubicin + cisplatin; J = carboplatin; Rec = recurrent

(50 mg/m^2 IV every 21 days), and 147 patients were treated with topotecan (.75 mg/m^2 IV during 30 minutes on days 1, 2, and 3 followed by cisplatin (50 mg/m^2 on day 1) repeated every 21 days. All regimens were administered for a maximum of 6 cycles for nonresponders or until disease progression or unacceptable toxicity prohibited additional chemotherapy. The complete response rate was 3% for cisplatin and 10% for the cisplatin-topotecan combination, and the complete and partial remission rates were 13% and 27%, respectively; the median progression-free survival was 2.9 and 4.6 months, respectively.

Palliative care

Palliation of the dying cervical cancer patient is difficult. Pain due to recurrent pelvic disease can be extreme and requires skillful use of combinations of narcotics, sedatives, and anxiolytics. Fistula from the bladder or rectum demands meticulous local skin care and occasionally surgical diversion procedures in patients with reasonable expected longevity. This patient population often has limited resources, with dependent children requiring careful social service planning. A small percentage has concurrent HIV infection, making the infectious disease specialist part of the palliative care team. The tripod of care in advanced cervical cancer is the judicious use of chemotherapy and radiation therapy, palliation of the symptoms of advancing disease, as well as emotional and social support for the patient and family members.

SUGGESTED READING

Eifel PJ, Winter K, Morris M, et al: Pelvic irradiation with concurrent chemotherapy versus pelvic and para-aortic irradiation for high-risk cervical cancer: An update of Radiation Therapy Oncology Group trial (RTOG) 90-01. J Clin Oncol 22:872–880, 2004.

Frazer IH: Prevention of cervical cancer through papillomavirus vaccination. Nature Rev Immunol 4:46–54, 2004.

Grigsby PW, Siegel BA, Dehdashti F, et al: Posttherapy surveillance monitoring of cervical cancer by FDG-PET. Int J Radiat Oncol Biol Phys 55:907–913, 2003.

Harper D, Franco E, Ferris D, et al: Efficacy of a bivalent L1 virus-like particle vaccine in prevention of infection with human papillomavirus types 16 and 18 in young women: A randomized controlled trial. Lancet 364:1757–1765, 2004.

Keys HM, Bundy BN, Stehman FB, et al: Cisplatin, radiation, and adjuvant hysterectomy compared with radiation and adjuvant hysterectomy for bulky stage IB cervical carcinoma. N Engl J Med 340:1154–1161, 1999.

Keys HM, Bundy BN, Stehman FB, et al: Radiation therapy with and without extrafascial hysterectomy for bulky stage IB cervical carcinoma: A randomized trial of the Gynecologic Oncology Group. Gynecol Oncol 89:343–353, 2003.

Kim RY, Alvarez RD, Omura GA: Advances in the treatment of gynecologic malignancies Part 1: Cancers of the cervix and vulva. Oncology 16:1510–1530, 2002.

Kochanski JD, Roeske JC, Mell LK, et al: Outcome of FIGO stage I-II cervical cancer patients treated with intensity modulated pelvic radiation therapy [abstract]. Proc Am Soc Clin Oncol 23:454, 2004.

Kuzuya K: Chemoradiotherapy for uterine cancer: Current status and perspectives. Int J Clin Oncol 9:458–470, 2004.

Lanciano R, Calkins A, Bundy BN, et al: Randomized comparison of weekly cisplatin or protracted venous infusion of fluorouracil in combination with pelvic radiation in advanced cervix cancer: A Gynecologic Oncology Group Study. J Clin Oncol 23:8289–8294, 2005.

Landoni F, Maneo A, Colombo A, et al: Randomised study of radical surgery versus radiotherapy for stage Ib-IIa cervical cancer. Lancet 350:535–540, 1997.

Lehman M, Thomas G: Is concurrent chemotherapy and radiotherapy the new standard of care for locally advanced cancer? Int J Gynaecol Oncol 11:87–99, 2001.

Long HJ 3rd, Bundy BN, Grendys EC Jr, et al: Randomized phase III trial of cisplatin with or without topotecan in carcinoma of the uterine cervix: A Gynecologic Oncology Group Study. J Clin Oncol 23:4626–4633, 2005.

Miller TR, Grigsby PW: Measurement of tumor volume by PET to evaluate prognosis in patients with advanced cervical cancer treated by radiation therapy. Int J Radiat Oncol Biol Phys 53:353–359, 2002.

Moore D, Blessing J, McQuellon R, et al: Phase III study of cisplatin with or without paclitaxel in stage IVB, recurrent, or persistent squamous cell carcinoma of the cervix: A Gynecologic Oncology Group study. J Clin Oncol 222:3113–3119, 2004.

Pearcey R, Brundage M, Drouin P, et al: Phase III trial comparing radical radiotherapy with and without cisplatin chemotherapy in patients with advanced squamous cell cancer of the cervix. J Clin Oncol 20:966–972, 2002.

Portelance L, Chao KS, Grigsby PW, et al: Intensity-modulated radiation therapy reduces small bowel, rectum, and bladder doses in patients with cervical cancer receiving pelvic and para-aortic irradiation. Int J Radiat Oncol Biol Phys 51:261–266, 2001.

Rose P, Bundy B, Watkins E, et al: Concurrent cisplatin-based radiotherapy and chemotherapy for locally advanced cervical cancer. N Engl J Med 340:1144–1153, 1999.

Rotman M, Sedlis A, Piedmonte MR, et al: A phase III randomized trial of postoperative pelvic irradiation in stage IB cervical carcinoma with poor prognostic features: Follow-up of a gynecologic oncology group study. Int J Radiat Oncol Biol Phys 65:169–176, 2006.

Thigpen T: The role of chemotherapy in the management of carcinoma of the cervix. Cancer J 9:425–432, 2003.

Tierney J: Neoadjuvant chemotherapy for locally advanced cervical cancer: A systematic review and meta-analysis of individual patient data from 21 randomized trials. Eur J Cancer 39:2470–2486, 2003.

Wright Jr TC, Schiffman M, Solomon D, et al: Interim guidance for the use of human papillomavirus DNA testing as an adjunct to cervical cytology for screening. Obstet Gynecol 103:304–309, 2004.

The authors would like to thank Dr. Xipeng Wang, Dr. Hye-Sook Chon, and Lora Lothringer for their assistance.

CHAPTER 21

Uterine corpus tumors

Kathryn M. Greven, MD, Maurie Markman, MD, and David Scott Miller, MD

ENDOMETRIAL CANCER

Carcinoma of the epithelial lining (endometrium) of the uterine corpus is the most common female pelvic malignancy. Factors influencing its prominence are the declining incidence of cervical cancer, longer life expectancy, and earlier diagnosis. Adenocarcinoma of the endometrium, the most prevalent histologic subtype, is currently the fourth most common cancer in women, with 39,080 new cases, ranking behind breast, lung, and bowel cancers. Endometrial adenocarcinoma is the eighth leading cause of death from malignancy in women, accounting for 7,400 deaths this year.

Epidemiology

Age Endometrial cancer is primarily a disease of postmenopausal women, although 25% of cases occur in premenopausal patients, with 5% of cases developing in patients < 40 years old.

Geography The incidence of endometrial cancer is higher in Western nations and very low in Eastern countries.

Immigrant populations tend to assume the risks of native populations, highlighting the importance of environmental factors in the genesis of this disease. Endometrial cancers tend to be more common in urban than in rural residents. In the United States, white women have a twofold higher incidence of endometrial cancer than black women.

Etiology and risk factors

Adenocarcinoma of the endometrium may arise in normal, atrophic, or hyperplastic endometrium. Two mechanisms are generally believed to be involved in the development of endometrial cancer. In approximately 75% of women, there is a history of exposure to unopposed estrogen, either endogenous or exogenous (type I). The tumors in these women begin as endometrial hyperplasia and progress to carcinomas, which usually are better differentiated and have a favorable prognosis.

In the other 25% of women, carcinomas appear spontaneously, are not clearly related to a transition from atypical hyperplasia, and rather arise in a background of atrophic or inert endometrium. These neoplasms tend to be associated with a more undifferentiated cell type and a poorer prognosis (type II).

Unopposed estrogen It has been hypothesized that long-term estrogenic stimulation of the endometrium unmodified by progesterone has a role in the development of endometrial carcinoma. This hypothesis derives from observations that women who are infertile or obese or who have dysfunctional bleeding due to anovulation are at high risk for this disease, as are women with estrogen-secreting granulosa theca cell ovarian tumors. Also, the recognition that atypical adenomatous (complex) hyperplasia is a precursor of cancer, and that it is associated with unopposed estrogen in women, underscores the importance of the association among risk factors, estrogens, and cancer. In the late 1970s and early 1980s, several case-control studies demonstrated that the risk of endometrial cancer is increased 4–15-fold in long-term estrogen users, as compared with age-matched controls.

It is well established that past use of oral contraceptive pills protects against endometrial cancer. Maxwell et al presented a retrospective review of the US Cancer and Steroid Hormone (CASH) study to determine the effects of progestin potency. They evaluated 417 endometrial cases and 2,452 controls. It appeared that there may be an increased benefit in the higher potency progestins (overall response = 0.3 [95% confidence interval (CI): 0.2–0.6]) vs lower potency progestins (overall response = 0.5 [95% CI: 0.3–0.6]), although these differences were not significant. They also suggested that in women with a higher body mass index (BMI), the higher potency progestins might be more protective. Higher progestin dose has a greater effect on decreasing risk.

Diet The high rate of occurrence of endometrial cancer in Western societies and the very low rate in Eastern countries suggest a possible etiologic role for nutrition, especially the high content of animal fat in Western diets. There may be a relationship between high-fat diets and the higher incidence of endometrial carcinoma in women with conditions of unopposed estrogen: Endogenous estrogens rise in postmenopausal women because of increased production of androstenedione or a greater peripheral conversion of this hormone to estrone. In obese women, the extraglandular aromatization of androstenedione to estrone is increased in fatty tissue.

Obesity Phenotypically, the majority of women who develop endometrial cancer tend to be obese. Women who are 30 pounds over ideal weight have a 3-fold increased risk of developing endometrial cancer, whereas those 50 pounds or more over ideal weight have a 10-fold increased risk.

Parity Nulliparous women are at 2 times greater risk of developing endometrial cancer, females who undergo menopause after age 52 are at 2.5 times greater risk, and those who experience increased bleeding at the time of menopause are at 4 times greater risk.

Other risk factors Other known risk factors for endometrial cancer include diabetes mellitus; hypertension; endometrial hyperplasia; and a family history of endometrial, breast, and/or colon cancer. Diabetic females have a 3-fold increased risk, and hypertensive patients have a 1.5-fold greater risk of endometrial cancer. Whereas patients found to have simple endometrial hyperplasia have a low risk of disease progression to cancer, 29% of those with complex atypical hyperplasia, if left untreated, will develop adenocarcinoma.

Tamoxifen exerts its primary effect by blocking the binding of estrogen to estrogen receptors. It also exerts mild estrogenic effects on the female genital tract. This weak estrogenic effect presumably accounts for an increased frequency of endometrial carcinoma observed in women receiving prolonged adjuvant tamoxifen therapy for breast carcinoma.

Initially reported in 1985, the increased frequency of endometrial carcinoma in patients treated with tamoxifen was characterized more fully in a study of 1,846 women recorded in the Swedish Cancer Registry. This study reported a 6.4-fold increase in the relative risk of endometrial carcinoma with a daily dose of 40 mg of tamoxifen. The greatest cumulative risk was observed after 5 years of tamoxifen use.

The National Surgical Adjuvant Breast and Bowel Project (NSABP) subsequently reported on the incidence of other cancers in 2,843 women with node-negative, estrogen-receptor–positive breast cancer treated with either tamoxifen or placebo in its B-14 randomized trial and an additional 1,220 patients treated with tamoxifen in another NSABP trial. The relative risk of endometrial carcinoma in the tamoxifen-treated patients was 7.5. The hazard rate was 0.2 per 1,000 cases with placebo and 1.6 per 1,000 cases with tamoxifen therapy. The mean duration of tamoxifen therapy for all patients was 35 months, and 36% of the cancers had developed by 2 years after the initiation of treatment. A more recent review of NSABP treatment and prevention trials revealed that the risk of uterine sarcomas was also increased with tamoxifen. The incidence of sarcomas was very low, however, with a rate of 0.17/1,000 women/year.

These data raise the question of whether tamoxifen should be used as adjuvant therapy for women at relatively low risk for breast cancer recurrence. First, it should be recognized that the endometrial cancers that develop in patients receiving tamoxifen exhibit the same stage, grade, and prognosis distribution as other endometrial cancers. There is some evidence that tamoxifen use is associated with an increased risk of uterine sarcoma; fortunately, this risk is low, and the cure rate should be high. Second, adjuvant tamoxifen reduces the cumulative rate of recurrence of breast cancer from 228 to 124 cases/1,000 women and the cumulative rate of second primary breast cancers from 40.5 to 23.5 cases/1,000 women.

When all of these facts are taken into account, there is an overall 38% reduction in the cumulative hazard rate for recurrence of breast cancer in tamoxifen-treated patients. Thus, the benefits of tamoxifen outweigh the risks of endometrial cancer.

The current recommendations for screening women on tamoxifen are to educate patients about the significance of abnormal spotting, bleeding, or discharge and to investigate promptly any of these abnormalities.

Some experts have proposed that tamoxifen-treated women be screened with transvaginal ultrasonography. However, recent data suggest a high false-positive rate and a low frequency of significant findings, leading to the conclusion that endometrial screening is not warranted.

Signs and symptoms

Postmenopausal women Symptoms of early endometrial carcinoma are few. However, 90% of patients complain of abnormal vaginal discharge, and 80% of these women experience abnormal bleeding, usually after menopause. In the general population, 15% of postmenopausal women presenting with abnormal bleeding will be found to have endometrial carcinoma. Signs and symptoms of more advanced disease include pelvic pressure and other symptoms indicative of uterine enlargement or extrauterine tumor spread.

Premenopausal women The diagnosis of endometrial cancer may be difficult to make in premenopausal patients. The physician must maintain a high index of suspicion in this group of patients and perform endometrial sampling in any women who complain of prolonged, heavy menstrual periods or intermenstrual spotting.

Screening and diagnosis

Screening There is no role for screening of asymptomatic patients for endometrial cancer.

Outpatient endometrial sampling procedures, such as endometrial biopsy or aspiration curettage coupled with endocervical sampling, are definitive if results are positive for cancer. The results of endometrial biopsies correlate well with endometrial curettings, and these biopsy procedures have the advantage of avoiding general anesthesia. However, if sampling techniques fail to provide sufficient diagnostic information or if abnormal bleeding persists, formal dilation and curettage is required.

Dilation and curettage is the gold standard for assessing uterine bleeding and diagnosing endometrial carcinoma. Before dilating the cervix, the endocervix should be curetted. Next, careful sounding of the uterus is accomplished. Dilation of the cervix is then performed, followed by systematic curetting of the entire endometrial cavity. Cervical and endometrial specimens should be kept separate and forwarded for pathologic interpretation.

The ACS recently concluded that there was insufficient evidence to recommend routine screening for endometrial cancer for average-risk women. However, the ACS recommends that at the time of menopause, all women should be informed about the risks and symptoms of endometrial cancer and strongly encouraged to report any unexpected bleeding or spotting to their physicians. Women at elevated risk for endometrial cancer from tamoxifen therapy should be informed about the risk and symptoms of endometrial cancer and strongly encouraged to report any unexpected bleeding or spotting to their physicians. In addition, results from three HNPCC (hereditary nonpolyposis colorectal cancer) registries have shown a 10-fold increased risk of endometrial cancer for women who carry the HNPCC genetic abnormality, with a cumulative risk for endometrial cancer of 43% by age 70. Women with or at risk for HNPCC can be offered endometrial screening annually beginning at age 35, but informed decision-making after a discussion of options, including benefits, risks, and limitations of testing, is appropriate. Additional investigation is needed to determine the appropriate monitoring for endometrial cancer in HNPCC carriers.

Pathology

Adenocarcinoma Endometrioid adenocarcinoma is the most common form of endometrial carcinoma, comprising 75%–80% of cases. It varies from well differentiated to undifferentiated. The former demonstrates well-preserved glands in at least 95% of the tumor, whereas in the latter, less than half of the neoplasm shows glandular differentiation. Squamous differentiation can be seen in 30%–50% of cases.

Adenoacanthoma Adenocarcinoma with benign squamous differentiation has been termed adenoacanthoma and generally has a good prognosis.

Adenosquamous carcinoma If the squamous component resembles squamous carcinoma, the tumor is designated an adenosquamous carcinoma. These lesions tend to have a worse prognosis due to their association with a poorly differentiated glandular component.

Serous carcinoma is an aggressive form of endometrial cancer that accounts for < 10% of these tumors. Serous cancer of the endometrium closely resembles serous carcinoma of the ovaries and fallopian tubes and is usually found in an advanced stage in older women.

Clear-cell carcinomas of the endometrium closely resemble their counterparts in the cervix, vagina, and ovaries. As with serous cancers, these tumors generally occur in older women and have a poor prognosis due to their propensity for early intraperitoneal spread.

Secretory adenocarcinoma is an uncommon endometrial cancer that resembles secretory endometrium with its associated progestational changes. These cancers tend to be of low grade and have a good prognosis.

Staging and prognosis

Two large prospective Gynecologic Oncology Group (GOG) surgical staging trials reported in 1984 and 1987 helped define the prognostic factors for endometrial carcinoma and the current treatment approach. In addition to evaluating the predictive value of such factors as age, race, and endocrine status, the studies confirmed that prognosis is directly related to the presence or absence of easily determined uterine and extrauterine risk factors.

Uterine prognostic factors include histologic cell type, tumor grade, depth of myometrial invasion, occult extension of disease to the cervix, and vascular space invasion.

Extrauterine prognostic factors include adnexal metastases, intraperitoneal spread of disease to other extrauterine structures, positive peritoneal cytology, pelvic lymph node metastases, and aortic node involvement.

Peritoneal cytology The current International Federation of Gynecology and Obstetrics (FIGO) staging system would classify the presence of malignant cells in the peritoneal fluid as stage IIIA disease, implying a worse prognosis, similar to that observed with cancer spread to the adnexa or serosa.

Tebeu et al compared the outcome of patients with stages I vs IIIA endometrial cancer and reported their results to the American Society of Clinical Oncology. The outcomes of the patients with stage IIIA disease were then reanalyzed by dividing the population into those based solely on the finding of a positive peritoneal cytology, "cytologic stage IIIA," and a group with histologic documentation of either serosal or adnexal involvement with cancer, "histologic stage IIIA."

The 5-year disease-specific survival for the patients with cytologic stage IIIA disease was 91%, remarkably similar to that of women in the series who presented with stage I endometrial cancer (92%). However, the 5-year disease-specific survival for the patients with histologic stage IIIA disease was only 50% ($P < .001$). This analysis was confirmed after controlling for other potential prognostic factors. These data raise the important question of whether the current endometrial cancer staging system, where the finding of a positive peritoneal cytologic result alone is considered a poor prognostic factor, should be reconsidered.

Uterine size was previously believed to be a risk factor and was part of the older clinical staging system. However, recent information indicates that uterine size is *not* an independent risk factor but rather relates to cell type, grade, and myometrial invasion.

Surgical staging Cell type and grade can be determined before hysterectomy, although in some series, grade, as determined by dilation and curettage, has an overall inaccuracy rate of 31% compared with grade in the hysterectomy specimen, and grade 3 tumors have an inaccuracy rate of 50%. Recognition of all of the other factors requires an exploratory laparotomy, peritoneal fluid sampling, and hysterectomy with careful pathologic interpretation of all removed tissue. This primary surgical approach led the FIGO to define endometrial cancer as a surgically staged disease in 1988, incorporating many of the prognostic factors into the staging process (Table 1).

Treatment

Surgery

Approximately 90% of patients with a diagnosis of endometrial cancer are medically able to undergo surgery. Preparation for this surgery should include evaluation of such concurrent medical problems as hypertension and diabetes, which are frequently found in patients with endometrial cancer.

TABLE 1: FIGO surgical staging for endometrial cancer

Stage	Grade	Characteristics
IA	G1,2,3	Tumor limited to the endometrium
IB	G1,2,3	Tumor invasion to less than half of the myometrium
IC	G1,2,3	Tumor invasion to more than half of the myometrium
IIA	G1,2,3	Endocervical glandular involvement only
IIB	G1,2,3	Cervical stromal invasion
IIIA	G1,2,3	Tumor invades serosa or adnexa or positive peritoneal cytology
IIIB	G1,2,3	Vaginal metastases
IIIC	G1,2,3	Metastases to pelvic or para-aortic lymph nodes
IVA	G1,2,3	Tumor invades the bladder and/or bowel mucosa
IVB		Distant metastases, including intra-abdominal and/or inguinal lymph nodes

Histopathology—Degree of differentiation[a]

G1	≤ 5% of a nonsquamous or nonmorular solid growth pattern
G2	6%-50% of a nonsquamous or nonmorular solid growth pattern
G3	> 50% of a nonsquamous or nonmorular solid growth pattern

FIGO = International Federation of Gynecology and Obstetrics

[a] Cases should be grouped by the degree of differentiation of the adenocarcinoma.

Open surgical procedure The operative procedure is performed through an adequate abdominal incision that allows for thorough intra-abdominal exploration and retroperitoneal lymph node removal if necessary. On entry into the peritoneal cavity, fluid samples are obtained for subsequent cytologic determination (intraperitoneal cell washings). Next, thorough intra-abdominal and pelvic exploration is undertaken, with biopsy or excision of any suspicious lesions. In particular, the uterus should be observed for tumor breakthrough of the serosal surface. The distal ends of the fallopian tubes are clipped or ligated to prevent possible tumor spillage during uterine manipulation.

These procedures should be followed by total extrafascial hysterectomy and bilateral salpingo-oophorectomy. The excised uterus is opened away from the operating table, and the depth of myometrial penetration is determined by clinical observation or microscopic frozen section. The depth of myometrial invasion can be accurately assessed in over 90% of cases.

Laparoscopic surgery An alternative method of surgically staging patients with clinical stage I endometrial cancer is gaining in popularity. This approach combines laparoscopically assisted vaginal hysterectomy with laparoscopic lymphadenectomy.

Laparoscopy-assisted surgical staging (LASS) is feasible in a select group of patients, as reported by Homesley et al. However, it is not yet known whether this approach is applicable to all patients with clinical stage I disease. In particular, patients who are overweight or have intra-abdominal adhesions may not be ideal candidates. Para-aortic lymphadenectomy is technically more difficult through the laparoscope. To obtain adequate exposure, it is necessary to elevate the small bowel mesentery into the upper abdomen, which becomes increasingly difficult as the patient's weight increases, especially when weight exceeds 180 pounds. Spirtos et al recently reported a feasibility trial by GOG on laparoscopic lymphadenectomy after incomplete surgical staging. A total of 69% of the women underwent complete endoscopic staging with photographic documentation, whereas 10% were incompletely staged. In addition, 20% needed laparotomy, of whom 6% had bowel complications and 11% were found to have more advanced disease. The safety, efficacy, and cost savings of LASS are currently being evaluated by GOG in a prospective randomized trial comparing LASS vs staging laparotomy.

Lymph node evaluation Any suspicious pelvic or para-aortic lymph nodes should be removed for pathologic evaluation. If there is no gross residual intraperitoneal tumor, pelvic and para-aortic lymph nodes should be removed for the following indications:

- invasion of more than one-half of the outer myometrium
- presence of tumor in the isthmus-cervix
- adnexal or other extrauterine metastases
- presence of serous, clear-cell, undifferentiated, or squamous types
- palpably enlarged lymph nodes.

Lymph nodes need not be removed in patients whose tumor is limited to the endometrium, regardless of grade, because < 1% of these patients have disease spread to pelvic or para-aortic lymph nodes. The decision of whether to perform lymph node sampling is less clear-cut for patients whose only risk factor is invasion of the inner half of the myometrium, particularly if the tumor grade is 1 or 2. This group has a ≤ 5% chance of node positivity.

Lymphadenectomy The extent of lymph node removal has been the subject of debate. Recently, GOG defined the extent of lymphadenectomy required for entry into its studies:

Pelvic lymphadenectomy

- The skin incision may be of the surgeon's choosing, including midline vertical, transverse, and lateral vertical. The procedure may be performed via laparoscopy or by a retroperitoneal approach.
- Identify the bifurcation of the common iliac, external iliac, and hypogastric arteries; veins; and the ureters bilaterally.
- Any enlarged or suspicious nodes will be excised or biopsied if unresectable.
- Remove bilaterally all nodal tissue and skeletonization of all vessels from the mid portion of the common iliac artery superiorly, to the circumflex iliac vein inferiorly.

■ Remove bilaterally all nodal tissue from the mid portion of the psoas muscle laterally to the ureters medially, including the hypogastric arteries and veins and from the obturator fossas anterior to the obturator nerves.

■ An adequate dissection requires that a minimum of four lymph nodes be demonstrated pathologically from each side (right and left) of the pelvis, preferably from multiple sites.

Para-aortic lymphadenectomy

■ The bifurcation of the aorta, the inferior vena cava, the ovarian vessels, the inferior mesenteric artery, the ureters, and duodenum should be identified.

■ The nodal tissue over the distal vena cava from the level of the inferior mesenteric artery to the mid right common iliac artery is removed.

■ The nodal tissue between the aorta and the left ureter from the inferior mesenteric artery to the left mid common iliac artery is removed.

■ An adequate dissection requires that lymphatic tissue be demonstrated pathologically from each side (right and left).

Surgical staging After these procedures, the patient is surgically staged according to the 1988 FIGO criteria. The overall surgical complication rate after this type of staging is approximately 20%. The rate of serious complications is 6%, and they include vascular, ureteral, and bowel injuries.

Grossly involved lymph nodes can often be completely resected. Havrilesky et al reported data for 96 patients with stage IIIC endometrial cancer and pelvic and/or aortic lymph node metastasis who underwent surgery between 1973 and 2002. Of these women, 45 had microscopic lymph node involvement and 51 had grossly enlarged nodes. Forty-four of the women with grossly involved lymph nodes underwent complete resection. Analysis revealed 5-year disease-specific survival rates of 50% in the patients with grossly positive lymph nodes who underwent complete resection, compared with 63% in those with microscopic metastatic disease, and 43% in the women with residual macroscopic lymph node metastasis.

Adjuvant radiation therapy

Following surgical staging, adjuvant radiation therapy is offered to patients based on prognostic factors found at the time of surgery. A pelvic recurrence rate of 7%–14% is predictable for all stage I patients after surgery alone, although certain subgroups with more risk factors may have a higher incidence of recurrence of endometrial carcinoma. Well-described prognostic factors include disease extent (cervical involvement, extrauterine involvement of the serosa, adnexa, lymph nodes, peritoneal fluid, or intra-abdominal spread), as well as histologic grade of the tumor, depth of myometrial penetration, pathologic subtype, and presence of lymphovascular space invasion.

Teletherapy Adjuvant irradiation has been delivered primarily using external-beam irradiation directed to the pelvis, which allows for treatment of the pelvic nodes.

A trial conducted by GOG compared the results of pelvic irradiation with those

Review of more than 21,000 patients from SEER data demonstrated improved overall and relative survival rates for those with stage IC endometrial cancer who were treated with adjuvant radiation therapy compared with surgery alone (*Lee CM, Szabo A, Shrieve DC, et al: JAMA 295:389-397, 2006*).

of observation following hysterectomy and lymphadenectomy. The estimated 2-year cumulative incidence of recurrence was 12% in the observation arm and 3% in those irradiated (P= .007). The treatment difference was particularly evident among a "high-intermediate risk" subgroup defined as those (1) with moderate to poorly differentiated tumor, presence of lymphovascular invasion, and outer-third myometrial invasion; (2) age 50 or older with any two risk factors previously listed; or (3) age of at least 70 with any risk factor previously listed, where the cumulative incidence of recurrence in the observed patients was 26% vs 6% in the treated patients. Overall survival rates at 3 years did not differ significantly between the two groups.

However, one-third of patients were found to be in a high-risk group that included patients who were older, had lymph-vascular space invasion, deep myometrial penetration, and high-grade disease. When outcomes were stratified by these factors, the addition of pelvic irradiation was found to reduce the recurrence and death rate from 36% to 17%, the cancer death rate from 17% to 10%, and the distant metastatic rate from 19% to 10%. This finding suggests that pelvic irradiation may not only influence pelvic recurrence in these patients, but that there is a subgroup of patients who may benefit in terms of distant metastasis and death. A larger trial with high-risk patients is needed to validate this assumption.

Of the 18 pelvic recurrences in the no adjuvant treatment arm, 13 were in the vagina. Thirteen other sites of recurrence were outside the pelvis. It has been speculated that vaginal irradiation alone could have controlled these vaginal recurrences, leading to interest in treatment with vaginal irradiation instead of pelvic irradiation.

The findings of a multicenter trial with 754 patients from the Netherlands called the Post Operative Radiation Therapy in Endometrial Carcinoma (PORTEC) study have been reported. Eligible patients had IC grade 1 (21%), IB or IC grade 2 tumors (69%), or IB grade 3 tumors (10%). After total abdominal hysterectomy without lymphadenectomy, patients were randomized to receive pelvic radiotherapy (46 Gy) or no further treatment.

Pelvic irradiation decreased the incidence of locoregional recurrence but did not affect survival. Patients with grade 3 histology demonstrated the highest risk of distant metastases and death caused by endometrial cancer. Most of the locoregional relapses were located in the vagina (30 of 40 cases). It is possible that vaginal brachytherapy could have prevented the majority of these cases. When patients were subdivided into a high-risk subgroup with two or three risk factors, including age $\geq$ 60, grade 3 histology, and myometrial depth $\geq$ 50%, the 10-year locoregional relapse rate was 4.6% in the radiotherapy group vs 23.1% in the control group.

TABLE 2: Recommendations for adjuvant pelvic irradiation

	Stage		
Histologic grade	**IA**	**IB**	**IC**
G1	–	–	–
G2	–	–	+[b]
G3	+[b]	+[b]	+[b]
Vascular space invasion[a]	+	+	+

[a] Any grade; +, irradiation recommended; –, irradiation not recommended

[b] After full lymphadenectomy, consider brachytherapy alone because of excess complications

Creutzberg et al registered patients on a prospective trial who had deep myometrial invasion and grade 3 histology. All patients were treated with pelvic irradiation following hysterectomy. Notably, these patients had a distant recurrence rate at 5 years of 31%, and a pelvic recurrence rate at 5 years of 14%. The information from this report as well as from the subgroup of patients in the GOG 99 trial suggests that there may be a role for systemic therapy as well as pelvic irradiation in this high-risk subgroup.

Straughn et al published a large retrospective study of the National Cancer Database, where there appeared to be a trend toward improved survival in patients with clinical stages IC and II disease who received adjuvant radiation therapy. However, a difference in recurrence rates or survival in patients with surgical stages IC and II disease who received adjuvant radiation therapy compared with observation was not demonstrated.

Brachytherapy A few reports have demonstrated excellent local control with vaginal irradiation alone. A review of the world literature included 1,800 patients with low- to intermediate-risk disease. Overall, the vaginal control rate was 99.3% following adjuvant high-dose rate vaginal brachytherapy.

In a randomized study from the Norwegian Radium Hospital, pelvic irradiation significantly decreased the incidence of locoregional recurrences compared with vaginal irradiation alone. Patients with deeply invasive, grade 3 tumors had lower death and recurrence rates when treated with pelvic plus vaginal irradiation than patients treated with vaginal irradiation alone.

Many women with endometrial cancer are being treated with lymphadenectomy at the time of hysterectomy. There has been some interest in using vaginal irradiation alone to treat women who have negative nodes but deep myometrial penetration or high-grade histology. Several small retrospective reports have demonstrated excellent outcomes for such patients. However, more experience is needed to determine whether vaginal irradiation alone is adequate. Fanning reported outcomes of 66 patients, with a follow-up of 4.4 years. These patients were treated with bilateral pelvic and para-aortic lymphadenectomy with hysterectomy and oophorectomy. Brachytherapy alone was given as adjuvant therapy. There were no pelvic recurrences. Major complications occurred in 6% of patients.

In general, vaginal irradiation alone is reserved for patients at low risk for pelvic node metastasis. Because of increased rectal and vaginal sequelae, treatment of the entire length of the vagina is usually not recommended.

Irradiation of the pelvis and vagina has been combined for the adjuvant treatment of some patients. Patients with cervical involvement or extrauterine disease, who may have an increased incidence of local failure, may benefit from the two treatments combined, although there are no data to suggest that the addition of brachytherapy improves outcome over external-beam irradiation alone. Patients with uterine-confined disease have excellent local control following treatment with either type of irradiation. Combining the two treatments has not been shown to benefit these patients.

Vaginal irradiation Vaginal irradiation can be delivered with high-dose rate (HDR) or low-dose rate (LDR) equipment. Both techniques have resulted in excellent local control rates and low morbidity when administered by experienced practitioners. Each technique has its advantages. HDR treatments require multiple insertions, generally with one insertion performed every week for 3–6 weeks. However, hospitalization is not required, and each insertion takes only a brief amount of time. LDR treatments are delivered once but require hospitalization for 2–3 days.

Stage I disease Current recommendations for the treatment of patients with pathologic stage I disease include adjuvant pelvic irradiation for women with deep myometrial penetration, grade 2 or 3 histology, or evidence of vascular space invasion (Table 2). Data support the use of vaginal irradiation alone for women with more superficial tumors and low-grade histology.

Radiation doses are generally 45–50 Gy with standard fractionation. The technique should include multiple fields treated daily, with attempts to protect the small bowel. Complications from adjuvant pelvic irradiation are related to technique and the extent of lymphadenectomy.

If full lymphadenectomy has been performed, the incidence of complications increases significantly with pelvic irradiation. For these patients, consideration should be given to adjuvant brachytherapy rather than pelvic irradiation.

Papillary serous histology The high rate of upper abdominal, pelvic, and vaginal recurrences in patients with uterine papillary serous cancers has led to the recommendation that they receive whole abdominal irradiation (WAI, with doses up to 30 Gy) and additional treatments to bring the pelvic dose to 50 Gy. A vaginal cylinder or colpostats may be used to boost the surface dose with 40 Gy. This treatment has resulted in a 5-year survival rate of 50%.

Stage II disease Patients whose endometrial cancer extends to the cervix usually represent a heterogeneous group with differing histologic grades and varying degrees of cervical involvement, myometrial penetration, and nodal involvement. Similar outcomes with preoperative and postoperative irradiation suggest that initial surgical treatment with tailored postoperative irradiation is a reasonable approach.

Current treatment recommendations frequently include adjuvant pelvic irradiation to a dose of 45–50 Gy, in addition to insertion of a vaginal cylinder or colpostats to raise the total dose to the vaginal surface to 80–90 Gy. This treatment should result in a 5-year disease-free survival rate of 80%, with a locoregional control rate of 90%. Of course, outcome varies with the extent of myometrial penetration, degree of cervical involvement, and histologic grade of tumor.

Extensive cervical involvement Patients who have a large amount of cervical involvement that precludes initial hysterectomy are candidates for preoperative irradiation. A multiple-field technique is used to deliver a dose of 40–45 Gy with standard fractionation. A midline block may be inserted for the last 20 Gy to protect the rectum.

Intracavitary insertion with a standard Fletcher applicator, consisting of a uterine tandem and vaginal colpostats, delivers 20–25 Gy to point A (defined as 2 cm caudally and 2 cm laterally to the cervical os). Hysterectomy should follow in approximately 4–6 weeks. The expected 5-year disease-free survival rate for patients with extensive disease is 70%–80%.

More favorable patients have an isolated extrauterine site (eg, adnexa or peritoneal cytology alone), low-grade histology, and/or disease confined to the pelvis. Greven et al reported that 17 patients with an isolated extrauterine site who had low-grade histology and received postoperative pelvic radiation therapy had a 100% disease-free survival rate. However, patients with grade 2 or 3 disease or more than one extrauterine site had progressively worse outcomes.

Isolated ovarian metastasis One subgroup found to have a relatively favorable prognosis includes women with isolated ovarian metastasis. Five-year disease-free survival rates ranging from 60%–82% have been reported in these women after hysterectomy and pelvic irradiation, depending on the histologic grade of the tumor and the depth of myometrial penetration. Pelvic irradiation usually includes a dose of 45–50 Gy using standard fractionation. A vaginal boost with a cylinder or colpostats may add 30–35 Gy to the vaginal surface.

Extension to pelvic and periaortic nodes Patients with pelvic node involvement alone have much better outcomes than patients with extension to periaortic nodes, despite the fact that they are both considered stage IIIC patients. Morrow et al demonstrated 5-year recurrence-free survival rates of 70% and 35% for patients with pelvic nodes compared with patients with para-aortic nodes, respectively. Patients with pelvic nodes and negative para-aortic nodes are generally treated with adjuvant pelvic radiation therapy. Those with para-aortic nodes are treated with extended-field irradiation, which includes 45–50 Gy to a volume encompassing the pelvic and periaortic regions.

Whole abdominal irradiation Because upper abdominal failures have been reported previously in patients with stage III disease, attention has focused on the role of WAI. Although subsets of patients have done well with WAI, it is unclear whether this more aggressive therapy has any benefit over pelvic irradiation. A GOG phase II trial of WAI demonstrated a 3-year disease progression-free survival rate of 35%. GOG has completed a trial of WAI compared with chemotherapy. (The outcomes from this trial are discussed in the chemotherapy section.) Unfortunately, because most studies have combined patients who have favorable stage III disease with patients who have unfavorable stage IV disease, it is impossible to determine whether there are some subgroups of patients who might best be managed with a particular therapy.

Combining radiation therapy with chemotherapy Because many of these patients are at increased risk of pelvic recurrence as well as distant recurrence, there is interest in combining pelvic radiation therapy with systemic therapy. RTOG (Radiation Therapy and Oncology Group) 9708 combined pelvic radiation therapy with cisplatin and followed it with cisplatin and paclitaxel. Toxicity was predominantly hematologic. Outcomes from this phase II trial are promising. GOG currently has a phase III trial open for patients with stage III/IV cancer that includes involved-field radiation therapy for all patients with randomization to two different chemotherapy regimens.

Definitive radiation treatment

For patients who are poor operative risks, definitive treatment with irradiation has produced excellent local control and survival rates. Such treatment is considered to be justified when the operative risk exceeds the 10%–15% uterine recurrence rate expected with irradiation alone.

A more favorable outcome with definitive irradiation is related to low clinical tumor stage, less aggressive histologic variant, and use of brachytherapy for at least part of the treatment. Five-year disease-specific survival rates as high as 87%, 88%, and 49% have been reported in patients with stages I, II, and III or IV disease, respectively. Ten-year local control rates in patients with stages I/II, III, and IV disease were 84%, 87%, and 68%, respectively.

Treatment techniques with irradiation alone for patients with early-stage disease and low-grade histology consist of uterine intracavitary insertions with Heyman or Simon capsules or an afterloading intrauterine tandem. Doses for intracavitary treatment range from 40–45 Gy prescribed to point A. Patients with more advanced disease, a large uterus, or aggressive histology generally receive both an intrauterine intracavitary insertion and external pelvic irradiation. External irradiation typically delivers 40–45 Gy to the pelvis, followed by intracavitary treatment that delivers 30–35 Gy to point A.

Complication rates Rates of serious complications attributable to irradiation range from 4%–5% with intracavitary treatment alone to 10%–15% with combined external and intracavitary irradiation.

Adjuvant systemic therapy

Only a few trials of adjuvant systemic therapy have been conducted in patients with early-stage endometrial cancer. At present, we believe that such therapy should not be recommended outside the clinical trial setting.

Endocrine therapy Early uncontrolled trials suggested that progestin therapy might prolong the disease progression-free interval and time to recurrence in patients with stages I and II lesions treated with initial surgery and irradiation. However, at least three subsequent randomized trials failed to show any survival benefit for progestins, and a meta-analysis has demonstrated no advantage of adjuvant progestin therapy.

Chemotherapy To date, there are emerging data suggesting a possible role for adjuvant chemotherapy. GOG compared doxorubicin with observation in 181 patients with high-risk, early-stage, endometrial carcinoma; at 5 years, there was no difference in recurrence rates. A subsequent phase II trial suggested a better outcome for 62 high-risk patients treated with adjuvant CAP (cyclophosphamide, Adriamycin [doxorubicin], and Platinol [cisplatin]) when compared with historic controls.

A Japanese Gynecologic Oncology Group study presented at the 2005 meeting of the American Society of Clinical Oncology (ASCO) has suggested that chemotherapy may also be employed as an alternative to radiotherapy in the treatment of more localized, intermediate-risk disease (> 50% myometrial invasion). Patients (n = 425) were randomized to receive either cisplatin/doxorubicin/cyclophosphamide or whole pelvic radiotherapy. The study revealed no difference between the two regimens with respect to risk of local recurrence (15% to 16%) or survival (progression-free or overall).

Results from a GOG trial comparing adjuvant chemotherapy (doxorubicin plus cisplatin) with WAI were reported by Randall et al. The patient population included patients with stages III and IV disease (75% and 25%, respectively) with 50% endometrioid histologies. Patients treated with WAI had significantly improved progression-free (38% vs 50%, respectively) and overall (42 % vs 55%) survival at 5 years. However, serious adverse effects were also more common in the chemotherapy group than the radiotherapy group, with treatment-related deaths twice as high in the former group, at 4% vs 2%. Pelvic and abdominal recurrences were the predominant pattern of recurrence for both treatment arms. Distant recurrences were slightly less frequent for patients treated with chemotherapy. This finding may support the concept of combining chemotherapy with involved-field irradiation. A GOG trial exploring this treatment strategy has recently closed to accrual. However, the results are not yet available.

Hormone replacement therapy (HRT) Whether HRT increases the likelihood of recurrence has been studied, with several retrospective reports showing no adverse outcomes. Thus, GOG undertook a large randomized placebo-controlled trial of HRT after treatment for earlier stage endometrial cancer. However, there were too few events, and it was closed after the findings of the Women's Health Initiative were released. In results presented by Barakat et al at the Society of Gynecologic Oncologists, HRT was not associated with a significant incidence of recurrent disease or mortality.

TABLE 3: Results of a phase III, dose-response trial of progestins in advanced or recurrent endometrial carcinoma

	Oral medroxyprogesterone	
Parameter	**200 mg/d (n = 145)**	**1,000 mg/d (n = 154)**
Response rate (%)	25	15
Complete response rate (%)	17	9
Median disease progression-free survival (mo)	3.2	2.5
Median survival (mo)	11.1	7.0

TREATMENT OF RECURRENT OR METASTATIC DISEASE

Patterns of recurrence

Recurrent endometrial cancer is initially confined to the pelvis in 50% of patients. The major sites of distant metastasis are the abdominal cavity, liver, and lungs.

Following diagnosis and initial treatment, periodic evaluation, including history, physical examination, and pelvic examination, is recommended at 3–6 month intervals for the first 5 years and yearly thereafter. The use in asymptomatic patients of more extensive and more costly procedures, such as chest x-ray, CT imaging, and marker studies, is of questionable value and is unlikely to have a major impact on survival. Symptomatic patients should be evaluated as is appropriate.

Radiation therapy

After hysterectomy alone for endometrial cancer, approximately 50% of recurrences are pelvic and 50% are extrapelvic. It is clear that locoregional recurrences can develop in isolation, without distant metastasis, and salvage can be accomplished with high-dose irradiation.

Pelvic recurrences Five-year disease-specific survival rates as high as 51% have been reported in patients with isolated locoregional recurrences treated with radiation therapy. Factors that have an adverse impact on outcome are increased size of tumor at recurrence, young age, pelvic vs vaginal involvement, and treatment of recurrence with external-beam irradiation only vs the addition of vaginal brachytherapy.

The PORTEC group has published its experience with salvage of vaginal recurrence in patients who did not receive adjuvant irradiation. At 5 years, the survival rate after vaginal relapse was 65% in the control group, compared with 43% in the irradiated group.

Radiation treatment for pelvic recurrence usually consists of external-beam irradiation with the addition of a brachytherapy boost that may include colpostats, a cylinder, interstitial needles, or seeds. Treatment must be individualized based on the location and size of the recurrence and the boost method selected. The tolerance of normal tissues must be respected, but combined doses > 60 Gy have been associated with improved local control.

Extrapelvic recurrences For patients with recurrences outside the pelvis, irradiation is effective in producing responses in localized symptomatic lesions. Therefore, irradiation may be effective for palliation of such lesions in the lymph nodes, brain, or bones. Doses and protocols vary, depending on the site of recurrence.

Pelvic exenteration for pelvic recurrences after irradiation

Isolated pelvic central recurrence after irradiation is rare. Selected patients in whom it does occur may benefit from pelvic exenterative surgery. No large series have been published, but some long-term survivors have been reported.

Barakat et al reported on 44 patients who underwent pelvic exenteration for recurrent endometrial cancer at Memorial Sloan-Kettering Cancer Center between 1947 and 1994. Primary therapy usually consisted of total abdominal hysterectomy and bilateral salpingo-oophorectomy, with most patients receiving either preoperative or postoperative radiotherapy. Prior to exenteration, 10 of 44 patients (23%) had never received any form of radiotherapy. The median interval between initial surgery and exenteration was 28 months (range, 2 to 189 months).

Exenteration was total in 23 patients, anterior in 20 patients, and limited to posterior in 1 patient. One vascular injury led to the only intraoperative death. Major postoperative complications occurred in 35 patients (80%) and included intestinal/urinary tract fistulas, pelvic abscess, septicemia, pulmonary embolism, and cerebrovascular accident. Median survival for the entire group of patients was 7.36 months, with 9 patients (20%) achieving long-term survival (> 5 years). Although the long-term survival rate after this procedure is only 20%, it remains the only potentially curative option for the few patients with central recurrence of endometrial cancer who have not responded to standard surgery and radiation therapy.

Endocrine therapy

Progestins produce complete and partial response rates of 15%–25% in patients with locoregional recurrence or distant metastases. The route, type, and dose of progestins do not appear to be related to response; hence, oral therapy is preferred.

In clinical practice, oral administration of 200 mg of medroxyprogesterone or 160 mg of megestrol produces blood levels similar to those achieved with parenteral therapy (400–1,000 mg of medroxyprogesterone IM weekly). A phase III trial conducted by GOG comparing 200 mg and 1,000 mg of medroxyprogesterone given orally daily found no differences between the two regimens, although it is noteworthy that the trends all favored the low-dose regimen (Table 3). Doses higher than 200 mg/d of medroxyprogesterone, therefore, are clearly not warranted.

Several factors are predictive of a favorable response to progestin therapy. Patients with well-differentiated lesions are more likely to respond than those with poorly differentiated tumors. A related observation is that a much higher percentage of grade 1 tumors have significant levels of estrogen and progesterone receptors; data show that lesions with higher receptor levels respond much more frequently to progestins than those with lower receptor levels. Response is almost always associated with better disease progression-free and overall survival.

The median time to disease progression for all patients treated with progestins is 3–4 months, and the median survival is 10 months.

Tamoxifen has a 0%–13% response rate, is not as active as progestins, and is of little value as second-line therapy in patients who do not respond to progestins.

GOG has evaluated combined therapy with tamoxifen plus a progestin given sequentially in the hope that tamoxifen may increase progesterone receptor expression and, thus, increase the likelihood of response to progestins. Whitney reported that continuous tamoxifen and medroxyprogesterone given every other week was an active treatment, with a 33% response rate. A subsequent study by Fiorica et al found a 27% response rate for alternating megestrol, with several prolonged responses. As with prior hormonal studies, patients with well-differentiated cancers were more likely to respond. Nevertheless, this trial was relatively unique in that 22% of patients with poorly differentiated tumors responded.

Other hormonal agents, such as gonadotropin-releasing hormone analogs and aminoglutethimide (Cytadren), have been studied to some extent in endometrial carcinoma. These agents do not appear to have sufficient activity to warrant further study.

Chemotherapy

Single agents Chemotherapy for advanced endometrial cancer focuses on three groups of agents with demonstrated activity: anthracyclines, platinum compounds, and taxanes.

Active agents The anthracyclines studied include doxorubicin and epirubicin (Ellence). In a total of 298 patients, doxorubicin produced a 27% response rate. Epirubicin, primarily in European studies including 27 patients, yielded a 26% response rate. Two platinum compounds have activity. Cisplatin, in 86 patients, elicited responses in 29%. Carboplatin (Paraplatin) produced a 31% response rate in 52 patients. Paclitaxel, in two GOG studies, yielded responses in 36% of chemotherapy-naive and 27% of previously treated patients.

For all of these studies, the disease progression-free interval ranged from 4–7 months, with an overall survival range of 8–12 months. Approximately one-third of the responses were clinical complete responses, with a substantially longer duration and better survival than partial responders.

Agents with limited activity Other agents studied have included alkylating agents (cyclophosphamide, ifosfamide [Ifex]), altretamine (Hexalen), fluorouracil (5-FU), methotrexate, mercaptopurine (Purinethol), vinblastine, etoposide, teniposide (Vumon), and mitoxantrone (Novantrone). All these agents exhibited insufficient activity to warrant further study.

Combination regimens A number of phase II trials of combination regimens have been conducted. The combination of carboplatin and paclitaxel has been demonstrated to be active in advanced endometrial cancer (50%–60% response rate). Further support for this approach was provided by a report from Sovak et al, who conducted a retrospective analysis of their experience with this combination chemotherapy regimen in endometrial cancer. The objective response rate in chemotherapy-naive patients was 47% (2% complete response rate), with a median progression-free survival of 4.2 months and median overall survival of 11 months. Ultimately, the relative merits of combination chemotherapy with carboplatin and paclitaxel must be judged in the context of the randomized trial that is being performed by GOG.

Following encouraging phase II results, Gallion et al reported on a phase III trial of circadian timed administration of cisplatin and doxorubicin and found no significant benefit. GOG then compared this two-drug (cisplatin [50 mg/m^2]/doxorubicin [60 mg/m^2]) regimen with a three-drug combination of cisplatin (50 mg/m^2), doxorubicin (45 mg/m^2), and paclitaxel (160 mg/m^2 as a 3-hour infusion), with G-CSF (granulocyte colony-stimulating factor, filgrastim [Neupogen]) support (GOG protocol 177). The three-drug combination of the paclitaxel-containing program produced a higher response rate (57% vs 35%) and an improved disease progression-free survival (8.3 vs 5.3 months). Overall survival was also modestly improved (15.3 vs 12.3 months; $P = .037$) with the three-drug program but with considerably greater toxicity, particularly peripheral neuropathy (grade 3, 12% vs 1%).

Chemotherapy plus progestins Combinations of chemotherapy plus progestins have been studied in a number of phase II trials. The only large, randomized trial evaluating this approach (GOG protocol 29) allocated patients with advanced or recurrent disease to receive either cyclophosphamide, doxorubicin, cisplatin, and megestrol or melphalan (Alkeran), 5-FU, and megestrol. In pilot studies, these two regimens had been reported to yield response rates of 75% and 94%, respectively. The randomized trial produced response rates of 36% and 38%, respectively, with no evident advantage of either combination over prior studies of single-agent doxorubicin with regard to response rate, disease progression-free interval, or overall survival. These results do not suggest any advantage for the combined use of chemotherapy and progestins.

Treatment recommendations

Patients who have advanced or recurrent endometrial carcinoma should be considered for systemic therapy. Patients should first be offered the opportunity to participate in a clinical trial. Those who are ineligible or who choose not to participate should be treated according to current evidence.

Patients who have a grade 1 tumor and/or known progesterone-receptor–positive disease clearly benefit from treatment with progestins (response rate, 40%;

median disease progression-free interval, 9 months; overall median survival, 14 months) and should be so treated. Those with a grade 2–3 tumor and/or known progesterone-receptor–negative disease do not do well with progestin therapy (response rate, 12%; median disease progression-free interval, 3 months; overall median survival, 10 months) and should be considered for initial treatment with single-agent chemotherapy (eg, paclitaxel, doxorubicin, carboplatin) or a combination regimen. Options include cisplatin/doxorubicin, cisplatin/paclitaxel, and carboplatin/paclitaxel. (It is difficult to justify the routine use of the three-drug paclitaxel-containing regimen noted previously despite the modest improvement in efficacy due to substantial toxicity.) Chemotherapy should also be considered for patients who do not respond to initial hormonal therapy.

Regimens that include both chemotherapy and hormonal therapy should not be considered outside a clinical trial because of the lack of data supporting any advantage of these combinations. Likewise, sequential use of tamoxifen and progestins is not indicated because of the absence of enhanced efficacy.

UTERINE SARCOMAS

Carcinosarcomas and other uterine sarcomas are uncommon tumors, accounting for less than 4% of all cancers of the uterine corpus. Carcinosarcomas, the most common histologic subtype, demonstrate both epithelial and stromal differentiation. Endometrial stromal sarcomas and leiomyosarcomas (LMSs) are characterized by differentiation toward one or more stromal tissues. LMSs occur at an earlier age than do carcinosarcomas, with a plateau observed in middle age. There is strong epidemiologic evidence that prior exposure to pelvic irradiation may increase the risk for the development of uterine sarcomas. Generally, these tumors are characterized by aggressive growth, with early lymphatic or hematogeneous spread. The overall survival rate is poor, with the majority of deaths occurring within 2 years of diagnosis.

Patterns of spread

Lymphatic metastases are a significant route of spread for carcinosarcoma, with a reported incidence of 40%–60% occurring with stage I disease. LMS has a propensity for extra-abdominal spread, often involving the lungs. For carcinosarcoma, the initial site for recurrence after surgical resection is likely to be the pelvis or abdomen, whereas LMSs tend to fail to recur distantly. In a prospective surgical staging trial by GOG, the recurrence rate for early-stage carcinosarcoma was 53% and for LMS was 71%.

Treatment

Surgery

Surgery is the mainstay of treatment for uterine sarcomas. For carcinosarcoma, this usually consists of total abdominal hysterectomy and bilateral salpingo-oophorectomy, with washings to be obtained for peritoneal cytology. The GOG prospective staging study reported a 17% incidence of nodal metastasis for this histologic subtype, so retroperitoneal nodes should be sampled as for poorly differentiated endometrial cancers. For patients with advanced/recurrent disease, aggressive surgical debulking does not appear to improve outcome.

Hysterectomy with oophorectomy is also standard therapy for uterine LMS. Retroperitoneal nodal sampling is not usually performed, because lymph node involvement is unusual. For late recurrences of LMS, surgery must be individualized. Five-year survival rates of 30%–50% have been reported following pulmonary resection for lung metastases. Patients with unilateral metastases have a significantly better prognosis than those with bilateral disease. Local and regional recurrences may also be amenable to surgical resection of disease.

Hysterectomy with oophorectomy is the standard of care for patients with low-grade endometrial stromal sarcomas. Removal of the ovaries was thought to be critical, as these tumors tend to have very high concentrations of estrogen and progesterone receptors and often respond to hormonal therapy. However, Li et al recently reviewed a multi-institutional experience and reported that bilateral salpingo-oophorectomy did not appear to affect time to recurrence or overall survival. Retention of ovarian function may be an option for premenopausal women with low-grade endometrial stromal sarcomas. Because these tumors have a tendency to spread via the lymphatics, resection of all disease, especially extension into the parametrium, should be attempted. This approach may require radical hysterectomy.

Adjuvant irradiation

Currently, there are no clear data suggesting improvement in outcome for patients with uterine sarcomas treated with adjuvant pelvic irradiation. Pelvic recurrence is a pattern of failure for most uterine sarcomas; isolated pelvic recurrences are uncommon. Adjuvant irradiation can decrease local recurrence, but there is no clear evidence that it improves survival. Patients will often experience recurrence distantly and treatment failure. Pelvic irradiation may be indicated for improvement of quality of life, however, because pelvic recurrence can be associated with pain, bleeding, and intestinal obstruction.

Adjuvant radiotherapy

Uterine sarcomas represent only 2%–5% of all uterine malignancies. These patients have a high incidence of distant, as well as pelvic, recurrences. In a nonrandomized prospective GOG study, patients with stages I and II mixed mesodermal sarcomas and LMSs had fewer pelvic recurrences following irradiation than did those patients who did not undergo pelvic irradiation. No difference in overall or disease-free survival was noted.

Several retrospective reports have suggested improved pelvic control rates following pelvic irradiation for stages I and II uterine sarcomas. Decreasing pelvic recurrences may improve symptom-free survival for these patients.

Currently, GOG has an open randomized study for patients with stages I–IV mixed mesodermal sarcomas. Following resection of gross disease, patients are randomized to receive WAI (30 Gy) with a pelvic boost (1,980 cGy) or chemotherapy alone with cisplatin, ifosfamide, and mesna (Mesnex).

Adjuvant chemotherapy

There is no proven role for adjuvant chemotherapy in stage I disease following complete surgical resection. A GOG study looking at adjuvant doxorubicin vs no further therapy showed no differences in recurrence rate, disease progression-free survival, or overall survival.

For patients with advanced/recurrent disease, single-agent chemotherapy can be used with a palliative intent. For carcinosarcomas, ifosfamide or paclitaxel appears to be the agent of choice. Doxorubicin has traditionally been used for LMSs. Look reported the GOG experience with gemcitabine (Gemzar) in patients previously treated for LMS, showing 20% of patients responded. Combination therapy with mitomycin (Mutamycin), doxorubicin, and cisplatin (Paraplatin; MAP) modestly increased the responses to 23% with increased toxicity. Hormonal agents, specifically progestins, are the treatment of choice for advanced/recurrent endometrial stromal sarcomas.

GESTATIONAL TROPHOBLASTIC DISEASES

Gestational trophoblastic diseases (GTDs) encompass a spectrum of neoplastic disorders that arise from placental trophoblastic tissue after abnormal fertilization. In the United States, GTDs account for less than 1% of gynecologic malignancies. Forty years ago, women with choriocarcinoma had a 95% mortality rate. Today, with the advent of effective chemotherapy and the development of a reliable tumor marker (β-subunit human chorionic gonadotropin [β-hCG]), the cure rate for choriocarcinoma is 90%–95%.

Clinical presentation

Complete mole

The classic signs of a molar pregnancy include the absence of fetal heart sounds, physical evidence of a uterus that is larger than expected for gestational age, and vaginal bleeding. Although an intact fetus may coexist with a partial mole, this occurs in fewer than 1 in 100,000 pregnancies.

The most common presenting symptom of molar pregnancy is vaginal bleeding, reported in up to 97% of patients. Intrauterine clots may undergo oxidation and liquefaction, producing pathognomonic prune juice-like fluid. Prolonged or recurrent bleeding may result in iron-deficiency anemia. Symptoms of anemia occur in approximately 50% of patients at the time of diagnosis. Early toxemia (hypertension, proteinuria, and edema) presenting during the first or second trimester is common (20%–30%) in molar pregnancy.

Hyperthyroidism is seen clinically in approximately 7% of molar pregnancies. An elevation of triiodothyronine (T_3) and thyroxine (T_4) levels is observed more commonly than are the clinical manifestations of tachycardia, sweating, weight loss, and tremor. These hormonal elevations are presumed to be secondary to the structural similarity of hCG to thyroid-stimulating hormone (TSH).

Partial mole

Patients with partial mole have different clinical features than those with complete mole. Fewer than 10% of patients with partial mole have uterine enlargement. Patients with partial mole do not have prominent theca-luteal cysts, hyperthyroidism, or respiratory insufficiency. They experience toxemia only rarely. The diagnosis of partial mole is usually made after histologic review of curettage specimens.

Gestational trophoblastic neoplasia

GTD develops in 6%–19% of patients after molar evacuation. Metastases sometimes have an identical histology to that of molar disease, but the vast majority are choriocarcinomas. Metastatic spread is hematogeneous. Because of its extensive vascular network, metastatic GTD often produces local, spontaneous bleeding. Berkowitz et al at the New England Trophoblastic Disease Center (NETDC) reported that the common metastatic sites of GTD are the lungs (80%); vagina (30%); pelvis (20%); liver (10%); brain (10%); and bowel, kidneys, and spleen (5% each).

Pulmonary metastases are common (80% of patients with metastatic disease) and occur when trophoblastic tissue enters the circulation via uterine venous sinuses. The radiologic features may be protean or subtle and include alveolar, nodular, and miliary patterns. Pleural effusions may also be present. Pulmonary metastases can be extensive and can cause respiratory failure and death.

Right upper-quadrant pain has been observed when hepatic metastases stretch Glisson's capsule. GI lesions may result in severe hemorrhage or in perforation with peritonitis, both of which require emergency intervention. Vaginal examination may reveal bluish metastatic deposits; these and other metastatic sites should not undergo biopsy because severe uncontrolled bleeding may occur.

CNS involvement from metastatic GTD suggests widespread disease and has a poor prognosis. CNS metastases are clinically evident in 7%–28% of patients with metastatic choriocarcinoma. Cerebral metastases tend to respond favorably to both radiotherapy and chemotherapy.

Diagnostic studies

Although the clinical presentation may suggest a diagnosis of GTD, certain laboratory studies, particularly a determination of the patient's β-hCG level, and radiographic studies are needed to confirm this diagnosis.

Laboratory studies Thyroid function studies should be performed in all patients with a clinical history or physical examination suggestive of hyperthyroidism. Abnormal thyroid function, manifested as an elevated T_4 level, is common in GTD. Metastatic deposits in the kidneys or GI tract may reveal themselves by hematuria or hematochezia.

Tumor markers A well-characterized glycoprotein hormone secreted by the syncytiotrophoblast, hCG is essential to maintaining normal function of the corpus luteum during pregnancy. Because all trophoblastic tumors secrete β-hCG, this hormone serves as an excellent marker for tumor activity in the nonpregnant patient. Serial β-hCG levels should be monitored during therapy to ensure adequate treatment. The level of β-hCG is roughly proportional to the tumor burden and inversely proportional to therapeutic outcome.

Radiologic studies A chest x-ray should always be performed because 70%–80% of patients with metastatic GTD have lung involvement. Although this x-ray usually demonstrates nodular metastases, the patterns of metastatic disease can range from atelectatic areas to subtle pleural abnormalities. A CT scan is often helpful in evaluating these nonspecific findings.

Since it has been demonstrated that 97%–100% of patients with CNS disease from choriocarcinoma have concomitant pulmonary metastases, a CNS work-up in asymptomatic patients with normal chest x-rays is not routinely warranted. If the chest x-ray is abnormal, or if β-hCG levels plateau or rise during treatment, a more thorough evaluation for metastatic disease is indicated. MRI of the brain, brain stem, and cerebellum as well as CT scans of the abdomen and pelvis should be performed to evaluate other likely sites of metastatic spread. The presence of intrauterine or ovarian disease also may be detected by MRI of the pelvis. Ultrasonography is a reliable, safe, economical, and relatively simple method for confirming the diagnosis of intrauterine GTD. It is also useful in identifying embryonic remnants.

The proposed FIGO 2000 anatomic staging system is a straightforward system based on anatomic criteria. In GTD, stage I disease is confined to the uterus; stage II disease is outside the uterus but limited to the genital structures; stage III disease extends to the lungs with or without known genital tract involvement; and stage IV disease includes all other metastatic sites. The FIGO 2000 scoring system is based on a method (adapted from the World Health Organization [WHO]) to identify patients at high risk for treatment failure. With the FIGO 2000 scoring system, patients are classified as being in a low-, middle-, or high-risk category. A total score of up to 4 is considered low risk; 5–7, middle risk; and 8 or greater, high risk. (Some centers recommend a low-risk score of 6 or less, a high-risk score of 7 or greater, and no middle-risk score.)

Treatment

The treatment strategy for GTD must be individualized for each patient. The stratification of risk groups enables physicians to direct an appropriate treatment strategy. Low-risk disease responds readily to single-agent chemotherapy and is virtually 100% curable. High-risk disease is not likely to be cured with single-agent therapy and therefore requires multidrug regimens.

Molar pregnancy

For patients with complete or partial hydatidiform mole, evacuation of the mole by suction and sharp curettage should be performed. Oxytocics also are given to produce uterine involution and to control bleeding. However, these agents should be used judiciously, as they may cause hyponatremia and fluid overload. A baseline chest x-ray and β-hCG measurement should be obtained prior to surgery. After molar evacuation, 80% of patients will need no further intervention.

Follow-up As mentioned previously, all patients with molar disease should obtain a baseline chest x-ray. Serial β-hCG levels should be obtained every 1–2 weeks until the level is normal for three consecutive assays. Complete remission is defined by three consecutive normal β-hCG levels. Once this has occurred, β-hCG levels should be checked monthly for 12 months, every 4 months for the following year, and then yearly for 2 years. However, Lavie et al recently showed that a single undetectable human chorionic gonadotropin level after evacuation is sufficient follow-up to ensure remission in patients with partial hydatidiform moles.

Although the use of oral contraceptives during the surveillance period remains controversial, strict contraception is required, because pregnancy would obviate the usefulness of β-hCG as a tumor marker. In general, once 12-month surveillance establishes a disease-free status, conception is acceptable. These women are always at high risk for future molar disease and will require close observation during future pregnancies. A pelvic ultrasonographic examination should be performed during the first trimester of all subsequent pregnancies to confirm that gestation is normal.

Chemotherapy is indicated when there is a plateau or increase in β-hCG levels on consecutive measurements, failure to reach normal levels by 16 weeks, or metastatic disease. Such patients are usually at low risk and will respond to single-agent chemotherapy. Methotrexate is the most commonly initiated single agent. Therapy is continued for one to two courses after a normal β-hCG level is achieved.

Low-risk metastatic disease

In more than 30 years of experience, single-agent chemotherapy with methotrexate has produced a high cure rate in patients with low-risk GTD. Likewise, methotrexate plus leucovorin induces remission in 90% of patients with low-risk metastatic disease with low toxicity. The use of dactinomycin (Cosmegen) in methotrexate-resistant patients increased the cure rate to more than 95%.

High-risk metastatic disease

The discovery that etoposide is an effective agent against trophoblastic disease led to the development of the EMA-CO regimen (etoposide, methotrexate, actinomycin D [dactinomycin], cyclophosphamide, Oncovin [vincristine]) by Bagshawe, who reported a survival rate of 83% in patients with high-risk choriocarcinoma.

EMA-CO is the preferred regimen for high-risk GTD. This regimen is also used for patients with middle-risk GTD, as defined by the FIGO 2000 criteria. EMA-CO is generally well tolerated, with no life-threatening toxic effects.

Alopecia occurs universally, and anemia, neutropenia, and stomatitis are mild. Reproductive function is preserved in approximately 75% of patients.

Within hours of receiving chemotherapy, patients with a significant tumor burden are at risk of hemorrhage into tumors and surrounding tissues. Thus, any acute organ toxicity that begins shortly after the induction of chemotherapy should be considered as possibly related to this phenomenon. Some researchers have advocated a reduction in dosage at the beginning of therapy in patients with large-volume disease to minimize these sequelae.

Salvage therapy

Unfortunately, about 25% of women with high-risk metastatic disease become refractory to EMA-CO and fail to achieve a complete remission. Currently, there is no standard salvage chemotherapy regimen for patients not responding to EMA-CO. However, salvage regimens that combine cisplatin, etoposide, vinca alkaloids, and bleomycin have been administered.

Early studies show cisplatin-based regimens to be an effective salvage therapy in GTD. A recent dose-intensive regimen, EMA-CE, utilizes cisplatin (100 mg/m^2) and etoposide (200 mg/m^2) combined with EMA, with favorable results.

Another alternative is to give cisplatin in the EMA-POMB regimen (Platinol [cisplatin], Oncovin [vincristine], methotrexate, bleomycin). POMB is administered as vincristine, 1 mg/m^2 IV, and methotrexate, 300 mg/m^2 IV (day 1); bleomycin, 15 mg IV over 24 h by continuous infusion (CI), and folinic acid, 15 mg bid for four doses (day 2); bleomycin, 15 mg IV over 24 h CI (day 3); and cisplatin, 120 mg/m^2 IV (day 4).

A new PEBA regimen (Platinol [cisplatin], etoposide, bleomycin, Adriamycin [doxorubicin]) was reported from China and was found to be effective in EMA-CO–resistant disease. A complete remission was achieved in 96% of the women, and 73% had a sustained complete remission that lasted at least 1 year. In a small study, ifosfamide alone and combined in the VIP regimen (VePesid [etoposide], ifosfamide, and Platinol [cisplatin]) showed promise as being an effective salvage drug in GTD. Lurain and Nejad reviewed the experience of the Brewer Trophoblastic Disease Center in patients with persistent or recurrent high-risk gestational trophoblastic neoplasia. They showed that those who develop resistance to methotrexate-containing treatment protocols should be treated with drug combinations employing a platinum agent and etoposide with or without bleomycin or ifosfamide.

Another consideration in the treatment of refractory GTD is the use of high-dose chemotherapy with autologous bone marrow transplantation.

SUGGESTED READING

ON ENDOMETRIAL CANCER

Barakat RR, Bundy BN, Spirtos NM, et al: A prospective randomized double-blind trial of estrogen replacement therapy vs placebo in women with stage I or II endometrial cancer: A Gynecologic Oncology Group Study. Proceedings of the Society of Gynecologic Oncologists' Annual Meeting; February 7–11, 2004; San Diego, California. Abstract 1.

Creutzberg CL, van Putten WL, Koper PC, et al: Survival after relapse in patients with endometrial cancer: Results from a randomized trial. Gynecol Oncol 89:201–209, 2003.

Creutzberg CL, van Putten WL, Warlam-Rodenhuis CC, et al: Outcome of high-risk stage IC, grade 3, compared with stage I endometrial carcinoma patients: The Postoperative Radiation Therapy in Endometrial Carcinoma Trial. J Clin Oncol 22:1234–1241, 2004.

Delin JB, Miller DS, Coleman RL: Other primary malignancies in patients with uterine corpus malignancy. Am J Obstet Gynecol 190:1429–1431, 2004.

Fiorica JV, Brunetto VL, Hanjani P, et al: Phase II trial of alternating courses of megestrol acetate and tamoxifen in advanced endometrial carcinoma: A Gynecologic Oncology Group Study. Gynecol Oncol 92:10–14, 2004.

Fleming GF, Brunetto VL, Cella D, et al: Phase III trial of doxorubicin plus cisplatin with or without paclitaxel plus filgrastim in advanced recurrent endometrial carcinoma: A Gynecologic Oncology Group Study. J Clin Oncol 22:2159–2166, 2004.

Fleming GF, Filiaci VL, Bentley RC, et al: Phase III randomized trial of doxorubicin + cisplatin versus doxorubicin + 24-h paclitaxel + filgrastim in endometrial carcinoma: A Gynecologic Oncology Group Study. Ann Oncol 15:1173–1178, 2004.

Gallion HH, Brunetto VL, Cibull M, et al: Randomized phase III trial of standard timed doxorubicin plus cisplatin in stage III and IV or recurrent endometrial carcinoma: A Gynecologic Oncology Group Study. J Clin Oncol 21:3808–3813, 2003.

Havrilesky LJ, Cragun JM, Calingaert B, et al: Resection of lymph node metastases influences survival in stage IIIC endometrial cancer. Gynecol Oncol 99:689–695, 2005.

Homesley HD, Boike G, Spiegel GW: Feasibility of laparoscopic management of presumed stage I endometrial carcinoma and assessment of accuracy of myoinvasion estimates by frozen section: A Gynecologic Oncology Group Study. Int J Gynaecol Cancer 14:341–347, 2004.

Keys HM, Roberts JA, Brunetto VL, et al: A phase III trial of surgery with or without adjunctive external pelvic radiation therapy in intermediate risk endometrial adenocarcinoma: A Gynecologic Oncology Group Study. Gynecol Oncol 92:744–751, 2004.

Lincoln S, Blessing JA, Lee RB, et al: Activity of paclitaxel as second-line chemotherapy in endometrial carcinoma: A Gynecologic Oncology Group Study. Gynecol Oncol 88:277–281, 2003.

Maxwell GL, Calingaert B, Risinger JI, et al: Progestin and estrogen potency of combination oral contraceptives and endometrial cancer risk. Proceedings of the Society of Gynecologic Oncologists' Annual Meeting; February 7–11, 2004; San Diego, California. Abstract 3.

Randall ME, Filiaci VL, Muss H, et al: Randomized phase III trial of whole-abdominal irradiation versus doxorubicin and cisplatin chemotherapy in advanced endometrial carcinoma: A Gynecologic Oncology Group Study J Clin Oncol 234:36–44, 2006.

Sagae S, Udagawa Y, Susumu N, et al: JGOG2033: Randomized phase III trial of whole pelvic radiotherapy vs cisplatin-based chemotherapy in patients with intermediate risk endometrial carcinoma (abstract). J Clin Oncol 23(suppl):455s, 2005.

Scholten AN, van Putten WL, Beerman H, et al; PORTEC Study Group: Postoperative radiotherapy for stage 1 endometrial carcinoma: Long-term outcome of the randomized PORTEC trial with central pathology review. Int J Radiat Oncol Biol Phys 63:834–838, 2005.

Sovak MA, Chuai S, Anderson S, et al: Paclitaxel and carboplatin (TP) for treatment of advanced or recurrent endometrial cancer: A retrospective study (abstract). J Clin Oncol 23(suppl):460s, 2005.

Spirtos NM, Eisekop SM, Boike G, et al: Laparoscopic staging in patients with incompletely staged cancers of the uterus, ovary, fallopian tube, and primary peritoneum: A Gynecologic Oncology Group (GOG) study. Am J Obstet Gynecol 193:1645–1649, 2005.

Straughn JM Jr, Numnum TM, Kilgore LC, et al: The use of adjuvant radiation therapy in patients with intermediate-risk stages IC and II uterine corpus cancer: A patient care evaluation study from the Amerian College of Surgeons National Cancer Data Base. Gynecol Oncol 99:530–535, 2005.

Tebeu PM, Popowski Y, Verkooijen HM, et al: Impact of positive peritoneal cytology on the survival of early stage endometrial cancer (abstract). Proc Am Soc Clin Oncol 23:455, 2004.

Thigpen E, Brady MF, Homesley HD, et al: Phase III trial of doxorubicin with or without cisplatin in advanced endometrial carcinoma: A Gynecologic Oncology Group Study. J Clin Oncol 22:3902–3908, 2004.

Whitney CW, Brunetto VL, Zaino RJ, et al: Phase II study of medroxyprogesterone acetate plus tamoxifen in advanced endometrial carcinoma: A Gynecologic Oncology Group Study. Gynecol Oncol 92:4–9, 2004.

ON GESTATIONAL TROPHOBLASTIC DISEASES

Allen JE, King MR, Farrar D, et al: Postmolar surveillance at a trophoblastic disease center that serves indigent women. Am J Obstet Gynecol 188:1151–1153, 2003.

Escobar PF, Lurain JR, Singh DK, et al: Treatment of high-risk gestational trophoblastic neoplasia with etoposide, methotrexate, actinomycin D, cyclophosphamide, and vincristine chemotherapy. Gynecol Oncol 91:552–557, 2003.

Lavie I, Rao GG, Castrillon DH, et al: Duration of human chorionic gonadotropin surveillance for partial hydatidiform moles. Am J Obstet Gynecol 192:1362–1364, 2005.

Lurain JR, Nejad B: Secondary chemotherapy for high-risk gestational trophoblastic neoplasia. Gynecol Oncol 97:618–623, 2005.

ON UTERINE SARCOMAS

Li AJ, Giuntoli RI 2nd, Drake R, et al: Ovarian preservation in stage I low-grade endometrial stromal sarcomas. Obstet Gynecol 106:1304–1308, 2005.

Look KY, Sandler A, Blessing JA, et al: Phase II trial of gemcitabine as second-line chemotherapy of uterine leiomyosarcoma: A Gynecologic Oncology Group Study. Gynecol Oncol 92:644–647, 2004.

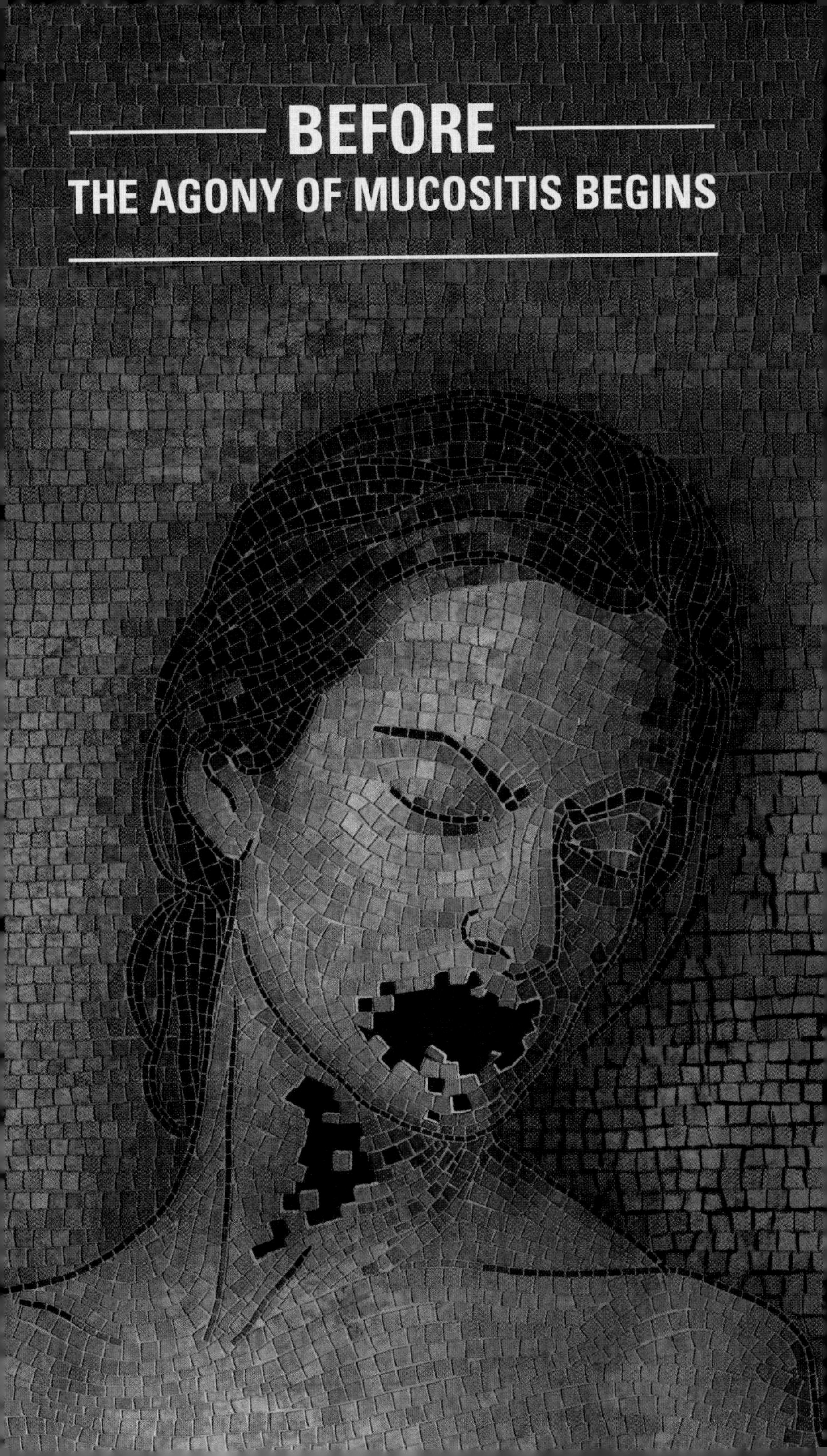
BEFORE
THE AGONY OF MUCOSITIS BEGINS

Kepivance®, the first and only epithelial growth factor, helps protect against the devastation of severe oral mucositis[1-3]

- **Offers the unique opportunity to shift the goal from symptom relief to protection.**[1-3]
  - — Proactively stimulates epithelial cell proliferation and differentiation to help provide cellular protection against mucosal injury.
- **Provides patients more days free from the devastation of oral mucositis.***†[1,2]
  - — Helps shift the severity to milder grades of oral mucositis.
  - — Results in a median of 6 fewer days of severe oral mucositis (Grade 3/4) and Grade 2/3/4 among patients overall.
  - — Reduces the median duration of Grade 3/4 by 3 days in patients who develop this severity.
  - — Reduces the incidence of Grade 4 by 68% and Grade 3/4 by 36%.
- **Helps patients continue to perform basic daily activities.***‡[1,2,4]
  - — Patients reported a 38% improvement in mouth and throat soreness and similar improvement in their abilities to eat, drink, swallow, and talk.

Kepivance® is indicated to decrease the incidence and duration of severe oral mucositis in patients with hematologic malignancies receiving myelotoxic therapy requiring hematopoietic stem cell support.

The safety and efficacy of Kepivance® have not been established in patients with non-hematologic malignancies.

Important Safety Information
In patients with hematologic malignancies, the most common serious adverse reaction in clinical trials attributed to Kepivance® was skin rash reported in less than 1% of patients. Other serious adverse reactions occurred at a similar rate in patients who received Kepivance® or placebo with the most frequent being fever, gastrointestinal events, and respiratory events. The most commonly reported adverse reactions attributed to Kepivance® were rash, erythema, edema, pruritus, dysesthesia, mouth/tongue thickness/discoloration, and taste alteration.

Please refer to the brief summary of Kepivance® prescribing information on next page.

*Results from a randomized, double-blind, placebo-controlled, phase 3 study (N = 212) in which patients with hematologic malignancies who were undergoing hematopoietic stem cell transplantation after myelotoxic therapy received either Kepivance® or placebo.[1,2]

†Analyses were performed in the overall patient population (patients who did not experience the event were assigned a duration of 0 days), and in a subset of patients who developed Grade 3/4 oral mucositis. Oral assessments were based on the World Health Organization oral toxicity scale.[2]

‡Mouth and throat soreness (MTS) and functional activity scores were collected with the use of a daily questionnaire and measured using a 5-point scale. MTS was a prespecified endpoint. Other functional activities were planned analyses.[2]

Kepivance®
(palifermin)

Shift to Protection

www.kepivance.com

References: 1. Kepivance® (palifermin) prescribing information, 2005. Amgen. **2.** Spielberger RS, Stiff P, Bensinger W, et al. Palifermin for oral mucositis after intensive therapy for hematologic cancers. *N Engl J Med.* 2004;351:2590-2598. **3.** Rubenstein EB, Peterson DE, Schubert M, et al. Clinical practice guidelines for the prevention and treatment of cancer therapy–induced oral and gastrointestinal mucositis. *Cancer.* 2004;100(suppl 9):2026-2046. **4.** Spielberger R, Emmanouilides C, Stiff P, et al. Use of recombinant human keratinocyte growth factor (palifermin) can reduce severe oral mucositis in patients with hematologic malignancies undergoing autologous peripheral blood progenitor cell transplantation after radiation-based conditioning. *J Support Oncol.* 2004;2(suppl 2):73-74.

Kepivance®
(palifermin)

BRIEF SUMMARY OF PRESCRIBING INFORMATION

CLINICAL PHARMACOLOGY

Special Populations

Results from a pharmacokinetics study in 24 subjects with varying degrees of renal impairment demonstrated that renal impairment has little or no influence on Kepivance® pharmacokinetics. No dose adjustment is recommended for patients with renal impairment.

INDICATIONS AND USAGE

Kepivance® is indicated to decrease the incidence and duration of severe oral mucositis in patients with hematologic malignancies receiving myelotoxic therapy requiring hematopoietic stem cell support.

The safety and efficacy of Kepivance® have not been established in patients with non-hematologic malignancies (see **PRECAUTIONS**).

CONTRAINDICATIONS

Kepivance® is contraindicated in patients with known hypersensitivity to *E coli*-derived proteins, palifermin, or any other component of the product.

PRECAUTIONS

Potential for Stimulation of Tumor Growth

The safety and efficacy of Kepivance® have not been established in patients with non-hematologic malignancies. The effects of Kepivance® on stimulation of KGF receptor-expressing, non-hematopoietic tumors in patients are not known. Kepivance® has been shown to enhance the growth of human epithelial tumor cell lines in vitro and to increase the rate of tumor cell line growth in a human carcinoma xenograft model.

Information for Patients

Patients should be informed of the possible adverse effects of Kepivance®, including muco-cutaneous adverse effects. These include rash, erythema, edema, pruritus, oral/perioral dysesthesia, tongue discoloration, tongue thickening, and alteration of taste. Patients should be instructed to report these adverse effects, or any other adverse reactions, to the prescribing physician (see **ADVERSE REACTIONS**).

The safety and efficacy of Kepivance® have not been established in patients with non-hematologic malignancies. Patients should be informed of the evidence of tumor growth and stimulation in cell culture and in animal models of non-hematopoietic human tumors.

Drug Interactions

No formal drug interaction studies have been conducted for Kepivance® with drugs that may be used in the intended patient population. Kepivance® has been shown to bind to heparin in vitro. Therefore, if heparin is used to maintain an IV line, saline should be used to rinse the line prior to and after Kepivance® administration.

Kepivance® should not be administered within 24 hours before, during infusion of, or within 24 hours after administration of myelotoxic chemotherapy (see **DOSAGE AND ADMINISTRATION**). In a clinical trial, administration of Kepivance® within 24 hours of chemotherapy resulted in increased severity and duration of oral mucositis.

Carcinogenesis, Mutagenesis, Impairment of Fertility

Carcinogenicity: The carcinogenic potential of Kepivance® has not been evaluated in long-term animal studies.

Mutagenicity: No clastogenic or mutagenic effects of Kepivance® were observed in the Ames or mammalian chromosomal aberration assays; however, such studies are generally not informative for biological products.

Impairment of Fertility: When Kepivance® was administered intravenously daily to male and female rats prior to and during mating, reproductive performance, fertility, and sperm assessment parameters were not affected at doses up to 100 mcg/kg/day. Systemic toxicity (clinical signs of toxicity and/or body weight effects), decreased epididymal sperm counts, and increased post-implantation loss were observed at doses ≥ 300 mcg/kg/day (5-fold higher than the recommended human dose). Increased pre-implantation loss and a decreased fertility index were observed at a Kepivance® dose of 1,000 mcg/kg/day.

Pregnancy Category C

Kepivance® has been shown to be embryotoxic in rabbits and rats when given in doses that are 2.5 and 8 times the human dose, respectively.

Increased post-implantation loss and decreased fetal body weights were observed when Kepivance® was administered to pregnant rabbits from days 6 to 18 of gestation at IV doses ≥ 150 mcg/kg/day (2.5-fold higher than the recommended human dose). However, treatment with these doses was also associated with maternal toxicity (clinical signs and reductions in body weight gain/food consumption). No evidence of developmental toxicity was observed in rabbits at doses up to 60 mcg/kg/day.

Increased post-implantation loss, decreased fetal body weight, and/or increased skeletal variations were observed when Kepivance® was administered to pregnant rats from days 6 to 17 or 19 of gestation at IV doses ≥ 500 mcg/kg/day (> 8-fold higher than the recommended human dose). Treatment with these doses was also frequently associated with maternal toxicity (clinical signs and body weight effects). No evidence of developmental toxicity was observed in rats at doses up to 300 mcg/kg/day.

There are no adequate and well-controlled studies in pregnant women. Kepivance® should be used during pregnancy only if the potential benefit to the mother justifies the potential risk to the fetus.

Lactating Women

It is not known whether Kepivance® is excreted in human milk. Because many drugs are excreted in human milk, caution should be exercised when Kepivance® is administered to a nursing woman.

Pediatric Use

The safety and effectiveness of Kepivance® in pediatric patients have not been established.

Geriatric Use

Clinical studies of Kepivance® did not include sufficient numbers of subjects age 65 years and over to determine whether they respond differently from younger subjects. Among 409 patients with hematologic malignancies who received Kepivance® in clinical studies, 9 (2%) were ≥ age 65.

ADVERSE REACTIONS

Please refer to the **PRECAUTIONS: Potential for Stimulation of Tumor Growth** section regarding the potential for tumor stimulatory effects in KGF receptor-expressing tumors.

Because clinical trials are conducted under widely varying conditions, adverse reaction rates observed in the clinical trials of a drug cannot be directly compared to rates in the clinical trials of another drug and may not reflect the rates observed in practice. The adverse reaction information from clinical trials does, however, provide a basis for identifying the adverse events that appear to be related to drug use and for approximating rates.

Safety data are based upon 409 patients with hematologic malignancies (NHL, Hodgkin's disease, AML, ALL, CML, CLL, or multiple myeloma) who received Kepivance® and 241 patients who received placebo in 3 randomized, placebo-controlled clinical studies and a pharmacokinetic study. Patients received Kepivance® either before, or before and after regimens of myelotoxic chemotherapy, with or without TBI, followed by PBPC support. The patients were predominantly between the ages of 41 and 60 years (median 48 yrs), male (62%), white (83%). NHL was the most common malignancy followed by Hodgkin's disease, multiple myeloma, and leukemia.

The most common serious adverse reaction attributed to Kepivance® was skin rash, which was reported in less than 1% (3/409) of patients treated with Kepivance®. Grade 3 skin rashes occurred in 14 patients, 9 of 409 (3%) receiving Kepivance® and 5 of 241 (2%) receiving placebo. In seven patients (5 Kepivance®, 2 placebo), study drug was discontinued due to skin rash. Other serious adverse reactions occurred at a similar rate in patients who received Kepivance® (20%) or placebo (21%). The most frequently reported serious adverse events in Kepivance® and placebo-treated patients were fever, gastrointestinal events, and respiratory events.

The most common adverse reactions attributed to Kepivance® were skin toxicities (rash, erythema, edema, pruritus), oral toxicities (dysesthesia, tongue discoloration, tongue thickening, alteration of taste), pain arthralgias, and dysesthesia. The median time to onset of cutaneous toxicity was 6 days following the first of 3 consecutive daily doses of Kepivance®, with a median duration of 5 days. In patients receiving Kepivance®, dysesthesia (including hyperesthesia, hypoesthesia, and paresthesia) was usually localized to the perioral region, whereas in patients receiving placebo dysesthesias were more likely to occur in extremities. Adverse events occurring more frequently in Kepivance®-treated patients as compared to placebo-treated patients (a higher incidence of ≥ 5%) are listed in Table 2.

Table 2. Adverse Events Occurring With ≥ 5% Higher Incidence in Kepivance® vs. Placebo

BODY SYSTEM Adverse Event	Kepivance® (n = 409)	Placebo (n = 241)
BODY AS A WHOLE		
Edema	28%	21%
Pain	16%	11%
Fever	39%	34%
GASTROINTESTINAL		
Mouth/Tongue Thickness or Discoloration	17%	8%
MUSCULOSKELETAL		
Arthralgia	10%	5%
SKIN AND APPENDAGES		
Rash	62%	50%
Pruritus	35%	24%
Erythema	32%	22%
SPECIAL SENSES		
Taste Altered	16%	8%
CNS/PNS		
Dysesthesia – Hyperesthesia/ hypoesthesia/paresthesia	12%	7%
METABOLIC		
Elevated serum lipase (Grade 3/4)	28% (11%)	23% (5%)
Elevated serum amylase (Grade 3/4)	62% (38%)	54% (31%)

Hypertension: In a phase 1 placebo-controlled study in patients undergoing hematopoietic transplantation and receiving Kepivance® (3 doses pre-myelotoxic therapy and 3 doses post-transplant), the proportion of Kepivance®-treated patients reporting an adverse event of hypertension in the 60- and 80-mcg/kg/day Kepivance® cohorts was greater than in the placebo group (2/15 patients [13%], 2/14 [14%], and 2/23 [9%], respectively). These events were transient and did not require treatment discontinuation in any patient. In an integrated analysis of adverse events across Kepivance® studies in the hematology transplant setting, hypertensive events were reported in 30/409 Kepivance® (7%) patients and 13/241 placebo (5%) patients.

Proteinuria: In a placebo-controlled study conducted in 145 patients with metastatic colorectal cancer receiving multi-cycle chemotherapy (5-FU/leucovorin), serial urine specimens were collected for 27 placebo-treated and 54 Kepivance®-treated patients. Among the 54 Kepivance®-treated patients, 9 patients with a baseline urinalysis negative for protein subsequently developed 2+ or greater proteinuria after treatment with Kepivance®. Among the 27 placebo-treated patients evaluated, none developed 2+ or greater proteinuria. Because of the study design, the number of cycles with urine analysis data collected was higher in the Kepivance®- treated patients. In addition, for the 9 patients with proteinuria, underlying medical conditions known to be associated with proteinuria were present at baseline. A causal relationship between Kepivance® and proteinuria has not been established.

Laboratory Values: Reversible elevations in serum lipase and amylase, which did not require treatment intervention, are shown in Table 2. In general, peak increases were observed during the period of cytotoxic therapy and returned to baseline by the day of PBPC infusion. Fractionation of amylase revealed it to be predominantly salivary in origin.

Immunogenicity

As with all therapeutic proteins, there is a potential for immunogenicity. The clinical significance of antibodies to Kepivance® is unknown but may include lessened activity and/or cross reactivity with other members of the FGF family of growth factors.

A sensitive electrochemiluminescence-based binding assay was performed on post-treatment sera from 645 patients treated with Kepivance® in clinical studies. Twelve (2%) of these 645 patients tested positive for antibodies to Kepivance® following treatment. None of the samples had evidence of neutralizing activity in a cell-based assay.

The incidence of antibody positivity is highly dependent on the specific assay and its sensitivity. Additionally, the observed incidence of antibody positivity in an assay may be influenced by several factors including sample handling, timing of sample collection, concomitant medications and underlying disease. For these reasons, comparison of the incidence of antibodies to Kepivance® with the incidence of antibodies to other products may be misleading.

OVERDOSAGE

The maximum amount of Kepivance® that can be safely administered in a single dose has not been determined. Single doses of 250 mcg/kg have been administered intravenously to 8 healthy volunteers without severe or serious adverse effects. Five of 14 patients receiving six doses of 80 mcg/kg/day administered intravenously over 2 weeks (three doses preceding and three doses following myeloablative chemotherapy/TBI) experienced serious or severe adverse events. These events were consistent with those observed at the recommended dose but were generally more severe.

DOSAGE AND ADMINISTRATION

The recommended dosage of Kepivance® is 60 mcg/kg/day, administered as an IV bolus injection for 3 consecutive days before and 3 consecutive days after myelotoxic therapy for a total of 6 doses.

Pre-myelotoxic therapy: The first 3 doses should be administered prior to myelotoxic therapy, with the third dose 24 to 48 hours before myelotoxic therapy (see **PRECAUTIONS: Drug Interactions**).

Post-myelotoxic therapy: The last 3 doses should be administered post-myelotoxic therapy; the first of these doses should be administered after, but on the same day of hematopoietic stem cell infusion and at least 4 days after the most recent administration of Kepivance® (see **PRECAUTIONS: Drug Interactions**).

No dose adjustment is recommended for patients with renal impairment (see **CLINICAL PHARMACOLOGY: Special Populations**).

Rx Only

This product, its production and/or its use may be covered by one or more US Patents, including US Patent Nos. 6,420,531 B1; 5,814,605; 5,824,643; and 5,677,278 as well as other patents or patents pending.

AMGEN®

Issue Date: 12/12/2005

Manufactured by:
Amgen Manufacturing, Limited,
a subsidiary of Amgen Inc.
One Amgen Center Drive
Thousand Oaks, CA 91320-1799
USA

Certain manufacturing operations have been performed by other firms.

www.kepivance.com

CHAPTER 22

Ovarian cancer

Stephen C. Rubin, MD, and Paul Sabbatini, MD

Despite the fact that it is highly curable if diagnosed early, cancer of the ovaries causes more mortality in American women each year than all other gynecologic malignancies combined. An estimated 22,430 new cases of this cancer will be diagnosed in the United States in 2007, and about 15,280 women will succumb to the disease.

Although the number of deaths from ovarian cancer continues to increase, notable advances in chemotherapy and surgery over the past several decades have begun to translate into improved survival. Long-term survival data reflecting these recent advances are expected to show further increases. According to American Cancer Society data, the overall 5-year survival rate from ovarian cancer has increased significantly, from 36% in the mid-1970s to 53% in the mid-1990s. Recent data from the National Cancer Institute show a similar increase in stage-specific survival. It is expected that data from the current decade, reflecting continued improvements in chemotherapy and surgery, will confirm even better survival.

This chapter will focus on epithelial cancers of the ovaries, which account for about 90% of ovarian malignancies.

Epidemiology

Age Ovarian cancer is primarily a disease of postmenopausal women, with the large majority of cases occurring in women between 50 and 75 years old. The incidence of ovarian cancer increases with age and peaks at a rate of 61.5 per 100,000 women in the 75–79-year-old age group.

Race The incidence of ovarian cancer appears to vary by race, although the effects of race are difficult to separate from those of environment related to culture, geography, and socioeconomic status. In the United States, the age-adjusted rate of ovarian cancer for Caucasians is estimated to be 17.9 per 100,000 population, which is significantly higher than 11.9 per 100,000 for the African-American population.

Geography There are distinct geographic variations in the incidence of ovarian cancer, with the highest rates found in industrialized countries and the lowest rates seen in underdeveloped nations. Japan, with an incidence of only about 3.0 per 100,000 population, is a notable exception to this observation. It has been postulated that geographic variations in the incidence of ovarian cancer are related, in part, to differences in family size.

Some of the highest rates are seen in women of Eastern European Jewish ancestry, who have an estimated incidence of 17.2 per 100,000 population, a probable result of the relatively high frequency of *BRCA1* and *BRCA2* mutations in this population.

Etiology and risk factors

The cause of epithelial ovarian cancer remains unknown. Although it now appears certain that, at the cellular level, ovarian cancer results from the accumulation of multiple discrete genetic defects, the mechanism(s) by which these defects develop have yet to be determined. Epidemiologic studies have identified a number of factors that may increase or decrease the risk of the disease. In addition, a small proportion of ovarian cancers in the United States, approximately 5%–10%, result from inherited defects in the *BRCA1* gene or other genes, including *BRCA2* and the hereditary nonpolyposis colorectal cancer *(HNPCC)* genes.

Diet It has been suggested that numerous dietary factors increase the risk of ovarian cancer, although the magnitude of the reported increase is relatively modest.

Fat Countries with a higher per capita consumption of animal fat tend to have higher rates of ovarian cancer.

Lactose Populations with a high dietary intake of lactose who lack the enzyme galactose-1-phosphate uridyltransferase have been reported to be at increased risk.

Coffee Conflicting reports have been published regarding the role of coffee consumption and the risk of ovarian cancer.

Environmental factors Various environmental risk factors also have been suggested.

Talc Exposure to talc (hydrous magnesium trisilicate) used as dusting powder on diaphragms and sanitary napkins has been reported in some studies to increase the risk of ovarian cancer, although other studies have failed to find an association.

Radiation Data on the association between exposure to ionizing radiation and the risk of ovarian cancer are also conflicting.

Viruses Several studies have examined the effect of viral agents, including mumps, rubella, and influenza viruses, on the risk of ovarian cancer. No clear relationship has been demonstrated.

Hormonal and reproductive factors In contrast to the conflicting data on dietary and environmental factors, some clear associations have been drawn between certain hormonal and reproductive factors and the risk of developing ovarian cancer.

Low parity and infertility Several analyses have documented that women with a history of low parity or involuntary infertility are at increased risk of ovarian cancer.

Ovulation-inducing drugs Evidence suggests that treatment with ovulation-inducing drugs, particularly for prolonged periods, may be a risk factor, although it is difficult to separate the increased risk related to the infertility itself from the risk carried by use of ovulation-inducing agents.

Hormone replacement therapy Although the data are not consistent, some studies have shown an association between the use of postmenopausal hormone replacement and the development of ovarian cancer. Data from the Women's Health Initiative randomized trial of estrogen plus progestin showed a slight increase in the risk of ovarian cancer in users of hormone replacement therapy, although it was not statistically significant.

Oral contraceptives Several large case-controlled studies have documented a marked protective effect of oral contraceptives against ovarian cancer. Women who have used oral contraceptives for at least several years have approximately half the risk of ovarian cancer as do nonusers, and the protective effect of oral contraceptives appears to persist for years after their discontinuation. It is estimated that the routine use of oral contraceptives may prevent nearly 2,000 cases of ovarian cancer yearly in the United States. Evidence suggests that the protective effect of oral contraceptives also applies to women carrying *BRCA* mutations.

Hereditary cancer syndromes There has been a fascinating evolution in our understanding of the role of hereditary factors in the development of ovarian cancer. It has been recognized for many years that women with a family history of cancer, particularly cancer of the ovaries or breasts, are themselves at increased risk of ovarian cancer. In the 1980s, Lynch and colleagues refined these observations by delineating several apparently distinct syndromes of hereditary cancer involving the ovaries, including breast-ovarian cancer syndrome, site-specific ovarian cancer syndrome, and Lynch II syndrome (HNPCC).

Epidemiologically, these syndromes appear to be inherited as an autosomal-dominant trait with variable penetrance. During the past decade, the specific genes responsible for HNPCC (*MSH1* and *MLH2*) and for most cases of hereditary ovarian cancer have been identified, allowing fundamental observations to be made regarding their molecular pathophysiology.

BRCA *mutations* The *BRCA1* gene is classified as a tumor suppressor, since mutations in this gene increase the risk of breast and ovarian cancers. Definitive identification of the function of the protein translated from this gene remains to be elucidated, although evidence suggests that it plays a role in the repair of oxidative damage to DNA. Part of the protein appears to contain a DNA-binding domain, suggesting that it also functions as a transcriptional regulator.

The frequency of *BRCA1* mutations in the general population is estimated at approximately 1 in 800 and in Jewish women of eastern European descent, 1 in 100.

Women carrying a germline mutation of *BRCA1* have a significantly elevated risk of both breast and ovarian cancers compared with the general population. The average population risk of developing breast cancer is about 12.5% (one in eight) and of developing ovarian cancer, 1.5%. However, in the presence of a germline *BRCA1* mutation and a strong family history of cancer, these risks rise to about 90% and 40% for breast and ovarian cancers, respectively.

It is important to recognize that these risk estimates are derived from families identified with multiple cases of breast and/or ovarian cancer. The risk for women with *BRCA1* mutations from families with less impressive family histories is probably lower for ovarian cancer, perhaps in the range of 15%–20%.

Although the presence of germline mutations in *BRCA1* is not limited to women with a strong family history of breast cancer, data from several laboratories suggest that *BRCA1* mutations usually are not a feature of sporadic ovarian cancer. Mutations in this gene appear to play a role in the development of approximately 50% of familial breast cancer cases and may account for the majority of hereditary ovarian cancers. Evidence from multiple studies suggests that *BRCA1*-related ovarian cancers may have a less aggressive clinical course than do sporadic ovarian cancers.

BRCA2 *mutations* Hereditary ovarian cancers not related to *BRCA1* are most often related to mutations in the *BRCA2* gene.

Signs and symptoms

Early-stage disease In the early stages, ovarian cancer may be an insidious disease, but nonspecific symptoms that may be clues to the diagnosis are present more often than previously thought. A prospective case-controlled study by Goff et al recently evaluated 1,709 women with the diagnosis of ovarian cancer and compared their self-reported symptoms with those of women without ovarian cancer who attended a primary care clinic. The combination of bloating, increased abdominal size, and urinary symptoms was found in 43% of those with cancer but in only 8% of those without cancer.

The impact of screening patients with serum CA-125 levels and transvaginal ultrasonography on mortality is being addressed in the Prostate, Lung, Colorectal, and Ovarian Trial (PLCO). In this study, 39,115 women were randomized to undergo screening. To date, screening has identified both early- and late-stage cancers, and the predictive value is low (3.7% for abnormal CA-125, 1.0% for abnormal transvaginal ultrasonography, and 23.5% for both). Follow-up is ongoing to determine whether there is an effect on mortality.

Early ovarian cancer also may be detected as a pelvic mass noted fortuitously at the time of a routine pelvic examination. Imaging with sonography, CT, or MRI will confirm the presence of a mass. The size, internal architecture, and blood flow of the mass can be used to make an educated guess as to whether it is benign or malignant, but imaging findings are not diagnostic in this regard. About half of patients with early ovarian cancers have an elevated serum CA-125 level.

Advanced-stage disease Patients may complain of abdominal bloating or swelling if ascites is present, and large pelvic masses may produce bladder or rectal symptoms. Occasional patients may have respiratory distress as a result of a large pleural effusion, which is more common on the right side. Infrequently, there may be a history of abnormal vaginal bleeding.

Most patients with advanced disease have ascites detectable by physical examination or imaging. Complex pelvic masses and an omental tumor cake may be present, and nodules can frequently be palpated in the pelvic cul-de-sac on rectovaginal examination. It should be noted that some patients with advanced ovarian cancer have essentially normal-sized ovaries. Approximately 80% of patients with advanced ovarian cancer will have an elevated CA-125 level.

Screening and diagnosis

Screening Unfortunately, no effective strategy exists for screening of the general population for ovarian cancer. Imaging techniques, including abdominal and transvaginal sonography, have been studied extensively, as has the serum marker CA-125. None of these techniques, alone or in combination, is specific enough to serve as an appropriate screening test, even in populations targeted by age.

Both the National Institutes of Health Consensus Conference (see full page of NIH guidelines) and the American College of Obstetricians and Gynecologists have issued statements advising against routine screening for ovarian cancer, which, due to its high false-positive rate, leads to an unacceptable amount of invasive interventions in women without significant disease.

The NIH Prostate, Lung, Colon, and Ovarian (PLCO) Screening Trial has accrued its full complement of 152,000 patients. Half are female and half are male. For the ovarian cancer segment of the trial, half of the women will be screened via physical examination, CA-125 level, and vaginal ultrasonography and the other half, via standard medical care. Since patients will be followed for 13 years or more, it will be many years before final results are available, but it is not expected that these screening modalities will be useful in the general population.

Recent studies using serum proteomics to screen for early ovarian cancer have yielded promising results. Work in this area is ongoing and may result in a clinically useful assay in the near future.

High-risk patients Management of women from families with hereditary ovarian cancer is controversial. Evidence suggests that surveillance of such women with serum markers and sonography is of limited benefit in early detection of ovarian cancer. Most experts recommend prophylactic excision of the ovaries after age 35 if the woman has completed childbearing, as several studies have shown that it will dramatically reduce the risk of ovarian cancer. Evidence also suggests that prophylactic oophorectomy substantially lowers the risk of breast cancer in women from high-risk families.

Preoperative evaluation Patients with suspected ovarian cancer should undergo a thorough evaluation prior to surgery. This assessment should include a complete history and physical examination and serum CA-125 level determination. In women younger than age 30, determinations of β-human chorionic gonadotropin (β-hCG) and α-fetoprotein (AFP) levels are useful, as germ-cell tumors are more common in this age group.

Abdominal CT and MRI In apparent early-stage cases, abdominal scanning by CT or MRI adds little to the diagnostic evaluation, and, thus, these studies are not routinely necessary. CT and MRI may be useful in providing a preoperative assessment of disease extent in probable advanced-stage cases.

Exploratory laparotomy The diagnosis of ovarian cancer is generally made by histopathologic study following exploratory laparotomy. The stage of the disease can only be determined by surgery, as discussed later.

Preoperative endometrial sampling Women with abnormal vaginal bleeding should undergo preoperative endometrial sampling.

Preoperative cytologic or histologic evaluation of effusions or tumor masses is neither necessary nor desirable. Often, patients with ascites and large pelvic masses, for whom exploration is necessary, are subjected to paracentesis or needle biopsy. These procedures only delay definitive management and may lead to seeding of tumor cells along needle tracks.

Pathology

The ovaries are notable for their ability to give rise to a large variety of neoplasms with distinct embryologic origins and differing histologic appearances.

Epithelial adenocarcinoma Approximately 90% of all ovarian malignancies are of epithelial origin, arising from the cells that invest the surface of the ovaries. These cells give rise to a variety of adenocarcinomas, including serous, mucinous, endometrioid, and clear-cell types. These tumors have benign counterparts of similar histologic appearance and can also exist as "borderline" cancers, also known as "tumors of low malignant potential." There is some prognostic significance to the cell type of the tumor, with clear-cell and mucinous varieties tending to be especially virulent.

Histologic differentiation Pathologists also classify adenocarcinomas according to the degree of histologic differentiation. Those tumors retaining clear-cut glandular features are considered grade 1, or well differentiated, whereas those that are largely composed of solid sheets of tumor are considered grade 3, or poorly differentiated. Tumors showing both glandular and solid areas are assigned to grade 2. The histologic grade seems to correlate roughly with biologic aggressiveness.

Stromal and germ-cell tumors Malignancies can also arise from the ovarian stroma or the primordial germ cells contained within the ovaries. Stromal tumors are often hormone-producing and include such types as the granulosa tumor, Sertoli-Leydig tumor, and several variants. Germ-cell tumors, which tend to be highly aggressive, include the dysgerminoma, endodermal sinus

NIH GUIDELINES ON SCREENING FOR OVARIAN CANCER

Until clinical trials gather enough information, no evidence supports routine screening for ovarian cancer in women without first-degree relatives affected by the disease, according to a consensus development panel convened by the NIH.

The panel did recommend that physicians take a comprehensive family history of their female patients. The panel also advised women to undergo routine annual rectovaginal pelvic examinations.

There are no conclusive data that screening is beneficial, even for women with two or more first-degree relatives with ovarian cancer, the panel stated. However, these women have a significant chance of having a hereditary ovarian cancer syndrome and should be counseled by a gynecologic oncologist or other qualified specialist regarding their individual risk.

Patients with hereditary ovarian cancer syndrome

Patients with hereditary ovarian cancer syndrome (assuming autosomal-dominant inheritance with 80% penetrance) have a 40% lifetime risk of developing ovarian cancer. Recent data suggest that screening these women reduces their mortality from ovarian cancer.

High-risk women

The three known hereditary syndromes that place a woman at exceedingly high risk are familial site-specific ovarian cancer syndrome, breast-ovarian cancer syndrome, and breast-ovarian-endometrial-colorectal cancer syndrome. Annual rectovaginal pelvic examinations, CA-125 level determinations, and transvaginal ultrasonography are recommended for these women until their childbearing is completed or until age 35, at which time prophylactic bilateral oophorectomy is recommended.

Prophylactic oophorectomy performed in women undergoing abdominal surgery for other indications, such as benign uterine disease, is also associated with a significant reduction in the risk of ovarian cancer. The appropriateness of hormonal replacement therapy is not straightforward given that many of these women are at higher risk for breast cancer. In addition, the report from the study by the Women's Health Initiative in postmenopausal women raised questions regarding the role of long-term hormonal replacement, particularly showing no benefit in terms of cardiovascular risk reduction. Women should discuss the potential for estrogen replacement vs other agents for the prevention of osteoporosis, for example, with their health care provider.

Other panel recommendations

Women with ovarian masses who have been identified preoperatively as having a significant risk of ovarian cancer should be advised to have their surgery performed by a gynecologic oncologist.

Aggressive attempts at cytoreductive surgery as the primary management of ovarian cancer will improve the chances for long-term survival.

Women with stage IA and IB, grade I ovarian cancer do not require postoperative adjuvant therapy, although many remaining patients with stage I disease do require chemotherapy. Subsets of stage I must be fully defined and ideal treatment determined.

Second-look laparotomy should not be employed as routine care for all patients but should be performed for patients enrolled in clinical trials or for patients in whom the surgery will affect clinical decision-making and the clinical course.

From Ovarian cancer: Screening, treatment and follow-up. NIH Consensus Statement. 12:1–30, 1994.

TABLE 1: FIGO staging system for ovarian cancer

Stage	Characteristics
I	Growth limited to the ovaries
IA	Growth limited to one ovary; no ascites; no tumor on the external surfaces, capsule intact
IB	Growth limited to both ovaries; no ascites; no tumor on the external surfaces, capsule intact
IC	Tumor either stage IA or IB but on the surface of one or both ovaries; capsule ruptured; ascites containing malignant cells present; or positive peritoneal washings
II	Growth involving one or both ovaries with pelvic extension of disease
IIA	Extension of disease and/or metastases to the uterus and/or fallopian tubes
IIB	Extension of disease to other pelvic tissues
IIC	Tumor either stage IIA or IIB but on the surface of one or both ovaries; capsule(s) ruptured; ascites containing malignant cells present; or positive peritoneal washings
III	Tumor involving one or both ovaries with peritoneal implants outside the pelvis and/or positive retroperitoneal or inguinal nodes; superficial liver metastasis equals stage III; tumor is limited to the true pelvis but with histologically verified malignant extension to the small bowel or omentum
IIIA	Tumor grossly limited to the true pelvis with negative nodes but with histologically confirmed microscopic seeding of abdominal peritoneal surfaces
IIIB	Tumor of one or both ovaries; histologically confirmed implants on abdominal peritoneal surfaces, none > 2 cm in diameter; nodes negative
IIIC	Abdominal implants > 2 cm in diameter and/or positive retroperitoneal or inguinal nodes
IV	Growth involving one or both ovaries with distant metastases; if pleural effusion is present, there must be positive cytologic test results to allot a case to stage IV; parenchymal liver metastasis equals stage IV

FIGO = International Federation of Gynecology and Obstetrics

tumor, malignant teratoma, embryonal carcinoma, and rare primary choriocarcinoma of the ovaries. Malignant germ-cell tumors occur primarily in younger patients, with an average age at diagnosis of about 19 years.

Staging and prognosis

Staging system

The staging system for ovarian cancer shown in Table 1, developed by the International Federation of Gynecology and Obstetrics (FIGO), is used uniformly in all developed countries. It is based on the results of a properly per-

TABLE 2: Procedures for surgical staging for apparent early ovarian cancer

Vertical incision
Multiple cytologic washings
Intact tumor removal
Complete abdominal exploration
Removal of remaining ovaries, uterus, fallopian tubes[a]
Omentectomy
Lymph node sampling
Random peritoneal biopsies, including the diaphragm

[a] May be preserved in selected patients who wish to preserve fertility

formed exploratory laparotomy, a fact that bears emphasis, since inadequate surgical staging has been and continues to be a significant problem.

Surgical staging The surgical staging of ovarian cancer is based on an understanding of the patterns of disease spread and must be conducted in a systematic and thorough manner. It should include a complete evaluation of all visceral and parietal surfaces within the peritoneal cavity, omentectomy, and biopsy of aortic and pelvic lymph nodes. It generally includes removal of the internal reproductive organs as well, although exceptions to this rule can be made for younger women with limited disease who may wish to retain fertility.

The issue of adequate surgical staging becomes particularly acute in just the patient population likely to be operated upon by individuals with no specialized training in gynecologic oncology: patients with adnexal masses that are not obvious cancers on preoperative evaluation. At the time of exploration, if the mass is shown to be malignant on frozen section and there is no obvious metastatic disease, a complete staging operation is essential to search for occult metastatic spread, which may be present in 20%–30% of such cases. Also, if the tumor is documented to be stage IA by thorough staging and the patient wishes to preserve the potential for future fertility, it may be appropriate to conserve the uterus and uninvolved ovaries and fallopian tube–an option often overlooked by the inexperienced surgeon.

The elements of surgical staging for apparent early ovarian cancer are listed in Table 2.

Prognostic factors

The prognosis of epithelial ovarian cancer depends on a number of factors.

Disease stage Of primary importance is the disease stage, which, when properly determined, is of strong prognostic significance. The distribution of ovarian cancer cases by stage follows: stage I, 26%; stage II, 15%; stage III, 42%; stage IV, 17%. For patients with advanced ovarian cancer, the amount of residual tumor at the conclusion of the initial operation is of major importance. Patients with stage III disease who have minimal or no residual tumor may have a 30%–50% chance of 5-year survival, whereas those patients with stage III disease left with bulky tumor masses have a 5-year survival rate of only about 10%.

Histologic grade and type Most studies have found the histologic grade of the tumor to have prognostic significance; the histologic cell type of the tumor is of less importance, although patients with clear-cell and possibly mucinous tumors may have a worse prognosis.

Molecular markers In recent years, a great deal of effort has been devoted to the identification of molecular markers of prognosis in ovarian cancer. Studies of HER2, *p53, ras,* and other oncogenes and tumor-suppressor genes have had varying results relative to prognostic significance. Currently, the assessment of molecular markers of prognosis has no clinical utility, although much work continues in this promising area, particularly with the development of high-throughput techniques for determining gene and protein expression.

Predictors of chemosensitivity Similarly, after 25 years of investigations assessing in vitro and in vivo methods to predict the sensitivity or resistance of ovarian cancers to various chemotherapeutic drugs, the clinical usefulness of such an approach remains under investigation. The American Society of Clinical Oncology (ASCO) recently reviewed the relevant literature on the subject and reached the same conclusion for cancers in general.

Treatment

Surgery plays a crucial role in all phases of the management of ovarian cancer and, when applied as part of a multidisciplinary approach, affords patients the highest likelihood of a favorable outcome. For most patients with ovarian carcinoma, surgery is not curative due to dissemination of tumor cells throughout the abdominal cavity. Therefore, successful management generally requires additional treatment.

The use of postoperative chemotherapy is standard for all patients with advanced-stage disease and for many patients with early-stage disease. Adjunctive chemotherapy significantly prolongs survival, with most current data supporting the use of platinum- and taxane-based regimens.

Despite a long history of the use of radiation therapy in ovarian carcinoma, opinions on its utility differ widely. Presumably, this controversy is due to the limited amount and adequacy of data comparing radiotherapy with modern chemotherapy regimens. Similarly, the role of radiotherapy as part of up-front combined-modality therapy, salvage treatment following chemotherapy, and palliative therapy remains unclear.

TREATMENT OF EARLY DISEASE

Clearly, comprehensive surgical staging is necessary to properly identify patients with stages I and II ovarian carcinoma. Beyond surgery, the need for adjuvant treatment with chemotherapy has been recently supported, with the exception of patients with stage I disease and well-differentiated histology.

Surgery

Suspicious adnexal masses should be excised intact and submitted for frozen section. If a malignancy is confirmed and there is no obvious metastatic spread, complete surgical staging should be undertaken. As discussed previously (see section on "Staging and prognosis"), it is of critical importance that surgical staging be performed in a systematic and complete manner. Inadequate staging may result in inappropriate postoperative treatment, which can severely compromise the chances for cure.

Data from the American College of Surgeons community hospital-based tumor registry show that almost 75% of the primary surgeries for ovarian cancer performed in this country are done so without the involvement of a gynecologic oncologist. This finding is particularly unfortunate given the fact that, with physical examination, measurement of CA-125 levels, and appropriate imaging tests, the majority of cases of ovarian cancer can be identified preoperatively. Results from other studies suggest that when a gynecologic oncologist is not present at the initial operation, staging is more often inadequate, cytoreduction is more often suboptimal, and long-term survival is poorer.

Conservation of reproductive organs In a woman of reproductive age with cancer limited to one ovary, it may be possible to conserve the uterus and opposite fallopian tube and ovary if she wishes to maintain the option of future fertility. To facilitate such intraoperative decision-making, it is essential that the surgeon's preoperative discussion with the patient and her family address the possibility of malignancy and review the surgical options for both benign and malignant diseases.

Operative laparoscopy Recent advances in the instrumentation for operative laparoscopy have led to an increase in the proportion of adnexal masses being managed with this technique. Physicians should exercise caution in selecting patients with adnexal masses for operative laparoscopic approaches. Unless the surgeon's laparoscopic skills are extraordinary, suspicious masses are best managed by laparotomy. For masses that are approached laparoscopically, the same surgical principles of removal without spill and complete surgical staging apply.

Systemic chemotherapy

The current management of patients with early-stage disease focuses on comprehensive surgical staging and the identification of high-risk features. Patients with stage IA or IB tumors with well-differentiated histology have excellent 5-year survival rates, and adjuvant chemotherapy is generally not used in such patients. High-risk features include moderately to poorly differentiated tumors, stage IC or II disease, and clear-cell histology.

The reported survival rates of 60%–80% in patients who have early-stage tumors with high-risk features suggested a potential role for adjuvant therapy. The Italian Inter-Regional Cooperative Group conducted two randomized trials to evaluate the role of adjuvant therapy in patients with stage I disease. The first trial compared cisplatin, 50 mg/m^2 q28d × 6, with observation in 85 patients with stage IA or IB, grade 2-3 disease. The 5-year disease-free survival rate was higher in patients treated with cisplatin than in those who were observed (83% vs 63%), but the 5-year overall survival rate was similar in the two groups (88% vs 82%).

The second trial compared cisplatin (same dose) to phosphorus-32 (P-32) administration in 161 patients with stage IA-IB, grade 2 or stage IC disease. The 5-year disease-free survival rate again favored the platinum arm (85% vs 65%), but the 5-year overall survival rate was unchanged and similar to that reported in the previous trial. P-32 administration was associated with more long-term toxicity.

More recent data have provided support for a survival benefit to the immediate use of adjuvant chemotherapy in patients with early-stage disease. The results of the ACTION (European Organization for Research on the Treatment of Cancer [EORTC] Adjuvant Treatment in Ovarian Neoplasm) and International Collaborative on Ovarian Neoplasm (ICON) trials were combined and reported. A 5-year survival rate improvement of 8% was reported for those receiving immediate chemotherapy compared with reserving chemotherapy for those who relapsed (74% vs 82%; 95% confidence interval [CI]: 2%–12%).

Improvements in the systemic chemotherapy for advanced ovarian cancer with associated improvements in survival are relevant to the design of regimens for early-stage disease. A Gynecologic Oncology Group trial (GOG 157) evaluated 3 vs 6 cycles of paclitaxel and carboplatin (Paraplatin) in patients with stage IA or IB, grade 2–3; stage IC; or stage II disease. The trial completed accrual in 1995, and final results showed no significant benefit to the longer regimen. The GOG replacement trial is evaluating 3 cycles of paclitaxel plus carboplatin with or without additional weekly paclitaxel (40 mg/m^2) in patients with early-stage disease.

In the absence of additional data, taxane- and platinum-based systemic chemotherapy should be considered the standard approach for patients who have early-stage disease with high-risk features. The optimal number of cycles is currently unclear, but 3 cycles were considered the standard arm in the GOG 157 trial.

Radiation therapy

Past GOG trials have established that patients with stage IA–IB, well-differentiated or moderately differentiated tumors have a 5-year survival rate of 90%–98%, which does not seem to improve with adjuvant chemotherapy. However, patients with less favorable neoplasms by virtue of higher grade or stage have poorer outcomes (80% 5-year survival rate among treated patients).

Whole-abdominal irradiation Externally administered whole-abdominal irradiation (WAI) has a number of theoretical and practical advantages over P-32 therapy. They include improved homogeneity of the radiation dose, treatment of pelvic and para-aortic lymph nodes, better coverage of all peritoneal surfaces, and lack of treatment restrictions due to postoperative adhesions.

However, late toxicity has been a legitimate concern. A retrospective study found that patients who received 6 cycles of cisplatin and cyclophosphamide with WAI administered between the third and fourth cycles had significantly better outcomes than those given single-agent cisplatin. The difference was particularly evident in patients with stage I or II, grade 3 tumors without gross residual disease.

A study by Hepp et al found WAI to be an effective adjuvant therapy in patients with optimally debulked tumors. In a series of 60 patients, the 5-year survival rate was 55%, with a median follow-up of 96.5 months. Patients who received chemotherapy (n = 41) fared slightly worse than those who received radiation therapy only. The abdominal control rate was 83%, and the grade 3 and 4 late toxicity rates were 7% and 3%, respectively.

The findings indicate that 5- and 10-year survival rates obtained with WAI are at least equivalent to results obtained using modern systemic agents. However, in view of the recognized limitations of these trials, more rigorously gathered data will be required to establish the role of WAI in these patients.

Collectively, existing data suggest that WAI should be studied further as a primary adjuvant treatment modality in patients thought to require treatment. Appropriate patients for trials including WAI are intermediate-risk patients, as defined by Dembo. The entire abdomen should be treated with an open-field technique using 100–150 cGy/d, to a total dose of 2,200–2,500 cGy. The utility of routine pelvic boosts is questionable in patients with completely debulked tumors.

TREATMENT OF ADVANCED DISEASE

Surgery

Typically, surgeons operating on patients with ovarian cancer find obvious evidence of widespread metastatic disease. Ascites is often present, with diffuse peritoneal tumor studding and extensive omental involvement. In such cases, it is still important to document the surgical stage (usually a substage of stage III) and carefully evaluate and describe the extent and location of tumor identified at both the beginning and conclusion of surgery.

Optimal cytoreduction The primary function of surgery in patients with advanced ovarian cancer is cytoreduction or debulking. When surgery is performed by experienced gynecologic cancer surgeons, at least 50% of patients with stage III ovarian cancer can be left with "optimal" residual tumor (ie, < 1 cm). The morbidity associated with such surgery is low, and operative mortality is rare.

Several benefits accrue to patients who can be left with optimal residual disease. These patients have an increased likelihood of achieving a complete clinical response to chemotherapy, and among those who achieve a complete response and have a second-look operation, a greater proportion will have no tumor detectable. In addition, the risk of relapse after negative second-look surgery is reduced in patients left with small-volume residual disease at the conclusion of their primary operation. Disease progression-free interval, median survival, and long-term survival are all improved in patients who have optimal cytoreduction.

Even among patients with suboptimal residual disease (> 1 cm) after primary surgery, those left with smaller tumor volumes (1–2 cm) have a survival advantage over those with a larger residuum. It is thus clear that aggressive surgical cytoreduction, if successful in reducing tumor to small volumes, improves several measures of outcome.

Interval cytoreduction In an EORTC trial, 299 patients with suboptimal advanced ovarian cancer were randomized to receive 6 cycles of cisplatin plus cyclophosphamide with or without interval surgical cytoreduction after the third cycle. Median survival for patients who underwent interval debulking surgery was 27 months, vs 19 months for patients who did not have interval debulking ($P = .01$). The GOG has recently completed a randomized trial of interval cytoreduction using a cisplatin-paclitaxel chemotherapy regimen. These results show no benefit for interval cytoreduction (median overall survival, 32 vs 33 months). The use of taxane-based chemotherapy and more standardized aggressive initial debulking by experienced gynecologic oncologists in the GOG trial have been offered as possible explanations for the discordant outcomes.

Chemotherapy

Primary treatment The results of two randomized trials support a survival advantage for patients treated with combinations of IV platinum and paclitaxel, as compared with those given a platinum plus cyclophosphamide. McGuire et al found a 37- vs 24-month median survival advantage for the platinum-paclitaxel arm. Similarly, an analysis of the intergroup trial by Piccart et al showed an improvement in median survival from 25 to 35 months ($P = .001$) in favor of the paclitaxel arm. In contrast, the initial analysis of the ICON 3 trial evaluating a control arm (carboplatin or CAP [cyclophosphamide, Adriamycin (doxorubicin), Platinol (carboplatin)] chemotherapy) vs paclitaxel and carboplatin has failed to show a survival advantage for the taxane-containing arm. Many factors in the study have been proposed to explain this difference, and for the present, taxane- and platinum-based therapy remains the standard.

A randomized trial (GOG 158) comparing paclitaxel (175 mg/m^2 via a 3-hour infusion) plus carboplatin (dosed to achieve an area under the curve [AUC] of 7.5) vs the standard regimen of paclitaxel (135 mg/m^2 via a 24-hour infusion) plus cisplatin (75 mg/m^2) in patients with optimally debulked disease showed the shorter schedule with carboplatin to be as effective as the older regimen. Due to its decreased toxicity and ease of administration, the shorter schedule with carboplatin is the preferred treatment.

In addition, preliminary results from the SCOTROC (Scottish Randomized Trial in Ovarian Cancer) suggested that, as primary treatment, docetaxel (Taxotere) and paclitaxel have similar efficacy when combined with carboplatin and that docetaxel produces less neuropathy.

A five-arm international randomized study of primary therapy for patients with stage III or IV disease has completed accrual, with results pending. This study

TABLE 3: Chemotherapy regimens for ovarian carcinoma

Drug/combination	Dose and schedule
Paclitaxel/carboplatin	
Paclitaxel	175 mg/m^2 IV infused over 3 hours on day 1
Carboplatin	Dose calculated by the Calvert formula to an AUC between 5.0 and 7.5 mg/mL/min IV infused over 30 minutes Carboplatin is given after paclitaxel
Repeat cycle every 21 days for six courses.	
PREMEDICATIONS: Dexamethasone, 20 mg PO, 12 and 6 hours prior to paclitaxel; as well as diphenhydramine, 50 mg IV, and ranitidine, 50 mg IV, both 30–60 minutes prior to paclitaxel.	
Coleman RL, Bagnell KG, Townley PM: Cancer J Sci Am 3:246–253, 1997.	
Single-agent topotecan[a] (refractory or recurrent disease)	
Topotecan	1.5 mg/m^2 IV over 30 minutes daily for 5 days
Repeat cycle every 21 days.	
Iva B, Ondrej B, Milan B, et al: Proc Am Soc Clin Oncol 19:1570a, 2000.	
Single-agent liposomal doxorubicin[a] (refractory or recurrent disease)	
Liposomal doxorubicin	50 mg/m^2 IV on day 1 at an initial rate of 1 mg/min and if tolerated complete administration over 1 hour
Repeat cycle every 4 weeks.	

[a]**NOTE:** Clinical experience is accumulating to suggest that liposomal doxorubicin (at doses of 40 mg/m^2 q 4 weeks) and topotecan (at 1.0 mg/m^2/d × 5 days or 4 mg/m^2/wk) are equally efficacious and better tolerated than these agents at initial phase II doses. Definitive trials are ongoing.
AUC = area under the curve

Muggia FM, Hainsworth JD, Jeffers S, et al: J Clin Oncol 15:987–993, 1997.

Table prepared by Ishmael Jaiyesimi, DO

will determine the optimal primary chemotherapy regimen among currently available standard agents (Table 3). It uses carboplatin and paclitaxel as the control arm and evaluates two triplets (carboplatin + paclitaxel with either gemcitabine [Gemzar] or liposomal doxorubicin [Doxil]) and two sequential doublets (topotecan [Hycamtin]/carboplatin + carboplatin/paclitaxel or carboplatin/gemcitabine + carboplatin/paclitaxel).

Intraperitoneal chemotherapy

A randomized, phase III study conducted by the Southwest Oncology Group (SWOG), Eastern Cooperative Oncology Group (ECOG), and GOG compared IV cisplatin (75 mg/m^2) and paclitaxel (135 mg/m^2 over 24 hours) with IV carboplatin (dosed to an AUC of 9) followed by IV paclitaxel (135 mg/m^2 over 24 hours) and intraperitoneal (IP) cisplatin (100 mg/m^2) in patients with optimally debulked disease. Results indicated superior recurrence-free survival in the patients treated with IP cisplatin (27.6 vs 22.5 months; $P = .020$), as well as an improvement in overall survival duration that was of borderline statistical significance (52.9 vs 47.6 months; $P = .056$). This trial is criticized because of the asymmetry of the experimental arms.

A more recent phase III study in patients with optimally debulked disease compared IV paclitaxel plus IV cisplatin as the standard treatment arm with IV paclitaxel (135 mg/m^2 over 24 hours [D1]), IP cisplatin (100 mg/m^2 [D2]), and IP paclitaxel (60 mg/m^2 [D8]). This study showed a progression-free (18.3 vs 23.8 months; $P = .05$) and median overall survival (49.7 vs 65.6 months; $P = .03$) advantage in favor of IP therapy. These results position IP treatment as the standard of care in selected women with optimally debulked stage III ovarian cancer. Grade 3-4 pain, fatigue, as well as hematologic, gastrointestinal, metabolic, and neurologic toxic effects were more common in the IP vs IV group ($P \leq .001$). Efforts at reducing toxicity, such as lowering IP cisplatin to 75 mg/m^2, are being investigated.

Consolidation therapy

Given the chemosensitive nature of ovarian cancer yet frequent relapse rate, many investigators are exploring consolidation strategies following primary surgery and chemotherapy. A phase III randomized trial of 12 vs 3 months of maintenance paclitaxel in patients who had achieved a clinically defined complete response to primary therapy showed a median disease progression-free interval of 28 vs 21 months in favor of the longer regimen ($P = .0023$). The trial met early stopping rules based on the disease progression-free survival difference, and thus the implications of this strategy with regard to overall survival are currently unknown. Enrollment into investigational consolidation studies remains a priority to advance the treatment of patients with ovarian cancer.

Recurrent disease Patients who respond to primary chemotherapy with paclitaxel and platinum agents and who relapse ≥ 6 months after the completion of treatment often have additional responses when retreated with the same agents. Response rates to repeat treatment with carboplatin are ~30% in those patients who relapse 12 months after primary therapy and 57% if the relapses occur > 24 months after primary therapy. In addition, a plethora of new agents have demonstrated modest phase II activity in patients with refractory disease.

Topotecan has received FDA (US Food and Drug Administration) approval for the treatment of patients with refractory disease (Table 3). An oral preparation is in phase III trials.

An open, randomized study compared topotecan (1.5 mg/m^2/d for 5 days) with paclitaxel (175 mg/m^2 q21d) in 226 women whose ovarian cancer had recurred after first-line platinum therapy. There were no statistically significant differences between the treatment groups with respect to response rate (20.5% vs 14.0%), response duration (25.9 vs 21.6 weeks), or median survival (63 vs 53 weeks).

Topotecan has efficacy comparable to that of paclitaxel in this setting and is being evaluated in combination with platinum and other agents.

Liposomal doxorubicin also has received FDA approval for the treatment of patients with metastatic platinum- and paclitaxel-refractory disease (Table 3). A randomized trial by Gordon et al compared liposomal doxorubicin with topotecan in this setting; similar response rates, time to disease progression, and overall survival (60.0 vs 56.7 weeks) were seen with these two agents.

Other agents Phase II trials have demonstrated the activity of other agents in patients with recurrent ovarian cancer. They include gemcitabine, vinorelbine, oral altretamine (Hexalen), and oral etoposide. In general, these agents have similar response rates, ranging from 10%–15% in patients with platinum-resistant disease and 30% in patients with platinum-sensitive disease, with a median duration of response ranging from 4 to 8+ months.

A recent randomized ICON 4/AGO-OVAR 2.2 study addressed the issue of using single-agent carboplatin vs paclitaxel with carboplatin for patients with platinum-sensitive recurrent disease (defined generally as patients relapsing more than 6 months from prior platinum therapy). Both disease progression-free (hazard ratio 0.76, 0.66–0.80; $P = .0004$) and 1-year overall survival (50% vs 40%) favored combination therapy. An AGO study evaluating carboplatin vs carboplatin with gemcitabine in a similar population was reported. This study likewise showed an improved response rate (47.2% vs 30.9%; $P = .0016$) and disease progression-free survival (8.6 months vs 5.8 months; $P = .0031$) favoring the combination. Other combinations such as topotecan or liposomal doxorubicin with carboplatin will also be investigated.

For many patients, ovarian cancer becomes a chronic disease characterized by a series of relapses followed by partial or complete remission. With the judicious selection and dosing of available agents to keep symptoms from disease and treatment to a minimum, a good quality of life can be maintained throughout much of the disease course.

High-dose chemotherapy

In a trial conducted largely in patients with platinum-resistant (66%) and bulky disease (61%), the median disease progression-free and overall survival intervals were short (7 and 13 months, respectively) in patients treated with high-dose chemotherapy and stem-cell support, suggesting no benefit. There is no role for high-dose chemotherapy in the standard management of patients with epithelial ovarian cancer.

Treatment recommendations and unresolved issues

For advanced ovarian cancer, current frontline management should incorporate a taxane with platinum-based therapy. Results also support the use of a taxane and platinum-based therapy in patients with high-risk early-stage disease.

Issues that are evolving include (1) the increasing evidence to support the role of intraperitoneal therapy in primary treatment; (2) the role of maintenance or consolidation treatment with standard chemotherapy or with novel agents following primary therapy; and (3) the optimal use of platinum vs nonplatinum agents, and whether used as single agents or in combination, for patients with recurrent disease.

Radiation therapy as a single modality

In a 1975 study from M. D. Anderson Hospital, 5-year survival rates with WAI and chemotherapy were similar, although toxicity and cost seemed to be lower with oral melphalan (Alkeran) than radiation therapy. A subsequent trial from Toronto randomized patients with advanced disease to receive either pelvic radiotherapy plus chlorambucil (Leukeran) or WAI. Although surgical staging and chemotherapy were less aggressive than current protocols, the survival advantage and altered failure patterns seen with the Canadian WAI regimen were provocative.

No prospective randomized trial has compared WAI, performed with modern techniques and equipment, with a modern chemotherapy regimen. However, published series document treatment outcomes with WAI that are at least comparable, if not superior, to outcomes with platinum-based chemotherapy regimens. The comparability of WAI to chemotherapy regimens including paclitaxel also is unknown.

Large-volume disease The ability of WAI to sterilize macroscopic deposits of ovarian carcinoma is limited. Patients with any site of residual disease > 1 cm have compromised outcomes, no matter what therapy they receive. However, given the limited radiation tolerance of the abdominal organs, patients with larger volumes of disease are not candidates for WAI as sole adjuvant treatment.

Chemotherapy plus radiation therapy

It is possible to identify patients for whom chemotherapy or radiotherapy is unlikely to be curative because of unfavorable histologic subtype, grade, and amount of residual disease following surgical cytoreduction. Combined-modality therapy incorporating various combinations and sequences of chemotherapy and radiation therapy has been studied in these patients.

Chemotherapy plus WAI Sequential combined-modality therapy (CMT) employing chemotherapy and irradiation has been shown to be feasible. There are a number of important differences between sequential CMT and salvage irradiation: (1) Planned sequential CMT permits the omission of second-look surgery in selected patients, possibly limiting late toxicity. (2) Clinical studies of CMT have often incorporated a reduction in the duration of chemotherapy, providing improved tolerance to radiation therapy; this approach permits appropriate radiation doses to be given and potentially limits the emergence of platinum-radiation therapy cross-resistance. (3) With CMT, many patients will have no demonstrable disease but are at high risk of recurrence, whereas with salvage WAI, all patients have clinical or pathologic evidence of disease.

In a European study, 64 of 94 patients with stages IC–IV disease who had undergone "radical" surgery and had no evidence of gross residual disease after 6 courses of chemotherapy (carboplatin, epirubicin [Ellence], and prednimustine [Sterecyt]) were randomized to receive either consolidation WAI (30 Gy), followed by a boost to the para-aortic region and pelvis (12.0 and 21.6 Gy, respectively), or no further therapy. Relapse-free survival rates were significantly higher in patients who received adjuvant chemoradiation therapy than in those who received adjuvant chemotherapy only (2- and 5-year relapse-free survival rates, 68% vs 56% and 49% vs 26%, respectively); the same was true of overall survival rates (2- and 5-year overall survival rates, 87% vs 61% and 59% vs 33%, respectively). The differences between the two treatment groups were more pronounced in patients with stage III disease (2- and 5-year relapse-free survival rates, 77% vs 54% and 45% vs 19%, respectively; 2- and 5-year overall survival rates, 88% vs 58% and 59% vs 26%, respectively).

Einhorn et al, from the Karolinska Hospital in Stockholm, treated 75 patients with stages IIB–IV ovarian carcinoma with combined surgery, chemotherapy, and WAI to 40 Gy, utilizing a "six-field" approach. Outcomes were compared with those of 98 patients treated in subsequent years with only surgery and chemotherapy. After different prognostic factors were controlled statistically, it was found that patients who received WAI had a significantly better survival rate than those who did not. The authors suggest that, given the results of this and other studies combined with the limited success of modern combination chemotherapy regimens, the role of abdominal radiation therapy should be further investigated in a prospective fashion.

Salvage and palliative radiotherapy after chemotherapy

Patients in whom microscopic disease is detected at surgical reassessment have been reported to have median overall and progression-free survival times of 27 and 19 months, respectively. Unfortunately, residual or recurrent disease following first-line chemotherapy is frequent, and salvage rates are dismal.

Patients with residual tumor detected at a planned surgical reassessment have a spectrum of disease, ranging from isolated positive cytology and/or microscopic serosal involvement to gross residual disease. In contrast, relapsing patients generally present with abdominal symptoms from advanced larger volume recurrences. The latter clinical situation is not particularly amenable to salvage radiotherapy. However, in the setting of small-volume residual disease detected immediately following chemotherapy, two radiotherapy approaches, external-beam irradiation and intraperitoneal radioisotopes, have been used with variable success. Most likely, this variability is related to significant differences in prognostic factors among treated patients. Unfortunately, there are only limited data that can be used to define subgroups that may or may not benefit from salvage WAI. Given the number of possible prognostic variables (Table 4), a clear consensus on this issue is unlikely to be reached.

Chemotherapy-refractory disease Favorable experiences with salvage radiation therapy in chemotherapy-refractory ovarian carcinomas continue to be reported. Sedlacek et al described 27 patients who had not responded to aggressive cytoreductive surgery followed by multiple-drug platinum-based chemotherapy and who received WAI (30–35 Gy at 100–150 cGy/fraction, with a pelvic boost to a total dose of 45 Gy). The 5-year survival rate was 15%. The extent of residual disease at the initiation of radiation therapy strongly correlated with the length of survival.

Baker et al analyzed the efficacy of salvage WAI in 47 patients with ovarian cancer who had not responded to one or more chemotherapy regimens. Actu-

TABLE 4: Possible prognostic factors for salvage radiation therapy following chemotherapy

Residual tumor before WAI	Lymph node status
Location of residual disease	Chemotherapy duration
Initial FIGO stage	Type of prior chemotherapy
Histologic grade	Completion of WAI
Disease bulk at diagnosis	Response to chemotherapy
Patient age	Histologic type
Disease-free interval from initial treatment to relapse	CA-125 level
	CA-125 level trend
Performance status	Parameters of WAI
Number of sites of residual disease	Interval debulking/second-look surgery

FIGO = International Federation of Gynecology and Obstetrics; WAI = whole-abdominal irradiation

arial 4-year survival and disease-free survival rates were 48% and 37%, respectively, in patients with microscopic residual disease, vs 11% and 5%, respectively, in patients with macroscopic residual disease. In addition, patients with disease limited to the pelvis after laparotomy (including gross disease) had a 4-year actuarial survival rate of 60% and disease-free survival rate of 54%, as compared with 16% and 4%, respectively, in patients with upper abdominal involvement.

This finding was confirmed by Firat and Erickson, who described their experience with selective radiotherapy in 28 patients with recurrent or persistent disease involving the vagina and/or rectum. Pelvic radiotherapy was uniformly successful in palliating vaginal bleeding. Furthermore, there were eight long-term survivors (five with no evidence of disease), implying that pelvic radiotherapy alone can be effective salvage therapy, particularly when there is no extrapelvic disease.

Fujiwara and colleagues reported high rates of objective and symptomatic responses using local radiotherapy in 20 patients (42 evaluable lesions) with recurrent ovarian cancer following chemotherapy. Lymph node metastases appeared to be particularly responsive.

Tinger et al reported an overall response rate of 73% in 80 patients with advanced and recurrent disease treated with palliative intent. Responses were maintained until death in all but 10 patients. Toxicity was limited, and there was no grade 4 toxicity. It was suggested that response rate, survival, and toxicity with palliative radiotherapy compared favorably with those of second- and third-line chemotherapy.

Based on these and other studies, certain treatment guidelines can be suggested:

- Patients with any site of residual disease > 0.5 cm will fare poorly with salvage WAI. However, salvage WAI can be considered in selected patients with microscopic residual disease following first-line chemotherapy.

- Irradiation-related morbidity can be minimized by limiting the abdominal dose to 25 Gy and abandoning WAI in patients who require treatment breaks of more than 1–2 weeks. In fact, randomized clinical trial data from Fyles et al show no benefit from WAI doses > 22.5 Gy.
- Patients with limited gross residual disease confined to the pelvis may constitute a prognostically favorable group in whom pelvic boosts or pelvic radiation therapy alone may be warranted.
- Localized radiation therapy to areas of symptomatic (and, in some cases, asymptomatic) recurrent disease is associated with high rates of durable responses with limited toxicity. In some cases, extended survival is possible.

The relative merits of salvage WAI compared with other treatments, such as intraperitoneal chemotherapy, second-line chemotherapy, and high-dose chemotherapy/bone marrow transplantation, can only be determined in a prospective, randomized, controlled trial.

SUGGESTED READING

Anderson GL, Judd HL, Kaunitz AM, et al: Effects of estrogen plus progestin on gynecologic cancers and associated diagnostic procedures: The Women's Health Initiative randomized trial. JAMA 290:1739–1748, 2003.

Armstrong DK, Bundy BN, Baergen R, et al: Randomized phase III study of IV paclitaxel and cisplatin vs IV paclitaxel, intraperitoneal (IP) cisplatin, and IP paclitaxel in optimal stage III epithelial ovarian cancer: A Gynecologic Oncology Group trial (GOG) 172 (abstract). Proc Am Soc Clin Oncol 21:201a, 2002.

Armstrong DK, Bundy B, Wenzel L, et al: Intraperitoneal cisplatin and paclitaxel in ovarian cancer. N Engl J Med 354:34-43, 2006.

Buys SS, Partridge E, Greene MH, et al: Ovarian cancer screening in the Prostate, Lung, Colorectal and Ovarian (PLCO) cancer screening trial: Findings from the initial screen of a randomized trial. Am J Obstet Gynecol 193:1630-1639, 2005.

Cardenes H, Randall ME: Integrating radiation therapy in the curative management of ovarian cancer: Current issues and future directions. Semin Radiat Oncol 10:61–70, 2000.

Eisen A, Rebbeck TR, Wood WC, et al: Prophylactic surgery in women with a hereditary predisposition to breast and ovarian cancer. J Clin Oncol 18:1980–1995, 2000.

Firat S, Erickson B: Selective irradiation for the treatment of recurrent ovarian carcinoma involving the vagina or rectum. Gynecol Oncol 80:213–220, 2001.

Fujiwara K, Suzuki S, Yoden E, et al: Local radiation therapy for localized, relapsed, or refractory ovarian cancer patients with or without symptoms after chemotherapy. Int J Gynecol Cancer 12:250–256, 2002.

Goff BA, Mandel LS, Melancon CH, et al: Frequency of symptoms of ovarian cancer in women presenting to primary care clinics. JAMA 291:2705–2712, 2004.

Gordon AN, Fleagle JT, Guthrie D, et al: Recurrent epithelial ovarian carcinoma: A randomized phase III study of pegylated liposomal doxorubicin versus topotecan. J Clin Oncol 19:3312–3322, 2001.

Hepp R, Baeza R, Olfos P, et al: Adjuvant whole abdominal radiotherapy in epithelial cancer of the ovary. Int J Radiat Oncol Biol Phys 53:360–365, 2002.

International Collaborative on Ovarian Neoplasm (ICON) Group: Paclitaxel plus carboplatin versus standard chemotherapy with either single agent carboplatin or cyclophosphamide, doxorubicin, and cisplatin in women with ovarian cancer: The ICON 3 randomized trial. Lancet 360:505–515, 2002.

ICON and AGO collaborators: Paclitaxel plus platinum based chemotherapy versus conventional platinum based chemotherapy in women with relapsed ovarian cancer: The ICON 4/AGO-OVAR 2.2 trial. Lancet 361:2099–2106, 2003.

ICON and EORTC-ACTION investigators: International Collaborative on Ovarian Neoplasm Trial 1 and Adjuvant Treatment in Ovarian Neoplasm Trial: Two parallel randomized phase III trials of adjuvant chemotherapy in patients with early stage ovarian cancer. J Natl Cancer Inst 95:105–112, 2003.

Kauff ND, Satagopan JM, Robson ME, et al: Risk-reducing salpingo-oophorectomy in women with BRCA1 or BRCA2 mutation. N Engl J Med 346:1609–1615, 2002.

Markman M, Liu PY, Wilczynski S, et al: Phase III randomized trial of 12 versus 3 months of maintenance paclitaxel in patients with advanced ovarian cancer after complete response to platinum and paclitaxel based chemotherapy: A Southwest Oncology Group and Gynecologic Oncology Group Trial. J Clin Oncol 21:2460–2465, 2003.

McGuire WP, Hoskins WJ, Brady MF, et al: Taxol and cisplatin improves outcome in patients with advanced ovarian cancer as compared to Cytoxan/cisplatin. N Engl J Med 334:1–6, 1996.

Ozols RF, Bundy BN, Greer E, et al: Phase III trials of carboplatin and paclitaxel compared with cisplatin and paclitaxel in patients with optimally resected stage III ovarian cancer: A Gynecologic Oncology Group Study. J Clin Oncol 21:3194–3200, 2003.

Pfisterer J, Plante M, Vergote I, et al: Gemcitabine/carboplatin (GC) vs carboplatin (C) in platinum-sensitive recurrent ovarian cancer (OVCA): Results of a Gynecologic Cancer Intergroup randomized phase III trial of the AGO OVAR, the NCIC CTG, and the EORTC GCG (abstract). Proc Am Soc Clin Oncol 23:449, 2004.

Piccart M, Bertelsen K, James K, et al: Randomized intergroup trial of cisplatin-paclitaxel versus cisplatin-cyclophosphamide in women with advanced epithelial ovarian cancer: Three-year results. J Natl Cancer Inst 92:699–708, 2000.

Randall TC, Rubin SC: Cytoreductive surgery for ovarian cancer. Surg Clin North Am 81:871–883, 2001.

Rose PG, Nerenstone S, Brady MF, et al: Secondary surgical cytoreduction for advanced ovarian carcinoma. N Engl J Med 351:2489–2497, 2004.

Suzuki M, Ohwara M, Sekiguchi I, et al: Radical cytoreductive surgery combined with platinums: Carboplatin and cisplatin chemotherapy for advanced ovarian cancer. Int J Gynaecol Cancer 9:54–60, 1999.

Tinger A, Waldron T, Peluso N, et al: Effective palliative radiation therapy in advanced and recurrent ovarian carcinoma. Int J Radiat Oncol Biol Phys 51:1256–1263, 2001.

Vasey PA, Jayson GC, Gordon A, et al; Scottish Gynaecological Cancer Trials Group: Phase III randomized trial of docetaxel-carboplatin versus paclitaxel-carboplatin as first-line chemotherapy for ovarian cancer. J Natl Cancer Inst 96:1682–1-691, 2004.

Vergote I, deWever I, Tjalma W, et al: Interval debulking surgery: An alternative for primary surgical debulking? Semin Surg Oncol 19:49–53, 2000.

Wong R, Milosevic M, Sturgeon J, et al: Treatment of early epithelial ovarian cancer with chemotherapy and abdominopelvic radiotherapy: Results of a prospective treatment protocol. Int J Radiat Oncol Biol Phys 45:657–665, 1999.

Writing Group for the Women's Health Initiative Investigators: Risks and benefits of estrogen plus progestin in healthy postmenopausal women: Principal results from the Women's Health Initiative randomized controlled trial. JAMA 288:321–333, 2002.

CHAPTER 23

Melanoma and other skin cancers

Eric H. Jensen, MD, Kim A. Margolin, MD, and Vernon K. Sondak, MD

Each year, more than 1 million people are diagnosed with skin cancer. The incidence of all other cancers combined is 1.3 million per year, meaning that skin cancer accounts for nearly 50% of all newly diagnosed cancers.

Melanoma represents approximately 4% of all skin cancers but is responsible for nearly three times the number of deaths as nonmelanoma skin cancers (approximately 7,910 vs 2,800). The incidence of melanoma has increased steadily since 1930 and continues to rise at a rate that has exceeded all other cancer types. Melanoma is now the fifth most common cancer in men and the sixth most common cancer in women.

SKIN

Advances in public awareness, surgical techniques, and adjuvant therapy have improved outcomes for patients with melanoma; however, it remains a highly morbid disease. Because of the relatively young age of onset, the toll of melanoma in terms of "life-years lost" is second only to leukemia among all malignancies in the United States

Epidemiology

Age Melanoma affects a broad range of age groups, including patients in their 20s and 30s, and even younger, with an average age of development of 55 years. Three-quarters of all cases will occur in individuals younger than 70 years of age. Age has been considered by some to be an independent predictor of long-term outcome, with decreasing survival noted in those patients diagnosed over 65 years of age. Paradoxically, emerging data suggest that younger patients are more likely to have involvement of regional lymph nodes with early-stage tumors.

Gender Men are slightly more likely to develop melanoma than women (1.2:1.0). Moreover, when compared stage for stage, men have a slightly worse prognosis than women. The most common site affected in men is the trunk, whereas the extremities are most affected in women. In the 25- to 29-year-old female population, melanoma is now the most common malignancy; it is surpassed only by breast cancer in the 30- to 35-year-old range.

Location Many studies have demonstrated that melanomas located on the head/neck, trunk, or back carry a worse prognosis than those on the extremities. It remains unclear whether that is due to delayed diagnosis of melanomas in more difficult to visualize sites or to an inherently poorer prognosis of melanomas in those sites. On the extremities, acral lentiginous and subungual melanomas carry a poor prognosis, with notably high local recurrence rates. In a small percentage of patients (< 10%), melanoma may arise in noncutaneous locations, including the pigmented cells of the retina and the mucous membranes of the oropharynx, vulva, and anal canal. These primary sites frequently go unnoticed until disseminated disease is present.

Geography Melanoma is most common in parts of the world where fair-skinned whites live in a sunny climate near the equator. Thus, Australia and Israel have among the highest melanoma incidences in the world (approximately 40 per 100,000 individuals per year). Whites in Hawaii and the southwestern United States also have a high incidence of melanoma, about 20–30 cases per 100,000 individuals annually, which equals or exceeds the incidence of colorectal cancer in those regions. The incidence of melanoma in the United States decreases with increasing latitude (ie, more northerly regions); overall, about 12 cases of melanoma are seen per 100,000 American whites.

Race Skin cancer is uncommon in African-American individuals, with an annual age-adjusted incidence of only 0.9% of that of whites. Asian and Hispanic individuals are similarly at low risk. It is important to recognize, however, that melanoma and other skin cancers do occur in these groups, and suspicious lesions should be appropriately evaluated.

The presentation of skin cancer may differ in African-Americans as well. For example, most melanomas in these patients occur in the less-pigmented skin of the palms and soles. Also, although basal cell carcinomas are rarely pigmented in fair-skinned individuals, they are almost always pigmented in blacks. Finally, the most common sites of squamous cell cancer in whites are the sun-exposed areas of the head/neck and arms, whereas less-exposed areas such as the legs are more common sites of origin in African-American patients.

Survival If detected at an early stage, most cutaneous melanomas and virtually all nonmelanoma skin cancers can be cured with surgical excision. The prognosis for patients with lymphatic dissemination decreases significantly, and few patients who develop metastatic disease will survive beyond 5 years.

Etiology and risk factors

All cancers arise through an interaction between environmental and genetic factors. The complex balance of these factors determines the likelihood of cancer development. It has been long recognized that there are environmental factors (most notably ultraviolet [UV] light exposure) that increase the risk of melanoma. Familial patterns of inheritance of dysplastic nevi and melanoma (variously called the B-K mole syndrome, dysplastic nevus syndrome, or familial atypical multiple mole and melanoma syndrome) were recognized in the 1970s. Recently, there has also been significant progress in identifying genetic factors that lead to a predisposition for the development of this disease.

Genetic predisposition Multiple genes have been implicated in the development and progression of melanoma. *CDKN2A* and *CDK4* are susceptibility genes located on chromosomes 9p21 and 12q14, which code for protein p16^{ink4A} (inhibitor of cyclin-dependent kinase 4A) and p14^{ARF} (alternate reading frame of the gene, *CDKN2A*), and cyclin-dependent kinase 4, respectively. Through their interactions with p53, Rb, and cyclins/cyclin-dependent kinases, the products of these genes are essential in the control of the cell cycle, and mutations with loss of function may be associated with melanomagenesis. The gene *p16* in particular plays a vital inhibitory role in maintaining cells at the G1/S interface through interactions with cyclin-dependent kinases 4 and 6, which control phosphorylation of the retinoblastoma family of proteins. With uninhibited phosphorylation of RB-1 protein, transcription factor E2F-1 is released, inducing S-phase genes. Therefore, mutations in *CDK* genes produce conditions of uninhibited progression of the cell cycle.

Although *CDKN2A* has been implicated in the development of melanoma, there are clearly multiple other factors involved, including intermittent UV light exposure. Germline mutations in *CDKN2A* have been identified in 40% of familial melanoma pedigrees. Additionally, the penetrance of these mutations has been shown to be highly dependent on geographic locations. Comparison of European, American, and Australian pedigrees reveals mutation penetrance by age 80 of 0.57, 0.7, and 0.91, respectively, indicating the importance of environmental factors in addition to genetic predisposition. Variants in the melanocortin-1 receptor gene may contribute to this environmental influence.

It has also been noted that 60% or more of melanoma cases contain a mutation in the B-*raf* gene, encoding a serine/threonine kinase involved in the mitogen-activated protein kinase (MAPK) pathway. A single transversion (T1799A) in exon 15 results in a missense mutation (V600E), which accounts for ≥ 85% of B-*raf* mutations. Similarly, the Ras family of genes (N-*ras* in particular) is being investigated for its role in melanomagenesis. The Raf and Ras kinase families act as mediators of intracellular signaling with particular importance in the regulation of cell growth.

The observation that B-*raf*–activating mutations can be found in a significant percentage of benign nevi as well as melanoma cell lines had initially led to the belief that these mutations were likely involved in the initiation of malignancy. More recently, it has been shown that only 10% of radial growth phase melanomas contain mutations, compared with 75% of vertical growth phase melanomas. This finding would indicate that B-*raf* may be more important as a determinant of malignant potential rather than an initiator of malignancy but also highlights the fact that much remains to be learned about the key events in the process of melanoma development.

UV light Melanoma and nonmelanoma skin cancers share a common causative factor—exposure to UV radiation in sunlight—although the precise mechanism of causation and the types of exposure most likely to cause each disease may vary. Most dangerous is UV-B radiation (wavelength, 290–320 nm), but UV-A radiation (320–400 nm) probably also has carcinogenic potential. Overall, skin cancer incidence rates are increasing, likely both because people spend more time in the sunlight and because the atmosphere's ability to screen out UV radiation has decreased (depletion of the ozone layer).

Chronic vs intermittent exposure Different types of skin cancer are associated with different patterns of sun exposure. Almost all basal cell and squamous cell cancers of the skin occur on chronically exposed areas of skin, such as the head, neck, and hands. There is a clear-cut association between cumulative sun exposure and the incidence of these nonmelanoma skin cancers.

On the other hand, exposure to intermittent solar radiation appears to be more important in most cases of melanoma. A number of studies have implicated sun exposure during childhood—particularly blistering sunburns—as a major risk factor. Melanoma is more common in indoor workers than outdoor laborers and occurs most often on parts of the body that are only occasionally exposed to the sun. The one exception to this principle is lentigo maligna melanoma, which occurs most frequently on the head and neck of older individuals with a long history of chronic sun exposure and evidence of actinic skin damage, as is the case for nonmelanoma skin cancer. Melanoma is rare on skin surfaces that are never exposed to the sun (the "bathing suit" or doubly covered areas).

Skin type and hair color Not everyone is at equal risk of developing skin cancer. As previously discussed, blacks are at lower risk than whites. Among whites, melanoma occurs most frequently in fair-skinned, light-haired individuals who sunburn easily and rarely or never tan.

Typical moles Typical or benign moles, also called melanocytic nevi, are small (< 6 mm), round, uniformly tan or brown, and symmetrical. They are generally raised above the skin surface, as opposed to freckles. Patients with many (> 25–50) melanocytic nevi are at increased risk of melanoma; most of these patients are also fair-skinned, light-haired individuals who burn easily and rarely tan.

Atypical moles, also called clinically atypical nevi or dysplastic nevi, are larger (generally > 6 mm), irregularly shaped, and have a pebbly surface. They are usually tan or brown but may have various shades of coloration within them.

At least 5% of the white population of the United States has at least one clinically atypical nevus. Otherwise healthy individuals with at least one clinically atypical nevus have a 6% lifetime risk of developing melanoma. This risk rises to as high as 80% in individuals who also have a family history of melanoma.

Some clinically atypical nevi eventually progress to melanoma. Even if every atypical mole is surgically removed, however, the patient remains at an increased risk of melanoma developing in the rest of the normal skin. Until such time, if ever, that genetic testing identifies those individuals with atypical moles who are at greatest risk of melanoma development, all individuals with clinically atypical

> Epidemiologic data demonstrate a difference in the association of sun exposure or dysplastic nevus with melanomas in different primary sites. Thus, primary melanoma of the head and neck origin, particularly lentigo maligna melanoma, is more closely correlated with chronic sun exposure, whereas superficial spreading or nodular melanoma of the trunk is more closely correlated with a large number of nevi *(Whiteman DC, Watt P, Purdie DM, et al: J Natl Cancer Inst 95:806-812, 2003).*

nevi should be carefully followed. Close follow-up is particularly important in those with a family history of melanoma.

Actinic keratoses are scaly, rough, erythematous patches that occur in chronically sun-exposed areas; they are both markers for and precursors to nonmelanoma skin cancer development. These lesions may progress to squamous cell cancers or, in some cases, regress spontaneously in response to prolonged avoidance of sun exposure. If few in number, actinic keratoses can be removed or destroyed with liquid nitrogen. For multiple lesions, topical fluorouracil (5-FU) and more recently imiquimod cream (Aldara) have been used successfully.

Burns Squamous cell cancers occasionally arise in burns or other scars. Burn scar cancers (so-called Marjolin's ulcers) may have a more aggressive clinical course than the usual nonmelanoma skin cancer.

Giant congenital nevi Congenital nevi are pigmented lesions actually present at birth, as opposed to developing months or years later. Even among known congenital nevi, however, only the giant (> 20 cm in diameter) congenital nevus, a rare lesion, is a documented precursor to melanoma. Most melanomas occurring in children younger than 10 years of age arise within these lesions. Whenever the cosmetic result permits, giant congenital nevi should be excised in early childhood. If complete excision is impossible, even with staged procedures, close follow-up is indicated.

Xeroderma pigmentosum, a rare congenital disorder in which patients lack the capacity to repair UV-induced DNA damage, is associated with the development of innumerable melanoma and nonmelanoma skin cancers at an early age.

Immunosuppression or prior hematologic malignancy Nonmelanoma skin cancers and to a much lesser degree melanomas are more common in patients who are immunosuppressed or have had previous hematologic malignancies. Furthermore, the aggressiveness of the skin tumors can be significantly greater in these patients.

Diagnosis

Although the vast majority of skin cancers are curable, a substantial number of skin cancer-related deaths occur each year. Since these cancers are visible on the skin, early detection should be the goal in every case.

Early diagnosis of melanoma

Differentiation from benign moles Early melanomas may be differentiated from benign moles by assessing the asymmetry, border irregularity, color, and diameter of the lesions (the so-called ABCDs; Table 1). Other signs of melanoma include itching, bleeding, ulceration, or changes in a preexisting benign mole.

Clinically atypical nevi have some, but not all, of the features of melanoma: They are > 6 mm, asymmetrical, and often show border irregularity. Significantly raised areas or regions of dark brown or black pigmentation in a known atypical nevus suggest the development of melanoma. Biopsy of any suspi-

TABLE 1: The 'ABCDs' for differentiating early melanomas from benign melanocytic nevi

Feature	Benign mole	Melanoma
Asymmetry	No	Yes
Border irregularity	No	Yes
Color	Uniform, tan/brown	Variegated, black
Diameter	< 6 mm	May be > 6 mm

cious skin lesion should be carried out (see section on "Biopsy techniques"). Patients with too many atypical nevi to excise require careful follow-up with frequent skin examinations.

Periodic total-body skin examinations combined with photographs of any atypical nevi and, most importantly, thorough patient education on the need to watch for changes in existing moles or the development of new lesions are essential components of the management of patients with atypical moles.

Differentiating nonmelanoma skin cancers

Nonmelanoma skin cancers usually are not confused with melanomas, since most (but not all) melanomas are pigmented and most (but not all) nonmelanoma skin cancers are not. Basal and squamous cell cancers may be more difficult to distinguish from one another, but certain features are more characteristic of one type than the other. Basal cell cancers often have a pearly, translucent appearance with a rolled border, whereas squamous cell cancers are often keratinized or ulcerated.

Actinic keratosis and squamous cell cancers likely represent a continuum of malignant progression. In general, actinic keratosis cancers are usually small (< 1 cm) and noted for their texture (the horn) rather than their appearance. Squamous cell cancers in situ are usually larger, bona fide plaques (Bowen's disease), with an appearance similar to plaques of psoriasis, for example. The clinical development of elevation/nodularity or induration heralds the presence of invasive disease because dermal extension produces lesion elevation.

Total-body skin examination

Total-body skin examination is a critical step in the initial evaluation and follow-up of a patient with a melanoma, nonmelanoma skin cancer, or clinically atypical nevus. Because of the common denominator of solar exposure in the causation of skin cancer, patients with one skin cancer are at significant risk of harboring or developing a second or even multiple skin cancers, often of a different histologic type. A complete skin examination is essential for patients with clinically atypical nevi, since they have an increased risk of developing melanoma on their entire skin surface, not just within recognized moles.

Fundamental to a thorough and complete skin examination is a well-lit room, a completely disrobed patient, and a relaxed and unhurried approach. Useful adjuncts in some cases include serial photography, both of individual lesions and whole skin areas, and special techniques of illumination and magnification, such as Wood's lamp ("black light") examination and epiluminescence microscopy (direct application of a magnifying lens to an area of the skin that has had oil applied to minimize reflectance), also called dermoscopy.

Examination of lymph nodes

Lymphatic spread is the most frequently encountered type of dissemination in both melanoma and nonmelanoma skin cancers. The regional lymph nodes should be carefully examined in all skin cancer patients at the time of presentation and at each follow-up visit. Since melanoma may also disseminate hematogenously to any lymph node basin in the body, all accessible node groups should be examined in melanoma patients.

Biopsy techniques

When the decision is made to biopsy a suspicious pigmented or nonpigmented skin lesion, several factors must be taken into consideration. Foremost among them is that the pathologist must receive adequate tissue in good condition to permit assessment of all relevant histologic features. Also critical is that the biopsy should not make subsequent surgical treatment more difficult.

Techniques to avoid Shallow shave biopsies, cryosurgery, or electrodesiccation do not allow for pathologic analysis of margins and depth of invasion and should be avoided.

Complete excision Most clinically suspicious skin lesions are best biopsied by complete excision using local anesthesia, taking a 1- to 2-mm margin of normal skin and including some subcutaneous fat.

Incisional or punch biopsy Unusually large lesions or those situated in cosmetically sensitive areas, such as the face, may be biopsied by incisional or punch biopsy. In these cases, the most abnormal area(s)—generally the most elevated portion(s) of the lesion—should be sampled.

Frozen-section analysis is not routinely employed for the diagnosis of skin lesions.

Biopsy of lymph nodes Palpably enlarged lymph nodes suspected of representing melanoma metastasis are best diagnosed using fine-needle aspiration (FNA). A positive aspiration cytology is grounds for performing a full lymph node dissection. If the cytology is nondiagnostic or negative, or if the node location precludes aspiration, an open biopsy is appropriate; only the enlarged node should be removed, with minimal dissection of the surrounding tissue. In this setting, frozen-section analysis may be employed and a full node dissection carried out during the same procedure.

Techniques for enhancing the detection of microscopic nodal metastases by applying more sensitive assay methods are under investigation. One such assay is the polymerase chain reaction (PCR) for the detection of mRNA sequences for tyrosinase, a protein that is specific for melanocytes. The prognostic and therapeutic implications of detecting micrometastases by these methods are under investigation in trials such as the Sunbelt Melanoma Trial.

Pathology

Histologic types of nonmelanoma skin cancer

Basal cell and squamous cell carcinomas The two most common types of nonmelanoma skin cancer are basal cell and squamous cell carcinomas. Bowen's disease is the name given to squamous cell carcinoma in situ involving the skin. Merkel's cell cancer is a rarer, more aggressive skin cancer, which presumably arises from the neuroendocrine cells of the skin. Wide excision is the primary treatment of Merkel's cell cancers, with radiation therapy frequently added to reduce local recurrence rates, although an additional survival benefit has never been shown.

Cancers arising in the skin appendages (eg, hair follicles, sweat glands) can be adenocarcinomas or apocrine cancers; they are exceedingly rare.

Sarcomas The most common primary sarcoma of the skin is dermatofibroma protuberans. Leiomyosarcoma, angiosarcoma, and malignant fibrous histiocytoma are much less common. Wide excision to negative margins is the standard of care for sarcomas of the skin. Adjuvant radiation therapy may be used to reduce local recurrence rates. Most cases of dermatofibroma protuberans are low grade and sensitive to imatinib (Gleevec) therapy, although this treatment is usually reserved for widespread disease.

Histologic types of cutaneous melanoma

Melanomas are classified into one of four subtypes (superficial spreading, nodular, lentigo maligna, and acral lentiginous) based on their clinical and histologic appearance as well as their anatomic location. Melanomas within a given subtype tend to behave similarly. Superficial spreading and nodular melanomas are by far the most frequent, comprising 85% of all melanomas. Melanoma progression is typified by an initial radial growth phase, during which time malignant cells spread horizontally, followed by a vertical growth phase, which is characterized by deep tumor invasion. The time course of radial to vertical growth phase transition appears to be a major variable among the different subtypes of melanoma. Because depth of tumor invasion is critical to prognosis, those tumors with an early transition to vertical growth phase have a worse prognosis than those with a prolonged radial growth phase.

Superficial spreading The defining characteristic of superficial spreading melanoma is an extended radial growth phase. Clinically, they appear flat in their early stages and may be large with heterogeneous pigmentation. These lesions may often be identified and removed prior to deep invasion and potential lymph node involvement. For these reasons, patients with superficial spreading melanoma can generally expect excellent survival rates.

Nodular Nodular melanomas are raised and often have relatively well-defined borders. Frequently, these lesions are darkly pigmented and may appear blue or black. Nodular melanomas demonstrate an early transition to vertical growth phase; thin lesions are rarely found to be nodular. Rather, most patients with nodular melanomas will present with intermediate or thick primary tumors at the time of diagnosis.

Lentigo maligna Elderly patients with extensive sun exposure are at high risk for lentigo maligna melanoma. These lesions are most common on the scalp and face and can be large and irregular; their removal often involves serious cosmetic considerations. In addition, melanoma in situ is frequently identified beyond the margins of the visible lesion, which adds to the difficulty of its removal.

Acral lentiginous The most common anatomic location for acral lentiginous melanomas is the sole of the feet; they may also be found on the palm or subungual region. In fair-skinned populations, they comprise about 2%–8% of all melanomas, whereas in African Americans, Hispanics, and Asians, they represent 40%–60% of all melanomas. They are often diagnosed at advanced stages, because they may be mistaken for benign entities such as trauma or infection. The treatment for lesions involving digits often requires amputation, whereas wide excision is performed for those on the palms and soles, often posing significant reconstructive challenges. Local recurrence rates are generally higher than for other melanoma subtypes.

Staging and prognosis of melanoma

A great deal of information is available regarding factors that correlate with clinical outcome in patients with melanoma. In the absence of known distant metastatic disease, the most important prognostic factor is regional lymph node involvement. Overall, however, 85% of melanoma patients present with clinically normal lymph nodes. In clinically node-negative patients, most investigators have found the microscopic degree of invasion of the melanoma, or microstaging, to be of critical importance in predicting outcome (Tables 2–4).

Microstaging

Two methods have been described for microscopic staging of primary cutaneous melanomas.

Clark's levels Wallace Clark and associates devised a system to classify melanomas according to the level of invasion relative to histologically defined landmarks in the skin. Although Clark's levels correlate with prognosis (lesions with deeper levels of invasion have a greater propensity for recurrence), the inherent problem with Clark's system is that the thickness of the skin—and hence the distance between the various landmark dermal layers—varies greatly in different parts of the body. Furthermore, except for Clark's level I (melanoma in situ), there is no scientific rationale for considering these landmarks to be biologic barriers to tumor growth. For example, there is no a priori reason to suspect that a lesion that reaches but does not invade the reticular dermis is

TABLE 2: TNM classification of melanoma

Primary tumor (T)	
Tx	Primary tumor cannot be assessed (eg, shave biopsy or regressed melanoma)
T0	No evidence of primary tumor
Tis	Melanoma in situ
T1	Melanoma ≤ 1.0 mm in thickness, with or without ulceration
T1a	Melanoma ≤ 1.0 mm in thickness and Clark's level II or III, no ulceration
T1b	Melanoma ≤ 1.0 mm in thickness and Clark's level IV or V or with ulceration
T2	Melanoma 1.01-2.0 mm in thickness, with or without ulceration
T2a	Melanoma 1.01-2.0 mm in thickness, no ulceration
T2b	Melanoma 1.01-2.0 mm in thickness, with ulceration
T3	Melanoma 2.01-4.0 mm in thickness, with or without ulceration
T3a	Melanoma 2.01-4.0 mm in thickness, no ulceration
T3b	Melanoma 2.01-4.0 mm in thickness, with ulceration
T4	Melanoma > 4.0 mm in thickness, with or without ulceration
T4a	Melanoma > 4.0 mm in thickness, no ulceration
T4b	Melanoma > 4.0 mm in thickness, with ulceration
Regional lymph nodes (N)	
Nx	Regional lymph nodes cannot be assessed
N0	No regional lymph node metastasis
N1	Metastasis in one lymph node
N1a	Clinically occult (microscopic) metastasis
N1b	Clinically apparent (macroscopic) metastasis
N2	Metastasis in two to three regional nodes or intralymphatic regional metastasis without nodal metastases
N2a	Clinically occult (microscopic) metastasis
N2b	Clinically apparent (macroscopic) metastasis
N2c	Satellite or in-transit metastasis without nodal metastasis
N3	Metastasis in four or more regional nodes, or matted metastatic nodes, or in-transit metastasis or satellite(s) with metastasis in regional node(s)
Distant metastasis (M)	
Mx	Distant metastasis cannot be assessed
M0	No distant metastasis
M1	Distant metastasis
M1a	Metastasis to skin, subcutaneous tissues, or distant lymph nodes
M1b	Metastasis to lungs
M1c	Metastasis to all other visceral sites or distant metastasis at any site associated with an elevated serum lactic dehydrogenase (LDH) level

From Greene FL, Page DL, Fleming ID, et al (eds): AJCC Cancer Staging Manual, 6th ed. New York, Springer-Verlag, 2002.

TABLE 3: Stage groupings for cutaneous melanoma

Clinical staging[a]				Pathologic staging[b]			
0	Tis	N0	M0	0	Tis	N0	M0
IA	T1a	N0	M0	IA	T1a	N0	M0
IB	T1b	N0	M0	IB	T1b	N0	M0
	T2a	N0	M0		T2a	N0	M0
IIA	T2b	N0	M0	IIA	T2b	N0	M0
	T3a	N0	M0		T3a	N0	M0
IIB	T3b	N0	M0	IIB	T3b	N0	M0
	T4a	N0	M0		T4a	N0	M0
IIC	T4b	N0	M0	IIC	T4b	N0	M0
III	Any T	N1	M0				
		N2					
		N3					
				IIIA	T1-4a	N1a	M0
					T1-4a	N2a	M0
				IIIB	T1-4b	N1a	M0
					T1-4b	N2a	M0
					T1-4a	N1b	M0
					T1-4a	N2b	M0
					T1-4a/b	N2c	M0
				IIIC	T1-4b	N1b	M0
					T1-4b	N2b	M0
					Any T	N3	M0
IV	Any T	Any N	Any M1	IV	Any T	Any N	Any M1

[a]Clinical staging includes microstaging of the primary melanoma and clinical/radiologic evaluation for metastases; by convention, it should be used after complete excision of the primary melanoma with *clinical* assessment for regional and distant metastases.

[b]Pathologic staging includes microstaging of the primary melanoma and pathologic information about the regional lymph nodes after partial or complete lymphadenectomy, except for pathologic stage 0 or stage 1A patients, who may not need pathologic evaluation of their lymph nodes.

Adapted from Balch CM, Buzaid AC, Soong SJ, et al: J Clin Oncol 19:3635–3648, 2001.

inherently less aggressive than a similar melanoma that penetrates the reticular dermis in an area where the skin is thinner.

Breslow's thickness An alternative microstaging method, described by Alexander Breslow, obviates some of the problems associated with Clark's levels. In this method, the thickness of the primary tumor is measured from the top of the granular layer of the epidermis to the deepest contiguous tumor cell at the base of the lesion using a micrometer in the microscope eyepiece.

Ulceration The presence of ulceration in a primary melanoma has been recognized as one of the strongest negative predictive factors for long-term survival. Ulceration is defined as the lack of a complete epidermal layer overlying

TABLE 4: Five-year survival rates of pathologically staged patients[a, b]

	IA	IB	IIA	IIB	IIC	IIIA	IIIB	IIIC
Ta: Nonulcerated	T1a	T2a	T3a	T4a	–	N1a	N1b	N3
melanoma	95%	89%	79%	67%	–	N2a	N2b	–
	–	–	–	–	–	67%	54%	28%
Tb: Ulcerated	–	T1b	T2b	T3b	T4b	–	N1a	N1b
melanoma	–	91%	77%	63%	45%	–	N2a	N2b
	–	–	–	–	–	–	–	N3
	–	–	–	–	–	–	52%	24%

[a] Adapted from Balch CM, et al: Melanoma of the skin, in Greene FL, Page DL, Fleming ID, et al (eds): AJCC Cancer Staging Manual, 6th ed. New York, Springer-Verlag, 2002.

[b] See Table 2 for staging details. N1 = 1 node; N2 = ≥ 2 nodes; Na = microscopic; Nb = macroscopic.

the melanocytic lesion. The presence of ulceration essentially upstages affected patients to the next highest T level. In other words, a patient with a 1.1–2-mm melanoma that is ulcerated will carry the same long-term prognosis as a patient with a 2.1–4-mm melanoma that does not have ulceration. The likelihood of finding ulceration is directly related to tumor depth: Patients with thin melanomas (≤ 1 mm) have a 6% rate of ulceration, whereas those with > 4-mm melanomas have a 63% incidence of ulceration. Along with tumor depth, ulceration is integral in determining a patient's long-term prognosis and is an independent predictor of patient outcome.

Many investigators have documented an inverse correlation between Breslow's tumor thickness and survival. More important, several studies have demonstrated that tumor thickness conveys more prognostic information than does Clark's level of invasion. In addition, the measurement of tumor thickness is generally more reproducible and less subjective than is the determination of Clark's level.

Occasionally, Breslow's thickness is impossible to determine and only the Clark's level is available for microstaging, usually because of technical factors related to the performance of the biopsy or the preparation of the histologic specimen. These situations, which inevitably result in the loss of important prognostic information, can be largely avoided by the performance of full-thickness (not shave) biopsies and by careful attention to detail when preparing specimens.

Regional lymph node involvement

In clinically localized disease, lymph node involvement is the strongest prognostic indicator in the staging of melanoma. Patients with nodal involvement at the time of their diagnosis have significantly decreased survival when compared with those who do not, independent of the primary lesion. There is a direct relationship between the depth of invasion of the primary lesion and the potential for lymph node involvement. The number of involved lymph nodes is inversely related to long-term survival. Patients with a single lymph node with metastatic disease have a better 5-year survival rate of approximately 60% than those who have multiple nodes (20%–25%). Also, patients with clinically enlarged or matted nodes at the time of diagnosis have a worse prognosis than those with microscopic disease.

An unknown primary

Melanoma of an unknown primary (MUP) is identified in up to 5% of patients who present with a newly diagnosed lesion. Lymphadenopathy is the most common presenting feature, followed by identification of visceral metastases and cutaneous nodules. In cases of MUP, consultations (such as ophthalmology, gastroenterology, otolaryngology, and gynecology) should be considered for appropriate evaluation of retinal and mucosal surfaces that may harbor a primary lesion. CT scan of the chest, abdomen, and pelvis should also be performed. PET scan may be considered, although its utility in the evaluation of melanoma is not yet clear. Surgical management of MUP should include lymphadenectomy for nodal disease and consideration of visceral resection if no other foci of disease are identified. Single dermal nodules with no identifiable primary lesion are typically treated in similar fashion to primary melanomas, with wide local excision and regional nodal evaluation (sentinel lymph node biopsy [SLNB]) if appropriate. If a primary lesion is identified, it should be excised widely. The prognosis for patients who present with MUP is similar to that for patients with metastatic disease from a known primary.

Clinical and pathologic staging

TNM staging system The melanoma staging committee of the American Joint Committee on Cancer (AJCC) has revised the TNM staging system to reflect more accurately the impact of statistically significant prognostic factors that were validated on a multi-institution sample of over 17,000 melanoma patients. The new system is shown in Tables 2 and 3.

For stages I and II (node-negative) melanoma, the most important prognostic factors are the Breslow depth (for thin melanomas < 1 mm; the Clark's level of invasion retains some prognostic value) and the presence or absence of ulceration (defined as the absence of an intact epidermis overlying a major portion of the primary melanoma). For stage III disease, the predictive factors are the number of nodes and extent of involvement (microscopic vs macroscopic), as well as the presence of satellite or in-transit deposits.

For patients with stage IV disease (distant metastases), there are few but significant differences in prognosis for disease limited to the skin, for subcutaneous and nodal sites vs visceral sites, and for levels of lactic dehydrogenase (LDH) in the serum.

Some of the most significant changes include new cutoff points for T classification (T1 = ≤ 1.0 mm, T2 = 1.01–2.0 mm, T3 = 2.01–4.0 mm, T4 = > 4 mm), inclusion of ulceration as a factor in T stage (a: no ulceration, b: ulceration), replacement of node size with node number for N stage, inclusion of node size (microscopic vs macroscopic) as a factor in N stage, and inclusion of LDH level as a factor in M stage. When incorporated into new clinical protocols, the new system will undoubtedly improve the value of data from clinical trials in this disease (Table 3).

Other prognostic factors

Age Overall, patients who are ≥ 65 years old have a survival rate that is decreased by 10%–15% compared with their younger counterparts. Although this trend has been demonstrated in numerous studies, whether age is truly an independent predictor of survival remains unclear. A different relationship between age and risk of lymph node involvement, however, is emerging. Data from the prospective Sunbelt Melanoma Trial and retrospective studies reveal that younger patients are significantly more likely to harbor nodal disease than older patients with similar lesions. Age, therefore, deserves consideration in management decisions regarding surgical evaluation of nodal basins.

Gender Many studies have identified a trend toward improved survival in women compared with men with melanoma. As an independent predictor of survival, however, this has frequently not reached statistical significance.

Anatomic location There is a correlation between anatomic location and prognosis of primary melanoma. Those with lesions on the back, upper arms, neck, and scalp (BANS area) have a worse prognosis than those with lesions on the extremities. This may be due to the simple fact that these lesions cannot be evaluated easily by the patient because of their inopportune location rather than a manifestation of true differences in tumor biology. In fact, location of the primary melanoma has not stood out as an independent predictor of prognosis in multivariate analysis. Men are more likely to develop truncal melanomas, whereas women are most likely to develop melanoma on their extremities. Acral lesions carry a worse prognosis than other extremity lesions.

Desmoplastic melanoma Desmoplastic melanomas represent a less common but clinically distinct spindle cell variant of melanoma with dense fibrosis and frequent neurotropism. Clinically, they are raised, firm nodules that are amelanotic in up to 40% of patients, leading to a common delay in diagnosis. Likely because of their neurotropism, these tumors have local recurrence rates as high as 40%, which has led many clinicians to advocate local radiation therapy following excision of these lesions. However, whether desmoplastic melanomas that lack neurotropism are truly at high risk for local recurrence, and whether radiation therapy helps control local recurrence if they are, remains an area of debate.

Additionally, although many of these lesions are deeply invasive at the time of diagnosis, desmoplastic melanomas are less likely to involve regional lymph node basins and more commonly develop distant metastases without lymphatic involvement. This observation should not deter sentinel lymph node biopsy in appropriate patients, as approximately 12% will harbor nodal disease. Despite these seemingly adverse prognostic factors, patients with desmoplastic and neurotropic melanomas tend to have overall survival rates that are slightly favorable compared with other melanomas.

Angiolymphatic invasion Defined as invasion of tumor cells into the wall and/or lumen of vessels or lymphatics of the dermis or deeper structures, angiolymphatic invasion is uncommon in malignant melanoma. However, this finding is clearly associated with more aggressive tumors and signifies likely poor outcomes for these patients. Multiple large studies have shown worsened long-term survival and more frequent lymph node involvement in patients with angioinvasive melanomas. In fact, risk of lymphatic involvement increases as much as threefold, whereas 5-year survival is reduced by as much as 50% when comparing matched patients with and without vascular invasion.

Regression The finding of regression represents host immune response to invasive melanoma. Areas where invasive cells may have once existed are replaced by inflammatory reaction and fibrosis, which may make it impossible to determine the precise depth of the initial lesion histologically. There is continuing debate regarding the prognostic importance of regression; however, many clinicians believe that thin lesions that show signs of regression should be given higher consideration for surgical nodal staging, given the fact that the initial lesion may have originally been more deeply invasive. Although some studies have shown that regressed lesions have a higher propensity for lymph node metastases than nonregressed primary tumors of the same thickness, this finding has not been universally observed.

Variable numbers of tumor infiltrating lymphocytes (TILs) are observed in melanoma. Tumors with a high number of TILs should carry an improved prognosis because of the active host response to tumor. In fact, many studies have shown this tendency.

Angiogenesis Studies have found angiogenesis to be an independent factor in long-term survival as well as local recurrence. More commonly identified as tumor depth increases, angiogenesis is a marker of invasive potential. Deep lesions with ulceration and high mitotic rates are typically associated with angiogenesis, and the combination of all of these factors is associated with poor outcome.

Treatment of melanomas

SURGICAL TREATMENT OF CUTANEOUS MELANOMA

Excision of the primary lesion

Margins of excision It was recognized over a century ago that tumor cells could extend within the skin for several centimeters beyond the visible borders of a melanoma, so that the risk of local recurrence relates to the width of normal skin excised around the primary tumor. Only much more recently was it realized that the thickness of the primary tumor influenced the likelihood of contiguous spread and that not all melanomas require the same excision margin. This realization prompted a number of randomized trials to determine the optimal excision margins for melanomas of different Breslow's thicknesses.

The Sunbelt Melanoma Trial is a multicenter prospective randomized trial involving 79 centers and more than 3,600 patients. In an evaluation of 961 patients, logistic regression analysis identified increasing Breslow thickness, ulceration, Clark level > III, and patient age ≤ 60 years as independent predictors for an increased risk of nodal disease. Currently, patients with melanoma ≥ 1 mm in Breslow depth are generally advised to undergo surgical staging of the nodes in conjunction with wide local excision. Selected patients with thin melanomas, < 1 mm in depth, may also be candidates for surgical staging of the nodes *(Sondak VK, Taylor JM, Sabel MS, et al: Ann Surg Oncol 11:247-258, 2004).*

Initially, a "one-size-fits-all" approach of taking a 5-cm margin around all cutaneous melanomas was adopted. With such wide margins, skin grafts were required after removal of melanomas on most parts of the body. Melanomas < 1 mm thick had low recurrence rates, however, even when less than the full 5-cm margin was excised.

A randomized trial found that when a 1-cm margin of normal skin was taken around a melanoma < 1 mm thick, the local recurrence rate was exceedingly low (< 1%), and patient survival was just as good as if 3-cm margins were taken. For melanomas 1–2 mm in thickness, patient survival was the same for both margins of excision, but the local recurrence rate was higher with the 1-cm margin (3.3% after 10-year follow-up).

Another randomized trial compared 2- vs 4-cm margins for all cutaneous melanomas between 1 and 4 mm in thickness. In this trial, both local recurrence and survival were the same regardless of whether 2- or 4-cm margins were taken. Skin grafts were less frequent and hospital stays shorter with the narrower margin.

In one phase III trial, 2-cm margins were compared with 5-cm margins for primary tumors ≤ 2 mm deep. Again, there was no difference in the local or distant relapse rate or overall survival.

Current recommendations Based on these three important studies, it is possible to make rational recommendations for excision margins for melanoma patients.

- For lesions > 1 mm in thickness, the recommended excision margin is 1 cm.
- For lesions 1–4 mm in thickness, a 2-cm margin is recommended.
- At least a 2-cm margin should be taken for lesions > 4 mm in thickness.

Several facts should be considered regarding these recommendations:

- Regardless of the recommended margin, a histologically negative margin is necessary. Thus, if a 2-cm margin is taken and the pathology report reveals melanoma cells or atypical melanocytic hyperplasia at the margins, further excision is indicated.
- When the anatomic location of the primary tumor precludes excision of the desired margin (eg, on the hands and feet or the face), at least 1 cm should be taken as long as the margins are histologically negative.
- If a minor compromise in excision margin can allow primary closure without a skin graft, it is worthwhile.

Management of regional lymph nodes

Physical examination is the primary screening tool for lymphatic involvement with melanoma. All potentially involved basins should be examined as part of a thorough history and physical examination. Patients who present with clinically negative nodes will have their further evaluation defined by the depth and characteristics of their primary melanoma. Currently, those patients with melanoma having Breslow depth ≥ 1 mm are candidates for surgical evaluation of nodal involvement using SLNB techniques. Patients with thinner melanomas may also be candidates for SLNB if adverse prognostic factors are identified in their primary tumor.

> Kesmodel et al recently identified mitotic rate (MR) as a predictor of sentinel lymph node (SLN) positivity in a review of 181 patients with thin (≤ 1 mm) melanomas who underwent SLN mapping and biopsy. Overall SLN positivity in this group was 5%. Mitotic figures were identified in 103 primary lesions, 9 of which had an associated positive SLN. No patient with an MR of 0 had a positive SLN. Univariate analysis identified MR and tumor thickness ≥ 0.76 mm as being associated with SLN positivity. Patients with a primary tumor ≥ 0.76 mm and an MR > 0 had a 12.3% risk of SLN involvement. The authors concluded that consideration should be given to performing SLN biopsy in patients with thin melanomas (0.76–1 mm) who also demonstrate an MR > 0 (*Kesmodel SB, Karakousis GC, Botbyl JD, et al: Ann Surg Oncol 12:449-458, 2005*).

Patients who have clinically positive (enlarged) lymph nodes will require evaluation to determine whether the nodes are in fact pathologically positive, in which case complete nodal dissection is indicated. The first step in evaluating palpable nodes is generally FNA. Positive cytology is sufficient to mandate complete nodal dissection. A negative or inadequate sample FNA may be repeated, with image guidance if necessary, or may lead directly to an open node biopsy, followed by complete lymphadenectomy in the event of a positive frozen section or touch-prep cytologic determination of metastasis.

Clinically enlarged nodes Melanoma patients with clinically enlarged nodes and no evidence of distant disease (AJCC stage III) should undergo complete regional lymphadenectomy. Physical examination may be inaccurate in its prediction of nodal involvement, however, and so other techniques may be utilized to identify positive nodes. FNA of palpable nodes may assist in further decision-making. If positive cytology is identified, lymphadenectomy should be performed. A negative FNA should not preclude further surgical evaluation. Touch-prep cytology may also be a useful adjunct for intraoperative evaluation of suspicious nodes during SLNB or open biopsy.

Clinically normal nodes The surgical management of clinically normal nodes is determined by the characteristics of the primary lesion. A direct relationship between thickness of the primary lesion and nodal involvement has long been recognized. In addition, the Sunbelt Melanoma Trial has identified additional prognostic factors that increase the risk of nodal disease.

Thin melanomas Patients with thin melanomas (< 1 mm Breslow depth) have a low risk of occult nodal involvement (< 5%) and therefore generally undergo wide excision with 1-cm margins and no nodal staging procedure. Some patients with

The Multicenter Selective Lymphadenectomy Trial (MSLT-I) randomly assigned patients with clinically localized melanoma to receive wide excision and sentinel lymph node (SLN) mapping and biopsy versus observation and subsequent complete lymph node dissection (CLND) with the development of clinically positive nodes. Preliminary data suggest that SLN positivity is the most important prognostic factor in early-stage melanoma. Positive SLNs were identified in 19.8% of patients undergoing immediate SLN biopsy, which was similar to the 20% who developed nodal disease while on observation. Analysis is ongoing to determine whether immediate completion lymphadenectomy following a positive SLN biopsy confers a survival advantage over delayed node dissection once clinically apparent disease is present. Ultrasonographic evaluation of nodal basins is currently being tested in the successor trial, MSLT-2, as a sensitive means to detect nodal recurrence. This trial will also evaluate the role of complete lymphadenectomy after a positive SLN biopsy.

melanomas 0.76–1 mm have a high enough risk of lymph node involvement to justify consideration of SLNB in addition to wide excision.

Multiple risk factors that confer an increased risk for lymph node metastases in patients with thin melanomas have been identified. If they are present, consideration may be given to SLNB in patients with thin melanomas (between 0.76 and 1 mm). Historically, Clark's level of IV or V was considered to be a significant prognostic indicator and continues to be included in the AJCC staging system. Emerging data, however, suggest that this criterion is probably the least satisfactory in discriminating those patients with thin melanomas who should undergo lymph node biopsy.

Intermediate-thickness melanomas Melanomas 1–4 mm in thickness are associated with an overall risk of occult lymph node involvement of 20%–25%. However, relative risk rises significantly with increasing depth of invasion. Patients with a 1-mm thick melanoma have approximately a 15% chance of involvement, whereas those with a 4-mm melanoma have up to a 55% risk of nodal metastases. For these reasons, wide excision of the primary tumor is generally accompanied by SLNB for evaluation of the nodal basin involved. An alternative approach of wide excision alone with observation and serial physical examination of nodal basins has been advocated by some clinicians and has not been shown to reduce long-term survival if complete lymph node dissection is performed at the identification of clinically positive nodes. The use of SLNB vs observation continues to be an area of intense debate.

Selective lymphadenectomy The identification and management of nodal disease have evolved significantly over the past 20 years. The evolution of SLNB has led to an improved ability to accurately stage patients earlier in their disease process. Historically, complete lymph node dissections were performed electively on patients with intermediate and thick melanomas with the belief that they would lead to a survival benefit. With elective node dissection, however, a significant percentage (80%–85%) of patients underwent complete lymphadenectomy only to find that their nodal basin was free of disease.

Currently, node dissection is used selectively, only on those melanoma patients who have been shown to have nodal involvement by SLNB. SLNB was described by Morton et al, who found that dermal injection of vital blue dye

(Lymphazurin) surrounding the primary melanoma site allowed for visualization of the draining lymphatics and the "sentinel" node, which was defined to be the first draining lymph node receiving lymph from the primary tumor bed. The original dye-based technique allowed for identification of the "sentinel" node in approximately 85% of cases.

> The current US cooperative group studies for stage III melanoma are divided into low- and high-risk categories for randomized trials of adjuvant therapy. Patients with high-risk disease, defined as stage IIIB or higher (Tables 2 and 3), are randomized to receive 1 year of high-dose IFN-α or 3 cycles of biochemotherapy containing dacarbazine, cisplatin, vinblastine, IFN-α, and IL-2. Patients with T3 or T4 primary melanoma and up to one microscopically involved node are randomized to receive 1 month of high-dose IFN-α or no systemic adjuvant therapy. The results of both of these studies may prove to raise more questions than are answered. For example, a result favoring biochemotherapy will raise the question of which component is essential for the adjuvant activity (see text and Table 5). A result favoring IFN-α would not definitively answer whether 1 month or 1 year of therapy is optimal for this uniquely selected group of patients.

To increase the success rate for sentinel node identification, technetium^{99m}–labeled sulfur colloid is injected into the primary site preoperatively, and the potentially involved lymph basins are identified with a gamma camera. The patient is then taken to the operating room, where a hand-held gamma probe is used to identify the sentinel node(s). This technique, in combination with the use of vital blue dye, has led to a success rate exceeding 99% in most large current trials.

The ability to accurately detect or rule out disease in the sentinel lymph node has allowed many patients to forego the higher morbidity of complete node dissection. In addition, patients can be more accurately staged and treated earlier in the course of their disease. The intuitive hope that this ability could lend itself to improved survival in patients who undergo SLNB remains to be determined in prospective, randomized trials. Even in the absence of a proven survival benefit, however, the staging advantages of SLNB are sufficiently compelling to justify its routine use in healthy patients with melanomas and a significant risk of nodal involvement. Current data also support the watch-and-wait approach to nodal evaluation, with lymph node dissection (LND) reserved for those who develop clinically positive nodes, which still has a place in the treatment of melanoma and likely does not negatively impact survival. The prospective clinical trials are currently investigating the role of complete lymphadenectomy following positive SLNB.

The evolution of reverse transcriptase-PCR (RT-PCR) has allowed for identification of submicroscopic metastatic nodal disease. It is unknown whether submicroscopic metastatic disease has clinical relevance in the long-term survival of patients with melanoma. These issues are currently being prospectively investigated in the Sunbelt Melanoma trial. Although a number of retrospective studies have suggested that RT-PCR analysis has a role to play in predicting outcome for patients with histologically negative sentinel nodes, a recent study with longer follow-up suggested that this prognostic value was lost over time. This observation stresses the importance of prospective evaluation of candidate prognostic tests such as RT-PCR.

Thick melanomas Primary melanomas > 4 mm in thickness are treated with a 2-cm excision margin. In addition, because deep melanomas harbor nodal metastases in up to 60% of patients, surgical evaluation of the nodal basin is generally pursued. Although elective LND has not proven beneficial in these patients, SLNB has been used extensively to guide diagnostic, prognostic, and therapeutic decision-making.

Isolation limb perfusion In-transit metastases—ie, cutaneous or subcutaneous nodules arising between the primary site and the regional lymph node basin—are a well-recognized, but fairly uncommon, site of failure in cutaneous melanoma. A surgical technique developed to treat in-transit metastases, isolation limb perfusion, involves cannulating the artery and vein to an extremity and connecting the cannulas to a cardiopulmonary bypass machine. This technique effectively isolates the blood flow to that extremity and allows for prolonged perfusion with cytotoxic and/or biologic agents.

Most commonly, the chemotherapeutic agent melphalan (Alkeran) has been used for isolation limb perfusion; this drug is generally heated to an elevated temperature (up to 41°C) and perfused for up to 90 minutes. Hyperthermic isolation perfusion with melphalan alone or combined with the investigational agent tumor necrosis factor-α (TNF-α) results in the regression of > 90% of cutaneous in-transit metastases. This approach is useful for limited clinical situations at centers experienced in the technique.

Hyperthermic isolation perfusion with melphalan has also been combined with wide excision in patients at high risk of recurrence of in-transit metastases. Adjuvant use of perfusion demonstrated no significant benefit in a large, international intergroup trial, however, and cannot be recommended.

SURGICAL TREATMENT OF NONCUTANEOUS MELANOMA

Noncutaneous melanomas generally present at a more advanced stage than cutaneous lesions. The site of the lesion greatly affects the approach to the primary tumor and regional lymph nodes.

Ocular melanomas generally do not have access to lymphatic channels, so the surgical principles outlined previously do not apply here. However, the unique propensity to metastasize hematogenously, often to the liver after a long relapse-free interval, warrants further study of this primary site's unique biology. Advances in understanding the biology of ocular melanomas may lead to adjuvant approaches different from therapies now under investigation for cutaneous primaries.

A diagnosis of ocular melanoma with no evidence of distant disease signifies that a decision must be made as to whether or not the eye can be spared. Some small melanomas situated peripherally in the retina can be excised with minimal loss of vision, but most cannot. For larger lesions, treatment options are enucleation (total removal of the eye) or implanted radiotherapy with a radioactive gold plaque fitted to the back of the eyeball immediately behind the tumor. A multi-institution, randomized trial comparing implanted radiotherapy with enucleation for local disease control and overall survival was completed by the Collaborative Ocular Melanoma Study Group; it appears that both techniques provide similar outcomes for all sizes of tumors.

Melanomas of the anus and vulva pose challenges in the treatment of both the primary lesion and regional nodes. Excision of primary tumors in these areas should not be overly radical: Abdominoperineal resection or radical vulvectomy is unnecessarily deforming and is not associated with improved survival compared with wide local excision. Abdominoperineal resection, with its attendant permanent colostomy, is indicated only for locally recurrent melanomas after prior sphincter-conserving excision or for melanomas with radiographic evidence of mesorectal node involvement.

Anal and vulvar melanomas often present with inguinal lymph node metastases; if there is no evidence of distant disease, both the primary site and regional nodes should be removed.

Nasal sinuses or nasopharyngeal melanomas Melanomas arising in the nasal or nasopharyngeal mucosa should be widely excised to include adjacent bony structures, if needed. Node dissection is reserved for patients who have proven nodal involvement. Radiation therapy should be considered for those patients whose primary tumor cannot be fully removed from this site with adequate margins.

ADJUVANT THERAPY FOR MELANOMA

The 10-year disease-free survival estimate for patients with T1a ($\leq$ 1 mm deep, no ulceration), T11a (1.01–2 mm deep, no ulceration), and T1b ($\leq$ 1 mm deep, with ulceration) is approximately 85%. However, fewer than half of patients with deep or intermediate-level primary tumors with ulceration (see AJCC system) and/or regional lymph node involvement will experience long-term disease-free survival.

Development of adjuvant therapy approaches that increase survival over surgery alone has been a long-standing goal of melanoma researchers.

Interferon-α (IFN-α) and adjuvant therapy for stage III melanoma

The epoch of effective adjuvant therapy for resected high-risk melanoma began with the publication of Eastern Cooperative Oncology Group (ECOG) protocol 1684 in 1996, which demonstrated a survival benefit associated with the administration of 1 year of "high-dose" IFN-α, consisting of 4 weeks of treatment, 5 days per week, at 20 mU/m^2 IV followed by 11 months of treatment, 3 times per week, at 10 mU/m^2 SC. The results of this practice-altering trial led to the approval of this drug for melanoma and to its established role as the comparator arm in several subsequent phase III adjuvant trials. The two subsequent large US cooperative group trials for high-risk resected local and regional melanoma confirmed the activity of high-dose IFN-α and the lack of benefit for less aggressive IFN-α regimens as well as for a ganglioside vaccine that had shown promise in this setting. Nearly all of the other trials, both before and after ECOG 1684 and predominantly in European centers, consisted of lower-dose, more prolonged administration of IFN-α. These regimens, although appearing to delay relapse in some cases, offered no survival benefit and have not been recommended for use outside clinical trials.

The most recent study is a multi-institution, randomized trial of polyethylene glycol IFN-α, a chemically modified molecule designed to prolong the exposure and decrease the frequency of administration. Although this agent is active for diseases that are responsive to low-dose IFN-α, such as chronic viral hepatitis and chronic myelogenous leukemia, it is not likely to prove beneficial for the adjuvant therapy of melanoma unless the chemical modification leads to beneficial alterations in the immunologic activity of the IFN-α. Even the role of high-dose IFN-α as a standard therapy or as a comparator for phase III trials has been questioned, since long-term follow-up of the original ECOG data suggests a gradual loss of the survival benefit over time. One approach currently under investigation is to use high-dose IFN-α as the platform upon which to build multiagent regimens for testing in the adjuvant setting; another approach is to use this agent as part of a vaccine strategy, as detailed later in this chapter.

The clinical toxicities of IFN-α are predominantly constitutional, consisting of fever and chills (which subside in most patients after the first few doses), nausea and anorexia, myalgias, and arthralgias. Fatigue, which may be progressive as therapy continues, is generally the most troublesome side effect and is often dose-limiting. CNS toxicity, ranging from mild difficulties with concentration to severe depression, is also related to the dose and duration of therapy.

The most common laboratory abnormalities consist of asymptomatic elevations in serum levels of transaminase and mild myelosuppression, as well as occasional nephrotoxicity. Virtually all of these effects are reversible and occur in dose- and schedule-dependent patterns that allow continued therapy with appropriate adjustments to the regimen.

Optimal adjuvant treatment of node-negative melanoma The best adjuvant intervention for patients with intermediate-risk melanoma has not yet been identified, but the goal of avoiding toxicity and the recognition that these patients may be the ideal candidates for immunotherapeutic interventions have justified the enrollment of these patients in trials of vaccines and low-dose IFN-α. Several trials outside the United States failed to demonstrate a survival benefit using IFN-α in various schedules and doses for patients with high-risk node-negative disease.

Radiation therapy

Radiation therapy is rarely employed after surgery for primary or nodal melanoma, although recent reports have demonstrated that the pessimistic impression that melanoma is a "nonradioresponsive" tumor is not justified. A study at M. D. Anderson Cancer Center suggested that postoperative radiation therapy to the neck after radical or modified radical neck dissection decreased regional recurrence rates in node-positive patients.

Formal investigation of the role of adjuvant irradiation in patients thought to be at uniquely high risk for locoregional disease has been hampered by technical challenges to protocol design and changes in the practical approach to these patients. Nevertheless, it seems reasonable to consider the use of postoperative radiation therapy in patients with multiple (≥ 10) involved lymph nodes or gross extracapsular extension, as these patients are at high risk of regional recurrence despite adequate lymph node dissection.

Since these patients are also candidates for IFN-α or investigational studies of adjuvant therapy, the optimal schedule for integrating radiation therapy with IFN-α will need to be determined. In the absence of definitive data, we defer the start of radiation therapy until after the completion of the initial month of IV IFN-α. One goal of the new agents is to provide radiosensitization, so radiation therapy can be a more useful adjunct either in the adjuvant setting, as addressed here, or in the advanced setting, as addressed later in the chapter.

TREATMENT OF ADVANCED MELANOMA

Chemotherapy

Single agents Among the numerous available chemotherapeutic agents, only dacarbazine, which has an 8%–10% objective response rate when given alone, is currently approved for the treatment of advanced melanoma. Most combination regimens in current use or under investigation include this agent. Temozolomide (Temodar), an oral alkylating agent approved for the treatment of malignant gliomas, has activity comparable to that of dacarbazine in advanced melanoma. Its mechanism of action is similar to that of dacarbazine, but its high oral bioavailability and penetration into the CNS make it ideal for consideration in treatment of this disease, with a high propensity for CNS metastasis. Although there are no adequate phase III data supporting this hypothesis, temozolomide has been substituted for dacarbazine in many combination regimens and is currently under investigation in combination with radiation therapy for patients with melanoma metastatic to the brain.

One important mechanism of resistance to dacarbazine and temozolomide is the removal of the chemotherapy-donated alkyl group from its target site on the guanine molecule by the enzyme alkyl guanyl transferase (ATase). Attempts to overcome this form of resistance involve the use of an inhibitor of ATase, O-6-benzyl guanine, or alternative administration schedules that downregulate cellular levels of ATase. Unfortunately, neither of these methods has proved to be effective so far, and the need remains acute for better cytotoxic agents and a greater understanding of potential targets for new drugs.

A number of other drugs have shown activity in early studies but have not been subjected to the rigorous testing required to define their possible role in current regimens. Thus, older regimens commonly included a nitrosourea, cisplatin, and a vinca alkaloid. More recently, the taxanes have been shown to possess some activity, supporting the development of potentially synergistic regimens with cisplatin. However, in view of their myelosuppression and the requirement for glucocorticoid prophylaxis, which could interfere with potential immunochemotherapeutic synergy, the taxanes have not been adopted for widespread use in melanoma.

TABLE 5: Randomized trials of biochemotherapy regimens in patients with metastatic melanoma

Regimen	No. of patients	No. of CRs	No. of PRs	OR rate (%)	Median survival (mo)
Falkson study					
DTIC	69	2	8	15	10
DTIC + IFN-α	68	6	8	21	9
DTIC + Tam	68	2	10	18	8
DTIC + IFN-α + Tam	66	3	10	19	10
Rosenberg study					
CDDP + DTIC + Tam	52	8	19	27	16
CDDP + DTIC + Tam + IFN-α ± IL-2	50	6	38	44	11
Ridolfi study					
CDDP + DTIC ± BiCNU	89	3	15	20	9.5
CDDP + DTIC ± BiCNU + IL-2 + IFN-α	87	3	19	25	11
Eton study					
CDDP + DTIC + Vlb	92	1	22	23	9.5
CDDP + DTIC + Vlb + IL-2 + IFN-α	91	6	38	44	11.8
Atkins study					
CDDP + Vlb + DTIC	201	6	17	11	8.7
CDDP + Vlb + DTIC + IL-2 + IFN	204	3	32	17	8.4
Del Vecchio study					
CDDP + Vnd + DTIC	69	0	15	21	12
CDDP + Vnd + IL-2 + IFN	70	2	18	27	11
Keilholz study					
DTIC + CDDP + IFN	180	7	34	23	9
DTIC + CDDP + IFN + IL-2	183	6	32	21	9

BiCNU = carmustine; CDDP = cisplatin; CR = complete response; DTIC = dacarbazine; IFN-α = interferon-α; IL-2 = interleukin-2; OR = overall response; PR = partial response; Tam = tamoxifen; Vlb = vinblastine; Vnd = vindesine

Combination regimens The principles of combination chemotherapy and potential drug synergy have been applied with limited success to the treatment of advanced melanoma (Table 5). Combinations based on the agents previously listed became popular when the group at M. D. Anderson Cancer Center demonstrated an encouraging response rate (in the 40% range) for a regimen containing dacarbazine, vinblastine, and cisplatin. When moderate doses of IFN-α and interleukin-2 (IL-2, aldesleukin, Proleukin) were added to this drug combination and given simultaneously, the overall objective response rates exceeded 50%, and complete responses occurred in 10% of patients. In a phase III study from the same institution, a small survival benefit of biochemotherapy over the same chemotherapeutic agents without IFN and IL-2 was achieved.

However, the attempt to reproduce these results in large, randomized cooperative group studies was disappointing, and the addition of the biologic agents was recently shown not to enhance the overall objective response rate and disease progression-free or overall survival. Similarly, disappointing results have been reported in other studies addressed at a similar question, as shown in Table 5. Thus, the role of biochemotherapy in advanced melanoma has not been defined and is not routinely recommended for use outside of investigational trials, since it rarely provides a durable complete remission. However, for young, otherwise healthy patients, particularly those who are symptomatic, biochemotherapy may be appropriate for the goal of achieving the highest likelihood of an initial response and symptom relief.

Melanomas often harbor a constitutively activating mutation in B-*raf* kinase, a signaling molecule involved in cell proliferation and survival. Sorafenib (also known as Bay 43-9006) is an investigational oral agent that inhibits the activity of this enzyme as well as that of other signaling molecules, including the receptor for vascular endothelial growth factor, suggesting it may have anti-angiogenic potential as well as direct antitumor activity. Although the single-agent activity of sorafenib was low among previously treated melanoma patients in a phase I trial (*Ahmad T, Marais R, Pyle L, et al: Proc Am Soc Clin Oncol [abstract] 23:708, 2004*), a combination of this agent with carboplatin and paclitaxel provided an objective response rate in the range of 30%, even in previously treated patients (*Flaherty KT, Brose M, Schuchter L, et al: Proc Am Soc Clin Oncol [abstract] 23:708, 2004*). A phase III trial of this combination with or without sorafenib is now under way.

The use of thalidomide (Thalomid) as an immunomodulator and/or inhibitor of angiogenesis has been studied extensively in melanoma, but the role for this agent remains undefined. Although initial trials suggested a remarkable level of activity for the combination of temozolomide (Temodar) with thalidomide, phase III trials to define the role of thalidomide remain to be completed. Although the appeal of an all-oral, fairly well-tolerated regimen supports the further development of this combination, the toxicities, particularly the increased risk of thromboembolic events, will require further study. It is possible that related drugs with a superior therapeutic index, such as lenalidomide (Revlimid, recently approved for myeloma), will have promising activity and may be better tolerated in combinations with other biologic agents, targeted small molecules, or cytotoxic agents for patients with advanced melanoma (*Bartlett JB, Michael A, Clarke IA, et al: Br J Cancer 90:955-961, 2004*).

Biologic therapies

IFN-α has been evaluated as a single agent in melanoma, and most of its experience is from older studies in which the methods of response assessment and confirmation of outcomes were less rigorous than in current studies. Although initial studies of IFN-α plus single or multiagent chemotherapy suggested activity superior to that expected from the single agents, randomized trials did not show a benefit. Thus, with the exception of its possible use in IL-2–containing biochemotherapy, IFN-α is not currently recommended as a single agent or in combination with available chemotherapy agents in advanced melanoma. It is possible that increased understanding of the biology and immunology of melanoma and the tu-

Investigators at the Cancer Institute Medical Group recently updated their phase II data on the use of biochemotherapy with maintenance biotherapy for responders (*O'Day SJ, Boasberg PD, Piro L, et al: Clin Cancer Res 8:2775-2781, 2002*) in a report to the American Society of Clinical Oncology in May 2005. A total of 133 patients with advanced melanoma were treated. The objective response rate was 44%, and 10% of patients enjoyed durable complete responses. The median survival was over 1 year, but the high rate of CNS relapse (nearly half of the time as the first site of relapse) emphasized the need for more effective prophylaxis and therapy for this "sanctuary" site. These investigators plan to study the ability of temozolomide (Temodar) and whole-brain irradiation to lower the CNS relapse rate in patients experiencing a systemic response, but more effective agents will undoubtedly be required to achieve this goal (*O'Day S, Atkins M, Weber J, et al: J Clin Oncol [abstract] 23[suppl]:710s, 2005*).

mor milieu will lead to the inclusion of IFN-α in new combinations, doses, and schedules for which there is a precise rationale for its use. The most valuable combinations of IFN-α for melanoma are likely to be in the adjuvant setting in carefully sequenced combinations with other immunotherapeutic agents such as peptide vaccine.

IL-2 is the only other recombinant biologic molecule with demonstrated antitumor activity against melanoma. The majority of published data come from trials of high doses of IL-2 (600,000–720,000 IU/kg IV every 8 hours for 14 doses, repeated after a 9-day rest period) given over limited treatment durations at toxicity levels requiring inpatient management. The most common toxicities, including hypotension with fluid retention, acidosis and renal insufficiency, neurotoxicity, and cardiovascular complications, can be life-threatening. Mucocutaneous and constitutional toxicities, including fever/chills, nausea/anorexia, and profound fatigue, may also limit the number of doses tolerated by patients. The generalized capillary leak syndrome may lead to multiorgan dysfunction, which requires skill and experience to administer the maximum number of doses tolerated while avoiding life-threatening toxicities. At these dose-intense levels, objective response rates of approximately 20% have been achieved, with about half of responding patients experiencing durable complete remissions lasting in excess of 5 years. Based on these favorable results, high-dose IL-2 was approved by the US Food and Drug Administration (FDA) in 1998 for the treatment of metastatic melanoma. Recently completed phase III trials have failed to demonstrate a significant reduction in toxicities or enhancement in the therapeutic efficacy of IL-2 using modulators chosen for their selective inhibitory effects on inflammatory pathways associated with the toxic effects of IL-2.

Although the frequency of durable complete responses to IL-2 therapy appears to be higher than that reported for other single agents and combination regimens, it is important to consider that patients selected for their ability to tolerate the serious multisystem toxicities of high-dose IL-2 may represent a more favorable group with a higher a priori likelihood of tumor response. Only limited data are available on the activity of outpatient, low-dose IL-2 regimens in patients with melanoma, and this form of therapy is not recommended outside a clinical trial.

IFN-α plus IL-2 IFN-α and IL-2 have been used together in the treatment of advanced melanoma, as well as other tumors. In addition to potential synergistic antitumor efficacy, the clinical advantage of this combination includes the relative lack of overlapping toxicities. Combinations of IFN-α and IL-2 at maximum doses in either the inpatient or outpatient setting have not, however, achieved a higher response rate than either agent alone in patients with metastatic melanoma and are not recommended for routine use.

> The effects of GM-CSF and IFN-α as vaccine adjuvants in combination with HLA-A2 peptides from Melan-A/MART-1, gp-100, and tyrosinase in HLA-A2–positive patients with advanced melanoma have been analyzed (*Kirkwood JM, Lee S, Land S, et al: Proc Am Soc Clin Oncol [abstract] 23:707, 2004*). The results suggested an association between immune responses and longer survival, but the potential benefit of peptide vaccine and GM-CSF in the adjuvant setting awaits the results of ECOG 4697, a trial designed for patients with metastatic melanoma that can be fully excised.

Melanoma vaccines Vaccines produced from allogeneic melanoma cell lines administered with one of several available nonspecific immunologic "adjuvants" (which stimulate antigen-presenting cells and enhance other aspects of immune recognition of antigens and response to target cells) have shown limited activity in patients with metastatic melanoma. These and related vaccine strategies, which are briefly summarized below, are likely to have greater promise in the adjuvant setting, where the effector-to-target ratios of immune cells to tumor cells are more favorable and the mechanisms of tumor resistance or escape from immune recognition and attack are not developed.

Canvaxin is a vaccine produced from two melanoma cell lines and administered with the bacille Calmette-Guerin (BCG) vaccine immune adjuvant. A large phase III trial comparing Canvaxin plus BCG vs BCG as a control for patients with stage III and IV melanoma was recently closed after interim analysis failed to identify any improvement in outcomes.

Tumor-specific antigens most critical to mediating an antimelanoma immune response and the most efficient methods to optimize the T-cell immune response, which is more promising than B-cell immunity against tumor antigens, remain the subject of ongoing investigations. Peptide vaccines that induce T-cell immunity to precisely defined immunodominant peptides contained in melanoma protein antigens have been developed and, in some cases, modified to enhance their presentation by HLA molecules on antigen-presenting cells and recognition by T lymphocytes. These vaccines may work well when administered directly to patients with an immune adjuvant, such as previously described, or may have enhanced immunostimulatory activity when administered as part of a dendritic cell vaccine. Dendritic cell-targeted therapy takes advantage of the dendritic cells' antigen-presenting function, involved in T-cell responses.

Under investigation are peptides from several known melanoma antigens, including the MAGE series, gp-100, tyrosinase, MART-1/Melan-A, and NY-ESO-1. Current studies are directed at the optimization of conditions for the production and administration of dendritic cells in addition to the source and delivery of tumor antigen. Clinical investigations are ongoing to study the best immu-

A promising area of vaccine investigation involves the use of CTLA4-Ab, a blocking antibody that inhibits the negative signals transmitted to T cells in the normal control of the immune response. Preliminary data in advanced melanoma patients suggest that this antibody, alone or in combination immunotherapy strategies, may "break immune tolerance," allowing the emergence of a beneficial immune response to tumor. Autoimmune complications of this therapy, including inflammatory events affecting the skin, liver, and intestinal mucosa, provide "proof of concept" that a potent immune response to melanoma cells leads to a cross-reactive immune attack on selected normal tissues. Further quantitation of these risks and the likely benefit of this approach are under evaluation in a large, multi-institutional, randomized trial of melanoma peptide vaccines and CTLA4-Ab in patients with advanced melanoma (*Sanderson K, Scotland F, Lee P, et al: J Clin Oncol 23:741-750, 2005; Hersh EM, Weber J, Powderly J, et al: Proc Am Soc Clin Oncol [abstract] 23:709, 2004*).

nologic adjuvant as well as combinations of peptide vaccines with cytokines (eg, GM-CSF [granulocyte-macrophage colony-stimulating factor, sargramostim, Leukine] and IL-2) that also enhance the T-cell response.

Gene therapy New advances in gene therapy have made possible the genetic modification of tumor cells as well as effector cells, such as dendritic cells and T cells. Some of the genetic modifications that have been studied include the transfection of genes for immunostimulatory cytokines, allogeneic HLA sequences, and accessory molecules critical for immune recognition. Continued efforts in this area will soon define the optimal system for the application of these laboratory techniques to the immunotherapy for human melanoma.

Treatment of CNS metastasis

Radiation therapy is the only treatment available for most patients with unresectable brain metastases, but meaningful responses are observed in less than 25% of treated patients. Alternative fractionation schedules have been investigated but have not proved to be superior to standard regimens of whole-brain irradiation. Recently, techniques of stereotactic irradiation have shown encouraging results in patients with melanoma metastatic to the CNS; this approach is currently recommended when the size, number, and location of metastases are amenable to stereotactic techniques. The median survival is only a few months. Corticosteroids are often given concomitantly with brain irradiation to minimize intracranial swelling and are tapered off rapidly after the completion of therapy. Because melanoma has limited responsiveness to radiotherapy and is often associated with intracranial hemorrhage, excision should be considered for brain metastases that can be removed safely. The benefit of adding whole-brain irradiation therapy to focal radiation or surgery for patients with brain metastases remains unproven and awaits new modulations of the available therapies, such as safe and effective radiosensitizers.

The lack of success in treating brain metastases clearly reflects both the relative radioresistance of this tumor and the lack of activity of available cytotoxic agents, including those that efficiently penetrate the CNS, such as nitrosoureas and temozolomide. Therapies with higher reported response rates have failed to reduce the rate of CNS metastatic disease, presumably due to their lack of CNS penetration and the emergence of metastases in a "sanctuary" site from a disease with a high propensity to seed the CNS. Thus, therapeutic success in this setting will require highly active combinations that can be used in the adjuvant setting before CNS metastases develop from recurrent disease, therapies with sufficient antitumor activity and CNS penetration, and agents with high antitumor activity and CNS penetration to treat those with established CNS metastatic disease.

Radiation therapy is occasionally of benefit in the palliative treatment of melanoma metastatic to bone or other symptomatic sites.

The importance of regulatory T cells in suppression of an antigen-specific immune response has recently been recognized, and efforts to address this mechanism of immune evasion in patients with advanced cancer include the use of lymphodepleting chemotherapy followed by infusion of cloned antigen-specific T cells and high-dose IL-2. Investigators at the National Cancer Institute recently showed this approach to be active in patients with advanced melanoma for whom prior therapy with cytokines had failed (Dudley ME, Wunderlich JR, Yang JC, et al: J Clin Oncol 23:2346-2357, 2005). The possibility that homeostatic reconstitution of lymphocytes following this type of chemotherapy may have similar activity to the more cumbersome and HLA-restricted process of reinfusing antigen-specific cloned T cells is currently undergoing evaluation in several other trials in patients with advanced melanoma.

Treatment of nonmelanoma skin cancer

Surgery

Margins of excision Most nonmelanoma skin cancers can be conservatively excised with much narrower margins than are required for cutaneous melanomas. Excision margins of 0.5–1.0 cm are adequate for most nonrecurrent basal cell and squamous cell cancers and yield local recurrence rates under 5%, provided that histologically negative margins are achieved. For most tumors in most anatomic sites, these excision margins can be achieved using standard surgical techniques with local anesthesia and primary closure.

Recurrent cancers and lesions in difficult sites More sophisticated techniques are required for recurrent skin cancers or those in cosmetically difficult areas, such as the tip of the nose or the eyelids. For these lesions, a variation of Mohs' micrographic surgery is frequently employed. Simply stated, this type of surgery is a controlled surgical excision in which the removed tissue is precisely oriented and carefully examined histologically, and serial re-excisions are performed wherever residual disease is noted.

Although Mohs' surgery may take much longer than routine surgical excision, the extra precision can be helpful for identifying the often asymmetric extensions of skin cancers, thus minimizing the amount of normal tissue resected. After Mohs' surgery has achieved complete excision, reconstruction is performed by whatever means is appropriate but often involves skin grafts or local flaps rather than primary closure.

More aggressive histologic types of skin cancers, particularly Merkel's cell cancers and sarcomas, generally require wider excision than do the more common basal cell and squamous cell cancers. Margins of 2–3 cm are usually taken, similar to those for a thick melanoma. In particular, dermatofibrosarcoma protuberans may spread in an eccentric fashion, with little extension in one direction but many centimeters of subclinical tumor growth in another.

Careful examination of the histologic status of the margins is essential. Mohs' surgery may be useful in some cases.

Radiation therapy

Radiation therapy is a potential treatment for skin cancers located in critical sites where surgical excision would be disfiguring. Primary basal cell and squamous cell cancers treated with radiation therapy have nearly identical cure rates (about 95%) to those treated with surgical excision.

Radiation therapy is also employed postoperatively to reduce local recurrence rates after excision of high-grade or recurrent sarcomas of the skin. It can also be used postoperatively in patients with basal cell or squamous cell carcinoma when margins are positive.

Topical and intralesional therapy

Topical therapy Occasionally, patients present with numerous skin cancers or tumors in essentially sensitive areas that would be impossible to resect completely. This scenario is particularly common in the immunosuppressed patient who is predisposed to skin cancer development. For these patients, topical therapy with 5-FU or imiquimod cream (a proinflammatory agent with immunostimulation and antitumor properties in superficial malignant lesisons) can dramatically reduce the number of excisions required.

Direct intralesional injection of IFN-α has been reported to treat basal cell cancers successfully. This technique may be particularly helpful for locally recurrent lesions after surgery and/or radiation therapy.

MANAGEMENT OF RECURRENT DISEASE

Local recurrence The vast majority of nonmelanoma skin cancers are successfully treated with surgery or primary irradiation, with fewer than 5% recurring locally. Of those that do recur locally, at least 80% are cured by further local treatment. Regional lymph node metastases develop in about 5% of patients with squamous cell cancers and $\leq$ 1% of patients with basal cell cancers. Nodal metastasis is somewhat more common in Merkel's cell cancers but is very unusual in sarcomas of the skin.

Regardless of the histologic type, whenever clinically obvious nodal enlargement occurs, a needle biopsy should be performed and a therapeutic LND performed if regional spread is documented. There is essentially no role for elective dissections of clinically normal nodes in any form of nonmelanoma skin cancer.

Distant metastasis occurs in about 2% of patients with squamous cell cancers and 0.1% of patients with basal cell cancers, most frequently after nodal recurrence. No effective therapy exists for metastatic nonmelanoma skin cancer, although a few reports of scattered temporary responses to chemotherapy exist. Lippman and colleagues described encouraging results with the combination of IFN-α and 13-*cis*-retinoic acid (isotretinoin [Accutane]).

SUGGESTED READING

ON SKIN CANCERS

Swetter SM, Geller AC, Kirkwood JM: Melanoma in the older person. Oncology 18:1187–1196, 2004.

Tsao H, Atkins MB, Sober AJ: Management of cutaneous melanoma. N Engl J Med 351:998–1012, 2004.

ON BIOLOGY AND EPIDEMIOLOGY OF MELANOMA

Chao C, McMasters KM: Relationship between age and other prognostic factors in melanoma. Am J Oncol Rev 3:446–454, 2004.

Curtin JA, Fridlyand J, Kgeshita T, et al: Distinct sets of genetic alterations in melanoma. N Engl J Med 353:2135–2147, 2005.

Demierre MF, Merlino G: Chemoprevention of melanoma. Curr Oncol Rep 6:406–413, 2004.

Kashani-Sabet M: Melanoma genomics. Curr Oncol Rep 6:401–405, 2004.

Tucker MA, Fraser MC, Goldstein AM, et al: A natural history of melanomas and dysplastic nevi: An atlas of lesions in melanoma-prone families. Cancer 94:3192–3209, 2002.

ON SURGICAL TREATMENT AND IMAGING

Ballo MT, Ang KK: Radiotherapy for cutaneous malignant melanoma: Rationale and indications. Oncology 18:99–108, 2004.

Bonnen MD, Ballo MT, Myers JN, et al: Elective radiotherapy provides regional control for patients with cutaneous melanoma of the head and neck. Cancer 100:383–389, 2004.

DuBay D, Cimmino V, Lowe L, et al: Low recurrence rate after surgery for dermatofibrosarcoma protuberans: A multidisciplinary approach from a single institution. Cancer 100:1008–1016, 2004.

Kammula US, Ghossein R, Bhattacharya S, et al: Serial follow-up and the prognostic significance of reverse transcriptase-polymerase chain reaction–Staged sentinel lymph nodes from melanoma patients. J Clin Oncol 22:3989–3996, 2004.

McMasters KM, Reintgen DS, Ross MI, et al: Sentinel lymph node biopsy for melanoma: Controversy despite widespread agreement. J Clin Oncol 19:2851–2855, 2001.

Mijnhout GS, Hoekstra OS, van Lingen A, et al: How morphometric analysis of metastatic load predicts the (un)usefulness of PET scanning: The case of lymph node staging in melanoma. J Clin Pathol 56:283–286, 2003.

Pawlik TM, Sondak VK: Malignant melanoma: Current state of primary and adjuvant treatment. Crit Rev Oncol Hematol 45:245–264, 2003.

Statius Muller MG, van Leeuwen PA, de Lange-de Klerk ES, et al: The sentinel lymph node status is an important factor for predicting clinical outcome in patients with stage I or II cutaneous melanoma. Cancer 91:2401–2408, 2001.

Thomas JM, Newton-Bishop J, A'Hern R, et al: Excision margins in high-risk malignant melanoma. N Engl J Med 350:757–766, 2004.

ON ADJUVANT THERAPY

Kirkwood JM, Manola J, Ibrahim J, et al: A pooled analysis of Eastern Cooperative Oncology Group and Intergroup trials of adjuvant high-dose interferon for melanoma. Clin Cancer Res 10:1670–1677, 2004.

ON SYSTEMIC THERAPY

Panelli MC, Wang E, Monsurro V, et al: Overview of melanoma vaccines and promising approaches. Curr Oncol Rep 6:414–420, 2004.

Ribas A, Butterfield LH, Glaspy JA, et al: Current developments in cancer vaccines and cellular immunotherapy. J Clin Oncol 21:2415–2432, 2003.

Rosenberg SA: Shedding light on immunotherapy for cancer. N Engl J Med 350:1461–1463, 2004.

Rosenberg SA, Dudley ME: Cancer regression in patients with metastatic melanoma after the transfer of autologous antitumor lymphocytes. Proc Natl Acad Sci 101(suppl 2):14639–14645, 2004.

The ABCDs of moles and melanomas

Concept and photographs:
Robert J. Friedman, MD, Darrell S. Rigel, MD, Alfred W. Kopf, MD, and the Skin Cancer Foundation

People at high risk of developing melanoma are those who have:

- A family history of melanoma, or who have had a melanoma in the past
- Unusual moles on the skin, or changing moles
- Fair skin, light hair and eye color, and who sunburn easily or tan with difficulty
- A record of painful or blistering sunburns as children or in their teenage years
- Indoor occupations and outdoor recreational habits

When you inspect moles, pay special attention to their sizes, shapes, edges, and color. A handy way to remember these features is to think of the A, B, C, and D of skin cancer–asymmetry, border, color, and diameter.

A
Asymmetry

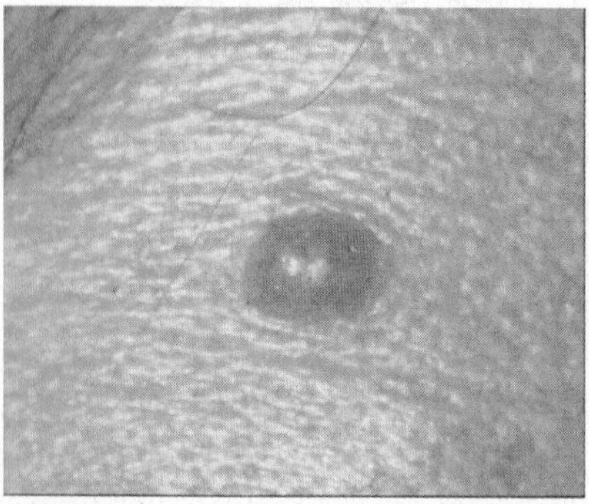

Benign **Symmetrical**

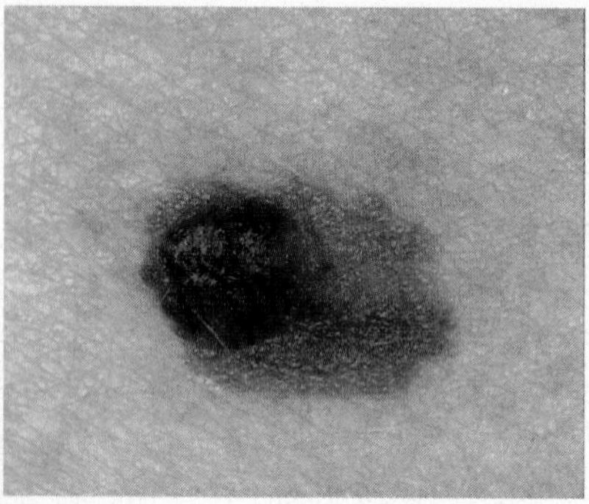

Malignant **Asymmetrical**

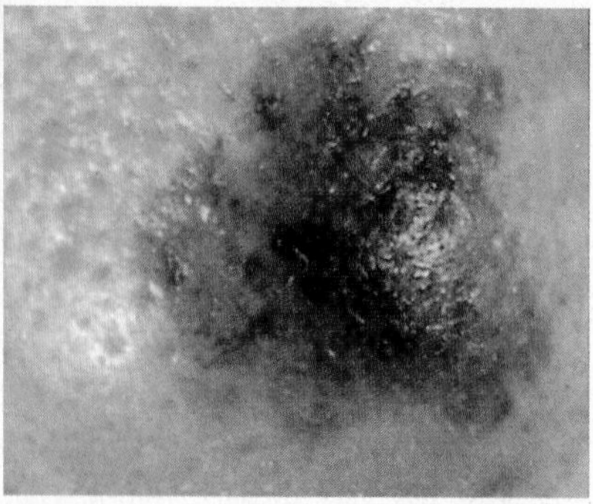

Malignant **Asymmetrical**

Some forms of early malignant melanoma are asymmetrical, meaning that a line drawn through the middle will not create matching halves. Moles are round and symmetrical.

B
Border

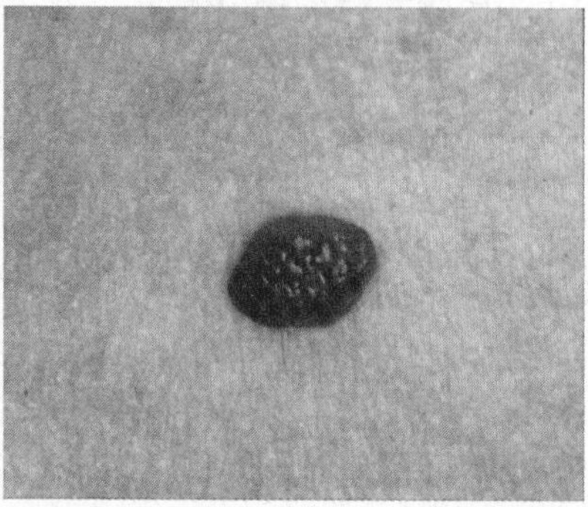

Benign **Even edges**

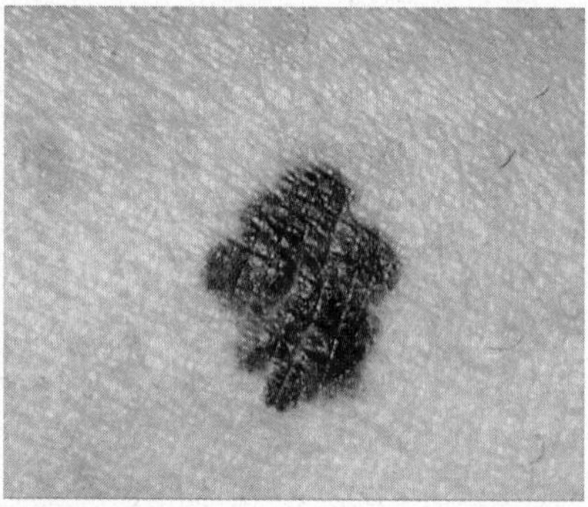

Malignant **Uneven edges**

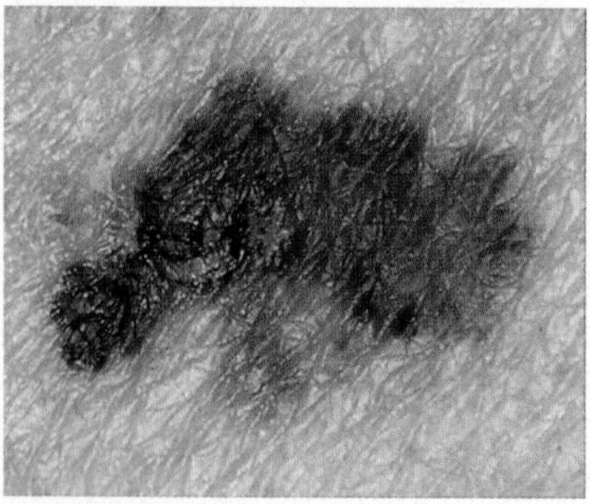

Malignant **Uneven edges**

The borders of early melanomas are frequently uneven, often containing scalloped or notched edges. Common moles have smooth, even borders.

C
Color

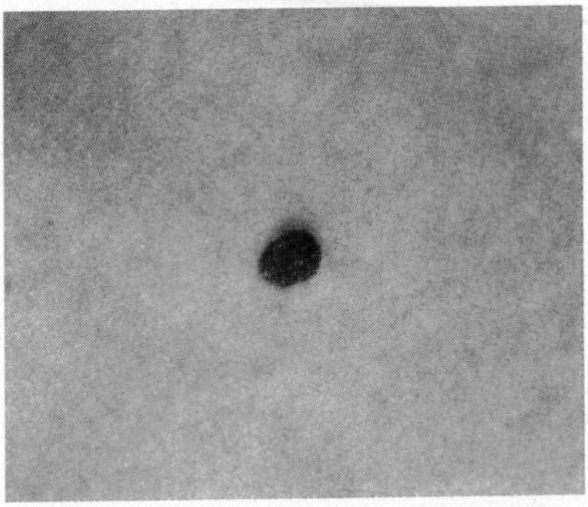
Benign One shade

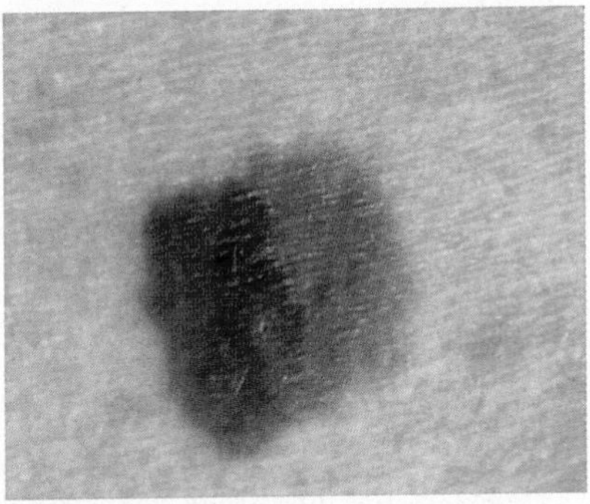
Malignant Two or more shades

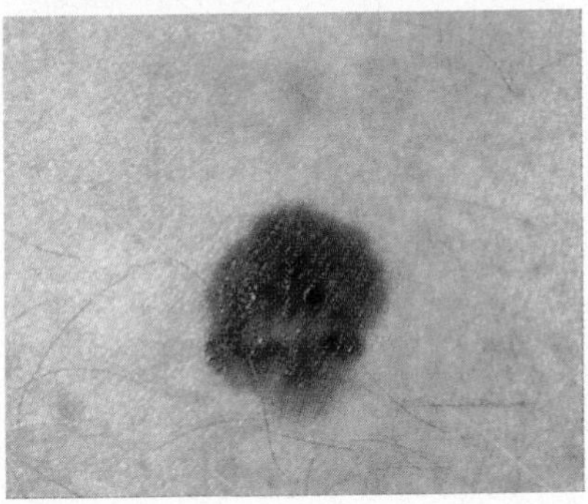
Malignant Two or more shades

Different shades of brown or black are often the first sign of a malignant melanoma. Common moles usually have a single shade of brown.

D
Diameter

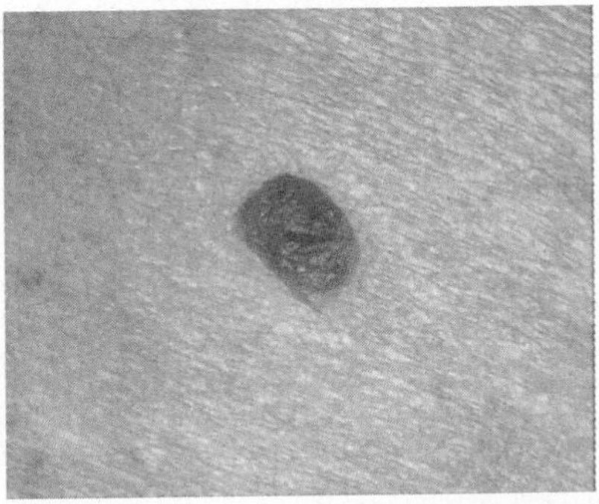
Benign Smaller than 6 mm

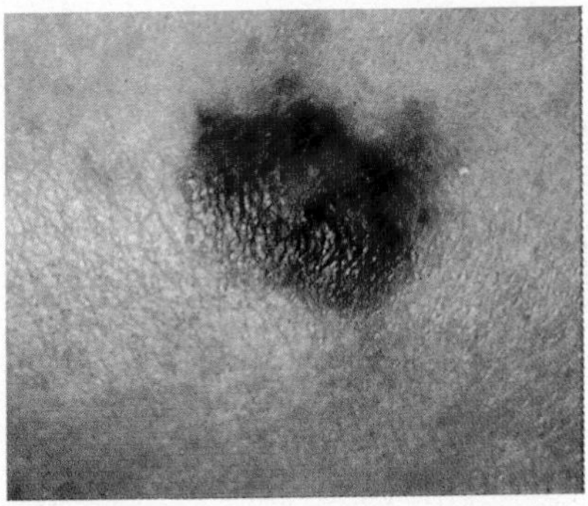
Malignant Larger than 6 mm

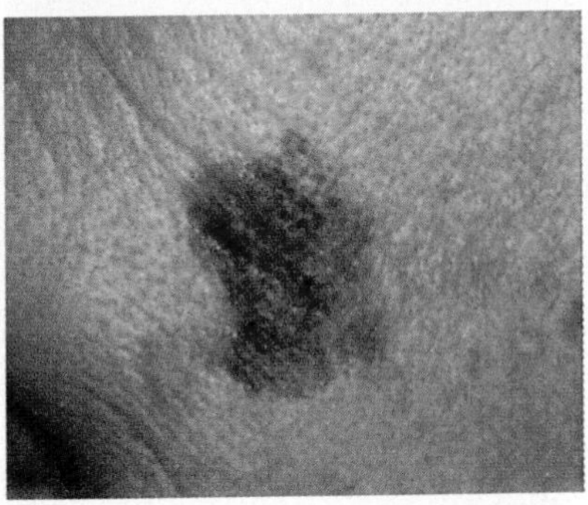
Malignant Larger than 6 mm

Common moles are usualy less than 6 mm in diameter (1/4 in.), the size of a pencil eraser. Early melanomas tend to be larger than 6 mm.

A color atlas of skin lesions

Prepared by Howard Koh, MD, and the
American Academy of Dermatology

COLOR ATLAS

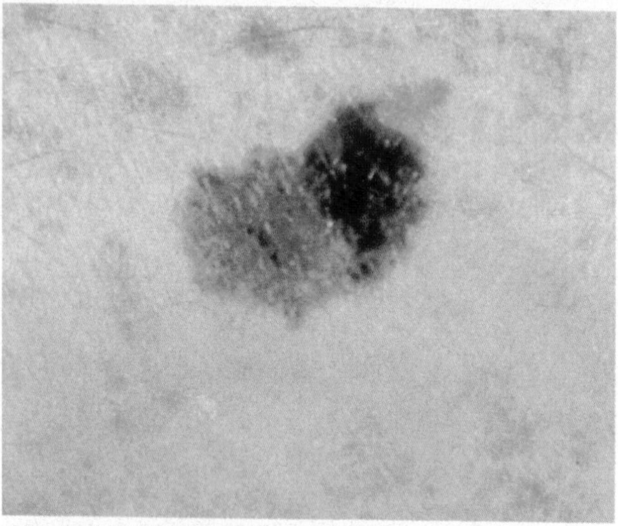

FIGURE 1: Malignant melanoma
The heterogeneous color and asymmetry of the lesion point to the diagnosis of melanoma. Particularly note the black color of the right side of the lesion. (Figures 1, 2, and 8 courtesy of the American Academy of Dermatology)

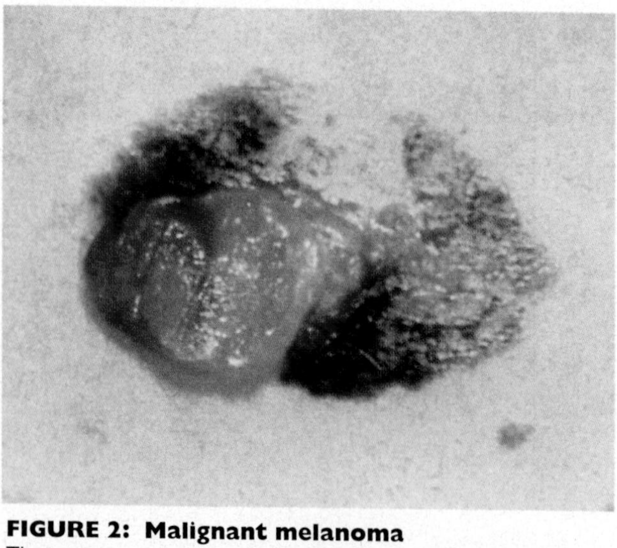

FIGURE 2: Malignant melanoma
There are several colors clearly visible in this lesion, consistent with melanoma. There are mottled black areas of the lesion, with central tumor growth that is eroded and less pigmented.

COLOR ATLAS

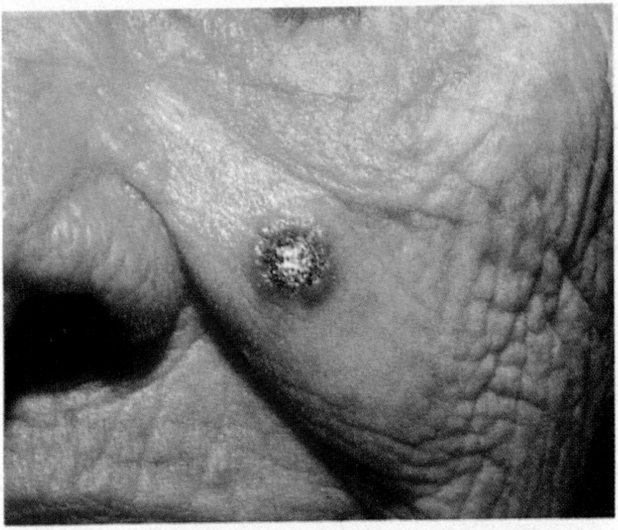

FIGURE 3: Pigmented basal cell epithelioma
While this lesion mimics melanoma, it has a slightly translucent appearance around the rim consistent with the diagnosis of basal cell cancer.

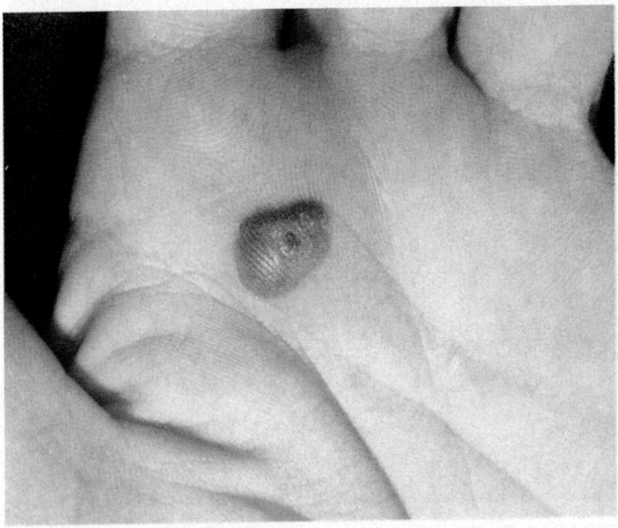

FIGURE 4: Blood blister
Although this lesion mimics melanoma, it is tense, fluid-filled, and benign. Normal skin markings are visible through much of the lesion.

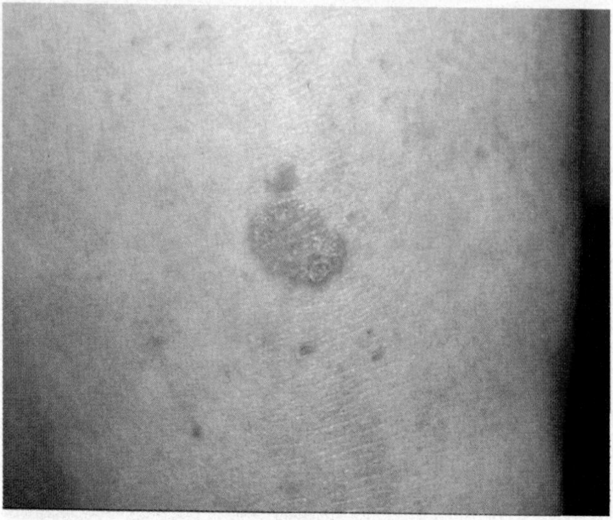

FIGURE 5: Bowen's disease
This sharply demarcated, slightly scaly plaque is typical of squamous cell cancer in situ.

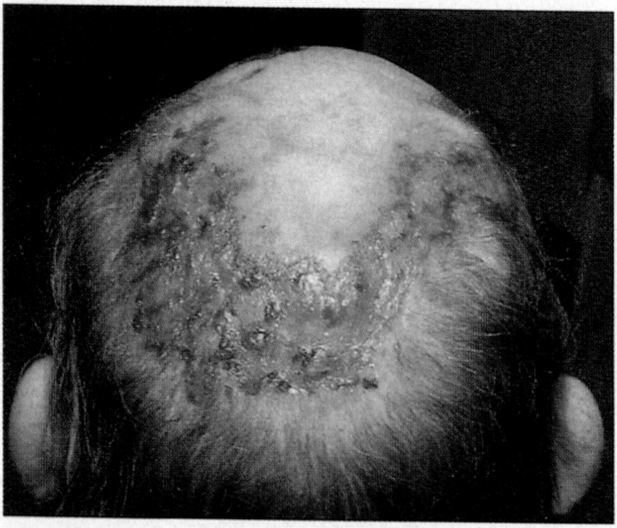

FIGURE 6: Basal cell carcinoma
This patient has extensive, ulcerative disease of the scalp. It is an unusual case that can be diagnosed only through biopsy and is associated with severe morbidity.

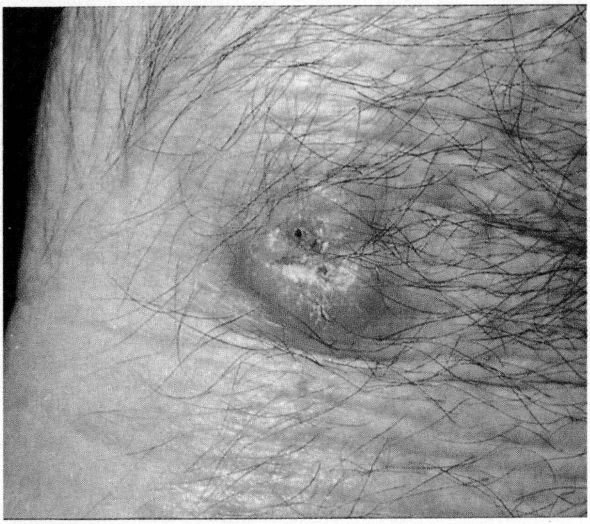

FIGURE 7: Squamous cell carcinoma
This infiltrated red plaque has central erosion and crust.

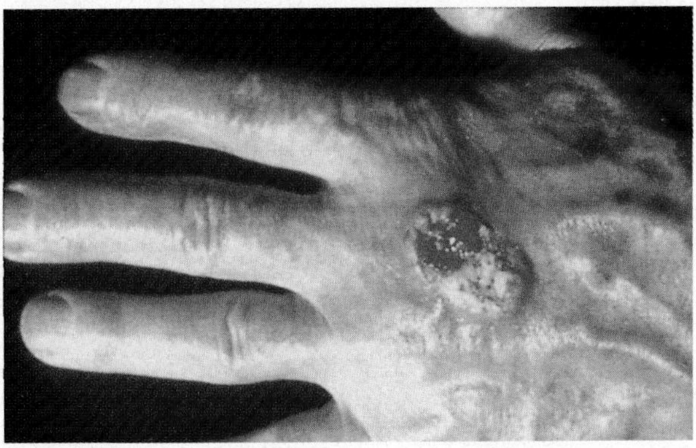

FIGURE 8: Squamous cell carcinoma
Erythematous and infiltrated lesion in a maximally sun-exposed area, with an erosive center.

CHAPTER 24

Bone sarcomas

Alan W. Yasko, MD, and Warren Chow, MD

Bone sarcomas are extremely rare neoplasms, which precludes determination of their true incidence. Approximately 2,760 new cases are identified annually in the United States. Population-based tumor registries seldom separate bone sarcomas into various histologic types.

Osteosarcoma is the most common malignant primary bone tumor (excluding multiple myeloma), comprising 30% of all such malignancies. The annual incidence of osteosarcoma is approximately 800 cases per year in the United States. Chondrosarcoma is the second most common malignant primary tumor of bone; its annual incidence is approximately half that of osteosarcoma. Ewing's sarcoma represents approximately 6% of all primary malignant bone tumors, with an annual incidence of 200 cases. Malignant fibrous histiocytoma (MFH) comprises < 1% of primary bone sarcomas.

Epidemiology

Gender The incidence of primary bone sarcomas is higher in males than in females regardless of histologic type. A low-grade variant of osteosarcoma (parosteal osteosarcoma) is observed more frequently in females.

Age Osteosarcoma and Ewing's sarcoma develop primarily in children and adolescents. A biphasic pattern of incidence of osteosarcoma has been observed; peaks in adolescents (rapid growth of long bones) and in the elderly (secondary tumors arising in association with Paget's disease or within previously irradiated tissue). Chondrosarcomas are rarely seen in skeletally immature patients. They usually develop in middle-aged and older adults. MFH is observed in adults.

Race No predilection has been noted in any particular race. However, Ewing's sarcoma is extremely rare in American and African blacks.

Disease site Any bone and any site within a given bone may be affected. Most osteosarcomas occur in the metaphyseal region of skeletally immature long bones (ie, distal femur, proximal tibia, and proximal humerus), which have the greatest growth potential. Ewing's sarcoma is classically described as a diaphyseal lesion but may arise in any region within an involved long bone. It commonly arises in the flat bones of the pelvis and scapula. Primary bone tumors of any histologic type are extremely rare in the spine and sacrum.

Survival Low-grade sarcomas are associated with the most favorable survival, which approaches 90% in patients with adequately treated tumors. With regard to high-grade sarcomas, survival has improved dramatically in patients with osteosarcoma or Ewing's sarcoma due to the advent of effective multiagent chemotherapy regimens. Survival has improved with multimodality therapy from historic rates of < 20% to current rates of 50%–75%.

Etiology and risk factors

For the majority of bone sarcomas, no specific etiology has been established. A few predisposing factors have been identified.

Genetic factors Children with familial retinoblastoma have a 13q chromosome deletion and an increased incidence of osteosarcoma. Li-Fraumeni syndrome is also associated with an increased risk of bone sarcomas, as well as other cancers such as breast, leukemia, soft-tissue sarcoma, brain, and adrenal cortical tumors. Li-Fraumeni syndrome results from a genetic loss of p53.

Radiation therapy Bone sarcomas constitute a rare but devastating consequence of therapeutic irradiation. Radiation-associated sarcomas develop within the radiation field, usually after a latent period of at least 3 years. The majority of these tumors are osteosarcomas. MFH and other histologies also can arise within a radiation field.

Chemotherapy Alkylating agents and anthracyclines administered for unrelated cancers have been implicated as etiologic factors in the development of second malignant neoplasms, particularly osteosarcoma.

Preexisting benign tumors/conditions Osteosarcomas can arise in association with Paget's disease and rarely in association with benign bone tumors (ie, fibrous dysplasia). Chondrosarcomas can develop in the cartilaginous component of osteochondromas (solitary and multiple hereditary exostosis) and in patients with enchondromatosis (Ollier's disease and Maffucci's syndrome). MFH can arise in association with bone infarcts.

Trauma A traumatic event often prompts medical intervention, at which time the bone sarcoma is detected. The short temporal relationship between the traumatic event and the diagnosis of the tumor usually rules out a causal relationship.

Orthopedic implants Case reports of bone sarcomas arising in the region in which a metallic prosthetic device has been implanted have been published. The rarity of these clinical situations relative to the vast number of devices implanted makes a causal relationship unlikely.

Signs and symptoms

Local symptoms Localized pain and swelling are the hallmark clinical features of bone sarcomas. The pain, which initially is insidious and transient, becomes progressively more severe and unremitting. Localized soft-tissue swelling, with or without associated warmth and erythema, may be present. A joint effusion may be observed, and range of motion of the adjacent joint may be limited and painful. Movement or weight-bearing of the involved extremity may exacerbate local symptoms.

Patients with tumors arising in the lower extremities can present with a painful limp. The neurovascular examination of the affected extremity is usually normal. Regional lymph nodes are rarely involved.

Pathologic fracture may also be a presenting sign, although a history of pain prior to fracture usually can be elicited.

Constitutional symptoms are rare in patients with bone sarcoma, but such symptoms as fever, malaise, and weight loss can be observed in those with Ewing's sarcoma.

Screening and diagnosis

Currently, there is no screening test for primary bone sarcomas. The diagnosis must be made by clinical and radiographic evaluations and confirmed by histopathologic analysis of biopsy-obtained tissue.

Physical examination should include an assessment of the local extent of the soft-tissue mass, if present, and its relationship to the adjacent joint.

Laboratory studies A CBC may demonstrate anemia and/or leukocytosis associated with Ewing's sarcoma, but, in general, results of these studies fall within the normal range. Alkaline phosphatase and lactic dehydrogenase (LDH) levels may be elevated in patients with osteosarcoma or Ewing's sarcoma. An abnormal glucose tolerance test may be observed in patients with chondrosarcomas.

X-rays Biplanar (AP and lateral) plain radiographs of the affected extremity provide critical information on the nature of the bone lesion. The specific site of involvement within the bone, pattern and extent of bone destruction, type of periosteal changes, presence of matrix mineralization within the tumor, and presence of soft-tissue extension may be gleaned from plain films.

CT Standard CT scans provide further delineation of many of these changes.

MRI is the imaging study of choice for the evaluation of the extent of an associated soft-tissue mass and the relationship of the tumor to the neurovascular structures, surrounding soft tissues, and the adjacent joint. The intramedullary extent of the tumor and presence of skip metastases within the bone are best demonstrated by MRI.

Bone scan A bone scan is performed to screen for distant osseous metastases.

Chest radiographic studies A plain film of the chest is required in any patient suspected of having a bone sarcoma. Once the diagnosis of malignancy has been established, a CT scan of the chest is a critical part of initial staging.

Biopsy With few exceptions, a biopsy must be obtained to confirm the diagnosis. Tissue may be obtained by percutaneous (closed) or surgical (open) techniques. The biopsy should be performed by personnel expert in percutaneous biopsy techniques who are familiar with bone tumors and their treatment.

TABLE 1: Surgical staging of bone sarcomas

Stage	Grade	Site
IA	Low	Intracompartmental
IB	Low	Extracompartmental
IIA	High	Intracompartmental
IIB	High	Extracompartmental
III	Any regional or distant metastasis	Any

Enneking WF, Spanier SS, Goodman MA: A system for the surgical staging of musculoskeletal sarcoma. Clin Orthop 153:106–120, 1980.

Biopsies performed at referring institutions have been reported to be associated with a higher incidence of misdiagnosis and complications, which may affect patient outcome. Optimally, the biopsy should be performed at the institution where definitive treatment will be given.

Pathology

Histologic subtypes Current histopathologic classification of bone neoplasms is based on the putative cell of origin. Malignant tumors may arise from any cellular constituent present in bone, including osteogenic (osteosarcoma), chondrogenic (chondrosarcoma), hematopoietic (multiple myeloma, lymphoma), vascular (angiosarcoma, hemangioendothelioma, leiomyosarcoma), lipogenic (liposarcoma), neurogenic (neurofibrosarcoma, chordoma), and histiocytic and fibrohistiocytic (MFH, Ewing's sarcoma) elements. Histologic subtyping is based on the predominant cellular pattern present within the tumor, degree of anaplasia, and relationship of the tumor to the bone (intramedullary vs surface).

A monoclonal antibody (CD99) that recognizes a cell-surface glycoprotein (p30/32MIC2) in human Ewing's sarcoma and peripheral neuroectodermal tumor (PNET) has been developed. There is strong immunoreactivity of CD99 in Ewing's sarcoma and PNET that aids in distinguishing these tumors from other small round-cell tumors of childhood and adolescence. Additional experience with CD99, however, demonstrates that it is not exclusively specific for Ewing's sarcoma and PNET.

Dedifferentiation Primary bone sarcomas can exhibit the phenomenon of "dedifferentiation." These neoplasms demonstrate a dimorphic histologic pattern, which is characterized by the presence of a borderline malignant or low-grade malignant tumor juxtaposed against a high-grade, histologically different sarcoma. Enchondromas, low-grade chondrosarcomas, low-grade variants of osteosarcoma (surface and intramedullary), and chordomas may all develop an area of high-grade spindle-cell tumor, usually MFH.

Metastatic spread Approximately 10%–20% of patients with osteosarcoma and 15%–35% of patients with Ewing's sarcoma have evidence of metastatic disease at initial presentation. In approximately 90% of patients with bone sarcomas, the initial site of distant metastasis is the lungs. Distant osseous sites, bone marrow, and viscera may also be involved as a manifestation of advanced disease, but involvement of these sites is less common and usually occurs after the development of pulmonary metastases. Regional lymph node involvement is rare.

Staging and prognosis

Staging system The staging system of the Musculoskeletal Tumor Society (MTS) is currently used (Table 1). This system is based on tumor grade (I = low or II = high), tumor extent (A = intraosseous involvement only or B = extraosseous extension), and presence of distant metastases, regardless of the extent of local disease (III). Patients with a localized tumor may have stage IA, IB, IIA, or IIB disease.

Prognostic factors Many studies have demonstrated that tumor response to preoperative chemotherapy, as determined by histologic analysis of the resected specimen, is the most powerful predictor of survival for patients with osteosarcoma. Adverse prognostic indicators, such as an axial primary tumor or elevated LDH and alkaline phosphatase levels, signal an even worse outcome.

Tumor size (low volume) and anatomic site (peripheral), absence of metastases at initial presentation, and good histologic response to chemotherapy are prognostic variables associated with better outcome in patients with osteosarcomas and Ewing's sarcoma. The translocation t(11;22), which results in the type 1 EWS-FLI1 fusion, is also a significant positive predictor of overall survival in Ewing's sarcoma.

For low-grade malignant tumors, adequacy of surgery is the most significant predictor of outcome.

Treatment

PRIMARY TREATMENT OF BONE SARCOMAS

Surgical excision is the mainstay of treatment for patients with low-grade sarcomas. For high-grade tumors, multimodality therapy is indicated. For most high-grade bone sarcomas, excluding chondrosarcoma, preoperative multiagent chemotherapy (3 to 4 cycles) is followed by surgical extirpation of the primary tumor. Chemotherapy is reinitiated postoperatively after wound healing has occurred (usually 2–3 weeks after surgery).

For patients with Ewing's sarcoma, the optimal therapy for local tumor control is less well defined. Historically, radiotherapy has been a mainstay of local treatment. However, there has been a recent trend toward surgery, with or without radiotherapy, to achieve local tumor control. No prospective, randomized studies have been performed to define the relative role of each of these treatment modalities, but several retrospective studies suggest improvements in local tumor control and patient survival when surgery is satisfactorily performed. Patients with unresectable tumors or microscopic or macroscopic residual disease following tumor excision clearly require adjuvant radiotherapy to consolidate their local treatment.

Surgical treatment strategy

The MTS recognizes wide excision, either by amputation or a limb-salvage procedure, as the recommended surgical approach for high-grade sarcomas. A wide excision removes the primary tumor en bloc along with its reactive zone and a cuff of normal tissue in all planes. Conceptually, this strategy is applicable to all high-grade sarcomas. Wide excision successfully controls local disease in ≥ 90% of patients.

The timing of surgery must be coordinated with the patient's chemotherapy schedule and with bone marrow recovery to minimize the period of systemic therapy. Generally, surgical intervention is postponed until the patient's absolute neutrophil count (ANC) has recovered to a level of ≥ 1,500/μL and platelet count, to a level of ≥ 70,000/μL.

Limb-salvage procedures

Wide tumor excision with limb preservation has supplanted amputation as the principal surgical method for eradicating local disease in patients with primary sarcomas of bone, regardless of histology or grade. Local tumor control and patient survival have not been compromised by this more conservative operative strategy. Refinements in surgical techniques and advances in bioengineering have increased the number of patients eligible for limb-salvage surgery. Currently, 75%–80% of patients may be treated with conservative surgery.

Successful limb-salvage surgery for the patient with a high-grade bone sarcoma is predicated on complete extirpation of the tumor, effective skeletal reconstruction, and adequate soft-tissue coverage. Planning for the operative procedure must begin far in advance to permit adequate time to procure the implant for reconstruction.

Types of resection Limb-sparing tumor resection falls into one of three types based on the anatomic site and extent of involved bone to be excised. Resection can involve (1) tumor-bearing bone and the adjacent joint (osteoarticular), (2) tumor-bearing bone only (intercalary), or (3) whole bone and adjacent joints (whole bone).

Since most bone sarcomas arise in the metaphysis of the long bone near the joint, the majority of procedures performed for these tumors involve resection of both the segment of tumor-bearing bone and the adjacent joint (osteoarticular resection). Most of these resections are performed through the adjacent joint (intra-articular). When the tumor extends along the joint capsule or ligamentous structures and/or invades the joint, the entire joint should be resected (extra-articular) to avoid violating areas that have tumor involvement.

Reconstruction Prosthetic arthroplasty is the most common method by which the skeletal defect and adjacent joint are reconstructed. Osteoarticular allografts, intercalary allografts, and vascularized and nonvascularized autografts are also used, depending on the extent of resection and requirements for successful reconstruction.

Tumors in the immature skeleton

Tumors arising in the immature skeleton pose a unique problem for the orthopedic oncologist, particularly in patients with substantial projected growth of the involved extremity. The surgical management of bone sarcomas in young patients, with few exceptions, has entailed amputation or rotationplasty.

Custom-manufactured expandable metallic joint prostheses can be implanted to allow for skeletal growth in those children deemed candidates for limb-salvage surgery. The long-term outcome of this technique has been promising. However, multiple operative procedures should be anticipated to maintain a functional extremity.

Soft-tissue coverage

Adequate soft-tissue coverage is critical to the success of any limb-salvage procedure. Local transposition muscle flaps and free tissue transfers are extremely useful for providing a healthy, well-vascularized soft-tissue envelope to cover the reconstruction and reduce the risk of deep infection.

SURGICAL TREATMENT OF METASTATIC DISEASE

The most common site of metastatic involvement for bone sarcoma is the lungs. Patients who present with pulmonary metastases (10%–20% of patients with osteosarcoma) have a poor prognosis (5-year survival rate < 15%). Approximately 30%–40% of patients who present with localized disease and who subsequently develop resectable pulmonary metastases can undergo salvage treatment with reinduction chemotherapy and metastasectomy (see section on "Treatment of advanced osteosarcoma"). Patients with extrapulmonary metastases or unresectable pulmonary metastases have a uniformly poor prognosis. The objective of any surgical intervention in these patients, therefore, would be palliative.

CHEMOTHERAPY FOR OSTEOSARCOMA

The probability of 5-year disease-free survival for patients with osteosarcoma of the extremities treated with either amputation or limb-salvage surgery alone is < 20%. Although the incidence of local recurrence is low, microscopic dissemination is likely to be present in 80% of patients at the time of diagnosis, leading to distant metastases, mostly in the lungs and bones, within the first 6–12 months. The incorporation of chemotherapy as part of the standard therapeutic plan for osteosarcoma (Table 2) has improved both relapse-free and overall survival.

Neoadjuvant/adjuvant chemotherapy

To achieve better systemic control and decrease the degree of functional defect following surgery, neoadjuvant (presurgical) treatment programs have been developed by several centers. Early trials incorporated high doses of metho-

TABLE 2: Chemotherapy regimens for bone sarcomas

Drug/combination	Dose and schedule
T-12 regimens	
Preresection:	
Methotrexate	8-12 g/m^2 IV on day 1 of week 0, day 8 of week 1, day 29 of week 4, and day 36 of week 5
Leucovorin	10-15 mg PO every 6 hours for 10 doses beginning 20 hours after each methotrexate dose and completed when the serum methotrexate level is $<$ 100 nmol/L. Additional leucovorin should be administered if elevated serum methotrexate levels are noted or if renal toxicity is present.
BCD regimen	
Bleomycin	15 U/m^2 IV bolus × 2 (on days 15 and 16 of week 2)
Cyclophosphamide	600 mg/m^2/d IV bolus × 2 days (on days 15 and 16 of week 2)
Dactinomycin	600 μg/m^2/d IV bolus × 2 days (on days 15 and 16 of week 2)
Preoperative chemotherapy is completed in 6 weeks and followed by definitive surgery between day 43 of week 6 and day 50 of week 7	
Postresection regimen for patients with primary tumor grades 1 and 2 (less necrosis):	
Doxorubicin	25 mg/m^2 IV continuous infusion over 3 days (on days 57, 58, 59 of week 8; days 106, 107, 108 of week 15; days 155, 156, 157 of week 22; days 190, 191, 192 of week 27; and days 225, 226, 227 of week 32)
Cisplatin	120 mg/m^2 IV on day 57 of week 8, day 106 of week 15, day 155 of week 22, day 190 of week 27, and day 225 of week 32
Methotrexate	As above on day 78 of week 11, day 99 of week 14, day 127 of week 18, and day 148 of week 21
BCD	Regimen as above on day 85 of week 12, day 134 of week 19, day 176 of week 25, and day 211 of week 30
Postresection regimen for patients with primary tumor grades 3 or 4 (more necrosis):	
Doxorubicin	As above on days 57, 58, 59 of week 8; days 106, 107, 108 of week 15; days 155, 156, 157 of week 22; and days 204, 205, 206 of week 29
Methotrexate	As above on day 78 of week 11, day 99 of week 14, day 127 of week 18, day 148 of week 21, day 176 of week 25, day 197 of week 28, day 225 of week 32, and day 246 of week 35
BCD	Regimen as above on days 85 and 86 of week 12, days 134 and 135 of week 19, days 183 and 184 of week 26, and days 232 and 233 of week 33

NOTE: Administering this protocol safely and successfully requires extensive experience and excellent supportive care.

Meyers PA, Gorlick R, Heller G, et al: J Clin Oncol 16:2452–2458, 1998.

Table prepared by Ishmael Jaiyesimi, DO

trexate, given weekly for 4 weeks with leucovorin rescue, prior to surgery. Subsequent modifications included the incorporation of bleomycin, dactinomycin (Cosmegen), and cyclophosphamide into the regimen, with the further addition of doxorubicin.

Long-term follow-up is necessary for patients treated for osteosarcoma. Late side effects of neoadjuvant chemotherapy for osteosarcoma were assessed in a retrospective review performed by investigators at the Rizzoli Institute in Italy. Of the 755 patients with localized osteosarcoma treated with 6 subsequent protocols, the following side effects were noted: symptomatic cardiomyopathy (1.7%), second malignant neoplasms (2.1% after a median of 7 years), permanent azoospermia (100% in men who received 60–75 g/m^2 of ifosfamide), subclinical renal impairment (48% in those who received > 60 g/m^2 of ifosfamide), and hearing impairment (40% of those who received cisplatin; *Longhi A, Ferrari S, Ferrari C, et al: J Clin Oncol [abstract] 24:522s, 2006*).

The next generation of trials adjusted the adjuvant (postoperative) chemotherapeutic regimen, depending on the degree of tumor necrosis found at the time of surgery. Patients who had a good tumor response (> 90% necrosis) were treated with additional cycles of the neoadjuvant regimen; those who had a poor response received cisplatin and doxorubicin. It remains controversial whether altering the adjuvant chemotherapeutic regimen for patients with poor histologic response truly changes their event-free survival.

The addition of ifosfamide (Ifex) did not improve survival in pediatric patients with osteosarcoma in a recent study. A Children's Oncology Group (COG) study reported no difference in outcome between a three-drug combination of cisplatin, doxorubicin, and high-dose methotrexate and a four-drug regimen of the same drugs plus ifosfamide. The European Osteosarcoma Intergroup (EOI) reported no difference in histopathologic response to preoperative chemotherapy and overall survival in patients randomized to receive a two-drug regimen with doxorubicin and cisplatin or a complex multidrug protocol containing doxorubicin, cisplatin, and high-dose methotrexate among other agents.

The EOI also investigated standard-dose vs increased-dose intensity (dose-dense) cisplatin and doxorubicin for patients with operable osteosarcoma of the extremity. The overall dose intensity was increased by 24% for cisplatin and 25% for doxorubicin. Good histologic response (≤ 10% viable tumor) was significantly higher in the intensified arm (51% vs 36%). Unfortunately, overall survival at 4 years was not significantly different (61% for standard and 64% for intensified).

The actuarial 5-year event-free survival rate in patients presenting with localized, primarily extremity osteosarcoma is > 70%. Regardless of the multidrug therapy used, event-free survival correlates with histologic response. Patients with > 90% tumor necrosis have a > 80% probability of 5-year event-free survival. Complete responses are more likely to occur in patients with the nonchondroblastic subtype and in those whose peak serum methotrexate levels are > 700 µmol/L. Chemosensitivity also seems to be diminished in patients with metastatic disease at presentation.

Poor responders Patients with poor tumor response may represent 30%–60% of the population with extremity osteosarcoma. For these patients, more effective treatment regimens, such as dose intensification using growth factors and stem-cell support, and newer agents need to be evaluated.

Alternative approaches One alternative approach to neoadjuvant therapy is adjuvant therapy. A randomized study of the Pediatric Oncology Group (POG) demonstrated no detectable difference in event-free survival whether chemotherapy was offered before or after surgery. The feasibility of safely performing limb-salvage surgery in these patients, however, has not been studied directly. Additionally, intra-arterial delivery of cytotoxic agents has shown no specific survival benefit but provides increased concentration of chemotherapy to the primary tumor, which may impact favorably on the extent of the resection for patients undergoing limb-salvage surgery.

Laboratory and clinical evidence has demonstrated synergistic cytotoxicity with sequential treatment of soft-tissue and bone sarcomas with gemcitabine (Gemzar) followed by docetaxel (Taxotere). This regimen resulted in an overall response rate of 43% in multiple types of soft-tissue sarcomas, osteosarcomas, and Ewing's sarcoma at the University of Michigan Comprehensive Cancer Center. These results have led to the development of a multi-institutional clinical trial of this regimen in patients with advanced osteogenic sarcoma (*Leu KM, Ostruszka LJ, Shewach D, et al: J Clin Oncol 22:1706-1712, 2004*).

TREATMENT OF ADVANCED OSTEOSARCOMA

Axial primary tumor For the 10%–15% of patients who present with axial primary osteosarcoma, neoadjuvant chemotherapy should be considered to reduce the tumor burden prior to surgery or radiation therapy. The Cooperative Osteosarcoma Study Group (COSS) reported that 11.4% of its patients treated before 1999 had proven metastases at diagnosis. Actuarial survival at 5 and 10 years was 29% and 24%, respectively, when treated with preoperative and postoperative multiagent chemotherapy as well as aggressive surgery for all resectable lesions. Multivariate Cox regression analysis demonstrated that multiple metastases at diagnosis and macroscopically incomplete surgical resection are significantly associated with inferior outcomes in patients with primary metastatic osteosarcoma.

Pulmonary metastasis Patients with metastatic disease to the lungs should be evaluated for resection. Following aggressive pulmonary metastasectomy, < 25% of patients will achieve prolonged relapse-free survival. Hence, these patients may also benefit from aggressive "secondary" adjuvant chemotherapy.

Chemotherapy should also be considered for patients whose pulmonary metastases are unresectable, with the intention of performing surgery in those who have a sufficient response; approximately 10% of such patients may become long-term survivors.

Poor-risk patients or patients with recurrent disease are candidates for clinical trials that evaluate chemotherapy dose intensification or newer therapeutic agents. Alternatively, the POG demonstrated stabilization of disease in patients with recurrent or refractory osteosarcoma employing the combination of cyclophosphamide and topotecan (Hycamtin), although objective responses were rare. Interestingly, investigators at the Mayo Clinic reported significant palliation of pain in osteosarcoma patients with symptomatic bone metastases who were treated with samarium-153-ethylene diamine tetramethylene phosphonate (^{153}Sm-EDTMP), a bone-seeking radiopharmaceutical, in conjunction with stem-cell rescue. Nonhematologic side effects were minimal.

The prognosis for patients who develop metachronous skeletal osteosarcoma has been considered grave compared with that for patients with relapse limited to the lungs. Investigators at Memorial Sloan-Kettering Cancer Center reported that in a small subset of patients who developed metachronous osteosarcoma at 24 months or more from the initial diagnosis (11 of 23 patients with osteosarcoma), combined-modality therapy with surgery and aggressive chemotherapy resulted in a 5-year postmetachronous survival rate of 83%, vs 40% for patients receiving monotherapy (usually surgery) only. These results refute an earlier pessimistic sentiment.

CHEMOTHERAPY FOR EWING'S SARCOMA

Prior to the availability of effective chemotherapeutic agents, < 10% of patients with Ewing's sarcoma survived beyond 5 years. The first intergroup Ewing's sarcoma study demonstrated an improved survival rate for patients receiving systemic therapy with the VACA regimen (vincristine, Actinomycin D [dactinomycin], cyclophosphamide, Adriamycin [doxorubicin]) for the first three drugs only and for patients receiving VAC plus bilateral pulmonary irradiation. In the future, selection of a specific therapeutic regimen may be influenced by the presence of molecular markers in addition to standard clinical criteria.

In the second intergroup study, the addition of doxorubicin to VAC, when given on an intermittent schedule and at a higher dose, improved the 5-year relapse-free survival rate to 73%; this rate was almost double that of the cohort of patients not receiving doxorubicin as part of their treatment. The worst results were observed in patients with pelvic, proximal extremity, and lumbar vertebral lesions.

In a phase III study, the addition of ifosfamide and etoposide to standard chemotherapy (doxorubicin, vincristine, cyclophosphamide, and dactinomycin) for patients with Ewing's sarcoma and PNET of the bone significantly improved overall survival for patients with localized disease (72% vs 61%), but it did not affect the outcome for patients with metastatic disease (overall survival 34% vs 35%). In addition to biologic adverse features at presentation (male sex, age, high LDH levels, anemia, fever, axial locations, non-type 1 fusion transcripts, and lack of feasibility of surgical resection), independent prognostic factors also include the type of chemotherapy and degree of tumor necrosis.

CHEMOTHERAPY FOR ADVANCED EWING'S SARCOMA

Aggressive combination chemotherapy and irradiation can lead to prolonged disease progression-free survival, even in patients with metastatic disease. The combination of ifosfamide (1.6 g/m^2) and etoposide (100 mg/m^2 given on days 1–5) results in high response rates of > 80%. Unfortunately, late recurrences are not uncommon.

Dose intensification of active chemotherapeutic compounds, including those employing autologous stem-cell rescue, has not been definitively shown to significantly improve survival of patients with poor-risk and metastatic Ewing's sarcoma and PNET. However, dose-dense chemotherapy is postulated to improve outcome in localized Ewing's sarcoma and is the focus of a randomized phase III trial of the COG. The arms studied were standard chemotherapy with growth factor support given every 3 weeks vs every 2 weeks. Newer therapeutic agents should be tested.

In patients with recurrent or refractory Ewing's sarcoma, the combination of cyclophosphamide and topotecan was shown to possess significant antitumor activity by the POG.

SUGGESTED READING

Anderson PM, Wiseman GA, Dispenzieri A, et al: High-dose samarium-153 ethylene diamine tetramethylene phosphonate: Low toxicity of skeletal irradiation in patients with osteosarcoma and bone metastases. J Clin Oncol 20:189–196, 2002.

Goorin AM, Schwartzentruber DJ, Devidas M, et al: Presurgical chemotherapy compared with immediate surgery and adjuvant chemotherapy for nonmetastatic osteosarcoma: Pediatric Oncology Group Study POG-8651. J Clin Oncol 21:1574–1580, 2003.

Grier HE, Krailo MD, Tarbell NJ, et al: Addition of ifosfamide and etoposide to standard chemotherapy in Ewing's sarcoma/primitive neuroectodermal tumor of bone. N Engl J Med 384:694–701, 2003.

Grimer RJ, Carter SR, Tillman RM, et al: Chondrosarcoma of bone: An assessment of outcome. J Bone Joint Surg Am 82:1203–1204, 2000.

Kager L, Zoubek A, Pötschger U, et al: Primary metastatic osteosarcoma: Presentation and outcome of patients treated on neoadjuvant Cooperative Osteosarcoma Study Group protocols. J Clin Oncol 21:2011–2018, 2003.

Ladanyi M: EWS-FLI1 and Ewing's sarcoma: Recent molecular data and new insights. Cancer Biol Ther 1:330–336, 2002.

Lewis IJ, Nooji M, for the European Osteosarcoma Intergroup: Chemotherapy at standard or increased dose intensity in patients with operable osteosarcoma of the extremity: A randomized controlled trial conducted by the European Osteosarcoma Intergroup (ISRCTN 86294690) (abstract). Proc Am Soc Clin Oncol 22:816, 2003.

Malawer MM, Chou LB: Prosthetic survival and clinical results with use of large-segment replacements in the treatment of high-grade bone sarcomas. J Bone Joint Surg Am 77:1154–1165, 1995.

Malo M, Davis AM, Wunder J, et al: Functional evaluation in distal femoral endoprosthetic replacement for bone sarcoma. Clin Orthop 389:173–180, 2001.

Meyers PA, Schwartz CL, Krailo M, et al: Osteosarcoma: A randomized, prospective trial of the addition of ifosfamide and/or muramyl tripeptide to cisplatin, doxorubicin, and high-dose methotrexate. J Clin Oncol 23:2004–2011, 2005.

Saylors RL, Stine KC, Sullivan J, et al: Cyclophosphamide plus topotecan in children with recurrent or refractory solid tumors: A Pediatric Oncology Group phase II study. J Clin Oncol 19:3463–3469, 2001.

Souhami RL, Craft AW, Van der Eijken JW, et al: Randomised trial of two regimens of chemotherapy in operable osteosarcoma: A study of the European Osteosarcoma Intergroup. Lancet 350:911–917, 1997.

CHAPTER 25

Soft-tissue sarcomas

Peter W. T. Pisters, MD, Mitchell Weiss, MD, Robert Maki, MD, PhD, and Gary N. Mann, MD

The soft-tissue sarcomas are a group of rare but anatomically and histologically diverse neoplasms. This is due to the ubiquitous location of the soft tissues and the nearly three dozen recognized histologic subtypes of soft-tissue sarcomas. In the United States, approximately 9,500 new cases of soft-tissue sarcoma are identified annually, and about 3,500 patients die of the disease each year. The age-adjusted incidence is 2 cases per 100,000 persons.

Epidemiology

Unlike the more common malignancies, such as colon cancer, little is known about the epidemiology of soft-tissue sarcomas. This, again, reflects the uncommon nature of these lesions.

Gender There is a slight male predominance, with a male-to-female ratio of 1.1:1.0.

Age The age distribution in adult soft-tissue sarcoma studies is < 40 years, 20.7% of patients; 40–60 years, 27.6% of patients; and > 60 years, 51.7% of patients.

Race Studies in large cohorts of patients demonstrate that the race distribution of soft-tissue sarcomas mirrors that of the American population (86% Caucasian, 10% African-American, 1% Asian-American, and 3% other).

Geography Studies have suggested that the incidence and mortality of soft-tissue sarcomas may be increasing in New Zealand. There are no currently available data addressing this possibility in the United States.

Etiology and risk factors

In the majority of cases of patients with soft-tissue sarcoma, no specific etiologic agent is identifiable. However, a number of predisposing factors have been recognized.

Radiation therapy Soft-tissue sarcomas have been reported to originate in radiation fields following therapeutic irradiation for a variety of solid tumors. Frequently, they are seen in the lower-dose regions at the edge of the radiation target volume. By definition, radiation-induced sarcomas arise no sooner than

3 years after radiation therapy and often develop decades later. The majority of these sarcomas are high-grade lesions (90%), and osteosarcoma is a predominant histology. Malignant fibrous histiocytoma (MFH), angiosarcoma, and other histologic subtypes have also been reported.

Chemical exposure Exposure to various chemicals in specific occupations or situations has been linked with the development of soft-tissue sarcoma. These chemicals include the phenoxy acetic acids (forestry and agriculture workers), chlorophenols (sawmill workers), Thorotrast (diagnostic x-ray technicians), vinyl chloride (individuals working with this gas, used in making plastics and as a refrigerant), and arsenic (vineyard workers).

Chemotherapy Soft-tissue sarcomas have been reported after previous exposure to alkylating chemotherapeutic agents, most commonly after treatment of pediatric acute lymphocytic leukemia. The drugs implicated include cyclophosphamide, melphalan (Alkeran), procarbazine (Matulane), nitrosoureas, and chlorambucil (Leukeran). The relative risk of sarcoma appears to increase with cumulative drug exposure.

Chronic lymphedema Soft-tissue sarcomas have been noted to arise in the chronically lymphedematous arms of women treated with radical mastectomy for breast cancer (Stewart-Treves syndrome). Lower-extremity lymphangiosarcomas have also been observed in patients with congenital lymphedema or filariasis complicated by chronic lymphedema.

Trauma and foreign bodies Although a recent history of trauma is often elicited from patients presenting with soft-tissue sarcoma, the interval between the traumatic event and diagnosis is often short; thus, a causal relationship is unlikely. Chronic inflammatory processes, however, may be a risk factor for sarcoma. Foreign bodies, such as shrapnel, bullets, and implants, have also been implicated.

Signs and symptoms

Signs and symptoms of soft-tissue sarcoma depend, in large part, on the anatomic site of origin. Due to the ubiquitous location of the soft tissues, these malignancies may arise at any site in the body where soft tissues are located. Since 50% of soft-tissue sarcomas arise in an extremity, the majority of patients present with a palpable soft-tissue mass. Pain at presentation is noted in only one-third of cases.

Extremity and superficial trunk Extremity and superficial trunk sarcomas account for 60% of all soft-tissue sarcomas. The majority of patients present with a painless primary soft-tissue mass.

Retroperitoneum Retroperitoneal sarcomas account for 15% of all soft-tissue sarcomas. Most patients (80%) present with an abdominal mass, with 50% of patients reporting pain at presentation. Due to the considerable size of the retroperitoneum and the relative mobility of the anterior intra-abdominal organs, these tumors often grow to substantial size before the patient's nonspecific complaints are evaluated or even before an abdominal mass is noted on physical examination.

Viscera Visceral soft-tissue sarcomas, which comprise 15% of all soft-tissue sarcomas, present with signs and symptoms unique to their viscus of origin. For example, GI leiomyosarcomas or gastrointestinal stromal tumors (GISTs) present with GI symptoms that are usually indistinguishable from those of the more common adenocarcinomas. Similarly, uterine leiomyosarcomas frequently present with painless vaginal bleeding, such as that often noted in patients with more common uterine malignancies.

Head and neck Head and neck sarcomas comprise 10% of all soft-tissue sarcomas. Although generally smaller than sarcomas in other sites, they may present with important mechanical problems related to compression or invasion of adjacent anatomy (eg, orbital contents, airway, or pharynx). In addition, their proximity to critical anatomy can pose management difficulties due to compromise in the delivery of both surgery and radiotherapy.

Pathology

Histopathologic classification As a consequence of the wide spectrum of soft tissues, a variety of histologically distinct neoplasms have been characterized. The current histopathologic classification is based on the putative cell of origin of each lesion. Such classification based on histogenesis is reproducible for the more differentiated tumors. However, as the degree of histologic differentiation declines, it becomes increasingly difficult to determine cellular origin.

In addition, many of these tumors dedifferentiate. This process results in a variety of overlapping patterns, making uniform classification difficult. Experienced soft-tissue pathologists frequently disagree as to the cell of origin of an individual tumor. Comparative studies have demonstrated concordance in histopathologic diagnosis in only two-thirds of cases. MFH used to be the most common histologic subtype of soft-tissue sarcoma. However, in one study, reanalysis histologically, immunohistochemically, and ultrastructurally allowed reclassification in 84% of tumors to a specific line of differentiation. GIST is now recognized as the most common form of sarcoma.

Assignment of a specific histologic subtype is of secondary importance. This is because, with the possible exceptions of certain small-cell sarcomas, rhabdomyosarcoma, fibrosarcoma, and some forms of angiosarcoma, histogenesis is not directly related to biologic behavior. The propensity for distant metastases and disease-related mortality are best predicted on the basis of histologic grade and tumor size.

TABLE 1: AJCC/UICC staging system for soft-tissue sarcomas

Primary tumor (T)

Tx	Primary tumor cannot be assessed
T0	No evidence of primary tumor
T1	Tumor ≤ 5 cm in greatest dimension
T1a	Superficial tumor[a]
T1b	Deep tumor[a]
T2	Tumor > 5 cm in greatest dimension
T2a	Superficial tumor[a]
T2b	Deep tumor[a]

Regional lymph nodes (N)

Nx	Regional lymph nodes cannot be assessed
N0	No regional lymph node metastasis
N1	Regional lymph node metastasis

Grade (G)

Gx	Grade cannot be assessed
G1	Well differentiated
G2	Moderately differentiated
G3	Poorly differentiated
G4	Poorly differentiated or undifferentiated (four-tiered systems only)

Stage grouping

Stage I	T1a-T2b	N0	M0	G1,2	G1	Low
Stage II	T1a-T2a	N0	M0	G3,4	G2,3	High
Stage III	T2b	N0	M0	G3,4	G2,3	High
Stage IV	Any T	N1	M0	Any G	Any G	High or low
	Any T	N0	M1	Any G	Any G	High or low

[a] Superficial tumor is located exclusively above the superficial fascia without invasion of the fascia; deep tumor is located either exclusively beneath the superficial fascia or superficial to the fascia with invasion of or through the fascia. Retroperitoneal, mediastinal, and pelvic sarcomas are classified as deep tumors.

AJCC = American Joint Committee on Cancer; UICC = International Union Against Cancer

From Greene FL, Page DL, Fleming ID, et al (eds): AJCC Cancer Staging Manual, 6th ed. New York, Springer-Verlag, 2002.

Staging and prognosis

AJCC/UICC staging system

The relative rarity of soft-tissue sarcomas, the anatomic heterogeneity of these lesions, and the presence of more than 30 recognized histologic subtypes of variable grade have made it difficult to establish a functional system that can accurately stage all forms of this disease. The revised staging system (6th edition) of the American Joint Committee on Cancer (AJCC) and the International Union Against Cancer (UICC) is the most widely employed staging classification for soft-tissue sarcomas (Table 1). All soft-tissue sarcoma subtypes are included, except dermatofibrosarcoma protuberans. Four distinct histologic grades are recognized, ranging from well differentiated to undifferentiated.

Histologic grade and tumor size are the primary determinants of clinical stage. Tumor size is further substaged as "a" (a superficial tumor that arises outside the investing fascia) or "b" (a deep tumor that arises beneath the fascia or invades the fascia).

The AJCC/UICC system is designed to optimally stage extremity tumors but is also applicable to torso, head and neck, and retroperitoneal lesions. It should not be used for sarcomas of the GI tract.

A major limitation of the current staging system is that it does not take into account the anatomic site of soft-tissue sarcomas. Anatomic site, however, is an important determinant of outcome. Patients with retroperitoneal, head and neck, and visceral sarcomas have a worse overall prognosis than do patients with extremity tumors. Although the anatomic site is not incorporated as a specific component of any current staging system, outcome data should be reported on a site-specific basis.

At Memorial Sloan-Kettering Cancer Center, a retrospective review of 369 patients with high-grade soft-tissue sarcoma of the extremity treated with postoperative radiation therapy was conducted to evaluate the influence of tumor site on local control and complications. The tumor site was upper extremity in 103 of patients (28%) and lower extremity in 266 patients (72%). With a median follow-up of 50 months, the 5-year actuarial rate of local control, distant relapse-free, and overall survival for the entire population was 82%, 61%, and 71%, respectively. The 5-year local control rates in patients with upper extremity lesions vs lower extremity lesions was 70% and 86%, respectively (P = .0004). On multivariate analysis, upper extremity site (P = .001) and positive resection margin (P = .02) were significant predictors of poor local control (*Alektiar KM, Brennan MF, Singer S: Int J Radiat Oncol Biol Phys 63:202-208, 2005*).

Prognostic factors

Understanding relevant clinicopathologic prognostic factors is important in treatment planning for patients with soft-tissue sarcoma. Several reports document the adverse prognostic significance of tumor grade, anatomic site, tumor size, and depth relative to the investing fascia (for extremity and body wall tumors). Patients with high-grade lesions, large (T2) sarcomas, a nonextremity subsite, or deep tumor location are at increased risk for disease relapse and sarcoma-specific death.

Sarcoma-specific nomogram Kattan and colleagues from Memorial Sloan-Kettering Cancer Center have developed a sarcoma-specific nomogram for estimation of sarcoma-specific 12-year survival. The nomogram takes into account pretreatment clinicopathologic factors, including anatomic site, histologic subtype, tumor size, histologic grade, tumor depth, and patient age. The nomogram is based on prospectively collected data and has been validated in a population of 2,136 patients with sarcoma. The nomogram can be found on www.nomograms.org and is available in a handheld personal digital assistant version. The sarcoma nomogram may be useful for patient stratification for clinical trials and for risk assessment and treatment planning for individual patients.

Prognostic factors for local vs distant recurrence Unlike other solid tumors, the adverse prognostic factors for local recurrence of a soft-tissue sarcoma differ from those that predict distant metastasis and tumor-related mortality. In other words, patients with a constellation of adverse prognostic factors for local recurrence are not necessarily at increased risk for distant metastasis or tumor-related death.

This concept has been validated by an analysis of the Scandinavian Sarcoma Group prospective database. In 559 patients with soft-tissue sarcomas of the extremities and trunk treated with surgery alone, inadequate surgical margin was found to be a risk factor for local recurrence but not for distant metastasis. Therefore, staging systems that are designed to stratify patients for risk of distant metastasis and tumor-related mortality using these prognostic factors (such as the AJCC/UICC system) do not stratify patients for risk of local recurrence.

Screening and diagnosis

Currently, there are no screening tests for soft-tissue sarcomas. Since the majority of patients with soft-tissue sarcoma have lesions arising in the extremities or superficial trunk, most of the comments here apply to soft-tissue lesions in those sites. A separate algorithm is usually employed for the evaluation of a primary retroperitoneal mass or visceral sarcoma.

Physical examination should include an assessment of the size of the mass and its mobility relative to the underlying soft tissues. The relationship of the mass to the investing fascia of the extremity (superficial vs deep) and nearby neurovascular and bony structures should be noted. Site-specific neurovascular examination and assessment of regional lymph nodes should also be performed.

Biopsy Any soft-tissue mass in an adult extremity should be biopsied if it is symptomatic or enlarging, is > 5 cm, or has persisted beyond 4–6 weeks.

Percutaneous approaches Percutaneous tissue diagnosis can usually be obtained with fine-needle aspiration (FNA) for cytology or by percutaneous core biopsy for histology. The needle track should be placed in an area to be excised or that can be encompassed in adjuvant radiotherapy fields if they are to be used. In most instances, when an experienced cytopathologist and/or histopathologist examines the specimen, a diagnosis of malignant soft-tissue sarcoma can be made. FNA is often viewed as a suboptimal method of establishing an initial diagnosis of soft-tissue sarcoma. Histology is usually preferred to cytology because more tissue is obtained, which allows for a more accurate delineation of tumor type and grade. Percutaneous tissue diagnosis is preferred to facilitate subsequent treatment planning and to permit surgical resection to be performed as a one-stage procedure.

Open biopsy In some cases, an adequate histologic diagnosis cannot be secured by percutaneous means. Open biopsy is indicated in these instances, with the exception of relatively small superficial masses, which can be easily removed by excisional biopsy with clear margins.

Biopsies should be incisional and performed with a longitudinal incision parallel to the long axis of the extremity. This approach facilitates subsequent wide local excision of the tumor and the incisional scar and results in minimal difficulties in wound closure. It also facilitates inclusion of any scars within the area of the tumor in adjuvant radiation fields without the excessive morbidity of large-field radiotherapy planning. The incision should be centered over the mass at its most superficial location. It is important to note that care should be taken not to raise tissue flaps. Meticulous hemostasis should be ensured after the biopsy to prevent dissemination of tumor cells into adjacent tissue planes by hematoma.

Retroperitoneal or intra-abdominal mass Biopsy of primary retroperitoneal soft-tissue masses is generally not required for radiographically resectable masses, nor is biopsy recommended for suspected GISTs. The circumstances under which percutaneous or preoperative biopsy of retroperitoneal masses should be strongly considered include:

- tissue diagnosis for radiographically unresectable disease
- clinical suspicion of lymphoma or germ-cell tumor
- tissue diagnosis for neoadjuvant treatment, including radiotherapy and/or chemotherapy
- suspected metastases from another primary tumor.

Primary tumor imaging Optimal imaging of the primary tumor depends on the anatomic site. For soft-tissue masses of the extremities, MRI has been regarded as the imaging modality of choice because it enhances the contrast between tumor and muscle and between tumor and adjacent blood vessels and also provides multiplanar definition of the lesion. However, a study by the Radiation Diagnostic Oncology Group that compared MRI and CT in 183 patients with malignant bone and 133 patients with soft-tissue tumors showed no specific advantage of MRI over CT from a diagnostic standpoint.

For pelvic lesions, the multiplanar capability of MRI may provide superior single-modality imaging. In the retroperitoneum and abdomen, CT usually provides satisfactory anatomic definition of the lesion. Occasionally, MRI with gradient sequence imaging can better delineate the relationship of the tumor to midline vascular structures, particularly the inferior vena cava and aorta. In the future, MRI-CT fusion techniques may facilitate treatment planning using conformal radiotherapy techniques.

More invasive studies, such as angiography and cavography, are almost never required for the evaluation of soft-tissue sarcomas.

Imaging for metastatic disease Cost-effective imaging to exclude the possibility of distant metastatic disease depends on the size, grade, and anatomic location of the primary tumor. In general, patients with low-grade soft-tissue sarcomas < 10 cm in size or intermediate-/high-grade tumors < 5 cm in diameter require only a chest x-ray for satisfactory staging of the chest. This reflects the fact that these patients are at comparatively low risk of presenting with pulmonary metastases. In contrast, patients with very large (≥ 10 cm) low-grade tumors or high-grade tumors ≥ 5 cm should undergo more thorough staging of the chest by CT.

Patients with retroperitoneal and intra-abdominal visceral sarcomas should undergo single-modality imaging of the liver to exclude the possibility of synchronous hepatic metastases. The liver is a common site for a first metastasis from these lesions.

Treatment

TREATMENT OF LOCALIZED DISEASE

Surgical resection is the cornerstone of therapy for patients with localized disease. Over the past 20 years, there has been a gradual shift in the surgical management of soft-tissue sarcoma of the extremities away from radical ablative surgery, such as amputation or compartment resection, and toward limb-sparing approaches combining wide local resection with preoperative or postoperative radiotherapy. The development of advanced surgical techniques (eg, microvascular tissue transfer, bone and joint replacement, and vascular reconstruction) and the application of multimodality approaches have allowed most patients to retain a functional extremity without any compromise in survival.

Surgery

The surgical approach to soft-tissue sarcomas depends on careful preoperative staging with MRI or CT for lesions of the extremities and a percutaneous histologic diagnosis and assessment of grade. In most instances, preoperative imaging studies allow for accurate prediction of resectability.

The surgical approach to soft-tissue sarcomas is based on an awareness that these lesions tend to expand and compress tissue planes, producing a pseudocapsule comprising normal host tissue interlaced with tumor fimbriae. Conservative surgical approaches in which the plane of dissection is immediately adjacent to this pseudocapsule, such as intracapsular or marginal excision, are associated with prohibitive local recurrence rates of 33%–63%.

Wide local resection encompassing a rim of normal tissue around the lesion has led to improvements in local control, with local recurrence rates of approximately 30% in the absence of adjuvant therapies. However, studies indicate that carefully selected patients with localized, small (T1), low-grade soft-tissue sarcomas of the extremity can be treated by wide resection alone, with local recurrence rates of < 10%. For example, in a cohort of 56 patients with primarily subcutaneous or intramuscular lesions treated with wide local excision without adjuvant irradiation, 4 local recurrences were noted.

The need for adjuvant irradiation in small (< 5 cm), high-grade lesions has been studied. A retrospective review of 204 patients with stage IIB soft-tissue sarcoma of the extremity treated at Memorial Sloan-Kettering Cancer Center has been completed. A total of 57% of patients did not receive adjuvant radiation therapy, whereas 43% received either brachytherapy or external-beam radiation therapy. With a median follow-up of 67 months, there was no significant difference in 5-year local control, distant relapse-free survival, or disease-specific survival when adjuvant irradiation was delivered.

Further studies will be required to define which subsets of patients with primary extremity sarcoma can be treated by wide excision surgery alone. Preoperative or postoperative radiotherapy should be employed for patients with primary T1 sarcomas in whom a satisfactory gross surgical margin cannot be attained without compromise of functionally important neurovascular structures.

Limb-sparing surgery plus irradiation Limb-sparing surgery employing adjuvant irradiation to facilitate maximal local control has become the standard approach for large (T2) soft-tissue sarcomas of the extremities. In most centers, upward of 90% of patients are treated with limb-sparing approaches. Amputation is reserved as a last-resort option for local control and is used with the knowledge that it does not affect survival. This approach was validated in a prospective National Cancer Institute (NCI) study, in which patients with a limb-sparing surgical option were randomized to receive limb-sparing surgery with postoperative radiation therapy or amputation. Both arms of the study included postoperative therapy with doxorubicin, cyclophosphamide, and methotrexate.

Surgical procedure The planned resection should encompass the skin, subcutaneous tissues, and soft tissues adjacent to the tumor, including the previous biopsy site and any associated drain sites. The tumor should be excised with a 2- to 3-cm margin of normal surrounding tissue whenever possible. Since good adjuvant approaches are available to facilitate local control, this ideal margin is sometimes compromised rather than attempting resection of adjacent, possibly involved bone or neurovascular structures that would result in significant functional loss. In the rare circumstance of gross involvement of neurovascular structures or bone, they can be resected en bloc and reconstructed.

Metal clips should be placed at the margins of resection to facilitate radiation field planning, when and if external irradiation is indicated. Drain sites should be positioned close to the wound to allow inclusion in radiation therapy fields. As noted earlier, avoidance of transverse incisions greatly facilitates the ability to include the tissues at risk in radiation target volume without unduly large fields.

Regional lymphadenectomy Given the low, 2%–3%, prevalence of lymph node metastasis in adult sarcomas, there is no role for routine regional lymphadenectomy. Patients with angiosarcoma, embryonal rhabdomyosarcoma, synovial sarcoma, and epithelioid histologies have an increased incidence of lymph node metastasis and should be carefully examined and radiographically imaged for lymphadenopathy. Clinically apparent lymphadenopathy should be treated with therapeutic lymphadenectomy. A recent analysis suggested that select patients undergoing lymphadenectomy, particularly in the absence of systemic metastases, may have a 5-year survival rate of 57%.

Radiotherapy

Scheduling Radiation therapy is usually combined with surgical resection in the management of patients with soft-tissue sarcomas of the extremities. The decision of whether to use preoperative (neoadjuvant) or postoperative (adjuvant) irradiation remains controversial and has been addressed in a phase III randomized trial.

Preoperative irradiation has a number of theoretic and practical advantages: (1) Smaller radiation portals can be utilized, as the scar, hematomas, and ecchymoses do not need to be covered. (2) Preoperative irradiation may produce tumor encapsulation, facilitating surgical resection from vital structures. (3) It is easier to spare a strip of skin and thereby reduce the risk of lymphedema. (4) The size of the tumor may be reduced, thus decreasing the extent of surgical resection. (5) Lower radiation doses can be utilized, as there are fewer relatively radioresistant hypoxic cells.

Preoperative irradiation also has several drawbacks, however. They include (1) the inability to precisely stage patients based on pathology due to downstaging and (2) increased problems with wound healing.

Studies of preoperative irradiation from the University of Florida, M. D. Anderson Cancer Center, and Massachusetts General Hospital demonstrated local control rates of 90% using doses of approximately 50 Gy. Survival depended on the size and grade of the primary tumor. Distant metastases were the primary pattern of failure.

Postoperative irradiation A number of retrospective reports, as well as a randomized trial from the NCI, have demonstrated that limb-sparing surgery plus postoperative irradiation produces local control rates comparable to those achieved with amputation. Five-year local control rates of 70%–90%, survival rates of 70%, and limb-preservation rates of 85% can be expected.

Equivocal or positive histologic margins are associated with higher local recurrence rates, and, therefore, adjuvant external-beam irradiation should be considered in all patients with sarcoma of the extremities with positive or close microscopic margins in whom reexcision is impractical. Postoperative doses of 60–65 Gy should be used.

Interstitial therapy with iridium-192 is used at some institutions as a radiation boost to the tumor bed following adjuvant external-beam irradiation. At Memorial Sloan-Kettering Cancer Center, adjuvant brachytherapy is often used in place of external irradiation. In a randomized trial, the 5-year local control rate was 82% in patients who received adjuvant brachytherapy, vs 69% in those treated with surgery alone. On subset analysis, the local control rate was found to be 89%, vs 66% for those patients with high-grade lesions. This study and further studies have indicated that brachytherapy has no impact on local control for low-grade lesions.

If an implant alone is used, the dose is 40–45 Gy to a volume that includes all margins; when a boost is combined with additional external-beam irradiation, a dose of 20–25 Gy is utilized. Some data suggest a higher rate of wound complications and a delay in healing when implants are afterloaded prior to the third postoperative day. Although some centers load implants sooner, this step must be performed with caution and strict attention to the incision site.

Over a 15-year period, 202 patients with high-grade sarcoma of the extremities underwent complete gross resection and adjuvant brachytherapy to a median dose of 45 Gy, delivered over 5 days. With a median follow-up of 61 months, the 5-year local control, distant relapse-free survival, and overall survival rates were 84%, 63%, and 70%, respectively. These rates compared favorably with data on external-beam irradiation. Morbidity of brachytherapy was considered acceptable, with reoperation rates of 12%, bone fractures in 3%, and nerve damage in 5%.

Comparison of irradiation techniques Comparable local control results (90%) are obtained with preoperative, postoperative, and interstitial techniques, although rates of wound complications are higher with preoperative techniques. Brachytherapy can offer a number of advantages. When brachytherapy is employed as the sole adjuvant, the entire treatment (surgery and irradiation) is completed in a 10- to 12-day period, compared with the 10–12 weeks required for typical external-beam irradiation (6–7 weeks) and surgery (4- to 6-week break before or after irradiation). Generally, smaller volumes can be irradiated with brachytherapy, which could improve functional results. However, smaller volumes may not be appropriate, depending on the tumor size, grade, and margin status.

The NCI of Canada Clinical Trials Group published 3-year median follow-up results of a randomized phase III trial comparing preoperative and postoperative radiotherapy for limb soft-tissue sarcoma (Figures 1A–1D). Wound complications were observed in 31 of 88 patients (35%) in the preoperative group and 16 of 94 patients (17%) in the postoperative group (difference, 18% [95% confidence interval: 5–30]; $P = .01$). Tumor size and anatomic site were also significant risk factors in multivariate analysis. Local control was identical in both arms of the trial. Five-year outcomes have been reported, and no difference in metastases, cause-specific survival, or overall survival was noted. Because preoperative radiotherapy is associated with a greater risk of wound complications than postoperative radiotherapy, but less late fibrosis and edema, the choice of regimen for patients with soft-tissue sarcoma should take into account the timing of surgery and radiotherapy and the size and anatomic site of the tumor.

Regardless of the technique employed, local control is a highly achievable and worthwhile endpoint, as demonstrated in a study of 911 patients treated by various techniques at Memorial Sloan-Kettering Cancer Center. Of the 116 patients who developed local recurrence, 38 patients subsequently developed metastases and 34 patients died. Metastases after local recurrence were predicted in patients with high-grade or large (> 5 cm) tumors.

Treatment recommendations Adjuvant radiotherapy should be employed for virtually all high-grade sarcomas of the extremities and larger (≥ 5 cm) low-grade lesions. If small (T1) lesions can be resected with clear margins, radio-

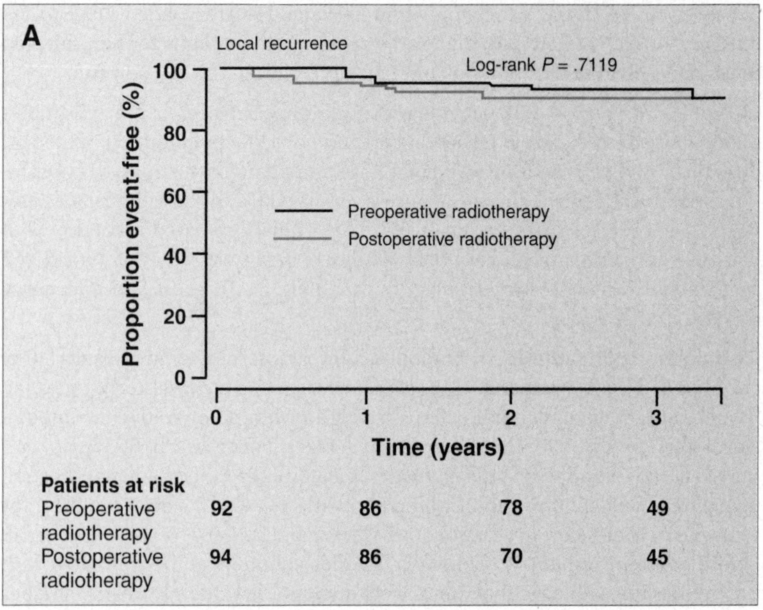

FIGURE 1A: Kaplan-Meier plots for probability of local recurrence in the National Cancer Institute of Canada Clinical Trials Group phase III trial.

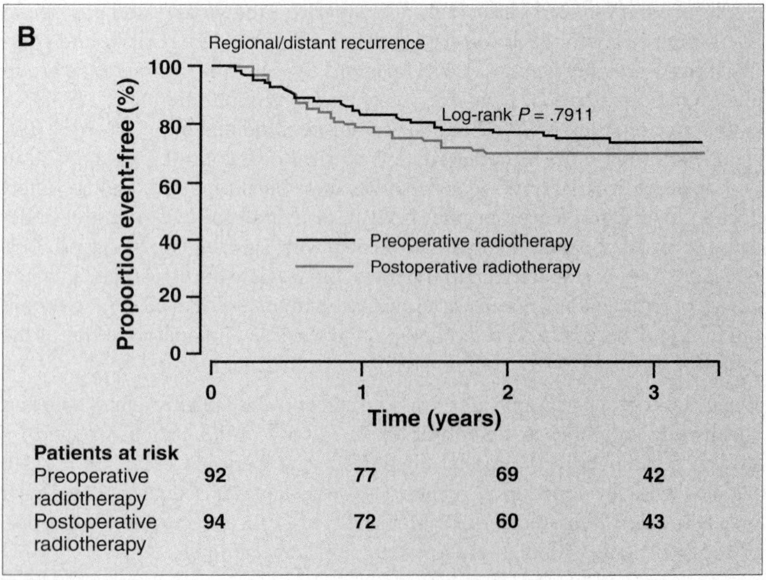

FIGURE 1B: Kaplan-Meier plots for probability of metastatic (regional and distant) recurrence in the National Cancer Institute of Canada Clinical Trials Group phase III trial.

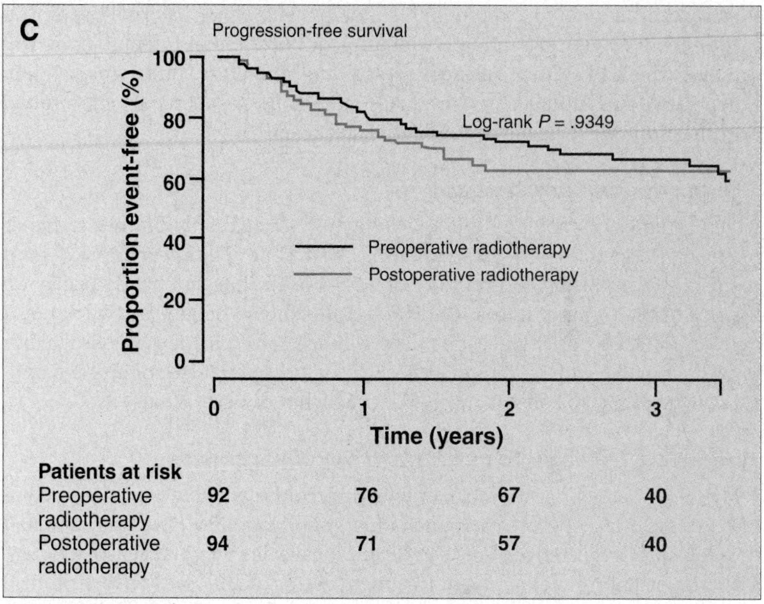

FIGURE 1C: Kaplan-Meier plots for probability of progression-free survival in the National Cancer Institute of Canada Clinical Trials Group phase III trial.

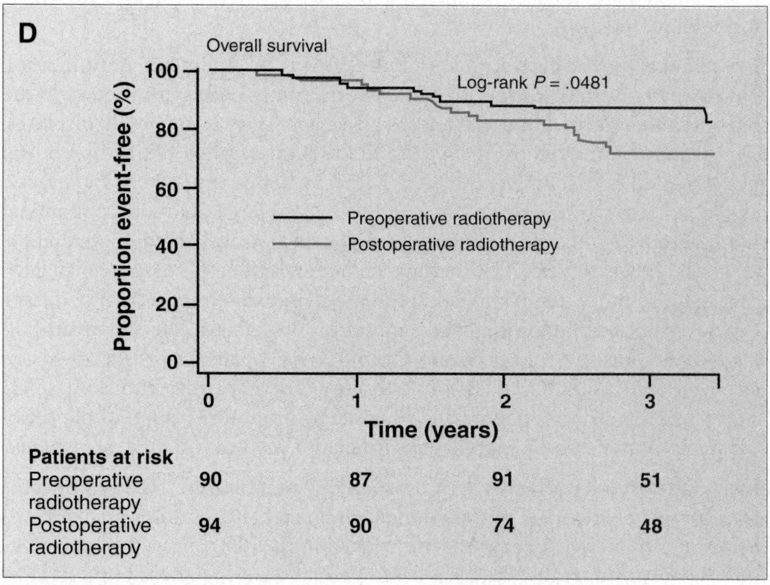

FIGURE 1D: Kaplan-Meier plots for probability of overall survival in the National Cancer Institute of Canada Clinical Trials Group phase III trial.

From O'Sullivan R, Davis AM, Turcotte R, et al: Lancet 359:2235–2241, 2002.

therapy can be omitted. Postoperative therapy with either external-beam irradiation (with or without an interstitial implant boost) or an implant alone will achieve a high likelihood of local control and, therefore, limb preservation. Preoperative irradiation, although equally efficacious, does carry a higher wound complication rate than the postoperative approach.

Primary radiation therapy

Several studies on radiation therapy alone in the treatment of unresectable or medically inoperable soft-tissue sarcomas have reported 5-year survival rates of 25%–40% and local control rates of 30%. Local control depends largely on the size of the primary tumor. Radiation doses should be at least 65–70 Gy, if delivery of such doses is feasible. The tumor's location may be particularly important in determining this dose because of the potential for damage to critical structures (eg, the spinal cord) with the higher doses normally used.

Radiation therapy in retroperitoneal sarcomas

Only 50% of patients with retroperitoneal sarcomas are able to undergo complete surgical resection. Of patients undergoing complete resection, one-half develop local recurrence. This significant local failure rate suggests a potentially important role for adjuvant treatment in all patients with retroperitoneal sarcomas. However, the role of radiation therapy for retroperitoneal sarcomas remains controversial due to the rarity of the tumor, the paucity of data, the retrospective nature of available studies, the low doses of radiation used in many studies, and the lack of consistent policies in determining the indications for radiation therapy.

Preoperative irradiation The advantages of preoperative radiotherapy have already been discussed for soft-tissue sarcomas of the extremities. In the retroperitoneum, an additional advantage is that bowel is frequently displaced significantly by the tumor. In contrast to the postoperative setting, the bowel being treated is also unlikely to be tethered by adhesions from prior surgery. These features significantly offset acute toxicity of large-field intra-abdominal radiotherapy (eg, nausea, vomiting, and diarrhea) as well as the potential for late-onset bowel toxicity. Conformal techniques capable of sparing normal tissues are also more easily applied in the preoperative setting, when the tumor can be visualized and the target area more readily defined. The American College of Surgeons Oncology Group (ACSOG) has opened a prospective, randomized trial (ACSOG 2 9031) investigating this very issue. In this phase III study, patients will be randomized to undergo surgical resection of the retroperitoneal tumor alone vs preoperative irradiation followed by surgical resection.

Intraoperative irradiation In a prospective trial from the NCI, 35 patients with completely resected retroperitoneal sarcomas were randomized to receive either intraoperative electron-beam irradiation (IORT) followed by low-dose (30–40 Gy) postoperative external-beam irradiation or high-dose postoperative external-beam irradiation (35–40 Gy plus a 20-Gy boost). Absolute local recurrence rates were significantly lower in the IORT group ($P < .05$), but disease-specific and overall survival rates did not differ between the two groups.

Similarly, a nonrandomized series from the Massachusetts General Hospital has suggested improved local control with IORT for patients with retroperitoneal sarcoma. In 16 patients who underwent irradiation, complete gross resection, and IORT, overall survival and local control rates were 74% and 83%, respectively. These numbers diminished to 30% and 61%, respectively, in the 13 patients treated with irradiation and complete gross resection without IORT. Although these local control results are encouraging, IORT remains investigational and cannot be advocated on a routine basis at this time.

Postoperative irradiation Two-year local control rates of 70% have been reported with the addition of postoperative irradiation. However, irradiation of the retroperitoneum/abdomen in doses that have effected local control in soft-tissue sarcoma of the extremities (50–65 Gy) is usually associated with significant GI toxicity. Obviously, the incidence of GI toxicity depends on the exact fields and technique used. However, as most retroperitoneal sarcomas are > 10–15 cm, the radiation fields employed are generally also quite large, and bowel is often located and/or tethered in the high-risk area. Three-dimensional treatment planning and conformal techniques can now be utilized to maximize the radiation dose to the tumor bed while minimizing the dose to the surrounding normal tissues.

Isolated limb perfusion

Recent studies have evaluated the role of isolated limb perfusion (ILP) in the management of sarcomas of the extremities. These studies have generally been extrapolations from protocols initially designed to treat locally advanced melanoma.

The agents most commonly employed for ILP have been melphalan (Alkeran) and tumor necrosis factor-alpha (TNF-α), with or without interferon-gamma (IFN-γ-1b [Actimmune]). The results of the largest series of ILP in patients with locally advanced soft-tissue sarcoma of the extremities were reported by Eggermont and colleagues. TNF-α has now been approved in Europe for ILP in patients with locally advanced, grade 2/3 soft-tissue sarcomas of the extremities.

The Netherlands Cancer Institute published its results in patients with unresectable soft-tissue sarcoma of the extremities who were perfused with melphalan and TNF-α. A total of 49 patients were treated and followed for a median of 26 months. One patient died shortly after perfusion, but 31 patients (63%) were able to undergo resection of the tumor. Based on clinical and pathologic grounds, an overall response was seen in 31 patients (63%), and a complete response was seen in 4 patients (8%). A total of 28 patients (57%) had local control with limb preservation. Toxicity was frequent but usually mild.

ROLE OF ADJUVANT CHEMOTHERAPY

The striking success of combined-modality therapy in children with osteogenic sarcoma, rhabdomyosarcoma, and the Ewing's sarcoma family of tumors has provided the stimulus for the use of aggressive combined-modality approaches in adults. The literature is replete with reports of the apparent benefit of combined-modality therapy in patients with resectable soft-tissue sarcoma. Yet most series are either retrospective or small nonrandomized trials.

Preoperative chemotherapy

Preoperative chemotherapy has been adopted at many centers for patients with large high-grade sarcoma. The specific regimens employed have evolved over the years but generally contain both an anthracycline and ifosfamide. Some investigators have added concurrent, sandwiched, or sequential preoperative radiation therapy in nonrandomized trials. European investigators have also explored combination chemotherapy with regional hyperthermia.

Aside from theoretic considerations, there are several pragmatic reasons to favor preoperative over postoperative treatment. First, a reduction in the size of a large lesion may permit surgical resection with less morbidity. Second, compliance may be better with preoperative therapy. One observation that supports the neoadjuvant approach is that response to preoperative chemotherapy, whether pathologic or radiographic, predicts improved tumor control and survival.

Neoadjuvant chemotherapy has been explored in a prospective randomized trial initiated by the EORTC (European Organization for Research on the Treatment of Cancer). The trial was open to patients who had a sarcoma measuring at least 8 cm (of any grade), a primary or recurrent intermediate- to high-grade (grade 2/3) sarcoma of any size, or a locally recurrent or inadequately excised grade 2/3 sarcoma. In spite of these broad eligibility criteria, accrual was slow, and the trial was closed after only 150 patients entered.

Patients were randomized to receive either immediate surgery, followed by radiation therapy for close or positive margins, or 3 cycles of chemotherapy with doxorubicin (50 mg/m^2 by IV bolus) plus ifosfamide (5 g/m^2 by 24-hour continuous infusion) with mesna. Among the 134 eligible patients, over 80% had primary tumors of the extremities, but only 4% had grade 2/3 lesions > 8 cm. Among 49 patients evaluable for response, 29% had major objective responses, including 4 complete responses. Only 18% had progression of disease before surgery. Chemotherapy was generally well tolerated and never prevented surgery. With a median follow-up of 7.3 years, the estimated 5-year survival rate was similar for both groups.

Trials have explored the role of neoadjuvant chemotherapy and radiation therapy to decrease the rate of distant failure and possibly impact survival. A study reported from Massachusetts General Hospital enrolled patients with high-grade soft-tissue sarcomas (8 cm or larger). Patients were treated with 3 cycles of preoperative chemotherapy consisting of MAID (mesna, doxorubicin [Adriamycin], ifosfamide, dacarbazine) interdigitated with 44 Gy of radiation therapy. This reigmen was followed by surgical resection and 3 cycles of postoperative MAID chemotherapy. In cases with positive surgical margins, an additional 16 Gy of radiation therapy was delivered.

This regimen resulted in a significant improvement in 5-year freedom from distant metastasis (75% vs 44%; $P = .0016$) when compared with historic control patients. Additionally, 5-year disease-free and overall survival rates were 70% vs 42% ($P = .0002$) and 87% vs 58% ($P = .0003$) for the MAID and control groups, respectively. There was a 29% rate of wound healing complications in the MAID group.

These data have been extended in a follow-up study of similar interdigitated chemotherapy/radiation therapy in a phase II study from the Radiation Therapy Oncology Group (RTOG). In this study, 66 patients with primary high-grade soft-tissue sarcoma ≥ 8 cm in diameter received a modified MAID regimen plus granulocyte colony-stimulating factor (G-CSF [Neupogen]) and radiation therapy, followed by resection and postoperative chemotherapy. Preoperative radiotherapy and chemotherapy were successfully completed by 89% and 79% of patients, respectively. Grade 4 hematologic and nonhematologic toxicities affected 80% and 23% of patients, respectively. Two patients developed late myelodysplasia. Delayed wound healing was noted in 31%. The estimated 3-year survival, disease-free survival, and local control rates were 75%, 55%, and 79%, respectively.

The M. D. Anderson Cancer Center conducted a phase I trial to define the maximum tolerated dose of continuous infusion doxorubicin administered with preoperative radiation therapy to a dose of 50 Gy. A total of 27 patients with intermediate- or high-grade sarcomas were enrolled in the trial. The maximum tolerated dose of doxorubicin was 17.5 $mg/m^2/wk$. Twenty-six patients underwent surgery, and all had a macroscopic complete resection (R0 or R1). Two patients had a pathologic complete response. These studies suggest that further investigation of a preoperative approach combining chemotherapy and radiation therapy is warranted.

Postoperative chemotherapy

A number of published trials have compared postoperative chemotherapy with observation alone in adults who had undergone resection of a primary or recurrent soft-tissue sarcoma. Most of these trials included fewer than 100 patients, and even the largest trial had inadequate statistical power to detect a 15% difference in survival. Other flaws confound the interpretation of many of the studies. Some trials included low-risk patients with small and/or low-grade sarcomas. In some trials, patient ineligibility rates were as high as 20%, and in none of the trials published before 2000 was ifosfamide part of the combination evaluated.

In five of the six trials in which doxorubicin monotherapy was studied, including one study limited to patients with uterine sarcoma, a significant improvement in survival could not be demonstrated. Among the trials of combination chemotherapy, most used the combination known as CyVADIC (cyclophosphamide, vincristine, doxorubicin [Adriamycin], dacarbazine). A significant survival advantage was seen in only one combination chemotherapy trial.

Nonetheless, some of the trials showed a trend or a statistically significant improvement in disease-free survival among patients who were administered adjuvant chemotherapy, especially among those with high-grade sarcomas of the extremities. Analyses of the pooled results of the published literature are consistent with this observation.

SMAC meta-analysis A formal meta-analysis of individual data from 1,568 patients who participated in randomized trials of postoperative adjuvant chemotherapy vs no chemotherapy control patients was performed by the Sarcoma Meta-Analysis Collaboration (SMAC). Although not all data were available for all patients, the analysis demonstrated a significant reduction in the risk of local or distant recurrence in patients who received adjuvant chemotherapy.

The overall hazard ratio for distant relapse-free survival was 0.70; ie, the risk of distant relapse (metastasis) was reduced by 30% in treated patients. The absolute benefit at 10 years was 10%, so the recurrence-free survival rate at 10 years was improved from 60% to 70%. Also, the hazard ratio for local recurrence-free survival was 0.73 (27% reduction in the risk of local recurrence), and the absolute benefit was 6%.

The hazard ratio for overall survival, however, was 0.89, which did not meet the criteria for statistical significance. The observed survival at 10 years was 54% for patients who received chemotherapy and 50% for those who did not. Subset analysis failed to show that the effects of chemotherapy differed by primary site, although the best evidence for an effect of adjuvant chemotherapy was seen in patients with sarcoma of the extremities.

Ifosfamide-containing trials Only one trial included in the meta-analysis used an ifosfamide-containing regimen; that trial involved only 29 patients. An attempt to conduct a large prospective trial of postoperative chemotherapy with the MAID regimen in the United States failed because of insufficient patient accrual.

An Italian cooperative group conducted a trial in which patients 18–65 years old with high-grade (≥ 5 cm) or any recurrent sarcoma of the extremities were randomized to receive postoperative chemotherapy or observation alone. The treatment consisted of 5 cycles of epirubicin (Ellence), 60 mg/m^2 on days 1 and 2, plus ifosfamide, 1.8 g/m^2 on days 1–5. G-CSF was used to support the granulocyte counts during therapy.

The trial had been planned for 200 patients but was interrupted after accrual of 104 patients, when an interim analysis showed a significant survival advantage for the chemotherapy-treated group. At 36 months after the last randomization, with a median follow-up of 59 months, median overall survival among the patients who received adjuvant chemotherapy was 75 months, vs 46 months for control patients ($P = .03$). In a longer-term follow-up analysis, survival was not improved on an intention-to-treat analysis, although 5-year overall survival rates still favored the patients receiving chemotherapy.

Two other randomized studies since the time of the original Italian study have been performed. They do not indicate a benefit for chemotherapy, but are underpowered to detect small differences in outcome.

Analyses of other collected prospective data regarding adjuvant chemotherapy from large referral centers have yielded somewhat conflicting data. In two analyses of patients with synovial sarcoma and one involving myxoid/round cell liposarcoma, chemotherapy appeared to improve overall survival. In a large analysis of two prospective databases, patients receiving chemotherapy initially had superior survival but then suffered inferior survival compared with those who received no adjuvant chemotherapy. Notably, patients were not randomized as part of their treatment. In fact, given this was a registry instead of a randomized study, there was by definition a bias to treat patients who had higher-risk tumors with chemotherapy, although this did not appear to correlate with a specific single variable in the analysis. Thus, if there is a benefit to adjuvant chemotherapy, it is a small one, and should be managed on a case-by-case basis.

Treatment recommendations

- Multidisciplinary treatment planning should precede the initiation of any therapy. An experienced multidisciplinary team should evaluate pathologic material and imaging studies and coordinate the integration of surgical resection, irradiation, and systemic therapy.
- Ideally, patients should be offered participation in clinical trials. Unfortunately, there are no active trials in the United States that will definitively answer the most important questions. Thus, a decision to treat must be made on an individual basis.
- Preoperative chemotherapy should be considered for fit, high-risk patients after a discussion of the risks and potential benefits. Older patients, especially those with cardiac or renal disease, are not optimal candidates for such treatment.
- Patients who do not receive preoperative chemotherapy may still be offered postoperative treatment. Adjuvant doxorubicin/ifosfamide combinations may improve relapse-free survival in carefully selected patients and can be considered for the treatment of those with tumor size > 5 cm, deep tumor location, and high histologic grade.
- For patients who opt for preoperative or postoperative chemotherapy, a regimen that includes doxorubicin (60–75 mg/m^2) or epirubicin (120 mg/m^2) plus ifosfamide (9–10 g/m^2), given for a total of 5 cycles, is a reasonable choice for subjects under age 60.
- Outside the context of a clinical trial, concurrent chemotherapy and irradiation should be avoided.

TREATMENT OF LOCAL RECURRENCE

Despite optimal multimodality therapy, local recurrence develops in 10%–50% of patients, with a median local recurrence-free interval of ~24 months. Local recurrence rates are a function of the primary site and are highest for retroperitoneal and head and neck sarcomas, for which adequate surgical margins are difficult to attain. In addition, high-dose adjuvant irradiation of these sites is often limited by the relative radiosensitivity of surrounding structures. These factors result in local recurrence rates of 40% for retroperitoneal sarcomas and up to 50% for head and neck sarcomas, which are substantially higher than the 10% proximity typically seen for extremity sarcomas.

A large retrospective analysis of patients with high-grade sarcoma of the extremities was reported from UCLA. Local recurrence required amputation in

38% of cases and was associated with a threefold decrement in survival. This finding accentuates the necessity for adequate local therapy for sarcomas presenting primarily as well as for multidisciplinary management of local recurrence.

Reoperation Following staging evaluation, patients with isolated local recurrence should undergo reoperation. The results of reoperation in this setting are good, with two-thirds of patients experiencing long-term survival.

Adjuvant radiation therapy If no prior radiation therapy was employed, adjuvant irradiation (50–65 Gy) should be used before or after surgery for locally recurrent disease. Radiation therapy (external-beam irradiation or brachytherapy) should be considered in patients for whom previous radiation doses were subtherapeutic or the previous radiation field design permitted additional treatment.

Reports from Memorial Sloan-Kettering Cancer Center, M. D. Anderson Cancer Center, and Princess Margaret Hospital suggest that patients who develop local recurrence following previous full-dose irradiation represent a difficult local control challenge. A report from Memorial Sloan-Kettering Cancer Center suggests that limb-sparing surgery combined with adjuvant brachytherapy may produce excellent local control and function in this group.

ILP Ongoing clinical investigations are defining the role of ILP in the management of patients with locally recurrent sarcoma.

TREATMENT OF LIMITED PULMONARY METASTASIS

Thoracotomy and metastasectomy The most common site of metastatic disease involvement of soft-tissue sarcoma is the lungs. Rates of 3-year survival following thoracotomy for pulmonary metastasectomy range from 23%–42%. This fact, combined with the limited efficacy of systemic therapy, is the basis for the recommendation that patients with limited pulmonary metastases and no extrapulmonary disease should undergo thoracotomy and metastasectomy.

Appropriate patient selection for this aggressive therapeutic approach to metastatic disease is essential. The following are generally agreed upon criteria: (1) the primary tumor is controlled or controllable; (2) there is no extrathoracic metastatic disease; (3) the patient is a medical candidate for thoracotomy; and (4) complete resection of all disease appears to be possible.

Preresection chemotherapy Chemotherapy is often recommended before resection of pulmonary metastases. However, there are no convincing data to support this approach.

CHEMOTHERAPY FOR UNRESECTABLE LOCALLY ADVANCED OR METASTATIC DISEASE

Single agents

Doxorubicin Early trials of doxorubicin reported major responses in approximately 30% of patients with advanced soft-tissue sarcoma. In more recent randomized series, however, the rate of response has been closer to 17%.

Subset analysis of patients with soft-tissue sarcoma from a broad phase II trial in which patients were randomized to receive various doses of doxorubicin demonstrated a steep dose-response relationship; patients treated with doses below 60 mg/m^2 rarely responded. Whether dose intensification of doxorubicin is associated with improved survival remains an open question (see section on "Intensifying chemotherapy").

Pegylated liposomal doxorubicin (Doxil in the United States, Caelyx in Europe) has demontrated limited activity in phase II trials, especially in patients whose disease is refractory to standard doxorubicin. In a randomized comparison among 95 previously untreated patients, however, the response rates to pegylated liposomal doxorubicin (50 mg/m^2 every 4 weeks; 10%) and to standard doxorubicin (75 mg/m^2 every 3 weeks; 9%) were similar, with no significant difference in time to disease progression or survival. Response rates improved to 14% and 12%, respectively, when GIST cases were excluded.

Ifosfamide In a randomized phase II trial conducted by EORTC, 18% of patients treated with ifosfamide (5 g/m^2) experienced major responses, in contrast to 12% of patients treated with cyclophosphamide (1.5 g/m^2), despite the greater myelosuppression with the latter agent. In a large American phase II trial, 17 of 99 patients with soft-tissue sarcoma responded to ifosfamide (8 g/m^2). All of the patients had been treated previously with doxorubicin-based therapy, suggesting a degree of non–cross-resistance.

Increasing ifosfamide dose Responses to ifosfamide ($\geq$ 12 g/m^2) have been observed in patients whose disease progressed while receiving lower doses, supporting the concept of a dose-response relationship.

In a randomized trial, the response to 9 g/m^2 of ifosfamide (17.5%) was superior to the 3% response observed among patients treated with 5 g/m^2. The reason for the low response to the lower dose was unclear. In a subsequent trial by the same investigators, the response to 12 g/m^2 was only 14%, however.

Among 45 evaluable patients enrolled in a Spanish phase II trial of ifosfamide (14 g/m^2 given by continuous infusion over 6 days), the response rate was 38%, but 47% of patients developed febrile neutropenia and 32%, grade 3 neurotoxicity.

At M. D. Anderson Cancer Center, ifosfamide (14 g/m^2 given by continuous infusion over 3 days) yielded responses in 29% of 37 patients with soft-tissue sarcoma and 40% of patients with bone sarcoma. Also within that report was a small cohort of patients in whom the response to the same total dose of ifosfamide was higher when the drug was given by an intermittent bolus rather than a continuous infusion; this finding led the authors to suggest that bolus therapy is more efficacious than continuous infusion. Pharmacokinetic studies, however, have shown no difference between a 1-hour infusion and bolus injection of ifosfamide with respect to the area under the curve for serum ifosfamide or its metabolites or the levels of ifosfamide metabolites in urine.

In an EORTC phase II trial, ifosfamide (12 g/m^2 given as a 3-day continuous infusion every 4 weeks) yielded a response rate of 17% among 89 chemotherapy-naive patients and 16% among 25 previously treated patients.

Ifosfamide doses as high as 14–20 g/m^2 have been given with hematopoietic growth factor support; reported response rates are high, but neurologic and renal toxicities often are dose-limiting. The available data suggest that synovial sarcoma is particularly sensitive to ifosfamide.

Dacarbazine The activity of dacarbazine in soft-tissue sarcoma has been recognized since the 1970s and was confirmed in a formal phase II trial. This marginally active agent has been used mostly in doxorubicin-based combinations. In particular, patients with leiomyosarcoma respond better to dacarbazine than do patients with other sarcoma subtypes.

Ecteinascidin (ET-743, trabectedin [Yondelis]), a novel compound derived from a marine organism, has demonstrated promising activity as well. In phase I trials, trabectedin demonstrated activity in heavily pretreated patients with advanced sarcoma. Three phase II trials of trabectedin (1,500 mg/m^2 over 24 hours every 3 weeks) in refractory non-GIST soft-tissue sarcoma have been reported.

In one trial, 2 partial responses and 4 minor responses were seen among 52 patients; 9 additional patients had stable disease for at least 6 months. Twenty-four percent of patients were free of disease progression at 6 months. The median survival was 12.8 months, with 30% of patients alive at 2 years.

In a second trial, responses were observed in 3 of 36 patients, with 1 complete response and 2 partial responses, for an overall response rate of 8% (95% confidence interval: 2–23). Responses, however, were durable, lasting up to 20 months.

Finally, a phase II study of patients treated in first line with the 24-hour infusion schedule of trabectedin demonstrated a 17% response rate. These data confirm that trabectedin is an active compound in the treatment of soft-tissue sarcomas, with a response rate similar to the 10%–30% range seen for either doxorubicin or ifosfamide. Phase I combination studies of trabectedin with other agents are pending. The predominant toxicities were neutropenia and elevation of transaminase levels. Two phase II trials of trabectedin in patients with GIST showed no therapeutic activity.

Other agents Gemcitabine (Gemzar) has demonstrated modest activity in several phase II trials, although results of a recent Southwest Oncology Group (SWOG) trial were disappointing. Taxanes, vinca alkaloids, and platinum compounds have demonstrated only marginal activity, however. It should be noted that the taxanes, gemcitabine, and vinorelbine have been observed to be active in angiosarcoma, especially involving the scalp and face.

Combination chemotherapy

Combination chemotherapy regimens have been used widely in the management of patients with soft-tissue sarcoma (Table 2). High response rates have been reported in a number of single-arm phase II trials. Most combination regimens include an anthracycline (either doxorubicin or epirubicin) plus an alkylating agent, dacarbazine, or both agents. Overall response rates are higher in these single-arm trials than when the same regimens are tested in larger, randomized studies.

CyVADIC and doxorubicin/dacarbazine regimens Combinations of doxorubicin with other agents have not proved to be superior to doxorubicin alone in terms of overall survival. Also, for over a decade, the CyVADIC regimen was widely accepted as the standard of care. In a prospective, randomized trial, however, CyVADIC did not prove to be superior to doxorubicin alone.

Doxorubicin (or epirubicin) plus ifosfamide Combinations of doxorubicin (or epirubicin) plus ifosfamide have consistently yielded responses in over 25% of patients in single-arm trials. In sequential trials conducted by the EORTC, doxorubicin at 75 mg/m^2 plus ifosfamide (5 g/m^2) was superior to doxorubicin at 50 mg/m^2 plus ifosfamide (5 g/m^2). A prospective randomized EORTC trial with 314 patients compared the two regimens. There was no difference in response rate or overall survival, but disease progression-free survival favored the more intensive regimen.

The strategy of intensifying the dosing of ifosfamide within the context of combination chemotherapy was explored in a randomized phase II trial. This study included both patients with localized disease treated with 4 cycles of preoperative chemotherapy as well as patients with metastatic disease. Overall, there was no survival benefit for patients treated with doxorubicin (60 mg/m^2) plus 12 g/m^2 of ifosfamide over those treated with doxorubicin (60 mg/m^2) plus 6 g/m^2 of ifosfamide. Also, there was no advantage to the patients with localized disease in terms of disease-free survival.

MAID regimen The MAID regimen yielded an overall response rate in 47% of patients in a large phase II trial. In a randomized comparison of AD (doxorubicin/dacarbazine) vs MAID regimens, the response to MAID was 32%, vs 17% with the two-drug regimen ($P < .002$). However, the price paid for the higher response was toxicity; of 8 toxic deaths reported in this trial, 7 occurred among the 170 patients treated with MAID. All treatment-related deaths occurred in patients > 50 years old. During the study, the doses of MAID were reduced to lessen toxicity. The median survival did not differ significantly between the two regimens, although a trend favoring the AD regimen was noted.

Combination chemotherapy vs single-agent doxorubicin Combination chemotherapy has been compared with single-agent doxorubicin in eight randomized phase III trials. Two trials were limited to patients with uterine sarcoma. Some of these studies showed superior response rates with combination chemotherapy, but none of the trials found a significant survival advantage. Kaplan-Meier plots of survival are virtually superimposable within each trial and from trial to trial.

It should be emphasized that approximately 20%–25% of patients entered into such trials are alive 2 years after therapy was initiated. Complete responses are uncommon and do not appear to translate into prolonged survival.

Gemcitabine plus docetaxel In a phase II study of 34 patients with unresectable leiomyosarcoma, mostly uterine in origin, 53% responded to a combination of gemcitabine (given by 90-minute infusion) plus docetaxel (Taxotere), with G-CSF support. An additional 20% had stable disease. Almost half of the patients had disease progression after anthracycline-based

TABLE 2: Chemotherapy regimens for soft-tissue sarcoma

Drug/combination	Dose and schedule
AIM	
Adriamycin (doxorubicin)	30 mg/m^2 IV on days 1 and 2 by rapid IV infusion
Ifosfamide	3,750 mg/m^2 on days 1 and 2 by IV infusion over 4 hours
Mesna	750 mg/m^2 IV infused immediately preceding and 4 and 8 hours after ifosfamide administration on days 1 and 2

Repeat cycle every 21 days.

NOTE: IV hydration at 300 mL/h beginning 3 hours before each treatment cycle and for 3 days at 100 mL/h after each day-1 ifosfamide infusion. Granulocyte colony-stimulating factor, 5 μg/kg subcutaneously, may be given starting 24-48 hours daily for 10 days or until a granulocyte count of 1,500/μL is reached. Appropriate supportive measures should be given.

Edmonson JH, Ryan LM, Blum RH, et al: J Clin Oncol 11:1269–1275, 1993.

Drug/combination	Dose and schedule
EIM	
Epirubicin	60 mg/m^2 IV infused on days 1 and 2, total dose of 120 mg/m^2 per cycle
Ifosfamide	1.8 g/m^2/d on days 1-5, total dose of 9 g/m^2 per cycle
Mesna	360 mg/m^2 IV infused immediately before and 4 and 8 hours after ifosfamide infusion

Repeat cycle every 3 weeks for a total of 5 cycles.

Granulocyte colony-stimulating factor, 300 μg subcutaneously given on days 8 through 15.

Hydration (1,500-2,000 mL) of fluids IV given after ifosfamide.

Frustaci S, Gherlinzoni F, De Paoli A, et al: J Clin Oncol 19:1238–1247, 2001.

Drug/combination	Dose and schedule
Gemcitabine and docetaxel*	
Gemcitabine	900 mg/m^2 IV on days 1 and 8
Docetaxel	100 mg/m^2 on day 8

Repeat cycle every 21 days.

NOTE: Granulocyte colony-stimulating factor is given subcutaneously on days 9 and 15. Patients who have undergone prior pelvic radiation therapy receive 25% dose reduction of both agents. Gemcitabine is delivered over 30 to 90 minutes in cycles 1 and 2 and by 90-minute infusion in all subsequent cycles.

* This regimen is still under study.

Hensley ML, Maki R, Venkatraman E, et al: J Clin Oncol 20:2824–2831, 2002.

Table prepared by Ishmael Jaiyesimi, DO

therapy. The median time to disease progression was 5.6 months, and grade 3-4 toxicity was uncommon. The activity of the gemcitabine-docetaxel combination was confirmed in a variety of other sarcoma subtypes in another study, which also confirmed the rationale for the sequence used in the study in vitro.

Intensifying chemotherapy Hematopoietic growth factors have facilitated the evaluation of dose-intensive chemotherapy in patients with sarcoma. The nonhematologic toxicities (cardiac, neurologic, and renal) of the agents most active in soft-tissue sarcoma prevent dramatic dose escalation.

Phase I and II trials of dose-intense anthracycline/ifosfamide regimens with hematopoietic growth factor support have shown that doxorubicin (70–90 mg/m²) can be used in combination with ifosfamide (10–12 g/m²) in selected patients. Response rates as high as 69% have been reported. Although toxicity increases, often dramatically, with these relatively modest dose escalations, the clinical benefit in terms of survival or palliation in patients with metastatic disease remains uncertain.

A prospective, randomized trial comparing gemcitabine-docetaxel with gemcitabine alone in a spectrum of histologic types of sarcoma has been completed. The response rates were 8% for gemcitabine alone and 16% for gemcitabine-docetaxel. Time to progression and overall survival were superior with gemcitabine-docetaxel (17.9 vs 11 months). Although this is one of the few studies in metastatic sarcoma to show a survival advantage, enthusiasm is tempered by toxicity, causing treatment discontinuation in up to 50% of patients after 6 months of gemcitabine-docetaxel chemotherapy. These data suggest that a dose reduction is needed in the off-study use of the therapy (*Maki RG, Hensley ML, Wathen JK, et al: J Clin Oncol [abstract] 24:523s, 2006*).

No randomized trial has demonstrated a survival advantage for patients treated with these more aggressive regimens. In one randomized trial, however, the French Federation of Cancer Centers Sarcoma Group demonstrated that, in comparison with standard doses, a 25% escalation in doses of MAID with G-CSF support did not improve outcome.

High-dose therapy with autologous stem-cell transplantation Most trials are small and presumably involve highly selected patients. In one trial involving 30 patients with metastatic or locally advanced sarcoma accrued over 6 years, more than 20% were free of disease progression at 5 years after high-dose therapy with stem-cell rescue. Complete response to standard induction chemotherapy predicted superior 5-year survival. Based on these favorable results, the investigators suggested a prospective randomized trial examining this approach. Although some groups are still exploring this approach, the appropriateness of generalizing these results to most patients with soft-tissue sarcoma remains speculative.

Prognostic factors for response to therapy Over the past 20 years, the EORTC has collected data on more than 2,000 patients with metastatic disease who participated in first-line anthracycline-based chemotherapy trials. Multivariate analysis of these data indicated that the patients most likely to respond to chemotherapy are those without liver metastases ($P < .0001$), younger patients, individuals with high histologic grade, and those with liposarcoma. In this Cox model, the factors associated with superior survival were good performance status, absence of liver metastases, low histologic grade, a long time to metastasis after treatment of the primary tumor, and young age.

The French Sarcoma Group has initiated a phase III randomized trial looking at intermittent vs continuous imatinib (Gleevec) therapy after completion of 1 year of continuous imatinib therapy. A total of 159 patients have enrolled in the trial. A partial or complete response was achieved in 52% of patients. Twenty-three patients were randomized to join the intermittent arm and 23, the continuous arm. After 3 months, 5 patients (21%) in the intermittent arm had evidence of disease progression, vs no patients in the continuous arm. Reintroduction of imatinib resulted in tumor control in all patients (*Blay JY, Berthaud D, Perol D, et al: J Clin Oncol [abstract] 22(14S):815, 2004*).

More recently, these same investigators have reported that the observed response rate is superior in patients who have pulmonary metastases only, as compared with those who have metastases to the lungs and other sites or to other sites only. These findings highlight the danger of reaching broad conclusions based on extrapolations from small trials that include highly selected patients. The EORTC data are also consistent with the observation that patients with metastatic GI sarcoma rarely respond to standard chemotherapy regimens. This increasingly recognized observation has been used to explain the low response rates seen in some trials.

Targeted therapy for GISTs

Advances in our understanding of the biology of GIST, and the availability of an effective therapy for patients with advanced disease, have resulted in intense interest in this entity and rapid expansion of this disease. Because this entity had not been recognized, the incidence of GIST was underappreciated. GIST is the most common nonepithelial tumor of the gastrointestinal tract, with an estimated annual incidence of 3,000–3,500 cases in the United States. Approximately 50%–60% of GISTs arise in the stomach and 25% in the small bowel. Other sites include the rest of the gastrointestinal tract, the omentum, mesentery, and retroperitoneum. These tumors may range in size from millimeters to huge masses. It is not clear how many of these GISTs become clinically relevant and how many are noted anecdotally at the time of endoscopic ultrasonography or other abdominal procedures.

The demonstration of the efficacy of imatinib (Gleevec) in GIST has been among the most dramatic and exciting observations in solid-tumor oncology. A randomized multicenter trial evaluated two doses of oral imatinib (400 vs 600 mg) in 147 patients with advanced GISTs. With a median follow-up of 288 days, 54% had a partial response, and 28% had stable disease, but there were no complete responses. Response was sustained, with a median duration over 6 months. Most patients had mild grade 1 or 2 toxicity, but only 21% had severe grade 3 or 4 toxicity. GI or intra-abdominal hemorrhage occurred in 5% of patients. There was no difference in response or toxicity between the two doses.

These observations were expanded in two parallel, multi-institution trials in which patients with GISTs were randomized to receive imatinib (400 or 800 mg daily). The results were remarkably similar. In the American trial, among 746 registered patients, the overall response rate was 43% for patients treated with 400 mg and 41% for those treated with 800 mg. There were no differences in survival between the two arms. At 2 years, disease progression-free and overall survival rates in the 400-mg arm were 50% and 78%, respectively. In the

800-mg arm, the rate of disease progression-free survival at 2 years was 53%, and the rate of overall survival was 73%.

In a large European trial, 946 patients were randomized to receive imatinib (400 mg daily or twice a day). Among the 615 patients whose response could be evaluated, there was no difference in response frequency (43%) or survival between the two arms. Complete responses were seen in 3% and 2% of the lower-dose and higher-dose patients, respectively. Sixty-nine percent of patients progressing on 400 mg of imatinib were allowed to cross over to the higher dose (800 mg). Further therapeutic activity was seen, with 26% of these patients free of disease progression at 1 year.

Based on these results, the EORTC, in conjunction with the Italian Sarcoma Group and the Australasian Gastrointestinal Group, has recently reported its results to further identify factors predicting early and late resistance to imatinib in patients with GIST. Initial resistance was defined as disease progression within 3 months of randomization, and late resistance was disease progression beyond 3 months. Initial resistance was noted in 116 of 934 patients (12%). Low hemoglobin level, high granulocyte count, and presence of lung and absence of liver metastases were independent predictors of initial resistance. Late resistance occurred in 347 of 818 patients. Independent predictors were high baseline granulocyte count, primary tumor outside the stomach, large tumor size, and low initial imatinib dose. The impact of the dose on late resistance was significant in patients with high baseline granulocyte counts and in patients with GI tumors originating outside the stomach and small intestine.

Among a group of 127 patients with advanced GISTs, activating mutations of KIT or PDGFRA (platelet-derived growth factor receptor-alpha) were identified in 87.4% and 3.9% of patients, respectively. In patients harboring an exon 11 mutation of KIT, the partial remission rate was 83.5%, whereas in patients without a discernible mutation in KIT or PDGFRA, the partial remission rate was 9.1%. The presence of an exon 11 mutation in KIT correlated with clinical response, decreased risk of treatment failure, and improved overall survival.

The National Comprehensive Cancer Network (NCCN) recently established a GIST Task Force to develop guidelines for the evaluation and treatment of patients with GIST. This group recommended 400 mg daily as the initial starting dose of imatinib. Dose escalation should be considered in patients who do not respond initially or who demonstrate unequivocal disease progression. Surgery remains the primary modality for treatment of primary GIST, but adjuvant and neoadjuvant trials are ongoing. The efficacy, dose, and duration of imatinib therapy in these settings have not been established, so participation of patients in such trials should be encouraged.

Recent data indicate that sunitinib malate (SU11248 [Sutent]) is an active agent in imatinib-refractory GIST. In both phase I/II and III studies, the response rate is on the order of 10%, with a greater than 60% chance of remaining on treatment for 6 months or longer. Notably, the patients with the most benefit were those with the converse c-kit genetic phenotype (exon 9 mutation or wild type c-kit) to that seen as sensitive to imatinib (exon 11 mutation). Nonetheless, imatinib remains the first line of therapy regardless of mutation type, since there is still a response rate seen for imatinib in patients with wild-type or exon 9 c-kit mutations and since overall imatinib is less toxic than sunitinib in its present schedule (4 weeks on at 50 mg by mouth daily, 2 weeks off). Some studies are examining new schedules of sunitinib (eg, 37.5 mg oral daily continuously), whereas other studies are evaluating the benefit of other small-molecule inhibitors of c-kit.

Assessment of response and treatment after disease progression on imatinib The use of standard (RECIST) response criteria in patients with GIST may be misleading. On CT or MR imaging, large tumor masses may become completely necrotic without a reduction in size for months in spite of dramatic clinical improvement. Indeed, such masses may actually increase in size. ^{18}F-FDG (^{18}F-fluorodeoxyglucose)-PET imaging may be extremely useful in selected patients, since response may be seen as early as 24 hours after a dose of imatinib. It should be noted that the survival of patients with stable disease parallels that of patients with major objective responses using RECIST criteria.

Surgery does not cure GIST that recurs after resection of primary disease and should be managed as metastatic disease. However, multimodality therapy should be considered in patients with limited sites of disease. It has also been recognized that patients with disease progression in limited sites of disease, occasionally with a growing nodule within a previously necrotic metastasis, may experience rapid disease progression of previously controlled areas. Thus, imatinib should be continued indefinitely in such patients, who should be referred for investigational therapy.

It is promising that other rare forms of sarcoma, such as dermatofibrosarcoma protuberans and desmoid tumors, have been reported to respond to imatinib, indicating the potential utility of these and many other kinase-targeted therapies now in phase I and II studies (PTK787, AMG706, sorafenib [BAY43-9006, Nexavar], temsirolimus [CCI-779], and everolimus [RAD001]). The finding of mTOR inhibitor AP23573 as effective for at least some sarcomas will spur further analysis of combinations of targeted agents as well as targeted agents with cytotoxic chemotherapy.

Recommendations for the treatment of metastatic sarcoma

- For patients with rapidly progressive disease or with symptoms, combination chemotherapy with an anthracycline/ifosfamide combination is indicated. For most patients, however, sequential single-agent therapy is less toxic and not inferior in terms of survival.
- The importance of histology relevant to selection of therapy is increasingly being appreciated. It is especially significant to distinguish GISTs from GI leiomyosarcomas. Patients with suspected GIST should be referred to subspecialty centers experienced in the multimodality management of this disease.
- Periods of watchful waiting may be appropriate for many patients with metastatic sarcoma who have no or only minimal symptoms.

SUGGESTED READING

Alektiar KM, Leung D, Zelefsky MJ, et al: Adjuvant brachytherapy for primary high-grade soft-tissue sarcoma of the extremity. Ann Surg Oncol 9:48–56, 2002.

Chawla SP, Sankhala KK, Chua V, et al: A phase II study of AP23573 (an mTOR inhibitor) in patients with advanced sarcomas (abstract). J Clin Oncol 23(16S):833s, 2005.

Coindre JM, Terrier P, Guillou L, et al: Predictive value of grade for metastasis development in the main histologic types of adult soft-tissue sarcomas: A study of 1,240 patients from the French Federation of Cancer Centers Sarcoma Group. Cancer 91:1914–1926, 2001.

Corless CL, Fletcher JA, Heinrich MC, et al: Biology of gastrointestinal stromal tumors. J Clin Oncol 22:3813–3825, 2004.

Cormier JN, Huang X, Xing Y, et al: Cohort analysis of patients with localized, high-risk, extremity soft tissue sarcoma treated at two cancer centers: Chemotherapy-associated outcomes. J Clin Oncol 22:4567–4574, 2004.

DeLaney TF, Spiro IJ, Suit HD, et al: Neoadjuvant chemotherapy and radiotherapy for large extremity soft-tissue sarcomas. Int J Radiat Oncol Biol Phys 56:1117–1127, 2003.

Demetri GD, van Oosterom AT, Blackstein M, et al: Phase 3, multicenter, randomized, double-blind, placebo-controlled trial of SU11248 in patients following failure of imatinib for metastatic GIST (abstract). J Clin Oncol 23(16S):308s, 2005.

Eilber FC, Eilber FR, Eckardt J, et al: The impact of chemotherapy on the survival of patients with high-grade primary extremity liposarcoma. Ann Surg 240:686–695, 2004.

Eilber FC, Rosen G, Nelson SD, et al: High-grade extremity soft-tissue sarcomas: Factors predictive of local recurrence and its effect on morbidity and mortality. Ann Surg 237:218–226, 2003.

Ferrari A, Gronchi A, Casanova M, et al: Synovial sarcoma: A retrospective analysis of 271 patients of all ages treated at a single institution. Cancer 101:627–634, 2004.

Fletcher JA, Corless CL, Dimitrijevic S, et al: Mechanisms of resistance to imatinib mesylate (IM) in advanced gastrointestinal stromal tumor (GIST) (abstract). Proc Am Soc Clin Oncol 22:815, 2003.

Fletcher CD, Gustafson P, Rydholm A, et al: Clinicopathologic re-evaluation of 100 malignant fibrous histiocytomas: Prognostic relevance of subclassification. J Clin Oncol 19:3045–3050, 2001.

Frustaci S, De Paoli A, Bidoli E, et al: Ifosfamide in the adjuvant therapy of soft tissue sarcomas. Oncology 65(suppl 2):80–84, 2003.

Garcia-Carbonero R, Supko JG, Maki RG, et al: Ecteinascidin-743 (ET-743) for chemotherapy-naive patients with advanced soft tissue sarcomas: Multicenter phase II and pharmacokinetic study. J Clin Oncol 23:5484–5492, 2005.

Gieschen HL, Spiro IJ, Suit HD, et al: Long-term results of intraoperative electron-beam radiotherapy for primary and recurrent retroperitoneal soft-tissue sarcoma. Int J Radiat Oncol Biol Phys 50:127–131, 2001.

Grobmyer SR, Maki RG, Demetri GD, et al: Neo-adjuvant chemotherapy for primary high-grade extremity soft tissue sarcoma. Ann Oncol 15:1667–1672, 2004.

Heinrich MC, Maki RG, Corless CL, et al: Sunitinib response in imatinib-resistant GIST correlates with *KIT* and *PDGFRA* mutation status (abstract). J Clin Oncol 24(18S):520s, 2006. 24(18S):520s, 2006.

Hensley ML, Maki R, Venkatraman E, et al: Gemcitabine and docetaxel in patients with unresectable leiomyosarcoma: Results of a phase II trial. J Clin Oncol 20:2824–2831, 2002.

Kattan MW, Leung DH, Brennan MF: Postoperative nomogram for 12-year sarcoma-specific death. J Clin Oncol 20:791–796, 2002.

Kraybill WG, Harris JH, Spiro I, et al: Radiation Therapy Oncology Group 95-14: A phase II study of neoadjuvant chemotherapy and radiation therapy in the management of high-risk, high grade, soft tissue sarcomas of the extremities and body wall (abstract). Proc Am Soc Clin Oncol 22:815, 2003.

Le Cesne A, Blay J, Judson I, et al: Phase II study of ET-743 in advanced soft tissue sarcomas: A European Organisation for the Research and Treatment of Cancer (EORTC) soft tissue and bone sarcoma group trial. J Clin Oncol 23:5276, 2005.

Le Cesne A, Judson I, Crowther D, et al: Randomized phase III study comparing conventional-dose doxorubicin plus ifosfamide vs high-dose doxorubicin plus ifosfamide plus recombinant human granulocyte-macrophage colony-stimulating factor in advanced soft-tissue sarcomas: A trial of the European Organization for Research on the Treatment of Cancer/Soft-Tissue and Bone Sarcoma Group. J Clin Oncol 18:2676–2684, 2000.

Leu KM, Ostruszka LJ, Shewach D, et al: Laboratory and clinical evidence of synergistic cytotoxicity of sequential treatment with gemcitabine followed by docetaxel in the treatment of sarcoma. J Clin Oncol 22:1706–1712, 2004.

Maki RG, Fletcher JA, Heinrich MC, et al: Results from a continuation trial of SU11248 in patients with imatinib-resistant gastrointestinal stromal tumor (GIST) (abstract). J Clin Oncol 23(16S):818s, 2005.

Noorda EM, Vrouenraets BC, Nieweg OE, et al: Isolated limb perfusion with tumor necrosis factor-alpha and melphalan for patients with unresectable soft tissue sarcoma of the extremities. Cancer 98:1483–1490, 2003.

O'Sullivan B, Bell RS, Bramwell VHC: Sarcomas of the soft tissues, in Souhami RL, Tannock I, Hohenberger P, et al (eds): Oxford Textbook of Oncology, 2nd ed, pp 2495–2523. Oxford, Oxford University Press, 2002.

O'Sullivan B, Davis A, Turcotte R, et al: Five-year results of a randomized phase III trial of preoperative vs post-operative radiotherapy in extremity soft tissue sarcoma (abstract). J Clin Oncol 22:(14S):9007, 2004.

O'Sullivan B, Davis AM, Turcotte R, et al: Preoperative versus postoperative radiotherapy in soft-tissue sarcoma of the limbs: A randomized trial. Lancet 359:2235–2241, 2002.

Pisters PW, Patel SR, Prieto VG, et al: Phase I trial of preoperative doxorubicin-based concurrent chemoradiation and surgical resection for localized extremity and body wall soft tissue sarcomas. J Clin Oncol 22:3375–3380, 2004.

Riad S, Griffin AM, Liberman B, et al: Lymph node metastasis in soft tissue sarcoma in an extremity. Clin Orthop Sep:129–134, 2004.

Rubin BP, Singer S, Tsao C, et al: KIT activation is a ubiquitous feature of gastrointestinal stromal tumors. Cancer Res 61:8118–8121, 2001.

Trovik CS, Bauer HC, Alvegard TA, et al: Surgical margins, local recurrence, and metastasis in soft-tissue sarcomas: Five hundred fifty-nine surgically treated patients from the Scandinavian Sarcoma Group Register. Eur J Cancer 36:710–716, 2000.

Van den Abbeele AD, Badawi RD Cliche J-P, et al: 18F-FDG-PET predicts response to imatinib mesylate (Gleevec) in patients with advanced gastrointestinal stromal tumors (GIST) (abstract). Proc Am Soc Clin Oncol 21:403a, 2002.

Wendtner C-M, Abdel-Rahman S, Krych M, et al: Response to neoadjuvant chemotherapy combined with regional hyperthermia predicts long-term survival for adult patients with retroperitoneal and visceral high-risk soft-tissue sarcomas. J Clin Oncol 20:3156–3164, 2002.

Zalcberg JR, Verweij J, Casali PG, et al: Outcome of patients with advanced gastrointestinal stromal tumours crossing over to a daily imatinib dose of 800 mg after progression on 400 mg. Eur J Cancer 41:1751-1757, 2005.

CHAPTER 26

Primary and metastatic brain tumors

Lisa M. DeAngelis, MD, Jay S. Loeffler, MD, and Adam N. Mamelak, MD

BRAIN TUMORS

Intracranial neoplasms can arise from any of the structures or cell types present in the cranial vault, including the brain, meninges, pituitary gland, skull, and even residual embryonic tissue. The overall annual incidence of primary brain tumors in the United States is 14 cases per 100,000 population.

The most common primary brain tumors are meningiomas, representing 27% of all primary brain tumors, and glioblastomas, representing 23% of all primary brain tumors; many of these tumors are clinically aggressive and high grade. Primary brain tumors are the most common of the solid tumors in children and the second most frequent cause of cancer death after leukemia in children.

Brain metastases occur in approximately 15% of cancer patients as a result of hematogenous dissemination of systemic cancer, and the incidence may be rising due to better control of systemic disease. Lung and breast cancers are the most common solid tumors that metastasize to the central nervous system (CNS). Melanoma and testicular and renal carcinoma have the greatest propensity to metastasize to the brain, but their relative rarity explains the low incidence of these neoplasms in large series of patients with brain metastases. Patients with brain metastases from nonpulmonary primaries have a 70% incidence of lung metastases. Although many physicians presume that all brain metastases are multiple, in fact, half are single and many are potentially amenable to focal therapies.

Epidemiology

Gender There is a slight predominance of primary brain tumors in men.

Age Primary brain tumors have a bimodal distribution, with a small peak in the pediatric population and a steady increase in incidence with age, beginning at age 20 years and reaching a maximum of 20 cases per 100,000 population between the ages of 75 and 84 years.

Etiology and risk factors

The cause of primary brain tumors is unknown, although genetic and environmental factors may contribute to their development.

> Epigenetic silencing of the MGMT (06-methylguanine-DNA methyltransferase) DNA-repair gene by promoter methylation is an independent prognostic factor in patients with glioblastoma and has been associated with longer survival in patients who received the alkylating agent temozolomide (Temodar; *Hegi ME, Diserens AC, Gorlia T, et al: N Engl J Med 352:997-1003, 2005).*

Genetic factors Clear heritable factors play a minor role in the genesis of primary brain tumors; less than 5% of patients with glioma have a family history of brain tumor. Several inherited diseases, such as tuberous sclerosis, neurofibromatosis type I, Turcot syndrome, and Li-Fraumeni cancer syndrome, predispose patients to the development of gliomas. However, these tumors tend to occur in children or young adults and do not account for the majority of gliomas that appear in later life.

Loss of heterozygosity (LOH) on chromosomes 9p and 10q and p16 deletions are frequently observed in high-grade gliomas, with low-grade gliomas having the fewest molecular abnormalities. In oligodendrogliomas, 1p and 19q LOH is associated with significantly improved survival.

Molecular markers of brain tumors can predict survival and will become increasingly important in the diagnosis and treatment of glioma.

Environmental factors Prior cranial irradiation is the only well-established risk factor for intracranial neoplasms.

Lifestyle characteristics Brain tumors are not associated with lifestyle characteristics such as cigarette smoking, alcohol intake, or cellular phone use.

Signs and symptoms

Brain tumors produce both nonspecific and specific signs and symptoms.

Nonspecific symptoms include headaches, which occur in about half of patients but are rarely an isolated finding of intracranial tumors, and nausea and vomiting, which are caused by an increase in intracranial pressure. Because of the widespread availability of CT and MRI, papilledema is now seen in < 10% of patients, even when symptoms of raised intracranial pressure are present.

Specific signs and symptoms are usually referable to the particular intracranial location of the tumor and are similar to the signs and symptoms of other intracranial space-occupying masses.

Lateralizing signs, including hemiparesis, aphasia, and visual-field deficits, are present in ~50% of patients with primary and metastatic brain tumors.

Seizures are a common presenting symptom, occurring in ~25% of patients with high-grade gliomas, at least 50% of patients with low-grade tumors, and 50% of patients with metastases from melanoma, perhaps due to their hemorrhagic nature. Otherwise, seizures are the presenting symptom in 15%-20% of patients with brain metastases. Seizures may be generalized, partial, or focal.

Stroke-like presentation Hemorrhage into a tumor may present like a stroke, although the accompanying headache and alteration of consciousness usually suggest an intracranial hemorrhage rather than an infarct. Hemorrhage is usually associated with high-grade gliomas, occurring in 5%-8% of patients with glioblastoma multiforme. However, oligodendrogliomas have a propensity to bleed, and hemorrhage occurs in 7%-14% of these low-grade neoplasms. Sudden visual loss and fatigue may be seen with bleeding into or infarction of pituitary tumors, termed *pituitary apoplexy*.

Altered mental status Approximately 75% of patients with brain metastases have impairment of consciousness or cognitive function. Some patients with multiple bilateral brain metastases may present with an altered sensorium as the only manifestation of metastatic disease; this finding can be easily confused with metabolic encephalopathy.

Screening for metastatic brain tumors

Screening for brain metastases is performed in only a few clinical situations.

Lung cancer Approximately 10% of patients with small-cell lung cancer (SCLC) have brain metastases at diagnosis, and an additional 20%-25% develop such metastases during their illness. Therefore, cranial CT or MRI is performed as part of the evaluation for extent of disease.

Occasionally, patients with non–small-cell lung cancer (NSCLC) undergo routine cranial CT or MRI prior to definitive thoracotomy, since the presence of brain metastases may influence the choice of thoracic surgical procedure. This approach is particularly valuable in patients with suspected stage IIB or III disease for whom thoracotomy is considered following neoadjuvant therapy. Screening for brain metastases is both clinically worthwhile and cost-effective.

Diagnosis

MRI The diagnosis of a brain tumor is best made by cranial MRI. This should be the first test obtained in a patient with signs or symptoms suggestive of an intracranial mass. MRI is superior to CT and should always be obtained with and without contrast material such as gadolinium (Figure 1).

High-grade or malignant primary brain tumors appear as contrast-enhancing mass lesions that arise in white matter and are surrounded by edema (Figure 2). Multifocal malignant gliomas are seen in ~5% of patients.

Low-grade gliomas typically are nonenhancing lesions that diffusely infiltrate and tend to involve a large region of the brain. Low-grade gliomas are usually best appreciated on T2-weighted or fluid-attenuated inversion recovery (FLAIR) MRI scans (Figure 3).

CT A contrast-enhanced CT scan may be used if MRI is unavailable or the patient cannot undergo MRI (eg, because of a pacemaker). CT is adequate to exclude brain metastases in most patients, but it can miss low-grade tumors or small lesions located in the posterior fossa. Tumor calcification is often better appreciated on CT than on MRI.

PET Body positron emission tomography (PET) scans performed for staging of systemic malignancies have a sensitivity of only 75% and a specificity of 83% for identification of cerebral metastases. Therefore, they are less accurate than MRI, which remains the gold standard.

Radiographic appearance of lesions On CT or MRI, most brain metastases are enhancing lesions surrounded by edema, which extends into the white matter (Figure 1). Unlike primary brain tumors, metastatic lesions rarely involve the corpus callosum or cross the midline.

The radiographic appearance of brain metastases is nonspecific and may mimic other processes, such as infection. Therefore, the CT or MRI scan must always be interpreted within the context of the clinical picture of the individual patient, particularly since cancer patients are vulnerable to opportunistic CNS infections or may develop second primaries, which can include primary brain tumors.

Other imaging tools Magnetic resonance spectroscopy and diffusion imaging can help differentiate low-grade from high-grade brain tumors but cannot distinguish different tumor types of the same grade.

Pathology

Glial tumors arise from astrocytes, oligodendrocytes, or their precursors and exist along a spectrum of malignancy. The astrocytic tumors are graded, using

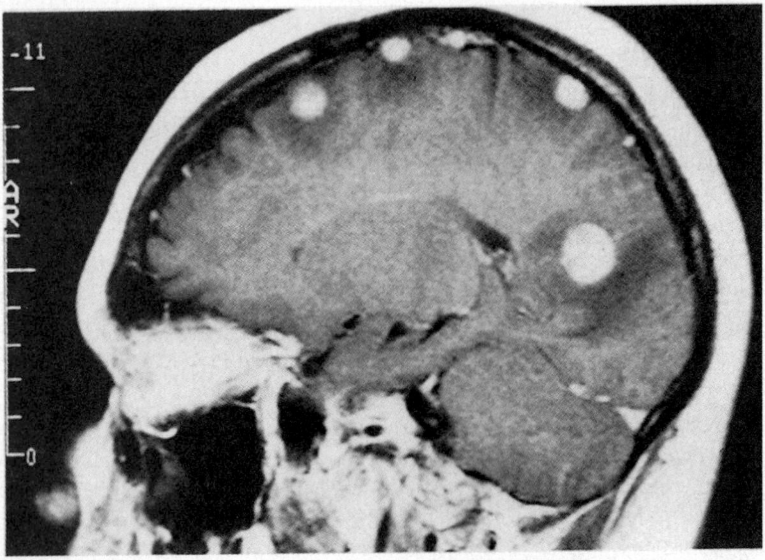

FIGURE 1: Gadolinium-enhanced MRI scan demonstrating multiple brain metastases. Note the edema surrounding each lesion.

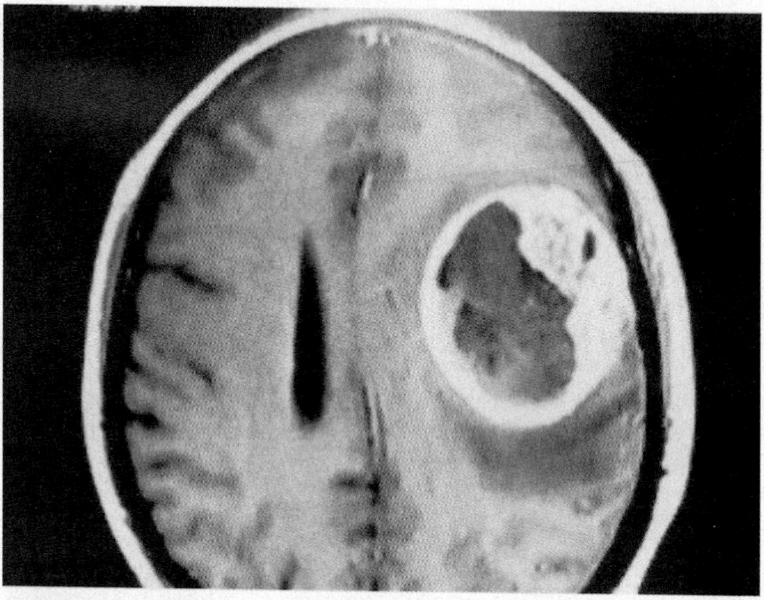

FIGURE 2: T1-weighted MRI with gadolinium contrast showing a typical appearance of a glioblastoma multiforme. Non–contrast-enhanced images of this lesion (not shown) revealed the presence of some hemorrhage.

the four-tier World Health Organization (WHO) system. Grade I tumors are localized tumors called pilocytic astrocytomas, which are usually found in children and may be associated with neurofibromatosis type I. Grade II tumors are low-grade diffuse fibrillary astrocytomas. Grade III (anaplastic astrocytoma) and IV (gliobastoma multiforme) tumors are high-grade malignant neoplasms. Grading is based on pathologic features, such as endothelial proliferation, cellular pleomorphism, mitoses, and necrosis.

Low-grade astroglial tumors (such as astrocytoma and oligodendroglioma) and mixed neuronal-glial tumors (such as ganglioglioma) grow slowly but have a propensity to transform into malignant neoplasms over time. Transformation is usually associated with progressive neurologic symptoms and the appearance of enhancement on MRI.

The high-grade gliomas include glioblastoma, gliosarcoma, anaplastic astrocytoma, and anaplastic oligodendroglioma. These tumors are extremely invasive, with tumor cells often found up to 4 cm away from the primary tumor.

Ependymomas Intracranial ependymomas are relatively rare, accounting for < 2% of all brain tumors. They are most frequently seen in the posterior fossa or spinal cord, although they may also arise in the supratentorial compartment. Ependymomas are typically low-grade histologically, but their high rate of recurrence indicates malignant behavior.

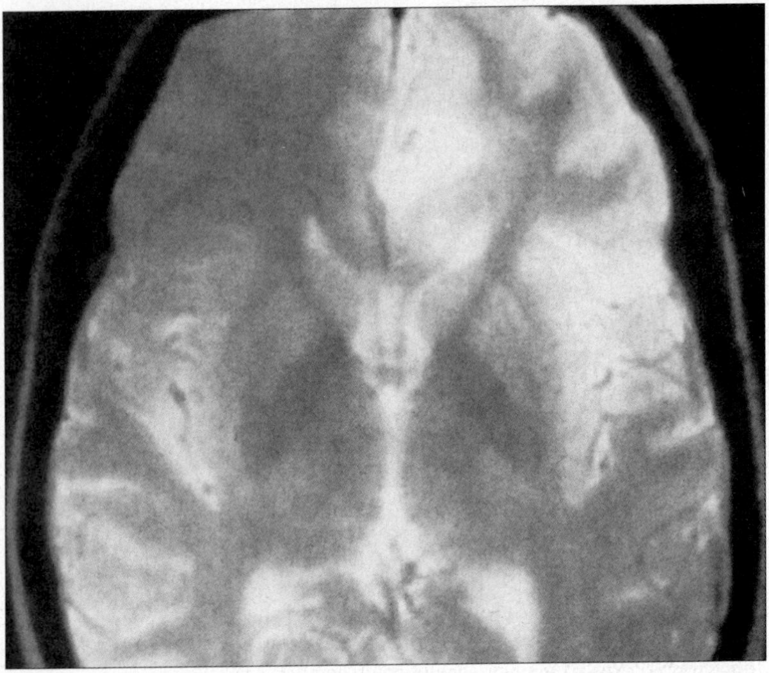

FIGURE 3: T2-weighted MRI demonstrating a diffusely infiltrating, low-grade oligodendroglioma involving the left frontal and temporal lobes. This lesion did not enhance with gadolinium.

Medulloblastomas are uncommon in adults but are one of the two most common primary brain tumors in children (the other being cerebellar astrocytomas). Medulloblastomas arise in the cerebellum and are always high-grade neoplasms.

Primitive neuroectodermal tumors (PNETs) are high-grade, aggressive tumors that usually occur in children. They include pineoblastoma and neuroblastoma. Histologically, they are identical to medulloblastomas, but their prognosis is usually worse than that for medulloblastomas. Thus, their biology is different, even though they may be similar pathologically.

Extra-axial tumors The most common extra-axial tumor is the meningioma. Meningiomas are usually benign tumors that arise from residual mesenchymal cells in the meninges. They produce neurologic symptoms by compressing the underlying brain. Meningiomas rarely are malignant or invade brain tissue.

Other common extra-axial tumors include pituitary adenoma, epidermoid or dermoid tumors, and acoustic neuroma (vestibular schwannoma). Most extra-axial tumors have a benign histology but can be locally invasive.

Metastatic brain tumors The pathology of metastatic brain lesions recapitulates the pathology of the underlying primary neoplasm. This feature often enables the pathologist to suggest the primary source in patients whose systemic cancer presents as a brain metastasis. However, even after a complete systemic evaluation, the site of the primary tumor remains unknown in 5%-13% of patients with brain metastases.

Staging and prognosis

Staging is not applicable to most primary brain tumors because they are locally invasive and do not spread to regional lymph nodes or distant organs. Staging with an enhanced complete spinal MRI and CSF evaluation is important for a few primary tumor types, such as medulloblastoma, ependymoma, and PNET, because they can disseminate via the CSF. All systemic cancers are stage IV when they present with brain metastasis.

Prognostic factors For patients with primary brain tumors, prognosis is inversely related to several important factors, including pathologic grade and patient age, and is directly related to the overall clinical condition at diagnosis. Several molecular markers that correlate well with prognosis have been identified recently, such as LOH on chromosomes 1p and 19q in anaplastic oligodendroglioma.

With conventional treatment, including surgical resection, radiotherapy, and chemotherapy, median survival is 3 years for patients with an anaplastic astrocytoma and 1 year for those with glioblastoma multiforme. In a population of patients with low-grade tumors, including astrocytoma and oligodendroglioma, median survival is 5-10 years; most of these individuals die of malignant transformation of their original tumor. Patients with low-grade oligodendroglioma can survive a median of 16 years in some series. Patients $\geq$ 40 years old with low-grade glioma generally have more aggressive disease; their median survival is usually < 5 years. Prognosis for patients with low-grade tumors is significantly better than for those with malignant tumors, with > 80% of patients experiencing long-term survival.

For a large proportion of patients with brain metastases, median survival is only 4-6 months after whole-brain radiotherapy. However, some patients (ie, those who are < 60 years old, have a single lesion, or have controlled or controllable systemic disease) can achieve prolonged survival, and these individuals warrant a more aggressive therapeutic approach. Furthermore, most of these patients qualify for vigorous local therapy for their brain metastases, such as surgical resection or, possibly, stereotactic radiosurgery. These approaches can achieve a median survival of 40 weeks or longer.

Treatment

Treatment of primary brain tumors and brain metastases consists of both supportive and definitive therapies.

SUPPORTIVE THERAPY

Supportive treatment focuses on relieving symptoms and improving the patient's neurologic function. The primary supportive agents are anticonvulsants and corticosteroids.

Anticonvulsants

Anticonvulsants are administered to ~25% of patients who have a seizure at presentation. Phenytoin (300-400 mg/d) is the most commonly used medication, but carbamazepine (600-1,000 mg/d), phenobarbital (90-150 mg/d), and valproic acid (750-1,500 mg/d) are equally efficacious. Doses of all these anticonvulsants can be titrated to the appropriate serum levels to provide maximal protection.

Newer anticonvulsants, such as levetiracetam (Keppra), gabapentin, lamotrigine (Lamictal), and topiramate (Topamax), are also effective. Most of these agents have the advantages of causing few cognitive side effects, and because they do not induce the hepatic microsomal system, they do not alter the metabolism of chemotherapeutic agents. These agents are rapidly replacing the older drugs as first-line antiepileptic therapy.

Prophylaxis Prospective studies have failed to show the efficacy of prophylactic anticonvulsants for patients with brain tumors who have not had a seizure. Consequently, prophylactic anticonvulsants should not be administered, except during the perioperative period, when their use may reduce the incidence of postoperative seizures; the drugs can be tapered off within 2 weeks of surgery. Increasingly, the new agents are being used for prophylaxis.

Corticosteroids

Corticosteroids reduce peritumoral edema, diminishing mass effect and lowering intracranial pressure. This effect produces prompt relief of headache and improvement of lateralizing signs. Dexamethasone is the corticosteroid of choice because of its minimal mineralocorticoid activity. The starting dose is ~ 16 mg/d, but this dose is adjusted upward or downward to reach the minimum dose necessary to control neurologic symptoms.

Long-term corticosteroid use is associated with hypertension, diabetes mellitus, a nonketotic hyperosmolar state, myopathy, weight gain, insomnia, and osteoporosis. Thus, the steroid dose in patients with a brain tumor should be tapered as rapidly as possible once definitive treatment has begun. Most patients can stop taking steroids by the time they have completed cranial irradiation. All patients taking corticosteroids for more than 6 weeks should be on antibiotic prophylaxis for *Pneumocystis carinii* pneumonia. Prophylaxis should continue for 1 month after the steroids have been discontinued.

DEFINITIVE THERAPY

Definitive treatment of brain tumors includes surgery, radiation therapy, and chemotherapy. The first step is to devise an overall therapeutic plan that should outline the sequence and elements of multidisciplinary therapy.

Surgery

Various surgical options are available, and the surgical approach should be carefully chosen to maximize tumor resection while preserving vital brain structures and minimizing the risk of postoperative neurologic deficits. The goals of surgery include (1) obtaining an accurate histologic diagnosis; (2) reducing tumor burden and associated mass effect caused by the tumor and/or peritumoral edema; (3) maintaining or re-establishing pathways for CSF flow; and, for primary brain tumors, (4) achieving potential "cure" by gross total removal. Surgery for metastatic brain tumor rarely achieves cure but can reduce tumor burden so that the tumor becomes more amenable to adjuvant irradiation or chemotherapy.

Surgical tools A variety of tools are available to help the neurosurgeon achieve these goals, including stereotactic and image-based guidance systems and electrophysiologic brain mapping.

Stereotactic frames provide a rigid, three-dimensional (3D) coordinate system for accurate targeting of brain lesions identified on CT or MRI scans and are particularly well suited for obtaining tissue for biopsy from tumors located in deep structures or in other sites where aggressive tissue removal would produce unacceptable neurologic deficits. A limitation of stereotactic biopsy is that small volumes of tissue are obtained, and tissue sampling errors may result in failure to reach a correct diagnosis. Stereotactic biopsy may be nondiagnostic in 3%-8% of cases and has a surgical morbidity of approximately 5%.

Image-based guidance system "Frameless" or "image-guided" stereotactic systems use computer technology to coregister preoperative imaging studies with intraoperative head position, thereby establishing stereotactic accuracy without the need for a frame. These systems are useful for achieving maximal resections of predefined tumor volumes and minimizing surgical morbidity. Intraoperative MRI accomplishes similar goals but is limited by a requirement for specialized operating suites.

Intraoperative brain mapping, also termed cortical mapping, uses electrical stimulation of the cortical surface to define the primary motor, sensory, or speech cortex. By identifying the exact location of these areas prior to tumor resection, the surgeon can avoid these structures, thereby preserving neurologic function. These tools enable the neurosurgeon to perform more complete removal of tumors with less morbidity.

Pathology-based surgical approach for primary brain tumors The surgical approach to an intracranial lesion is strongly influenced by the suspected or previously confirmed pathology. Guidelines for the management of the most common tumors are discussed.

Meningiomas and other extra-axial tumors Benign extra-axial tumors, such as meningiomas, usually have a well-defined plane separating them from the surrounding brain parenchyma. In general, total extirpation can be achieved by open craniotomy, particularly when the tumor is located over the convexity. Firm attachment of the tumor to the dura, cranial nerves, vascular structures, or skull base may make this impossible. Subtotal resections that preserve neural or vascular structures while reducing mass effect are often favored for extensive skull base tumors.

The surgical management of other benign extra-axial tumors, such as acoustic neuroma, pineocytoma, choroid plexus papilloma, and pituitary adenoma, closely parallels that of meningiomas. Gross total resection is generally curative and should be attempted whenever safe.

Low-grade gliomas Gross total resection, whenever possible, is the goal of surgery for low-grade gliomas and mixed neuronal-glial tumors (eg, astrocytoma, oligodendroglioma, pilocytic astrocytoma, and ganglioglioma). Long-term survival is generally considered better in patients who have undergone a gross total resection than in those who have had a subtotal resection (5-year survival rates > 80% for gross total resection vs ~50% for subtotal resection).

If a radiographically proven gross total resection is attained, postoperative irradiation or chemotherapy can often be withheld until there is evidence of tumor progression (see section on "Radiation therapy"). If a postoperative scan reveals a small but surgically accessible residual lesion, immediate reoperation should be considered, particularly in children or in those with pilocytic astrocytomas (WHO grade I).

When low-grade tumors are found in patients with medically refractory chronic epilepsy, surgical management should be oriented toward curing the epilepsy, as well as achieving total tumor removal.

Ependymomas Gross total resection is the goal of surgery whenever possible for ependymomas. Because ependymomas arise in the ventricular system, they can disseminate in the CSF. Therefore, all patients should be assessed for subarachnoid metastases with complete cranial and spinal MRI performed with gadolinium.

High-grade gliomas More extensive resections improve the quality of life and neurologic function of patients with high-grade gliomas (glioblastoma multiforme, anaplastic astrocytoma, and anaplastic oliogodendroglioma) by reducing mass effect, edema, and steroid dependence. Resection of > 98% of the remaining tumor volume prolongs survival relative to subtotal or partial resections, but extensive subtotal resections do not appear to confer any survival advantage over biopsy alone or limited resection. For this reason, most neurosurgeons attempt to achieve maximal resection while minimizing risk to critical areas of the brain.

Recurrent or progressive tumors When a brain tumor recurs or enlarges, reoperation is often necessary to reduce mass effect. Although rarely curative, these procedures can improve quality of life and modestly extend survival. In general, reoperation is not considered in patients with a Karnofsky performance status (KPS) score ≤ 60 or in those patients who are not candidates for adjuvant therapy following initial surgery. Recurrent tumor cannot be distinguished from radiation necrosis on routine MRI. Both disorders may cause severe mass effect and edema, and resection is the optimal treatment for both. However, PET or magnetic resonance spectroscopy (MRS) can often distinguish tumor from treatment effect.

Initial resection or reoperation followed by intracavitary or intraparenchymal administration of chemotherapy, immunotherapy, or liquid I-125 radiotherapy (GliaSite) is being explored but is still investigational. Carmustine (BiCNU)-impregnated wafers (Gliadel) are the only form of intracavitary chemotherapy currently approved by the US Food and Drug Administration (FDA) for glioblastoma.

Surgical approach for metastatic tumors Resection followed by whole-brain irradiation significantly prolongs survival compared with whole-brain irradiation alone in patients with a solitary brain metastasis, and some patients achieve long-term disease-free survival. Most patients with brain metastases have a life expectancy of < 6 months, but the majority who undergo resection of a solitary metastatic lesion followed by irradiation will die of systemic rather than intracranial disease.

Excision of metastatic brain tumors is rarely curative, however, as microscopic cells may be left behind. Nevertheless, the reduced tumor burden becomes more amenable to adjuvant irradiation and/or chemotherapy.

Criteria The decision whether to recommend surgery for metastatic brain tumors should be based on the following factors:

Extracranial oncologic status A comprehensive work-up of the patient's extracranial oncologic status is necessary. Extensive critical organ metastases preclude surgery in favor of palliative irradiation as the sole therapy. Brain surgery should not be performed in patients with limited expected survival (3-6 weeks) based on extracranial disease.

Number of metastases In general, only patients harboring a single metastasis are considered for resection. Occasionally, a large tumor will be removed in the presence of multiple smaller nodules if the edema and mass effect of this lesion are causing a substantial neurologic deficit that could be improved by tumor removal.

If brain metastasis is the presenting sign of systemic cancer and no clear primary source can be identified with routine staging, surgery may also be required to establish a tissue diagnosis and plan further therapy.

In addition, surgical removal of a brain metastasis often reverses the neurologic deficits caused by compression of local structures by tumor and reduces intracranial hypertension.

Three studies have concluded that when multiple (up to three distinct locations) metastases are resected, either with or without radiotherapy, survival times are identical to those in patients with surgically resected solitary metastases and almost twice as long as those in patients treated by radiation therapy or radiosurgery alone. These studies suggest that a more aggressive surgical approach may be justified in patients with multiple brain metastases who have stable systemic disease.

Recurrence of solitary metastases Up to 20% of solitary metastases may recur in long-term survivors. In these cases, a second operation may be warranted to remove the recurrent lesion and confirm the histologic diagnosis (ie, exclude radionecrosis).

Radiation therapy

Radiation therapy plays a central role in the treatment of brain tumors in adults. It is the most effective nonsurgical therapy for patients with malignant gliomas and also has an important role in the treatment of patients with low-grade gliomas and metastatic brain tumors.

Whole-brain vs partial-brain irradiation Whole-brain irradiation is reserved for multifocal lesions, lesions with significant subependymal or leptomeningeal involvement, and metastatic brain tumors. For the majority of patients with unifocal disease, limited-field treatment results in less morbidity and appears to produce equal, albeit poor, overall survival.

CT-based treatment planning, or 3D conformal radiation therapy, is a relatively new method of treatment planning that utilizes CT information and powerful computer technology to optimize delivery of external-beam radiotherapy to tumors. Recent studies demonstrate that the predominant failure pattern of high-grade gliomas treated with high-dose (90 Gy) conformal radiation therapy remains local. Conformal treatments do not increase the risk of marginal or distant recurrences, but they can decrease the late effects of radiotherapy by reducing the volume of normal brain irradiated.

Radiation therapy for low-grade gliomas Retrospective studies suggest a limited radiation dose response in low-grade gliomas. However, selection bias may play a role in these studies.

Several recently completed randomized studies addressed the question of optimal timing and dose of radiotherapy in patients with low-grade gliomas. An American intergroup randomized trial compared 50.4 vs 64.8 Gy of radiation in patients with low-grade glioma. A European Organization for Research on the Treatment of Cancer (EORTC) trial compared 45.0 vs 59.4 Gy of radiation in patients with low-grade astrocytoma. Both studies confirmed the superiority or equivalent efficacy of the lower radiation dose.

A second EORTC trial tested immediate vs delayed radiotherapy in individuals with low-grade glioma. Although immediate radiotherapy significantly improved 5-year disease progression-free survival, overall survival was identical in the two treatment arms. Furthermore, quality of life was better in patients whose radiotherapy was deferred until clinical or radiographic disease progression was evident.

Recommended treatment approach for low-grade astrocytomas The role of postoperative radiotherapy in the management of incompletely resected low-grade astrocytomas has not been firmly established. However, based on the available data, the following principles appear to be reasonable:

- A complete surgical resection of hemispheric astrocytomas should be attempted.
- If a complete surgical resection has been attained, radiation therapy can be withheld until MRI or CT studies clearly indicate a recurrence that cannot be approached surgically.

- When a complete surgical resection is not performed, postoperative irradiation may be recommended, depending upon the patients' clinical condition. Patients with controlled seizures and no neurologic deficit can be followed and radiation therapy deferred until clinical or radiographic disease progression occurs. Patients with progressive neurologic dysfunction, such as language or cognitive difficulties, require immediate therapy. Astrocytomas must be treated with radiotherapy, but oligodendrogliomas or mixed gliomas may benefit from chemotherapy as initial treatment (see later in this chapter).
- Radiation therapy should be delivered, using a megavoltage machine, in 1.7- to 2.0-Gy daily fractions, to a total dose of about 50 Gy. The treatment fields should include the primary tumor volume only, as defined by MRI, and should not encompass the whole brain.
- In low-grade astrocytomas, radiation therapy can be expected to produce a 5-year survival rate of 50% and a 10-year survival rate of 20%. Patients with low-grade oligodendrogliomas survive even longer.
- Cognitive impairment may develop in long-term survivors of low-grade gliomas treated with radiotherapy.

Radiation therapy for high-grade gliomas An analysis of three studies of high-grade gliomas performed by the Brain Tumor Study Group (BTSG) showed that postoperative radiotherapy doses > 50 Gy were significantly better in improving survival than no postoperative treatment and that 60 Gy resulted in significantly prolonged survival compared with 50 Gy. On the other hand, an American intergroup protocol, which randomized patients to receive 60 Gy of whole-brain irradiation, with or without a local boost of 10 Gy, demonstrated no survival benefit in the group receiving treatment with a total radiation dose of 70 Gy. These results may have been confounded by the competing morbidity of whole-brain radiotherapy given at a dose of 60 Gy.

Based on these data, involved-field radiotherapy to 60 Gy in 30-33 fractions is standard treatment for high-grade histologies; this amount corresponds to a dose just above the threshold for radionecrosis. Patients older than age 60 with glioblastoma have identical survival rates after an abbreviated course of radiotherapy (40 Gy in 15 fractions) as after the standard regimen. Reducing treatment time with this approach is a reasonable option for older patients. About half of patients with anaplastic astrocytomas exhibit radiographic evidence of response following 60 Gy of radiation, compared with 25% of patients with glioblastoma multiforme. Complete radiographic response is rare in either case.

Radiation therapy for metastatic brain tumors For symptomatic patients with brain metastases, median survival is about 1 month if untreated and 3-6 months if whole-brain radiation therapy is delivered, with no significant differences among various conventional radiotherapy fractionation schemes (20 Gy in 5 fractions, 30 Gy in 10 fractions, 40 Gy in 20 fractions). A more protracted schedule is used for patients who have limited or no evidence of systemic disease or for those who have undergone resection of a single brain metastasis, since these patients have the potential for long-term survival or even cure. The use of hypofractionated regimens is associated with an increased risk of neurologic toxicity.

The addition of the radiosensitizer motexafin gadolinium to whole-brain radiotherapy (130 Gy) did not improve survival or time to neurologic disease progression in a randomized phase III trial. Subgroup analysis suggested prolonged time to neurocognitive disease progression in patients with brain metastases from lung cancer.

Relief of neurologic symptoms The major result of whole-brain radiation therapy is an improvement in neurologic symptoms, such as headache, motor loss, and impaired mentation. The overall response rate ranges from 70% to 90%. Unfortunately, symptomatic relief is not permanent, and symptoms recur with intracranial tumor progression.

Solitary lesion Postoperative whole-brain radiation therapy significantly improves control of CNS disease after resection of a single brain metastasis but has no impact on overall survival. Postoperative whole-brain radiation therapy may be withheld, therefore, in selected patients, such as elderly individuals or those with highly radioresistant primaries (eg, renal cancer), because these patients are vulnerable to the toxic effects of cranial irradiation without reaping the potential benefits.

Multiple lesions Patients with multiple lesions are generally treated with whole-brain radiation therapy alone. Retreatment with a second course of whole-brain radiation therapy can provide further palliation for patients with progressive brain metastases (who have at least a 6-month or longer remission of symptoms after the initial course of cranial irradiation).

Concomitant steroid therapy Since the radiographic and clinical responses to whole-brain irradiation take several weeks, patients with significant mass effect should be treated with steroids during whole-brain radiation therapy. Dexamethasone (16 mg/d) is started prior to therapy, and the dose may be tapered as tolerated during treatment. Occasionally, higher doses are necessary to ameliorate neurologic symptoms. However, most patients can be safely tapered off corticosteroids at the completion of whole-brain radiotherapy.

Alternatives to conventional radiotherapy

The results of standard radiation treatment in patients with malignant gliomas are poor. Patients with glioblastoma multiforme have a median survival of 9-12 months, whereas patients with anaplastic astrocytomas survive a median of 3 years. In an attempt to improve these poor results, a number of new approaches have been tried, including hyperfractionated radiotherapy (HFRT), focal dose escalation with interstitial brachytherapy, and radiosurgery, but none improve survival. Brachytherapy and HFRT have been abandoned.

Radiosurgery Over the past several years, there has been growing interest in the use of radiosurgery for the treatment of primary and recurrent malignant brain tumors. Radiosurgery is currently performed with one of three technologies: high-energy photons produced by linear accelerators; the gamma knife; or, less frequently, charged particles, such as protons or other ions produced by cyclotrons or synchrotrons.

The survival rates, patterns of recurrence, and rates of complications (including radionecrosis) of radiosurgery and brachytherapy are similar. Radiosurgery is more appealing than brachytherapy for the management of highly focal malignant gliomas because it is a noninvasive, single-day procedure that can usually be performed in an outpatient setting.

A Radiation Therapy Oncology Group (RTOG) trial comparing external-beam radiotherapy and BiCNU vs external-beam radiotherapy, BiCNU, and radiosurgery revealed there was no survival advantage for patients treated with a radiosurgery boost. Based on the results of this phase III trial, radiosurgery cannot be recommended as part of the initial treatment for patients with glioblastoma multiforme. However, radiosurgery for focally recurrent disease is occasionally appropriate.

Radionecrosis Both brachytherapy and stereotactic radiosurgery can induce focal radionecrosis. This complication produces symptoms of mass effect in about 50% of patients with malignant glioma, requiring resection to remove the necrotic debris. (Fewer than 5% of patients with other lesions [eg, brain metastases] require reoperation for radionecrosis.) Occasionally, treatment with corticosteroids can control the edema around the radionecrotic area, but often the patient becomes steroid-dependent, with all of the attendant complications of chronic steroid use. Radionecrosis can be a significant limitation of the focal radiotherapy techniques.

Additional radiotherapeutic approaches

A new technology has been developed to fill a surgical cavity with an inflatable balloon that contains radioactive iodine (GliaSite). The temporary source of radiation appears to increase local control without leading to radionecrosis.

Recommended approach for extra-axial tumors Surgery alone is curative in the vast majority of patients with benign tumors. However, in certain subsets of patients, postoperative radiotherapy may control further growth of these lesions.

Pituitary adenomas For hormonally inactive pituitary adenomas that persist or recur after surgery, 45-50 Gy is delivered in 25-28 fractions to the radiographic boundaries of the tumor. For Cushing disease and acromegaly, higher doses are required for biochemical remission. Coronal-enhanced MRI is critical for treatment planning, since CT often does not visualize the skull base and the entire extent of disease.

The most common indications for radiotherapy are invasion of the cavernous sinus or the suprasellar space and incomplete resection of macroadenomas (> 1.5 cm). Most pituitary lesions do not grow following radiotherapy, and hormonally active tumors usually demonstrate a hormonal response with a reduction in hormone hypersecretion in 1-3 years. Following radiation therapy, 20%-50% of patients develop panhypopituitarism, requiring hormone replacement therapy. Other significant complications (ie, damage to the visual apparatus) are rare today.

Meningiomas are readily curable with complete surgical resection. However, base of skull lesions and lesions involving a patent venous sinus often cannot be resected completely. For some patients with these lesions, a course of postoperative radiotherapy is indicated. In general, 54 Gy is delivered in 30 fractions to the radiographic tumor region utilizing 3D treatment planning. Malignant meningiomas always require postoperative radiotherapy, even after gross total resection. Radiosurgery may also be useful in treating meningiomas, and doses of 13-18 Gy are associated with a high rate of control at 10 years following therapy.

Acoustic neuroma has classically been considered a surgical disease. Following total resection, recurrence rates are < 5%. When only subtotal resection is possible, disease recurs in at least 60% of patients.

Radiosurgery has been used as an alternative to surgery for acoustic neuroma. Control rates of > 80% at 20 years have been reported. For patients with useful hearing prior to radiosurgery, that function is preserved in < 50%. After radiosurgery, 10% of patients experience facial weakness and 25%, trigeminal neuropathy. The risk of cranial neuropathies is related to the size of the lesion treated.

Radiosurgery for metastatic brain tumors

Radiosurgery has been used as sole therapy, as a boost to whole-brain radiation therapy, or for recurrent lesions in patients with brain metastases. Radiosurgery has the advantage of delivering effective focal treatment, usually in a single dose, without irradiating the normal brain. Radiosurgery of brain metastases ≤ 1 cm achieves 1- and 2-year local control rates of 86% and 78%, respectively, significantly better than 56% and 24% for lesions > 1 cm. It is particularly useful for patients who have one to three lesions, each < 4 cm in diameter. Patients with numerous lesions are not good candidates for radiosurgery because some of the ports may overlap, and, more importantly, these patients likely harbor other microscopic lesions in the brain that are not being treated effectively with such focal therapy.

Brain metastases are particularly amenable to treatment with radiosurgery. Metastatic tumors do not infiltrate the brain and tend to have well-circumscribed borders; therefore, they can be targeted effectively with highly focused irradiation techniques that maintain a sharp delineation between the enhancing tumor seen on neuroimaging and normal brain. Furthermore, radiosurgery does not have the operative morbidity that may be associated with resection of a brain metastasis. Consequently, it can be used safely in many patients who are not surgical candidates, and it can even treat lesions in surgically unapproachable locations such as the brainstem.

Radiosurgery can achieve crude local control rates of 73%-98% over a median follow-up of 5-26 months. Radiosurgery was initially used primarily as a boost after treatment with whole-brain radiotherapy. Three randomized trials have reported on the value of radiosurgery in addition to whole-brain radiotherapy for patients with multiple brain metastases. Although all three studies show a local control advantage and an improvement in quality-of-life endpoints with the addition of a radiosurgery boost, none shows a statistical advantage in survival. For patients with multiple brain metastases, adding radiosurgery to whole-brain radiotherapy only offers an improved neurologic quality of life with no impact on survival.

A prospective, randomized RTOG trial compared whole-brain radiotherapy alone vs whole-brain radiotherapy plus radiosurgery in patients with one to three metastases. Local control, neurologic function, and steroid doses were improved in patients with a single lesion treated with radiosurgery. Although there was no statistical improvement in overall survival in the two arms of the trial, a subset analysis showed improved survival for those patients with a single lesion.

Radiosurgery is often considered an alternative to standard surgical resection, but it is unclear whether they are equivalent. Most retrospective studies suggest that the two techniques produce similar results; however, some reports indicate that surgery offers improved local control, whereas others suggest that radiosurgery is superior.

Increasingly, radiosurgery is being used as sole therapy for one to three brain metastases. A prospective randomized trial is currently under way to determine outcome with radiosurgery with or without whole-brain radiotherapy, but most investigators expect the results to be similar to those observed in the phase III trial of surgical resection of a single brain metastasis with or without radiotherapy: improved local control but no survival benefit. There is growing evidence from large retrospective series that radiosurgery alone may be as effective as radiosurgery plus whole-brain irradiation for the control of CNS disease; however, some series point to a higher incidence of brain recurrence if whole-brain radiotherapy is withheld. Radiosurgery alone substantially shortens treatment time and eliminates the risk of cognitive impairment associated with whole-brain irradiation, particularly in elderly patients.

Median survival from the time of radiosurgery is 6–15 months, and some patients can live for years without recurrence. Most patients exhibit clinical improvement and decreased steroid requirement after radiosurgery, and only 11%–25% of patients eventually die of neurologic causes.

Treatment recommendations for metastatic brain tumors

In patients with one to three brain metastases, aggressive local therapy (surgical resection or radiosurgery) produces superior survival and quality of life than does whole-brain radiation therapy alone. Radiosurgery may be the optimal choice for elderly patients at greater risk for surgical morbidity. Whole-brain radiotherapy does not contribute to survival after surgical resection and probably not after radiosurgery. Increasingly, we are reserving it for use at CNS recurrence and not following a complete resection or radiosurgery with routine whole-brain irradiation.

Bevacizumab combined with irinotecan was well tolerated in 32 patients with recurrent malignant glioma. Response rate was 63% and median progression-free survival was 24 weeks *(Vrendenburgh JJ, Desjardins A, Herndon II JE, et al: Proc Am Soc Clin Oncol 24:59s, 2006).*

Chemotherapy

Malignant gliomas Chemotherapy has a limited benefit in the treatment of patients with malignant gliomas. In studies using nitrosoureas, it does not significantly lengthen median survival in all patients, but a subgroup seems to have prolonged survival with the addition of adjuvant chemotherapy to radiotherapy. Prognostic factors (age, KPS score, and histology) do not predict which patients will benefit from chemotherapy.

In a large phase III trial, patients with newly diagnosed glioblastoma were randomized to receive radiotherapy alone or radiotherapy with concurrently administered temozolomide followed by adjuvant temozolomide (Temodar). A total of 573 patients were studied, and median survival was significantly prolonged from 12.1 months to 14.6 months with the addition of temozolomide to radiotherapy. The 2-year survival rate was only 10.4% in those treated with radiotherapy alone compared with 26.5% in those who received radiotherapy plus temozolomide. The combined-modality regimen was well tolerated and associated with minimal additional toxicity. This regimen has now become the standard for all newly diagnosed patients with glioblastoma and combines the potential radiosensitizing effect of concurrent temozolomide with the benefit of adjuvant chemotherapy.

Although this study demonstrates clear benefit in patients with glioblastoma, many investigators have extrapolated this regimen for use in patients with gliomas of all grades. This regimen is currently under study in patients with grade III glioma, but until those data are available, we recommend a standard course of radiotherapy followed by adjuvant temozolomide for patients with anaplastic gliomas.

Despite initial treatment, virtually all malignant gliomas recur. At relapse, patients may benefit from re-resection, focal radiotherapy techniques (such as radiosurgery), or different chemotherapeutic agents. Most patients will have received temozolomide as part of initial therapy so procarbazine (Matulane) or a nitrosourea would be a reasonable conventional choice at recurrence. Hydroxyurea and imatinib mesylate may also provide durable antitumor activity in some patients. Clinical trials employing signal transduction inhibitors, epidermal growth factor receptor inhibitors, or antiangiogenic agents may also be available at tumor relapse.

There has been considerable interest in the potential use of antiangiogenic agents in malignant gliomas. Thalidomide (Thalomid) is a weak antiangiogenic drug and as a single agent, it has produced few responses, but stable disease was seen in one-third of patients. Preliminary data on bevacizumab (Avastin) and chemotherapy in patients with recurrent malignant glioma demonstrate a 60% response rate with prolonged survival. This highly promising result is under further study.

Astrocytomas Chemotherapy has no role in the initial treatment of low-grade astrocytomas, and usually they have progressed to malignant tumors at the time of recurrence.

Oligodendroglioma In contrast, the oligodendroglioma is now recognized as a particularly chemosensitive primary brain tumor. This finding was first observed with the anaplastic oligodendroglioma but has recently been seen with the more common low-grade oligodendroglioma. Chemosensitivity of anaplastic and low-grade tumors is associated with loss of chromosomes 1p and 19q.

> Newly diagnosed patients with anaplastic oligodendroglioma were randomized to receive radiotherapy alone vs preradiotherapy PCV (procarbazine, lomustine [CeeNu], and vincristine) followed by radiotherapy. Preradiotherapy PCV prolonged progression-free survival (1.9 yrs vs 2.6 yrs, $P = .053$) but did not affect survival. PCV was associated with grade 3/4 toxicity in 64% of patients (*Cairncross G, Seiferheld W, Shaw E, et al: Proc Am Soc Clin Oncol [abstract] 23:1500, 2004*).

Several alkylating agents are active, but the best studied regimen is procarbazine, lomustine (CeeNu), and vincristine (PCV), which produces response rates of 75% and 90% in malignant and low-grade oligodendrogliomas, respectively. Consequently, chemotherapy is an important therapeutic modality and may be used as initial treatment in patients with low-grade tumors who require therapeutic intervention. This approach defers or eliminates the late cognitive toxicity associated with cranial irradiation in patients with low-grade tumors who can have relatively prolonged survival. Patients with malignant oligodendrogliomas require radiotherapy with or without chemotherapy for initial treatment.

Most chemotherapy trials in patients with oligodendrogliomas used standard PCV or an intensified form of the regimen (Table 1). The intensified regimen is cycled every 6 weeks, whereas the standard regimen is cycled every 8 weeks. It is not clear which regimen has greater efficacy, but the intensive regimen is associated with more myelosuppression. Temozolomide has activity against oligodendroglial tumors either at diagnosis or recurrence, even in those previously treated with PCV. It is much better tolerated than PCV and has replaced PCV as the initial chemotherapeutic agent of choice.

Metastatic brain tumors Chemotherapy usually has a limited role in the treatment of brain metastases and has not proven to be effective as an adjuvant therapy after irradiation or surgery. However, it may have some efficacy in patients with recurrent brain metastases who are not eligible for further whole-brain radiation therapy or stereotactic radiosurgery. In addition, a recent phase III trial of chemotherapy with early vs delayed whole-brain radiotherapy in NSCLC patients with brain metastases showed an identical intracranial response rate and survival. Thus, systemic chemotherapy had some efficacy against brain metastases.

A recently completed phase II trial of temozolomide (75 mg/m^2/d) and concurrent whole-brain radiotherapy (40 Gy in 20 fractions) vs whole-brain radiotherapy alone demonstrated improved response rates and neurologic improvement in the combined-modality arm.

TABLE 1: Chemotherapeutic regimens for gliomas

Regimen	Dose	Route and frequency
Single-agent BiCNU		
BiCNU	200 mg/m^2 (maximum cumulative dose, 1,500 mg/m^2)	IV q8wk
Single-agent temozolomide		
Temozolomide	150-200 mg/m^2	PO on days 1-5
Repeat cycle every 28 days.		
Standard PCV		
Procarbazine	60 mg/m^2/d	PO on days 8-21
Lomustine (CeeNu)	110 mg/m^2	PO on day 1
Vincristine	1.4 mg/m^2 (maximum dose, 2 mg)	IV on days 8 and 29
Repeat cycle every 6-8 weeks, optimally for 6 cycles.		
Intensified PCV[a]		
Procarbazine	75 mg/m^2/d	PO on days 8-21
Lomustine (CeeNu)	130 mg/m^2	PO on day 1
Vincristine	1.4 mg/m^2 (no dose limit)	IV on days 8 and 29
Repeat cycle every 6 weeks.		

[a] Sometimes used in patients with oligodendrogliomas

Brain metastases from chemosensitive primary tumors Brain metastases from primary tumors that are chemosensitive, such as SCLC, choriocarcinoma, and breast cancer, may be responsive to systemic therapy. Single drugs or drug combinations should be selected based on their expected activity against the primary tumor. Temozolomide has activity against recurrent brain metastases, particularly from NSCLC and melanoma.

SUGGESTED READING

ON PRIMARY INTRACRANIAL TUMORS

Black PMCL, Loeffler JS: Cancer of the Nervous System. Philadelphia, Lippincott Williams & Wilkins, 2004.

Chang SM, Parney IF, Huang W, et al: Patterns of care for adults with newly diagnosed malignant glioma. JAMA 293:557–564, 2005.

Forsyth PA, Weaver S, Fulton D, et al: Prophylactic anticonvulsants in patients with brain tumour. Can J Neurol Sci 30:106–112, 2003.

Laws ER, Parney IF, Huang W, et al: Survival following surgery and prognostic factors for recently diagnosed malignant glioma: Data from the Glioma Outcomes Project. J Neurosurg 99:467–473, 2003.

Liau LM, Prins RM, Kiertscher SM, et al: Dendritic cell vaccination in glioblastoma patients induces systemic and intracranial T-cell responses modulated by the local central nervous system tumor microenvironment. Clin Cancer Res 11:5515–5525, 2005.

Megyesi JF, Kachur E, Lee DH, et al: Imaging correlates of molecular signatures in oligodendrogliomas. Clin Cancer Res 10:4303–4306, 2004.

Pope WB, Lai A, Nghiemphu P, et al: MRI in patients with high-grade gliomas treated with bevacizumab and chemotherapy. Neurology 66:1258-1260, 2006.

Reardon DA, Egorin MJ, Quinn JA, et al: Phase II study of imatinib mesylate plus hydroxyurea in adults with recurrent glioblastoma multiforme. J Clin Oncol 23:9359-9368, 2005.

Reijneveld JC, van der Grond J, Ramos LM, et al: Proton MRS imaging in the follow-up of patients with suspected low-grade gliomas. Neuroradiology Aug 20, 2005 [Epub ahead of print].

Roa W, Brasher PM, Bauman C, et al: Abbreviated course of radiation therapy in older patients with glioblastoma multiforme: A prospective randomized clinical trial. J Clin Oncol 22:1583–1588, 2004.

Shai R, Shi T, Kremen TJ, et al: Gene expression profiling identifies molecular subtypes of gliomas. Oncogene 22:4918–4923, 2003.

Souhami L, Seiferheld W, Brachman D, et al: Randomized comparison of stereotactic radiosurgery followed by conventional radiotherapy with carmustine to conventional radiotherapy with carmustine for patients with glioblastoma multiforme: Report of RTOG 93-05 protocol. Int J Radiat Oncol Biol Phys 60:853–860, 2004.

Stupp R, Mason WP, van den Bent MJ, et al: Radiotherapy plus concomitant and adjuvant temozolomide for glioblastoma. N Engl J Med 352:987–996, 2005.

Taphoorn MJ, Klein M: Cognitive deficits in adult patients with brain tumours. Lancet Neurol 3:159–168, 2004.

Tatter SB, Shaw EG, Rosenblum ML, et al: An inflatable balloon catheter and liquid ^{125}I radiation source (GliaSite Radiation Therapy System) for treatment of recurrent malignant glioma: Multicenter Safety and Feasibility Trial. J Neurosurg 99:297–303, 2003.

Tsao MN, Mehta MP, Whelan TJ, et al: The American Society for Therapeutic Radiology and Oncology (ASTRO) evidence-based review of the role of radiosurgery for malignant glioma. Int J Radiat Oncol Biol Phys 63:47–55, 2005.

ON PRIMARY EXTRA-AXIAL TUMORS

Bassiouni H, Hunold A, Asgari S, et al: Tentorial meningiomas: Clinical results in 81 patients treated microsurgically. Neurosurgery 55:108–116, 2004.

Whittle IR, Smith C, Navoo P, et al: Meningiomas. Lancet 363:1535–1543, 2004.

ON METASTATIC BRAIN TUMORS

Andrews PW, Scott CB, Sperduto PW, et al: Whole brain radiation therapy with or without stereotactic radiosurgery boost for patients with one to three brain metastases: Phase III results of the RTOG 95-08 randomised trial. Lancet 363:1665–1672, 2004.

Antonadou D, Paraskevaidis M, Sarris G, et al: Phase II randomized trial of temozolomide and concurrent radiotherapy in patients with brain metastases. J Clin Oncol 17:3644–3650, 2003.

Hasegawa T, Kondziolka D, Flickinger JC, et al: Brain metastases treated with radiosurgery alone: An alternative to whole-brain radiotherapy? Neurosurgery 52:1318–1326, 2003.

Lassman AB, DeAngelis LM: Brain metastases. Neurol Clin 21:1–23, 2003.

Lutterbach J, Cyron D, Henne K, et al: Radiosurgery followed by planned observation in patients with one to three brain metastases. Neurosurgery 52:1066–1073, 2003.

Mehta MP, Rodrigus P, Terhaard CHJ, et al: Survival and neurologic outcomes in a randomized trial of motexafin gadolinium and whole-brain radiation therapy in brain metastases. J Clin Oncol 21:2529–2536, 2003.

Mehta MP, Tsao MN, Whelan TJ, et al: The American Society for Therapeutic Radiology and Oncology (ASTRO) evidence-based review of the role of radiosurgery for brain metastases. Int J Radiat Oncol Biol Phys 63:37–46, 2005.

Nguyen T, DeAngelis LM: Treatment of brain metastases. J Support Oncol 2:405–416, 2004.

O'Neill BP, Iturria NJ, Link MJ, et al: A comparison of surgical resection and stereotactic radiosurgery in the treatment of solitary brain metastases. Int J Radiat Oncol Biol Phys 55:1169–1176, 2003.

Pollock BE, Brown PD, Foote RL, et al: Properly selected patients with multiple brain metastases may benefit from aggressive treatment of their intracranial disease. J Neurooncol 61:73–80, 2003.

Rohren EM, Provenzale JM, Barboriak DP, et al: Screening for cerebral metastases with FDG-PET in patients undergoing whole-body staging of non-central nervous system malignancy. Radiology 226:181–187, 2003.

Sheehan JP, Sun MH, Kondziolka D, et al: Radiosurgery in patients with renal cell carcinoma metastasis to the brain: Long-term outcomes and prognostic factors influencing survival and local tumor control. J Neurosurg 98:342–349, 2003.

Varlotto JM, Flickinger JC, Niranjan A, et al: The impact of whole-brain radiation therapy on the long-term control and morbidity of patients surviving more than one year after gamma knife radiosurgery for brain metastases. Int J Radiat Oncol Biol Phys 62:1125–1132, 2005.

Win T, Laroche CM, Groves AM, et al: The value of performing head CT in screening for cerebral metastases in patients with potentially resectable non-small cell cancer: Experience from a UK cardiothoracic centre. Clin Radiol 59:935–938, 2004.

CHAPTER 27

AIDS-related malignancies

Ronald T. Mitsuyasu, MD, and Jay S. Cooper, MD

Malignancies have been detected in approximately 40% of all patients with acquired immunodeficiency syndrome (AIDS) sometime during the course of their illness. These cancers have been both a primary cause of death in some patients and also a source of considerable morbidity. In the current era of protease inhibitors and highly active antiretroviral therapy (HAART), patients infected with the human immunodeficiency virus (HIV) are surviving longer than ever. HAART appears to have substantially reduced the incidence of Kaposi's sarcoma (KS) and non-Hodgkin lymphoma (NHL) and may enhance the efficacy of treatment for those patients who do develop these tumors. Unfortunately, HAART has not shown a similar effect on the development of other types of neoplasms, and the need to care for patients who develop malignancies in the setting of HIV remains a challenge. Furthermore, HAART is not available universally, with many patients in resource-poor developing countries not having access to antiretroviral drugs.

In a prospective observation study of the causes of death of HIV-infected patients in France in the year 2000, of 964 deaths, 269 (28%) were attributable to malignancies, with 105 of them being non-Hodgkin lymphoma. Malignant disease was the most common cause of death in this group of HIV-infected adults in the era of highly active antiretroviral therapy (HAART). The increased proportion of solid tumors as the cause of death (> 10% of all deaths) may be due to the decreasing incidence of AIDS-defining malignancies since the widespread use of HAART, longer life expectancies of patients with HIV, and the aggressive and poor prognostic nature of these tumors in HIV patients *(Bonnet F, Lewden C, May T, et al: Cancer 101:317-324, 2004).*

KAPOSI'S SARCOMA

KS has been the most common tumor associated with HIV infection, but it currently develops in < 10% of homosexual men with AIDS in the United States and 1%–2% of other HIV-infected persons. The incidence of KS has declined substantially, from 4.8 per 100 person-years in 1990 to 1.5 per 100 person-years in 1997. In 2003, a European study found that the incidence of KS among HIV-infected individuals was less than 10% of the incidence seen a decade earlier in 1994.

Epidemiology

Gender Among AIDS patients in the United States, the incidence of KS is higher in males than in females. There is also a higher incidence of KS in men than in women in Africa (male-female ratio, 2:1), despite the equal prevalence of HIV infection among men and women.

Age The age distribution of AIDS-related KS follows the distribution of HIV infection. As such, AIDS-related KS can occur in all age groups. In American adult males, the most common age of onset of AIDS-related KS is 30–40 years old. No peak age has been reported.

Race No racial or ethnic differences in the incidence of AIDS-related KS have been observed.

Geography In the United States, KS is seen in < 10% of homosexual men with AIDS. The proportion of KS among AIDS-defining diagnoses is lower in parts of Europe, where there are proportionately fewer male homosexual AIDS cases (eg, 6.8% of Italian AIDS patients), and higher in parts of Africa, where KS is endemic in the non–HIV-infected population. Among AIDS cases in the United States, the proportion of patients with KS has declined from the beginning of the AIDS epidemic, possibly as a result of changes in high-risk sexual behavior among homosexual men and the wider use of more effective antiretroviral combination regimens.

Etiology and risk factors

In the United States, the observation that KS occurs predominantly in homosexual men and the epidemiologic evidence that KS has declined among AIDS patients in parallel with the declining incidence of sexually transmitted diseases (STDs) among homosexual men support the theory that a sexually transmitted agent may be involved in the development of AIDS-related KS.

Viruses In 1994, unique viral DNA sequences were identified in tumor tissues from patients with AIDS-related KS, which led to the identification of a new virus called KS-associated herpesvirus (KSHV) or human herpesvirus type 8 (HHV-8). HHV-8 has been found in > 90% of AIDS-KS tumors, as well as in classic KS, endemic African KS, and post–organ transplant-related KS. It has also been identified in body cavity-based lymphoma/primary effusion lymphoma, multicentric Castleman's disease, and angio-immunoblastic lymphadenopathy with dysproteinemia (AILD) in HIV-infected patients.

HHV-8 may be transmitted through sexual contact, blood products, or organ transplantation. The seroprevalence of HHV-8 in AIDS-related KS is nearly 100%. HHV-8 has been found in high concentration in saliva in KS patients.

HHV-8 is critical in the pathogenesis of AIDS-related KS. The mechanism by which HHV-8 induces KS in susceptible individuals is the subject of intense current investigations.

Environmental and host factors Various environmental and host factors, including HIV- and HHV-8–induced cytokines, AIDS-associated infections, the host's hormonal milieu, immunosuppression, and antiretroviral therapy, may induce or suppress the development of KS and alter its growth.

Signs and symptoms

The manifestations of KS in patients with AIDS are variable and range from small innocuous-looking cutaneous lesions to symptom-producing visceral or oral lesions, which may be troublesome and even life-threatening. Although just about every internal organ can occasionally be involved with KS, it is rarely seen in the bone marrow or CNS.

Skin lesions KS tumors typically begin as flat or raised lesions that may progress to plaquelike or nodular tumors. Lesions vary in size and shape but are generally nonpruritic and painless. They range in color from light pink to red to deep purple. KS lesions may be cosmetically disfiguring and may result in social stigmatization that far exceeds any actual physical impairment.

Dermal and lymphatic infiltration with tumor can result in edema of the extremities, periorbital areas, and genitals and may be complicated by skin breakdown and bacterial cellulitis. Edema can be marked and may prevent patients from wearing shoes and/or walking.

Lesions on the feet can cause pain and hamper walking.

Oral lesions are often asymptomatic but can produce pain and swallowing difficulties.

GI tract involvement with KS is seen in up to 50% of patients. Most lesions are asymptomatic; however, obstruction, bleeding, or enteropathy can occur occasionally.

Pulmonary KS usually presents as dyspnea without fever and may become severely debilitating and rapidly fatal if untreated.

Screening and diagnosis

Currently, there are no screening tests for KS. Although most KS lesions are readily recognized, early lesions may be difficult to diagnose, and the lesions of other diseases (eg, bacillary angiomatosis) may mimic those of KS. Once clinically suspected, the diagnosis of KS is made by biopsy and histologic examination of skin lesions, an excised lymph node, or other tissue or by presumptive diagnosis based on the bronchoscopic or endoscopic appearance of a visceral lesion.

GI KS has a typical red, raised appearance and is difficult to diagnose by biopsy because of the submucosal location of many lesions.

Pulmonary KS In patients with pulmonary KS, chest radiographs typically demonstrate diffuse, reticular-nodular infiltrates, mediastinal enlargement, and, sometimes, pleural effusion. Bronchoscopy may reveal extensive endobronchial involvement with tumor. Definitive diagnosis requires transbronchial or open-lung biopsy. Transbronchial biopsies, however, often yield negative results. A presumptive diagnosis of pulmonary KS may be made, in the absence of fever, based on typical radiographic and endobronchial findings of KS-appearing lesions and after the exclusion of infections.

Thallium and technetium-99m scanning may help differentiate KS from other pulmonary diseases. Patients with KS have been found to have thallium– and technetium–avid scans, whereas pulmonary lymphomas and infections are more typically gallium–avid.

Pathology

Cutaneous KS is a lesion of the dermis composed of a proliferation of aberrant vascular structures lined by abnormal-appearing, spindle-shaped endothelial cells and with extravasated erythrocytes and leukocytes within the structures. These spindle cells are generally sparse in early stages but become more numerous and "stack up" between the vascular structures as the tumor advances. Infiltration of mononuclear leukocytes, including plasma cells, T cells, and monocytes, is more prominent in earlier lesions. The histologic appearance of KS in AIDS patients is similar to that seen in non–HIV-infected patients.

Cell of origin The KS tumor cell is believed to be of mesenchymal, endothelial origin. Several endothelial cell markers are positive in KS, including stains for *Ulex europaeus*, CD31, CD34, and EN-4. In addition, the tumor stains with factor VIIIa, CD68, and α-actin but not with PAL-E.

Staging and prognosis

Prognostic factors Although it is difficult to predict from the initial presentation which patients are most likely to have rapidly progressive tumors, several retrospective studies have shown a correlation of survival with the degree of T-cell immunodeficiency, as reflected in the absolute number of T-helper cells. Prior opportunistic infections or the presence of such symptoms as fevers, night sweats, and weight loss (B symptoms) also portend a poor prognosis. Patients who develop KS or whose tumor growth accelerates after an opportunistic infection often have a more aggressive clinical course. Patients with pulmonary involvement generally have a poor prognosis.

Staging system A tumor classification system has been proposed for AIDS-related KS by the oncology committee of the AIDS Clinical Trials Group (ACTG). This system segregates patients into good or poor prognostic groups based on tumor characteristics, immune system function, and systemic illness (the TIS system; see Table 1). A retrospective analysis of 294 patients with AIDS-related KS has shown that the TIS system is a valid predictor for survival.

Gauging response to therapy Given the heterogeneity and unpredictable growth of this tumor, it is often difficult to gauge objective responses. The peculiarities of this multicentric tumor make some subjectivity almost inevitable in gauging treatment responses.

Treatment

The treatment of AIDS-related KS requires an individualized approach, based on the extent and location of the lesions, the wishes and treatment needs of the patient, the presence of tumor-associated symptoms (eg, pain, bleeding, edema), the presence of other AIDS-associated illnesses, and the patient's tolerance of medications. Nevertheless, the following general statements can be made:

- Patients with widespread symptomatic disease or life-threatening visceral involvement require prompt, cytoreductive treatment with one or more chemotherapeutic drugs.
- Even in the absence of symptomatic visceral disease, the disfigurement and emotional distress of having these visible reminders of AIDS may mandate treatment for psychological reasons.
- For patients with asymptomatic indolent lesions, aggressive treatment is not mandatory, but these patients may derive substantial benefits from local treatment or investigational therapies that are directed against HIV or HHV-8 or that may interrupt the pathogenesis of KS and/or restore immune competence.

TABLE 1: Staging classification for AIDS-related KS[a]

	Risk status	
Characteristic	Good risk (0)	Poor risk (1)
	All of the following:	Any of the following:
Tumor (T)	Tumor confined to skin and/or lymph nodes and/or minimal oral disease[b]	Tumor-associated edema or ulceration; extensive oral KS; GI KS; KS in other non-nodal viscera
Immune system (I)	CD4 cells $\geq$ 150/mm^3	CD4 cells < 150/mm^3
Systemic illness (S)	No history of opportunistic infection or thrush; no B symptoms[c]; performance status $\geq$ 70 (Karnofsky scale)	History of opportunistic infection and/or thrush; B symptoms; performance status < 70 (Karnofsky scale); other HIV-related illness (eg, neurologic disease, lymphoma)

Adapted from Krown SE, Metroka C, Wernz JC: J Clin Oncol 7:1201, 1989, as modified by Krown SE, et al: J Clin Oncol 15:3085, 1997.

[a] Patients are assigned a disease state TXIXSX, where X corresponds to the risk designation (0 or 1) for each risk category

[b] Minimal oral disease is non-nodular KS confined to the palate

[c] B symptoms: unexplained fever, night sweats, > 10% involuntary weight loss, or diarrhea persisting for more than 2 weeks

Treatment options

With the introduction of protease inhibitors and non-nucleoside reverse transcriptase inhibitors for HIV, cases of KS regression with combination antiretroviral therapy have been reported. Because KS seems to be influenced by the state of HIV infection, we believe that all patients with AIDS-related KS should have their HIV infection under optimal control. There is no one best anti-HIV regimen, and oncologists should consult with infectious disease specialists familiar with the treatment of HIV infection. Occasionally, a flare in KS tumor progression may be seen when antiretroviral therapy is initiated. Eventually, even with good anti-HIV therapy, many patients with AIDS-related KS will require some form of treatment for their tumor.

Local treatments, including cryotherapy, topical retinoic acid, intralesional chemotherapy and other sclerosing agents, and local irradiation, can produce good local control of tumors. Interferon-alfa (IFN-α [Intron A, Roferon-A]) and cytotoxic chemotherapy are effective systemic treatments for patients with more extensive or symptomatic disease. Single-agent or combination chemotherapy is effective in controlling tumors, even in patients with extensive disease and severe immune deficiencies (Table 2). The use of hematopoietic growth factors has facilitated the administration of myelosuppressive treatments, such as IFN-α and chemotherapy.

IFN-α

The first treatment licensed for AIDS-related KS was recombinant IFN-α. Tumor responses have been seen in approximately 30% of patients treated with SC interferon given either daily or 3 times weekly. Current practice is to administer IFN-α 3 times weekly by SC injection. Unmaintained response durations in trials of IFN-α monotherapy have ranged from 12 to 24 months in complete responders and from 8 to 12 months in partial responders.

Duration of therapy The optimal duration of IFN-α treatment is unknown; however, many patients relapse within a few months after discontinuation of therapy. Reinduction of second responses with IFN-α after relapse may be unreliable and often is of short duration. It is therefore generally recommended that treatment with IFN-α be continued for as long as drug tolerance and tumor responses continue.

Dose The optimal dose of IFN-α also has not been clearly established. IFN-α is generally administered at either 3 or 5 million units SC 3 times weekly together with antiretroviral therapy.

Major dose-limiting toxicities of IFN-α include fever, chills, rigor, and other flu-like symptoms. They are dose related and often observed at the initiation of treatment but lessen somewhat with continued use. Neutropenia, elevation of transaminase levels, depression, peripheral neuropathy, and other neuropsychiatric abnormalities may also occur.

Other side effects include headaches, cognitive impairments, paresthesias, and mild thrombocytopenia. As the subjective side effects of IFN-α are also common in HIV-related or other conditions, care must be taken to avoid ascribing all of these symptoms to drug toxicity and overlooking treatable infections and other conditions.

Retinoids

Alitretinoin gel 0.1% (9-*cis*-retinoic acid [Panretin]) has received approval of the US Food and Drug Administration (FDA) for the topical treatment of localized cutaneous KS. This compound inhibits the growth of KS and induces apoptosis of KS cells by binding to retinoic acid receptors on the cell surface.

Phase II clinical trials comparing 3–4 times daily application of alitretinoin vs placebo gel demonstrated a 35% rate of complete and partial responses in the alitretinoin-treated patients, as compared with a rate of 18% in controls.

The median time to response to alitretinoin was 29–34 days, with a median duration of response of 12–16 weeks. Responses were seen in both previously untreated and previously treated KS patients and were not dependent on patients' CD4 cell count.

Local cutaneous adverse reactions to alitretinoin include erythema, skin irritation, skin cracking, flaking, peeling, and desquamation. The severity of these reactions can be mitigated by less frequent dosing, thinner application, or use of topical vitamin E.

TABLE 2: Chemotherapy for AIDS-related KS

Regimen	Dose	Response rate[a] (%)
Vincristine	2 mg/wk IV	20-60
Vinblastine	0.05-0.1 mg/kg/wk IV	25-30
Doxorubicin	20 mg/m^2 IV every other wk	50-60
Etoposide	150 mg/m^2 IV every d × 3 q3-4wk	75
Vinorelbine	30 mg/m^2 IV q2wk	47
Liposomal daunorubicin	40 mg/m^2 IV q2-4wk	25-70
Liposomal doxorubicin	20 mg/m^2 IV q2-4wk	58-63
Paclitaxel	100-135 mg/m^2 IV over 3 h q2-4 wk	60-72
Irinotecan	150 mg/m^2 IV days 1-10	75
Vincristine + vinblastine	2 mg IV vincristine alternating with 0.1 mg/kg IV vinblastine every other wk	45
Vincristine + bleomycin	2 mg IV vincristine + 10 mg/m^2 IV bleomycin q2wk	23-70
Doxorubicin + bleomycin + vincristine	10 mg/m^2 IV doxorubicin + 10 mg/m^2 IV bleomycin + 1-2 mg IV vincristine q2wk	87

[a] Complete responses plus partial responses

Alitretinoin should be reserved for patients who do not require systemic treatment for visceral disease. However, it may be used in conjunction with other treatments for cutaneous disease.

Oral 9-*cis*-retinoic acid has been investigated in patients with AIDS-related KS and found to have a 37% response rate.

Bexarotene (Targretin), an oral retinoid X receptor (RXR)-selective agonist, has been studied in patients with AIDS-related KS, with an overall response rate of 33% in one study.

Chemotherapy

For patients with more widely disseminated, rapidly progressive, or symptomatic disease, systemic chemotherapy is generally warranted. Chemotherapy drugs are included in Table 2.

Antiretroviral drugs A total of 21 anti-HIV drugs have received FDA approval, and more are in various stages of clinical development. When evaluated by an oncologist, the majority of HIV-infected individuals will be taking some anti-HIV drugs. The interactions between cytotoxic chemotherapy and the various anti-HIV drugs have not been fully studied. Thus, oncologists treating patients with AIDS-related KS should continue to monitor them frequently for side effects. Withholding antiretroviral therapy during chemotherapy and then immediately restarting it after giving the chemotherapy drugs may avoid some toxic effects of drug interactions, especially with high-dose therapy.

Combination regimens The two most frequently utilized combination chemotherapy regimens are Adriamycin (doxorubicin), bleomycin, and vincristine (ABV) and bleomycin and vincristine (BV). These regimens were initially reported to yield tumor response rates in excess of 70%–90%, with good palliation of symptoms, including decreased edema, decreased pain, and, in patients with pulmonary KS, respiratory improvement and alleviation of obstructive symptoms. A beneficial effect of these combinations on survival has not been clearly demonstrated, however.

Early reports of a high response rate with these combination regimens have not been reproduced by later multicenter trials. A conservative response rate of 50%–60% has been reported in more contemporary phase III trials. The discrepancy in response rates most likely stems from differences in the response criteria used.

Liposomal anthracyclines (eg, liposomal doxorubicin [Doxil] and liposomal daunorubicin [DaunoXome]) are also effective in inducing tumor regression in KS. Clinical trials have shown that liposomal anthracyclines as single agents can achieve a response rate equal to or better than that obtained with the ABV combination regimen. As such, the liposomal anthracyclines have become first-line chemotherapy for AIDS-related KS.

The dose-limiting toxicity is neutropenia, and many patients will require the use of granulocyte colony-stimulating factor (G-CSF, filgrastim [Neupogen]) after several cycles of treatment. Other common side effects include nausea, fatigue, anemia, and thrombocytopenia. A palmar-plantar syndrome, characterized by acute painful erythematous swelling of the hands and feet, has been reported with the use of liposomal doxorubicin. Once the symptoms resolved, readministration of liposomal doxorubicin did not necessarily reproduce the syndrome. Neither of the liposomal anthracyclines has been reported to depress left ventricular function.

A retrospective analysis of 111 patients treated for HIV-related primary CNS lymphoma in 5 Australian hospitals concluded that the provision of HAART and radiation therapy (at least 30 Gy) improves survival *(Newell ME, Hoy JF, Cooper SG, et al: Cancer 100:2627-2636, 2004).*

Paclitaxel has been shown to produce responses in both chemotherapy-naive KS patients and patients with refractory tumors, including those refractory to liposomal anthracyclines. Dosage is typically 100-135 mg/m^2 IV given over 3 hours every 2–4 weeks. This agent is widely considered the primary second-line chemotherapy for KS.

The dose-limiting toxicity is neutropenia. Other reported toxicities include anemia, stomatitis, alopecia, and fatigue. Neuropathy has not been a major problem with this low-dose approach.

Investigational agents Other drugs under investigation for the treatment of KS include Col-3 and other antiangiogenesis compounds. Studies of compounds that may affect HHV-8 gene expression (eg, valproic acid) or signal transduction pathways in KS-infected cells (eg, imatinib [Gleevec]) are also in development or in early clinical testing in KS patients. Cidofovir (Vistide) does not appear to be clinically active.

Radiation therapy

Although radiation therapy can easily produce sufficient regression of KS to be useful for palliation of symptomatic disease or cosmetic improvement of disfiguring lesions, this practice has become less common as HAART has changed the natural history of AIDS. More than 90% of lesions will respond (complete responses [CRs] and partial responses [PRs]). Local radiation therapy commonly alleviates pain and bleeding, lessens edema, and shrinks obstructing lesions.

Treatment technique For most superficial lesions, a single, shaped, en face beam of relatively limited penetration (approximately 100 kV) works well. A relatively low-energy electron beam (eg, 6 MeV) often can be used with shielding as an alternative to superficial x-rays.

Large lesions For large lesions, electron beams are used more often, due to the limited penetration of kilovoltage x-ray beams and the limited width of the treatment cones attached to most superficial x-ray units. For patients with more widespread tumors of the legs with edema, parallel opposed megavoltage x-ray beams and overlying bolus material are often used to provide homogeneous irradiation to the entire area.

Dose fractionation regimens Several dose fractionation regimens have proven effective in AIDS-related KS. As this tumor is radiosensitive, almost any dose

In a prospective trial conducted in Zimbabwe, between 1994 and 1999, 495 patients (470 evaluable) who had AIDS-related KS received supportive care and local radiotherapy to symptomatic localized disease but not HAART. In addition, patients were randomly assigned to receive no additional care; oral etoposide; hemi- or full-body radiotherapy; or dactinomycin, vincristine, and bleomycin. There was no significant survival difference between the groups; however, based on physical and psychological scales, the best quality of life was associated with the group receiving etoposide *(Olweny CL, Borok M, Gudza I, et al: Int J Cancer 113:632-639, 2005)*.

of radiation therapy can produce some response. Interestingly, in vitro irradiation of KS cell cultures induces the cells to produce interleukin-6 (IL-6) and oncostatin M (OSM), which, in turn, make the cells more sensitive to radiation therapy.

For most cutaneous lesions, a single treatment of 800 cGy will produce a short-term response. For lesions on sensitive structures (eg, penis, hands, conjunctivae), some radiation oncologists attenuate treatment to a total dose of 2,000 cGy administered in 300 cGy increments (accepting a 50% decrease in CR rate), whereas 3,000 cGy delivered over 2 weeks is more typically used for lesions in general.

Prospectively acquired data clearly demonstrate a dose-response relationship for radiation therapy in AIDS-related KS. A dose of 4,000 cGy delivered in 20 fractions over 4 weeks was significantly more effective than 2,000 cGy in 10 fractions or 800 cGy in 1 fraction, as measured by a higher response rate, longer duration of tumor control, and the absence of residual hyperpigmentation. However, the short- and medium-term effects of moderately intense but briefer regimens, such as 3,000 cGy in 10 fractions over 2 weeks, probably are equivalent to those of higher total dose, more protracted regimens, and the moderately intense regimens require only half the time to deliver.

For patients with an anticipated survival of < 3 months, in whom the response duration may be of less overall importance, a single fraction of 800 cGy is likely to provide the same benefit as the more intensive regimens. In contrast, small lesions in patients who are expected to survive for at least 1 year should be treated with fractionated radiation therapy, such as 3,000 cGy in 10 fractions over 2 weeks.

NON-HODGKIN LYMPHOMA

The incidence of NHL is 60 times higher in individuals with HIV infection than in the general population. The overall occurrence of lymphoma as a manifestation of AIDS has declined somewhat as treatment of HIV has improved.

Although NHL currently comprises < 5% of all initial AIDS-defining conditions, it accounts for as many as 15% of all AIDS-related deaths. The majority of patients present with advanced-stage, high- or intermediate-grade, B-cell lymphoma and have a high frequency of extranodal involvement. Primary CNS lymphoma occurs in approximately 0.5% of patients with AIDS.

The majority of patients with AIDS-related lymphoma have advanced HIV disease. Median CD4 cell counts in patients with systemic lymphoma range from 100 to 200 cells/mm^3, whereas CD4 cell counts < 50 cells/mm^3 are found in nearly all patients with primary CNS lymphoma.

Epidemiology

At-risk groups NHL occurs with approximately equal frequency in all population groups infected by HIV, including IV drug users, homosexual-bisexual men, transfusion recipients, and patients with hemophilia.

Gender and race AIDS-related NHL is seen more frequently in men than in women and occurs more often in whites than in blacks.

Age The age distribution of AIDS-related NHL follows the distribution of HIV infection. Primary CNS lymphoma occurs with the same frequency in all age groups.

Geography Current data do not indicate any geographic differences in the incidence of AIDS-related NHL.

Etiology and risk factors

AIDS-related NHL is believed to arise as a consequence of continued stimulation of B-cell proliferation as a result of HIV, Epstein-Barr virus (EBV), and other infections, all of which occur in the setting of profound T-cell immunodeficiency. An association between the polyomavirus, simian virus 40 (SV40), and diffuse large B-cell and follicle-type lymphoma has been detected. HIV also induces the expression of a number of cytokines (eg, IL-6 and IL-10) that can further increase B-cell activation.

Small noncleaved lymphomas Genetic errors are increased in the setting of chronic B-cell proliferation, and a variety of chromosomal translocations resulting in oncogene activation can lead to polyclonal and monoclonal B-cell expression. Other molecular biological abnormalities associated with small noncleaved lymphomas include expression of an abnormal TP53 (alias p53) tumor-suppressor gene and the c-*myc* or *ras* oncogene.

Immunoblastic lymphoma The pathogenesis of AIDS-related immunoblastic lymphoma appears to be distinct from that of small noncleaved lymphoma and is more likely related to EBV infection without c-*myc* dysregulation. Clonal integration of EBV within tumor cells, with expression of various latent EBV proteins, has been demonstrated in essentially all cases of AIDS-related primary CNS lymphoma and in as many as two-thirds of systemic lymphomas.

Diffuse large cell lymphoma The specific molecular aberrations described in patients with AIDS-related diffuse large cell lymphoma appear distinct as well, with recent descriptions of abnormal *bcl-6* expression in approximately 40% of cases.

Body cavity–based lymphoma/primary effusion lymphoma appears to be highly associated with HHV-8 and EBV. The tumor cells stain positive for CD45. The disease appears to occur predominantly in males and may coexist with KS in patients with AIDS.

Signs and symptoms

B symptoms (ie, fever, weight loss, and night sweats) are seen in approximately 80% of patients with systemic AIDS-related NHL. In these patients, it is mandatory to exclude the presence of occult opportunistic infections before ascribing B symptoms to the lymphoma itself.

Extranodal involvement Advanced-stage disease is expected in the majority of patients, with extranodal involvement reported in 60%–90% of patients in most series. Common sites of extranodal involvement include the CNS (occurring in approximately 30% of patients), GI tract (25%), and bone marrow (25%). Essentially any other site in the body can also be involved, including the rectum, soft tissue, oral cavity, lungs, and heart.

CNS lymphoma Patients with primary CNS lymphoma often present with focal neurologic deficits, seizures, and/or altered mental status. Any site in the brain may be involved, and one to four space-occupying lesions are usually seen on MRI or CT scan.

Other sites Changes in bowel habits, GI bleeding, weight loss, pain, and hepatomegaly are common presenting symptoms in patients with GI involvement. Pancytopenia may indicate bone marrow involvement.

Primary effusion lymphoma Patients usually present with pleural or pericardial effusion without an identifiable mass. Pain, shortness of breath, and B symptoms are the main initial complaints.

Screening and diagnosis

Diagnosis of NHL in patients with AIDS requires histologic confirmation by biopsy with immunophenotypic and/or molecular gene rearrangement studies.

A complete staging evaluation should be done. This should include:

- CT or MRI of the head and chest/abdomen/pelvis
- bone marrow aspiration and biopsy
- liver function studies
- spinal fluid analysis.

Assessing spinal fluid for EBV The presence of EBV DNA in CSF, as determined by polymerase chain reaction (PCR), appears to have a high specificity and sensitivity for the diagnosis of primary CNS lymphoma. The use of thallium single-photon emission computed tomography (SPECT) may further increase the diagnostic yield.

Pathology

Common tumor types Over 95% of AIDS-related NHL cases are of B-lymphocyte origin. Most AIDS-related NHL tumors are high-grade types, including the immunoblastic and small noncleaved lymphomas. Diffuse large cell lymphoma constitutes up to 30% of AIDS lymphomas.

Less common tumor types Although not considered part of the AIDS epidemic, several cases of T-cell lymphoma occurring in HIV-infected patients have been described. In addition, cases of Ki-1–positive, large cell anaplastic lymphoma have been reported in HIV-infected patients. The clinical and pathologic characteristics of these forms of lymphoma are similar to those seen in non–HIV-infected individuals.

CNS lymphomas are typically of the immunoblastic or large cell type.

GI and oral cavity lymphomas Large cell or immunoblastic lymphomas are also more likely to involve the GI tract and oral cavity than are small noncleaved lymphomas.

Primary effusion lymphoma The cells are large and pleomorphic with prominent nucleoli and immunoblastic morphology. Clonal immunoglobulin DNA rearrangement demonstrates clonality of the tumor cells but not surface immunoglobulin expression.

Staging and prognosis

Staging system Staging of AIDS-related NHL is the same as that for non–AIDS-related NHL. The Ann Arbor classification system for staging of NHL is utilized (see chapter 30), and the staging work-up includes imaging studies, as well as bone marrow and CNS evaluation for lymphomas.

Prognostic factors Four factors have been shown to correlate most closely with shorter survival in patients with systemic AIDS-related NHL:

- a history of opportunistic infection prior to the lymphoma
- CD4 cell count < 100 cells/mm^3
- Karnofsky performance score < 70
- stage IV disease, especially if due to bone marrow or meningeal involvement.

In patients without these findings, the median survival is typically 11–12 months, as compared with a median survival of approximately 4–5 months in those with one or more of these adverse prognostic features.

Three factors correlate with *better* survival in patients with primary CNS lymphoma:

- Karnofsky performance score > 70
- age < 35 years
- adequate dose of radiation therapy.

Type of lymphoma To date, no major differences have been seen in response or survival among the various pathologic types of sys-

> The International Prognostic Index (IPI) for lymphoma was evaluated along with a number of other clinical and laboratory prognostic variables for lymphoma or HIV in a cohort of 111 patients with AIDS–non-Hodgkin lymphoma treated after the era of potent antiretroviral therapy (HAART). Regression modeling revealed only two independent predictors for death: the IPI score and the CD4 cell count. These variables were used to establish four internally validated risk strata that predicted 1-year survival and might be useful in guiding therapeutic options (*Bower M, Gazzard B, Mandalia S, et al: Ann Intern Med 143:265-273, 2005*).

TABLE 3: Chemotherapy for AIDS-related NHL

Regimen	Drugs and dosage	Cycle length	CR rate (%)	Median survival
m-BACOD	Methotrexate, 500 mg/m^2 IV on day 15, with leucovorin, 25 mg PO q6h × 4, after completion of methotrexate	q28d	41	35 wk
	Bleomycin, 4 U/m^2 IV on day 1			
	Adriamycin (doxorubicin), 25 mg/m^2 IV on day 1			
	Cyclophosphamide, 300 mg/m^2 IV on day 1			
	Oncovin (vincristine), 1.4 mg/m^2 IV on day 1 (maximum, 2 mg)			
	Dexamethasone, 3 mg/m^2 PO on days 1-5			
CDE	Cyclophosphamide, 800 mg/m^2/96 h IV	q28d	46	8.2 mo
	Doxorubicin, 50 mg/m^2/96 h IV			
	Etoposide, 240 mg/m^2/96 h IV			
EPOCH	Etoposide, 200 mg/m^2/96 h IV	q3-4wk	79	53 mo+
	Prednisone, 60 mg/m^2 PO on days 1-6			
	Oncovin (vincristine), 1.6 mg/m^2/96 h IV			
	Cyclophosphamide, 187 mg/m^2 IV on day 5 (if CD4 cell count < 100 cells/mm^3) or 375 mg/m^2 IV on day 5 (if CD4 cell count ≥ 100 cells/mm^3)*			
	Doxorubicin, 40 mg/m^2/96 h IV			
CEOP	Cyclophosphamide, 750 mg/m^2 IV on day 1	q3-4wk	47	10 mo
	Epirubicin, 50 mg/m^2 IV on day 1			
	Oncovin (vincristine), 2 mg IV on day 1			
	Prednisone, 100 mg PO on days 1-5			
CHOP	Cyclophosphamide, 750 mg/m^2 IV on day 1	q21d	63	9 mo
	Doxorubicin, 50 mg/m^2 IV on day 1			
	Oncovin (vincristine), 1.4 mg/m^2 IV on day 1 (maximum, 2 mg)			
	Prednisone, 60 mg PO on days 1-5			

CR = complete response; * With dose escalation as tolerated with each subsequent cycle, to a maximum of 750 mg/m^2

temic AIDS-related NHL. Patients with polyclonal lymphomas appear to have better tumor responses to chemotherapy and better survival. Patients with primary CNS lymphoma have an extremely poor prognosis, with a median survival of only 2–3 months despite therapy; treatment with potent antiretroviral therapy does seem to improve survival. Prognosis for patients with primary effusion lymphoma is also poor, with a median survival of only 5 months.

Treatment

TREATMENT OF SYSTEMIC NHL

Chemotherapy

The mainstay of treatment for patients with systemic AIDS-related NHL is chemotherapy. As the likelihood of dissemination is great, AIDS patients who develop NHL must be assumed to have widespread disease at presentation and should be treated with systemic chemotherapy, even if dissemination is not confirmed on routine staging evaluation.

Some of the commonly used regimens designed for AIDS-related NHL are listed in Table 3. No regimen appears to be superior to any other, although early findings show that the EPOCH regimen (etoposide, prednisone, Oncovin [vincristine], cyclophosphamide, doxorubicin) gives the best results to date.

CNS prophylaxis with either intrathecal cytarabine (Ara-C; 50 mg) or intrathecal methotrexate (10–12 mg) every week for four treatments has been shown to be effective in reducing the incidence of CNS relapse.

In an Italian study, rituximab (Rituxan), an anti-CD 20 monoclonal antibody, also has been studied in combination with CDE (cyclophosphamide, doxorubicin, etoposide) at lower doses and has been shown to have an overall response rate of 86% and an actuarial 2-year survival rate of 80%.

Dose intensity Standard-dose chemotherapy (eg, CHOP [cyclophosphamide, doxorubicin, Oncovin, prednisone]) is generally recommended for most patients with AIDS-related NHL. Results from trials using continuous infusion therapy (eg, EPOCH or CDE) have shown better CR rates and long disease progression-free and overall survival.

Certain subsets of patients with high CD4 cell counts (> 100 cells/mm^3), no B symp-

> To determine whether the addition of rituximab (Rituxan) to CHOP resulted in better outcomes in patients with AIDS-related NHL, 149 patients were randomized (2:1) to receive CHOP with rituximab (days 1 and 3 of each cycle) or CHOP alone. Three monthly maintenance doses of rituximab were administered to the rituximab group following completion of chemotherapy. CR rates were similar (58% vs 48%), as were median times to response (11.0 vs 10.5 weeks, respectively). More grade 4 neutropenia (61% vs 48%) was seen in the rituximab group. Death due to infection occurred in 14 of 95 (10%) of those in the rituximab group vs 1 of 50 (2%) of those in the CHOP-alone group. No response benefit was seen from the addition of rituximab to CHOP for the initial treatment of AIDS-related NHL, and the high incidence of infections and death raises concern in this population *(Kaplan LD, Lee J, Ambinder RF, et al: Blood 106:1538-1543, 2005).*

Patients with high-risk or relapsed AIDS-related non-Hodgkin lymphoma after first-line chemotherapy underwent peripheral blood stem-cell (PBSC) collection. Patients with chemosensitive disease received carmustine, etoposide, cytarabine, and melphalan (BEAM) and PBSC transplantation. Highly active antiretroviral therapy (HAART) was maintained throughout treatment, and prophylactic treatment with ciprofloxacin, fluconazole, and acyclovir was maintained until 30 days after engraftment. All 14 patients received PBSC transplantation, with prompt engraftment and no opportunistic or other infections. Complete response was achieved in 10 of 11 patients. Three patients died after PBSC: two from lymphoma progression and one from liver failure. Eight patients are disease free at a median of 28 months after treatment. High-dose therapy plus PBSC transplantation appears feasible and active in patients with AIDS lymphoma (*Serrano D, Carrion R, Balsalobre P, et al: Exp Hematol 33:487-494, 2005*).

toms, lower disease stage at presentation (stage I or II), and good performance status (0 or 1) may enjoy prolonged survival (> 2 years) when treated with either a standard-dose or intensive, high-dose regimen. However, until more data are available to identify these patient subsets, the intensive, high-dose approach is not recommended outside clinical trial settings.

Growth factor support The major dose-limiting toxic effect of multiagent chemotherapy regimens is myelosuppression. Studies of m-BACOD (methotrexate with leucovorin, bleomycin, Adriamycin [doxorubicin], cyclophosphamide, Oncovin [vincristine], dexamethasone) or CHOP chemotherapy demonstrated that coadministration of myeloid hematopoietic growth factors enhanced patient tolerance of these regimens.

Salvage chemotherapy Patients in whom initial treatment fails or relapse after initial remission rarely achieve a prolonged second remission. Studies of various salvage regimens with or without autologous stem-cell support are in progress. Mitoguazone (MGBG), given at a dose of 60 mg/m^2 on days 1 and 8 and then every 2 weeks, achieved a CR in 11.5% of patients with primary refractory or relapsed disease. The median survival for the whole group was 2.6 months, whereas a median survival of 21.5 months was noted in the complete responders.

Second-line chemotherapy (eg, ESHAP [etoposide, methylprednisolone, high-dose Ara-C, Platinol (cisplatin)]) has been shown to have a CR of up to 31% and a PR of 23%, with a median survival of 7.1 months, in patients with refractory or relapsed AIDS-related NHL.

Radiation therapy

The role of radiotherapy in systemic lymphoma is limited to consolidation of the effects of chemotherapy. Treatment principles are similar to those used for aggressive NHL in the non-HIV setting and typically involve the use of involved or extended fields only.

Lymphomatous meningitis For patients with lymphomatous meningitis and/or radiographically detectable cerebral deposits, "step-brain" irradiation (including the covering meninges) is administered along with intrathecal chemotherapy to control microscopic spinal disease. Focal radiation therapy may be required for known tumor deposits in the spine. Unfortunately, many such patients develop multiple deposits anywhere along the spinal axis, either synchronously or metachronously.

Fractionated doses of 3,000–4,500 cGy may be used to control local lymphoma deposits in nodal areas. Patients who have lymphomatous meningitis typically have a poor prognosis and are best treated with regimens that do not unduly occupy their time (eg, 3,000 cGy in 10 fractions over 2 weeks).

TREATMENT OF PRIMARY CNS LYMPHOMA

An effective therapy for patients with AIDS-related CNS lymphoma has not yet been found.

Radiation therapy

The conventional standard of treatment is step-brain irradiation, which can result in response rates of 50% and improve survival, as compared with untreated patients, even when adjusted for antiretroviral therapy, CD4 cell count, and time to diagnosis. Treatment is directed to the entire cranial contents, including the meninges down to C2.

Doses equivalent to 3,900 cGy (or more) delivered at 200 cGy/fraction appear to be associated with increased survival. Better Karnofsky performance scores and younger age at the time of treatment are also associated with longer survival. Mean survival ranges from 2 to 6 months, with death often due to complicating opportunistic infections.

HAART

By itself, HAART appears to have some activity against CNS lymphoma. Observers have reported anecdotal instances of regression of biopsy-proven, AIDS-related CNS lymphoma after the institution of HAART along with ganciclovir and IL-2.

Chemotherapy

As HAART has changed the biologic behavior of AIDS, there has been more interest in using high-dose methotrexate in CNS lymphoma based on evidence of activity in non–AIDS-associated disease. Studies to evaluate short courses of combination chemotherapy or the use of less myelosuppressive single agents followed by whole-brain irradiation are currently in progress. Although these approaches appear to be efficacious in non–HIV-infected patients with primary CNS lymphoma, the available data do not suggest that this approach is superior to CNS irradiation alone in AIDS patients.

CERVICAL CARCINOMA

Cervical carcinoma in the setting of HIV infection has been recognized as an AIDS-defining malignancy since 1993. Unfortunately, in some women, cervical carcinoma may be the first indication that they have HIV infection.

Cervical intraepithelial neoplasia (CIN) is also seen in association with HIV infection. These premalignant lesions, also known as squamous intraepithelial lesions (SILs), may foretell a higher incidence of cervical carcinoma among HIV-infected women. SILs have been associated with human papillomavirus (HPV), particularly those subtypes with greater oncogenic potential, such as serotypes 16, 18, 31, 33, and 35.

Epidemiology

Prevalence of HIV infection and cervical abnormalities The risk of HIV infection in women with an abnormal Pap smear varies with the prevalence of HIV infection in the given population. Screening in clinics in high-prevalence areas has yielded HIV-positivity rates of between 6% and 7% (and up to 10% in parts of Africa). In such high-prevalence areas, among women younger than age 50 with cervical carcinoma, up to 19% of women were found to be HIV positive. HIV-positive women have up to a 10-fold increased risk of abnormal cervical cytology. Several centers have reported abnormal cytology rates of 30%–60% in HIV-positive women and Pap smears consistent with cervical dysplasia in 15%–40%. The prevalence of cervical dysplasia increases with declining CD4 cell counts in HIV-infected women.

Nationwide, invasive cervical carcinoma was found in 1.3% of women with AIDS. In New York, invasive cervical carcinoma constitutes 4% of AIDS-defining illnesses in women. Recent findings from linkage studies in the US and Italy clearly have shown increased rates of cervical cancer in women with HIV.

Race and geography The prevalence of invasive cervical carcinoma among American Hispanic and black women is lower than that in white women. However, this difference may stem from a difference in access to health care. The southern and northeastern sections of the United States have a higher reported number of cases of HIV-associated invasive cervical carcinoma.

Etiology and risk factors

The severe cellular immunodeficiency associated with advanced HIV infection may allow oncogenic viruses to flourish and may also compromise the body's immunologic defenses that control the development of these tumors.

HPV There is abundant evidence that HPV infection is related to malignant and premalignant neoplasia in the lower genital tract. HPV serotypes 16, 18, 31, 33, and 35 are the most oncogenic strains and have been associated with invasive cervical carcinoma and progressive dysplasia. The prevalence of cervical SILs among HIV-infected women may be as high as 20%–30%, with many having higher cytologic and histologic grade lesions.

Signs and symptoms

The majority of cervical SILs are detected on routine cytologic evaluation of Pap smears in women with HIV infection.

Advanced invasive disease Postcoital bleeding with serosanguineous and/or foul-smelling vaginal discharge is usually the first symptom of more advanced invasive disease. Lumbosacral pain or urinary obstructive symptoms may indicate advanced disease.

Screening and diagnosis

Because the majority of patients with cervical dysplasia or early invasive cancer are asymptomatic, frequent cytologic screening of women at risk for HIV infection must be undertaken. The role of newly developed HPV vaccines in preventing HPV infection or disease progression in HIV-infected women has yet to be determined.

Screening of HIV-positive women Current screening recommendations call for women with HIV infection to have pelvic examinations and cytologic screening every 6 months. Pap smears indicating cervical SILs must be taken seriously, and abnormalities justify immediate colposcopy. Although abnormalities are sometimes missed by relying solely on cytologic screening, recommendations for routine colposcopy have not yet been established.

Screening of women with a history of cervical SILs For women who have a history of cervical SILs, more frequent reevaluation and cytologic screening should be undertaken. Since these women are at high risk for recurrence or development of lesions in other areas of the lower genital tract, post-therapy surveillance with repeat colposcopy also is warranted.

Work-up of women with invasive carcinoma For women with invasive carcinoma, complete staging should be undertaken; this should include pelvic examination, CT of the pelvis and abdomen, chest x-ray, and screening laboratory tests for hepatic and bone disease. In addition, full evaluation and treatment for HIV and related complications should be initiated.

Pathology

Squamous cell carcinoma Most cases of cervical carcinoma are of the squamous cell type.

Staging and prognosis

The staging classification for cervical carcinoma (see chapter 20), as adopted by the International Federation of Gynecology and Obstetrics (FIGO), also applies to AIDS patients.

Cervical dysplasia in HIV-infected women is often of higher cytologic and histologic grade. These women are more likely to have CIN II-III lesions with extensive cervical involvement, multisite (vagina, vulva, and anus) involvement, and endocervical lesions.

HIV-infected women with cervical carcinoma typically present with more advanced disease and appear to have a more aggressive clinical course. Tumors are typically high grade with a higher proportion of lymph node and visceral involvement at presentation. Mean time to recurrence after primary treatment is short, and many patients have persistent disease after primary therapy. The median time to death in one series was 10 months in HIV-infected women, as compared with 23 months in HIV-negative patients.

Treatment

TREATMENT OF PREINVASIVE DISEASE

Cryotherapy, laser therapy, cone biopsy, and loop electrosurgical excision procedure (LEEP) have all been used to treat preinvasive disease in HIV-infected patients. Short-term recurrence rates of 40%–60% have been reported.

Determinants of recurrence Immune status of the patient seems to be the most important determining factor for recurrence. Close surveillance after initial therapy is critical, and repetitive treatment may be necessary to prevent progression to more invasive disease.

TREATMENT OF CERVICAL CARCINOMA

The same principles that guide oncologic management of the immunocompetent patient with cervical carcinoma (see chapter 20) are utilized in AIDS patients with this cancer.

Surgery can be undertaken for the usual indications, and surgical decisions should be based on oncologic appropriateness and not on HIV status.

Radiation therapy As most AIDS patients with cervical cancer present with advanced disease, radiation therapy is indicated more often than surgery. If the patient's overall physical condition permits, treatment regimens are identical to those used for the same stage disease in uninfected individuals (see chapter 20). It is important to note that the standard of care for advanced carcinoma of the cervix (stages III-IV, without hematogeneous dissemination) now includes a combination of irradiation and concurrent cisplatin-based chemotherapy. At present, there is insufficient evidence to suggest that irradiation or other treatments for cervical carcinoma in AIDS patients is any less effective than in similar non–HIV-infected individuals.

Chemotherapy regimens, such as cisplatin (50 mg/m^2) or carboplatin (Paraplatin; 200 mg/m^2), bleomycin (20 U/m^2; maximum, 30 U), and vincristine (1 mg/m^2), have been used in patients with metastatic or recurrent disease. Vigorous management of side effects and complications of these treatments and of AIDS itself must be provided.

ANAL CARCINOMA

Although anal carcinoma is not currently an AIDS-defining illness, the incidence of this tumor is increasing in the population at risk for HIV infection. The incidence of anal carcinoma in homosexual men in a San Francisco study was estimated at between 25–87 cases per 100,000, compared with 0.7 case per 100,000 in the entire male population.

Etiology and risk factors

HPV Precursor lesions of anal intraepithelial neoplasia (AIN), also known as anal SILs, have been found to be associated with HPV infection, typically with oncogenic serotypes, eg, types 16 and 18. Cytologic abnormalities occur in nearly 40% of patients, especially those with CD4 cell counts < 200 cells/mm^3. Abnormal cytology may predict the later development of invasive carcinoma.

Other STDs and sexual practices Individuals with a history of perianal herpes simplex, anal condylomas, or practice of anal-receptive behavior with multiple sexual partners are at higher risk of developing this tumor than those without such a history.

Signs and symptoms

Rectal pain, bleeding, discharge, and symptoms of obstruction or a mass lesion are the most frequent presenting symptoms.

Screening and diagnosis

Studies to evaluate the usefulness of anoscopy with frequent anal cytology have been undertaken to determine whether early detection of AIN may result in interventions that would prevent the development of invasive tumors.

Work-up of patients with anal carcinoma For patients with anal carcinoma, determination of the extent of local disease, as well as full staging for dissemination, should be undertaken (see chapter 16).

Pathology

Squamous cell carcinoma The majority of anal carcinomas are of the squamous cell type.

Histologic grading The grading for AIN is similar to that for CIN, with AIN-1 denoting low-grade dysplasia and AIN-2 and AIN-3, higher grade dysplastic lesions. The gross appearance of lesions on anoscopy does not predict histologic grade. Higher grade dysplastic lesions are seen in patients with lower CD4 cell counts.

Staging and prognosis

The staging of squamous cell carcinoma of the anus in HIV-infected individuals is the same as that in non–HIV-infected patients (see chapter 16). Patients with severe immunosuppression, ie, CD4 cell counts < 50 cells/mm^3, may present with more advanced, more aggressive disease. The true natural history of this tumor in the AIDS population has yet to be defined, however.

Treatment

TREATMENT OF AIN AND CARCINOMA IN SITU

Treatment of patients with local AIN is similar to that of women with CIN. Ablative therapy may be used.

TREATMENT OF INVASIVE ANAL SQUAMOUS CELL CARCINOMA

Anal cancer can be controlled with chemotherapy and radiation therapy despite HIV infection. However, patients who have low CD4 cell counts appear to be more likely to experience severe toxicity and to require colostomy for salvage therapy than those with higher CD4 cell counts. For patients with squamous cell carcinoma of the anus, chemotherapy with mitomycin (Mutamycin; 10 mg/m^2 on day 1) and fluorouracil (5-FU; 1,000 mg/m^2 by continuous infusion on days 1–4) combined with radiation therapy can produce high rates of complete remission.

Concomitant radiation therapy, 5-FU, and mitomycin have been reported to produce a CR in 9 of 11 patients with AIDS-associated invasive anal carcinoma (median CD4 cell count at diagnosis of 209 cells/mm^3) and a 60% 2-year actuarial survival rate. Two patients remain alive more than 8 years following treatment, but severe toxicity (three grade 3 hematologic, one grade 3 dermatologic, one grade 4, and one grade 5 gastrointestinal toxicity) and one death resulted from treatment.

Recent evidence appears to suggest that 5-FU plus cisplatin may be superior to 5-FU plus mitomycin. Tolerance to treatment seen in patients who have relatively intact immune systems is similar to that seen in HIV-infected patients. The role of cetuximab (Erbitux) and other target therapies in this disease population also has not yet been determined. However, the appropriate dose of radiation therapy for patients with anal carcinoma in the context of HIV infection remains unsettled. Patients who are unable to tolerate chemoradiation therapy and those in whom treatment fails (defined as a positive biopsy after CR) should be considered for abdominoperineal resection.

OTHER NON–AIDS-DEFINING MALIGNANCIES

Case reports and small reported series of other malignant tumors occurring in HIV-infected individuals include Hodgkin lymphoma (HL), nonmelanomatous skin cancers, lung cancer, germ-cell tumors, myeloid or lymphoid leukemias, multiple myeloma, renal cell carcinoma, breast cancer, head and neck cancer, brain tumors, squamous tumor of the conjunctiva, and leiomyosarcoma in pediatric patients. Most of these case reports describe only a few affected individuals, and there are insufficient numbers of patients to confirm an increased risk of developing these malignancies among HIV-infected individuals, with the possible exceptions of HL, nonmelanomatous skin cancers, lung cancer, conjunctival cancer, seminoma, and pediatric leiomyosarcoma.

Rates of other non–AIDS-defining cancers appear to be increasing among HIV-infected individuals. In an Australian cancer data base, 196 cases of non–AIDS-defining cancers were noted in 13,067 individuals (1.5%) among 8,351 HIV-infected-only patients and 8,118 patients with AIDS.

As HIV-infected individuals are surviving longer with currently available combination anti-HIV drugs, clinicians should anticipate seeing the development of more tumors in these patients. Greater vigilance for these tumors is warranted.

HL Most of the studies showing a possible increased incidence of HL in HIV-infected individuals are from European countries, especially Italy and Spain. The most common histology is mixed cellularity and lymphocyte-depleted. Male predominance, a higher prevalence of B symptoms, and more extranodal disease on presentation are the main characteristics of HL in HIV patients.

Chemotherapy is recommended for this group of patients, due to the high proportion of stage III or IV disease. Standard treatments include ABVD (Adriamycin, bleomycin, vinblastine, and dacarbazine) or ABVD alternating with MOPP (mechlorethamine [Mustargen], Oncovin [vincristine], procarbazine [Matulane], and prednisone). More recently, early results with BEACOPP [bleomycin, etoposide, doxorubicin (Adriamycin), cyclophosphamide, Oncovin (vincristine), procarbazine, prednisone] and the Stanford V regimen look promising.

The Stanford V regimen and concomitant HAART appear to be well tolerated in patients with HL and HIV infection, producing a 53% CR rate with a median overall survival of 11 months and a 55% 2-year disease-free survival rate in one study. However, patients with high initial prognostic scores (above 2) fare significantly worse than patients with lower initial prognostic scores.

Radiation therapy appears useful in approximately 50% of cases of HIV-associated HL. Of 14 patients treated at M. D. Anderson Cancer Center (stage I: 1; stage II: 3; stage III: 4; and stage IV: 6), 1 patient received radiation therapy alone and 7 received both chemotherapy and irradiation. The projected overall 5-year survival (64-month median follow-up) was 54%. A greater proportion of patients died because of other HIV-related causes than because of HL.

Nonmelanomatous skin cancers As in the general population, basal cell carcinoma is more common than squamous cell carcinoma in the setting of HIV infection. The risk factors for the development of these tumors are the same as in the general population: namely, fair skin, history of sun exposure, and family history. A study from San Francisco demonstrated that these skin cancers can be treated successfully with standard local therapy, with a recurrence rate indistinguishable from that of the general population (approximately 6%).

Lung cancer Patients with HIV appear to have a higher relative risk of developing lung cancer than do age-matched controls (relative risk = 4.5; 95%; confidence interval = 4.2-4.8). These tumors tend to present at later stages than do tumors with similar histologic distribution in the general population.

Pediatric leiomyosarcoma Cases of aggressive leiomyosarcoma developing in HIV-positive children have been reported. Leiomyosarcoma is a rare tumor, occurring in < 2 cases per 10 million non–HIV-infected children. However, a much higher than expected frequency of leiomyosarcoma has been reported in HIV-infected children. Visceral sites are commonly involved, eg, the lungs, spleen, and GI tract.

Acknowledgment: Supported, in part, by grants from the State of California, University-wide Task Force on AIDS to the UCLA California Collaborative HIV/AIDS Research Center (CHOS-LA-608) and USPHS, NIH grants AI-27660, CA-70080, and RR00865.

SUGGESTED READING

ON KAPOSI'S SARCOMA

Aversa SM, Cattelan AM, Salvagno L, et al: Treatments of AIDS-related Kaposi's sarcoma. Crit Rev Oncol Hematol 53:253–265, 2005.

Kigula-Mugambe J, Kavuma A: Epidemic and endemic Kaposi's sarcoma: a comparison of outcomes and survival after radiotherapy. Radiother Oncol 76:59–62, 2005.

Krown SE: Highly active antiretroviral therapy in AIDS-associated Kaposi's sarcoma: Implications for the design of therapeutic trials in patients with advanced, symptomatic Kaposi's sarcoma. J Clin Oncol 22:399–402, 2004.

Levine AM, Quinn DI, Gorospe G, et al: Phase I trial of vascular endothelial growth factor-antisense (VEGF-AS, Veglin) in relapsed and refractory malignancies (abstract). Blood 102(suppl):#418, 2003.

Mocroft A, Kirk O, Clumeck N, et al: The changing pattern of Kaposi sarcoma in patients with HIV, 1994-2003: The EuroSIDA study. Cancer 100:2644–2654, 2004.

Vaccher E, di Gennaro G, Simonelli C, et al; Italian Cooperative Group on AIDS Tumors (GICAT): Evidence of activity of irinotecan in patients with advanced AIDS-related Kaposi's sarcoma. AIDS 19:1915–1916, 2005.

ON NON-HODGKIN LYMPHOMA

Bower M, Gazzard B, Mandalia S, et al: A prognostic index for systemic AIDS-related non-Hodgkin lymphoma treated in the era of highly active antiretroviral therapy. Ann Intern Med 143:265–273, 2005.

Kaplan LD, Lee JY, Ambinder RF, et al: Rituximab does not improve clinical outcome in a randomized phase III trial of CHOP with or without rituximab in patients with HIV-associated non-Hodgkin lymphoma: AIDS Malignancy Consortium Trial 010. Blood 106:1538–1543, 2005.

Newell ME, Hoy JF, Cooper SG, et al: Human immunodeficiency virus-related primary central nervous system lymphoma: Factors influencing survival in 111 patients. Cancer 100:2627–2636, 2004.

Re A, Cattaneo C, Michieli M, et al: High-dose therapy and autologous peripheral-blood stem-cell transplantation as salvage treatment for HIV-associated lymphoma in patients receiving highly active antiretroviral therapy. J Clin Oncol 21:4423–4427, 2003.

Robotin MC, Law MG, Milliken S, et al: Clinical features and predictors of survival of AIDS-related non-Hodgkin's lymphoma in a population-based case series in Sydney, Australia. HIV Med 5:377–384, 2004.

Serrano D, Carrion R, Balsalobre P, et al; Spanish Cooperative Groups GELTAMO and GENSIDA: HIV-associated lymphoma successfully treated with peripheral blood stem cell transplantation. Exp Hematol 33:487–494, 2005.

Sparano JA, Lee S, Chen MG, et al: Phase II trial of infusional cyclophosphamide, doxorubicin, and etoposide in patients with HIV-associated non-Hodgkin's lymphoma: An Eastern Cooperative Oncology Group Trial (E1494). J Clin Oncol 22:1491–1500, 2004.

ON CERVICAL AND ANAL CARCINOMAS

Ahdieh-Grant L, Li R, Levine AM, et al: Highly active antiretroviral therapy and cervical squamous intraepithelial lesions in human immunodeficiency virus-positive women. J Natl Cancer Inst 96:1070–1076, 2004.

Berry JM, Palefsky JM, Welton ML: Anal cancer and its precursors in HIV-positive patients; Perspectives and management. Surg Oncol Clin N Am 13:355–373, 2004.

Stadler RF, Gregorecyk SG, Euhus DM, et al: Outcome of HIV-infected patients with invasive squamous-cell carcinoma of the anal canal in the era of highly active antiretroviral therapy. Dis Colon Rectum 47:1305–1309, 2004.

Wilkin TJ, Palmer S, Brudney KF, et al: Anal intraepithelial neoplasia in heterosexual and homosexual HIV-positive men with access to antiretroviral therapy. J Infect Dis 190:1685–1691, 2004.

ON NON–AIDS-DEFINING MALIGNANCIES

Bonnet F, Lewden C, May T, et al: Malignancy-related causes of death in human immunodeficiency virus-infected patients in the era of highly active antiretroviral therapy. Cancer 101:317–324, 2004.

Burgi A, Brodine S, Wegner S, et al: Incidence and risk factors for the occurrence of non-AIDS-defining cancers among human immunodeficiency virus-infected individuals, Cancer 104:1505–1511, 2005.

Grulich AE, Li Y, McDonald A, et al: Rates of non–AIDS-defining cancers in people with HIV infection before and after AIDS diagnosis. AIDS 16:1155–1161, 2002.

Hartmann P, Rehwald U, Salzberger B, et al: BEACOPP therapeutic regimen for patients with Hodgkin's disease and HIV infection. Ann Oncol 14:1562–1569, 2003.

Lim ST, Levine AM: Non-AIDS-defining cancers and HIV infection. Curr HIV/AIDS Rep 2:146–153, 2005.

Spina M, Gabarre J, Rossi G, et al: Stanford V regimen and concomitant HAART in 59 patients with Hodgkin disease and HIV infection. Blood 100:1984–1988, 2002.

CHAPTER 28

Carcinoma of an unknown primary site

John D. Hainsworth, MD, and Lawrence M. Weiss, MD

Carcinoma of an unknown primary site is a common clinical syndrome, accounting for approximately 3% of all oncologic diagnoses. Patients in this group are heterogeneous, having a wide variety of clinical presentations and pathologic findings. A patient should be considered to have carcinoma of an unknown primary site when a tumor is detected at one or more metastatic sites, and routine evaluation (see below) fails to define a primary tumor site.

Although all patients with cancer of an unknown primary site have advanced, metastatic disease, universal pessimism and nihilism regarding treatment are inappropriate. Subsets of patients with specific treatment implications can be defined using clinical and pathologic features. In addition, trials of empiric chemotherapeutic regimens incorporating new antineoplastic agents have suggested improved response rates and survival in unselected groups of patients with carcinoma of an unknown primary site.

Epidemiology

Gender Unknown primary cancer occurs with approximately equal frequency in men and women and has the same prognosis in the two genders.

Age As with most epithelial cancers, the incidence of unknown primary cancer increases with advancing age, although a wide age range exists. Some evidence suggests that younger patients are more likely to have poorly differentiated histologies.

Disease sites Autopsy series performed prior to the availability of CT resulted in the identification of a primary site in 70%-80% of patients. Above the diaphragm, the lungs were the most common primary site, whereas various GI sites (pancreas, colon, stomach, liver) were most common below the diaphragm. Several frequently occurring cancers, particularly breast and prostate cancers, were rarely identified in autopsy series.

With improved radiologic diagnosis, the spectrum of unknown primary cancer has probably changed. Limited recent autopsy data suggest a lower percentage of primary sites identified, particularly in patients with poorly differentiated histology.

TABLE 1: Immunohistochemical studies useful in the differential diagnosis of carcinoma vs another neoplasm

	Immunoperoxidase stains			
Tumor type	Pan-keratin	CD45 and other markers	S-100 protein	Vimentin
Carcinoma	+	–	–	–/+
Malignant lymphoma	–	+	–	–/+
Malignant melanoma	–	–	–/+	+
Sarcoma	–	–	–	+

Signs and symptoms

Patients with unknown primary cancer usually present with symptoms related to the areas of metastatic tumor involvement.

Sites of metastatic involvement include the lungs, liver, and skeletal system; therefore, symptoms referable to these areas are common.

Constitutional symptoms such as anorexia, weight loss, weakness, and fatigue are common.

Physical findings include peripheral adenopathy, pleural effusions, ascites, and hepatomegaly.

Pathologic evaluation

Optimal pathologic evaluation is critical in the evaluation of patients with carcinoma of an unknown primary site and can aid with the following:

- distinguishing carcinoma from other cancer types
- determining histologic type
- identifying the primary site
- identifying specific characteristics that may direct specific treatments.

Initial approach Although cytologic evaluation, including fine-needle aspiration biopsy, can often determine whether a lesion is malignant, a tissue biopsy will probably be needed to further evaluate the neoplasm. Tissue is required for paraffin-section immunohistochemistry, which is currently the usual methodology of choice in the work-up. Electron microscopy, which optimally requires glutaraldehyde fixation, is usually no longer required. Nucleic acid microarray analysis represents a technology of the future, as it lacks an FDA-approved platform.

TABLE 2: Most useful organ-specific markers

Organ or type of cancer	Antibody
Breasts	GCDFP-15, estrogen receptor
Lung	TTF-1
Gastrointestinal carcinoma	CDX-2
Stomach	CDX-2 + Hep-Par
Colon	CDX-2 + CK20
Liver	Hep-Par
Pancreas	CK17
Kidneys	CD10
Prostate	Prostate-specific antigen
Serous/endometrioid gynecologic	ER
Urinary bladder	CK7, CK20, CK5/6
Seminoma/embryonal carcinoma	OCT-4
Mesothelioma	Calretinin
Thyroid	TTF-1 + thyroglobulin

Carcinoma vs other neoplasms It is important to rule out the possibility of malignant lymphoma, malignant melanoma, and sarcoma. A battery of antibodies is utilized in an attempt to distinguish carcinoma from other types of neoplasms, as summarized in Table 1. The staining result obtained with any single marker is unreliable, as exceptions may occur for each individual antibody. For example, although keratin is a relatively reliable marker of carcinoma, some carcinomas (eg, adrenal cortical carcinoma or undifferentiated carcinoma of the thyroid) may be keratin-negative, whereas some types of sarcoma are characteristically keratin-positive (eg, epithelioid sarcoma).

Determination of histologic type There may be clues on initial histologic examination. For example, the presence of gland formation or mucin production would indicate an adenocarcinoma, whereas the presence of keratinization would indicate a squamous cell carcinoma. Evidence of neuroendocrine differentiation may be suggested by the presence of a characteristic relatively fine chromatin pattern. Immunohistochemistry can also be of use, as expression of keratin subtypes 7 and 20 would favor adenocarcinoma, and expression of keratin subtypes 5/6 and 14 would favor squamous cell carcinoma. Reliable neuroendocrine markers include chromogranin A and synaptophysin.

Identification of specific treatment target characteristics Even if the primary site is not determined, characteristics of the carcinoma may suggest specific treatment options or impart prognostic information. Examples of the former may include determination of estrogen or progesterone receptors or expression of members of the epidermal growth factor receptor family (eg, HER2/neu). Examples of the latter may include Ki-67, which is a surrogate marker of the proliferation rate of a neoplasm.

Clinical evaluation

After a biopsy has established metastatic carcinoma, a relatively limited clinical evaluation is indicated to search for a primary site. Recommended evaluation includes a complete history, physical examination, chemistry profile, CBC, chest radiograph, and CT scan of the abdomen.

Symptomatic areas Specific radiologic and/or endoscopic evaluation of symptomatic areas should be pursued. In addition, mammography, ultrasonography, and breast MRI should be performed in women with clinical features suggestive of metastatic breast cancer (eg, estrogen receptor-positive tumor and/or specific metastatic involvement including axillary nodes, bones, or pleura), and serum prostate-specific antigen (PSA) level should be measured in men with features suggestive of prostate cancer (eg, blastic bone metastasis; Table 2). In young men with poorly differentiated carcinoma, serum human chorionic gonadotropin (hCG) and alpha-fetoprotein (AFP) levels should always be measured.

Asymptomatic areas In general, radiologic or endoscopic evaluation of asymptomatic areas is not productive and should be avoided. Positron emission tomography (PET) scanning has identified primary sites in 20%-30% of patients in several small series; although further evaluation is necessary, this procedure should be considered for patients with carcinoma of an unknown primary site. Several reports have documented that superfluous testing is frequently performed in these patients, and several thousand dollars can be spent in a futile search for the primary tumor site.

Cervical lymphadenopathy Metastatic squamous carcinoma in cervical lymph nodes usually involves upper or mid-cervical locations. All patients should undergo a thorough search for a primary site in the head and neck region, including direct endoscopic examination of the oropharynx, hypopharynx, nasopharynx, larynx, and upper esophagus. Any suspicious areas should be biopsied. Fiberoptic bronchoscopy should be considered in patients with involvement of low cervical or supraclavicular nodes. This type of evaluation will identify a primary site, usually in the head and neck, in 85%-90% of these patients. Further evaluation with PET scanning can identify a primary site in 15%-30% of the remaining patients and should be considered.

Inguinal lymphadenopathy Patients with metastatic squamous cell cancer presenting in inguinal lymph nodes almost always have an identifiable primary site in the perineal area. Women should undergo careful examination of the vulva, vagina, and cervix; men should have careful inspection of the penis. Anoscopy should be performed to exclude lesions in the anorectal area.

TABLE 3: Recommended treatment for recognized clinicopathologic subsets

Histopathology	Clinical subset	Treatment
Adenocarcinoma	Women with isolated axillary adenopathy	Treat as stage II breast cancer
	Women with peritoneal carcinomatosis	Treat as stage III ovarian cancer
	Men with blastic bone metastases or elevated serum PSA level	Treat as metastatic prostate cancer
	Single metastatic site	Local excision and/or radiation therapy
Squamous cell carcinoma	Cervical adenopathy	Treat as head/neck primary (combined-modality therapy)
	Inguinal adenopathy	Node dissection ± radiation therapy
Poorly differentiated carcinoma	Young men with a mediastinal/retroperitoneal mass	Treat as extragonadal germ-cell tumor
	Neuroendocrine features by immunoperoxidase staining or electron microscopy	Treat with platinum/etoposide-based regimen
	All others with good performance status	Treat with taxane/platinum or platinum/etoposide-based regimen
Neuroendocrine carcinoma	Well differentiated (low grade)	Treat as advanced carcinoid tumor
	Poorly differentiated or small cell	Treat with platinum/etoposide-based regimen

PSA = prostate-specific antigen

Treatment

Table 3 summarizes the recommended treatment for various recognized clinicopathologic subsets.

Adenocarcinoma

When evaluating patients with adenocarcinoma of an unknown primary site, several clinical subsets should be identified and treated specifically. Empiric therapy for patients not included in any of these subsets is outlined in the final section of this chapter.

Women with isolated axillary adenopathy Treatment appropriate for stage II breast cancer should be administered. Mastectomy reveals an occult primary cancer in 50%-60% of these patients, even when physical examination and mammography are normal. Axillary dissection with breast irradiation is also a reasonable treatment, although there are no definitive comparisons of this approach vs mastectomy. Adjuvant systemic therapy, following standard guidelines for stage II breast cancer, is also indicated.

Women with peritoneal carcinomatosis Often, the histopathology in these patients suggests ovarian cancer (ie, serous cystadenocarcinoma or papillary adenocarcinoma). However, all women with this syndrome should be treated as if they had stage III ovarian cancer. Initial cytoreductive surgery should be followed by chemotherapy with a taxane/platinum combination, as recommended for advanced ovarian cancer. In these patients, serum CA-125 can often be used as a tumor marker.

Men with bone metastasis Metastatic prostate cancer should be suspected and usually can be diagnosed with either an elevated serum PSA level or positive tumor staining for PSA. In such patients, androgen deprivation therapy, as recommended for advanced prostate cancer, is often of palliative benefit.

Patients with a single metastatic site Surgical resection or radiation therapy should be administered to patients who present with clinical evidence of a single metastasis. Prior to proceeding with local therapy in these patients, PET scanning should be considered to rule out additional metastatic sites. Thyroid cancer and squamous head and neck or lung cancer should also be considered. Some of these patients have prolonged survival after local therapy, particularly those who present with a sole metastasis in an isolated peripheral lymph node group. For the patient with a metastastic squamous cell cancer involving a cervical lymph node with no known primary, see the discussion of "Unknown Head and Neck Primary Site" in chapter 4 on "Head and Neck Tumors." The role of "adjuvant" systemic therapy is undetermined in these patients.

Squamous cell carcinoma

Squamous cell cancer accounts for only 10% of light microscopic diagnoses in patients with unknown primary cancer. Isolated cervical adenopathy is the most common presentation for squamous cell carcinoma of an unknown primary site; other patients have isolated inguinal adenopathy at presentation. Specific management is essential for both of these subgroups, since both have the potential for long-term survival following treatment.

Patients with cervical lymphadenopathy in whom no primary site is identified should be treated as if they had a primary site in the head and neck. Concurrent treatment with chemotherapy and radiation therapy has recently proved superior to local treatment alone and to these treatment modalities used sequentially. Radiation therapy doses and techniques should be identical to those used in treating patients with known head and neck primaries. In addition to the involved neck, the nasopharynx, oropharynx, and hypopharynx should be included in the radiation field. Radical neck dissection should be considered in patients who have any evidence of residual cancer following combined-modality therapy.

Five-year survival rates with combined-modality therapy are 60%-70% and appear superior to results with local modalities alone (30%-50%). The extent of cervical lymph node involvement is the most important prognostic factor.

Patients with inguinal lymphadenopathy Identification of a primary site in the perineal area is important in patients with inguinal lymphadenopathy, as curative therapy is available for some patients, even after metastasis to inguinal lymph nodes. In the uncommon patient for whom no primary site is identified, inguinal node dissection, with or without radiation therapy, can result in long-term survival. Although limited data exist on this uncommon subgroup, the demonstrated superiority of combined-modality therapy vs local treatment alone for primary squamous cell cancers in the perineal area (eg, cervix, anus) has led to a suggestion that the addition of platinum-based chemotherapy may improve treatment results.

Poorly differentiated carcinoma

This heterogeneous group includes a minority of patients with highly responsive neoplasms and therefore requires special attention in initial clinical and pathologic evaluations. Specialized pathologic techniques can identify some patients with tumor types known to be treatable; these patients should be treated using standard guidelines for the appropriate tumor type.

In the remaining patients, several investigators have documented an increased responsiveness to platinum-based chemotherapy when compared with patients with adenocarcinoma of an unknown primary site. In addition, several series have described a small cohort of long-term survivors following platinum-based treatment. Patients with poorly differentiated adenocarcinoma have usually been included in this group when making treatment decisions. Although most patients in this group should receive an empiric trial of treatment, several specific subsets can be recognized.

Men with extragonadal germ-cell cancer syndrome Young men with a predominant tumor location in the mediastinum and retroperitoneum and/or high levels of serum hCG or AFP should be treated as if they had a poor prognosis germ-cell tumor (ie, four courses of chemotherapy with cisplatin/etoposide/bleomycin, followed by surgical resection of residual radiographic abnormalities).

Molecular genetic analysis can identify an i(12p) chromosomal abnormality diagnostic of a germ-cell tumor in some of these patients, even when the diagnosis cannot be made by any other pathologic evaluation. Patients with germ-cell tumors diagnosed in this manner have been shown to be as responsive to treatment as patients with extragonadal germ-cell tumors of typical histology.

Patients with poorly differentiated neuroendocrine carcinoma With the improved immunoperoxidase stains now available, neuroendocrine fea-

TABLE 4: Results of empiric chemotherapy for carcinoma of an unknown primary site[a]

Regimen	Number of patients	Response rate (%)	Median survival (mo)
Old regimens			
FAM	120	20	8
AM	197	29	5
CAF/CMeF	72	17	5
Cisplatin/5-FU–based	186	24	6
Other cisplatin-based	90	30	5
New regimens			
Paclitaxel/carboplatin/etoposide	71	46	11
Paclitaxel/carboplatin	72	41	12
Docetaxel/platinum	76	24	8
Paclitaxel/carboplatin/gemcitabine	120	25	9
Gemcitabine/cisplatin	40	42	8
Gemcitabine/docetaxel	35	40	10

F = 5-FU (fluorouracil); A = Adriamycin (doxorubicin); M = mitomycin; C = cyclophosphamide; Me = methotrexate

[a]Reported series using similar regimens have been compiled; response rates and median survivals are averages.

tures are recognized more frequently in patients with poorly differentiated carcinoma. These tumors are distinct in biology and therapeutic implications from well-differentiated neuroendocrine tumors (eg, carcinoid tumors, islet-cell tumors) of an unknown primary site, which almost always present with multiple liver metastases. In contrast to typical carcinoid tumors, poorly differentiated neuroendocrine tumors are difficult to recognize by light microscopic examination alone, although some of the latter tumors have neuroendocrine or “small-cell” features.

Patients with poorly differentiated neuroendocrine carcinoma of an unknown primary site should receive a trial of chemotherapy with a regimen containing a platinum and etoposide. In a group of 51 such patients, the complete response rate was 28% following treatment with cisplatin and etoposide, with or without bleomycin; the overall response rate was 71%. Eight patients (16%) had durable complete remissions.

More recently, the combination of paclitaxel, carboplatin (Paraplatin), and etoposide has shown a high level of efficacy in the treatment of poorly differentiated neuroendocrine tumors (see section on “Empiric chemotherapy”). The substitution of carboplatin for cisplatin makes this regimen better tolerated than cisplatin/etoposide.

Although the identity of most poorly differentiated neuroendocrine tumors remains unknown, this group of chemotherapy-responsive patients can be reliably identified using specialized, but widely available, pathologic evaluation.

Other patients with poorly differentiated carcinoma Most patients with poorly differentiated carcinoma do not have neuroendocrine features or clinical features of germ-cell tumor. Patients in this group should receive an empiric trial of chemotherapy, unless an extremely poor performance status precludes this possibility. In a group of 220 such patients treated with cisplatin-based regimens effective for germ-cell tumor at a single institution, the overall response rate was 64%, with 27% complete responses. Median survival of this group was 20 months, and 13% of patients have been disease free for more than 8 years and are considered cured. Although the young median age of 39 years indicates that this was a select patient group, the extreme chemosensitivity of some patients in this large, heterogeneous group is clearly demonstrated.

Empiric chemotherapy

Systemic therapy for patients not included in any specific treatable subgroup has been difficult. Unfortunately, this group includes the majority of patients with adenocarcinoma of an unknown primary site; some patients with poorly differentiated carcinoma and no "favorable" clinical features also respond poorly to current therapy.

'Old' regimens Table 4 summarizes results compiled from phase II trials of empiric chemotherapy. Most patients in these trials had adenocarcinoma, but 5%-10% had poorly differentiated carcinoma. In general, the most extensively tested empiric regimens as well as various cisplatin-based regimens have been those effective for GI malignancy and breast cancer. Most tested regimens have produced response rates of 20%-35% and median survival durations of 5-8 months. There is little evidence of prolongation of median survival or long-term complete remission with any of these regimens, and none is considered "standard treatment" in this group of patients.

Regimens incorporating new agents The recent availability of several new antineoplastic agents with broad-spectrum activity has renewed interest in the empiric therapy of carcinoma of an unknown primary site. The taxanes, gemcitabine (Gemzar), and the topoisomerase I inhibitors are all agents with potential efficacy in the treatment of an unknown primary cancer.

Most experience to date has been with taxane/platinum-based regimens. Results of phase II trials suggest higher response rates and longer median survivals along with a moderate decrease in toxicity with these regimens vs previous cisplatin-based regimens (Table 4). Long-term follow-up of patients treated with paclitaxel/carboplatin/etoposide shows actual 2-year and 3-year survival rates of 20% and 14%, respectively. Recently, other combinations of new agents (eg, gemcitabine/cisplatin and gemcitabine/docetaxel) have also shown substantial activity, but further experience is required before comparisons are possible. At present, paclitaxel/carboplatin, with or without etoposide, should be considered for empiric therapy for patients with adenocarcinoma of an unknown primary site and good performance status.

SUGGESTED READING

Culine S, Lortholary A, Voigt J, et al: Cisplatin in combination with either gemcitabine or irinotecan in carcinomas of unknown primary site: Results of a randomized phase II study. Trial for the French Study Group in Carcinomas of Unknown Primary (GEFCAPI 01). J Clin Oncol 21:3479–3482, 2003.

Grau C, Johansen LV, Jakobsen J, et al: Cervical lymph node metastases from unknown primary tumours. Radiother Oncol 55:121–129, 2000.

Greco FA, Burris HA 3rd, Litchy S, et al: Gemcitabine, carboplatin, and paclitaxel for patients with carcinoma of unknown primary site: A Minnie Pearl Cancer Research Network study. J Clin Oncol 20:1651–1656, 2002.

Greco FA, Gray J, Burris HA 3rd, et al: Taxane-based chemotherapy for patients with carcinoma of unknown primary site. Cancer J 7:203–212, 2001.

Miranda FT, Spigel DR, Hainsworth JD, et al: Paclitaxel/carboplatin/etoposide therapy for advanced proorly differentiated neuroendocrine carcinoma: A Minnie Pearl Cancer Research Network phase II trial (abstract). Proc Am Soc Clin Oncol 23:322S, 2005.

Pouessel D, Culine S, Becht C, et al: Gemcitabine and docetaxel as front-line chemotherapy in patients with carcinoma of an unknown primary site. Cancer 100:1257–1261, 2004.

Smith SM, Argiris A, Stenson K, et al: Combined modality therapy with chemoradiation for squamous cell carcinoma of the head and neck from an occult primary (abstract). Proc Am Soc Clin Oncol 21:235, 2002.

CHAPTER 29

Hodgkin lymphoma

Joachim Yahalom, MD, and David Straus, MD

In the year 2007, approximately 8,190 new cases of Hodgkin lymphoma (HL) will be diagnosed in the United States. Over the past 4 decades, advances in radiation therapy and the advent of combination chemotherapy have tripled the cure rate of patients with HL. In 2007, more than 80% of all newly diagnosed patients can expect a normal, disease-free life span.

Epidemiology

Gender The male-to-female ratio of HL is 1.3:1.0.

Age The age-specific incidence of the disease is bimodal, with the greatest peak in the third decade of life and a second, smaller peak after the age of 50 years.

Race HL occurs less commonly in African-Americans (2.3 cases per 100,000 persons) than in Caucasians (3.0 per 100,000 persons).

Geography The age-specific incidence of HL differs markedly in various countries. In Japan, the overall incidence is low and the early peak is absent. In some developing countries, there is a downward shift of the first peak into childhood.

Etiology and risk factors

The cause of HL remains unknown, and there are no well-defined risk factors for its development. However, certain associations have been noted that provide clues to possible etiologic factors.

Familial factors For example, same-sex siblings of patients with HL have a 10 times higher risk for the disease. Patient-child combinations are more common than spouse pairings. Higher risk for HL is associated with few siblings, single-family houses, early birth order, and fewer playmates—all of which decrease exposure to infectious agents at an early age. The monozygotic twin sibling of a patient with HL has a 99 times higher risk of developing HL than a dizygotic twin sibling of a patient with HL. These associations suggest a genetic predisposition and/or a role for an infectious or environmental agent during childhood or early adolescence in the etiology of the disease.

Viruses Familial aggregation may imply genetic factors, but other epidemiologic findings mentioned previously suggest an abnormal response to an infective agent. Both factors may play a role in the pathogenesis of the disease. The

The prognostic significance of the presence of Epstein-Barr virus (EBV) in classic HL tumor cells remains unclear. The Scotland and Newcastle Epidemiological Study of Hodgkin Disease, a population-based case control study, found that EBV association with classic HL was linked to a significantly shorter overall and disease-specific survival for patients 50 years of age or older, but not for younger patients (*Jarrett RF, Stark GL, White J, et al: Blood 106: 2444-2451, 2005*). Among children and adolescents treated on German-Austrian pediatric multicenter trials for HL, a small, but statistically significant, difference in overall, but not failure-free, survival was found for patients whose tumors were associated with EBV as compared with those whose tumors were not. In subset analyses, this difference was seen in patients with advanced disease, and with a subset of nodular sclerosis. HL is associated with an increased number of Reed-Sternberg cells (*Claviez A, Tiemann M, Luders H, et al: J Clin Oncol 23:4048-4056, 2005*).

Epstein-Barr virus (EBV) has been implicated in the etiology of HL by both epidemiologic and serologic studies, as well as by the detection of the EBV genome in 20%-80% of tumor specimens.

There have been no conclusive studies regarding the possible increased frequency of HL in patients with human immunodeficiency virus (HIV) infection. However, HL in HIV-positive patients is associated with an advanced stage and poor therapeutic outcome. (For further discussion of HL in patients with HIV infection, see chapter 27.)

Signs and symptoms

HL is a lymph node-based malignancy and commonly presents as an asymptomatic lymphadenopathy that may progress to predictable clinical sites.

Location of lymphadenopathy More than 80% of patients with HL present with lymphadenopathy above the diaphragm, often involving the anterior mediastinum; the spleen may be involved in about 30% of patients. Less than 10%–20% of patients present with lymphadenopathy limited to regions below the diaphragm. The commonly involved peripheral lymph nodes are located in the cervical, supraclavicular, and axillary areas; para-aortic pelvic and inguinal areas are involved less frequently. Disseminated lymphadenopathy is rare in patients with HL, as is involvement of Waldeyer's ring and occipital, epitrochlear, posterior mediastinal, and mesenteric sites.

Systemic symptoms About 30% of patients experience systemic symptoms. They include fever, night sweats, or weight loss (so-called B symptoms) and chronic pruritus. These symptoms occur more frequently in older patients and have a negative impact on prognosis (see section on "Staging and prognosis").

Extranodal involvement HL may affect extranodal tissues by direct invasion (contiguity; the so-called E lesion) or by hematogenous dissemination (stage IV disease). The most commonly involved extranodal site is the lungs. Liver, bone marrow, and bone may also be involved.

Diagnosis

The initial diagnosis of HL can only be made by biopsy. Because reactive hyperplastic nodes may be present, multiple biopsies of a suspicious site may be necessary. Needle aspiration is inadequate because the architecture of the lymph node is important for diagnosis and histologic subclassification.

Pathology

Reed-Sternberg cell

In a biopsied lymph node, the Reed-Sternberg (R-S) cell is the diagnostic tumor cell that must be identified within the appropriate cellular milieu of lymphocytes, eosinophils, and histiocytes. HL is a unique malignancy pathologically in that the tumor cells constitute a minority of the cell population, whereas normal inflammatory cells are the major cell component. As a result, it may be difficult to identify R-S cells in some specimens. Also, other lymphoproliferations may have cells resembling R-S cells.

The R-S cell is characterized by its large size and classic binucleated structure with large eosinophilic nucleoli. Two antigenic markers are thought to provide diagnostic information: CD30 (Ber-H2) and CD15 (Leu-M1). These markers are present on R-S cells and their variants but not on background inflammatory cells. It is also important to obtain a stain for CD20, since it may be positive in minority of patients with classic HL (nodular sclerosis or mixed cellularity). The prognostic significance of CD20-positive R-S cells in classic HL is controversial.

Recent studies have confirmed the B-cell origin of the R-S cell. Single-cell polymerase chain reaction (PCR) analysis of classic R-S cells shows a follicular center B-cell origin for these cells with clonally rearranged but crippled V heavy-chain genes, presumably leading to inhibition of apoptosis. Also, high levels of the nuclear transcription factor-kappa-B (NF-kB) have been found in R-S cells; these high NF-kB levels may play a role in pathogenesis by interfering with apoptosis. A molecular link between R-S cells and tumor cells of mediastinal diffuse large B-cell lymphoma has been recently found in gene-profiling studies.

Histologic subtypes

According to the Rye classification (based on the number and appearance of R-S cells, as well as the background cellular milieu), there are four histologic subtypes of HL.

Nodular sclerosis, the most common subtype, is typically seen in young adults (more commonly in females) who have early-stage supradiaphragmatic presentations. Its distinct features are the presence of (1) broad birefringent bands of collagen that divide the lymphoid tissue into macroscopic nodules and (2) an R-S cell variant, the lacunar cell.

Mixed cellularity is the second most common histology. It is more often diagnosed in males, who usually present with generalized lymphadenopathy or extranodal disease and with associated systemic symptoms. R-S cells are frequently identified; bands of collagen are absent, although fine reticular fibrosis may be present; and the cellular background includes lymphocytes, eosinophils, neutrophils, and histiocytes.

> The expression of the antiapoptotic protein bcl-2 in tissue microarrays from patients with classic HL has recently been found to be an independent predictor of shortened failure-free survival, with a trend toward shortened overall survival. This finding could be associated with resistance to treatment-induced programmed cell death or apoptosis (*Sup SJ, Alemany CA, Pohlman B, et al: J Clin Oncol 23:3773-3779, 2005*).

Lymphocyte-predominant HL is an infrequent form of HL in which few R-S cells or their variants may be identified. The cellular background consists primarily of lymphocytes in a nodular or sometimes diffuse pattern. The R-S variants express a B-cell phenotype (CD20-positive, CD15-negative). B-cell clonality has also been demonstrated by PCR of the immunoglobulin heavy-chain genes in single R-S variant cells in biopsy material from patients with lymphocyte-predominant HL.

This finding has led investigators to propose that lymphocyte-predominant HL is a B-cell malignancy with a mature B-cell phenotype, distinct from the other three histologic types of HL. Lymphocyte-predominant HL is often clinically localized, is usually treated effectively with irradiation alone, and may relapse late (a clinical feature reminiscent of low-grade lymphoma). The 15-year disease-specific survival is excellent (> 90%).

The World Health Organization (WHO) classification recognizes a new subtype of lymphocyte-rich classic HL that has morphologic similarity to nodular lymphocyte-predominant HL. However, the R-S cells have a classic morphology and phenotype (CD30-positive, CD15-positive, CD20-negative), and the surrounding lymphocytes are reactive T cells. This disease subtype does not show a tendency toward late relapse and should be managed like other classic HL histologies.

Lymphocyte depletion is a rare diagnosis, particularly since the advent of antigen marker studies, which led to the recognition that many such cases represented T-cell non-HLs (NHLs). R-S cells are numerous, the cellular background is sparse, and there may be diffuse fibrosis and necrosis. Patients usually have advanced-stage disease, extranodal involvement, an aggressive clinical course, and a poor prognosis.

Staging and prognosis

Precise definition of the extent of nodal and extranodal involvement with HL according to a standard staging classification system is critical for selection of the proper treatment strategy.

Staging system

The staging system is detailed in Table 1, and the anatomic regions that provide the basis for the staging classification are illustrated in Figure 1. The assignment of stage is based on:

- the number of involved sites
- whether lymph nodes are involved on both sides of the diaphragm and whether this involvement is bulky (particularly in the mediastinum)

- whether there is contiguous extranodal involvement (E sites) or disseminated extranodal disease
- whether typical systemic symptoms (B symptoms) are present.

In defining the disease stage, it is important to note how the information was obtained, since this fact reflects on remaining uncertainties in the evaluation for extent of disease. Clinical staging refers to information that has been obtained by initial biopsy, history, physical examination, and laboratory and radiographic studies only. A pathologic stage is determined by more extensive surgical assessment of potentially involved sites, eg, by surgical staging laparotomy and splenectomy.

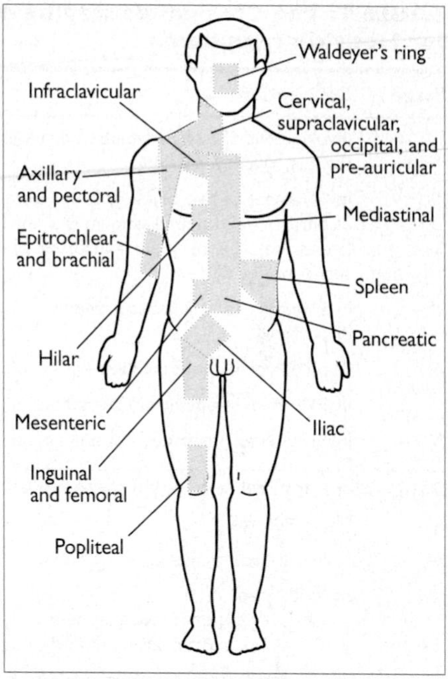

FIGURE 1: Anatomic regions for staging of Hodgkin lymphoma

Also, various designations relating to the presence or absence of B symptoms or bulky disease (see Table 1) can be applied to any disease stage. For example, a patient with no B symptoms but with a bulky mediastinal mass and involvement of the cervical lymph nodes would be defined as having CS IIAX disease. A patient with axillary disease and fever who underwent a staging laparotomy that revealed involvement of the para-aortic lymph nodes and spleen would be staged as PS III_2B.

Most recent studies in stage I/II disease distinguish between favorable and unfavorable early-stage disease, according to the European Organization for Research and Treatment of Cancer (EORTC) definitions outlined in Table 2.

Clinical staging evaluation

Disease-associated symptoms As mentioned previously, disease-associated symptoms may occur in up to one-third of patients. They may include B symptoms, pruritus, and, less commonly, pain in involved regions after ingestion of alcohol. In each anatomic stage, the presence of B symptoms is an adverse prognostic indicator and may strongly affect treatment choices. B symptoms are carefully defined in the staging system. Unexplained fever should be > 38°C and recurrent during the previous month, night sweats should be drenching and recurrent, and unexplained weight loss should be significant only if > 10% of body weight has been lost within the preceding 6 months. Although pruritus is no longer considered to be a B symptom, the presence of general-

TABLE 1: The Cotswald's staging classification for Hodgkin lymphoma

Stage	Description
I	Involvement of a single lymph node region or lymphoid structure (eg, spleen, thymus, Waldeyer's ring)
II	Involvement of two or more lymph node regions on the same side of the diaphragm (ie, the mediastinum is a single site, hilar lymph nodes are lateralized). The number of anatomic sites should be indicated by a subscript (eg, II_2).
III	Involvement of lymph node regions or structures on both sides of the diaphragm:
	III_1: With or without involvement of splenic, hilar, celiac, or portal nodes
	III_2: With involvement of para-aortic, iliac, or mesenteric nodes
IV	Involvement of extranodal site(s) beyond that designated E
Designations applicable to any disease stage[a]	
A	No symptoms
B	Fever, drenching sweats, weight loss
X	Bulky disease: > 1/3 the width of the mediastinum > 10 cm maximal dimension of nodal mass
E	Involvement of a single extranodal site, contiguous or proximal to a known nodal site
CS	Clinical stage
PS	Pathologic stage

[a] For examples of how these designations are applied to disease stage, see text discussion.

ized itching may be considered to be an adverse prognostic symptom.

Certain combinations of B symptoms are more prognostically significant than others. For example, the combination of fever and weight loss has a worse prognosis than do night sweats alone.

Physical examination should carefully determine the location and size of all palpable lymph nodes. Inspection of Waldeyer's ring, detection of splenomegaly or hepatomegaly, and evaluation of cardiac and respiratory status are important.

Laboratory studies should include a CBC with WBC differential and platelet count, the erythrocyte sedimentation rate (ESR), tests for liver and renal function, and assays for serum alkaline phosphatase and lactate dehydrogenase (LDH). A moderate to marked leukemoid reaction and thrombocytosis are common, particularly in symptomatic patients, and usually disappear with treatment.

ESR The ESR may provide helpful prognostic information. At some centers, treatment programs for patients with early-stage disease are influenced by the

TABLE 2: EORTC prognostic definition of early-stage disease

Favorable	CS I and II (maximum 3 involved areas) and < 50 years *and* ESR < 50 mm/h (no B symptoms) *or* ESR < 30 mm/h (B symptoms present) *and* MT ratio < 0.33
Unfavorable	CS II ≥ 4 nodal areas involved *or* age ≥ 50 years *or* ESR ≥ 50 mm/h (no B symptoms) *or* ESR ≥ 30 mm/h (B symptoms present) *or* MT ratio ≥ 0.33

CS = Cotswald's staging; EORTC = European Organization for Research and Treatment of Cancer; ESR = erythrocyte sedimentation rate; MT = mediastinal/thoracic

degree of ESR elevation. In addition, changes in the ESR following therapy may correlate with response and relapse.

Abnormalities of liver function studies should prompt further evaluation of that organ, with imaging and possible biopsy.

Alkaline phosphatase An elevated alkaline phosphatase level may be a nonspecific marker, but it may also indicate bone involvement that should be appropriately evaluated by a radionuclide bone scan and directed skeletal radiographs.

Patients at low risk for bone marrow involvement by Hodgkin lymphoma have been recently defined in a clinical prediction model. They include patients with stage IA/IIA disease without anemia and leukopenia, patients with stage IA/IIA disease who are younger than 35 years old with either anemia or leukopenia but no iliac or inguinal nodal involvement, and patients with stage IIIA/IVA disease without any of these four risk factors (*Vassilakopoulos TP, Angelopoulou MK, Constantinou N, et al: Blood 105:1875-1880, 2005*).

Imaging studies Radiologic studies should include a chest x-ray and CT scan of the chest, abdomen, and pelvis with IV contrast. In most patients, PET scan will provide important information on the extent of disease, and a baseline for evaluation of response to treatment is highly recommended. Radionuclide bone scan, MRI of the chest or abdomen, and CT scan of the neck are contributory only under special circumstances.

Evaluation for supradiaphragmatic disease The thoracic CT scan details the status of intrathoracic lymph node groups, the lung parenchyma, pericardium, pleura, and chest wall. Since the chest CT scan may remain abnormal for a long time after the completion of therapy, the evaluation of pretreatment involvement and response to therapy is assisted by the use of a PET or gallium scan. ^{18}F-fluorodeoxyglucose (FDG)-PET scanning provides more information and better resolution than does a gallium scan.

Evaluation of the abdomen and pelvis A CT scan and PET are the basic imaging studies for evaluation of the abdomen and pelvis.

Recently, highly significant associations have been reported between PET scanning performed during chemotherapy for Hodgkin lymphoma after 2 or 3 cycles and progression-free and overall survival at 2 years (*Hutchings M, Mikhaeel NG, Fields PA, et al: Ann Oncol 16:1160-1168, 2005*). The predictive value of PET scanning after 2 cycles of chemotherapy is currently being investigated in early-stage HL.

TABLE 3: Results of prospective randomized studies with short chemotherapy followed by IFRT for early-stage HL

Study (# of patients)	Prognostic group	Treatment	RFS or FFTF	OS (median follow-up)
Milan (133)	Favorable and unfavorable	ABVD (4) + IFRT (36 Gy)	94%	94% (12 years)
GHSG HD8 (1,064)	Unfavorable	COPP/ABVD (4) + IFRT (30 Gy + 10 Gy to bulk)	84%	92% (5 years)
EORTC H8U (995)	Unfavorable	MOPP/ABV (4) + IFRT (36 Gy)	96%	93% (4 years)
GHSG HD10 (1,131)	Favorable	ABVD (2 or 4) + IFRT (20 or 30 Gy)	97%	99% (2 years)
GHSG HD11 (1,363)	Unfavorable	ABVD (4) or BEACOPP (4) + IFRT (20 or 30 Gy)	90%	97% (2 years)

Abbreviations: For chemotherapy, see Table 4

EORTC = European Organization for Research and Treatment of Cancer; FFTF = freedom from treatment failure; GHSG = German Hodgkin's Study Group; HL = Hodgkin lymphoma; IFRT = involved-field radiation therapy; OS = overall survival; RFS = relapse-free survival

Bone marrow biopsy Bone marrow involvement is relatively uncommon, but because of the impact of a positive biopsy on further staging and treatment, unilateral bone marrow biopsy should be part of the staging process of patients with stage IIB disease or higher.

Lymphangiography and staging laparotomy

These two old methods of staging have been replaced by modern imaging techniques using high-resolution CT scanning and FDG-PET.

Treatment

HL is sensitive to radiation and many chemotherapeutic drugs, and, in most stages, there is more than one effective treatment option. Disease stage is the most important determinant of treatment options and outcome. All patients, regardless of stage, can and should be treated with curative intent.

TREATMENT OF STAGE I/II DISEASE

The treatment of choice for favorable and unfavorable early-stage classic HL is brief chemotherapy followed by involved-field radiotherapy (IFRT). Most of the experience that yielded excellent treatment results with low toxicity was with ABVD (Adriamycin [doxorubicin], bleomycin, vinblastine, and dacarbazine) for 4 cycles and IFRT of 30 to 36 Gy. Table 3 summarizes data from randomized studies that reported on the combination of short chemotherapy (4 or even only 2 cycles) followed by IFRT. The three top randomized studies have also indicated that adding extended-field radiotherapy to chemotherapy is not necessary and the small involved field is adequate.

> Updates on the results of German Hodgkin's study group randomized twin trials in favorable (HD 10) and unfavorable (HD 11) early-stage HL were recently presented by Muller RP (*Int J Radiat Oncol Biol Phys [abstract] 63:[suppl 1]:51, 2005*) and Diehl (*Klimm BC, Engert A, Brillant C, et al: J Clin Oncol [abstract] 23[suppl]:561s, 2005*). HD10 was designed to test how far the treatment may be reduced. In HD10, 1,370 patients with favorable early-stage HL were randomized up front into 4 arms: ABVD x 4 or ABVD x 2, and each group was followed by IFRT of 30 or 20 Gy. At 4 years, freedom from treatment failure (FFTF) was similar in all groups (94%), and overall survival was 97%. Reducing chemotherapy appeared safe, and at this point, there was no difference between the RT doses. HD11 targeted patients with unfavorable early-stage disease and randomized them to recieve either ABVD x 4 or BEACOPP x 4, both programs were followed by either 20 or 30 Gy to the involved field. The interim analysis at 2 years has not shown a difference between the arms, with a FTTF rate of 90%.

The most recent (and as yet not fully mature) excellent results are with shortening the duration of chemotherapy to only 2 cycles of ABVD in favorable patients and reducing the IFRT dose to 20 Gy (Table 3). If the excellent results obtained by the German Hodgkin's Study Group prevail with additional follow-up, brief ABVD and low-dose IFRT will become the standard of care for favorable early-stage HL.

Subtotal lymphoid irradiation (ie, treatment of the mantle and para-aortic fields only) remains an adequate alternative treatment of clinically or pathologically staged favorable (nonbulky and without B symptoms) early-stage HL (stage I/II). Yet this option is no longer the treatment of choice due to the risk of second tumors and (to a lesser degree) coronary artery disease in long-term survivors of extensive radiotherapy alone as practiced in the past. In classic (non–lymphocyte predominant) HL, subtotal lymphoid irradiation is adequate for patients who are not candidates for a chemotherapy-containing strategy.

In patients who underwent pathologic staging (laparotomy) and were treated with primary irradiation alone, several large series reported a 15- to 20-year survival rate of nearly 90% and a relapse-free survival rate of 75%–80%. Most relapses (75%) occurred within 3 years after the completion of therapy; late relapses were uncommon. More than half of the patients who relapsed after radiotherapy alone were still curable with standard chemotherapy.

Canadian and European studies have reported excellent overall survival results in patients selected for radiotherapy on the basis of clinical prognostic

In the recent EORTC/GELA study H9, 1,591 patients with stage I-II HL were enrolled into two trials based on four prognostic factors: age, symptoms, number of involved areas, and mediastinal mass to thoracic ratio. The H9-F trial compared 36 Gy IFRT vs 20 Gy IFRT vs no RT in patients in complete remission after 6 cycles of EBVP. In the H9-F trial for favorable patients, of the 783 patients enrolled, 619 (79%) achieved a CR and were randomized to receive treatment. After a median follow-up of 33 months, the 4-year event-free survival rates were 87% in the 36 Gy and 84% in the 20 Gy arms; it was 69% in the 0 Gy arm ($P <$ .001). The 4-year overall survival rate was 98% in all three arms. The group concluded that in patients with favorable HL who achieved CR after 6 cycles of EBVP, omission of IFRT leads to an unacceptable failure rate; in contrast, an IFRT dose reduced to 20 Gy provides equivalent early results to an IFRT dose of 36 Gy (*Noordijk EM, Thomas J, Ferme C, et al: J Clin Oncol [abstract] 23[suppl]:561s, 2005*).

factors alone. Thus, irradiation alone can be safely offered to clinically staged patients with favorable prognostic factors who are not candidates for combined-modality treatment.

Chemotherapy alone In two prospective, randomized studies, radiotherapy alone was as effective as or superior to MOPP (mechlorethamine [Mustargen], Oncovin [vincristine], procarbazine [Matulane], and prednisone) chemotherapy in improving the survival of patients with early-stage disease. Although the relapse rate after chemotherapy is similar to that after radiotherapy, conventional-dose salvage chemotherapy used after failure of chemotherapy produces poor results, which translates into an inferior overall survival.

More recently, five prospective randomized studies compared chemotherapy alone with chemotherapy followed by IFRT or regional radiotherapy in patients with early-stage HL. The Children's Cancer Group (CCG) tested the role of radiation therapy in young patients (< 21 years old) who attained a complete response with risk-adapted chemotherapy (mostly COPP [cyclophosphamide, Oncovin (vincristine), procarbazine, and prednisone)/ABV [Adriamycin (doxorubicin), bleomycin, and vinblastine], 4 to 6 cycles). They enrolled 829 patients into the study (68% had early-stage disease); 501 patients who achieved a complete response were then randomized to receive either low-dose (21 Gy) IFRT or no further treatment. The accrual was stopped earlier than planned because of a significantly higher number of relapses on the no-radiotherapy arm. The 3-year event-free survival rate with an intent-to-treat analysis was 92% for patients randomized to receive radiotherapy and 87% for those randomized to receive no further treatment ($P =$ .057).

The EORTC/Groupe d'Etude des lymphomes de l'adulte (GELA) conducted a large randomized trial in patients with favorable early-stage classic HL. All patients received 6 cycles of EBVP (epirubicin [Ellence], bleomycin, vinblastine, and prednisone). Only patients who achieved a complete response were randomized to receive either IFRT of 36 Gy, IFRT of 20 Gy, or no irradiation. After an interim analysis, the EORTC/GELA groups closed the entry to the no-radiotherapy arm because of the excessive number of relapses. It should be noted that in previous EORTC studies, EBVP with IFRT was found to be inferior to MOPP/ABV with IFRT hybrid in patients with unfavorable disease but provided excellent results when combined with radiotherapy and was compared with radiotherapy alone in patients with favorable disease.

The National Cancer Institute of Canada and the Eastern Cooperative Oncology Group (ECOG) included 405 patients with nonbulky stage I/II disease. They were randomized to receive either "standard therapy," namely, subtotal nodal irradiation (STNI) for favorable patients, and ABVD (2 cycles) followed by STNI for unfavorable (B, elevated ESR, ≥ 3 sites, age ≥ 40, mixed cellularity histology) patients or experimental therapy consisting of 6 cycles or 4 cycles (if complete response was attained after 2 cycles) of ABVD and no radiotherapy. At a median follow-up of 4.2 years, progression-free survival with ABVD alone was significantly inferior ($P = .006$; hazard ratio = 2.6; 5-year estimates of disease progression-free survival, 87% vs 93%). At 5 years, no event-free or overall survival difference has been detected. The study was planned for 12 years' analysis of survival.

The Memorial Sloan-Kettering Cancer Center trial included 152 patients with nonbulky early-stage HL. Patients were randomized up front to receive either ABVD × 6 alone or ABVD × 6 followed by radiotherapy. At 60 months, the duration of complete response and freedom from disease progression for ABVD and radiotherapy vs ABVD alone were 91% vs 87% ($P = .61$) and 86% vs 81% ($P = .61$), respectively. Overall survival was 97% with ABVD and radiotherapy vs 90% with ABVD alone ($P = .08$). Although the differences between the outcome of the two treatment groups were not statistically significant, the study was not powered to detect differences between the treatment strategies that were smaller than 20%, due to the small number of patients and events.

In a prospectively randomized study reported from India, patients with HL who achieved a complete response after ABVD were randomized to receive either IFRT or no further therapy. The 8-year event-free and overall survival rates were significantly better for the patients who received consolidation with IFRT than for those who received ABVD alone. Subset analysis indicated that the benefit from added IFRT was more prominent in advanced-stage than in early-stage disease.

The National Comprehensive Cancer Network (NCCN) guidelines recommend combined-modality therapy as the treatment of choice for favorable or unfavorable classic HL. Opinions differ as to the use of chemotherapy alone, and it remains highly controversial.

TECHNICAL ASPECTS OF RADIATION THERAPY

Involved-field radiotherapy

In a combined-modality setting, irradiation of the involved lymph node chain, with or without adjacent sites, and tailoring of the field borders to the postchemotherapy tumor volume (in critical areas such as the mediastinum) are recommended. IFRT is the most appropriate irradiation approach after chemotherapy. IFRT or regional radiotherapy alone is used for lymphocyte-predominant HL. Recommendations for IFRT for HL are detailed in an article by Yahalom and Mauch.

Extended radiation fields

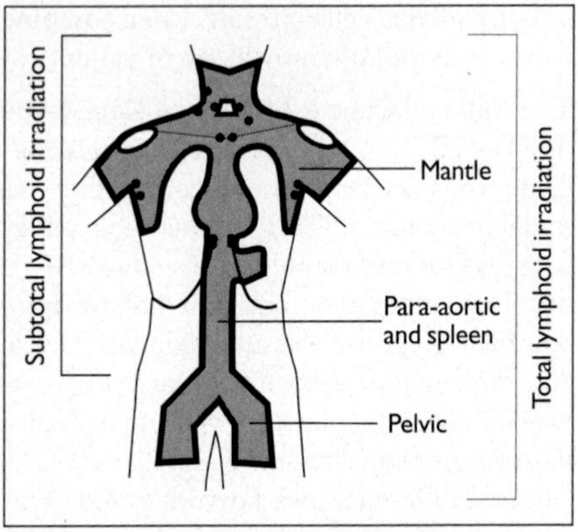

FIGURE 2: Extended radiation fields used for treatment of classic Hodgkin lymphoma with irradiation alone

Successful therapy with irradiation alone in classic HL requires treatment of all clinically involved lymph nodes and all nodal and extranodal regions at risk for subclinical involvement (Figure 2). The HL radiation fields were designed to conform to the philosophy of treating regions beyond the immediately involved area while accounting for normal tissue tolerance and the technical constraints of field size. The extended radiation fields are inappropriate when radiation is administered as consolidation following chemotherapy and thus are rarely used today.

Dose considerations

When irradiation alone is used to treat HL, the standard total dose to each field is 3,600 cGy, delivered in daily fractions of 180 cGy over 4 weeks. In addition, clinically involved areas are given a boost of 360–540 cGy in 2–3 fractions to bring the total dose to these areas up to 3,960–4,140 cGy. Patients who receive irradiation as consolidation after chemotherapy receive a total dose of 2,000–3,600 cGy in 150–180-cGy fractions. We normally use opposed anterior and posterior fields that are evenly weighted and treat both fields daily. Three-dimensional conformal radiotherapy and intensity-modulated radiation therapy (IMRT) are employed for selected cases.

SIDE EFFECTS AND COMPLICATIONS OF RADIOTHERAPY

Side effects of radiotherapy depend on the irradiated volume, dose administered, and technique employed. They are also influenced by the extent and type of prior chemotherapy, if any, and by the patient's age.

Acute effects The potential acute side effects of involved fields in the upper body include mouth dryness, change in taste, pharyngitis, nausea, dry cough, dermatitis, and fatigue. These side effects are usually mild and transient.

The main potential side effects of subdiaphragmatic irradiation are loss of appetite, nausea, and increased bowel movements. These reactions are usually mild and can be minimized with standard antiemetic medications.

Irradiation of more than one field, particularly after chemotherapy, can cause myelosuppression, which may necessitate treatment delays.

Delayed effects Delayed side effects may develop anywhere from several weeks to several years after the completion of radiotherapy.

Lhermitte's sign Approximately 15% of patients who receive the full dose of radiation to the neck may note an electric shock sensation radiating down the backs of both legs when the head is flexed (Lhermitte's sign) 6 weeks to 3 months after mantle-field radiotherapy. Possibly secondary to transient demyelinization of the spinal cord, Lhermitte's sign resolves spontaneously after a few months and is not associated with late or permanent spinal cord damage.

Pneumonitis and pericarditis During the same period, radiation pneumonitis and/or acute pericarditis may occur in < 5% of patients who receive large fields of radiation to the mediastinum; these side effects occur more often in those who have extensive mediastinal disease. Both inflammatory processes have become rare with modern radiation techniques.

Herpes zoster infection Patients with HL, regardless of treatment type, have a propensity to develop herpes zoster infection within 2 years after therapy. Usually, the infection is confined to a single dermatome and is self-limited. If the cutaneous eruption is identified promptly, treatment with systemic acyclovir will limit its duration and intensity.

The largest series of HL survivors was reported at the 2005 ASCO meeting. Of 8,270 deaths (excluding HL), the NCI-International HL Group compared age-, gender- and calendar year-specific mortality rates with those in the general population based on 14 registries. The overall relative risk of mortality was 2.5. Significant excess deaths were due to second cancers and noncancer causes and remained significantly elevated for more than 30 years following HL diagnosis. Significantly increased risks were observed for deaths due to cardiovascular, respiratory, infectious, and hematologic diseases; risks were significantly elevated in both sexes, four age groups, and three calendar year periods. Risk of death from ischemic heart disease, pneumonia, bacterial infection, viral infection, and hematologic disorders was significantly elevated in all treatment groups. *(Dores G, Schonfeld S, Chen J, et al: J Clin Oncol [abstract] 23[suppl]:562s, 2005).*

Subclinical hypothyroidism Radiotherapy of the neck can induce subclinical hypothyroidism in about one-third of patients. This condition is detected by elevation of thyroid-stimulating hormone (TSH). Thyroid replacement with levothyroxine (T_4) is recommended, even in asymptomatic patients, to prevent overt hypothyroidism and decrease the risk of benign thyroid nodules.

Infertility Irradiation of the pelvis may have deleterious effects on fertility. In most patients, this problem can be avoided by appropriate gonadal shielding. In females, the ovaries can be moved into a shielded area laterally or inferomedially near the uterine cervix. Irradiation fields that spare the pelvis do not increase the risk of sterility.

Secondary malignancies Patients with HL who were cured with radiotherapy and/or chemotherapy have an increased risk of secondary solid tumors (most commonly, lung, breast, and stomach cancers, as well as melanoma) and NHL 10 or more years after treatment. Chemotherapy combinations that do not include alkylating agents or a new brief program (such as Stanford V) as well as the smaller involved fields and lower doses are less likely to have the increased risk observed with extended fields and/or MOPP or MOPP-like chemotherapy.

Lung cancer Patients who are smokers should be strongly encouraged to quit the habit because the increase in lung cancer that occurs after irradiation or chemotherapy with alkylating agents has been detected mostly in smokers. Alkylating agents (such as in the MOPP regimen) and radiation therapy were associated with an increased risk of lung cancer in an additive and dose-dependent fashion. These effects were multiplied by tobacco use (see Suggested Reading).

Breast cancer The increase in breast cancer risk is inversely related to the patient's age at HL treatment; no increased risk has been found in women irradiated after 30 years of age. The risk of breast cancer is increased with higher radiation breast dose and is reduced in patients who received chemotherapy or ovarian irradiation that induced early menopause. In a case-controlled study performed at The Netherlands Cancer Institute, 48 women with breast cancer after HL were matched with 175 women with HL and no breast cancer. The study demonstrated that women who received chemotherapy followed by radiation therapy had a significantly decreased relative risk (RR) of developing breast cancer as compared with patients treated with irradiation alone (RR = 0.45; P = .005). For patients treated with irradiation alone, the risk of breast cancer increased significantly with increasing radiation dose to the breast (P trend = .01). Reaching menopause before the age of 35 years after treatment with chemotherapy and irradiation was associated with a markedly reduced risk of breast cancer (RR = 0.06; P = .001). The risk reduction with combined-modality treatment indicates the importance of ovarian function in the tumorigenesis process of radiation-induced breast cancer. A larger international case-controlled study of 105 breast cancer patients and 266 controls had similar findings.

In most situations, modern IFRT should spare the breast. Breast cancer is curable in its early stages, and early detection has a significant impact on survival. Breast examination should be part of the routine follow-up for women cured of HL, and routine mammography should begin about 8 years after treatment.

Cardiovascular disease An increased risk of cardiovascular morbidity has been reported among patients who have received mediastinal irradiation. In a retrospective study evaluating the cardiac risks of 450 patients cured of HL with radiotherapy alone or in combination, 42 patients (10%) developed coronary artery disease (CAD) at a median of 9 years after treatment, 30 patients (7%) developed carotid and/or subclavian artery disease at a median of 17 years after treatment, and 25 patients (6%) developed clinically significant valvular dysfunction at a median of 22 years after treatment. The most common valve lesion was aortic stenosis, which occurred in 14 valves. The only treatment-related factor associated with the development of CAD was use of a radiation technique that resulted in a higher total dose to a portion of the heart (RR = 7.8; 95% confidence interval [CI] = 1.1–53.2; P = .04). No specific treatment-related factor was associated with carotid or subclavian artery disease or valvular dysfunction. Freedom from cardiovascular morbidity was 88% at 15 years and 84% at 20 years.

To reduce this hazard, radiation fields should conform to the involved postchemotherapy volume, and the dose should be reduced to 20–30 Gy if possible. Patients who have received radiation to the mediastinum should be monitored and advised about other established CAD risk factors, such as smoking, hyperlipidemia, hypertension, and poor dietary and exercise habits. Cholesterol levels should be monitored and treated if elevated.

Effects on bone and muscle growth In children, high-dose irradiation will affect bone and muscle growth and may result in deformities. Current treatment programs for pediatric HL are chemotherapy-based; radiotherapy is limited to low doses.

TREATMENT OF STAGE III/IV DISEASE

Chemotherapy has become curative for many patients with advanced stages of HL. MOPP has been the primary effective combination chemotherapy regimen for advanced-stage disease since the 1960s. Over the past several years, ABVD has been shown to be more effective and less toxic than MOPP, particularly with respect to sterility and secondary leukemia.

Combination chemotherapy regimens

Doxorubicin-containing regimens A doxorubicin-containing regimen, such as ABVD (Table 4), is the treatment of choice for patients presenting with stage III or IV disease, as demonstrated by a randomized phase III trial undertaken by the Cancer and Leukemia Group B (CALGB). This trial showed higher complete response rates with ABVD and ABVD/MOPP (82% and 83%, respectively) than with MOPP alone (65%).

One reason for the improved response rate in the groups treated with doxorubicin-containing regimens was the higher percentage of patients who were able to receive ≥ 85% of the expected chemotherapy dose, particularly in the ABVD group. In addition, rates of significant and life-threatening neutropenia were higher in patients treated with the MOPP-containing regimens than in those treated with other regimens.

Subsequent trials compared ABVD, alternating MOPP/ABVD, and a MOPP/ABV hybrid. Alternating MOPP/ABVD and the MOPP/ABV hybrid were found to be equally effective in treating advanced-stage HL. However, a recent intergroup study that compared ABVD with MOPP/ABV hybrid (without irradiation) was closed early because of concerns of excess treatment-related deaths and second malignancies (mostly acute myelogenous leukemia and lung cancer) in the MOPP/ABV hybrid arm. ABVD and MOPP/ABV hybrid yielded similar 5-year failure and overall survival rates.

Shortened dose-intense regimens Recently, shortened dose-intense regimens have shown promise. For example, the 12-week Stanford V regimen (see Table 4) combined with IFRT produced a 5-year overall survival rate of 96% and a freedom from disease progression rate of 89%. The freedom-from-disease-progression rate was significantly superior among patients with a prognostic score of 0–2, compared with those with a score of 3 and higher (94% vs 75%; $P = .0001$). Of interest, in 142 patients from Stanford, no secondary leukemia was observed, and 42 pregnancies were reported.

TABLE 4: Chemotherapeutic regimens used for the treatment of Hodgkin lymphoma

Regimen	Dosage and schedule	Frequency
MOPP		
Mechlorethamine	6 mg/m^2 IV on day 1	
Oncovin	1.4 mg/m^2 IV on day 1 (maximum dose, 2.0 mg)	
Procarbazine	100 mg/m^2 PO on days 1-7	*Repeat cycle*
Prednisone[a]	40 mg/m^2 PO on days 1-14	*every 28 days.*
ABVD		
Adriamycin	25 mg/m^2 IV on days 1 and 15	
Bleomycin	10 mg/m^2 IV on days 1 and 15	
Vinblastine	6 mg/m^2 IV on days 1 and 15	*Repeat cycle*
Dacarbazine	375 mg/m^2 IV on days 1 and 15	*every 28 days.*
BEACOPP		
Bleomycin	10 mg/m^2 IV on day 8	
Etoposide	100 mg/m^2 (200 mg/m^2)[d] IV on days 1-3	
Adriamycin	25 mg/m^2 (35 mg/m^2)[d] IV on day 1	
Cyclophosphamide	650 mg/m^2 (1,200 mg/m^2)[d] IV on day 1	
Oncovin	1.4 mg/m^2[e] IV on day 8	
Procarbazine	100 mg/m^2 PO on days 1-7	
Prednisone	40 mg/m^2 PO on days 1-14	*Repeat cycle*
G-CSF from day 8		*every 21 days*
Stanford V		
Doxorubicin	25 mg/m^2 IV on days 1 and 15	*Repeat cycle*
Vinblastine[b]	6 mg/m^2 IV on days 1 and 15	*every 28 days for*
Mechlorethamine	6 mg/m^2 IV on day 1	*a total of 3 cycles.*
Vincristine[b]	1.4 mg/m^2 IV[c] on days 8 and 22	*Radiotherapy to*
Bleomycin	5 U/m^2 IV on days 8 and 22	*initial sites ≥ 5 cm*
Etoposide	60 mg/m^2 IV on days 15 and 16	*(dose: 36 cGy).*
Prednisone	40 mg/m^2 PO every other day (maximum dose, 2.0 mg)	

[a] In the original report, prednisone was given only in cycles 1 and 4.

[b] Vinblastine dose was decreased to 4 mg/m^2 and vincristine dose to 1 mg/m^2 during cycle 3 for patients ≥ 50 years of age.

[c] Tapered by 10 mg every other day starting at week 10

[d] Increased dose for BEACOPP

[e] Maximal dose of 2 mg

G-CSF = granulocyte colony-stimulating factor

An escalated dose version of BEACOPP (bleomycin, etoposide, Adriamycin [doxorubicin], cyclophosphamide, Oncovin [vincristine], procarbazine, and prednisone) was found to have a statistically significant superior freedom from treatment failure at 5 years compared with standard-dose BEACOPP and alternating monthly COPP and ABVD for patients with advanced stages of HL. Short-term hematologic toxicity was greatest for escalated BEACOPP, and a significant increased risk for secondary acute leukemias was also seen as compared with standard-dose BEACOPP and COPP/ABVD.

In a recent update of the Stanford V chemoradiotherapy program, 256 patients with classic HL were treated on prospective trials with the weekly Stanford V (see Table 4) regimen ± radiotherapy (RT). In all patients, freedom from disease progression was 91% at 8 years and 89% at 12 years, and overall survival rates were 95% at 8 and 12 years. Among 24 patients with disease progression, 16 (67%) were successfully treated with second-line therapy. No cases of secondary myelodysplasia/ leukemia or non-HL have occurred. To date, 72 post-treatment conceptions (excluding pretreatment semen or embryo cryopreservation) were recorded, with 65 live births (plus 4 current pregnancies) among 34 men and 30 women. An intergroup CALGB randomized study is currently comparing the Stanford V combined-modality regimen with ABVD for 6 cycles (and radiotherapy only for bulky disease) in patients with advanced-stage HL. This study is still open for accrual. *(Horning SJ, Hoppe RT, Advani R, et al: Blood 104:abstract 308, 2004).*

Combined-modality therapy

Although the role of consolidation radiotherapy after induction chemotherapy remains controversial, irradiation is routinely added in patients with advanced-stage disease who present with bulky disease or who remain in uncertain complete remission after chemotherapy. Retrospective studies have demonstrated that adding low-dose radiotherapy to all initial disease sites after chemotherapy-induced complete response decreases the relapse rate by ~25% and significantly improves overall survival.

Interpretation of the impact of irradiation in prospective studies has been controversial. However, a Southwest Oncology Group (SWOG) randomized study of 278 patients with stage III or IV HL suggested that the addition of low-dose irradiation to all sites of initial disease after a complete response to MOP-BAP (mechlorethamine, Oncovin [vincristine], prednisone, bleomycin, Adriamycin [doxorubicin], and procarbazine) chemotherapy improves the duration of remission in patients with advanced-stage disease. An intention-to-treat analysis showed that the advantage of combined-modality therapy was limited to patients with nodular sclerosis. No survival differences were observed.

A recent meta-analysis demonstrated that the addition of radiotherapy to chemotherapy reduces the rate of relapse but did not show a survival benefit for the combined-modality approach.

The EORTC conducted a randomized trial in patients with stages III and IV HL in which those achieving a complete remission with MOPP/ABV hybrid were randomized to receive either low-dose IFRT or no radiotherapy. Of the 739 patients enrolled, 421 achieved a complete remission. The median follow-up was 79 months. There was no statistically significant difference in 5-year

TABLE 5: Toxicities associated with combination chemotherapy and radiation therapy

Acute toxicities	
Alopecia Nausea and vomiting Diarrhea Mucositis Paresthesias and neuropathies CNS confusion	Anemia, leukopenia, and thrombocytopenia Disulfiram-like reaction following alcohol while taking procarbazine
Delayed toxicities	
Secondary malignancies Acute myelogenous leukemia Acute lymphocytic leukemia Non-Hodgkin lymphoma Melanoma Sarcoma Breast, gastric, lung, and thyroid cancers	Pulmonary complications Bleomycin-related lung toxicity Pulmonary fibrosis Cardiac complications Cardiomyopathy Accelerated atherosclerotic heart disease Pericardial fibrosis
Endocrine complications Infertility Hypothyroidism	

event-free or overall survival. Partial responders received low-dose IFRT, and their event-free and overall survival rates were similar to those patients who achieved a complete remission.

LONG-TERM TOXICITIES OF COMBINATION CHEMOTHERAPY

The CALGB trial and the intergroup trials mentioned previously (see section on "Combination chemotherapy regimens") noted differences in the long-term toxicities of various combination chemotherapeutic regimens (Table 5).

Myelodysplasia and acute leukemia MOPP therapy is known to be related to the development of myelodysplastic syndromes (MDS) and acute leukemia. These secondary hematologic malignancies begin 2 years following therapy and decline by 10 years, with the maximum risk between 5 and 9 years. Patients with these malignancies have a poor prognosis.

The incidence of secondary leukemia appears to increase with cumulative doses of chemotherapy, age > 40 years when receiving chemotherapy for HL, and splenectomy. It is controversial whether combined-modality therapy increases the risk of leukemia compared with chemotherapy alone.

Cytogenetic studies of secondary leukemias reveal a loss of the long arm of chromosome 5 and/or 7. Less frequently, there is a loss of chromosome 18 or rearrangement of the short arm of chromosome 17. A balanced rearrangement of 11q23 and 21q22 also has been described with etoposide therapy.

Other malignancies also are being observed with increasing frequency after chemotherapy (most regimens included alkylating agents), particularly for lung cancer and NHL. These malignancies have a longer latency period and usually are not observed until 15 years after therapy.

Infertility is another long-term complication seen with combination chemotherapy. At least 80% of males are found to have permanent azoospermia or oligospermia following more than 3 cycles of MOPP chemotherapy; < 10% of men will have recovery of spermatogenesis within 1–7 years following the end of chemotherapy. The risk of infertility with ABVD chemotherapy is significantly lower than that with MOPP chemotherapy, approximately 15%–25%. All men who desire childbearing potential following therapy should be counseled regarding sperm banking.

In females, there is a 50% rate of primary ovarian failure overall. The risk is 25%–30% in patients treated at age 25 or younger but increases to 80%–100% in women older than age 25. Many women who do maintain ovarian function during chemotherapy will have premature menopause following therapy.

Pulmonary complications have been reported with ABVD chemotherapy and are related to bleomycin-induced lung toxicity. In a Memorial Sloan-Kettering Cancer Center study of 60 patients with early-stage HL receiving ABVD chemotherapy with or without mediastinal irradiation, 53% reported dyspnea on exertion or cough during chemotherapy and 37% had a significant decline in pulmonary function. Bleomycin was discontinued in 23% of patients. Following ABVD therapy, there was a significant decline in median forced vital capacity (FVC) and diffusing capacity of the lungs for carbon monoxide (DLCO). Radiotherapy following ABVD chemotherapy resulted in a further decrease in FVC but did not significantly affect functional status. At longer follow-up, only 1 of 60 patients reported persistent dyspnea on minimal exertion.

In the CALGB trial, there were 3 fatal pulmonary complications in 238 patients; all 3 patients were older than age 40.

Pulmonary fibrosis has also been described after combined-modality therapy.

A total of 141 patients were treated with bleomycin-containing chemotherapy for newly diagnosed HL. Bleomycin pulmonary toxicity (BPT) was defined by the presence of pulmonary symptoms, bilateral interstitial infiltrates, and no evidence of an infectious etiology. BPT was observed in 18% of patients. Increasing age; doxorubicin, bleomycin, vinblastine, and dacarbazine as initial therapy; and granulocyte colony-stimulating factor use were associated with the development of BPT. Patients with BPT had a median 5-year overall survival rate of 63% vs 90% (*P* = .001) in unaffected patients. The mortality rate from BPT was 4.2% in all patients and 24% in patients who developed the pulmonary syndrome. The incidence of and mortality from BPT were highest in patients older than 40 years. The omission of bleomycin had no impact on obtaining a complete remission, progression-free survival, or overall survival. The authors concluded that BPT results in a significant decrease in 5-year overall survival in patients who are treated for HL. Age > 40 years seems to add substantially to the risk (*Martin WG, Ristow KM, Habermann TM, et al: J Clin Oncol 23:7614-7620, 2005*).

Pulmonary function testing usually reveals a decreased diffusion capacity and restrictive changes prior to the onset of symptoms.

Cardiomyopathy is a recognized complication of doxorubicin therapy but is not commonly seen in patients receiving ABVD chemotherapy. Patients who are treated with 6 cycles of ABVD chemotherapy receive a total doxorubicin dose of 300 mg/m^2; cardiac toxicity is rarely seen in patients who receive a total dose ≤ 400 mg/m^2.

MANAGEMENT OF RELAPSED DISEASE

Relapse after radiation therapy

Patients with early-stage HL who relapse after initial therapy with irradiation alone have excellent complete remission rates and 50%–80% long-term survival rates when treated with MOPP or ABVD. The dose regimens used for salvage therapy are the same as those outlined in Table 4.

Relapse after combination chemotherapy

Among patients with advanced-stage HL, 70%–90% will have complete response to treatment; however, up to one-third of patients with stage III or IV disease will relapse, usually within the first 3 years after therapy.

Various studies have identified the following poor prognostic factors for response to first-line chemotherapy: B symptoms, age > 45 years, bulky mediastinal disease, extranodal involvement, low hematocrit, high ESR, high levels of CD30, and high levels of serum interleukin-10 and soluble IL-2 receptor.

An International Prognostic Index (IPI) has been devised for advanced HL based on a retrospective analysis of 1,618 patients from 25 centers. In the final model, seven factors were used: albumin < 4 g/dL, hemoglobin < 10.5 g/dL, male gender, stage IV disease, age ≥ 45 years, WBC ≥ 15,000/μL, and lymphocytes < 600/μL (or 8% of the WBC count). The worst prognostic group (7%) had a 5-year overall survival rate of 56% and a failure-free survival rate of 42%.

In a comparison of seven well-known prognostic models for HL applied retrospectively to a population of patients with advanced-stage disease, three were found to be the most predictive of outcome. One was the IPI, men-

> Schmitz et al from the European Bone marrow transplant group (EBMT) updated the results of 161 patients with biopsy-proven relapse of HL who were randomized to 2 cycles of dexamethasone (DEXA), BCNU, etoposide, cytarabine, and melphalan (Dexa-BEAM) followed by 2 further cycles of Dexa-BEAM (arm A) or 2 cycles of high-dose BEAM+ASCT (arm B). Only chemosensitive patients were eligible for analysis. A total of 150 chemosensitive patients were needed to show an improvement of 20% in 2-year freedom from treatment failure (FFTF) with a power of 0.8. With comparable baseline characteristics and a median follow-up of 83 months, 7-year FFTF was 32% in arm A and 49% in arm B. Subgroup analysis for 7-year FFTF favored arm B in both early/late first relapse but not in multiple relapse. Overall survival did not significantly differ between the groups (*Schmitz N, Haverkamp H, Josting A, et al: J Clin Oncol [abstract] 23[suppl]:562s, 2005*).

tioned previously. The other two were the Memorial Sloan-Kettering Cancer Center model (employing age, LDH, hematocrit, inguinal nodal involvement, and mediastinal mass bulk) and the Database on Hodgkin Lymphoma model (employing stage, age, B symptoms, albumin, and gender). Integration of the three models in a linear model improved their predictive power.

High-dose therapy with autologous stem-cell transplantation The preferred salvage method for patients who relapsed after combined-modality therapy or chemotherapy alone or remained refractory to those programs is high-dose chemoradiotherapy with autologous stem-cell transplantation (ASCT).

Two randomized studies (from Great Britain and Germany) demonstrated an event-free survival advantage with the high-dose therapy approach. Although a significant survival advantage was not observed due to the crossover design of the studies, most patients with refractory disease or postchemotherapy relapse are currently managed with high-dose chemoradiation therapy and ASCT.

No standard conditioning regimen has been used in this setting, as patients have had prior treatment with a variety of combinations of chemotherapy and radiation therapy. Although most patients who have received bone marrow have been treated with several regimens or have had poorly responsive disease from initial diagnosis, the complete response rate has ranged from 50%–80%, with approximately 40%–80% of responding patients achieving durable remission.

Recent analysis of prognostic factors in patients receiving high-dose salvage therapy indicated that B symptoms at relapse, extranodal disease, and short (< 1 year) remission or no remission are factors associated with a poor outcome.

A recent study from Memorial Sloan-Kettering Cancer Center reported the results of high-dose chemotherapy with ASCT in 65 patients with relapsed or refractory HL. At a median follow-up of 43 months, overall survival was estimated to be 73% and event-free survival was estimated to be 58% by intent-to-treat analysis. In a multivariate logistic regression model, there were three adverse prognostic factors: extranodal sites of relapse or refractory disease, complete remission duration of less than 1 year or refractory disease, and B symptoms. Patients with no or one adverse factor had an overall survival of 90% and an event-free survival of 83%; those with two adverse factors had an overall survival of 57% and an event-free survival of 27%; and those with three adverse factors had an overall survival of 25% and an event-free survival of 10%. A follow-up study of a risk-adapted approach based on the study previously described suggested that patients with adverse prognostic factors may benefit from further augmentation of high-dose programs, including a “double-transplant” for selected patients.

TARCEVA® (erlotinib) TABLETS BRIEF SUMMARY
Please see the Tarceva package insert for full prescribing information.
INDICATIONS AND USAGE Non-Small Cell Lung Cancer TARCEVA monotherapy is indicated for the treatment of patients with locally advanced or metastatic non-small cell lung cancer after failure of at least one prior chemotherapy regimen. Results from two, multicenter, placebo-controlled, randomized, Phase 3 trials conducted in first-line patients with locally advanced or metastatic NSCLC showed no clinical benefit with the concurrent administration of TARCEVA with platinum-based chemotherapy [carboplatin and paclitaxel or gemcitabine and cisplatin] and its use is not recommended in that setting. **Pancreatic Cancer** TARCEVA in combination with gemcitabine is indicated for the first-line treatment of patients with locally advanced, unresectable or metastatic pancreatic cancer. **CONTRAINDICATIONS** None. **WARNINGS Pulmonary Toxicity** There have been infrequent reports of serious Interstitial Lung Disease (ILD)-like events, including fatalities, in patients receiving TARCEVA for treatment of NSCLC, pancreatic cancer or other advanced solid tumors. In the randomized single-agent NSCLC study (see **CLINICAL STUDIES** section), the incidence of ILD-like events (0.8%) was the same in both the placebo and TARCEVA groups. In the pancreatic cancer study–in combination with gemcitabine–(see **CLINICAL STUDIES** section), the incidence of ILD-like events was 2.5% in the TARCEVA plus gemcitabine group vs. 0.4% in the placebo plus gemcitabine group. The overall incidence of ILD-like events in approximately 4900 TARCEVA-treated patients from all studies (including uncontrolled studies and studies with concurrent chemotherapy) was approximately 0.7%. Reported diagnoses in patients suspected of having ILD-like events included pneumonitis, radiation pneumonitis, hypersensitivity pneumonitis, interstitial pneumonia, interstitial lung disease, obliterative bronchiolitis, pulmonary fibrosis, Acute Respiratory Distress Syndrome and lung infiltration. Symptoms started from 5 days to more than 9 months (median 39 days) after initiating TARCEVA therapy. In the lung cancer trials most of the cases were associated with confounding or contributing factors such as concomitant/prior chemotherapy, prior radiotherapy, pre-existing parenchymal lung disease, metastatic lung disease, or pulmonary infections. In the event of an acute onset of new or progressive, unexplained pulmonary symptoms such as dyspnea, cough, and fever, TARCEVA therapy should be interrupted pending diagnostic evaluation. If ILD is diagnosed, TARCEVA should be discontinued and appropriate treatment instituted as needed (see **ADVERSE REACTIONS** and **DOSAGE AND ADMINISTRATION - Dose Modifications** sections). **Myocardial infarction/ischemia:** In the pancreatic carcinoma trial, six patients (incidence of 2.3%) in the TARCEVA/gemcitabine group developed myocardial infarction/ischemia. One of these patients died due to myocardial infarction. In comparison, 3 patients in the placebo/gemcitabine group developed myocardial infarction (incidence 1.2%) and one died due to myocardial infarction. **Cerebrovascular accident:** In the pancreatic carcinoma trial, six patients in the TARCEVA/gemcitabine group developed cerebrovascular accidents (incidence: 2.3%). One of these was hemorrhagic and was the only fatal event. In comparison, in the placebo/gemcitabine group there were no cerebrovascular accidents. **Microangiopathic Hemolytic Anemia with Thrombocytopenia:** In the pancreatic carcinoma trial, two patients in the TARCEVA/gemcitabine group developed microangiopathic hemolytic anemia with thrombocytopenia (incidence: 0.8%). Both patients received TARCEVA and gemcitabine concurrently. In comparison, in the placebo/gemcitabine group there were no cases of microangiopathic hemolytic anemia with thrombocytopenia. **Pregnancy Category D** Erlotinib has been shown to cause maternal toxicity with associated embryo/fetal lethality and abortion in rabbits when given at doses that result in plasma drug concentrations of approximately 3 times those in humans (AUCs at 150 mg daily dose). When given during the period of organogenesis to achieve plasma drug concentrations approximately equal to those in humans, based on AUC, there was no increased incidence of embryo/fetal lethality or abortion in rabbits or rats. However, female rats treated with 30 mg/m^2/day or 60 mg/m^2/day (0.3 or 0.7 times the clinical dose, on a mg/m^2 basis) of erlotinib prior to mating through the first week of pregnancy had an increase in early resorptions that resulted in a decrease in the number of live fetuses. No teratogenic effects were observed in rabbits or rats. There are no adequate and well-controlled studies in pregnant women using TARCEVA. Women of childbearing potential should be advised to avoid pregnancy while on TARCEVA. Adequate contraceptive methods should be used during therapy, and for at least 2 weeks after completing therapy. Treatment should only be continued in pregnant women if the potential benefit to the mother outweighs the risk to the fetus. If TARCEVA is used during pregnancy, the patient should be apprised of the potential hazard to the fetus or potential risk for loss of the pregnancy. **PRECAUTIONS Drug Interactions** Co-treatment with the potent CYP3A4 inhibitor ketoconazole increases erlotinib AUC by 2/3. Caution should be used when administering or taking TARCEVA with ketoconazole and other strong CYP3A4 inhibitors such as, but not limited to, atazanavir, clarithromycin, indinavir, itraconazole, nefazodone, nelfinavir, ritonavir, saquinavir, telithromycin, troleandomycin (TAO), and voriconazole (see **DOSAGE AND ADMINISTRATION - Dose Modifications** section). Pre-treatment with the CYP3A4 inducer rifampicin decreased erlotinib AUC by about 2/3. Alternate treatments lacking CYP3A4 inducing activity should be considered. If an alternative treatment is unavailable, a TARCEVA dose greater than 150 mg should be considered for NSCLC patients, and greater than 100 mg considered for pancreatic cancer patients. If the TARCEVA dose is adjusted upward, the dose will need to be reduced upon discontinuation of rifampicin or other inducers. Other CYP3A4 inducers include, but are not limited to, rifabutin, rifapentine, phenytoin, carbamazepine, phenobarbital and St. John's Wort (see **DOSAGE AND ADMINISTRATION - Dose Modifications** section). **Hepatotoxicity** Asymptomatic increases in liver transaminases have been observed in TARCEVA treated patients; therefore, periodic liver function testing (transaminases, bilirubin, and alkaline phosphatase) should be considered. Dose reduction or interruption of TARCEVA should be considered if changes in liver function are severe (see **ADVERSE REACTIONS** section). **Patients with Hepatic Impairment** *In vitro* and *in vivo* evidence suggest that erlotinib is cleared primarily by the liver. Therefore, erlotinib exposure may be increased in patients with hepatic dysfunction (see **CLINICAL PHARMACOLOGY - Special Populations - Patients with Hepatic Impairment** and **DOSAGE AND ADMINISTRATION - Dose Modification** sections). **Elevated International Normalized Ratio and Potential Bleeding** International Normalized Ratio (INR) elevations and infrequent reports of bleeding events including gastrointestinal and non-gastrointestinal bleedings have been reported in clinical studies, some associated with concomitant warfarin administration. Patients taking warfarin or other coumarin-derivative anticoagulants should be monitored regularly for changes in prothrombin time or INR (see **ADVERSE REACTIONS** section). **Carcinogenesis, Mutagenesis, Impairment of Fertility** Erlotinib has not been tested for carcinogenicity. Erlotinib has been tested for genotoxicity in a series of *in vitro* assays (bacterial mutation, human lymphocyte chromosome aberration, and mammalian cell mutation) and an *in vivo* mouse bone marrow micronucleus test and did not cause genetic damage. Erlotinib did not impair fertility in either male or female rats. **Pregnancy Pregnancy Category D** (see **WARNINGS** and **PRECAUTIONS - Information for Patients** sections). **Nursing Mothers** It is not known whether erlotinib is excreted in human milk. Because many drugs are excreted in human milk and because the effects of TARCEVA on infants have not been studied, women should be advised against breast-feeding while receiving TARCEVA therapy. **Pediatric Use** The safety and effectiveness of TARCEVA in pediatric patients have not been studied. **Geriatric Use** Of the total number of patients participating in the randomized NSCLC trial, 62% were less than 65 years of age, and 38% of patients were aged 65 years or older. The survival benefit was maintained across both age groups (see **CLINICAL STUDIES** section). In the pancreatic cancer study, 53% of patients were younger than 65 years of age and 47% were 65 years of age or older. No meaningful differences in safety or pharmacokinetics were observed between younger and older patients in either study. Therefore, no dosage adjustments are recommended in elderly patients. **Information for Patients** If the following signs or symptoms occur, patients should seek medical advice promptly (see **WARNINGS, ADVERSE REACTIONS** and **DOSAGE AND ADMINISTRATION - Dose Modification** sections). • Severe or persistent diarrhea, nausea, anorexia, or vomiting • Onset or worsening of unexplained shortness of breath or cough • Eye irritation. Women of childbearing potential should be advised to avoid becoming pregnant while taking TARCEVA (see **WARNINGS - Pregnancy Category D** section). **ADVERSE REACTIONS** Safety evaluation of TARCEVA is based on 856 cancer patients who received TARCEVA as monotherapy, 308 patients who received TARCEVA 100 or 150 mg plus gemcitabine, and 1228 patients who received TARCEVA concurrently with other chemotherapies. There have been reports of serious events, including fatalities, in patients receiving TARCEVA for treatment of NSCLC, pancreatic cancer or other advanced solid tumors (see **WARNINGS,** and **DOSAGE AND ADMINISTRATION - Dose Modifications** sections). **Non-Small Cell Lung Cancer** Adverse events, regardless of causality, that occurred in at least 10% of patients treated with single-agent TARCEVA at 150 mg and at least 3% more often than in the placebo group in the randomized trial of patients with NSCLC are summarized by NCI-CTC (version 2.0) Grade in Table 5. The most common adverse reactions in patients receiving single-agent TARCEVA 150 mg were rash and diarrhea. Grade 3/4 rash and diarrhea occurred in 9% and 6%, respectively, in TARCEVA-treated patients. Rash and diarrhea each resulted in study discontinuation in 1% of TARCEVA-treated patients. Six percent and 1% of patients needed dose reduction for rash and diarrhea, respectively. The median time to onset of rash was 8 days, and the median time to onset of diarrhea was 12 days.

Table 5: Adverse Events Occurring in ≥10% of Single-Agent TARCEVA-treated Non-Small Cell Lung Cancer Patients (2:1 Randomization of TARCEVA to Placebo)

	TARCEVA 150 mg N=485			Placebo N=242		
NCI CTC Grade	**Any Grade**	**Grade 3**	**Grade 4**	**Any Grade**	**Grade 3**	**Grade 4**
MedDRA Preferred Term	**%**	**%**	**%**	**%**	**%**	**%**
Rash	75	8	<1	17	0	0
Diarrhea	54	6	<1	18	<1	0
Anorexia	52	8	1	38	5	<1
Fatigue	52	14	4	45	16	4
Dyspnea	41	17	11	35	15	11
Cough	33	4	0	29	2	0
Nausea	33	3	0	24	2	0
Infection	24	4	0	15	2	0
Vomiting	23	2	<1	19	2	0
Stomatitis	17	<1	0	3	0	0
Pruritus	13	<1	0	5	0	0
Dry skin	12	0	0	4	0	0
Conjunctivitis	12	<1	0	2	<1	0
Keratoconjunctivitis sicca	12	0	0	3	0	0
Abdominal pain	11	2	<1	7	1	<1

Liver function test abnormalities (including elevated alanine aminotransferase (ALT), aspartate aminotransferase (AST) and bilirubin) were observed in patients receiving single-agent TARCEVA 150 mg. These elevations were mainly transient or associated with liver metastases. Grade 2 (>2.5–5.0 x ULN) ALT elevations occurred in 4% and <1% of TARCEVA and placebo treated patients, respectively. Grade 3 (>5.0–20.0 x ULN) elevations were not observed in TARCEVA-treated patients. Dose reduction or interruption of TARCEVA should be considered if changes in liver function are severe (see **DOSAGE AND ADMINISTRATION - Dose Modification** section). **Pancreatic Cancer** Adverse events, regardless of causality, that occurred in at least 10% of patients treated with TARCEVA 100 mg plus gemcitabine in the randomized trial of patients with pancreatic cancer are summarized by NCI-CTC (version 2.0) Grade in Table 6. The most common adverse reactions in pancreatic cancer patients receiving TARCEVA 100 mg plus gemcitabine were fatigue, rash, nausea, anorexia and diarrhea.

In the TARCEVA plus gemcitabine arm, Grade 3/4 rash and diarrhea were each reported in 5% of TARCEVA plus gemcitabine-treated patients. The median time to onset of rash and diarrhea was 10 days and 15 days, respectively. Rash and diarrhea each resulted in dose reductions in 2% of patients, and resulted in study discontinuation in up to 1% of patients receiving TARCEVA plus gemcitabine. The 150 mg cohort was associated with a higher rate of certain class-specific adverse reactions including rash and required more frequent dose reduction or interruption.

Table 6: Adverse Events Occurring in ≥10% of TARCEVA-treated Pancreatic Cancer Patients: 100 mg cohort

	TARCEVA + Gemcitabine 1000 mg/m² IV N=259			Placebo + Gemcitabine 1000 mg/m² IV N=256		
NCI CTC Grade	**Any Grade**	**Grade 3**	**Grade 4**	**Any Grade**	**Grade 3**	**Grade 4**
MedDRA Preferred Term	%	%	%	%	%	%
Fatigue	73	14	2	70	13	2
Rash	69	5	0	30	1	0
Nausea	60	7	0	58	7	0
Anorexia	52	6	<1	52	5	<1
Diarrhea	48	5	<1	36	2	0
Abdominal pain	46	9	<1	45	12	<1
Vomiting	42	7	<1	41	4	<1
Weight decreased	39	2	0	29	<1	0
Infection*	39	13	3	30	9	2
Edema	37	3	<1	36	2	<1
Pyrexia	36	3	0	30	4	0
Constipation	31	3	1	34	5	1
Bone pain	25	4	<1	23	2	0
Dyspnea	24	5	<1	23	5	0
Stomatitis	22	<1	0	12	0	0
Myalgia	21	1	0	20	<1	0
Depression	19	2	0	14	<1	0
Dyspepsia	17	<1	0	13	<1	0
Cough	16	0	0	11	0	0
Dizziness	15	<1	0	13	0	<1
Headache	15	<1	0	10	0	0
Insomnia	15	<1	0	16	<1	0
Alopecia	14	0	0	11	0	0
Anxiety	13	1	0	11	<1	0
Neuropathy	13	1	<1	10	<1	0
Flatulence	13	0	0	9	<1	0
Rigors	12	0	0	9	0	0

*Includes all MedDRA preferred terms in the Infections and Infestations System Organ Class

In the pancreatic carcinoma trial, 10 patients in the TARCEVA/gemcitabine group developed deep venous thrombosis (incidence: 3.9%). In comparison, 3 patients in the placebo/gemcitabine group developed deep venous thrombosis (incidence 1.2%). The overall incidence of grade 3 or 4 thrombotic events, including deep venous thrombosis, was similar in the two treatment arms: 11% for TARCEVA plus gemcitabine and 9% for placebo plus gemcitabine. No differences in Grade 3 or Grade 4 hematologic laboratory toxicities were detected between the TARCEVA plus gemcitabine group compared to the placebo plus gemcitabine group. Severe adverse events (≥grade 3 NCI-CTC) in the TARCEVA plus gemcitabine group with incidences < 5% included syncope, arrhythmias, ileus, pancreatitis, hemolytic anemia including microangiopathic hemolytic anemia with thrombocytopenia, myocardial infarction/ischemia, cerebrovascular accidents including cerebral hemorrhage, and renal insufficiency (see **WARNINGS** section). Liver function test abnormalities (including elevated alanine aminotransferase (ALT), aspartate aminotransferase (AST) and bilirubin) have been observed following the administration of TARCEVA plus gemcitabine in patients with pancreatic cancer. Table 7 displays the most severe NCI-CTC grade of liver function abnormalities that developed. Dose reduction or interruption of TARCEVA should be considered if changes in liver function are severe (see **DOSAGE AND ADMINISTRATION - Dose Modification** section).

Table 7: Liver Function Test Abnormalities (most severe NCI-CTC grade) in Pancreatic Cancer Patients: 100 mg Cohort

	TARCEVA + Gemcitabine 1000 mg/m² IV N=259			Placebo + Gemcitabine 1000 mg/m² IV N=256		
NCI CTC Grade	**Grade 2**	**Grade 3**	**Grade 4**	**Grade 2**	**Grade 3**	**Grade 4**
Bilirubin	17%	10%	<1%	11%	10%	3%
ALT	31%	13%	<1%	22%	9%	0%
AST	24%	10%	<1%	19%	9%	0%

NSCLC and Pancreatic Cancer Indications During the NSCLC and the combination pancreatic cancer trials, infrequent cases of gastrointestinal bleeding have been reported, some associated with concomitant warfarin or NSAID administration (see **PRECAUTIONS - Elevated International Normalized Ratio and Potential Bleeding** section). These adverse events were reported as peptic ulcer bleeding (gastritis, gastroduodenal ulcers), hematemesis, hematochezia, melena and hemorrhage from possible colitis (see **PRECAUTIONS** section). Cases of Grade 1 epistaxis were also reported in both the single-agent NSCLC and the pancreatic cancer clinical trials. NCI-CTC Grade 3 conjunctivitis and keratitis have been reported infrequently in patients receiving TARCEVA therapy in the NSCLC and pancreatic cancer clinical trials. Corneal ulcerations may also occur (see **PRECAUTIONS - Information for Patients** section). In general, no notable differences in the safety of TARCEVA monotherapy or in combination with gemcitabine could be discerned between females or males and between patients younger or older than the age of 65 years. The safety of TARCEVA appears similar in Caucasian and Asian patients (see **PRECAUTIONS - Geriatric Use** section). **OVERDOSAGE** Single oral doses of TARCEVA up to 1,000 mg in healthy subjects and up to 1,600 mg in cancer patients have been tolerated. Repeated twice-daily doses of 200 mg single-agent TARCEVA in healthy subjects were poorly tolerated after only a few days of dosing. Based on the data from these studies, an unacceptable incidence of severe adverse events, such as diarrhea, rash, and liver transaminase elevation, may occur above the recommended dose (see **DOSAGE AND ADMINISTRATION** section). In case of suspected overdose, TARCEVA should be withheld and symptomatic treatment instituted. **DOSAGE AND ADMINISTRATION Non-Small Cell Lung Cancer** The recommended daily dose of TARCEVA is 150 mg taken at least one hour before or two hours after the ingestion of food. Treatment should continue until disease progression or unacceptable toxicity occurs. There is no evidence that treatment beyond progression is beneficial. **Pancreatic Cancer** The recommended daily dose of TARCEVA is 100 mg taken at least one hour before or two hours after the ingestion of food, in combination with gemcitabine (see the gemcitabine package insert). Treatment should continue until disease progression or unacceptable toxicity occurs. **Dose Modifications** In patients who develop an acute onset of new or progressive pulmonary symptoms, such as dyspnea, cough or fever, treatment with TARCEVA should be interrupted pending diagnostic evaluation. If ILD is diagnosed, TARCEVA should be discontinued and appropriate treatment instituted as necessary (see **WARNINGS - Pulmonary Toxicity** section). Diarrhea can usually be managed with loperamide. Patients with severe diarrhea who are unresponsive to loperamide or who become dehydrated may require dose reduction or temporary interruption of therapy. Patients with severe skin reactions may also require dose reduction or temporary interruption of therapy. When dose reduction is necessary, the TARCEVA dose should be reduced in 50 mg decrements. In patients who are being concomitantly treated with a strong CYP3A4 inhibitor such as, but not limited to, atazanavir, clarithromycin, indinavir, itraconazole, ketoconazole, nefazodone, nelfinavir, ritonavir, saquinavir, telithromycin, troleandomycin (TAO), or voriconazole, a dose reduction should be considered should severe adverse reactions occur. Pre-treatment with the CYP3A4 inducer rifampicin decreased erlotinib AUC by about 2/3. Alternate treatments lacking CYP3A4 inducing activity should be considered. If an alternative treatment is unavailable, a TARCEVA dose greater than 150 mg should be considered. If the TARCEVA dose is adjusted upward, the dose will need to be reduced upon discontinuation of rifampicin or other inducers. Other CYP3A4 inducers include, but are not limited to rifabutin, rifapentine, phenytoin, carbamazepine, phenobarbital and St. John's Wort. These too should be avoided if possible (see **PRECAUTIONS - Drug Interactions** section). Erlotinib is eliminated by hepatic metabolism and biliary excretion. Therefore, caution should be used when administering TARCEVA to patients with hepatic impairment. Dose reduction or interruption of TARCEVA should be considered should severe adverse reactions occur (see **CLINICAL PHARMACOLOGY - Special Populations - Patients With Hepatic Impairment, PRECAUTIONS - Patients With Hepatic Impairment**, and **ADVERSE REACTIONS** sections). **HOW SUPPLIED** The 25 mg, 100 mg and 150 mg strengths are supplied as white film-coated tablets for daily oral administration. TARCEVA® (erlotinib) Tablets, 25 mg: Round, biconvex face and straight sides, white film-coated, printed in orange with a "T" and "25" on one side and plain on the other side. Supplied in bottles of 30 tablets (NDC 50242-062-01). TARCEVA® (erlotinib) Tablets, 100 mg: Round, biconvex face and straight sides, white film-coated, printed in gray with "T" and "100" on one side and plain on the other side. Supplied in bottles of 30 tablets (NDC 50242-063-01). TARCEVA® (erlotinib) Tablets, 150 mg: Round, biconvex face and straight sides, white film-coated, printed in maroon with "T" and "150" on one side and plain on the other side. Supplied in bottles of 30 tablets (NDC 50242-064-01). **STORAGE** Store at 25°C (77°F); excursions permitted to 15°–30°C (59°–86°F). See USP Controlled Room Temperature.

Manufactured for: OSI Pharmaceuticals Inc., Melville, NY 11747
Manufactured by: Schwarz Pharma Manufacturing, Seymour, IN 47274
Distributed by: Genentech, Inc., 1 DNA Way, South San Francisco, CA 94080-4990
For further information please call 1-877-TARCEVA (1-877-827-2382)
or visit our website www.tarceva.com.

℞ ONLY

Genentech BIOONCOLOGY™ | (OSI)™ oncology

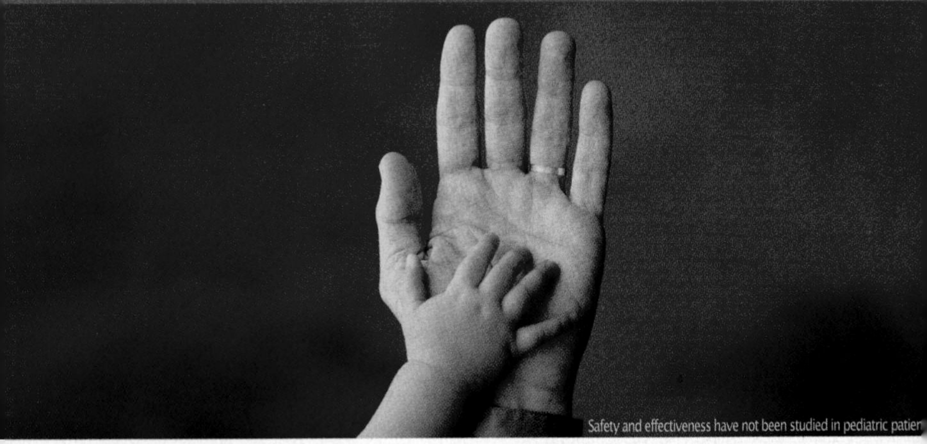
Safety and effectiveness have not been studied in pediatric patien

A therapeutic advance in second-line NSCLC

Proven to prolong your patient's lifeline

Tarceva significantly improved overall survival by 37%[1]
Increased median survival by 42.5% and increased 1-year survival by 45%[1]

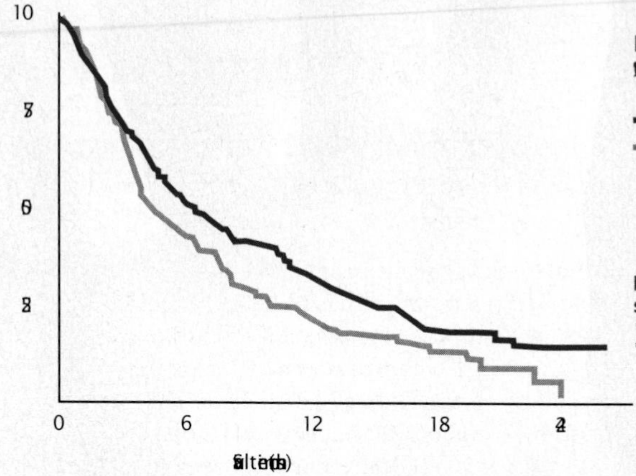

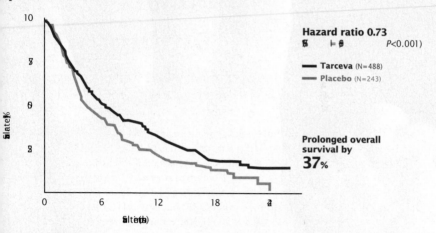

Hazard ratio 0.73
P<0.001)

Tarceva (N=488)
Placebo (N=243)

Prolonged overall survival by 37%

- Tarceva met all secondary endpoints in the analysis: progression-free survival, tumor response and response duration.[1,2]

Tarceva improved survival in good performance status patients in the second-line setting[2]

	PS 0–1					
	Median survival (months)		1-year survival		Overall survival HR (95% CI)	*P*-value
	Tarceva	Placebo	Tarceva	Placebo		
2nd line	9.4 (n=156)	6.7 (n=82)	40%	30%	0.68 (0.50–0.94)	0.018
3rd line	7.9 (n=164)	6.9 (n=84)	35%	26%	0.76 (0.57–1.01)	0.059

	PS 2–3					
	Median survival (months)		1-year survival		Overall survival HR (95% CI)	*P*-value
	Tarceva	Placebo	Tarceva	Placebo		
2nd line	3.4 (n=87)	3.3 (n=39)	18%	8%	0.83 (0.56–1.24)	0.365
3rd line	4.3 (n=81)	3.2 (n=38)	20%	8%	0.70 (0.46–1.06)	0.091

Stratification factor as demonstrated at baseline; distribution differs slightly from values reported at time of randomization.[1]

Please see accompanying brief summary on previous pages.

Tarceva®
erlotinib
tablets

Proven to prolong survival

References: 1. Tarceva® (erlotinib) full prescribing information, OSI Pharmaceuticals, Inc., 2005. **2.** Data on file, OSI Pharmaceuticals, Inc. **3.** Hidalgo M, Siu LL, Nemunaitis J, et al. Phase I and pharmacologic study of OSI-774, an epidermal growth factor receptor tyrosine kinase inhibitor, in patients with advanced solid malignancies. *J Clin Oncol.* 2001;19:3267-3279.

37% of NHLs in patients between the ages of 35 and 64 years at diagnosis but for only 16% of cases in those younger than age 35.

NHL

Race Incidence varies by race, with whites at higher risk than blacks and Asian-Americans (incidence rates increased 40%–70% in whites compared with blacks). Most histologies, particularly low-grade small lymphocytic and follicular lymphomas, are more common in whites than in blacks. Only peripheral T-cell lymphoma, mycosis fungoides, and Sézary syndrome are more common in blacks than in whites.

Geography NHL is most common in developing countries, with the United States having the highest rate worldwide. The lowest NHL rates are found in China and Thailand (2–3 per 100,000 population). Certain endemic geographic factors appear to influence the development of NHL in specific areas.

HTLV-1–associated NHL Human T-cell lymphotrophic virus-1 (HTLV-1)–associated adult T-cell lymphoma/leukemia (ATLL) occurs more frequently where HTLV-1 is endemic, in southern Japan and the Caribbean, and occurs sporadically in Brazil, sub-Saharan Africa, the Middle East, and the southeastern United States. The seroprevalence in southwest Japan is 16%, although the lifetime risk of ATLL for these persons is 2%–6%.

Burkitt lymphoma in Africa The incidence (per 100,000 population) of Burkitt NHL in Africa (Nigeria and Tanzania) is 6–8, as compared with 0.1 in the United States. The clinical features of Burkitt lymphoma in Africa differ from those of cases reported to the American Burkitt Lymphoma Registry. Etiologic endemic factors include malaria as a source of chronic B-cell antigenic stimulation and Epstein-Barr virus (EBV)-induced immortalization of B lymphocytes.

Immunoproliferative small intestinal disease (α-chain disease) Heavy-chain disease is a disorder of B-lymphoid cells characterized by diffuse thickening of the small intestine due to a lymphoplasmacytic infiltrate with secretion of incomplete IgA heavy chains. This clinicopathologic entity is rarely encountered in individuals other than those of Mediterranean ethnic origin.

Follicular lymphomas are more common in North America and Europe but are rare in the Caribbean, Africa, China, Japan, the Middle East, and Latin America.

Peripheral T-cell lymphomas are more common in Europe and China than in North America. They represent 7%–12% of lymphomas in Western countries.

Disease site Malignant lymphomas are a heterogeneous group of neoplasms that usually arise or present in lymphoid tissues, such as lymph nodes, spleen, and bone marrow, but they may arise in almost any tissue. The most frequent sites for extranodal lymphomas, which constitute about 20%–30% of all lymphomas (peripheral T-cell NHL 80%; extranodal, follicular 9%), are the stomach, skin, oral cavity and pharynx, small intestine,

A recently reported population-based study of the familial risk for NHL revealed significant increases in risk for parents and siblings, especially for diffuse large B-cell lymphoma and follicular lymphoma. Overall, there was little difference in the degree of risk for the various histopathologic subtypes (*Altieri A, Bermejo JL, Hemminki K: Blood 106:668-672, 2005*).

and central nervous system (CNS). Although primary CNS lymphoma is rare, there has been a threefold increase in incidence, even if patients with HIV infection and other types of immunosuppression are excluded.

Survival The 5-year relative survival rate of patients with NHL increased from 28% between 1950 and 1954 to 55% between 1992 and 1998. These improvements in survival occurred mainly in patients with intermediate/high-grade histologies. The potential for cure varies among the different histologic subtypes and is directly related to stage at presentation and response to initial therapy. The natural history (survival rates) for indolent lymphomas has been unchanged from the 1950s to the early 1990s, although a recent analysis from Iowa of Surveillance, Epidemiology, and End Results (SEER) data (1979–1999) shows improving survival rates of patients with follicular lymphoma.

Etiology and risk factors

Chromosomal translocations and molecular rearrangements Nonrandom chromosomal and molecular rearrangements play an important role in the pathogenesis of many lymphomas and correlate with histology and immunophenotype (Table 1). The most commonly associated chromosomal abnormality in NHL is the t(14;18)(q32;q21) translocation, which is found in 85% of follicular lymphomas and 28% of higher grade NHLs. This translocation results in the juxtaposition of the *bcl-2* apoptotic inhibitor "oncogene" at chromosome band 18q21 to the heavy-chain region of the immunoglobulin locus within chromosome band 14q32.

The t(11;14)(q13;q32) translocation results in overexpression of *bcl-1* (cyclin D1/PRAD 1), a cell-cycle–control gene on chromosome 11q13, and has a diagnostic, nonrandom association with mantle cell lymphoma. The t(3;16)(q27;p11) translocation makes the gene for the IL-2 (interleukin-2) receptor a partner of *bcl-6*, which is expressed in diffuse large cell lymphoma.

Chromosomal translocations involving 8q24 lead to c-*myc* deregulation and are frequently seen in Burkitt and Burkitt-like lymphomas, including those associated with HIV infection.

Environmental factors also may play a role in the development of NHL.

Occupations Certain workers have a slightly increased risk of developing NHL, including farmers; pesticide applicators; grain (flour) millers; meat workers; wood and forestry workers; chemists; painters; mechanics; machinists; printers; and workers in the petroleum, rubber, plastics, and synthetics industries.

Chemicals that have been linked to the development of NHL include a vari-ety of pesticides and herbicides (2,4-D-organophosphates, chlorophenols), solvents and organic chemicals (benzene, carbon tetra-chloride), wood pre-servatives, dusts (wood, cotton), and some components in hair dye.

Chemotherapy and radiotherapy Patients who receive chemotherapy and/or radiation therapy are also at increased risk of developing NHL.

Viruses Several viruses have been implicated in the pathogenesis of NHL,

TABLE 1: Correlation of chromosomal abnormalities in NHL with histology, antigen rearrangements, and oncogene expression

Cytogenetic abnormality	Histology	Antigen rearrangement	Oncogene expression
B-cell lymphoma			
t(14;18)(q32;q21)	Follicular lymphoma, diffuse large B-cell lymphoma	IgH	*bcl-2*
	MALT lymphoma	IgH	MALT-1
t(11;14)(q13;q32)	Mantle cell	IgH	*bcl-1*
t(1;14)(p22;q32)	MALT lymphoma	IgH	*bcl-10*
t(11;18)(q21;q21)	MALT lymphoma		API-2 on chromosome II MALT-1on chromosome 18
t(9;14)(p13;q32)	Lymphoplasmacytic lymphoma	IgH	*PAX-5*
t(14;19)(q32;q13)	B-CLL	IgH	*bcl-3*
8q24 translocations	Burkitt lymphoma and variants		c-*myc*
t(8;14)(q24;q32)		IgH	
t(2;8)(p11-12;q24)		Ig-λ	
t(8;22)(q24;q11)		Ig-κ	
(3;22)(q27;q11)	Diffuse (large cell, small cleaved cell)	Ig-κ	*bcl-6 (LAZ-3)*
Trisomy 12	Small lymphocytic, B-CLL		
T-cell lymphoma			
14q11 abnormalities			
inv 14(q11;q32)	Variable	TCR-δ	*tcl-1*
t(11;14)(p13;q11)	T-ALL	TCR-δ	*tcl-2*
t(10;14)(q24;q11)	Variable	TCR-δ	*hox-11* (*tcl-3*)
t(1;14)(p32;q11)	T-ALL	TCR-δ	*tcl* (*tal1*, *tcl-5*)
7q35 abnormalities			
t(7;9)(q34-36;q32)	T-ALL or lymphoblastic lymphoma	TCR-β	*tcl-4*
t(7;14)(q34-36;q11)	Variable	TCR-β	
t(7;19)(q34-36;q13)	T-ALL	TCR-β	*lyl-1*
t(2;5)(p23;q35)	Anaplastic large cell (Ki-1positive)		*npm*, *alk*

alk = anaplastic lymphoma kinase gene; B-CLL = B-cell chronic lymphocytic leukemia; IgH = immunoglobulin heavy chain; Ig-κ = immunoglobulin kappa light chain; Ig-λ = immunoglobulin lambda light chain; *LAZ-3* = *LAZ-3* transcription factor gene; MALT = mucosa-associated lymphoid tissue; *npm* = nucleophosmin gene; T-ALL = T-cell acute lymphocytic leukemia; TCR = T-cell antigen receptor; API-2 = apoptosis inhibitor 2; MALT-1 = MALT lymphoma gene 1 including EBV; HTLV-1; Kaposi's sarcoma–associated herpesvirus (KSHV, also known as human herpesvirus 8, or HHV-8); and hepatitis C virus (HCV). Meta-analyses have shown 13%–15% HCV seroprevalence in certain geographic regions among persons with B-cell NHL.

EBV is a DNA virus that has been associated with Burkitt lymphoma, particularly in endemic areas of Africa; Hodgkin lymphoma; lymphomas in immunocompromised patients (ie, organ transplantation and HIV infection); sinonasal lymphoma (Asia and South America); and sporadically in other B- and T-cell lymphomas. In contrast to studies performed in European patients, Mexican patients with intestinal lymphomas show a high frequency of EBV positivity; this finding is not limited to T-cell NHLs but rather includes a significant portion of B-cell NHLs. EBV can transform lymphocytes in culture. B lymphocytes from normal EBV-positive subjects grow as tumors in mice with severe combined immunodeficiency.

HTLV-1 is a human retrovirus that establishes a latent infection via reverse transcription in activated T-helper cells. A minority (5%) of carriers develop ATLL. An HTLV-1–like provirus has been detected in some patients with mycosis fungoides, although conflicting findings have been reported.

KSHV or HHV-8: KSHV-like DNA sequences are frequently detected in primary effusion lymphomas in patients with HIV infection and in those with multicentric (plasma cell variant) Castleman's disease.

HCV infection is associated with the development of clonal B-cell expansions and certain subtypes of NHL, particularly in the setting of essential (type II) mixed cryoglobulinemia. HCV may predispose B cells to malignant transformation by enhancing signal transduction upon binding to the CD81 (TAPA-1) molecule.

Bacterial infections Infection with *Borrelia burgdorferi*, the etiologic agent in Lyme disease, has been detected in about 35% of patients with primary cutaneous B-cell lymphoma in Scotland. A near-complete clinical and histologic remission of a primary marginal zone B-cell lymphoma was observed after eradication of *B burgdorferi* with antibiotic treatment. Gastric mucosa-associated lymphoid tissue (MALT) lymphoma is seen most frequently, but not exclusively, in association with *Helicobacter pylori* infection. Recent studies indicate that *Campylobacter jejuni* and immunoproliferative small intestinal disease (α-chain disease) are related.

Chlamydial infections A report noted an association between infection with *Chlamydia psittaci* and ocular adnexal lymphoma. The infection was found to be highly specific and does not reflect a subclinical infection widespread among the general population. Responses to antibiotics have been reported. Attempts to confirm this association in the Western hemisphere have been unsuccessful.

Immunodeficiency Patients with congenital and acquired states of immunosuppression that are at increased risk include ataxia-telangiectasia, Wiskott-Aldrich syndrome, common variable hypogammaglobulinemia, X-linked lymphoproliferative syndrome, and severe combined immunodeficiency.

Acquired immunodeficiency states, such as HIV infection (relative risk of NHL is 150–250 increased among patients with AIDS, usually high grade and extranodal), iatrogenic immunosuppression (ie, organ or blood stem-cell transplantation recipients, long-term survivors of Hodgkin lymphoma), and a variety of collagen vascular and autoimmune diseases (eg, Sjögren's syndrome, rheumatoid vasculitis and Felty's syndrome, systemic lupus erythematosus, chronic lymphocytic thyroiditis, and angioimmunoblastic lymphadenopathy) also pose an increased risk of NHL.

Autoimmunity An increased incidence of GI lymphomas is seen in patients with celiac (nontropical) sprue and inflammatory bowel disease, particularly Crohn's disease. An aberrant clonal intraepithelial T-cell population can be found in up to 75% of patients with refractory celiac sprue prior to the development of overt T-cell lymphoma using immunophenotyping and T-cell receptor gamma gene rearrangement PCR (polymerase chain reaction) techniques. Systemic lupus erythematosus and rheumatoid arthritis have been associated with B-cell lymphoma.

Signs and symptoms

Fever, weight loss, and night sweats, referred to as systemic B symptoms, as well as fatigue and weakness, are more common in advanced or aggressive NHL but may be present in all stages and histologic subtypes.

Low-grade lymphomas Painless, slowly progressive peripheral adenopathy is the most common clinical presentation in patients with low-grade lym-phomas. Patients sometimes report a history of waxing and waning adenopa-thy before seeking medical attention. Spontaneous regression of enlarged lymph nodes can occur and can cause a low-grade lymphoma to be confused with an infectious condition.

Primary extranodal involvement and B symptoms are uncommon at presentation; however, both are common in advanced or end-stage disease. Bone marrow is frequently involved, sometimes in association with cytopenias. Splenomegaly is seen in about 40% of patients, but the spleen is rarely the only involved site at presentation.

Intermediate- and high-grade lymphomas The clinical presentation of intermediate- and high-grade lymphomas is more varied. Although the majority of patients present with adenopathy, more than one-third present with extranodal involvement, the most common sites being the GI tract (including Waldeyer's ring), skin, bone marrow, sinuses, genitourinary (GU) tract, thyroid, and CNS. B symptoms are more common, occurring in about 30%–40% of patients.

Lymphoblastic lymphoma often presents with an anterior superior mediastinal mass, superior vena cava syndrome, and leptomeningeal disease with cranial nerve palsies.

American patients with Burkitt lymphoma often present with a large abdominal mass and symptoms of bowel obstruction.

Screening and diagnosis

A recent study from Arizona documented the low sensitivity (including often associated histologic misclassification) of fine-needle aspiration (FNA) for the diagnosis of patients with newly diagnosed and relapsed NHL and Hodgkin lymphoma. When directly compared, only 12% of 67 FNA diagnoses correlated with subsequent excisional biopsy results (including immunophenotyping). When morphology alone was analyzed, only 2% of 43 FNA diagnoses correlated with subsequent excisional biopsy diagnosis (*Hehn ST, Grogan TM, Miller T: J Clin Oncol 22:3046-3052, 2004*).

No effective methods are available for screening or identifying populations at high risk of developing NHL. A definitive diagnosis can be made only by biopsy of pathologic lymph nodes or tumor tissue. It is critical to perform an excisional node biopsy (fine-needle aspirations are insufficient for diagnostic purposes) to avoid false-negative results and inaccurate histologic classification. When clinical circumstances make surgical biopsy of involved lymph nodes or extranodal sites prohibitive, a core biopsy obtained under CT or ultrasonographic guidance may suffice but often requires the integration of histologic examination and immunophenotypic and molecular studies for diagnosis. A formal review by an expert hematopathologist is mandatory. Additional studies, such as immunophenotyping and genotyping, are often necessary.

Initial diagnostic evaluation of patients with lymphoproliferative malignancy should include the following:

- Careful history (night sweats, weight loss, fever; neurologic, musculoskeletal, or GI symptoms)
- Physical examination (lymph nodes, including submental, infraclavicular, epitrochlear, iliac, femoral, and popliteal nodes; pericardial rub, pleural effusion, distended neck and/or upper extremity veins in superior vena cava syndrome; breast masses; hepatosplenomegaly, bowel obstruction, renal mass, and testicular or ovarian mass; focal neurologic signs, such as plexopathy, spinal cord compression, nerve root infiltration, and meningeal involvement; skin lesions)
- Biopsy of peripheral lymphadenopathy (excisional biopsy)
- Chest x-ray (mediastinal or hilar adenopathy, pleural effusions, parenchymal lesions)
- CT scan of the chest (mediastinal, hilar, or parenchymal pulmonary disease)
- CT scan of the abdomen and pelvis (enlarged lymph nodes, splenomegaly, filling defects in liver and spleen)
- Bilateral bone marrow biopsy and aspirate
- PET scans (selected cases: B-cell follicular and aggressive histologies) for staging at diagnosis, response, assessment, and relapse
- CBC with differential and platelet count (peripheral blood

TABLE 2: Immunophenotypic and histochemical diagnosis of B-cell lymphomas/leukemias

Marker	Follicular	CLL	Mantle	MZL/MALT	PLL*	DLBCL	HCL	BL/BLL
SIg	+	dim+	+	+/+	+	+(–)	+	+
CD5	–	+	+	–/–	–(+)	–	–	–
CD10	+	–	–	–/–	–	–(+)	–	+
CD20	+	dim+	+	+/+	+	+	+	+
CD23	–(+)	+	–	–/–	+(–)	–	–	–
CD43	–	+	+	–(+)/–(+)	–	–(+)	+	–
CD103	–	–	–	+/–	–	NA	+	NA
Cyclin D1	–	–	+	–/–	–	–	–(+)	–

+, > 90% positive; +(–), > 50% positive; –(+), < 50% positive; –, < 10% positive; MZL/MALT=splenic marginal zone/mucosa-associated lymphoid tissue; CLL = chronic lymphocytic leukemia; PLL = prolymphocytic leukemia; HCL = hairy cell leukemia; BL/BLL = Burkitt lymphoma/Burkitt-like lymphoma, DLBCL = Diffuse large B-cell lymphoma; SIg = surface immunoglobulin

* A T-cell variant is present in approximately 20%–30% of PLL cases.

lymphocytosis with circulating malignant cells is common in low-grade and mantle cell lymphomas). Bone marrow and peripheral blood involvement may be present, and the distinction between leukemia and lymphoma is difficult to make in some cases.

- General chemistry panel (lactic dehydrogenase [LDH] level determination) is mandatory.
- HIV serology in at-risk patients with diffuse large cell and other aggressive and Burkitt histologies; HTLV-1 serology in select patients with cutaneous T-cell lymphoma, especially if they have hypercalcemia
- Cytogenetic and molecular analyses of lymph node, bone marrow, and peripheral blood (selected cases)
- Immunophenotyping can be of particular benefit in distinguishing B-cell chronic leukemia/small lymphocytic lymphoma from other lymphomas (Table 2).
- Examination of CSF and consideration of intrathecal chemotherapy prophylaxis in patients with (1) diffuse aggressive NHL with bone marrow, epidural, testicular, paranasal sinus, breast, or multiple extranodal sites; (2) high-grade lymphoblastic lymphoma and Burkitt lymphoma and its variants; (3) primary CNS lymphoma if no evidence of increased intracranial pressure
- Upper GI endoscopy and/or GI series with small bowel follow-through in patients with head and neck involvement (tonsil, base of tongue, nasopharynx) and those with a GI primary; mantle cell lymphoma is associated with a high incidence of occult GI involvement.

- Ultrasonography of opposite testis in patients with a testicular primary
- Spinal MRI scan for epidural disease when clinically indicated (useful in the evaluation of suspected spinal cord compression).

Pathology

The Working Formulation was proposed in 1982 as a modification of the Rappaport classification of NHL based on morphology and biologic aggressiveness. Although many subtypes were not recognized, including T-cell lineage lymphomas, a revised European-American classification of lymphoid neoplasms (REAL classification) was introduced in 1994 incorporating T-cell malignancies, subtypes of Hodgkin lymphoma and newer defined lymphoma-proliferative disorders. The WHO (World Health Organization) classification for lymphomas (introduced in 1999) uses the principles of the REAL classification and defines each entity according to morphologic features, immunophenotype, genetic features, postulated normal counterpart, and clinical features. The WHO classification is similar to the REAL classification, with some modifications and reassessments based on current data (Table 3).

WHO CLASSIFICATION

The most frequently occurring clinical entities recognized by the REAL/WHO classification are diffuse large B-cell lymphoma (DLBCL, 31%), follicular lymphoma (22%), lymphoma of MALT type (8%), small lymphocytic lymphoma (7%), mantle cell lymphoma (6%), peripheral T-cell lymphoma (7%), primary mediastinal large B-cell lymphoma (2%), anaplastic large T-/null-cell lymphoma (2%), lymphoblastic lymphoma of T- or B-cell lineage, marginal zone (monocytoid) B-cell lymphoma (2%), lymphoplasmacytic lymphoma (2%), Burkitt lymphoma (2%), and other (9%).

The WHO modification of the REAL classification includes three types of follicular lymphoma (grades 1–3). Grades 1 and 2 correspond to follicular small-cleaved cell and follicular mixed small-cleaved and large cell lymphoma, which are considered to be low-grade lymphomas by the Working Formulation. Grade 3 corresponds to follicular large cell lymphoma, which is considered an intermediate-grade NHL in the Working Formulation, and is generally treated as a large cell lymphoma. The WHO/REAL classification considers B-cell small lymphocytic lymphoma to be synonymous with chronic lymphocytic leukemia.

Other indolent lymphomas recognized by the WHO/REAL classification, but not by the Working Formulation, include lymphoplasmacytic lymphoma, splenic marginal zone B-cell lymphoma, extranodal marginal zone lymphoma of MALT type, and nodal marginal zone B-cell lymphoma.

The REAL and WHO classifications have recognized marginal zone lymphomas (MZLs) as unique clinical and pathologic entities, ie, extranodal (MALT), nodal, and splenic NHL subtypes. MALT NHL is extremely indo-

TABLE 3: WHO classification of lymphoid neoplasms

- B-cell neoplasms
  - Precursor B-cell neoplasm
    - *Precursor B-lymphoblastic leukemia/lymphoma (precursor B-cell acute lymphoblastic leukemia)*
  - Mature (peripheral) B-cell neoplasms
    - *B-cell chronic lymphocytic leukemia/small lymphocytic lymphoma*
    - B-cell prolymphocytic leukemia
    - Lymphoplasmacytic lymphoma
    - Splenic marginal zone B-cell lymphoma (± villous lymphocytes)
    - Hairy cell leukemia
    - *Plasma cell myeloma*/plasmacytoma
    - Extranodal marginal zone B-cell lymphoma of MALT type
    - Nodal marginal zone B-cell lymphoma (± monocytoid B cells)
    - *Follicular lymphoma*
    - *Mantle cell lymphoma*
    - *Diffuse large B-cell lymphoma*
      - Mediastinal large B-cell lymphoma
      - Primary effusion lymphoma
    - *Burkitt lymphoma/Burkitt-like lymphoma*
- T-cell and NK-cell neoplasms
  - Precursor T-cell neoplasm
    - *Precursor T-lymphoblastic lymphoma/leukemia (precursor T-cell acute lymphoblastic leukemia)*
  - Mature (peripheral) T-cell neoplasms
    - T-cell prolymphocytic leukemia
    - T-cell granular lymphocytic leukemia
    - Aggressive NK-cell leukemia
    - Adult T-cell lymphoma/leukemia (HTLV-1+)
    - Extranodal NK/T-cell lymphoma, nasal type
    - Enteropathy-type T-cell lymphoma
    - Hepatosplenic γ/δ T-cell lymphoma
    - Subcutaneous panniculitis-like T-cell lymphoma
    - *Mycosis fungoides*/Sézary syndrome
    - Anaplastic large cell lymphoma, T-/null-cell, primary cutaneous type
    - Peripheral T-cell lymphoma, not otherwise characterized
    - *Angioimmunoblastic T-cell lymphoma*
    - *Anaplastic large cell lymphoma, T-/null-cell, primary systemic type*
- Hodgkin lymphoma (Hodgkin disease)
  - Nodular lymphocyte-predominant Hodgkin lymphoma
  - Classic Hodgkin lymphoma
    - *Nodular sclerosis Hodgkin lymphoma (grades 1 and 2)*
      - Lymphocyte-rich classic Hodgkin lymphoma
    - *Mixed cellularity Hodgkin lymphoma*
      - Lymphocyte-depletion Hodgkin lymphoma

Italic type denotes more common clinical entities. WHO = World Health Organization; MALT = mucosa-associated lymphoid tissue; NK = natural killer; HTLV-1 = human T-cell lymphotrophic virus-1

TABLE 4: Ann Arbor staging classification for NHL[a]

Stage	Area of involvement
I	One lymph node region
I_E	One extralymphatic organ or site
II	Two or more lymph node regions on the same side of the diaphragm
II_E	One extralymphatic organ or site (localized) in addition to criteria for stage II
III	Lymph node regions on both sides of the diaphragm
III_E	One extralymphatic organ or site (localized) in addition to criteria for stage III
III_S	Spleen in addition to criteria for stage III
III_{SE}	Spleen and one extralymphatic organ or site (localized) in addition to criteria for stage III
IV	One or more extralymphatic organs with or without associated lymph node involvement (diffuse or disseminated); involved organs should be designated by subscript letters (P, lung; H, liver; M, bone marrow)

[a]Class A patients experience no symptoms; class B patients experience unexplained fever of ≥ 101.5°F; unexplained, drenching night sweats; or loss of >10% body weight within the previous 6 months.

lent and presents as localized stage I–II disease, rarely disseminating. The stomach is the most frequent site, but low-grade NHLs (and former pseudolymphomas) of the lungs, thyroid, salivary gland, and orbit are of this type.

Staging and prognosis

Determining the extent of disease in patients with NHL provides prognostic information and is useful in treatment planning. However, histologic sub-classification (WHO classification) is the primary determinant of survival and potential for cure. Compared with patients with limited disease, those with extensive disease usually require different therapy, and certain extranodal sites of involvement, such as the CNS and testes, require specific treatment modalities.

Ann Arbor system Although initially devised for Hodgkin lymphoma, the Ann Arbor system has been routinely applied to NHL (Table 4). Because Hodgkin lymphoma commonly spreads via contiguous lymph node groups, this system is based primarily on the distribution of lymphatic involvement with respect to the diaphragm and the presence of extralymphatic organ involvement. The Ann Arbor system does not reflect the noncontiguous nature of disease spread in NHL, does not discriminate well between stage III and IV intermediate-grade disease, and fails to account for tumor bulk or number of extranodal sites.

Some trials in Burkitt and Burkitt-like lymphoma use the St. Jude/Murphy staging system (Table 5), in part to more completely describe the extent of extranodal

TABLE 5: St. Jude/Murphy staging system for Burkitt lymphoma

Stage		Description
I		A single tumor (extranodal) or a single anatomic area (nodal) with the exclusion of the mediastinum or abdomen
II		A single extranodal tumor with regional node involvement
		Two single extranodal tumors on the same side of the diaphragm with or without regional node involvement
		Primary gastrointestinal tumor with or without involvement of associated mesenteric nodes only
		Two or more nodal areas on the same side of the diaphragm
	IIR	Completely resected intra-abdominal disease
III		Two single extranodal tumors on opposite sides of the diaphragm
		All primary intrathoracic tumors (mediastinal, pleural, thymic)
		All paraspinal or epidural tumors, regardless of other tumor sites
		All extensive primary intra-abdominal diseases
		Two or more nodal areas on opposite sides of the diaphragm
	IIIA	Localized but nonresectable intra-abdominal disease
	IIIB	Widespread multiorgan abdominal disease
IV		Any of the above with initial CNS and/or bone marrow involvement (less than 25% involvement; greater than 25% involvement is defined as L3 A/LL)

disease. Unlike the current WHO classification, this staging system recognizes Burkitt leukemia as a separate entity. Moreover, this system was developed when surgery was used for diagnostic and therapeutic purposes. Patients are then also typically stratified into two risk groups, with low-risk patients defined as having a normal LDH level and a single focus of disease measuring less than 10 cm and all others considered to be high risk.

Prognostic factors Histology and morphology remain the major determinants of treatment outcome and prognosis, but gene expression signatures are likely to be the principal determinants in the future. Some patients with slow-growing low-grade lymphoma may remain well for many years with minimal or no initial therapy, whereas survival of patients with some types of high-grade lymphoma is measured only in weeks unless aggressive treatment is initiated promptly. The biologic and clinical behaviors of these disorders vary among the different histologic subtypes.

The International Prognostic Index (IPI) was developed by 16 institutions and cooperative groups in the United States, Europe, and Canada as a prognostic factor model for aggressive NHL treated with doxorubicin-containing regimens. Clinical features that have been independently predictive of survival are included in Table 6.

TABLE 6: International Prognostic Index

Parameter	Adverse factor
Age	≥ 60 years
Ann Arbor stage	III or IV
Serum LDH level	Above normal
Number of extranodal sites of involvement	≥ 2
Performance status	≥ ECOG 2 or equivalent

LDH = lactic dehydrogenase; ECOG = Eastern Cooperative Oncology Group

From International non-Hodgkin's Lymphoma Prognostic Factors Project: N Engl J Med 329:987–994, 1993.

This index appears to be a useful guide for selecting treatment for patients with aggressive diffuse large cell NHL by identifying subsets of patients in whom intensified primary therapy may be warranted. Because younger and older patients have markedly different prognoses and younger patients are more likely to be considered for more intensive investigational regimens, an age-adjusted model for patients ≤ 60 years old has been proposed. In younger patients, stage (III or IV), high LDH level, and nonambulatory performance status are independently associated with decreased survival. Persons with no or one risk factor have a predicted 5-year overall survival of 73%, compared with 26% for high-risk patients with four or five risk factors.

The IPI also appears to be useful in predicting outcome in patients with low-grade lymphoma, mantle cell lymphoma, and relapsed or refractory large B-cell lymphoma in patients undergoing autologous stem-cell transplantation (SCT).

A new prognostic factor model has been devised based on a study of 919 cases of follicular lymphoma, known as the Follicular Lymphoma IPI (FLIPI; Table 7). Multivariate analysis showed that age (> 60 vs ≤ 60 years), Ann Arbor stage (III–IV vs I–II), number of extranodal sites (> 4 vs ≤ 4), LDH level (above

TABLE 7: Follicular Lymphoma International Prognostic Index

Parameter	Adverse factor
Age	> 60 years
Ann Arbor stage	III or IV
Hemoglobin level	< 120 g/L
Serum LDH level	> ULN
Number of nodal sites	> 4

Low risk: 0–1 factors; intermediate risk: 2–3 factors; high risk: 4–5 factors

LDH = lactic dehydrogenase; ULN = upper limit of normal

From Solal-Celigny P, Roy P, Colombat P, et al: Follicular Lymphoma International Prognostic Index. Blood 104:1258–1265, 2004.

A companion trial to the US Intergroup comparison of rituximab–CHOP to CHOP and maintenance rituximab to observation in diffuse large B-cell lymphoma demonstrated that the addition of rituximab to CHOP reduced treatment failures and death in patients with bcl-6–negative disease but not in patients with bcl-6–positive DLBCL *(Winter JN, Weller EA, Horning SJ, et al: Blood 107(11):4207-4213,2006.).*

normal vs normal/below normal), and hemoglobin level (< 120 g/L vs ≥ 120 g/L) were predictors of overall survival. In follicular lymphoma, the majority of cases are designated as low risk by IPI; the FLIPI distinguishes among these lower-risk cases.

Treatment-related factors Time to complete remission has been identified as an important treatment-related prognostic factor in aggressive NHL. Pa-tients who require more than 5 cycles of standard chemotherapy to achieve remission have a high risk of relapse. Similarly, patients with gallium-avid tumors who have persistent gallium uptake at the midpoint of treatment are less likely to have durable remissions. Sequential PET scanning has demonstrated similar results.

Immunobiologic factors Various immunobiologic factors have been sug-gested as predictors of outcome in NHL.

Immunophenotype Several studies have suggested that patients with aggressive nonanaplastic T-cell NHL have a higher relapse rate and decreased overall survival than do patients with B-cell disease. These observations have been confirmed in updated REAL/WHO studies involving large numbers of patients.

Tumor cell proliferation Studies using the Ki-67 antibody, a marker of nuclear proliferation, have shown that increased tumor cell proliferation is a poor prognostic factor in diffuse large cell lymphoma.

Cytogenetic abnormalities and oncogene expression Patients with lymphomas with abnormalities involving chromosomes 1, 7, and 17 have a worse prognosis than do patients with other lymphomas of similar stage and bulk that do not exhibit these changes. Mutations of *p53* are associated with histologic transformation in follicular NHL, which is a phenomenon frequently associated with a poor prognosis. Expression of *bcl*-2 or CD5 in diffuse large cell lymphoma has also been associated with inferior survival, whereas *bcl-6* expression is a marker of germinal center derivation, a powerful predictor of a favorable outcome.

Molecular profiling DNA microarray technology for gene expression profiling has identified distinct prognostic subgroups in DLBCL and follicular NHL. Studies with malignant DLBCL cells have characterized patients into the following subgroups: germinal center B-like DLBCL, activated B-like DLBCL, and a heterogeneous subgroup termed type-3 DLBCL. Patients with germinal center B-like DLBCL have a significantly improved overall survival compared with the other molecular profiles. Recent studies in follicular NHL have identified two gene expression signatures that also predicted survival: immune-response 1 and immune-response 2. Interestingly, the genes that defined the prognostic signatures were not expressed in the tumor cells but were expressed by the nonmalignant tumor-infiltrating cells (primarily T cells, macrophages, and dendritic cells).

TABLE 8: Chemotherapeutic regimens for NHL

Regimen	Dose	Route and frequency
CVP ± rituximab		
Cyclophosphamide	750-1,000 mg/m^2	IV on day 1
Vincristine	1.4 mg/m^2	IV on day 1 (maximum, 2 mg)
Prednisone	100 mg or 100 mg/m^2	PO on days 1-5
Rituximab	375 mg/m^2	IV on day 1
Repeat treatment every 21 days.		
CHOP ± rituximab		
Cyclophosphamide	750 mg/m^2	IV on day 1
Doxorubicin	50 mg/m^2	IV on day 1
Oncovin (vincristine)	1.4 mg/m^2	IV on day 1 (maximum, 2 mg)
Prednisone	40 mg/m^2 or 100 mg/d or 100 mg/m^2/d	PO on days 1-5
Rituximab	375 mg/m^2	IV on day 1
Repeat treatment every 21 days or every 14 days (with granulocyte colony-stimulating factor).		
CHOEP ± rituximab		
Cyclophosphamide	750 mg/m^2	IV on day 1
Doxorubicin	50 mg/m^2	IV on day 1
Etoposide	100 mg/m^2	IV on days 1-3
Oncovin (vincristine)	1.4 mg/mL	IV on day 1 (maximum, 2 mg)
Prednisone	100 mg	PO on days 1-5
Rituximab	375 mg/m^2	IV on day 1
Repeat treatment every 21 days.		
FND		
Fludarabine	25 mg/m^2	IV on days 1-3
Novantrone	10 mg/m^2	IV on day 1
Dexamethasone	20 mg	PO/IV on days 1-5
Repeat treatment every 21-28 days depending on hematologic recovery.		

Treatment

The therapeutic approach for NHL differs for each subtype. Chemotherapy remains the most important modality (Tables 8 and 9). However, in select instances, radiation therapy or surgical resection plays a critical role. Biologic approaches, including interferons, monoclonal antibodies (Table 10), and recombinant toxins have shown significant activity and are now incorporated into treatment paradigms. Autologous and allogeneic SCTs, traditionally reserved for recurrent or refractory disease, are being evaluated as part of initial therapy in high-risk settings. This section will be organized by NHL subtype to best illustrate the biologic characteristics and therapeutic considerations that determine the management strategy for individual patients. Common NHLs

TABLE 9: Commonly used salvage regimens for NHL

Regimen	Dose	Route and frequency
EPOCH[a]		
Etoposide	50 mg/m^2/d	Continuous 96-h IV infusion on days 1-5
Oncovin (vincristine)	0.4 mg/m^2/d	Continuous 96-h IV infusion on days 1-5
Doxorubicin	10 mg/m^2/d	Continuous 96-h IV infusion on days 1-5
Cyclophosphamide	750 mg/m^2	IV on day 6
Prednisone	60 mg	PO on days 1-6
New cycle begins on day 21.		
DHAP[a]		
Platinol (cisplatin)	100 mg/m^2	Continuous 24-h IV infusion on day 1
Cytarabine	2 g/m^2	3-h IV infusion q12h for 2 doses on day 2
Dexamethasone	40 mg	IV on days 1-4
CEPP[a]		
Cyclophosphamide[b]	600 mg/m^2	IV on days 1 and 8
Etoposide[c]	70 mg/m^2	IV on days 1-3
Procarbazine	60 mg/m^2	IV on days 1-10
Prednisone	60 mg	PO on days 1-10
ESHAP[a]		
Etoposide	40 mg/m^2	1-h IV infusion on days 1-4
Solu-Medrol (MPS)	250-500 mg	15-min IV infusion on days 1-5
Cytarabine	2 g/m^2	2-h IV infusion on day 5
Platinol (cisplatin)	25 mg/m^2	Continuous 96-h IV infusion on days 1-4 (total dose, 100 mg/m^2)
MINE[a]		
Mesna	1,333 mg/m^2	IV on days 1-3
Mesna	500 mg	PO 4 h post ifosfamide
Ifosfamide	1,333 mg/m^2	IV (over 1 h) on days 1-3
Novantrone	8 mg/m^2	IV (over 15 min) on day 1
Etoposide	65 mg/m^2	IV (over 1 h) on days 1-3
ICE[a]		
Ifosfamide	5,000 mg/m^2	Continuous IV × 24 h on day 2
Mesna	5,000 mg/m^2	Continuous IV × 24 h on day 2
Carboplatin	AUC 5 mg/mL/min IV on day 2	
Etoposide	100 mg/m^2	IV on days 1-3

[a] ± Rituximab [b] Escalate 50 mg/m^2 as allowed [c] Escalate 15 mg/m^2 as allowed
AUC = area under the curve; MPS = methylprednisolone

will be covered in depth, whereas less frequent entities will be described in more limited detail.

FOLLICULAR LYMPHOMA

Follicular lymphoma comprises 22% of all NHLs; only DLBCL is more common. The clinical presentation may be nodal or extranodal, and bone marrow involvement occurs in the majority of cases. Extensive intra-abdominal adenopathy without peripheral node enlargement is not uncommon. Clinical behavior is variable, reflecting the heterogeneity of the underlying biology; some

TABLE 10: Monoclonal antibodies for lymphoid malignancies

Antigen	Antibody	Type	Investigational status
CD20	Rituximab (Rituxan)	Chimeric	FDA approved
	Ibritumomab (Zevalin)	Y-90-murine	FDA approved
	Tositumomab (Bexxar)	I-131 murine	FDA approved
CD52	Alemtuzumab (Campath)	Humanized	FDA approved
CD22	Epratuzumab	Humanized	Phase II/III
HLA-DR	Hu1D10 (Remitogen)	Humanized	Phase II
CD80	Galiximab (IDEC-114)	Primatized	Phase II
CD23	Lumiliximab (IDEC-152)	Primatized	Phase I

FDA = Food and Drug Administration

patients survive decades, whereas others progress rapidly to resistant disease or transform to a more aggressive histology. There are rare spontaneous remissions. Transformation is common, occurring in 3%–6% of patients each year and ultimately 30%–50% of all patients. Although generally responsive to treatment, the clinical course is characterized by repeated relapses. Median survival for advanced-stage disease is 6 years. Although there was no improvement in survival for patients with follicular lymphoma for many years, there is new evidence that outcomes have improved, independent of the introduction of rituximab (Rituxan).

It is crucial to distinguish between reactive follicular hyperplasia and follicular lymphoma, as the former is a benign condition. Morphologic features as well as the absence of Bcl-2 staining within the follicle and the absence of CD10 and/or Bcl-6 protein expression in the interfollicular areas help to distinguish reactive follicular hyperplasia from follicular lymphoma. Follicular lymphoma is graded according to the number of admixed centroblasts within the neoplastic follicles. Grade 3 follicular lymphoma, previously known as follicular large cell lymphoma, is now subdivided into two subtypes: Grade 3a is characterized by a mixture of centrocytes and centroblasts within the follicle, whereas grade 3b has only sheets of centroblasts with no residual centrocytes. The neoplastic lymphocytes in follicular lymphoma express the pan-B markers CD19, CD20, CD22, and CD79a and antigens of the germinal center (including CD10 and Bcl-6). Most follicular lymphomas express Bcl-2 protein, which is highly correlated with the t(14;18)(q32;q21), the cytogenetic hallmark of the disease. This translocation results in the juxtaposition of the *bcl-2* oncogene into the immunoglobulin H heavy-chain locus on chromosome 14, resulting in its constitutive expression. Follicular lymphoma grade 3b with *bcl-6* rearrangement but no t(14;18)(q32;21) may be more closely related to DLBCL than to other follicular lymphomas.

As previously mentioned, the FLIPI is a prognostic index designed specifically for follicular lymphomas based on five adverse prognostic factors (Table 7). Age is the most important factor. Three risk categories have been defined, each consisting of approximately one-third of patients. More than two-thirds of low-risk patients but only one-third of high-risk patients survive 10 years. Whereas clinical parameters are surrogates for biologic characteristics, DNA expression profiling using microarray technology may soon supersede clinical prognostic indicators such as the FLIPI.

A recent report from the National Cancer Institute (NCI) describes two gene expression signatures associated with vastly different clinical outcomes in follicular lymphoma. These two signatures represent the expression of immunoregulatory genes in the nonmalignant cells infiltrating the malignant lymphoma at the time of diagnosis. Others have found that the number of macrophages/high-powered field was an independent predictor of overall survival in follicular lypmphoma, also underscoring the importance of host response in follicular lymphoma.

Treatment of early-stage disease For the relatively small number of patients with stage I or II follicular lymphoma, radiotherapy continues to be the standard of care. A recent update from the Princess Margaret Hospital's series of involved-field radiotherapy (IFRT) for early-stage disease showed cumulative relapse rates of 54% and 56% at 15 and 25 years, with only a 2% risk of relapse beyond 15 years. Combined-modality therapy has also resulted in excellent disease control, and a randomized trial comparing IFRT with combined-modality therapy is ongoing. Use of functional imaging with PET may improve the results of IFRT by more accurately identifying patients with truly localized disease.

For clinical stage I and IIA low-grade follicular lymphoma, irradiation alone is directed to the entire involved lymphoid region, as defined by the Rai and Ann Arbor staging classifications, or the involved region plus one additional uninvolved region on each side of the involved nodes. The recommended dose is approximately 30 Gy for nonbulky disease showing prompt regression and 36 Gy for bulky or slowly regressive disease, in 1.75 to 1.8 Gy daily fractions. As the majority of subsequent relapses occur outside previous radiation fields, often in adjacent or distal lymph nodes, extended-field or total lymphoid irradiation has been used to try to improve cure rates. Clinical series have shown improvement in freedom from relapse only, with no significant difference in long-term survival.

Treatment of advanced-stage disease

Watch and wait The standard management of asymptomatic patients with follicular lymphoma has been a "watch-and-wait" approach. Treatment is delayed until symptoms or cytopenias intervene or there is impending compromise of vital organs. Multiple phase III randomized trials comparing immediate chemotherapy with observation for asymptomatic patients with advanced-stage follicular lymphoma have shown no difference in outcome. In fact, for patients older than age 70, the chances of not requiring chemotherapy were 40% at 10 years in a recently published trial. The median time to first systemic therapy for patients randomized to the observation arm was 2.6 years. Complete remission rates, however, were higher in the patients treated immediately after diagnosis than in those who were observed and later treated (63% vs 27%). The achievement of a complete remission may prove to be important if the ultimate goal is to administer postremission therapy (eg, vaccine) that is likely to be most effective in the presence of minimal residual disease. A phase III trial comparing the watch-and-wait approach with rituximab therapy for asymptomatic advanced-stage disease is ongoing in Europe.

Irradiation Irradiation for clinical stage III and IV, low-grade, extensive-stage NHL is used locally for palliation of symptomatic sites of disease and is extremely effective. Abbreviated fractionated schedules (25 to 30 Gy in 2.5 to 3 Gy daily fractions, respectively) are often used. Total-body irradiation, usually consisting of 12 Gy in 2 Gy fractions twice a day, is used as part of preparative regimens for bone marrow transplantation.

Rituximab For patients with symptoms or other reasons for treatment, there are many treatment options, including single or multiagent chemotherapy, monoclonal antibodies or radioimmunoconjugates, combinations of chemotherapy and immunotherapy with anti-idiotype vaccines, and new agents such as bortezomib (Velcade). Treatment with rituximab results in overall response rates of nearly 50%, with a median response duration of approximately 1 year, in relapsed or refractory indolent lymphomas. In previously untreated patients, however, the overall response rate was 80% and the median disease progression-free survival is 18 months in one trial from France. Of note, 28% of all treated patients and 34% of all complete and partial responders maintained their responses for 5 or more years. Similar results have been reported by the US North Central Cancer Treatment Group (NCCTG).

To improve on response rates and duration of response, additional doses of rituximab have been administered as "maintenance therapy." The median event-free survival is prolonged with this approach, especially for

> The Eastern Cooperative Oncology Group randomized responding patients induced with CVP (cyclophosphamide, vincristine, and prednisone) to receive either maintenance rituximab (Rituxan) or observation. Maintenance rituximab following CVP induction improved disease progression-free and overall survival in patients with follicular lymphoma; overall survival at 4 years was 88% in the maintenance rituximab group compared with 72% in the observation group (*P* = .03; *Hochster HS, Weller E, Gascoyne RD, et al: Blood [abstract] 106:106a, 2005*).

previously untreated patients. In previously treated patients, the total duration of benefit from rituximab appears to be the same whether patients receive maintenance rituximab on a scheduled basis or reinduction with rituximab only at the time of disease progression. A confirmatory trial (ECOG 4402) in untreated patients is in progress in patients with a low tumor burden. Maintenance regimens have varied, and the impact of the frequency of administration on the duration of response is unknown. Questions also remain regarding the impact of maintenance rituximab on the quality of life and the cost of care.

Interferon-α The use of interferon (IFN)-α in follicular lymphoma has been extensively investigated both in combination with chemotherapy and as maintenance therapy, with varying results. In most studies, IFN-α was associated with a prolongation of remission but not overall survival. A notable exception was the GELF86 (Group d'Etude des Lymphomes Folliculaires) trial, in which overall survival was prolonged. The Southwestern Oncology Group (SWOG) recently reported the results of a large phase III trial in which patients with indolent lymphomas were randomized to receive IFN-α or observation following induction with an intensive anthracycline-containing regimen and in some cases radiotherapy. Postremission therapy did not prolong disease progression-free or overall survival. Although the results of randomized trials in follicular lymphoma and toxicities associated with IFN-α have led many physicians to abandon its use altogether, a large phase III study is currently ongoing in Germany comparing standard vs intensive dose maintenance.

Chemotherapy with and without rituximab Studies comparing single-agent chemotherapy with multiagent therapy in patients with advanced-stage follicular lymphoma have not shown meaningful differences in outcomes. Fludarabine, identified in the 1980s as an active agent in follicular lymphoma, has been incorporated into combination regimens with high response rates (including molecular remissions) but has not been shown to prolong the duration of remission when compared with other multiagent regimens. Secondary myelodysplastic syndromes and acute leukemias have now been associated with the fludarabine, mitoxantrone (Novantrone), dexamethasone (FND) regimen. High response rates and durable remissions have resulted when rituximab was combined with CHOP chemotherapy in a small number of patients with follicular lymphoma, some of whom were treatment-naive. Four phase III trials comparing combinations of chemotherapy and rituximab with chemotherapy alone in previously untreated patients have now been reported. Overall response rates and either median time to treatment failure or event-free survival were superior in the chemoimmunotherapy arm in every series.

> A reported analysis of the phase III trial comparing cyclophosphamide, vincristine, and prednisone with and without rituximab (Rituxan) in untreated patients with follicular lymphoma (FL) showed that time to disease progression was prolonged in the rituximab-containing arm regardless of baseline FLIPI score or histology. This finding suggests that rituximab may overcome adverse prognostic factors in FL patients treated with chemotherapy (*Imrie K, Belch A, Pettengell R, et al: J Clin Oncol [abstract] 23[suppl]:566s, 2005*).

Radioimmunotherapy The anti-CD20 radioimmunoconjugates Y-90 ibritumomab tiuxetan (Zevalin) and I-131 tositumomab (Bexxar) both deliver ionizing radiation to target cells and their neighbors and have proven to be relatively easy to administer, safe, and effective. Response rates are higher and remissions more durable when radioimmunoconjugates are used early in the clinical course. Both agents are likely to have their greatest impact when used in previously untreated patients.

Unlike patients with diffuse large B-cell lymphoma, patients with follicular lymphoma benefit from rituximab (Rituxan) maintenance following induction with rituximab plus chemotherapy. The German Lymphoma Study Group recently reported that response duration is prolonged with maintenance rituximab compared with observation after rituximab plus fludarabine, cyclophosphamide, and mitoxantrone (Novantrone) in a phase III trial. The median response duration was not reached at 3 years following maintenance, whereas it was 10 months for the observation arm (*P* = .02; *Hiddemann W, Forstpointer R, Dreyling M, et al: J Clin Oncol [abstract] 23[suppl]:566s, 2005*).

In previously treated patients, Y-90 ibritumomab tiuxetan, a high-energy beta-emitter, yielded an overall response rate of 80% for relapsed or refractory follicular or transformed CD20+ B-cell NHL, with a median duration of response of 14 months. For patients refractory to rituximab, response rates with Y-90 ibritumomab tiuxetan are high (74% overall response rate), but the median duration of response is relatively short (6.4 months; range 0.5–25+ months). The dose-limiting feature of this approach is hematologic toxicity. Short-lived myelosuppression occurs 7–9 weeks post treatment. Dosing is based on weight (0.4 mCi/kg), with a reduction (0.3 mCi/kg) for those with mild thrombocytopenia (< 100,000/mL).

I-131 tositumomab is both a gamma- and beta-emitter and is individually dosed on the basis of dosimetry to deliver 75 cGy of total-body irradiation. Similar to Y-90 ibritumomab tiuxetan, it is effective in both heavily pretreated relapsed and refractory patients. Heavily pretreated patients with refractory low-grade or transformed NHL had an overall response rate of 65% (20% complete response rate), with a median duration of response of 6.5 months. These rates were notable in view of a response rate of only 28% in the preceding chemotherapy regimen. Like Y-90 ibritumomab tiuxetan, I-131 tositumomab is associated with predictable myelosuppression. Secondary myelodysplasia and leukemia have occurred in patients treated with radioimmunotherapy, but only in patients previously treated with chemotherapy and thereby already at risk. In previously untreated patients, the complete response rate was 75%, with a 5-year disease progression-free survival of 59%. These data must be interpreted carefully, as this study enrolled a relatively young patient population (median age, 49 years), with low bulk disease, a group that some physicians would choose to observe rather than treat.

I-131 tositumomab has been used to consolidate responders following induction with CHOP chemotherapy. In a phase II trial of previously untreated patients with follicular lymphoma, the percentage of complete response/unconfirmed complete response increased from 39% following CHOP chemotherapy to 60% following consolidation with I-131 tositumomab. At 2 years, approximately 80% of patients remain disease free. Based on these phase II

The National Cancer Institute (NCI) initiated a phase III randomized multi-institution trial to assess the effects of patient-specific vaccines with lymphoma-derived idiotypes in patients with newly diagnosed, previously untreated, low-grade stage III or IV follicular lymphoma. Patients who achieve a complete remission after prednisone, Adriamycin (doxorubicin), cyclophosphamide, and etoposide (PACE) are randomized to receive a carrier-conjugated autologous idiotype vaccine in combination with GM-CSF (granulocyte-macrophage colony-stimulating factor, complete vaccine) or vaccine consisting of carrier plus GM-CSF only. Two-thirds of randomized patients will receive the complete vaccine. Accrual is ongoing.

results and the encouraging outcome of patients treated with rituximab-CHOP (R-CHOP), the US Intergroup is currently comparing CHOP followed by I-131 tositumomab with R-CHOP in treatment-naive patients.

Anti-idiotype vaccines Lymphoma-specific idiotypes serve as tumor-specific antigens in follicular lymphoma and constitute the basis for vaccine therapy. In early vaccine trials, immunized patients who generated an anti-idiotype response experienced longer remissions than those who failed to mount a response. Anti-idiotype vaccine has been shown to clear minimal residual disease detectable only by PCR after intensive chemotherapy. In phase I trials, vaccination resulted in tumor shrinkage in some patients. One phase III placebo-controlled trial investigating this strategy is still accruing patients, whereas two others have completed enrollment. While we await the results of these important studies, alternative methodologies, including DNA vaccines and dendritic cell-based vaccination, are under investigation.

Novel agents New agents targeting specific molecular targets such as the ubiquitin-proteasome pathway have shown promise in the treatment of follicular lymphoma. In recently reported phase II trials, bortezomib (Velcade) has shown activity in follicular lymphoma as well as in mantle cell lymphoma. New combinations including bortezomib are now being investigated. Bendimustine is a novel alkylator with activity in both rituximab-refractory and rituximab-sensitive indolent NHL.

Other new agents are also showing activity, including the histone deacetylase inhibitor suberoylanilide hydroxamic acid (SAHA) and a mammalian target of rapamycin (mTOR) inhibitor (CCI-779). Novel antibodies such as anti-CD80 and combinations of antibodies have also shown promise in the treatment of follicular lymphoma.

SCT The natural history of follicular lymphoma is characterized by response to therapy but repeated relapses and progressively shorter and shorter remissions, ultimately resulting in death from progressive disease. Autologous and allogeneic SCTs are alternative strategies often associated with durable remissions that may impact overall survival. Unfortunately, immediate and long-term toxicities are significant and must be considered when assessing the appropriate role of transplantation in the overall treatment plan for individual patients. The only phase III trial to address the role of autologous SCT in patients with relapsed follicular lymphoma closed prematurely because of poor accrual. Nonetheless, disease progression-free and overall survival were significantly longer with high-dose chemotherapy (HDCT) and autologous SCT (with purged or unpurged autografts) than with conventional alkylator therapy. Whether any of the new therapeutic strategies will prove to be as effective as autologous SCT in the relapsed setting remains to be seen.

The ubiquitin-proteasome pathway plays a critical role in regulating cell-cycle progression, transcription factor activation, apoptosis, and cell trafficking. The results of an expanded multicenter phase III trial of bortezomib (Velcade), including 19 patients with follicular lymphoma, were recently reported. The overall response rate was 60% in this histologic subset, with a disease progression-free survival of 18 months in responders (*O'Connor OA, Wright J, Moskowitz C, et al: Ann Oncol [abstract] 16[suppl 5]:66, 2005*).

Several groups have investigated the role of autologous SCT as consolidation therapy for patients in first complete or partial remission. Although disease progression-free survival may be prolonged, an impact on survival has not been demonstrated consistently. Contemporary trials evaluating the role of autologous SCT for follicular lyphoma in first remission induced with rituximab-containing regimens are needed. The results of a German Lymphoma Study Group trial comparing interferon maintenance with myeloablative chemotherapy with autologous SCT after induction with CHOP or R-CHOP are awaited. An increased incidence of secondary myelodysplasia following autologous SCT in first remission has reduced enthusiasm for this approach.

Single-institution studies as well as analysis of registry data suggest that a tumor-free graft is an important determinant of outcome in follicular lymphoma. Administration of rituximab during stem-cell mobilization provides an "in vivo" purge, reducing contamination of the autograft with malignant lymphocytes. The long-term benefit of such an approach has not yet been demonstrated.

Allogeneic SCT has been investigated primarily in young patients with HLA-identical sibling donors and extensive disease and/or marrow involvement. Low relapse rates suggest that this approach is potentially curative but is associated with high treatment-related morbidity and mortality. Reduced-intensity transplantation is based on the assumption that a graft-vs-lymphoma effect is operative and has the potential to cure follicular lymphoma. Whether this approach will reduce toxicity while maintaining the low relapse rates associated with standard myeloablative allotransplants remains to be established. A randomized trial comparing this strategy with autologous SCT in relapsed follicular lymphoma has been initiated in the United States.

Overall treatment strategy Whereas treatment choices were once limited to single or combination alkylator-based treatment, we now are faced with choosing among a wide variety of strategies. There are many unanswered questions that can only be addressed through well-designed clinical trials. Hence, whenever possible, every patient should be enrolled in prospective clinical studies. In the absence of symptoms or other indications for treatment, patients should be observed. A combination of rituximab and chemotherapy is suggested in the absence of a clinical trial. Selected patients with comorbidities may be best served with rituximab alone. Radioimmunotherapy is recommended at the time of relapse, with transplantation reserved for selected patients in first or subsequent relapse.

CHRONIC LYMPHOCYTIC LEUKEMIA/ SMALL LYMPHOCYTIC LYMPHOMA

CLL/SLL is a malignancy of small, round, B lymphocytes involving peripheral blood, bone marrow, and lymph nodes. The term "SLL" is reserved for cases in which there are no circulating malignant lymphocytes. SLL generally presents with lymph node and splenic involvement. Involvement of the bone marrow and peripheral blood may develop later in the course of disease. At the time of presentation, patients may be asymptomatic, complain of only fatigue, or have symptoms related to cytopenias (including autoimmune hemolytic anemia, lymphadenopathy, or splenomegaly). The immunophenotype helps to distinguish CLL/SLL from other B-cell leukemias/lymphomas, including mantle cell and leukemic forms of follicular lymphoma. Typically, the malignant lymphocytes stain weakly with surface immunoglobulin, CD20, CD22, and CD79b; they are CD5+, CD23+, and FMC7–. Cytogenetic abnormalities are detected in the majority of cases when fluorescence in situ hybridization (FISH) analysis is used. Trisomy 12, deletions at 13q14, and deletions at 11q22-23 are common. Many molecular markers of prognosis have been studied in CLL, including Zap-70, but their value in SLL is unknown.

Given the relatively small numbers of patients with SLL, they have generally been included in clinical trials of "indolent lymphoma." Conventional alkylator-based regimens as well as fludarabine, pentostatin (Nipent), and cladribine and combinations thereof have been used when patients become symptomatic. Anthracyclines have not been shown to benefit patients with SLL/CLL. When compared with follicular lymphoma, CLL/SLL is less likely to respond to rituximab as a single agent. Alemtuzumab (Campath), a potent therapy for CLL, is less effective in treating nodal disease than peripheral blood and bone marrow involvement. SCT, both autologous and allogeneic, has been studied in selected patient populations but should be reserved for relapsed young patients with good performance status.

SPLENIC MARGINAL ZONE LYMPHOMA

Splenic marginal zone lymphoma (SMZL) is a rare disorder comprising less than 1% of NHLs. Clinically, this lymphoma most often presents as splenomegaly with splenic hilar node involvement but without peripheral adenopathy. The bone marrow is commonly involved, and malignant villous lymphocytes may be detected in the peripheral blood. Sometimes confused with CLL or mantle cell lymphoma, SMZL may be distinguished by its immunophenotype. Typically, cells are CD20+, CD79a+, CD5–, CD10–, CD23–, and CD43–. Staining for cyclin D1 is negative, excluding mantle cell lymphoma. The absence of CD103 helps to exclude hairy cell leukemia. Allelic loss of chromosome 7q21-32 is common. The clinical course is indolent. Cytopenias respond to splenectomy with long-lasting remissions. Anecdotal remissions have been seen following rituximab therapy. Transformation to more aggressive histologies may occur.

NODAL MARGINAL ZONE LYMPHOMA

Nodal marginal zone lymphoma (NMZL) is a primary nodal B-cell disorder that resembles lymph nodes involved by marginal zone lymphomas of extranodal or splenic origin without extranodal or splenic involvement. Lymphadenopathy (either localized or generalized) is the presenting complaint in most cases. Extranodal lymphoma may be uncovered in the evaluation of many cases of suspected NMZL. The clinical course is usually indolent, similar to that of other MZLs.

Extranodal marginal zone B-cell lymphoma of MALT type

MALT lymphomas comprise only 7%–8% of B-cell lymphomas but nearly 50% of all gastric lymphomas. Although the GI tract is most often involved, other common sites include the lungs, head and neck, ocular adnexae, skin, thyroid, and breasts. There often is an associated history of autoimmune disorders, such as Sjögren's syndrome or Hashimoto's thyroiditis or chronic inflammatory processes secondary to infectious agents (*H pylori*, *B burgdorferi*, or *C psittaci*). A form of MALT involving the small bowel (immunoproliferative small intestinal disease, previously known as α-chain disease) has recently been associated with *C jejuni*. The majority of patients present with stage I or II disease. The frequency of bone marrow involvement appears to differ depending on the primary site of involvement. Multiple extranodal sites may be involved at the time of presentation. Transformation to a high-grade lymphoma may occur in approximately 8% of cases.

The malignant lymphocytes of MALT lymphoma are typically CD20+, CD79a+, CD5–, CD10–, and CD23–. The t(11;18)(q21;q21) is characteristic of MALT lymphomas, particularly those involving the stomach or lungs. The translocation creates a fusion between the MALT-1 gene, which is an essential regulator of *bcl-10*–mediated NF-kB signaling, and the AP12 gene, which inhibits apoptosis. This genetic abnormality is a marker of MALT lymphomas that do not respond to antibiotic therapy for *H pylori* infection, are associated with a more advanced stage, and do not transform into more aggressive histologic subtypes. This translocation has not been associated with nodal or splenic MZLs or other types of lymphoma.

Treatment of *H pylori* infection with triple therapy (eg, omeprazole [Prilosec], metronidazole, and clarithromycin [Biaxin]) results in regression in the majority of early lesions.

Researchers from France have reported an association between Campylobacter and immunoproliferative small intestinal disease. Five of seven patients studied had evidence of *C jejuni* in frozen tissue using molecular techniques. The index patient was treated with triple antimicrobial therapy because of similarities with *Helicobacter pylori*-linked mucosa-associated lymphoid tissue (MALT) lymphoma and experienced a complete remission that persisted at the time of publication, 1 year later (*Lecuit M, Abachin E, Martin A, et al: N Engl J Med 350:239-248, 2004*).

However, tumors invading beyond the submucosa and lesions with t(11;18) are associated with a failure to respond to *H pylori* eradication, deep penetration, and distant spread.

Localized MALT gastric lymphoma that does not respond to antibiotics may be cured with local irradiation, with a field including the stomach and perigastric lymph nodes. This treatment is safe, extremely effective, and preserves the stomach. A single-institution experience reported a 96% complete response rate and a 90% freedom-from-treatment-failure rate, at a median follow-up of 4 years. If local irradiation fails, chemotherapy or rituximab, and in some instances surgery, can be used. Alkylator-based therapy or purine analogs have been used with success for persistent or disseminated disease. The typical dose of radiotherapy is 30 Gy in 20 fractions directed to the stomach and perigastric lymph nodes.

LYMPHOPLASMACYTIC LYMPHOMA/WALDENSTRÖM'S MACROGLOBULINEMIA

Lymphoplasmacytic lymphoma/Waldenström's macroglobulinemia is a disorder of small B lymphocytes, plasmacytoid lymphocytes, and plasma cells, typically involving the bone marrow, lymph nodes, and spleen. It is usually associated with a serum monoclonal protein (usually IgM) with associated hyperviscosity or cryoglobulinemia. The clinical presentation is usually related to hyperviscosity with visual symptoms, stroke, or congestive heart failure. Peripheral neuropathies occur in approximately 10% of patients related to reactivity of the IgM with myelin-associated glycoprotein or gangliosides. An association with HCV infection has been demonstrated. Characteristically, the immunophenotypic analysis reveals surface and cytoplasmic immunoglobulin, usually IgM type, and B-cell–associated antigens (such as CD19, 20, 22, and 79a). The malignant cells are CD5–, CD10–, and CD23–.

The clinical course is generally indolent. Asymptomatic patients may be observed. Plasmapheresis may be appropriate first therapy for those who present with hyperviscosity. The clinical status of the patient, not the level of the protein, determines when treatment is initiated. Choice of therapy depends on many individual factors, including age, comorbidities, and the particular indication for therapy. Rituximab and nucleoside analogs (cladribine and fludarabine) as well as the traditional oral alkylators have shown efficacy. Combinations of these agents are also under study. Bortezomib has shown activity in Waldenström's macroglobulinemia. SCT, both autologous and allogeneic, is being investigated in younger patients with relapsed or refractory disease.

DIFFUSE LARGE B-CELL LYMPHOMA

Clinical presentation DLBCL makes up about one-third of the cases of NHL and is generally classified as a mature peripheral B-cell neoplasm by the WHO classification and an intermediate-grade lymphoma by the REAL classification. The clinical presentation is variable, but generally patients present with either peripheral lymphadenopathy (neck, axillae) or enlarged nodes in the

TABLE 11: International Prognostic Index (IPI) in diffuse large B-cell lymphoma

Risk group	No. of risk factors	% of patients	Overall survival (2 yr)	Overall survival (5 yr)
Low	0, 1	35%	84%	73%
Low-intermediate	2	27%	66%	51%
High-intermediate	3	22%	54%	43%
High	4, 5	16%	34%	26%

mediastinum, the mesenteric region, or the retroperitoneum. These sites predict symptoms, which may include chest pain; facial swelling and suffusion of the eyelids (superior vena cava [SVC] syndrome from mediastinal disease); abdominal discomfort, ascites (mesenteric), or back pain; or renal obstruction (retroperitoneal presentations). More than 30% of patients present with disease in extranodal sites, such as the GI tract (including Waldeyer's ring), skin, bone marrow, sinuses, GU tract, thyroid, and CNS. B symptoms, consisting of fever, sweats, and weight loss, are more common in DLBCL than in the indolent lymphomas and occur in about 30% of patients. The median age at presentation is 60 years.

Once the diagnosis is clearly established, staging studies are carried out to determine treatment and define parameters for follow-up. Generally, imaging studies of the chest, abdomen, and pelvis are obtained, and CT scans provide the most accurate anatomic information. Recently, functional imaging using PET scans (which have largely replaced gallium scans) has shown promise as a means of distinguishing between residual scar and active disease after treatment. Further, some investigators have shown that early response by PET scan (after 2 to 3 cycles) is a good prognostic indicator. In addition to CT and PET scans, bone marrow aspirate and biopsy, serum LDH level, and serum beta-2 microglobulin level have been described as important predictors of outcome.

Pathology/immunology The diagnosis should be made by incisional or excisional biopsy of an available lymph node, with adequate tissue for immunologic studies, such as flow cytometry or immunohistochemistry (IHC), to identify the characteristic B-cell clonality (kappa or lambda restriction). In many cases of DLBCL, CD10 is present, indicating a germinal center origin. The CD20 antigen is present in almost all cases of B-cell

Analysis of 146 cases of lymphoplasmacytic lymphoma salvaged with autologous stem-cell transplantation (SCT) has been reported by the European Bone Marrow Transplant Registry. Actuarial overall survival was 90% at 1 year, 79% at 3 years, and 69% at 5 years. Autologous SCT is safe, even in multiply relapsed patients, and results in sustained disease-free survival in significant numbers of patients (*Kyriakou CA, Goldstone AH, Sureda A, et al: Blood [abstract] 104:7a, 2004*).

lymphomas and on almost all normal B cells. In addition, markers for *bcl*-2 and *bcl*-6 offer prognostic information and are part of most diagnostic evaluations of DLBCL. The use of fine-needle aspiration (FNA) or core biopsy should be discouraged and is acceptable only when tissue cannot be safely obtained by other means and only if flow cytometry is used to help classify the disease and distinguish it from epithelial malignancies that can masquerade as lymphoma.

Prognostic factors Clinical predictors of response have been identified and are now widely used to help design therapeutic plans and clinical trials. These predictors include patient age (< or > age 60), performance status (0, 1 vs 2–4), number of extranodal sites (more than two), Ann Arbor stage (I or II vs III or IV), and serum LDH level (> normal; Table 6). Older patients, higher stage, poorer performance status, higher number of extranodal sites, and higher LDH level all predict a worse outcome, and this model has been validated in more than 3,000 patients. These parameters have been called the IPI; this index is used to plan therapy and clinical trials in the United States and abroad and may be used to predict survival (Table 11).

More recently, genomics have been used to help predict outcome based on molecular signature (see section on Molecular profiling). This molecular system provides prognostic information independent of the IPI. Several investigators using similar statistical methodologies have yielded comparable results, and recently these analyses have been extended to other lymphomas.

Treatment Prior to the 1970s, most patients with stage I/II large cell lymphoma (intermediate grade in the Working Formulation) were treated with irradiation alone, with overall cure rates of 40%–50%. Patients with pathologically favorable stage I/II disease had even better outcomes, but relapse rates, even in these patients, were still 20%–30%. Pathologic staging, therefore, selected a group suitable for irradiation alone. This approach is no longer appropriate, in view of the success of chemotherapy and irradiation in clinically staged patients.

Currently, Coiffier et al found that the addition of rituximab improved results in elderly patients with DLBCL, and recent data confirm these observations for younger patients as well. For patients with clinical stage I or II disease (by the Ann Arbor criteria), most studies suggest that chemotherapy (CHOP and most would add rituximab) for 3 to 4 cycles followed by localized radiation therapy is preferred. Excellent local and systemic control is obtained with combined-modality therapy.

In an ECOG phase III trial, Horning et al showed that 8 cycles of CHOP and irradiation produced a 10-year disease-free survival rate of 57%, compared with 46% with CHOP alone ($P = .04$). Overall survival was 64% vs

Miller et al compared 68 patients with limited diffuse large B-cell NHL from SWOG 8736 treated with CHOP (3) plus involved-field radiotherapy (RT) with 62 patients from SWOG 0014 treated with rituximab (Rituxan), CHOP(3), and involved-field RT. Disease progression-free and overall survival rates measured at 2 years were 94% and 95% for the rituximab group and 85% and 93% for the other group, respectively. Three patients in the rituximab group have died and 5 patients in the other group have died, whereas 4 and 10 relapses occurred, respectively, within the first 2 years (*Miller TP, Unger JM, Spier C, et al: Blood [abstract] 104:158, 2004*).

60%, respectively ($P = .23$), and time to disease progression was 73% vs 63%, respectively ($P = .07$).

Miller et al showed that CHOP (3 cycles of CHOP and irradiation) produced a disease progression-free survival at 5 years of 77%, vs 64% for 8 cycles of CHOP alone ($P = .03$). Overall survival at 5 years was 82% vs 72%, respectively ($P = .02$). A recent update of this SWOG study was reported by Miller et al, with an 8.2-year median follow-up. The 5-year estimates for CHOP (3 cycles plus irradiation) vs CHOP (for 8 cycles) remained unchanged. Kaplan-Meier estimates now show overlapping curves at 7 years for failure-free survival and 9 years for overall survival. The treatment advantage for CHOP (for 3 cycles plus irradiation) for the first 7–9 years was diminished because of excess late relapses and NHL deaths occurring between 5 and 10 years. Patients with good IPI risk factors had a 5-year overall survival of 94%; patients with one adverse risk factor had an overall survival of 70%; those with three adverse risk factors had a 5-year survival of 50%.

These results were confirmed by a single-arm (doxorubicin-containing chemotherapy) approach followed by IFRT conducted by the British Columbia Cancer Agency. However, two recent reports from European investigators question the value of consolidation irradiation in early-stage disease. These studies did not use rituximab or ^{18}fluorodeoxyglucose (FDG)-PET staging, and details on the irradiation technique used are not available.

Until further studies define the optimal therapy for stage IA–IIA DLBCL (nonbulky), many investigators consider 3 to 4 cycles of CHOP with rituximab and IFRT the initial treatment of choice. For patients with bulky disease, a minimum of 6 cycles of CHOP is typically administered. Irradiation doses of 30–36 Gy, delivered in 1.75–1.8 Gy over 3–4 weeks after completion of systemic therapy, appear to be adequate. Radiation fields usually include involved lymph node sites or an involved extranodal site and its immediate lymph node drainage areas. Furthermore, the disease should be easily encompassed in a radiation field with acceptable toxicity.

Disease site or potential toxicities may influence the treatment plan:

- Lymphomas of the head and neck may be managed with chemotherapy alone to avoid the acute mucositis and long-term xerostomia associated with radiation therapy fields that are large and include both parotid glands.

- Fully resected gastric or small intestinal lymphoma may be treated with chemotherapy alone. Patients at high risk of perforation or life-threatening hemorrhage may require surgical resection. Alternatively, chemotherapy followed by local irradiation may allow gastric preservation in some patients.

For patients with more advanced stage (III or IV) disease, CHOP has been the standard (now with rituximab) for 6 to 8 cycles or 2 cycles beyond remission. Recent data suggest an advantage to "dose-dense" therapy, shortening the interval between cycles from 3 to 2 weeks with growth factor support. More data

> Wolf et al reported relapse rates in 234 patients with aggressive NHL treated on two Australasian Leukemia and Lymphoma Group studies. These patients reached complete remission after anthracycline-based chemotherapy. At a median follow-up of 7.5 years, 69 patients (41%) had relapsed, with 70% of relapses including original sites of disease and 35% solely so (*Wolf M, Morgan SJ, Wirth A, et al: Blood [abstract] 104:4587, 2004*).

are needed to validate these results. Many studies now suggest an advantage to the addition of immunotherapy in the form of rituximab, and in almost every study, the combination of rituximab and chemotherapy has improved the response rate and disease-free survival. There appears to be no advantage to maintenance therapy with rituximab in this setting, however, as long as rituximab is included in the induction. Responses are seen in upward of 80% of patients, and approximately 50%–60% achieve a complete remission. It appears that 50% of these patients (30%–50% overall) are likely cured.

For patients who either do not have a complete remission or who relapse, alternative therapies are possible, but long-term responses have been seen mostly with autologous or allogeneic SCT. Patients who do not have responsive disease prior to SCT generally do poorly. The IPI has been used to predict outcome for transplantation in DLBCL. The role of autologous SCT for high-risk patients remains open to debate. A randomized clinical trial of early versus delayed high-dose therapy for patients with high- and high-intermediate risk diffuse aggressive lymphoma conducted by the US Intergroup is just completing accrual. If this trial confirms the benefit of early SCT in poor-risk patients with chemosensitive diffuse aggressive NHL, subsequent studies will focus on increasing the number of patients who become eligible for transplant consolidation. Investigational treatments include novel antibodies, radioimmunotherapy, and single-agent chemotherapy drugs. Nonmyeloablative SCT is being evaluated in patients with recurrent or refractory disease.

Some investigators believe that irradiation for stage III and IV (advanced or extensive) DLBCL may be added after the completion of definitive chemotherapy if there is localized residual disease to improve local control. Irradiation may also be delivered after chemotherapy to areas of initially bulky disease, again to enhance local control. These recommendations are based on the observation that when DLBCL relapses after definitive chemotherapy, it usually does so in initially involved or bulky areas of disease. The benefits and potential side effects of irradiation should be weighed against the use of alternative chemotherapy salvage regimens.

MANTLE CELL LYMPHOMA

Clinical presentation By comparison with low-grade NHL, patients with mantle cell lymphoma are older (median age is 64 years), mostly male (75%), and more likely to have peripheral blood involvement (about 30%) and extranodal involvement (mostly the GI tract and CNS, as discussed below). The clinical course in mantle cell lymphoma is characterized by the worst features of the aggressive lymphomas (an aggressive course) and the indolent lymphomas (frequent recurrences). The disease is often widespread at diagnosis, and marrow involvement and splenomegaly are common. GI tract involvement is also common, and many centers suggest evaluation of the GI tract at the time of diagnosis. CNS recurrences are frequent (up to 20%), but isolated CNS disease is a rare occurrence. Leukemic presentations have been described.

Pathology/immunology This disorder was originally classified as diffuse, small, cleaved lymphoma by the REAL classification and represents less than 10% of all NHLs. In this disease, a homogeneous population of small lymphoid cells with irregular nuclear borders arises from and expands the mantle zone surrounding the germinal centers of the lymph nodes, spreading diffusely through the node as the germinal centers are overrun. The lymphocytes express IgM or IgD, as in CLL, but in much greater density. It was recognized that the cells carry a translocation of the long arms of chromosomes 11 and 14 notated as t(11;14)(q13;q23). This molecular event juxtaposes the *bcl-1* gene on chromosome 11 to the immunoglobulin heavy-chain gene on chromosome 14, leading to overexpression of *bcl-1*. This gene encodes the cell-cycle regulatory protein cyclin D1, which is believed to play a role in checkpoint control in DNA synthesis. The immunophenotype is characteristic, and mantle cell lymphomas are usually CD5+, CD20+, CD10−, CD23−, and FMC7+. This immunophenotype is similar to that seen with CLL/SLL, except that CD23 is most often expressed in CLL/SLL but usually is not expressed in mantle cell lymphoma. The key to the diagnosis is the demonstration in tumor tissue or peripheral blood of the t(11;14) by FISH or the cyclin D1 protein by IHC. Inactivation of the *ATM* gene has been described in mantle cell lymphoma.

Treatment Responses to aggressive chemotherapy (CHOP or R-CHOP) are seen, but patients relapse frequently, and median survival is short. Recent data suggest an advantage to SCT while patients are in remission, but more data are required to validate these results. Patients who have relapsed after autologous SCT have been "rescued" by allogeneic SCT.

The National Comprehensive Cancer Network (NCCN) guidelines recommend clinical trials for patients with mantle cell lymphoma (there is no "standard" therapy), and ongoing trials are investigating a short course of R-CHOP followed by radioimmunotherapy with ibritumomab tiuxetan. Investigators have found that aggressive hyperfractionated chemotherapy with rituximab (R-hyper-CVAD) may result in long-term responses in patients with mantle cell lymphoma (Table 12). Anti-idiotype vaccine studies are also underway in this disease, and novel chemotherapy regimens/agents designed to take advantage of the molecular biology of this disease (flavopiridol, bortezomib) are being tested.

BURKITT AND BURKITT-LIKE LYMPHOMA

Clinical presentation These diseases present as three distinct clinical entities: endemic, sporadic, and immunodeficiency-related types. Endemic Burkitt lymphoma most often presents in young children or adolescents with large nodes in the neck, often involving the maxilla or mandible. These cases are most often seen in equatorial Africa and follow the distribution of endemic malaria, hence its designation as "endemic Burkitt lymphoma." In American, or sporadic, Burkitt or Burkitt-like lymphomas, the disease presents in the abdomen and extranodal sites, especially in the GI tract. Sporadic Burkitt lymphoma accounts for 1%–2% of all adult lymphomas in Western Europe and the United States. The immunodeficiency type is seen in the setting of HIV infection but can be seen in patients with CD4 cell counts > 200 cells/mL. In both endemic and sporadic Burkitt and in Burkitt-like lymphomas, males are affected more often than females.

The LDH level is often elevated, owing to the high turnover rate of these cells and the bulk of disease. The bone marrow and CNS are often involved, and if not involved initially, they are at risk, so CNS prophylaxis is needed. A staging system for Burkitt and Burkitt-like lymphomas has been developed by Murphy and associates (Table 5).

Pathology/immunology These lymphomas are characterized by small, round noncleaved cells. They are the most rapidly proliferating NHLs but make up less than 1% of cases of NHL in adults in the United States. Under the microscope, it is difficult to distinguish Burkitt from Burkitt-like lymphomas and either from the B-cell French-American-British (FAB) L3 variant of acute lymphoblastic leukemia. Indeed, the WHO classification recognizes the lymphoma and leukemic phases as a single entity, a mature B-cell neoplasm. The disease is characterized by medium-sized cells with an abundant basophilic cytoplasm with lipid vacuoles. There are round nuclei with clumped chromatin and multiple nucleoli; a diffuse pattern of infiltration is seen and is classic for Burkitt lymphoma. The numerous macrophages that are usually seen in the lymph node biopsy specimens give rise to the so-called starry-sky appearance.

The proliferative rate of this tumor is high, and there are frequent apoptotic cells. In the Burkitt-like variant, there is greater pleomorphism in nuclear size and shape, and the nuclei have fewer nucleoli. There is a low level of concordance among pathologists (about 53%) when they attempt to distinguish Burkitt from Burkitt-like lymphomas, and even by clinical criteria, that distinction is difficult. The cells express surface IgM, CD19, CD20, CD22, CD10, and CD79a and do not express CD5, CD23, and TdT. Bcl-6, a zinc finger protein, is usually expressed. The major consideration in the differential diagnosis is precursor B-cell lymphoma/leukemia, which in contrast expresses TdT; surface immunoglobulin is mostly negative. CD20 may also be negative in this disorder. In Burkitt lymphoma, the expression of CD10 and Bcl-6 protein suggests that these cells originate from the germinal center, and indeed, this is confirmed by sequence analysis of the immunoglobulin variable heavy-chain and light-chain genes. Somatic hypermutation of these genes has been described.

Genetics The almost constant genetic abnormality in Burkitt lymphoma is overexpression of the c-*myc* oncogene; in 80% of cases, this abnormality results from a balanced translocation between chromosomes 8 and 14, notated as t(8;14), where the c-*myc* oncogene on chromosome 8 is juxtaposed to immunoglobulin heavy-chain enhancer elements on chromosome 14. In the remaining 20% of cases, there are other translocations, including t(2;8)(p12;q24) and t(8;22)(q24;q11). There have been different breakpoints identified in Burkitt lymphoma, and they have been associated with the sporadic and immunodeficiency subtypes.

TABLE 12: M. D. Anderson regimen (hyper-CVAD/Ara-C–MTX) for mantle cell lymphoma, lymphoblastic lymphoma, and acute lymphoblastic leukemia

Agent	Dose and frequency
Cyclophosphamide	300 mg/m^2 infused over 3 h q12h × 6 doses (days 1-3) with mesna
Doxorubicin	50 $mg/m^2/d$ on day 4
Vincristine	1.4 mg/m^2 (max 2 mg) IV on days 4 and 11
Dexamethasone	40 mg/d days 1-4 and 11-14
	Alternate every 21 days with
Methotrexate (MTX)	1 g/m^2 continuous infusion over 24 h (day 1)
Ara-C	3 g/m^2 over 2 h q12h × 4 doses (days 2 and 3)
Leucovorin rescue	50 mg PO at the end of MTX infusion and then 25 mg PO q6h × 48 h

Aggressive supportive care, including administration of cytokines, fluconazole (Diflucan), acyclovir, and trimethoprim-sulfamethoxazole, is strongly recommended.

EBV One cannot discuss these highly aggressive NHLs without discussing the role of EBV. This virus, a member of the herpesvirus family, has the ability to infect resting B cells and transform them into proliferating blasts, most likely by bypassing antigens on lymphocytes and activating signaling molecules. By contrast, certain viruses (HCV) and bacteria (*H pylori*) may cause lymphoma by activating lymphocytes in an antigen-specific manner. EBV infection results in a polyclonal proliferation of lymphoblasts that are latently infected with the virus, as opposed to the infection seen in infectious mononucleosis, which is a lytic infection. This process is regulated by the expression of up to 9 latent viral proteins, which are under the control of the transcription factor EBV nuclear antigen 2 (EBNA-2). It appears that the type and result of EBV infection in lymphoid tissue are controlled by various "growth programs," each causing expression of different viral proteins, which then determine the fate of the infected cell. These in vitro events are different from what occurs in healthy carriers of EBV (up to 90% of the population has been exposed), where the viral proteins are not expressed because all of the latently infected cells are resting memory B cells. It is in the germinal center of the lymph node, however, that virally infected cells can transform into memory B cells, as the viral proteins are expressed within the B cells of the germinal center.

Although EBV was found in patients with Burkitt lymphoma over 40 years ago, the role of EBV in the disease still remains uncertain. In Burkitt lymphoma, a consistent lesion is the overexpression of the c-*myc* oncogene, which results from a reciprocal translocation between chromosomes 8 and 14 [t(8;14)]. The exact role of c-*myc* overexpression in the pathogenesis of the disease is not known, but c-*myc* is known to play a role in cell-cycle progression and cellular

TABLE 13: Cyclophosphamide, vincristine, doxorubicin, high-dose methotrexate (CODOX-M) regimen

Day	Drug	Dose	Method	Time
1	Cyclophosphamide	800 mg/m^2	IV	–
	Vincristine	1.5 mg/m^2 (max 2 mg)	IV	–
	Doxorubicin	40 mg/m^2	IV	–
	Cytarabine	70 mg/m^2	IT	–
2-5	Cyclophosphamide	200 mg/m^2	IV	Daily
3	Cytarabine	70 mg	IT	–
8	Vincristine	1.5 mg/m^2 (max 2 mg)	IV	–
10	Methotrexate	1,200 mg/m^2	IV	Over 1 h
		240 mg/m^2	IV	Each hour over 23 h
11	Leucovorin	192 mg/m^2	IV	At hour 36
		12 mg/m^2	IV	Every 6 h until methotrexate level is < 5 x 10^{-8} M
13	G-CSF	5 μg/kg (or 1 x 263 μg ampule)	SC	Daily until AGC 1 x 10^9/L
15	Methotrexate	12 mg	IT	–
16	Leucovorin	15 mg	PO	24 h after IT methotrexate
Ifosfamide, etoposide, and high-dose cytarabine (IVAC) regimen[a]				
1-5	Etoposide	60 mg/m^2	IV	Daily over 1 h
	Ifosfamide	1,500 mg/m^2	IV	Daily over 1 h
	Mesna	360 mg/m^2 (mixed with ifosfamide)	IV	Over 1 h
		then 360 mg/m^2	IV	3 h (7 doses/ 24 h)
1 & 2	Cytarabine	2 g/m^2	IV	Over 3 h, 12 hourly (total of four doses)
5	Methotrexate	12 mg	IT	–
6	Leucovorin	15 mg	PO	24 h after IT methotrexate
7	G-CSF	5 μg/kg	SC	Daily until AGC > 1.0 x 10^9/L

[a] Commence next cycle (CODOX-M) on the day that the unsupported AGC is > 1.0 x 10^9/L, with an unsupported platelet count of > 75 x 10^9/L.

AGC = absolute granulocyte count; G-CSF = granulocyte colony-stimulating factor; IT = intrathecal; IV = intravenous; PO = oral; SC = subcutaneous transformation. EBV is found in over 95% of cases of "endemic Burkitt lymphoma," which occurs in Africa, but its role in the pathogenesis of the disease is still not clear. It appears that none of the growth-promoting latent genes is expressed in Burkitt lymphoma, and the only latent protein of the virus that is present is EBNA-1. The possibility then exists that although associated with Burkitt lymphoma, EBV may only be a passenger rather than an etiologic agent. The reason therapy with antiviral agents (ganciclovir or acyclovir) cannot be used to treat EBV-associated lymphomas is that the required thymidine kinase (TK) gene is not expressed in latent EBV infection. Recent studies using the small molecule arginine butyrate to upregulate the TK gene and protein expression with concomitant antiviral antibiotics have met with some success.

Treatment Patients must be treated quickly after diagnosis, which should be made on a full biopsy so that adequate tissue is obtained. Tumor lysis syndrome occurs most often with Burkitt lymphoma, and attempts to reduce uric acid production with allopurinol or to degrade it with the enzyme rasburicase (Elitek) should be part of the management, as should aggressive hydration. Patients should be managed in a facility with access to support such as urgent dialysis, since it may be necessary if tumor lysis syndrome occurs.

Treatment includes aggressive chemotherapy, with anthracyclines and cyclophosphamide as the cornerstone. Regimens incorporating hyperfractionated cyclophosphamide such as hyper-CVAD, developed by Murphy and adopted by the M. D. Anderson group, have been used: CODOX-M/IVAC (cyclophosphamide, vincristine, doxorubicin, high-dose methotrexate/ifosfamide [Ifex], etoposide, and high-dose cytarabine; Table 13) and the French regimen incorporate intensive therapy given weekly in various combinations and intrathecal chemotherapy of high-dose methotrexate or high-dose cytarabine to facilitate CNS penetration. In children, the results are excellent, and about 80% of patients can be cured. In adults, the outcome is not as favorable, but with newer more intensive regimens, 40%–60% of patients survive 5 years without disease. New approaches using rituximab and early SCT are being investigated, as are new agents (flavopiridol and an analog of resveratrol) with unique mechanisms of action, which may have relevance to Burkitt and Burkitt-like lymphoma.

PRIMARY MEDIASTINAL LARGE B-CELL LYMPHOMA

Clinical presentation Primary mediastinal large B-cell lymphoma (PMLBCL) occurs most often in young women (female:male ratio is 2:1) who present with mediastinal masses only. These masses are usually bulky and often invade surrounding structures, such as the pleura, lungs, pericardium, and chest wall, but rarely is disease found outside the chest cavity. At recurrence, however, extranodal sites such as the lungs, adrenal glands, liver, or kidneys may be involved. Because of the location and bulk of the disease, patients complain of chest pain, cough, shortness of breath, and are often found to have SVC. This can be subtle, with unexplained breast enlargement the only symptom in some cases. The diagnosis can be delayed if the clinician does not recognize the signs and symptoms of SVC. This clinical presentation is similar to classic Hodgkin lymphoma, and indeed, that is the primary differential diagnostic consideration when these patients are evaluated.

Pathology/immunology PMLBCL with sclerosis is a distinct clinical, pathologic, and molecular abnormality, which has evolved to be recognized as different from other lymphomas. The pathology is characterized by a diffuse proliferation of large cells with clear cytoplasm, often accompanied by extensive sclerosis. The cells are mostly of B-cell origin and express CD20 and other B-cell markers but do not express surface immunoglobulin (Ig). Indeed, the discordant expression of CD79a and Ig expression are distinguishing features of PMLBCL. There are data that describe gains of chromosomal material in tissue specimens, most often 2p, 9p, 12q, and Xq. The *rel*, *mal*, and *fig1* (interleukin-4 [IL-4] gene) oncogenes are overexpressed in tissue specimens. Ig genes have a high level of somatic hypermutation. All of these observations suggest that this entity is unique, especially compared with B-cell lymphomas that arise in peripheral nodes. IL-13 expression and downstream effectors of IL-13 signaling pathways are overexpressed, along with TNF family members and TNF receptor-associated factor-1.

The overexpression of the *rel* oncogene, previously described, has been associated almost exclusively with the nucleus, consistent with NF-κB pathway activation, and the *mal* overexpression has been confirmed in these gene array studies. These data help us to reorder our thinking about these clinically unique lymphomas and to begin to build a molecular story that is consistent with the clinical observation that PMLBCL is more like classic Hodgkin lymphoma than like DLBCL. Further, the observations that certain signaling pathways are involved provide a rationale to attack these pathways specifically in a targeted approach.

Treatment The clinical course is variable; some report a poor outcome with conventional, CHOP-based chemotherapy regimens and irradiation, and some report an excellent outcome. It seems clear that bulk of disease and LDH level are important prognostic factors and that prediction of the outcome by the IPI is useful. A variety of chemotherapy regimens have been evaluated, including CHOP and MACOP-B/VACOP-B (methotrexate or etoposide, Adriamycin, cyclophosphamide, Oncovin, prednisone, bleomycin), and more recently rituximab has been incorporated into the management. Usually, radiation therapy is a part of the initial treatment. In general, in 2006, patients receive anthracycline-containing chemotherapy with rituximab and after 4 to 6 courses, radiation therapy is given to patients with bulky disease. There are no randomized trials comparing radiation therapy with no radiation therapy in this setting. PET scanning may influence the use of consolidation radiation therapy in the future.

PERIPHERAL T-CELL LYMPHOMA, NOT OTHERWISE CHARACTERIZED

Peripheral T-cell lymphoma, not otherwise characterized (PTCL-noc) is predominantly a nodal lymphoma that represents the most common T-cell lymphoma subtype in Western countries, comprising approximately 50%–60% of

T-cell lymphomas and 5%–7% of all NHLs. PTCL-noc usually affects male adults (5:1 male-to-female ratio) with a median age of 61 years (range, 17–90) with 25% of patients presenting in stage I or IIE, 12% in stage III, and 63% in stage IV. Patients with PTCL-noc from this study commonly presented with unfavorable characteristics, including B symptoms (40%), elevated LDH level (66%), bulky tumor ≥ 10 cm (11%), nonambulatory performance status (29%), and extranodal disease (56%), leading to the majority of patients (53%) falling into the unfavorable IPI category (score of 3 to 5).

Most T-cell NHL patients are treated in the same manner as intermediate-grade B-cell patients, with anthracycline-based combination chemotherapy such as CHOP. Randomized trials comparing CHOP with other combination regimens confirmed CHOP as a standard regimen for intermediate-grade B-cell NHL; unfortunately, these trials do not allow for subset analysis of T-cell patients. Rituximab should not be included in the treatment of PTCL-noc (unless other conditions such as immune thrombocytopenic purpura exist), as CD20 is not expressed. Other therapeutic agents tested in T-cell NHL include purine and pyrimidine analogs, denileukin diftitox (Ontak), and a retinoic acid/IFN-α combination.

Denileukin diftitox is a novel recombinant fusion protein consisting of peptide sequences for the enzymatically active and membrane translocation domains of diphtheria toxin with recombinant IL-2 (CD25 receptor); it has been studied mostly in cutaneous T-cell NHL, although clinical benefit has been reported in other T-cell NHL patients. Recently, the histone deacetylase inhibitors SAHA and depsipeptide have shown significant activity against PTCL-noc.

ANGIOIMMUNOBLASTIC T-CELL LYMPHOMA

Angioimmunoblastic T-cell lymphoma (AITL), also known as angioimmunoblastic lymphadenopathy with dysproteinemia, is one of the more common T-cell lymphomas, accounting for 15%–20% of cases and 4%–6% of all lymphomas. The mean age at presentation is 57 to 65 years, with a slight male predominance, and the majority of patients present with stage III or IV disease. AITL is commonly a systemic disease with nodal involvement with various associated disease features, such as organomegaly, B symptoms (50%–70%), skin rash, pruritus, pleural effusions, arthritis, eosinophilia, and varied immunologic abnormalities (positive Coombs' test, cold agglutinins, hemolytic anemia, antinuclear antibodies, rheumatoid factors, cryoglobulins, and polyclonal hypergammaglobulinemia).

Spontaneous disease regression is seen on rare occasions, although AITL typically follows an aggressive clinical course. Treatment with anthracycline-based combination chemotherapy results in complete remission (CR) rates of 50%–70% of AITL patients, although only 10%–30% of patients are long-term survivors. One prospective, nonrandomized multicenter study treated newly diagnosed "stable" AITL patients with single-agent prednisone and combination chemotherapy for relapsing/refractory patients or initially if "life-threatening" disease was present at diagnosis. CR was 29% with single-agent prednisone, whereas CR for relapsed/refractory patients or patients treated initially with combination chemotherapy was 56% and 64%, respectively. With a median follow-up of 28 months (range, 7 to 53), the overall and disease-free survival rates were 40.5% (confidence interval [CI], 24% to 56%) and 32.3% (CI, 17%–47%), respectively, although the median overall survival was 15 months. There are anecdotal reports of relapsed AITL patients who have responded to immunosuppressive therapy, such as low-dose methotrexate/prednisone, as well as reported responses to purine analog treatment. Furthermore, cyclosporine has demonstrated activity in relapsed AITL patients in case reports, and the Eastern Cooperative Oncology Group (ECOG) is evaluating this agent in a prospective study.

ANAPLASTIC LARGE-CELL LYMPHOMA, T-/NULL-CELL, PRIMARY SYSTEMIC TYPE

Anaplastic large-cell lymphoma (ALCL), primary systemic type, accounts for approximately 2%–3% of all NHLs. This disease mainly involves lymph nodes, although extranodal sites may be involved (not exclusively the skin; see section on ALCL, CD30+ cutaneous type). This disease may be divided in part based on the expression of the tyrosine kinase anaplastic lymphoma kinase (ALK), created from a balanced chromosomal translocation t(2;5). When heterogeneous patient populations are analyzed, the prevalence of ALK positivity in primary systemic ALCL cases is 50%–60%. ALK-positive ALCL is typically diagnosed in men prior to age 35 (male-to-female ratio, 3:0), with frequent systemic symptoms and extranodal and advanced-stage disease. ALK-negative patients are usually older (median age, 61 years), with a male-to-female ratio of 0:9, with a similar high incidence of extranodal disease. In addition to the prognostic importance of ALK positivity, the IPI has been identified as an independent prognostic factor within the group of ALK-positive ALCL patients, with a reported 5-year overall survival of 94% vs 41% for IPI 0 or 1 and 2 to 4, respectively. This better prognosis is apparent despite ALK-positive patients more commonly presenting with poorer performance status and more advanced-stage disease compared with ALK-negative patients.

Therapy for pediatric ALCL is often based on prognostic risk factors, with treatment regimens modeled after high-grade B-cell NHL protocols. Following a brief cytoreductive prephase, short, intensified polyagent chemotherapy is administered, with the number of cycles dependent on the stage of disease. Therapy for adult ALCL, systemic type, has commonly included anthracycline-based regimens such as CHOP. Autologous hematopoietic SCT in first complete remission for ALK-negative ALCL has been advocated by some groups, although this approach warrants prospective validation.

HEPATOSPLENIC T-CELL LYMPHOMA

Hepatosplenic T-cell lymphoma (HSTCL) is an uncommon T-cell lymphoma that is seen mainly in young males (median age, 35) presenting with B symptoms, prominent hepatosplenomegaly, mild anemia, neutropenia, thrombocytopenia (commonly severe), significant peripheral blood lymphocytosis, and rare lymphadenopathy and is associated with an aggressive clinical course (median survival, 12 to 14 months).

The tumor cells are usually negative for CD4 and CD8 (85%); positive for CD2, CD3, and CD7 (negative for CD5); and express CD56 in 70%–80% of cases. TIA-1 is present in almost all cases, but commonly granzyme B and perforin are not present, an indication of a nonactivated cytotoxic T-cell phenotype. Cells usually express the γ/δ T-cell receptor (Vd1+/Vd2–/Vd3–) but are negative for EBV.

Historically, patients have been treated with CHOP-like regimens. Early autologous SCT has been favored by some investigators based on anecdotal cases. A recent report described activity with the purine analog pentostatin in relapsed HSTCL patients. Approximately 10%–20% of HSTCL cases arise in immunocompromised patients, predominantly in the solid-organ transplant setting.

EXTRANODAL NK/T-CELL LYMPHOMA, NASAL AND NASAL-TYPE

Extranodal NK/T-cell lymphoma, nasal and nasal-type, formerly known as angiocentric lymphoma, is rare in Western countries, being more prevalent in Asia and Peru. The disease commonly presents in men at the median age of 50 years. This entity is associated with EBV and is typically characterized by extranodal presentation and localized stage I/II disease but with angiodestructive proliferation and an aggressive clinical course. These tumors have a predilection for the nasal cavity and paranasal sinuses ("nasal"), although the "nasal-type" designation encompasses other extranodal sites of NK/T-cell lymphomatous disease (skin, GI, testis, kidneys, upper respiratory tract, and rarely orbit/eye).

Combined-modality therapy incorporating doxorubicin-based chemotherapy (minimum of 6 cycles for patients with stage III or IV disease), IFRT (median dose, 50 Gy; range, 30–67 Gy), and intrathecal prophylaxis is recommended for patients with extranodal NK/T-cell lymphoma, nasal, although the benefit of the addition of chemotherapy to radiation therapy has not been confirmed for limited-stage disease.

Patients with systemic disease have poor long-term survival (5-year overall survival, 20%–25%), with high locoregional (over 50%) and systemic failure rates (over 70%).

ENTEROPATHY-TYPE INTESTINAL T-CELL LYMPHOMA (EITCL)

Enteropathy-type intestinal T-cell lymphoma (EITCL; also known as intestinal T-cell lymphoma) is a rare T-cell lymphoma of intraepithelial lymphocytes that commonly presents with multiple circumferential jejunal ulcers in adults with a brief history of gluten-sensitive enteropathy. EITCL accounts for less than 1% of NHLs, according to the International Lymphoma Study Group, and has been recognized to have a poor prognosis, with reported 5-year overall and disease-free survival rates of 20% and 3%, respectively. This finding is in part related to many patients presenting with a poor performance status and varied complications of locally advanced disease by the time a diagnosis of EITCL has been confirmed.

EITCL may present without an antecedent celiac history, but most patients have abdominal pain and weight loss. Evidence of celiac serologic markers such as positive antigliadin antibodies and/or HLA types such as DQA1*0501/DQB1*0201/DRB1*0304 may be present at diagnosis of EITCL. Moreover, these genotypes may represent celiac patients at higher risk for development of EITCL. Small bowel perforation or obstruction, GI bleeding, and enterocolic fistulae are recognized complications of this disease. The immunophenotype consists of pan–T-cell antigens, usually CD8+, and the mucosal lymphoid antigen CD103 is often expressed.

Following diagnosis of EITCL, doxorubicin-based combination chemotherapy should be considered for each patient, and aggressive nutritional support with parenteral or enteral feeding is critical in the care of these patients. Patients with known celiac disease should adhere to a gluten-free diet.

ADULT T-CELL LEUKEMIA/LYMPHOMA

The retrovirus HTLV-1 has been documented to be critical to the development of adult T-cell leukemia/lymphoma (ATL). HTLV-1 is known to cause diseases other than ATL, including tropical spastic paraparesis/HTLV-1–associated myelopathy, infective dermatitis, and uveitis. In endemic areas in Japan, approximately 10%–35% of the population is infected with HTLV-1. Among these carriers, the overall risk of ATL is approximately 2.5% in patients who live to age 70. Of the Caribbean population, 2%–6% are HTLV-1 carriers, whereas less than 1% of the population in lower-risk areas, such as the United States and Europe, are seropositive. HTLV-1 is transmitted through sexual intercourse, transfused blood products (products containing white blood cells, not fresh frozen plasma), shared needles, breast milk, and vertical transmission. Transfusion of HTLV-1–contaminated blood products results in seroconversion in approximately 30%–50% of patients, at a median of 51 days.

The clinical features of 187 ATL patients included a median age at onset of 55 years, lymphadenopathy (72%), skin lesions (53%), hepatomegaly (47%), splenomegaly (25%), and hypercalcemia (28%) present at diagnosis. The differential diagnosis between cutaneous ATL and mycosis fungoides is often difficult. ATL is separated into four subtypes divided by clinicopathologic features and prognosis: acute, lymphoma, chronic, and smoldering. Shimoyama and colleagues reported on the characteristics of 818 ATL patients in 1991. Patients with acute-type ATL present with hypercalcemia, leukemic manifestations, and tumor lesions and have the worst prognosis, with a median survival of approximately 6 months. Patients with lymphoma-type ATL present with low circulating abnormal lymphocytes (< 1%) and nodal, liver, splenic, CNS, bone, and GI disease; the median survival is 10 months. Patients with the chronic type present with > 5% abnormal circulating lymphocytes and have a median survival of 24 months, whereas the median survival of patients with the smoldering type has not yet been reached.

ATL is an aggressive neoplasm with resistance to conventional chemotherapy, in part due to the viral protein tax-mediated resistance to apoptosis and overexpression of *p*-glycoprotein (the product of the multidrug resistance-1 gene). Patients may initially respond to combination chemotherapy, but unfortunately, response durations are brief (5 to 7 months). El-Sabban and colleagues combined arsenic trioxide (Trisenox) with IFN-α, which induced cell-cycle arrest and apoptosis. Response rates of 70%–90% to combination IFN-α and zidovudine (Retrovir) therapy have been demonstrated in ATL, with associated increased median survival rates compared with those of historic control (11 to 18 vs 4 to 8 months, respectively). A recent clinical trial that investigated initial cytoreductive therapy with CHOP followed by antinucleoside, IFN-α, and oral etoposide therapy demonstrated encouraging results. Other agents with anecdotal activity in ATL include irinotecan (Camptosar) and the purine analogs (pentostatin and 2-chlorodeoxyadenosine), although pentostatin did not appear to improve outcomes when added to combination chemotherapy. Future research should include the investigation of recombinant toxins and antibodies, such as denileukin diftitox and alemtuzumab.

CUTANEOUS T-CELL LYMPHOMAS

Cutaneous T-cell lymphomas (CTCLs) constitute a group of cutaneous NHLs with clonal expansion of T lymphocytes into the skin. Several entities are recognized by classification systems such as the European Organization for Research and Treatment of Cancer (EORTC) and the WHO classification, which are based on morphologic, histopathologic, and molecular features (Table 14).

External superficial irradiation is well tolerated and effective for local control of CTCL. Radiation prescriptions are similar to those for the other lymphomas already discussed.

MYCOSIS FUNGOIDES/SÉZARY SYNDROME

Mycosis fungoides represents the most common type of CTCL, comprising 50% of CTCLs with a male predominance of approximately 2:1 and a predominance of African-American patients of 1.6:1. It has a yearly incidence of 0.36 cases per 100,000 population that has remained constant over the past decade. Clinical and histologic diagnosis of mycosis fungoides has proved to be difficult, since in early stages, it may resemble other dermatoses such as eczematous dermatitis, psoriasis, and parapsoriasis.

Clinically, mycosis fungoides is characterized by erythematous patches, evolving into plaques or tumors; however, the progress is variable. It is classified as an indolent lymphoma by the EORTC. Sézary syndrome is the aggressive, leukemic, and erythrodermic variant of CTCL, which is characterized by circulating, atypical, malignant T lymphocytes with cerebriform nuclei (Sézary cells), and lymphadenopathy. For staging purposes, the tumor node metastasis (TNM) system is most commonly used.

Treatment of early-stage disease At present, CTCLs are regarded as incurable. In early CTCL, the cell-mediated immune response is usually normal.

TABLE 14: WHO-EORTC classification of cutaneous lymphomas with primary cutaneous manifestations

Cutaneous T-cell and NK-cell lymphomas

Mycosis fungoides

Mycosis fungoides variants and subtypes

- Folliculotropic mycosis fungoides
- Pagetoid reticulosis
- Granulomatous slack skin

Sézary syndrome

Adult T-cell leukemia/lymphoma

Primary cutaneous CD30+ lymphoproliferative disorders

- Primary cutaneous anaplastic large cell lymphoma
- Lymphomatoid papulosis

Subcutaneous panniculitis-like T-cell lymphoma

Extranodal NK/T-cell lymphoma, nasal type

Primary cutaneous peripheral T-cell lymphoma, unspecified

- Primary cutaneous aggressive epidermotropic CD8+ T-cell lymphoma (provisional)
- Cutaneous γ/δ T-cell lymphoma (provisional)
- Primary cutaneous CD4+ small/medium-sized pleomorphic T-cell lymphoma (provisional)

Cutaneous B-cell lymphomas

Primary cutaneous marginal zone B-cell lymphoma

Primary cutaneous follicle center lymphoma

Primary cutaneous diffuse large B-cell lymphoma, leg type

Primary cutaneous diffuse large B-cell lymphoma, other

- Primary cutaneous intravascular large B-cell lymphoma

Precursor hematologic neoplasm

CD4+/CD56+ hematodermic neoplasm (formerly blastic NK-cell lymphoma)

EORTC = European Organization for Research and Treatment of Cancer; WHO = World Health Organization

Therefore, the majority of these cases can be treated successfully with topical modalities. Early aggressive therapy does not improve the prognosis of patients with CTCL. The skin-targeted modalities include psoralen plus ultraviolet A (PUVA); narrow-band–ultraviolet B (NB-UVB); skin electron-beam radiation therapy; as well as topical preparations of steroids, retinoids, carmustine, or nitrogen mustard (Table 15).

Treatment of advanced-stage disease A limited number of patients progress to more aggressive and advanced disease with either cutaneous or extracutaneous tumor manifestations. Treatment goals in advanced stages should be to reduce the tumor burden, relieve symptoms, and decrease the risk of transformation into aggressive lymphoma. Established treatment options include mono- or polychemotherapy including COP or CHOP regimens, extracorporeal photopheresis, interferons, retinoids, monoclonal antibodies (alemtuzumab), and recombinant toxins (denileukin diftitox). Combinations are frequently used (Table 15).

In mycosis fungoides, stage IA and IIA, only the skin is treated with low-energy electrons. The target volume does not exceed a depth of 5 mm. Significant myelotoxicity is therefore unusual. Irradiation may consist of local or total skin, depending on the extent of disease. The standard dose for total-skin electron-beam therapy is 36 Gy delivered by dual fixed-angle, six-field methods 4 days a week. Electron-beam therapy results in a complete response rate of 56%–96% in patients with stage IA–IIA disease. There is a high relapse rate in extensive cases after total skin electron-beam therapy without adjuvant therapy, such as topical chemotherapy and PUVA. Consequent relapse-free survival for patients with stage IA disease is 33%–52% at 10 years.

LYMPHOMATOID PAPULOSIS

Lymphomatoid papulosis is most commonly associated with mycosis fungoides, CD30+ large T-cell lymphoma, and Hodgkin lymphoma. Three histologic types have been identified, characterized as types A, B, and C. Types A and C consist of large lymphocytes resembling Reed-Sternberg cells. Type A cells are embedded in a dense inflammatory background, whereas type C cells form large sheets imitating CD30+ large T-cell lymphoma. Type B simulates classic features of mycosis fungoides, with epidermotropism and a dermal band-like infiltrate composed of small to medium cells. Lymphomatoid papulosis lesions occasionally exhibit clonal gene rearrangements.

Lymphomatoid papulosis represents a benign, chronic recurrent, self-healing, papulonodular, and papulonecrotic CD30+ skin eruption. However, 10%–20% of patients may develop a lymphoid malignancy, but the prognosis for patients with lymphomatoid papulosis is otherwise excellent, with a 100% 5-year survival. There is no curative treatment available. Lymphomatoid papulosis is managed by observation, intralesional steroid injection, topical bexarotene (Targretin), ultraviolet light therapy, or low-dose methotrexate.

ALCL, CD30+ CUTANEOUS TYPE

Primary systemic CD30+ ALCL and primary cutaneous CD30+ ALCL represent identical morphologic entities, but they are clinically distinct diseases.

The neoplastic cells of primary cutaneous CD30+ large T-cell lymphoma (CD30+ LTCL) are of the CD4+ helper T-cell phenotype with CD30 expression. It represents 9% of CTCLs and typically presents with solitary or localized nodules. This tumor has an excellent prognosis, as confirmed in several studies, in contrast to the transformation of mycosis lymphoma to a CD30– large cell variant. It shows histologic and immunophenotypic overlap with lymphomatoid papulosis. In most cases, tumor cells show anaplastic features, less commonly a pleomorphic or immunoblastic appearance. However, there is no difference in the prognosis and survival rate. Primary cutaneous CD30+ LTCLs

TABLE 15: Initial treatment options for cutaneous T-cell lymphoma by stage

Stage	Clinical features	Treatment options
IA	Limited patch, plaque (< 10% BSA)	Topical steroids, nitrogen mustard, or BiCNU, bexarotene gel[a], spot electron-beam irradiation, PUVA
IB-IIA	Extensive patch, plaque (> 10% BSA)	Topical nitrogen mustard or BiCNU, PUVA, bexarotene gel[a], total skin electron-beam irradiation, methotrexate, IFN, PUVA + IFN, bexarotene capsules, PUVA + bexarotene capsules
IIB	Tumors	Spot electron-beam irradiation, PUVA ± IFN, methotrexate, bexarotene capsules, denileukin diftitox
III	Erythroderma without Sézary cells	PUVA, total skin electron-beam irradiation, topical Sézary cells, nitrogen mustard, or BiCNU, bexarotene capsules, IFN, PUVA + IFN, alemtuzumab, methotrexate, purine analogs, photopheresis
III	Erythroderma with Sézary cells	Extracorporeal photopheresis, PUVA + IFN, bexarotene capsules ± PUVA, methotrexate, purine analogs, denileukin diftitox, alemtuzumab
IV	Lymph node or visceral organ	Bexarotene capsules, IFN, denileukin diftitox, purine analogs, visceral involvement cytotoxic chemotherapy ± skin-directed therapies

[a]Topical bexarotene may cause irritation if applied to a large body surface area.

BSA = body surface area; BiCNU = carmustine; PUVA = psoralen plus ultraviolet A; IFN = interferon

rarely carry the t(2;5) translocation and are usually ALK-negative. These lesions may undergo spontaneous regression, as do the lesions of lymphomatoid papulosis. The mechanism of tumor regression remains unknown.

Spot radiation therapy or surgical excision is the preferred treatment, with systemic chemotherapy reserved for cases with large tumor burden and extracutaneous involvement. More recently, there has been reported efficacy of recombinant IFN-γ-1b (Actimmune) and combined treatment with bexarotene and IFN-α-2a (Roferon-A).

LTCL, CD30– CUTANEOUS

Primary cutaneous CD30– large T-cell lymphomas (CD30– LTCL) do not produce T-helper 2 (Th2) cytokines and do not express CD30. Microscopically, a dense nodular or diffuse infiltrate characterized by pleomorphic medium or large cells and immunoblastic lymphocytes is present. Large cells comprise over 30% and might resemble classic mycosis fungoides undergoing large cell transformation.

These lymphomas are aggressive neoplasms, with an estimated 15% 5-year survival rate. Patients present with solitary, localized, or generalized plaques, nodules, or tumors without spontaneous regression. Multiagent systemic chemotherapy is recommended in most cases, with radiotherapy limited to localized disease.

PLEOMORPHIC T-CELL LYMPHOMAS WITH SMALL/MEDIUM CELLS

The small/medium pleomorphic CTCL type appears clinically with single erythematous to violaceous nodules or tumors and accounts for less than 3% of CTCL cases. Most cases have an unfavorable prognosis, with a median survival of ≤ 24 months; however, the CD3+, CD4+, CD8–, CD30– subtype with limited lesions might be associated with a better prognosis, with a reported 45% 5-year survival rate.

The optimal therapy for pleomorphic T-cell lymphomas with small/medium cells has not been defined. Localized lesions have been treated with radiation therapy or surgical excision. Only short-term outcome has been reported. Patients with generalized skin disease or progression have been treated effectively with systemic treatments, including multiagent chemotherapy, retinoids, interferons, and monoclonal antibodies.

SUBCUTANEOUS PANNICULITIS-LIKE T-CELL LYMPHOMA

Subcutaneous panniculitits-like T-cell lymphoma (SCPTCL) is a rare T-cell lymphoma that infiltrates the subcutaneous fat without dermal and epidermal involvement, causing erythematous to violaceous nodules and/or plaques. Systemic symptoms are frequent and include weight loss, fever, and fatigue. The disease may be complicated by the hemophagocytic syndrome. SCPTCL may be preceded by a benign-appearing panniculitis for years. The infiltrate is pleomorphic and associated with inflammation and necrosis. The T-cell phenotype is α/β^+ with $CD4^{(+/-)}$, $CD8^+$, and $CD56^{(-/+)}$. Standard treatment includes CHOP-like chemotherapy, local radiation treatment, and/or steroids. Five-year survival rates exceed 80%.

CUTANEOUS γ/δ T-CELL LYMPHOMA

Cutaneous γ/δ T-cell lymphoma is a rare panniculitis presenting with disseminated (ulcerated) plaques, nodules, or tumors. Involvement of mucosal or extranodal sites is common. Systemic symptoms, including weight loss, fever, and fatigue, are almost always present. The hemophagocytic syndrome is often noted. The γ/δ^+ T cells are characteristically $CD2^+$, $CD3^+$, $CD4^-$, $CD5^-$, $CD7^{(-/+)}$, $CD8^{(-/+)}$, and $CD56^+$. Aggressive chemotherapy is indicated, with consideration of autologous or allogeneic SCT incorporated into the initial treatment schema. The median survival is less than 2 years.

CUTANEOUS B-CELL LYMPHOMAS

Primary cutaneous B-cell lymphomas (CBCLs) are rare entities. They constitute up to 25% of all cutaneous lymphomas. However, the incidence of CBCLs has been underestimated due to the absence of immunologic and molecular markers. In addition, their terminology and classification remain controversial, with until recently separate and distinct terminology promoted by the WHO and the EORTC. Primary CBCLs are distinct from nodal lymphomas, and the majority of them have an excellent prognosis. Several types are recognized, with the most common types being follicle center cell lymphoma (FCCL) and MZL.

Follicle center cell lymphoma FCCL is defined as a proliferation of centrocytes (small to large cleaved cells) and centroblasts (large round cells with prominent nuclei), showing a nodular or diffuse infiltrate in the majority of cases and presenting only rarely a true follicular pattern. FCCL is the most common subtype, comprising 40% of CBCLs. It is classified as DLBCL in the WHO classification. FCCL shows a predilection for the head, neck, and trunk in elderly patients, with a median age of 60 years and a male predominance of approximately 1.5:1. The clinical course is usually indolent, with an excellent overall survival of up to 97%. However, relapses occur frequently. The large round cell morphology might be associated with a higher rate of disease progression and poorer prognosis.

Small centrocytes predominate in low-grade FCCL, whereas an increased number of large cells occur in high-grade FCCL; however, lesions with pure high-grade disease may behave indolently and should not by themselves drive the treatment administered. In contrast to their nodal counterpart, *bcl*-2 is usually not expressed in neoplastic cells, and the t(14;18) translocation is rarely detected. More recently, low rates of *bcl*-2 expression have been reported. In addition to CD10+ and *bcl*-6+ expression, FCCL also has an aberrant expression of CD45 RA and CD43 and thus provides a helpful clue to distinguish it from pseudolymphomas. Radiation therapy is often the preferred therapy for solitary or localized group lesions. Surgical excision can be considered for small lesions. Chemotherapy, though effective, rarely results in cure. Rituximab has proven to be effective for palliation. Observation is a reasonable alternative in many instances.

Immunocytoma/marginal zone lymphoma IC/MZL is a recently recognized low-grade lymphoma and represents the second most common subtype of CBCL. It predominantly occurs on the upper and lower extremities. The median age at presentation is 55 years, and females are affected more often than males. The reported survival rates are 97%–100%, although relapses commonly occur. Histologically, IC/MZL has features of MALT lymphomas and shows a nodular or diffuse dermal infiltrate with a heterogeneous cellular infiltrate of small lymphocytes, lymphoplasmacytoid cells, plasma cells, intranuclear inclusions (Dutcher bodies), and reactive germinal centers that may be infiltrated by neoplastic cells. Diagnosis can be difficult, because of the variable composition of the infiltrate that may be interpreted as a reactive process or as FCCL. In contrast to FCCL, MZL is negative for *bcl*-6 and CD10. In 50% of cases, CD43 is highly expressed. Large cell transformation and a head and neck presentation may be associated with a worse prognosis. Therapeutic alternatives are similar to those described for FCCL.

LARGE B-CELL LYMPHOMA OF THE LEG (LBCLL)

Primary cutaneous large B-cell lymphoma of the leg (LBCLL) forms a separate category in the WHO–EORTC classification, as a more aggressive type confined to elderly patients, with a median age of 76 years at diagnosis and a female predominance of 7:2. Most cases have a follicle center cell origin, and histologic evaluation shows a diffuse dermal infiltrate with predominance in large B cells with multilobulated nuclei, comprised of centroblasts and immunoblasts, with presence of small, cleaved cells and a minor admixed infiltrate component. Eosinophilic intranuclear (Dutcher body) or intracytoplasmic (Russell body) inclusions of immunoglobulin are common. Unlike FCCL, LBCLLs consistently express *bcl-2*, although they are not associated with the t(14;18) translocation.

The prognosis is less favorable for LBCLL than for other CBCLs, with a 5-year survival rate of 50%-60%. Prognostic factors identified with a poor outcome include the predominance of round cells (centroblasts/immunoblasts) over cleaved cells (centrocytes) in the tumor infiltrate, MUM-1 expression, and multiple lesions at presentation. The use of an IPI-based model is required to investigate whether LBCLL is associated with a poorer prognosis. These lymphomas should be treated as systemic DLBCL with anthracycline-based chemotherapy. In patients presenting with a single, small skin tumor, radiotherapy is a consideration. Rituximab has also been incorporated into combination regimens.

Intravascular large B-cell lymphoma The WHO–EORTC has proposed intravascular large B-cell lymphoma (IVLBCL) or angiotropic B-cell lymphoma as a provisional entity. This subtype is rare and corresponds to the proliferation of malignant lymphocytes within lumina of small vessels, involving most frequently the skin and CNS. It was previously considered a vascular tumor and referred to as malignant angioendotheliomatosis. Although the majority of cases are of B-cell origin, few cases of T-cell lineage have been reported. The reason for intravascular localization is not clear, but association with an unknown surface receptor or dysfunction of lymphocyte-endothelial interaction affecting adhesion molecules has been suspected.

IVLBCL is clinically characterized by tender erythematous, purpuric, indurated patches and plaques located on the trunk and thighs, where it can resemble panniculitis. Cases of generalized telangiectasia over normal skin have been reported. Cytomorphology reveals intravascular occlusion of small vessels, filled with large atypical centroblast-like B lymphocytes. IHC shows CD19, CD20, CD45, and CD79a expression. Genotypic analysis has demonstrated clonality, although it may not be positive in every case. Generally, the prognosis of this aggressive type of lymphoma is poor despite the use of combination chemotherapy, because of the initial or secondary CNS involvement. Prognosis appeared better in some reports, if isolated cutaneous involvement was present. However, no large series permitting a precise prognosis to be determined are available.

PLASMACYTOMA

Primary cutaneous involvement of plasmacytoma is uncommon and generally develops as a consequence of direct spread from an underlying multiple myeloma. It represents 4% of extramedullary plasmacytomas and affects predominantly elderly men with a median age of 60 years at diagnosis. It is characterized by a monoclonal proliferation of mature plasma cells. Cutaneous plasmacytomas are potentially curable, with a 5-year survival rate of > 90%. However, the presentation of multiple lesions is an important adverse prognostic factor. Histopathology shows a dense monomorphous dermal infiltrate of plasma cells with a varying degree of maturation and atypia, admixed with few lymphocytes and histiocytes. Neoplastic plasma cells express clonal immunoglobulin, CD38, and CD79a but are negative for CD20. Rarely, amyloid deposition within the tumor is demonstrated, which is more common in secondary cutaneous involvement of plasmacytoma. A recent organized workshop on plasma cell dyscrasias questioned whether these cases are true cutaneous plasmacytomas, represent reactive B-cell infiltrates associated with an infectious etiology, or represent a variant of MZL with a predominant population of plasma cells. Diagnosis may rely on demonstration of monoclonality by restriction of Ig light-chain expression. Excision or radiation treatment is most commonly used.

B-CELL PSEUDOLYMPHOMA

The distinction between a true CBCL and B-cell pseudolymphoma is often difficult; however, IHC and molecular techniques make a distinction more likely. B-cell pseudolymphoma involves most commonly the face and chest, with a female predominance. Precipitating stimuli may be arthropod bites, drugs, tattoos, and injections. In Europe, an association with *B burgdorferi* infection has been reported. Microscopically, there is a dense polymorphous infiltrate with various numbers of eosinophils, plasma cells, T lymphocytes, and histiocytes. Histologic features may resemble IC/MZL. A transformation into malignant B-cell lymphoma has been observed.

HIV-RELATED LYMPHOMAS

Most lymphomas seen in patients who have HIV infection are of an aggressive histology and advanced stage at presentation. Extranodal disease is common, with unusual sites of presentation, including the rectum, CNS, and multiple soft-tissue masses. Some patients present with primary CNS lymphoma. Poor-risk factors include a high LDH level, large tumor bulk, extranodal disease, and low CD4 cell counts (< 100 cells/mL). Because of their increased risk of opportunistic infections and impaired hematologic reserve, historically many patients with HIV-related lymphomas have been unable to tolerate aggressive chemotherapy regimens. Current antiviral medications have allowed for the use of more traditional regimens, including R-CHOP and R-CHOEP (R-CHOP with etoposide; see Table 8), with results comparable to those of other NHL patients with similar histologies and presentations.

CNS prophylaxis with intrathecal chemotherapy is necessary to prevent meningeal dissemination. (For a more detailed discussion of HIV-related NHL, see chapter 27.)

Post-transplantation NHL Post-transplantation lymphoproliferative disorders (PTLDs) comprise a histologic spectrum, ranging from hyperplastic-appearing lesions to frank NHL or multiple myeloma histology. The incidence varies from 1% in renal transplant recipients to 8% in lung transplant recipients, who require more potent immunosuppressive therapy. The use of anti–T-cell therapies or T-cell depletion in recipients of SCT will increase the risk of PTLD. More than 90% of tumors are associated with EBV. Reduction of immunosuppression can lead to disease regression. In anatomically limited PTLD, resection or targeted radiation treatment can be effective. Traditional chemotherapy has been associated with significant toxicity but can result in long-term disease-free remissions or cure. Biologic agents including IFN and more recently rituximab have shown significant promise. In vitro expanded EBV-specific cytotoxic T cells have been used for treatment and prophylaxis for PTLD following allogeneic SCT.

Primary CNS lymphoma Primary CNS lymphoma is a rare form of NHL, arising within and confined to the CNS. Histologically, primary CNS lymphomas are indistinguishable from systemic NHLs. More than 40% of patients have evidence of leptomeningeal dissemination, and 15% have ocular disease at presentation. A stereotactic needle biopsy is the procedure of choice for histopathologic diagnosis. Resection does not appear to improve survival. Modern management includes high-dose methotrexate alone or combined with agents that penetrate the CNS (high-dose cytarabine, vincristine, and procarbazine [Matulane]). Whole-brain radiotherapy has been considered a standard component of treatment; however, long-term neurotoxicity remains a concern, and, therefore, alternative approaches are being explored.

Treatment complications

Tumor lysis syndrome is a common complication after treatment of high-grade, bulky NHLs (due to their exquisite sensitivity to therapy and high proliferative capacity). The syndrome is characterized by renal failure, hyperkalemia, hyperphosphatemia, and hypocalcemia.

Measures to prevent this complication include aggressive hydration; allopurinol; alkalinization of the urine; and frequent monitoring of electrolytes, uric acid, and creatinine. Dialysis is sometimes required. Rasburicase, a recombinant urateoxidase enzyme, is now available for the prevention and treatment of hyperuricemia. (For a more comprehensive discussion of the tumor lysis syndrome, see chapter 45.)

Follow-up of long-term survivors

Relapse The most important risk to patients with NHL is relapse. Among patients with diffuse aggressive lymphomas, most recurrences are seen within the first 2 years after the completion of therapy, although later relapses may occur.

Physical examination and laboratory testing at 2- to 3-month intervals and follow-up CT scans (with or without PET scan) at 6-month intervals for the first 2 years following diagnosis are recommended.

Early detection of recurrent disease is important because these patients may be candidates for potentially curative high-dose therapy and SCT. Patients with advanced low-grade NHL are at a constant risk of relapse, and late recurrence of disease may be seen, sometimes after more than a decade-old remission.

Secondary malignancies Long-term survivors are at increased risk of second cancers. In a survey of 6,171 patients with NHL who survived 2 or more years, nearly 1,000 patients lived 15 or more years after diagnosis. Second cancers were reported in 541 subjects, with significant excesses seen for all solid tumors; acute myelogenous leukemia; melanoma; Hodgkin lymphoma; and cancers of the lungs, brain, kidneys, and bladder. The actuarial risk of developing a second malignancy at 3–20 years after diagnosis of NHL was 21%, compared with a population-expected cumulative risk of 15%.

Treatment complications With the decline in the role of irradiation as part of the initial therapy for NHL, the risk of certain radiation-induced complications has been reduced or eliminated in more recently diagnosed patients. Nevertheless, total-body irradiation is often used as a component of myeloablative conditioning regimens. Also, transplant recipients are at increased risk of secondary myelodysplasia and acute myeloid leukemia, regardless of whether they received a radiation-containing conditioning regimen. All individual chemotherapy agents have their own potential long-term morbidity.

Long-term survivors need continued follow-up for possible treatment-related complications. Some of these toxicities may still be unknown. Careful documentation of late complications will be important in the design of future treatment strategies aimed at preserving or improving response rates and the duration of remission while reducing toxicity.

SUGGESTED READING

Arneshna KM, Smith P, Norton A, et al: Long-term effect of a watch and wait policy versus immediate systemic treatment for asymptomatic advanced-stage non-Hodgkin lymphoma: A randomized controlled trial. Lancet 362:516–522, 2003.

Bendandi M: The role of idiotype vaccines in the treatment of human B-cell malignancies. Expert Rev Vaccines 3:163–170, 2004.

Chiu B, Weisenburger DD: An update of the epidemiology of non-Hodgkin's lymphoma. Clin Lymphoma 4:161–168, 2003.

Coiffier B, Lepage E, Briere J, et al: CHOP chemotherapy plus rituximab compared with CHOP alone in elderly patients with diffuse large B-cell lymphoma. N Engl J Med 346:235–242, 2002.

Czucman MS, Weaver R, Alkuzweny B, et al: Prolonged clinical and molecular remission in patients with low-grade or follicular non-Hodgkin's lymphoma treated with rituximab plus CHOP chemotherapy: 9-year follow-up. J Clin Oncol 22:4711–4716, 2004.

Dave SS, Wright G, Tan B, et al: Prediction of survival in follicular lymphoma based on molecular features of tumor-infiltrating immune cells. N Engl J Med 351:2159–2169, 2004.

Goy AH, Younes A, McLaughlin P, et al: Phase II study of proteasome inhibitor bortezomib in relapsed or refractory B-cell non-Hodgkin's lymphoma. J Clin Oncol 23:667–675, 2005.

Hainsworth JD, Litchy S, Burris HA III, et al: Rituximab as first-line and maintenance therapy for patients with indolent non-Hodgkin's lymphoma. J Clin Oncol 20:4261–4267, 2002.

Hamlin PA, Zelenetz AD, Kewalramani T, et al: Age-adjusted International Prognostic Index predicts autologous stem cell transplantation outcome for patients with relapsed or primary refractory diffuse large B-cell lymphoma. Blood 102:1989–1996, 2003.

Lossos IS, Czerwinski DK, Alizadeh AA, et al: Prediction of survival in diffuse large-B-cell lymphoma based on the expression of six genes. N Engl J Med 350:1828–1837, 2004.

Milpied N, Deconinck E, Gailland T, et al: Initial treatment of aggressive lymphoma with high-dose chemotherapy and autologous stem cell support. N Engl J Med 350:1287–1295, 2004.

O'Connor OA, Wright J, Moskowitz C, et al: Phase II clinical experience with the novel proteasome inhibitor bortezomib in patients with indolent non-Hodgkin's lymphoma and mantle cell lymphoma. J Clin Oncol 23:676–685, 2005.

Orlowski RZ, Stinchcombe TE, Mitchell BS, et al: Phase I trial of the proteasome inhibitor PS-341 in patients with refractory hematologic malignancies. J Oncol 20:4420–4427, 2002.

Petersen PM, Gospodarowicz M, Tsang R, et al: Long-term outcome in stage I and II follicular lymphoma following treatment with involved field radiation therapy alone (abstract). Proc Am Soc Clin Oncol 23:561, 2004.

Querfeld C, Guitart J, Kuzel TM, et al: Primary cutaneous lymphomas: A review with current treatment options. Blood Rev 17:131–142, 2004.

Rodriguez J, Caballero MD, Gutierrez A, et al: Autologous stem-cell transplantation in diffuse large B-cell non-Hodgkin's lymphoma not achieving complete response after induction chemotherapy: The GEL/TAMO experience. Ann Oncol 15:1504–1509, 2004.

Rosado MF, Byrne GE Jr, Ding F, et al: Ocular adnexal lymphoma: A clinicopathologic study of a large cohort of patients with no evidence for an association with *Chlamydia psittaci*. Blood 107:467–472, 2006.

Rosenwald A, Wright G, Leroy K, et al: Molecular diagnosis of primary mediastinal B cell lymphoma identifies a clinically favorable subgroup of diffuse large B cell lymphoma related to Hodgkin lymphoma. J Exp Med 198:851–862, 2003.

Savage KJ, Monti S, Kutok JL, et al: The molecular signature of mediastinal large B-cell lymphoma differs from that of other diffuse large B-cell lymphomas and shares features with classical Hodgkin lymphoma. Blood 102:3871–3879, 2003.

Schouten HC, Quan W, Kvaloy S, et al: High-dose therapy improves progression-free survival and survival in relapsed follicular non-Hodgkin's lymphoma: Results from the randomized European CUP trial. J Clin Oncol 21:3918–3927, 2003.

Solal-Celigny P, Roy P, Colombat P, et al: Follicular Lymphoma International Prognostic Index. Blood 104:1258–1265, 2004.

Waters JS, Webb A, Cunningham D, et al: Phase I clinical and pharmacokinetic study of bcl-2 antisense oligonucleotide therapy in patients with non-Hodgkin's lymphoma. J Clin Oncol 18:1812–1823, 2000.

Willemze R, Jaffe ES, Burg G, et al: WHO–EORTC classification for cutaneous lymphomas. Blood 105:3768–3785, 2005.

Wilson WH, Grossbard ML, Pittaluga S, et al: Dose-adjusted EPOCH chemotherapy for untreated large B-cell lymphomas: A pharmacodynamic approach with high efficacy. Blood 99:2685–2693, 2002.

Winter JN, Gascoyne RD, Van Besien K: Low grade lymphoma. In: Broudy VC, Berliner N, Larson RA, et al (eds): Hematology 2004, pp 203–220. Washington, DC, American Society of Hematology, 2004.

CHAPTER 31

Multiple myeloma and other plasma cell dyscrasias

Sundar Jagannath, MD, Paul Richardson, MD, and Nikhil C. Munshi, MD

MYELOMA

MULTIPLE MYELOMA

Multiple myeloma is a disseminated malignancy of monoclonal plasma cells that accounts for 8% of all hematologic cancers. In the year 2007, an estimated 19,900 new cases will be diagnosed in the United States, and 10,790 Americans will die of this disease. Incidence rates for myeloma (5.3 in men and 3.5 in women) and mortality rates (3.7 in men and 2.5 in women) per 100,000 population have remained stable for the past decade.

Epidemiology

Gender Men are affected more frequently than women (1.4:1.0 ratio).

Age The median age at presentation is 71 years, according to most tumor registries, although the median age reported in studies is approximately 60 years.

Race The annual incidence per 100,000 population is 6.4 among white men and 4.1 among white women. Among black men and women, the frequency doubles to 12.7 and 10.0, respectively, per 100,000 population. This racial difference is not explained by socioeconomic or environmental factors and is presumably due to unknown genetic factors.

Geography There is no clear geographic distribution of multiple myeloma. In Europe, the highest rates are noted in the Nordic countries, the United Kingdom, Switzerland, and Israel. France, Germany, Austria, and Slovenia have a lower incidence, and developing countries have the lowest incidence. This higher relative incidence in more developed countries probably results from the combination of a longer life expectancy and more frequent medical surveillance.

Survival The 5-year survival rate for all patients treated with conventional therapy is approximately 25%–30%. The 5-year survival rate is lower among patients ≥ age 65 (20%–25%) than in those < age 65 (30%–35%).

Etiology and risk factors

No predisposing factors for the development of multiple myeloma have been confirmed.

Environment Some causative factors that have been suggested include radiation exposure (radiologists and radium dial workers), occupational exposure (agricultural, chemical, metallurgical, rubber plant, pulp, wood and paper workers, and leather tanners), and chemical exposure to formaldehyde, epichlorohydrin, Agent Orange, hair dyes, paint sprays, and asbestos. None of these associations has proven to be statistically significant, and all have been contradicted by negative correlations. The initial report that survivors of the atomic bombings in Japan had an increased risk of developing myeloma has been refuted by longer follow-up.

Viruses A preliminary report in a limited number of patients noted the presence of herpesvirus 8 in the dendritic cells of patients with multiple myeloma. However, further evaluation by a number of investigators has failed to confirm this result. Patients with myeloma also do not appear to have a significant immune response against this virus.

Cytogenetics Karyotypic abnormalities in myeloma are complex, with both numeric and structural abnormalities. DNA aneuploidy is observed in more than 90% of cases, predominantly hyperdiploid, and less than 10% have hypodiploidy, which carries a poor prognosis. Recurrent nonrandom structural abnormalities have been identified and linked to the pathogenesis and prognosis of myeloma. The immunoglobulin heavy-chain gene at 14q32 is frequently involved in translocations with partner chromosomes 4, 6, 8, 11, and 16. The location and oncogenes involved are shown in Table 1. Translocations involving chromosomes 4 and 16 as well as del1q and del17p13 (p53) have been associated with a poor prognosis. Del13q or monosomy 13 is observed in 15%–20% of patients with conventional cytogenetics and also carries a poor prognosis across standard and high-dose therapies. Interphase fluorescence in situ hybridization (FISH) with a specific probe for chromosome 13q34 (retinoblastoma gene, *Rb 1*) identifies this abnormality in up to 50% of patients, with a less clear prognostic implication.

Genetic factors Although multiple myeloma is not an inherited disease, there have been numerous case reports of multiple incidence in the same family. However, a case-control study revealed no significant increase in the incidence among relatives of patients who had multiple myeloma, other hematologic malignancies, or other cancers.

> Interactions between multiple myeloma (MM) cells and their microenvironment, the extracellular matrix and the bone marrow stromal cells (BMSCs), allow MM cells to survive, grow, migrate, and resist apoptosis induced by traditional chemotherapies. These effects are partially mediated through adhesion-mediated signalling and partly through various cytokines, including IL-6, VEGF, IGF-1, and IL-2. The molecular signals mediating the proliferative effects include the *ras/raf* MAPK pathway, whereas the PI3K/Akt pathway provides cell survival and drug resistance signals. Improved understanding of these interactions and the molecular mechanisms mediating them has now allowed us to evaluate novel therapies that directly target MM cells as well as act on the bone marrow microenvironment.

TABLE 1: The location and oncogenes involved in multiple myeloma

Locus	Oncogene	Incidence
11q13	Cyclin D1	15%-20%
6p21	Cyclin D3	5%
4p16.3	FGFR3 and MMSET	12%
16q23	c-*maf*	5%-10%
8q24	c-*myc*	< 10%
6p25	MUM1/IRF4	5%
20q11	MAFB	5%
1q21-34	*bcl*-9, IL-6R, *mcl*-1	Frequent

Monoclonal gammopathy of unknown significance (MGUS) Patients with MGUS develop myeloma, macroglobulinemic lymphoma, or amyloidosis at a rate of 1% per year.

Signs and symptoms

The clinical features of multiple myeloma are variable. Findings that suggest the diagnosis include lytic bone lesions, anemia, azotemia, hypercalcemia, and recurrent infections. Approximately 30% of patients are free of symptoms and are diagnosed by chance.

Bone disease Bone pain, especially from compression fractures of the vertebrae or ribs, is the most common symptom. At diagnosis, 70% of patients have lytic lesions, which are due to accelerated bone resorption. These changes are induced by factors modulating osteoclastic activity and produced by the bone marrow microenvironment and, to a lesser extent, myeloma cells. These factors include interleukin (IL)-1B, tumor necrosis factor (TNF)-α, and IL-6 as well as newly identified factors such as osteoprotogerin, TNF-related activation-induced cytokine (TRANCE), and receptor activator of nuclear factor kappa B (RANK) ligand. DKK-1 has been described as a soluble factor produced by multiple myeloma cells inhibiting osteoblastic activity.

Anemia Normocytic, normochromic anemia is present in 60% of patients at diagnosis. It is due primarily to the decreased production of RBCs by marrow, infiltration with plasma cells, and the suppressive effect of various cytokines. Patients with renal failure may also have decreased levels of erythropoietin, which may worsen the degree of anemia.

Hypercalcemia Among newly diagnosed patients, 20% have hypercalcemia (corrected serum calcium level, > 11.5 mg/dL) secondary to progressive bone destruction, which may be exacerbated by prolonged immobility. Hypercalcemia should be suspected in patients with myeloma who have nausea, fatigue, confusion, polyuria, or constipation. It may suggest high tumor burden. It should be considered an oncologic emergency and promptly treated.

Renal failure Approximately 20% of patients present with renal insufficiency and another 20% develop this complication in later phases of the disease. Light-chain cast nephropathy is the most common cause of renal failure. Additional causes include hypercalcemia, dehydration, and hyperuricemia. Uncommonly, amyloidosis, light-chain deposition disease, nonsteroidal anti-inflammatory agents taken for pain control, intravenous radiographic contrast administration, and calcium stones may contribute to renal failure. More recently, bisphosphonate therapy has been associated with renal failure.

Infections Many patients with myeloma develop bacterial infections that may be serious. In the past, gram-positive organisms (eg, *Streptococcus pneumoniae, Staphylococcus aureus*) and *Haemophilus influenzae* were the most common pathogens. More recently, however, gram-negative organisms have become frequent. The increased susceptibility of patients with myeloma to bacterial infections, specifically with encapsulated organisms, has been attributed to impairments of host-defense mechanisms, such as hypogammaglobulinemia, granulocytopenia, and decreased cell-mediated immunity.

Screening and diagnosis

No screening measures for multiple myeloma have demonstrated any benefit.

The diagnosis usually requires the presence of bone marrow plasmacytosis and a monoclonal protein in the urine and/or serum (Table 2). One immunoglobulin class is produced in excess, whereas the other immunoglobulin classes are usually depressed.

Initial work-up The initial work-up for patients suspected of having a plasma cell dyscrasia should include:

- CBC with differential count and platelet count
- routine serum chemistry panel (eg, calcium, BUN, creatinine)
- bone marrow aspirate and biopsy to assess plasmacytosis
- serum protein electrophoresis and immunofixation to define protein type
- 24-hour urine protein, electrophoresis, and immunofixation
- quantitative immunoglobulin levels
- skeletal survey (bone scans contribute little since isotope uptake is often low in purely lytic bone disease)
- cytogenetics, including FISH.

The recently available serum free light-chain assay is useful in patients with light-chain–only disease, oligo- or nonsecretory myeloma, renal failure, and amyloidosis.

MRI is an excellent tool for evaluation of spinal cord compression/impinge-

TABLE 2: Common laboratory features of plasma cell dyscrasias

Multiple myeloma
Marrow plasmacytosis > 10%
Monoclonal immunoglobulin peak (usually > 3.0 g/dL)
Suppressed uninvolved immunoglobulins
Clonal plasma cells
Presence of Bence Jones protein
Lytic bone lesions or diffuse osteopenia
Related organ or tissue impairment
Smoldering myeloma
Same as multiple myeloma but without symptoms and
Hemoglobin > 10.5 g/dL
Monoclonal immunoglobulin peak (< 4.5 g/dL)
Normal serum calcium and creatinine levels
No lytic bone lesions
Solitary plasmacytoma of bone (SPB)
Solitary bone lesion due to plasma cell tumor
Normal skeletal survey and MRI of the skull, spine, and pelvis
Normal bone marrow plasmacytosis
No anemia, hypercalcemia, or renal disease
Preserved levels of uninvolved immunoglobulins
Monoclonal gammopathy of unknown significance (MGUS)
Monoclonal immunoglobulin level < 3.0 g/dL
Bone marrow plasma cells < 10%
No bone lesions
No symptoms due to plasma cell dyscrasia
Usually preserved levels of uninvolved immunoglobulins
No related organ or tissue impairment
Amyloidosis without myeloma
Same as MGUS plus evidence of amyloidosis on biopsy

ment. In addition, MRI identifies generalized signal abnormalities and focal lesions that can be monitored after therapy. MRI is especially useful in staging nonsecretory disease presenting as macrofocal lesions.

In addition, prognostic factors, such as β_2-microglobulin (β2M), serum albumin, C-reactive protein, lactic dehydrogenase (LDH) levels, plasma cell labeling index, and ploidy, may provide additional useful data.

Laboratory and pathologic features

Peripheral blood The peripheral blood smear may reveal a normocytic, normochromic anemia with rouleaux formation. Plasma cells may also be seen.

Bone marrow Bone marrow examination usually reveals an increased number of plasma cells. These cells are strongly positive for CD38, CD138, and cytoplasmic immunoglobulin (cIg). The majority of myeloma cells also express CD40 and CD56. Myeloma cells are negative for CD5, CD20, and surface immunoglobulin (sIg) expression. Whereas normal plasma cells express CD19, malignant plasma cells lose its expression. CD10 expression is generally negative but has sometimes been noted in advanced disease. Monoclonality may be demonstrated by immunoperoxidase staining with κ and λ antibodies.

The pattern of bone marrow involvement in plasma cell myeloma may be macrofocal. As a result, plasma cell count may be normal when an aspirate misses the focal aggregates of plasma cells that are better visualized radiographically or on direct needle biopsy.

Monoclonal proteins The types of monoclonal protein produced are IgG (60%), IgA (20%), IgD (2%), IgE (< 0.1%), or light-chain κ or λ only (18%). Biclonal elevations of myeloma proteins occur in < 1% of patients, and < 5% of patients are considered to have nonsecretory disease because their plasma cells do not secrete detectable levels of monoclonal immunoglobulin.

Staging and prognosis

The Durie-Salmon staging system is employed most frequently to stage multiple myeloma (Table 3). However, the variability in interpretation of staging criteria has resulted, in part, from imprecise quantification of the extent of bone lesions and from factors other than myeloma that contribute to hypercalcemia (eg, immobility) or anemia (eg, renal failure). Additionally, this staging system has not been predictive of response or survival in the studies using high-dose therapy or novel agents. An alternate staging system is proposed using simple laboratory measurements of serum β2M and albumin (International Staging System [ISS]).

Prognosis

Cytogenetic abnormalities Chromosomal abnormalities, especially loss of whole chromosome 13 (monosomy) or deletions of parts of chromosome 13 (13q), with hypodiploid have been associated with inferior survival after both standard chemotherapy and high-dose therapy. Primary translocations involving 14q32 and 6p21 (cyclin D3), 4p16 (FGFR3), and 16q23 (c-*maf*) in multivariate analysis have been shown to be important predictors of survival.

β2M Serum β2M level is an important and convenient prognostic indicator. When cytogenetic changes are not studied, β2M is consistently the most important prognostic indicator on multivariate analysis. As β2M is excreted by the kidneys, high levels are observed in patients with renal failure; in this setting, the interpretation of an elevated value is unclear.

LDH High LDH levels also have been associated with plasmablastic disease, extramedullary tumor, plasma cell leukemia, plasma cell hypodiploidy, drug resistance, and shortened survival.

Other indicators of shortened survival include elevated C-reactive protein, DNA hypodiploidy, high plasma cell labeling indices, and plasmablastic histology. Patients with DNA hypodiploidy are also less likely to respond to chemotherapy.

TABLE 3: Durie-Salmon staging system for multiple myeloma

Stage	Criteria	Myeloma cell mass ($\times 10^{12}$ cells/m^2)
I	Hemoglobin > 10 g/dL	< 0.6 (low)
	Serum calcium level ≤ 12 mg/dL (normal)	
	Normal bone or solitary plasmacytoma on x-ray	
	Low M-component production rate:	
	IgG < 5 g/dL	
	IgA < 3 g/dL	
	Bence Jones protein < 4 g/24 h	
II	Not fitting stage I or III	0.6-1.2 (intermediate)
III	Hemoglobin < 8.5 g/dL	> 1.2 (high)
	Serum calcium level > 12 mg/dL	
	Multiple lytic bone lesions on x-ray	
	High M-component production rate:	
	IgG > 7 g/dL	
	IgA > 5 g/dL	
	Bence Jones protein > 12 g/24 h	

Subclassification	Criterion
A	Normal renal function (serum creatinine level < 2.0 mg/dL)
B	Abnormal renal function (serum creatinine level ≥ 2.0 mg/dL)

Treatment response criteria

Since the criteria for treatment response in patients with multiple myeloma have varied among institutions, response rates have been difficult to compare in the past. Bence Jones protein is reduced more rapidly in responders than is serum myeloma protein because of the rapid renal catabolism of light chains.

IBMTR (EBMT) Response Criteria:

Complete response requires all of the following:

- No serum/urine M protein by immunofixation electrophoresis for ≥ 6 weeks
- < 5% plasma cells in bone marrow aspirate
- No increase in the size or number of lytic bone lesions
- Disappearance of soft-tissue plasmacytomas.

Partial response requires all of the following:

- > 50% reduction in serum M protein ≥ 6 weeks
- ≥ 90% reduction in 24-hr urinary light chain excretion
- ≥ 50% reduction in soft-tissue plasmacytomas
- No increase in the size or number of lytic bone lesions.

Treatment

Exciting advances in the understanding of tumor biology and microenvironment–and their potential interaction–have helped to identify unique targets for rational therapeutic intervention to enhance outcome, which has not improved with conventional chemotherapy over the past 3 decades. Until recently, only 5%–10% of patients with multiple myeloma lived longer than 10 years, and cure remains elusive.

NEWLY DIAGNOSED PATIENTS

Chemotherapy

Dexamethasone/thalidomide Thalidomide (Thalomid) has been employed alone and in combination with dexamethasone as initial therapy in newly diagnosed patients. When employed alone, response (50% reduction in paraprotein) was observed in 36% of patients; when it was used along with dexamethasone, the response rate was higher (72% and 64% in two studies), including a 16% complete response rate in one study. The results of a randomized Eastern Cooperative Oncology Group (ECOG) trial showed that the combination of thalidomide and dexamethasone was superior to dexamethasone alone (63% vs 41%; $P = .001$) and comparable to VAD (vincristine, Adriamycin [doxorubicin], and dexamethasone). This combination does not damage stem cells and allows adequate stem-cell collection. A definite increase in thrombotic episodes has been observed with this combination, prompting prophylactic administration of aspirin, coumadin, or low molecular weight heparin.

VAD or VDD (vincristine, liposomal doxorubicin [Doxil], and dexamethasone) regimens spare stem cells and do not impair stem-cell collection (Table 4). Such regimens produced a response rate of approximately 45–55% in untreated patients, without improvement in overall survival over MP (melphalan [Alkeran] and prednisone). Responses occurred more rapidly with VAD-based regimens than with MP; these rapid responses may provide an advantage in patients with hypercalcemia, renal failure, or severe bone pain. No dosage adjustment is necessary for renal failure. Use of this combination has decreased since the introduction of dexamethasone/thalidomide and other combinations due to the need for a central line, the inconvenience of IV administration, and attendant toxicities.

Pulse dexamethasone alone has also been used in older patients and patients who need vertebral radiotherapy for spinal cord compression or for painful vertebral compressions, as this approach avoids severe myelosuppression (Table 4).

TABLE 4: Proposed standard treatment of multiple myeloma

Disease or patient status	Treatment approach
Initial therapy	
Candidates for high-dose therapy	
Dexamethasone	40 mg on days 1-4, 9-12, and 17-20 every 35 days or on days 1-4 every 2 weeks
Dexamethasone/thalidomide	Dexamethasone as above or at a lower dose if clinically indicated with thalidomide (up to 200 mg/d)
VAD	Vincristine (0.5 mg/d IV) + Adriamycin (10 $mg/m^2/d$ IV), both given as continuous infusion on days 1-4, along with dexamethasone (40 mg) on days 1-4, 9-12, and 17-20 every 35 days
Clinical trials	High-dose melphalan and SCT following induction therapy Bortezomib with dexamethasone Bortezomib with thalidomide and dexamethasone Lenalidomide and dexamethasone Bortezomib with liposomal doxorubicin
Noncandidates for high-dose therapy	
Above options or	
MP	Melphalan (8 $mg/m^2/d$ PO) + prednisone (100 mg/d PO) on days 1-4 every 4-5 weeks
Clinical trials	MP with cyclophosphamide MP with bortezomib
Relapsed myeloma	
Conventional chemotherapy	Dexamethasone and thalidomide Alkylating-agent combination (MP, VBMCP) Cyclophosphamide, etoposide, DCEP
High-dose chemotherapy	Melphalan (200 mg/m^2) and autotransplant (if previously not transplanted) mini-allogeneic transplant
Novel agents	Bortezomib (1.3 mg/m^2) on days 1, 4, 8, and 11 every 3 weeks with or without dexamethasone, liposomal doxorubicin, or thalidomide Bortezomib with cyclophosphamide Bortezomib with melphalan Lenalidomide with dexamethasone
Clinical trials	Lenalidomide with bortezomib Melphalan, arsenic trioxide, ascorbic acid (MAC) Other phase II novel agents

DCEP = dexamethasone, cyclophosphamide, etoposide, and cisplatin; SCT = stem-cell transplantation; VBMCP = vincristine, BiCNU, melphalan, cyclophosphamide, prednisone

MP The combination of melphalan and prednisone has been used over the past 30 years, and other combinations of multiple alkylating agents have not been found to be superior to MP. A meta-analysis of 18 published randomized trials comparing MP with other combination regimens arrived at the same conclusion. Approximately 40% of patients have responded to the MP regimen, with a median remission duration of 18 months and an overall median survival of 3 years. The MP regimen should be avoided in patients considered to be transplant candidates.

MP and thalidomide (MPT) In a prospective, randomized trial in patients older than age 65, MPT produced an overall response rate of 78%, including a 28% rate of near complete response, compared with a response rate of 44% and a near complete response rate of 5% with MP. MPT offers a possible alternative for older people who generally are not candidates for high-dose therapy.

Melphalan and other alkylating agents damage bone marrow stem cells, affecting the ability to mobilize an adequate number of cells for high dose-therapy. Extensive use of alkylating agents may also predispose patients to the subsequent development of myelodysplastic syndrome (MDS) or acute myeloid leukemia (AML). These limitations have now substantially reduced the use of MP in newly diagnosed patients.

High-dose therapy following induction

High-dose therapy employed after induction therapy improves the response rate as well as event-free and overall survival. The impressive improvement in event-free (median, 28 vs 18 months) and overall survival (57 vs 42 months) reported in a randomized trial (IFM 90) has been confirmed by another large randomized trial (median overall survival, 54.8 vs 42.3 months; MRC VII). Most of these studies enrolled patients < 65 years old. Older individuals (< age 70) may tolerate high-dose therapy with peripheral stem-cell support well, without excess mortality. Moreover, outcome, in terms of event-free and overall survival, is comparable to that in matched cohorts < 65 years old, making older individuals (≥ 65 years old) also candidates for high-dose therapy. More recently, older patients (> age 70) receiving intermediate-dose melphalan (100 mg/m^2) with stem-cell support have been shown to have a better outcome than matched controls receiving conventional therapy.

A high-dose alkylating agent, most commonly melphalan at 200 mg/m^2 with peripheral blood stem-cell support, is a standard conditioning regimen. Addition of total-body irradiation (TBI) does not improve the outcome but increases morbidity and results in higher mortality. Interestingly, in a randomized study, Fermand et al have confirmed an equivalent survival benefit between up-front high-dose therapy vs high-dose therapy as a salvage regimen at relapse following initial induction therapy.

Tandem transplants Improved outcome reported after tandem transplants in large cohorts of patients in single-institution studies has been confirmed in a mature randomized study. Seven years after initiation of therapy, the event-free (42% vs 21%) and overall survival (20% vs 10%) rates were superior for patients receiving tandem transplants (IFM 94). Another randomized trial with a shorter follow-up has confirmed the superior event-free survival (median, 34 vs 25 months) for patients receiving tandem transplants. However, the added benefit of the second transplant was not seen in a subset of patients with a complete response or a very good partial response (> 90% paraprotein reduction) after the first transplant.

Radiotherapy

Higher doses of radiotherapy (40–50 Gy) are employed for local control and cure of solitary plasmacytoma involving bone and extramedullary sites. Lower doses (20–30 Gy) may be employed for palliation of local bone pain from tumor infiltration, pathologic fractures, and spinal cord compression. It should be emphasized that excellent pain relief may be obtained by prompt institution of high-dose corticosteroid therapy, especially in newly diagnosed patients.

Radiotherapy should be employed sparingly, as irradiation of multiple sites may impair stem-cell mobilization in patients who are candidates for high-dose therapy. Employment of high doses of radiation to the spine may preclude the subsequent use of TBI as a conditioning regimen for high-dose therapy.

REMISSION MAINTENANCE

Alkylating agents Maintenance therapy with alkylating agents has not prolonged survival, compared with no maintenance therapy. This approach is no longer recommended.

Steroids for maintenance Two large randomized trials have shown glucocorticoid maintenance prolongs the duration of remission and life expectancy. The first trial by the Southwest Oncology Group (SWOG) used prednisone (50 mg) every other day, whereas the maintenance regimen in the National Cancer Institute (NCI)-Canada trial contained dexamethasone (40 mg) daily for 4 days every 4 weeks.

Thalidomide Patients responding to thalidomide and achieving maximal response have received lower dose thalidomide (50–100 mg) with or without added dexamethasone (40 mg for 4 days every month) as maintenance therapy. In the MPT regimen, continued administration of thalidomide prolongs the duration of remission. The IFM 99-06 study evaluated maintenance therapy with thalidomide plus pamidronate compared with pamidronate alone compared with observation only following tandem autologous transplantation. Superior event-free survival (EFS) and overall survival were reported in the cohort receiving thalidomide plus pamidronate.

α-Interferon Twenty-four randomized trials have investigated α-interferon as maintenance therapy and reported no consistent significant benefit. A recent larger intergroup trial also reported no benefit of interferon maintenance therapy after conventional therapy and autotransplantation.

Novel agents Bortezomib is currently under study as a maintenance strategy. In the APEX study, bortezomib administered weekly proved efficacious and was well tolerated in responding patients who had successfully completed initial treatment. Lenalidomide is also under study as maintenance post-transplant, given at a low dose (10 mg/d).

REFRACTORY OR RELAPSING DISEASE

Approximately 10%–30% of patients with newly diagnosed multiple myeloma are unresponsive to chemotherapy. Moreover, virtually all patients who respond initially will relapse. Of patients who relapse after an unmaintained remission, approximately 60% achieve a second remission or stable disease with resumption of the original therapy.

Conventional chemotherapy

Alkylating agents, alone or in combination, have been effective in approximately one-third of patients with VAD-refractory disease. IV melphalan (70–100 mg/m^2) and the combination of high-dose cyclophosphamide and etoposide are two examples of such regimens (Table 4).

Thalidomide has an established role in therapy for refractory/relapsed multiple myeloma, with 30% of patients achieving at least 50% reduction in paraprotein levels. Remissions obtained are durable: In a large cohort of patients with multiple myeloma receiving thalidomide, 2-year event-free survival rates of ~25% have been observed. Initially, thalidomide was employed in a dose-escalating schedule, starting at 200 mg and achieving a maximal dose of 800 mg. Recently, lower doses have been employed in combination with steroids (Table 4).

High-dose chemotherapy High-dose melphalan and stem-cell rescue should be offered to patients who have deferred the transplant initially. A randomized trial on early vs late transplantation has shown that a survival benefit is conferred on the patients undergoing salvage transplantation.

Novel agents

Lenalidomide (Revlimid, also known as CC-5013) is a small molecule, thalidomide analog with immunomodulatory effects. It has greater potency than thalidomide in preclinical studies and is better tolerated, with less neurotoxicity, somnolence, or constipation. In a phase II trial, lenalidomide (30 mg daily for 3 weeks on and 1 week off) induced minimal responses or better in 25% of patients with relapsed or refractory myeloma. The addition of dexamethasone in 68 patients who either progressed or remained stable on lenalidomide monotherapy resulted in additional response in 29%.

Two large multicenter phase III trials of lenalidomide with dexamethasone compared with dexamethasone and placebo in relapsed multiple myeloma have demonstrated a significant improvement in response rate (partial response, 59% vs 21%, respectively) and time to disease progression (11.1 vs 4.7 months, respectively) in the cohort receiving the lenalidomide combination in one study and almost identical results in the second study. Deep vein thrombosis was a significant complication of this combination, occurring in approximately 15% of patients.

TABLE 5: Supportive therapies for multiple myeloma

Problem	Therapy
Chronic anemia (especially with renal impairment)	Erythropoietin
Prolonged neutropenia with infection	G-CSF
Recurrent infections with IgG < 400 mg/dL	Gamma globulin
Osteoporosis	Bisphosphonates

G-CSF = granulocyte colony-stimulating factor

Proteasome inhibition Bortezomib (Velcade, PS-341) is a first-in-class, potent, selective, and reversible small molecule inhibitor of the proteasome. The proteasome plays a key role in the degradation of ubiquinated proteins, which in turn have important functions in controlling tumor cell growth and survival both in vitro and in vivo.

A large multi-institution phase II trial of bortezomib (given IV at a dose of 1.3 mg/m^2 on days 1, 4, 8, and 11 every 21 days) demonstrated remarkable activity in a heavily treated, relapsed and refractory patient population, including patients in whom transplantation failed and patients not responding to thalidomide, with durable responses in about 35% receiving bortezomib alone (with a number of complete responses). Side effects related to the drug were predominantly gastrointestinal in nature, with neuropathy, fatigue, and reversible cytopenias also noted. Toxicities were generally manageable with supportive care and dose reduction. Patients who did not respond to bortezomib monotherapy (progressive disease after 2 cycles or stable disease after the first 4 cycles) were permitted to receive combination bortezomib and dexamethasone. Combination therapy induced additional responses in 18% of patients (13 of 74).

The results of a large, randomized phase III trial of bortezomib monotherapy compared with high-dose dexamethasone enrolled 669 patients with relapsed multiple myeloma and showed significant improvement in the median time to disease progression (5.7 vs 3.6 months, respectively; $P < .0001$) and median overall survival (29.8 vs 23.7 months, respectively; $P = .027$). Response rates to bortezomib as a single agent were impressive at 38%. The most commonly reported adverse events for bortezomib were gastrointestinal events, fatigue, pyrexia, and thrombocytopenia; for dexamethasone, they were fatigue, insomnia, and anemia.

Clinical studies are ongoing with bortezomib in combination with pegylated liposomal doxorubicin, thalidomide, melphalan, and lenalidomide, and have shown impressive disease control in refractory myeloma. In patients with relapsed or refractory multiple myeloma, the objective response rate for bortezomib plus pegylated liposomal doxorubicin (30 mg/m^2 on day 4) in a phase I dose-escalation study was 77%. When bortezomib (1.0 or 1.3 mg/m^2) was administered with thalidomide (in doses ranging from 50 to 200 mg starting at cycle 2), 86% of patients with relapsed or refractory disease achieved a complete or partial response. A phase I trial combining bortezomib with lenalidomide has recently been completed and results have revealed less neuropathy than that seen with thalidomide. Remarkable activity has been reported with approximately 60% of patients achieving response despite having received multiple prior therapies, including both agents separately before study entry.

Arsenic trioxide (Trisenox), administered as a daily IV infusion dosed at 0.15 mg/kg in a phase II study, has shown response in 3 of 14 patients with relapsed refractory disease. Adverse effects included cytopenia requiring G-CSF (granulocyte colony-stimulating factor, filgrastim, Neupogen) support. Based on preclinical data suggesting synergism between arsenic trioxide, dexamethasone, and ascorbic acid, a phase II evaluation of this combination is in progress, as are studies with melphalan.

Allogeneic transplantation For younger patients with resistant relapse or poor-prognosis disease (ie, deletion of chromosome 13), allogeneic transplantation may be an important option. However, high treatment-related mortality (30%–50%) with myeloablative allogeneic transplantation has discouraged the use of allografts in early-phase myeloma. New nonmyeloablative transplantation procedures that reduce mortality and exploit a graft-vs-tumor effect are being studied. In one study, 34 patients, including patients with relapsed or refractory disease, received melphalan at 200 mg/m^2 with autografting and then (40–120 days later) received allograft after nonmyeloablative conditioning. Treatment-related mortality at day 100 was 6%, with 53% of patients achieving complete response. With a median follow-up of 328 days after allografting, the overall survival rate was 81%, but chronic graft-vs-host disease remains a major challenge, occurring in up to two-thirds of patients.

Supportive therapies

Various supportive therapies may be beneficial in patients with multiple myeloma (Table 5).

Chronic anemia Patients with chronic symptomatic anemia may benefit from a trial of epoetin alfa (Epogen, Procrit), 40,000 U given by SC injection once weekly. Darbepoetin alfa (Aranesp), dosed at 200 to 300 μg by SC injection every 2 to 3 weeks, is an alternative approach.

Infection Serious infection with encapsulated organisms is encountered by patients with myeloma due to their inability to mount successful antibody production (and lack of opsonization). Prompt institution of antibiotics is therefore recommended in the face of systemic infection. Antibiotic prophylaxis is also recommended whenever high-dose glucocorticoids are used for treatment. Patients with recurrent serious infections may benefit from monthly gamma globulin. Shingles is not uncommon in these patients, and prophylaxis following transplantation and during bortezomib therapy is advised.

Bone pain or imminent fracture Therapy with bisphosphonates, such as pamidronate, alendronate (Fosamax), or zoledronic acid (Zometa), may prevent or delay bone pain or recurrent or imminent pathologic fracture in patients with stage III disease and at least one bone lesion. Pamidronate administered over the long term (21 monthly treatments) to patients with stage III multiple myeloma with at least one lytic lesion has been shown to reduce skeletal events and decrease the need for irradiation. Moreover, patients without lytic lesions also show a decrease in bone mineral density, and this decrease persists despite chemotherapy. These patients may also benefit from therapy with pamidronate. Several clinical and preclinical studies suggest that pamidronate may have an antimyeloma effect.

Zoledronic acid, a more potent bisphosphonate, has comparable efficacy and safety to pamidronate in treatment of skeletal lesions. The ease of administration of a 4-mg dose, which reduces the infusion time to 15 minutes compared with 2 hours for pamidronate, has led to approval of zoledronic acid by the US Food and Drug Administration (FDA) for prevention of bone-related complications in myeloma. Caution should be exercised with long-term use of bisphosphonates, as renal impairment and osteonecrosis of the jaw bones have been reported.

Percutaneous vertebroplasty provides pain relief that is not only rapid but sustained, and it also strengthens the vertebral bodies. Kyphoplasty is a safer procedure that involves insertion of a balloon followed by injection of polymethyl methacrylate, the principal component of bone cement, in the balloon. It is performed with the patient under local anesthesia. Transient worsening of pain and fever may occur and is responsive to nonsteroidal anti-inflammatory agents.

Smoldering myeloma

Smoldering myeloma is an asymptomtic plasma cell dyscrasia that is diagnosed by the chance finding of an elevated serum protein concentration during a screening examination.

Laboratory features Features of low tumor mass are usually present, without renal disease, hypercalcemia, or lytic bone lesions (Table 2). Marrow plasma cytosis occurs in less than 30% of patients, and anemia, if present, is mild (hemoglobin value > 10.5 g/dL).

Treatment Chemotherapy should be withheld until there is clear disease progression or a risk of a complication. The role of bisphosphonates and thalidomide in this setting is under investigation.

Prognostic factors Recent studies have helped define prognostic criteria for groups at high risk of early disease progression (eg, cytogenetic changes [especially chromosome 13], labeling index of plasma cells [> 0.4%], β2M levels [4 mg/L], and diffuse disease activity or multiple focal lesions on MRI evaluation). Such criteria, along with the presence of lytic lesions, serum myeloma protein > 5 g/dL, and Bence Jones protein > 500 mg/24 h, identify patients at high risk of disease progression, in whom the early commencement of chemotherapy may be beneficial.

OTHER PLASMA CELL DYSCRASIAS

Other plasma cell dyscrasias include MGUS, solitary plasmacytoma of bone (SPB), solitary extramedullary plasmacytoma, Waldenström's macroglobulinemia, amyloidosis, POEMS (polyneuropathy, organomegaly, endocrinopathy, monoclonal gammopathy, and skin changes) syndrome, and heavy-chain diseases.

Monoclonal gammopathy of unknown significance

MGUS occurs in 1% of normal individuals > 40 years old, and its frequency rises progressively with age.

Laboratory features Common laboratory features of MGUS are listed in Table 2.

Treatment Approximately 25% of patients with this disorder develop multiple myeloma, macroglobulinemia, or non-Hodgkin lymphoma over 20 years. The initial concentration of serum monoclonal protein > 1.5 g/dL, non-IgG-type paraprotein, and abnormal serum free light chain ratio are significant predictors of disease progression at 20 years. The long period of stability supports annual monitoring with serum electrophoresis and blood counts and suggests that chemotherapy may be withheld until there is evidence of a serious disorder.

Solitary plasmacytoma of bone

Approximately 3% of patients with myeloma have SPB.

Laboratory features All patients have either no myeloma protein or very low levels in serum or urine (Table 2). MRI may reveal abnormalities not detected by bone survey and may upstage patients to multiple myeloma. Persistence of monoclonal protein for more than 1 year after irradiation predicts early progression to multiple myeloma.

Treatment of SPB consists of radiation therapy (at least 45 Gy). Multiple myeloma becomes evident in most patients over time, so only 20% of patients remain free of disease for more than 10 years. The median time for disease progression is 2–3 years.

Solitary extramedullary plasmacytoma

In contrast to SPB, solitary extramedullary plasmacytoma is often truly localized and can be cured in up to 50% of patients with localized radiation therapy (45–50 Gy) and/or resection.

Waldenström's macroglobulinemia

This uncommon disease is characterized by lymphoplasmacytic bone marrow and tissue infiltrate in addition to elevated IgM production. The mutation pattern analysis suggests that final transformation occurs in the postgerminal center IgM memory B cell. Corresponding with variation in cell morphology, there is variation in the immunophenotype. Mature plasma cells exhibit CD38 antigen; however, lymphoid cells are typically CD19, CD20, CD22, and FMC7 positive.

Waldenström's macroglobulinemia usually affects people in the fifth to seventh decades of life and can cause symptoms due to tumor infiltration (marrow, lymph nodes, and/or spleen), circulating IgM (hyperviscosity, cryoglobulinemia, and/or cold agglutinin hemolytic anemia), and tissue deposition of IgM (neuropathy, glomerular disease, and/or amyloidosis).

Hyperviscosity syndrome With hyperviscosity syndrome, patients may have visual symptoms, dizziness, cardiopulmonary symptoms, decreased consciousness, and a bleeding diathesis. Neuropathy is usually due to an IgM antibody reacting with a myelin-associated glycoprotein (MAG).

Therapy for hyperviscosity consists of plasmapheresis followed by chemotherapy to control the malignant proliferation. Patients with poor performance status and elderly patients unable to tolerate chemotherapy may be maintained with periodic plasmapheresis.

Treatment Alkylating agents in combination with steroids or purine analogs remain the mainstay of therapy. Alkylating agents alone or in combination with steroids effect a 50% reduction in paraprotein in about half of patients, and the median survival time is around 5 years. The purine analogs fludarabine and cladribine (2-CdA) elicit a more rapid response than other agents, with a response rate of more than 75% observed in small series of patients. Preliminary results of a large, American multi-institution evaluation of fludarabine reported partial responses in only 33% of patients.

Purine analog therapy may result in significant myelosuppression in later cycles of therapy and prolonged immunosuppression with increased opportunistic infections. Purine analogs are effective salvage options in patients refractory to or relapsing following alkylator therapy. Patients refractory to one purine analog are rarely salvaged by a different purine analog. Patients with resistant relapse are less likely to benefit (response rate, 18%) and should be considered for more intensive intervention, including high-dose therapy.

Other treatment options Rituximab (Rituxan), an anti-CD20 monoclonal antibody, is effective in Waldenström's macroglobulinemia because the CD20 antigen is usually present on the lymphoid cell component of macroglobulinemia. Preliminary results indicate that about 30% of previously treated patients (refractory or relapsing off therapy) may benefit from rituximab.

Striking activity of thalidomide in multiple myeloma has prompted its use in Waldenström's macroglobulinemia. In a series of 20 patients receiving thalidomide, 25% achieved a 50% reduction in paraprotein. Higher doses of thalidomide were not well tolerated in an elderly cohort of patients. Interestingly, preliminary results of bortezomib-based therapy in relapsed Waldenström's macroglobulinemia have been promising.

High-dose therapy with autologous bone marrow or blood stem-cell rescue has been effective in achieving 50% reduction in paraprotein in almost all patients in small pilot trials.

Amyloidosis

Amyloidosis occurs in 10% of patients with multiple myeloma. This infiltrative process results from organ deposition of amyloid fibrils, which consist of the NH_2 terminal amino acid residues of the variable portion of the light-chain immunoglobulin molecule. The abnormal protein is produced by clonal plasma cells.

Clinical features include the nephrotic syndrome, cardiomyopathy, hepatomegaly, neuropathy, macroglossia, carpal tunnel syndrome, and periorbital purpura.

Laboratory features Serum and urine immunofixation studies show a monoclonal immunoglobulin in approximately 80% of patients. The light chain is more frequently of the λ than κ type. Diagnosis can be made by the presence of apple-green birefringence on polarized light examination of subcutaneous fat aspirates stained with Congo red.

Treatment of AL (monoclonal protein–associated) amyloidosis Survival of patients with amyloidosis is variable. Patients with congestive heart failure have a median survival of only 4 months. Oral MP extends the median survival to 17 months, compared with 13 months in untreated patients. Complete hematologic response is rare; similarly, reversal of organ damage is uncommon.

In a large cohort of patients receiving high-dose melphalan with stem-cell support, a complete hematologic response was observed in 47% of patients with at least 1 year of follow-up. However, the transplant-related mortality is high with high-dose therapy (14%–37%). Complete hematologic response was associated with improved clinical response (improved organ function) and survival. Complete hematologic response in the absence of cardiac involvement predicted excellent outcome (1-year survival, 91%).

Patients with the overlap syndrome of myeloma and AL amyloidosis should be treated aggressively for myeloma; response can be seen in terms of both myeloma and resolution of amyloid symptoms.

POEMS syndrome

Clinical features and course The POEMS syndrome is a rare plasma cell dyscrasia that presents with peripheral, usually sensorimotor, neuropathy; monoclonal gammopathy (IgA λ being more common); sclerotic bone lesions, noted in nearly all patients; and organomegaly, endocrinopathy, and skin changes.

Other features include hyperpigmentation, hypertrichosis, thickened skin, papilledema, lymphadenopathy, peripheral edema, hepatomegaly, splenomegaly, and hypothyroidism. Diabetes mellitus is not part of this syndrome.

Compared with patients with symptomatic myeloma, individuals with POEMS syndrome are younger (median age, 51 years) and live longer (median, 8 years). The clinical course is commonly characterized by progressive neuropathy.

Treatment Plasmapheresis does not appear to be of benefit in POEMS syndrome, and patients are often treated similarly to those with myeloma. Patients presenting with isolated sclerotic lesions may have substantial resolution of neuropathic symptoms after local therapy for plasmacytoma with surgery and/or radiotherapy. Autologous SCT has been pursued in selected patients and has been associated with prolonged progression-free survival.

Heavy-chain diseases

Heavy-chain diseases are plasma cell dyscrasias characterized by the production of heavy-chain immunoglobulin molecules (IgG, IgA, IgM) that lack light chains.

α Heavy-chain disease results from lymphocyte and plasma cell infiltration of the mesenteric nodes and small bowel and has features of malabsorption, such as diarrhea, weight loss, abdominal pain, edema, and nail clubbing. The heavy-chain molecule may be detected in serum, jejunal secretions, and urine.

γ Heavy-chain disease Patients with γ heavy-chain disease may present with fever, weakness, lymphadenopathy, hepatosplenomegaly, and involvement of Waldeyer's ring. Eosinophilia, leukopenia, and thrombocytopenia are common. Treatment with regimens similar to those used for non-Hodgkin lymphoma may be effective.

μ Heavy-chain disease is seen exclusively in patients with chronic lymphocytic leukemia (CLL). Vacuolated plasma cells are common in the marrow, and many patients have κ light chains in the urine. Therapy is similar to that used for CLL (see chapter 34).

SUGGESTED READING

ON MULTIPLE MYELOMA

Attal M, Harousseau JL, Facon T, et al: Single versus double autologous stem-cell transplantation for multiple myeloma. N Engl J Med 349:2495–2502, 2003.

Badros A, Barlogie B, Morris C, et al: High response rate in refractory and poor-risk multiple myeloma after allo-transplantation using a nonmyeloablative conditioning regimen and donor lymphocyte infusions. Blood 97:2574–2579, 2001.

Barlogie B, Desikan R, Eddlemon P, et al: Extended survival in advanced and refractory myeloma after single-agent thalidomide: Identification of prognostic factors in a phase II study of 169 patients. Blood 98:492–494, 2001.

Berenson JR, Crowley JJ, Grogan TM, et al: Maintenance therapy with alternate-day prednisone improves survival in multiple myeloma patients. Blood 99:3163–3168, 2002.

Facon T, Avet-Losieau H, Guillerm G, et al: Chromosome 13 abnormalities identified by FISH analysis and serum b_2-microglobulin produce a powerful myeloma staging system for patients receiving high-dose therapy. Blood 97:1566–1571, 2001.

Fermand JP, Ravaud P, Chevret S, et al: High-dose therapy and autologous peripheral blood stem cell transplantation in multiple myeloma: Up-front or rescue treatment? Results of a multicenter sequential randomized clinical trial. Blood 92:3131–3136, 1998.

Hideshima T, Richardson P, Chauhan D, et al: The proteasome inhibitor PS-341 inhibits growth, induces apoptosis, and overcomes drug resistance in human multiple myeloma cells. Cancer Res 61:3071–3076, 2001.

Jagannath S, Durie BG, Wolf J, et al: Bortezomib therapy alone and in combination with dexamethasone for previously untreated symptomatic multiple myeloma. Br J Haematol 129:776–783, 2005.

Kyle RA, Rajkumar SV: Multiple myeloma. N Engl J Med 351:1860–1873, 2004.

Munshi NC, Hideshima T, Carrasco D, et al: Identification of genes modulated in multiple myeloma using genetically identical twin samples. Blood 103:1799–1806, 2004.

Rajkumar SV, Blood E, Vesole D, et al: Phase III clinical trial of thalidomide plus dexamethasone compared with dexamethasone alone in newly diagnosed multiple myeloma: A clinical trial coordinated by the Eastern Cooperative Oncology Group. J Clin Oncol 24:431–436, 2006.

Richardson PG, Schlossman RL, Weller E, et al: Immunomodulatory derivative of thalidomide CC-5013 overcomes drug resistance and is well tolerated in patients with relapsed multiple myeloma. Blood 100:3063–3067, 2002.

Richardson PG, Sonneveld P, Schuster MW, et al, for the Assessment of Proteasome Inhibition for Extending Remissions (APEX) Investigators: Bortezomib or high-dose dexamethasone for relapsed multiple myeloma. N Engl J Med 352:2487-2498, 2005.

Rosen LS, Gordon D, Antonio BS, et al: Zoledronic acid vs pamidronate in the treatment of skeletal metastases in patients with breast cancer or osteolytic lesions of multiple myeloma: A phase III, double-blind, comparative trial. Cancer J 7:377–387, 2001.

ON OTHER PLASMA CELL DYSCRASIAS

Dhodapkar MV, Jacobson JL, Gertz MA, et al: Prognostic factors and response to fludarabine therapy in Waldenström's macroglobulinemia: Results of US intergroup trial (Southwest Oncology Group S9003). Blood 98:41–48, 2001.

Dimopoulos MA, Zomas A, Viniou NA, et al: Treatment of Waldenström's macroglobulinemia with thalidomide. J Clin Oncol 19:3596–3601, 2001.

Sanchorawala V, Wright DG, Seldin DC, et al: An overview of the use of high-dose melphalan with autologous stem-cell transplantation for the treatment of AL amyloidosis. Bone Marrow Transplant 28:637–642, 2001.

Weber D, Treon SP, et al: Uniform response criteria in Waldenstrom's macroglobulinemia: Consensus panel recommendations for the Second International Workshop on Waldenstrom's macroglobulinemia. Semin Oncol 30:127–131, 2003.

CHAPTER 32

Acute leukemias

Margaret R. O'Donnell, MD

Hematopoietic malignancies account for 6%-8% of new cancers diagnosed annually. In the year 2007, an estimated 44,240 new cases of leukemia will be diagnosed, and 21,790 deaths will be attributable to leukemias of all types. The total age-adjusted incidence of leukemia, including both acute and chronic forms, is 9.6 per 100,000 population; the incidence of acute lymphoblastic leukemia (ALL) is 1.5 per 100,000 and of acute myelogenous leukemia (AML) is 2.7 per 100,000 population.

Epidemiology

Gender The incidence of both ALL and AML is slightly higher in males than in females.

Age The age-specific incidence of AML is similar to that of other solid tumors in adults, with an exponential rise after age 40. With regard to ALL, 60% of cases are seen in children, with a peak incidence in the first 5 years of life and a subsequent drop in incidence until age 60, when a second peak emerges.

Race and ethnicity The incidence of acute leukemia is slightly higher in populations of European descent. Also, a report from the University of Southern California indicates that acute promyelocytic leukemia (APL) is more common in Hispanic populations than in other ethnic groups.

Etiology and risk factors

There is wide diversity in the behavior of the various subsets of acute leukemias. Thus, it is unlikely that there is one common etiology for these aberrant cellular proliferations. There are, however, some accepted risk factors for leukemogenesis.

Chemical exposure Increased incidence of AML and myelodysplasia (preleukemia) has been reported in persons with prolonged exposure to benzene and petroleum products. The interval between exposure and the onset of leukemia is long (10–30 years). Chromosomal damage is common.

Pesticide exposure also has been linked to some forms of AML. The incidence of AML is beginning to rise in developing countries, as industrialization and pollution increase.

Other environmental exposures Exposure to hair dyes, smoking, and non-ionic radiation may also increase the risk of leukemia.

Prior chemotherapy or irradiation Use of alkylating agents, such as cyclophosphamide and melphalan (Alkeran), in the treatment of lymphomas, myelomas, and breast and ovarian cancers has been associated with the development of AML, usually within 3–5 years of exposure and often preceded by a myelodysplastic phase. Cytogenetic abnormalities, particularly monosomy 5, 7, 11, and 17, are common. Concurrent radiation exposure slightly increases the risk of leukemogenesis posed by alkylating agents.

Topoisomerase II inhibitors (etoposide, teniposide [Vumon], doxorubicin and its derivatives, and mitoxantrone [Novantrone]), used to treat ALL, myeloma, testicular cancer, and sarcomas, have also been implicated in leukemogenesis. These agents, in contrast to alkylators, are associated with a short latency period without antecedent myelodysplasia and with cytogenetic abnormalities involving chromosome 11q23 or 21q22 in the malignant clone.

Genetic disorders An increased incidence of AML is seen in patients with Down syndrome, Bloom syndrome, or Fanconi's anemia, as well as in individuals with ataxia-telangiectasia or Wiskott-Aldrich syndrome. In identical twins younger than age 10, if one child develops leukemia (usually ALL), there is a 20% chance that the other twin will develop leukemia within a year; subsequently, the risk falls off rapidly and joins that of nonidentical siblings, which is three to five times that of the general population.

Signs and symptoms

Effects on hematopoiesis Leukemia manifests symptomatically by its impact on normal hematopoiesis. Thus, easy fatigability, bruising, or bleeding from mucosal surfaces, fever, and persistent infection are all reflections of the anemia, thrombocytopenia, and decrease in functional neutrophils associated with marrow replacement by malignant cells. Bone pain is common in children with ALL (occurring in 40%–50%) but is less common in adults with acute leukemias (5%–10%).

WBC count elevation and pancytopenia Whereas a marked elevation in WBC count is the classic hallmark of leukemia, pancytopenia is more common, particularly in patients of all ages with ALL or in elderly patients with AML, who may have had preexisting marrow dysfunction (myelodysplasia). Only 10% of newly diagnosed patients with either AML or ALL present with leukocyte counts > 100,000/μL. These patients, however, constitute a poor prognostic group and are at increased risk of CNS disease, tumor lysis syndrome, and leukostasis due to impedance of blood flow from intravascular clumping of blasts, which are "stickier" than mature myeloid or lymphoid cells.

Leukostasis may manifest as an alteration in mental status; intermittent or persistent cranial nerve palsies, particularly those involving extraocular muscles; priapism; dyspnea; or pleuritic chest pain, due to small leukemic emboli in the pulmonary vasculature.

Physical findings in AML are usually minimal. Pallor, increased ecchymoses or petechiae, retinal hemorrhage, gingival hypertrophy, and cutaneous involvement are more common with monocytic (M4 or M5) variants of AML than with other variants of AML.

Hepatosplenomegaly and lymphadenopathy Mild hepatosplenomegaly and lymphadenopathy are seen in many cases, particularly in childhood ALL. Massive hepatosplenomegaly occurs infrequently and should raise the suspicion of a leukemia evolving from a prior hematologic disorder, such as chronic myelogenous leukemia (CML) or myelodysplasia. Mediastinal adenopathy is seen in 80% of cases of T-cell ALL, is less common in other ALLs, and is rare in AML.

Visceral involvement is also rare, occurring as an initial manifestation of AML in < 5% of cases, but it may be more frequent during subsequent relapses. These focal collections of blasts, called chloromas or granulocytic sarcomas, can present as soft-tissue masses, infiltrative lesions of the small bowel and mesentery, or obstructing lesions of the hepatobiliary or genitourinary system.

CNS involvement is uncommon at presentation in adult AML (< 1%) and adult ALL (3%–5%). In most instances, CNS involvement is detected by screening lumbar puncture in high-risk patients who are asymptomatic at the time of the puncture. Symptoms, when they do occur, include headache, diplopia, cranial nerve palsies, radicular pain, and/or weakness in a particular nerve root distribution. CNS involvement usually is restricted to leptomeninges; parenchymal mass lesions are uncommon.

Testicular involvement Like the CNS, the testes appear to be a "sanctuary" for isolated relapses in pediatric but not adult ALL. Signs of testicular involvement include painless, asymmetrical enlargement.

Metabolic effects of acute leukemia relate primarily to the rate of cell death.

Hyperuricemia with possible interstitial or ureteral obstruction is seen predominantly in AML with moderate leukocytosis; this condition may be exacerbated by a rapid response to chemotherapy and the "tumor lysis syndrome" (hyperuricemia with renal insufficiency, acidosis, hyperphosphatemia, and hypocalcemia), which may occur within the first 24–48 hours after initiating chemotherapy. To prevent this complication, all patients should receive allopurinol and urine alkalinization before marrow-ablative chemotherapy is initiated. In patients with high tumor burden, renal insufficiency, or acidosis prior to initiation of chemotherapy, rasburicase may offer a more rapid treatment for hyperuricemia. (For a more detailed discussion of hyperuricemia and tumor lysis syndrome, see chapter 45.)

Coagulopathies can also complicate the hemostatic defects associated with thrombocytopenia. Disseminated intravascular coagulation (DIC) is most often seen in APL (French-American-British Cooperative group [FAB] subtype M3) due to release of procoagulants from the abnormal primary granules, which activate the coagulation cascade, leading to decreased factors II, V, VIII, and X, and fibrinogen, as well as rapid platelet consumption. Lysozyme released from monoblasts in M4 and M5 subtypes of AML can also trigger the clotting cascade. Finally, DIC can occur following asparaginase (Elspar) chemotherapy for ALL.

TABLE 1: WHO classification of AML

AMLs with recurrent cytogenetic translocations	
	AML with t(8;21)(q22;q22), AML1(CBF-alpha)/ETO
	APL [APL with t(15;17),(q22;q11-12] and variants, PML/RAR-alpha
	AML with abnormal bone marrow eosinophils [inv(16)(p13;q22) or t(16;16)(p13;q11), CBFβ/MYH11X]
	AML with 11q23 (mixed-lineage leukemia) abnormalities
AML with multilineage dysplasia	
	With prior myelodysplastic syndrome (MDS)
	Without prior MDS
AML and MDS, therapy-related	
	Alkylating agent-related
	Epipodophyllotoxin-related (some may be lymphoid)
	Other types
AML not otherwise categorized	
	AML minimally differentiated (M0)
	AML without maturation (M1)
	AML with maturation (M2)
	Acute myelomonocytic leukemia (M4)
	Acute monocytic leukemia (M5)
	Acute erythroid leukemia (M6)
	Acute megakaryocytic leukemia (M7)
	Acute basophilic leukemia
	Acute panmyelosis with myelofibrosis
Acute biphenotypic leukemias	

AML = acute myelogenous leukemia; APL = acute promyelocytic leukemia; WHO = World Health Organization

Vardiman JW, Harris NL, Brunning RD: Blood 100:2292–2302, 2002.

Diagnosis

Abnormalities on the CBC raise the possibility of leukemia. The diagnosis is substantiated pathologically by a bone marrow examination.

All patients should have cytochemistry, immunophenotyping by fluorescent-activated cell sorter (FACS) using monoclonal antibodies directed at leukemia-specific antigens and cytogenetic analysis of the marrow or peripheral blood blasts at diagnosis. Other tests used to evaluate metabolic abnormalities (electrolytes, creatinine, and liver function tests) and coagulopathies are also needed at diagnosis. A lumbar puncture should be performed at diagnosis in all pediatric patients with ALL and in all patients with neurologic symptoms regardless of age and pathology.

Pathology and cytogenetics

Acute leukemias comprise a group of clonal disorders of maturation at an early phase of hematopoietic differentiation. Morphology and cytochemical stains designed to detect intracellular myeloperoxidase or esterases have been the traditional methods used to classify acute leukemias into either myeloid or lymphoid derivations.

TABLE 2: WHO classification of ALL

Precursor B-cell acute lymphoblastic leukemia (cytogenetic subgroups)	
	t(9;22)(a34;q11); *BCR/ABL*
	t(v;11q23); *MLL* rearranged
	t(1;19)(q23;p13) *E2A/PBX1*
	t(12;21)(p12;q22) *ETV/CBF*-alpha
Precursor T-cell acute lymphoblastic leukemia	
Burkitt-cell leukemia [t(8;14) or t(8;22)]	

ALL = acute lymphoblastic leukemia; WHO = World Health Organization
Harris NL, Jaffe ES, Diebold J, et al: J Clin Oncol 17:3835–3849, 1999.

Coupling these traditional methods with cytogenetic analysis and highly specific monoclonal antibodies directed against cell-surface antigens has led to the detection of new prognostic factors and has provided an approach to detect minimal residual disease.

In 1997, a panel of hematopathologists met to update the FAB classification of hematologic malignancies, which was based on morphology and cytochemistry alone. They proposed a new classification, incorporating immunophenotyping, cytogenetics, and clinical disease features, which has been adopted by the World Health Organization (WHO; Tables 1 and 2).

Myeloid leukemias

The new WHO classification retains the morphologic subgroups of the FAB system in the subgroup of "AML not otherwise categorized" but has created new categories that recognize the importance of certain cytogenetic translocations as predictors of response to therapy. In this category are AML with t(8;21)(q22;q22), AML with abnormal eosinophils and inv(16)(p13;q22) or t(16;16)(p13;q11), AML with 11q23 mixed-lineage leukemia abnormalities, and APL with t(15;17)(q22;q11-12) variants (Table 1).

The WHO classification also attempts to deal with the evidence that, in many older patients, marrow dysfunction antedates the onset of acute leukemia. These myelodysplastic syndromes (MDSs) are characterized by ineffective hematopoietic production and disrupted maturation of one or more cell lines. These abnormalities are often accompanied by loss of chromosomal material, particularly loss of chromosomes –5 or –5q, –7 or –7q, and –3 or –20. As the bone marrow becomes more dysfunctional, increasing numbers of blasts are seen in the marrow.

In the FAB classification, the demarcation line between myelodysplasia and AML was 30% marrow blasts. However, patients with 20%–29% blasts (previously classified as refractory anemia with excess blasts in transition [RAEB-t]) have a biologic behavior and poor survival similar to those of patients with AML. WHO recommended lowering the threshold for the diagnosis of AML to 20% marrow blasts and deleting the FAB category of RAEB-t. In addition, patients with 5%–20% blasts who have t(15;17), t(18;21), or inv(16) are considered to have AML rather than MDS and should receive AML treatment.

The WHO system further subdivides the AML patients with dysplastic maturation into those with or without antecedent cytopenias (usually 3 months prior to diagnosis had been the arbitrary cutoff point) and those with a history of prior exposure to chemotherapy agents (alkylating agents, epipodophyllotoxins, or others). In 2003, the International Working Group for the Diagnosis and Standardization of Response Criteria accepted the WHO classification as the standard for AML diagnosis.

The genetic profile of malignant cells has been found to vary widely from normal, with many genes being either overexpressed or suppressed. DNA microarray techniques allow the simultaneous analysis of thousands of genes that are being studied in AML and ALL for their predictive ability to define cohorts of patients with similar outcomes; this process may in turn allow the selection of candidate genes that can be used as therapeutic targets in the future.

Lymphoblastic leukemias

Lymphoblastic leukemias can arise from either B-cell or T-cell progenitors that arrest at an early stage of maturation and then proliferate. Marrow involvement of > 25% lymphoblasts is used as the demarcation line between lymphoblastic lymphoma, in which the preponderance of tumor bulk is in nodal structures, and ALL. Approximately 75% of adult ALLs are B cell in derivation and 25% are T cell.

Precursor B-cell ALL Most B-cell leukemias are early or "pre-B" cell, expressing CD19 and CD10 (the common acute leukemia antigen [cALLa]) but lacking surface or cytoplasmic immunoglobulin; this group of early B-cell leukemias has a more favorable prognosis than that of B-cell leukemias in which the cells have a more mature phenotype. Chromosomal rearrangements juxtaposing an oncogene with a promoter region are often seen in this disease category. A small fraction (2%) of patients with precursor B-cell ALL lack CD10 expression. Patients with CD10 disease have a high incidence of *MLL* gene expression (83%) and a very poor disease-free survival (12%) at 2 years. The new WHO classification identifies these cytogenetic subgroups (Table 2).

Mature B-cell ALL The more mature B-cell ALL, or Burkitt-cell leukemia, is associated with translocations of the c-*myc* gene on chromosome 8 and the immunoglobulin heavy-chain gene on chromosome 14q32 in 80% of cases or with the light-chain genes of chromosome 2p11 or 22q11 in the other 20%. Burkitt-cell leukemia has increased in frequency recently, as it is one of the lymphoproliferative disorders that occur in individuals infected with the human immunodeficiency virus (HIV); leukemia may appear early in the course of the HIV infection, before the onset of opportunistic infections or severe T-cell deficiency (see chapter 27).

T-cell ALL is frequently associated with translocations of T-cell receptor genes on chromosome 14q11 or 7q34 with other gene partners. T-cell ALL had been associated with a poor prognosis when treated with conventional ALL regimens but now is associated with a better prognosis if treated with aggressive antimetabolite therapy. Precursor T-cell ALL has a poorer outcome.

Infection with human T-cell leukemia virus-1 (HTLV-1) should be looked for in patients with T-cell ALL presenting with hypercalcemia and lytic bone lesions. HTLV-1 infection is endemic in southern Japan, the southern Pacific basin, the Caribbean basin, and sub-Saharan Africa. High infection rates are also seen in parts of Iran, India, and Hawaii. Recent immigrants from endemic areas retain a risk of infection similar to that of their point of origin. However, fewer than 0.1% of persons carrying HTLV-1 will develop T-cell leukemia.

ALL with myeloid antigen expression vs undifferentiated leukemia

A subset of patients with leukemia exhibit features of both myeloid and lymphoid differentiation. These patients were originally classified as having mixed-lineage leukemia. Patients with a leukemic clone that expresses two or more ALL antigens and one myeloid antigen comprise 20% of adult ALL cases. Although expression of myeloid antigen is considered to be a poor-risk feature in children, it does not constitute a distinct poor-risk feature in adults.

Immunophenotyping has also helped define a group of patients with undifferentiated myeloid leukemia (M0) who previously were likely to be treated as if they had ALL. These leukemias have a primitive morphology and lack myeloperoxidase. On immunophenotyping, they express at least one early myeloid antigen, usually CD13 or CD33, and no T- or B-cell markers. Based on immunophenotyping, undifferentiated leukemias are treated in the same manner as myeloid malignancies.

ALL prognostic factors

Cytogenetic abnormalities have a significant impact on the prognosis of patients with ALL. Approximately half of patients with ALL have cytogenetic abnormalities; they usually take the form of translocations of genetic information, rather than deletions of genetic material, which are seen more commonly in AML.

Philadelphia chromosome The most ominous cytogenetic abnormality in ALL is the translocation of the *abl* gene from chromosome 9 to the breakpoint cluster region on chromosome 22, forming a new gene product (BCR-ABL) with tyrosine kinase activity. This translocation, referred to as the Philadelphia chromosome (Ph), is found in 95% of cases of CML and in 20%–30% of newly diagnosed adults with ALL.

The fusion protein produced by the Bcr-Abl translocation in Ph+ ALL (p190) differs from the product seen in CML (p210); the p190 product is a smaller protein than the p210 product and has higher tyrosine kinase activity. Use of polymerase chain reaction (PCR) techniques that target only the p210 product will significantly underestimate the incidence of Ph+ ALL. In a recent update of the German ALL trials, 37% of patients were Ph+, with 77% showing the p190 product vs 23% showing the p210 product.

Although patients with Ph+ ALL may attain a morphologic remission with conventional chemotherapy (82%), almost all such patients will have persistent molecular evidence of disease. Patients who do achieve a molecular remission have a longer duration of remission than those who continue to express p190 or p210 activity (30 vs 12 months).

Recently, the GIMEMA group published outcomes data of a large trial of adult patients with ALL in which both cytogenetic data and molecular probes for specific gene products were combined to define prognostic groups. The molecular abnormalities that were evaluated were t(9;22) BCR-ABL, t(4;11)/MLL-AFA, t(1;19) E_2A/PBX_1, 9p/p15-p16 deletions, and 6q deletions. Categories based primarily on classic karyotypes were normal, hyperdiploid, and miscellaneous structural abnormalities of uncertain significance.

The use of molecular probes was particularly informative in patients with failed karyotypic analysis or normal cytogenetics. The use of the BCR-ABL probe increased the number of cases with a t(9;22) abnormality from 64 to 104 (26% of patients in the trial); more than 50% of add(9p)/p15-p16 abnormalities were detected only by molecular testing. Patients with t(9;22), t(4;11), and t(1;19) had disease-free intervals of 0.4–0.6 years, whereas those with del(6q), hyperdiploid, or pseudodiploid karyotypes had intermediate disease-free survival of 1.3–1.6 years; those with a normal karyotype or del(9p)/p15-p16 had better outcomes (2.9 and 4 years, respectively).

Other translocations Translocations involving the mixed-lineage leukemia gene at chromosome 11q23 are partnered with several other chromosomes, including 4q21, 9q22, and 19q13. Translocations involving chromosome 11q23 are frequently seen in secondary leukemias, particularly those arising after chemotherapy with etoposide or teniposide. Although most of these translocations are associated with AML, ALL has also arisen in this setting. All the 11q23 translocations, as well as the more common (1;19) translocation, are associated with poorer outcomes when compared with similar immunophenotypes coupled with normal cytogenetics.

Treatment strategy

Treatment for patients with ALL and AML can be subdivided into two or three phases. Induction chemotherapy is the initial treatment designed to clear the marrow of overt leukemia. This phase usually involves multiple drugs that cause pancytopenia for 2–3 weeks.

The purpose of consolidation therapy is to further reduce the residual leukemic burden in patients who are in morphologic remission. Molecular markers of residual disease can often be detected after induction chemotherapy, which indicates the need for further treatment. The intensity of consolidation therapy varies, depending on the risk of relapse (based primarily on cytogenetic risk groups) and patient age.

Maintenance chemotherapy using low-dose oral chemotherapy for 18–24 months has been shown to prolong relapse-free survival in pediatric patients with ALL and in adults with APL. Its value is less clear in adults with ALL; maintenance is rarely used in AML.

TREATMENT OF ALL

Although 70%–80% of pediatric patients with ALL can anticipate a prolonged remission or cure of disease with combination chemotherapy, the overall long-term disease-free survival for adults with ALL is 35%–50%. Poorer outcomes in adults are attributed to a higher incidence of unfavorable cytogenetic abnormalities [t(9;22), t(8;14), or t(4;11)t(1;19)] or coexpression of myeloid antigens, as well as to higher WBC counts at diagnosis.

Adults also have poorer tolerance for some of the chemotherapeutic agents used in treatment, such as asparaginase, as well as higher rates of infection and comorbid disease, all of which result in increased end-organ toxicity and frequent treatment delays.

Recent reports have emphasized a difference in outcomes for adolescents and young adults dependent upon treatment using pediatric or adult ALL protocols. In a comparison of 177 adolescents (15 to 20 years old) treated on the French pediatric trial vs adult regimens, the complete remission (CR) rate was 98% vs 81% and the 5-year event-free survival rate was 67% vs 41%. The pediatric regimen had significantly higher doses of asparaginase and prednisone and had much higher thresholds for dose reductions and interruption of therapy.

Induction therapy

The initial goal of therapy is to rapidly reduce the leukemic burden to a level undetectable by conventional methods of light microscopy and flow cytometry, a state that is deemed a CR. Two standard induction regimens have been used in adults with ALL—the Hoelzer regimen, developed by the Berlin-Frankfurt-Munster (BFM) multicenter group, and the Larson regimen, developed by the Cancer and Leukemia Group B (CALGB). Along with the standard induction schemas, two newer regimens, the Hyper-CVAD regimen from M. D. Anderson and the Linker regimen (2002 version), which have a similar induction drug dosing as the older regimens but include much higher doses of antimetabolites (cytarabine and methotrexate) and etoposide for dose-dense consolidations, are outlined in Table 3 along with the standard induction schemas. Overall, complete remissions are obtained in 80%–94% for adults younger than age 60 treated with any of these regimens.

The addition of an anthracycline to the standard pediatric leukemia induction regimen of vincristine, prednisone, and asparaginase increased the CR rate in adults from 50%–60% to 70%–85% in several series. In a recent CALGB study, the use of cytokines, ie, granulocyte colony-stimulating factor (G-CSF, filgrastim [Neupogen]), during induction in patients older than 60 years of age reduced treatment-related mortality from 31% to 5% when compared with placebo-treated controls.

The US Food and Drug Administration (FDA) recently approved pegaspargase (Oncaspar) as a component of a multiagent chemotherapy regimen for the first-

TABLE 3: ALL induction and consolidation therapy

Induction	Consolidation	CNS prophylaxis	Maintenance
BFM REGIMEN			
Phase I	**Phase I**[a]	**Weeks 5-8**	6-MP 60 mg/m² PO on weeks 10-18 and 29-130
VCR 2 mg IV on days 1, 8, 15, 22	VCR 2 mg IV on days 1, 8, 15, 22	MTX 10 mg IT on days 31, 38, 45, 52	
DNR 25 mg/m² IV on days 1, 8, 15, 22	Adria 25 mg/m² IV on days 1, 8, 15, 22		
PSE 60 mg/m² PO on days 1-28	Dex 10 mg/m² PO on days 1-28	Cranial RT[b] 2,400 cGy (given along with phase II induction)	MTX 20 mg PO or IV weekly on weeks 10-18 and 29-130
L-Asp 5,000 IU/m² IV on days 1-14			
Phase II	**Phase II**		
CTX 650 mg/m² IV on days 29, 43, 57 (maximum, 1,000 mg)	CTX 650 mg/m² IV on day 29		
	Ara-C 75 mg/m² IV on days 31-34, 38-41		
Ara-C 75 mg/m² IV on days 31-34, 38-41, 45-48, 52-55	6-TG 60 mg/m² PO on days 29-42		
6-MP 60 mg/m² IV on days 29-57			

Adria = Adriamycin (doxorubicin); ALL = acute lymphoblastic leukemia; Ara-C = cytarabine; BFM = Berlin-Frankfurt-Munster; CTX = cyclophosphamide; Dex = dexamethasone; DNR = daunorubicin; Dox = doxorubicin; L-Asp = L-asparaginase; 6-MP = mercaptopurine; MTX = methotrexate; PSE = prednisone; RT = radiation therapy; 6-TG = thioguanine; VCR = vincristine

[a] Begin week 20

[b] Cranial RT dose for prophylaxis is reduced to 1,800 cGy if patient is being considered for allogeneic BMT while in first complete remission

Induction and early intensification	CNS prophylaxis and interim maintenance	Late intensification	Prolonged maintenance
CALGB REGIMEN			
Course I: Induction (4 wk)	**Course III: CNS prophylaxis and interim maintenance[e] (12 wk)**	**Course IV: Late intensification[f] (8 wk)**	**Course V: Prolonged maintenance[g]**
CTX 1,200 mg/m^2 IV on day 1[c]	Cranial RT 2,400 cGy on days 1-12	Dox 30 mg/m^2 IV on days 1, 8, 15	VCR 2 mg IV on day 1 of q4wk
DNR 45 mg/m^2 IV on days 1-3[c]	MTX 15 mg IT on days 1, 8, 15, 22, 29	VCR 2 mg IV on days 1, 8, 15	PSE 60 mg/m^2/d on days 1-5 of q4wk
VCR 2 mg IV on days 1, 8, 15, 22	6-MP 60 mg/m^2/d PO on days 1-70	Dex 10 mg/m^2/d PO on days 1-14	MTX 20 mg/m^2 PO on days 1, 8, 15, 22
PSE 60 mg/m^2/d PO/IV on days 1-21[c]	MTX 20 mg/m^2 PO on days 36, 43, 50, 57, 64	CTX 1,000 mg/m^2 IV on day 29	6-MP 80 mg/m^2/d PO on days 1-28
L-Asp 6,000 IU/m^2 SC on days 5, 8, 11, 15, 18, 22		6-TG 60 mg/m^2/d PO on days 29-42	
		Ara-C 75 mg/m^2/d SC on days 29, 32, 36-39	
Course II: Early intensification[d] (4 wk; repeat once)			
MTX 15 mg IT on day 1			
CTX 1,000 mg/m^2 IV on day 1			
6-MP 60 mg/m^2/d PO on days 1-14			
Ara-C 75 mg/m^2/d SC on days 1-4, 8-11			
VCR 2 mg IV on days 15, 22			
L-Asp 6,000 IU/m^2 SC on days 15, 18, 22, 25			

[c]For patients > 60 years old, modify doses as follows: CTX, 800 mg/m^2 on day 1; DNR, 30 mg/m^2 on days 1-3; PSE, 60 mg/m^2 on days 1-7

[d] Weeks 5-12 [e] Weeks 13-25 [f] Begin week 26 [g] Until 24 months from diagnosis

TABLE 3: ALL induction and consolidation therapy *(continued)*

Induction/consolidation	Dosage
LINKER REGIMEN	
Induction 1A (DVPAsp)	
Daunorubicin	60 mg/m^2 IV on days 1-3 (and day 15 if day 14 bone marrow had residual leukemia)
Vincristine	1.4 mg/m^2 IV on days 1, 8, 15, and 22 (capped at 2.0 mg if age > 40 years)
Prednisone	60 mg/m^2 PO on days 1-28
Asparaginase	6,000 IU/m^2 SC on days 17-28
Consolidation 1B, 2B (HDAC/etoposide)	
Cytarabine	2,000 mg/m^2 IV over 2 h on days 1-4
Etoposide	500 mg/m^2 IV over 3 h on days 1-4
Consolidation 2A (DVPAsp)	
Daunorubicin	60 mg/m^2 IV on days 1-3
Vincristine	1.4 mg/m^2 IV on days 1, 8, and 15 (capped at 2.0 mg if age > 40 years)
Prednisone	60 mg/m^2 PO on days 1, 21
Asparaginase	6,000 IU/m^2 SC 6 doses over 2 weeks
Consolidation 1C, 2C, 3C (HDMTX/6-MP)	
Methotrexate	220 mg/m^2 IV bolus, then 60 mg/m^2/h x 36 h on days 1-2, 15-16
Leucovorin	50 mg/m^2 IV every 6 h for 3 doses, then oral leucovorin until methotrexate < 0.05 μmol/L
Mercaptopurine	75 mg/m^2 PO on days 1-28
Maintenance[h]	
Methotrexate	20 mg/m^2 weekly
Mercaptopurine	75 mg/m^2 daily

DVPAsp = daunorubicin, vincristine, prednisone, and asparaginase; HDAC = high-dose cytarabine + Ara-C); HDMTX = high-dose methotrexate; 6-MP = mercaptopurine

[h]Beginning after hematologic recovery from cycle 3C and continuing until 30 months from complete response

TABLE 3: ALL induction and consolidation therapy *(continued)*

Induction/consolidation	Dosage
M. D. ANDERSON (HYPER-CVAD) REGIMEN	
Cyclophosphamide	300 mg/m^2 infused over 3 h q12h × 6 doses (days 1-3)
Doxorubicin	25 $mg/m^2/d$ continuous infusion over 24 h × 2 days to begin 12 h after last cyclophosphamide dose (days 4 and 5)
Vincristine	1.4 mg/m^2 (max 2 mg) IV on days 4 and 11
Dexamethasone	40 mg/d days 1-4 and 11-14
Alternate q21d with	
MTX	1 g/m^2 continuous infusion over 24 h (day 1)
Cytarabine	3 g/m^2 over 2 h q12h × 4 doses (days 2 and 3)
Leucovorin rescue	50 mg PO at end of MTX infusion and then 25 mg PO q6h × 48 h
Methylprednisolone	50 mg IV twice daily (days 1–3)

All patients received a minimum of 4 doses of interthecal methotrexate for CNS prophylaxis. All patients received maintenance therapy twice a year with 6-MP (150 mg/d), methotrexate (20 g/m^2 oral weekly), vincristine (2 mg/month IV), and prednisone (200 mg oral daily for 5 days along with vincristine).

DVPAsp = daunorubicin, vincristine, prednisone, and asparaginase; HDAC = high-dose cytarabine + Ara-C; MTX = methotrexate; 6-MP = mercaptopurine line treatment of patients with ALL. The drug had originally been approved only for ALL patients who were allergic to native forms of asparaginase.

T-cell ALL There is evidence that patients with T-cell ALL may benefit from early treatment with cytarabine (Ara-C) and cyclophosphamide. Pharmacologic studies show high levels of Ara-C triphosphate accumulation in T lymphoblasts and synergy between cyclophosphamide and Ara-C in cell lines of T-cell malignancies. T lymphocytes also have a lower expression of polyglutamate synthetase than pre-B blasts. Randomized trials in children with T-cell ALL showed that the use of high-dose methotrexate (up to 5 g/m^2) improved outcome.

Mature B-cell ALL Patients with the more mature B-cell ALL (Burkitt-cell leukemia) experienced an improvement in survival when high doses of cyclophosphamide, methotrexate, and Ara-C were incorporated early in the treatment course. The probability of leukemia-free survival improved from 35% with standard ALL induction to 60%–70% with these newer regimens.

Consolidation therapy

The BFM, CALGB, Linker (2002), and Hyper-CVAD consolidation regimens for ALL are outlined in Table 3. As yet, no randomized trials have compared these regimens. However, in sequential studies from Memorial Sloan-Kettering Cancer Center and the BFM group, as well as the Linker study, use of multiple cycles of non–cross-resistant drugs for 3 to 8 cycles after remission followed by maintenance with methotrexate and mercaptopurine (Purinethol) resulted in overall long-term disease-free survival rates of 38%–52%.

Long-term outcome data of 288 patients treated with Hyper-CVAD showed an 81% CR rate after 1 cycle and a 92% rate after 1 cycle each of A&B (see Table 3); a 5% overall death rate during induction was noted, although treatment-related mortality reached 15% in patients older than age 60 despite the use of G-CSF. At a median follow-up of 63 months, the 5-year disease-free survival was 38%, similar to that reported in the BFM and CALGB trials. In this series, adverse prognostic factors for disease-free survival were age ≥ 45 years, poor performance status, WBC > 50,000/μL, Ph+ cytogenetics, more than 1 cycle to achieve a CR, or > 5% residual blasts at day 14. Patients with none or one of these factors had a 52% 5-year disease-free survival rate, vs 37% for patients with 2 or 3 factors and only 10% for patients with ≥ 4 risk factors.

In the 2002 Linker trial, which intensifies the consolidation with alternating cycles of higher dose Ara-C (HDAC) and etoposide alternating with cycles of high-dose methotrexate, the 5-year relapse-free survival rate was 52% overall and 60% for patients with standard-risk features. Prognostic features that were associated with a poor outcome in this study included pre-B ALL with > 100,000/μL WBC count at diagnosis, cytogenetic abnormalities involving chromosome 11q23 or t(9;22), and time to remission > 30 days. Without either allogeneic or autologous transplantation, all high-risk patients relapsed within a short (1–9 month) time.

The French LALA-94 trial of 922 patients was designed to look at postremission therapy that was stratified by risk of relapse. The standard-risk patients who achieved CR with 1 cycle of induction therapy were randomized to receive either conventional cyclophosphamide, Ara-C, and mercaptopurine or early intensification with intermediate-dose Ara-C (1 g/m^2 × 8 doses) and mitoxantrone.

In this group, there was no difference in 5-year disease-free survival (33% conventional vs 37% early intensification, with an overall survival at 5 years of 44%). High-risk patients included those with defined cytogenetic risks (excluding Ph+), WBC > 30,000/μL, and CNS disease at diagnosis or who required more than 35 days to achieve CR. Patients with a sibling donor received allogeneic transplant in CR, with the remainder randomized to receive either the early intensification chemotherapy or autologous transplant. The 5-year disease-free survival was 45% for those receiving allogeneic transplant and 23% for those without a donor.

There was no significant difference in overall survival with chemotherapy vs autologous transplant, but there was a different pattern of relapse, with fewer late relapses in the autologous patients (disease-free survival 25% vs 13% for chemotherapy only). The patients with Ph+ disease were randomized to receive allogeneic transplant with either a sibling or unrelated donor or autologous transplant. Although allogeneic transplant resulted in a significantly better 3-year disease-free survival (34%) than autologous transplant (15%); these outcomes indicate the need for improved consolidation strategies.

Prognostic factors for relapse In all the large European and American trials, there are several common factors associated with poor outcome. The most consistent factor is the presence of t(9;22), t(4;11), or (1;19) cytogenetic abnormalities. Increasing age and higher leukocyte counts at presentation are also poor-risk features. A recent international trial involving more than 1,500 patients confirmed prior observations that in Ph-negative patients, age (> 35 years), WBC count > 30,000/μL for precursor B-cell ALL and > 100,000/μL for T-cell ALL and lineage itself are prognostic factors of overall and disease-free survival. Younger patients with low WBC counts had a 55% 5-year disease-free survival rate vs 34% for patients with either the age or WBC parameters listed above and 5% for patients with poor-risk features. In addition, the rapidity of response has been an important prognostic factor for outcome, with the time point for expectation of clearance of marrow blasts shortening from 28 days in the BFM trial to 14–17 days with the Linker regimen and day 8 in both with the most recent French (LALA 94) trial and the pediatric ALL trials.

Molecular techniques, such as PCR amplification of leukemia-specific sequences of RNA or DNA, have been used in research settings to reveal residual leukemia cells. These sensitive techniques can detect the persistence of cells with the leukemic phenotype at a sensitivity of 1 cell in 10^4 normal cells in patients who are deemed to be in CR by conventional techniques. In two pediatric studies, detection of leukemia-specific gene rearrangements (≥ 1 cell in 10^4 normal cells) 5–6 months after initiation of treatment was associated with a high relapse rate.

A confirmatory study in adults with standard-risk ALL using a combination of aberrant immunophenotyping and PCR amplification of T-cell receptor or immunoglobulin gene rearrangements was recently reported. Patients who had no detectable residual disease by day 11 from the start of induction therapy had a 3-year disease-free survival rate of 92% compared with 65% for those with no residual disease by week 16. Patients who had detectable minimal residual disease beyond that point had a 3-year disease-free survival of only 12%.

High-risk patients Although the BFM regimen is now standard therapy for good-prognosis patients, high-risk patients are being selected for dose-intensive therapies, including HDAC and methotrexate or etoposide, high-dose methotrexate, and asparaginase.

For patients with Ph+ ALL, several centers have begun combining imatinib (Gleevec) with induction and consolidation chemotherapy. In series from both Japan and the United States, the addition of imatinib during induction has resulted in a CR rate of 95%–100% after 1 cycle of induction, and patients have achieved molecular remission documented by PCR in 50%–60% of patients within 2 months.

Transplantation Recent series have reported a disease-free survival rate of 55%–68% for "high-risk" patients with ALL undergoing transplantation during first CR. When treated with conventional-dose chemotherapy prior to the discovery of imatinib, patients with Ph+ ALL had a disease-free survival rate of < 10% regardless of other risk factors and a median time to relapse of 12 months. These patients should be referred for allogeneic or matched-unrelated donor (MUD) transplantation expeditiously upon attaining a CR. Several centers are incorporating imatinib along with conventional consolidation chemotherapy in patients with Ph+ ALL to try to reduce the leukemic burden further before transplantation, primarily in patients awaiting an unrelated donor transplant. Trials using imatinib post allogeneic transplantation to reduce relapse rates are also in progress. (Strategies for the most effective use of the various transplant options are discussed in chapter 36.)

CNS prophylaxis

CNS relapse occurs at a much higher frequency in patients with ALL compared with those with AML. The rate of CNS relapse was 20% in the first year in a pediatric ALL trial in which the CNS therapy was attenuated to a subtherapeutic level.

Patients with ALL require preemptive therapy for occult CNS disease with either (1) intrathecal methotrexate and/or Ara-C combined with cranial irradiation or (2) high-dose systemic Ara-C or methotrexate combined with intrathecal therapy.

Maintenance therapy

Maintenance therapy with daily mercaptopurine and weekly methotrexate for 18–24 months beyond consolidation remains the standard of care for children with ALL. In adults, the benefit of maintenance therapy is less certain. In low-risk adults, who may have an outcome more similar to that in the pediatric population, maintenance therapy would appear to be justified (see Table 3 for maintenance regimens). In individuals who have mature B-cell ALL, it is unlikely that maintenance therapy has any effect. In other high-risk adult populations, more than half of patients relapse while on maintenance therapy, indicating the need for other strategies to eradicate minimal residual disease.

Treatment of relapse

Treatment of relapsed adult ALL is a major challenge. Since most protocols for initial treatment incorporate 6 to 11 agents with different cytotoxic mechanisms, a selection process for drug resistance has occurred. The overall remission rate for relapse therapy is 30%–40%, with a median duration of remission of 6 months.

Salvage strategies include reinduction with the initial regimen in patients with late relapse or high-dose antimetabolites (Ara-C or methotrexate [see hyper-CVAD regimen, Table 3]) in those who relapse early. Recent experimental approaches include monoclonal antibodies directed against leukemia-specific antigens conjugated to either radionuclides or toxins, tyrosine kinase inhibitors, allogeneic or autologous transplantation, or new agents. In clinical trials, Ara-C has produced a CR in 53% of T-cell ALL induction failures on first relapse and in 27% in second relapse in children; responses of 25% have been reported in adults.

Clofarabine (Clolar) has been approved for treatment of relapsed refractory ALL in children. Of 25 patients, 5 achieved a CR, including children who had relapsed following allogeneic transplantation. The maximum tolerated dose was 52 mg/m^2 infused over 1 hour daily for 5 days. Significant toxic effects include capillary leak syndrome, hepatotoxicity, and skin rash.

In individuals with Ph+ ALL or CML in lymphoid blast crisis, imatinib can induce remissions in up to 30% of patients. These remissions are short-lived, but imatinib may control the leukemia long enough for a donor to be identified, thus providing an option for an allogeneic transplant in second remission, which carries a better outcome than a transplant performed with active disease. In patients with relapsed Ph+ ALL, the addition of interferon-alfa-2a (Roferon-A) to imatinib has shown durable remissions (> 18 months) in five of six patients who were not candidates for transplantation.

Dasatinib (Sprycel), recently approved by the FDA for imatinib-resistant Ph+ leukemias, can provide short-term salvage therapy for patients whose disease progresses while receiving combinations of imatinib and chemotherapy.

Nelarabine (Arranon) has also recently been approved for the treatment of T-cell lymphoblastic disease. In a recommended dose of 1,500 mg/m^2 on days 1, 3, and 5, this agent has produced response rates of 30%–50% in heavily pretreated patients.

TREATMENT OF AML

Although the chemotherapeutic agents used in the initial therapy for AML have not changed much in the past 30 years, our knowledge of the biology of

TABLE 4: AML induction and consolidation therapy

Induction		Consolidation	
AML			
Ara-C	200 mg/m^2 IV as continuous infusion × 7 d	Ara-C[b]	3 g/m^2 q12h IV as 2- to 3-h infusion on days 1, 3, and 5; repeat q28d × 4 cycles
IDA[a]	12 mg/m^2 IV on days 1-3		
ALSG regimen			
Ara-C[b]	3 g/m^2 IV q12h as 2- to 3-h infusion on days 1, 3, 5, and 7 (8 doses)	Ara-C	100 mg/m^2 IV as continuous infusion × 5 d
		Daun	50 mg/m^2 IV × 2 d
Daun	45–60 mg/m^2 IV on days 1-3	VP-16	75 mg/m^2 IV × 5 d
VP-16	75 mg/m^2 IV × 7 d		

ALSG = Australian Leukemia Study Group; AML = acute myelogenous leukemia; Ara-C = cytarabine; Daun = daunorubicin; IDA = idarubicin; VP-16 = etoposide

[a] Idarubicin has been substituted for daunorubicin, 45 mg/m^2, which had been the prevalent anthracycline used in clinical trials prior to 1993. Mitoxantrone, 10 mg/m^2 × 5 days, has also been used as an alternative.

[b] For patients < 60 years of age

leukemia has increased. The identification of prognostic factors can provide more realistic expectations of response to standard treatment and can define the population for whom investigational therapy is appropriate early in the course of disease.

Prognostic factors Cytogenetic abnormalities and mutation of the fetal liver tyrosine kinase (FLT_3) gene are the major predictors of remission and risk of relapse for patients with AML. Patients with translocation of genetic materials involving core binding regions [t(15;17), t(8;21) inv(16), or t(16;16)] have a good prognosis, with remission rates of 88% and 5-year disease-free survival rates of 55%–90%, whereas patients with loss of genetic material from chromosome 5 or 7 (−5 or −5q, −7 or −7q) and complex karyotypic abnormalities (defined as more than three abnormalities) have lower rates of CR (30%–40%) and disease-free survival (5%) at 5 years. Patients with either normal or intermediate cytogenetic abnormalities have a CR rate of 67% and a 5-year disease-free survival rate of 25%, based on data from a large CALGB trial.

Internal duplication of FLT_3 can be found in one-third of patients with normal cytogenetics or in patients with t(15;17) (APL) but is uncommon in either poor-risk karyotypes or non-APL translocations. This abnormality does not appear to have an impact on remission, but it is a predictor for relapse (74% relapse rate in FLT_3 patients with a normal karyotype vs 46% for patients without FLT_3).

Mutations of nucleophosmin protein (NPM1), which shuttle nucleic acids and proteins from the nucleus to the cytoplasm as well as binding *p53*, are a newly reported common abnormality, most prevalent (47%) in patients with a normal karyotype. Although there is frequent overlap with FLT_3 mutations, patients with an isolated NMP1 mutation and a normal karyotype have a 60% disease-free survival versus 40% for those with either wild-type or mutations of both FLT_3 and NMP1 and 20% for those with an isolated FLT_3 mutation.

Poor-risk cytogenetics, antecedent MDS, and a high incidence of multidrug resistance (MDR-1) protein are found more commonly in patients older than age 60, which accounts for the lower CR rates (30%–55%) seen in older individuals compared with their younger counterparts (remission rates, 60%–80%). Many older patients with preexisting MDS may clear marrow blasts with antileukemic treatment but may still have impaired hematopoiesis and persistent cytopenias, since they may have no normal residual stem cells to repopulate the marrow.

Induction therapy

For the majority of patients with AML, induction chemotherapy is initiated before cytogenetic information is available; the notable exception is with APL-FAB-M_3, which has a distinctive morphology and clinical presentation. The gene product of the t(15;17) translocation can be rapidly confirmed by PCR when the clinical diagnosis is suspected. Since the therapy for APL differs significantly from that for the other AML subtypes, it is important to make this distinction.

Ara-C and an anthracycline such as daunorubicin or idarubicin (Idamycin) have been the standard drugs used for AML induction chemotherapy for 30 years (Table 4). Depending on the prognostic groups, remission rates of 60%–80% are seen in younger (< age 60) patients and of 35%–55% in patients older than age 60. Other agents such as mitoxantrone and etoposide also have antileukemic activity, but no significant increase in remission rates or relapse-free survival have been seen when mitoxantrone was substituted for an anthracycline or etoposide was added to infusional Ara-C and daunorubicin. Mitoxantrone and etoposide were compared with Ara-C and daunorubicin as induction for patients older than age 55 in SWOG (Southwest Oncology Group) trials; CR rates were 44% for Ara-C and daunorubicin and 33% for mitoxantrone and etoposide, and median survival was 8 and 6 months, respectively.

Gemtuzumab ozogamicin (Mylotarg), an anti-CD_{33} antibody conjugated to the drug calicheamicin, was originally approved for the treatment of relapsed AML in older patients. Currently, there are two clinical trials in Great Britain and the United States evaluating the addition of gemtuzumab ozogamicin to standard Ara-C and daunorubicin or fludarabine, idarubicin, Ara-C, and G-CSF. Preliminary reports from the British trial showed a CR rate of 86%.

Gemtuzumab ozogamicin has also been used as a single agent for induction in patients > 61 years who were considered too frail for conventional therapy with Ara-C and daunorubicin. A CR rate of 33% was achieved in 18 patients aged 61 to 75 years; no benefit was seen in 22 patients older than age 75 due to high early mortality (7 of 22 patients).

TABLE 5: AML relapse therapy

Ara-C	2-3 g/m^2 IV q12h as 3-h infusion × 8 doses	*plus*	Mitox	12 mg/m^2 IV on days 1-3[a] *or*
			Daun	60 mg/m^2 IV on days 5 and 6 *or*
			VP-16	100 mg/m^2 IV daily × 5 d[a]
Topo	1.25 mg/m^2 q24h continuous infusion × 5 d	*plus*	Ara-C	1 g/m^2 over 2 h on days 1-5 *and*
			Amif	200 mg/m^2 qod starts day 6 until ANC > 1,500/μL
Ara-C	2 g/m^2/d IV × 5 d	*plus*	FdURD	300 mg/m^2/d × 5 d + G-CSF[a] ± Ida 10 mg/m^2/d on days 1-3
Mitox	10 mg/m^2 IV	*plus*	VP-16	100 mg/m^2 IV as 2-h infusion daily × 5 d
Gemtuz	4-9 mg/m^2 on days 1 and 14			

Amif = amifostine; AML = acute myelogenous leukemia; ANC = absolute neutrophil count; Ara-C = cytarabine; Daun = daunorubicin; FdURD = fludarabine: G-CSF = granulocyte colony-stimulating factor; Gemtuz = gemtuzumab; Ida = idarubicin; Mitox = mitoxantrone; Topo = topotecan; VP-16 = etoposide

[a] Also used for relapsed acute lymphoblastic leukemia

Another strategy to improve remission rates has been to use higher doses of Ara-C during induction. Both the Australian Leukemia Study Group (ALSG) and the SWOG compared standard Ara-C and daunorubicin (and etoposide in the ALSG trial) with high-dose Ara-C in patients < 50 years (Table 4). The CR rates were 71% and 74% for standard vs high-dose therapy in the ALSG study and 55% vs 58% in the SWOG trial. In both studies, there was a significantly higher disease-free survival for the high-dose arm at 5 years and (48% vs 25% for ALSG and 33% vs 22% for SWOG) but no difference in overall survival due to increased early toxicity.

Subgroups of patients may benefit from high-dose Ara-C. In the SWOG trial, patients with CD34+ blasts had a low CR rate of 36% with standard Ara-C but an equivalent rate to those with CD34– blasts (58%) when treated with high-dose Ara-C. There was a strong correlation between CD34 positivity and MDR-1 expression is this cohort, leading to the inference that high-dose Ara-C might help overcome drug resistance.

However, a recent 1,700-patient German trial showed no difference in disease-free survival when two cycles of high-dose Ara-C and mitoxantrone (HAM) were compared with one cycle of standard Ara-C-containing regimen followed by HAM. The overall disease-free survival was 40% for both arms in patients younger than age 60 and 29% for those older than age 60; 80% of young patients received both cycles, while only one-third of patients over 60 received cycle 2 irrespective of dose intensity of the initial cycle.

Therapy-related AML has a particularly poor prognosis. At best, only 50% of patients will achieve a remission, usually of brief duration (median, 5 months), despite the use of aggressive drug combinations. Allogeneic or unrelated-donor transplants appear to offer the only curative option in these patients, achieving a 3-year disease-free survival rate of 25% in two studies of allogeneic transplantation.

GM-CSF An Eastern Cooperative Oncology Group (ECOG) study showed that granulocyte-macrophage colony-stimulating factor (GM-CSF, sargramostim [Leukine]), used following completion of induction chemotherapy in older patients (55–70 years old), shortened the duration of neutropenia by 6 days and, thus, decreased treatment-related mortality, leading to both an improved CR rate and longer survival. The FDA approved GM-CSF for use in this setting. However, other trials using different cytokines in younger patients have not shown a survival benefit.

Consolidation therapy

Once remission of AML is attained, consolidation chemotherapy is required to achieve a durable remission or cure. Standard consolidation regimens are listed in Table 4.

Increased dose intensity In a CALGB study, 596 patients in CR were assigned to receive four courses of postremission Ara-C in one of three dosages: 100 mg/m^2 as a continuous infusion for 5 days, 400 mg/m^2 as a continuous infusion for 5 days, or 3 g/m^2 as a 3-hour infusion every 12 hours on days 1, 3, and 5. For patients ≤ 60 years old, the percentage of patients in CR at 4 years was significantly higher in the HDAC group (44%) than in either the 400-mg/m^2 or 100-mg/m^2 group (29% and 24%, respectively). For patients > 60 years old, consolidation dose intensity had no impact on disease-free survival, with all groups plateauing at a rate of 16% by 2 years.

Other approaches to consolidation include 1 to 3 cycles of consolidation followed by autologous or allogeneic bone marrow transplantation. Both of these approaches also tend to be limited to patients < 60 years old and have produced long-term disease-free survival rates of 45%–60% in several studies. (See chapter 36 for a more detailed discussion of transplantation approaches.) Long-term disease-free survival is strongly influenced by cytogenetic abnormalities present at diagnosis, and transplant options should be considered for patients with high-risk features while in first remission due to poor outcomes with conventional chemotherapy.

CNS prophylaxis

Routine CNS prophylaxis is recommended only for adult patients with AML at high risk of CNS recurrence, ie, patients with a WBC count > 50,000/µL at presentation or those with myelomonocytic or monocytic AML (FAB M4 or M5). Patients receiving HDAC (≥ 7.2 g/m^2) for induction or consolidation therapy achieve therapeutic drug levels in the CSF, obviating the need for intrathecal therapy. Patients given conventional Ara-C doses may be treated with intrathecal methotrexate (12 mg IT) or Ara-C (30 mg IT). Both agents can be combined with hydrocortisone (30 mg IT) for patients with active CNS disease.

TREATMENT OF REFRACTORY OR RELAPSED AML

Patients who do not respond to initial therapy or who relapse within 6 months of attaining a CR, as well as those with antecedent myelodysplasia or therapy-related AML, are considered to have relatively resistant disease.

Efforts to overcome drug resistance have focused on (1) HDAC-containing regimens, (2) new agents, (3) targeted therapy using leukemia-specific monoclonal antibodies conjugated with radionuclides or toxins, and (4) nonchemotherapeutic agents to block the drug efflux pump associated with MDR-1 gene expression.

HDAC High doses of Ara-C (2–3 g/m^2 for 8-12 doses) paired with mitoxantrone, etoposide, methotrexate, or fludarabine have produced short-lived CRs in 40%–60% of relapsed patients with AML (see Table 5 for dosage regimens). Response rates were higher in patients who had received standard-dose Ara-C for induction and who had subsequently relapsed than in those in whom induction therapy had failed. The median duration of remission was 4–6 months.

Combinations of mitoxantrone and etoposide have been reported to produce a 40%–50% CR rate in patients who had relapsed or for whom standard dose Ara-C and anthracycline had failed, again with a median duration of remission of 4–6 months. Combinations of intermediate-dose Ara-C (1 g/m^2/d for 6 days) with mitoxantrone and etoposide produced CR rates of 79% in relapsed patients and 46% in those who did not respond to induction therapy or had AML evolving from MDS, with a median CR duration of 8 months.

New agents Topotecan (Hycamtin) in combination with Ara-C has been reported to produce a CR in 35%–70% of patients with high-grade myelodysplasia.

Nucleoside analogs, such as cladribine (2-CdA) and fludarabine, showed activity in pediatric AML. A British trial reported a 61% CR rate for a combination of fludarabine, Ara-C, G-CSF, and idarubicin, with a median CR duration of 7 months. The combination of gemcitabine (Gemzar; 600 mg/m^2/hr, with infusion durations escalating from 6–12 hours) and mitoxantrone (12 mg/m^2/d × 3 days) beginning on day 1 was used to treat 26 patients with relapsed or refractory AML and 8 patients with MDS or CML blast crisis. Five CRs and six partial remissions (PRs) were seen in the patients with AML and four CRs and one PR were seen in the MDS/CML group. The maximum tolerated duration of gemcitabine infusion was 12 hours, with stomatitis and esophagitis being the nonhematologic toxicities in 50% of patients. Another nucleoside analog, clofarabine, showed a 16% remission rate in a phase I-II trial in patients with relapsed AML.

Another class of chemotherapeutic agents that are being evaluated are farnesyl transferase inhibitors, which target signal transduction pathways. One of these agents, tipifarnib (Zarnestra), showed a 29% response rate as a single agent in patients with relapsed or refractory AML. Currently, SWOG is evaluating two different doses and schedules of this drug in patients at least 70 years old with newly diagnosed AML. Temozolomide (Temodar), an oral alkylating agent currently approved for the treatment of astrocytoma, has been shown to have activity against myeloid malignancy, with a 20% clearance of marrow blasts in 18 patients with high-risk myeloid malignancy following a 7-day course of medication. Prolonged marrow aplasia was the dose-limiting toxicity.

Another approach being studied in older patients is the use of hypomethylating agents, such as decitabine or azacitidine, either alone or in combination with histone deacetylase inhibitors, such as valproic acid, for the initial treatment of older patients with AML. Response rates of 15%–25% have been reported.

Targeted therapy Gemtuzumab ozogamicin has been approved by the FDA for the treatment of relapsed AML in older patients (Table 5). Aggregate data from three trials involving 277 patients, with a median age of 61, showed a 26% complete response rate, with a median remission duration of 6.4 months.

Treatment-related toxicity was low; the only infusional side effects were fever/chills and slow platelet plus granulocyte recovery (≥ 5 weeks). No cardiac or cerebellar toxicities were reported. Liver function abnormalities were reported in 25%–30% of patients. The median CR duration for responding patients was 9 months.

Multidrug resistance modification Cyclosporine is a potent inhibitor of *p*-glycoprotein–mediated drug efflux. A SWOG trial compared HDAC, 3 g/m^2/d × 5 d, followed by daunorubicin, 45 mg/m^2/d as a continuous infusion on days 6-8, either alone (arm 1) or together with cyclosporine, 16 mg/m^2/d as a continuous infusion on days 6–8 (arm 2) in 226 patients with relapsed or refractory AML. Although the CR rates were similar for arms 1 and 2 (33% vs 40%), the relapse-free survival rates favored patients treated with the MDR modifier (9% for arm 1 vs 34% for arm 2 at 2 years; $P = .03$). The overall survival rate was also superior (12% for arm 1 vs 22% for arm 2 at 2 years; $P = .04$). Survival and induction response improved with increasing concentrations of daunorubicin intracellularly in cyclosporine-treated patients, suggesting that cyclosporine enhanced anthracycline cytotoxicity. Trials substituting the cyclosporine analog valspodar (PSC-833, Amdray) have not demonstrated a significant improvement in CR rate or survival.

Transplantation Although none of the previous options currently offers more than a 10%–15% chance of long-term disease-free survival, they do provide temporary cytoreduction sufficient to permit further high-dose treatment strategies, such as bone marrow transplantation using sibling, unrelated donor or purged autologous marrow. Allogeneic bone marrow transplantation achieves a 30%–40% disease-free survival rate at 5 years in patients transplanted during first relapse or second remission. Autologous bone marrow transplantation also has curative potential for patients beyond first CR, with most large series reporting disease-free survival rates of 30%–35% in selected patients (usually those with good-risk cytogenetics or initial CR duration longer than 1 year).

Reduced-intensity conditioning regimens are being explored as treatment options in older patients and in those with comorbidity that would otherwise preclude full-dose allogeneic transplantation. Preliminary results from several centers have shown 1- and 2-year disease-free survival rates of 50% for patients

TABLE 6: APL induction and consolidation therapy

Induction		Consolidation		Maintenance	
French APL 93 trial					
ATRA	45 mg/m^2 PO daily in 2 divided doses for a minimum of 45 d and a maximum of 90 d	**Cycle 1** Repeat induction doses of Ara-C and Daun		ATRA	45 mg/m^2/d $\times$ 15 d every 3 months
				±	
Ara-C	100 mg/m^2 IV as a continuous infusion $\times$ 7 d	**Cycle 2**		MTX	15 mg/m^2/wk PO
		Ara-C	2 g/m^2 IV infused over 1 h q12h $\times$ 8 doses (days 1-4)	6-MP	50 mg/m^2/d PO
		6-MP	90 mg/m^2/d PO + MTX 15 mg/m^2/wk PO $\times$ 2 years		
		± ATRA	45 mg/m^2/d for 15 d every 3 months		
Daun	60 mg/m^2 IV $\times$ 3 d	Daun	45 mg/m^2 IV on days 1-3		
or					
AIDA study		**Cycle 1**		ATRA	45 mg/m^2/d x 15 d every 3 months
ATRA	45 mg/m^2 PO daily	Ara-C	1 g/m^2 IV infused over 6 h daily $\times$ 4 d		
IDA	12 mg/m^2 IV on days 2, 4, 6, and 8	*plus* IDA	5 mg/m^2/d IV $\times$ 4 d (3 h after end of Ara-C infusion)	MTX	15 mg/m^2 q wk
				6-MP	50 mg/m^2/d
		Cycle 2			
		Mitox	10 mg/m^2/d IV on days 1-5		
		plus VP-16	100 mg/m^2 $\times$ 5 d by 1-h infusion 12 h after Mitox		
		Cycle 3			
		IDA	12 mg/m^2 IV on day 1		
		plus Ara-C	150 mg/m^2 SC q8h $\times$ 5 d		
		plus			
		6-TG	70 mg/m^2 PO q8h $\times$ 5 d		

APL = acute promyelocytic leukemia; Ara-C = cytarabine; ATRA = all-*trans*-retinoic acid; Daun = daunorubicin; IDA = idarubicin; Mitox = mitoxantrone; MTX = methotrexate; 6-TG = thioguanine;

aged 55 to 70 years receiving reduced-intensity allogeneic transplantation for consolidation of first remission.

New methods of marrow purging and post-transplant immune stimulation also are being explored to decrease relapse-related mortality.

TREATMENT OF APL

APL represents a uniquely homogeneous subset of AML defined by its cytogenetic abnormality, t(15;17), which results in fusion of the retinoic acid receptor (RAR) α-gene on chromosome 17 with the promyelocytic leukemia (PML) gene on chromosome 15. This abnormality yields the PML/RAR-α fusion protein, detectable by PCR techniques, which is useful for both diagnosis and evaluation of minimal residual disease (MRD). Most (80%) patients with APL have characteristic hypergranular blasts; laboratory evidence of DIC is present in 70%–90% of patients at diagnosis or shortly after. Although low-dose heparin (5–15 U/kg/h) and factor replacement are used as supportive adjuncts during chemotherapy, hemorrhagic events contribute 10%–15% excess mortality during induction chemotherapy for APL compared with other AML subtypes.

Because of the unique biology and specific clinical features of APL, induction and consolidation regimens for APL differ from strategies used for other FAB types.

Involvement of the RAR-α gene in the pathogenesis of APL suggested the use of retinoids as therapy. A study from Shanghai showed CR rates of 85% with all-*trans*-retinoic acid (ATRA, tretinoin, Vesanoid). ATRA offered the advantages of a shorter neutropenic period (2 weeks) and slightly faster resolution of DIC (4 vs 7 days), as compared with standard chemotherapy with Ara-C and daunorubicin. Normalization of marrow morphology and cytogenetics requires 30–60 days of ATRA.

APL syndrome Approximately 25% of patients with APL develop "differentiation syndrome" (formerly known as ATRA syndrome). Symptoms of this syndrome are fever, respiratory distress with pulmonary infiltrates or pleural effusions, and cardiovascular collapse. Temporary pseudotumor cerebri is a fairly common (10%) side effect of ATRA. Although these symptoms most often correlate with leukocytosis (WBC count > 10,000/μL), many patients develop symptoms with WBC counts between 5,000 and 10,000/μL. The syndrome is seen in patients treated with ATRA as well as in those treated with arsenic trioxide (Trisenox).

Treatment of this syndrome involves prompt use of high-dose steroids, initiation of either hydroxyurea or conventional Ara-C/daunorubicin chemotherapy to control leukocytosis, and temporary discontinuation of ATRA or arsenic trioxide.

Initial treatment options

Standard-dose Ara-C and daunorubicin produced CR rates of 70%–80% within disease-free survival rates of 40%–50%. WBC and platelet counts at presentation correlate with the risk of relapse. Patients with a WBC < 10,000/μL and a platelet count > 40,000/mL have a disease-free survival of 97%; those with a WBC

< 10,000/μL and a platelet count < 40,000/mL have a disease-free survival of 86%; those with a WBC > 10,000/μL have a disease-free survival of 78%.

Three large studies have shown that ATRA in combination with anthracycline-based chemotherapy results in an improved long-term disease-free survival. The French APL 93 trial compared sequential ATRA followed by chemotherapy with concomitant ATRA plus chemotherapy (see Table 6, first regimen). Patients achieving CR received 2 cycles of consolidation therapy and then were randomized to receive 1) intermittent ATRA (2 weeks every 3 months for 2 years), 2) low-dose oral chemotherapy (mercaptopurine and methotrexate for 2 years), 3) both, or 4) observation. The CR rate in both induction arms was 92%. However, relapse rates were 6% for the ATRA plus chemotherapy arm vs 16% for ATRA followed by chemotherapy ($P = .04$).

A total of 289 patients were randomized to receive maintenance treatment. Relapse rates at 2 years were 30% for patients who received no maintenance treatment, 18% for patients receiving ATRA maintenance therapy alone, 14% for patients receiving chemotherapy without ATRA, and 7% for patients receiving chemotherapy plus ATRA. Overall survival was significantly better in patients receiving maintenance chemotherapy with or without ATRA for 2 years.

The Italian AIDA study used only ATRA and idarubicin for induction. The CR rate was 95%, with only 5% mortality during induction, suggesting that Ara-C is not required to achieve remission (Table 6). However preliminary reports from the French APL 2000 study, which compared daunorubicin (60 mg/m^2 for 3 days) and ATRA alone with a regimen that also used infusional Ara-C during induction and consolidation, showed a reduction in the relapse rate (3.8% vs 11.9%) for the arm with Ara-C and a disease-free survival rate of 94% vs 83%.

Small single-institution series have reported favorable remission and disease-free survival rates in patients induced with arsenic trioxide alone (86% complete response) or combined with ATRA (95% for low- and intermediate-risk patients). High-risk patients had poorer response rates (75% complete response) despite the addition of gemtuzumab ozogamicin (9 mg/m^2) on day 1 of induction therapy.

New agents Arsenic trioxide is now the standard reinduction therapy for patients with APL who are refractory to, or have relapsed from, retinoid and anthracycline chemotherapy. As a single agent, arsenic trioxide has produced a CR in 34 of 40 patients (85%) with relapsed APL, with 86% of patients achieving molecular remission. Relapsed patients who achieved a molecular remission with arsenic trioxide alone had a median relapse-free survival of 18 months; those who received arsenic trioxide followed by autologous transplantation have had relapse-free survivals in excess of 70% at 2 years. Allogeneic transplantation should be reserved for those who do not achieve a molecular remission.

Although liver toxicity was reported with the use of arsenic trioxide in the original Chinese studies, the most significant toxicities in the US multicenter trial were the "APL syndrome," ventricular arrhythmia in patients with prolongation of the AT/QTc interval on ECG, and peripheral neuropathy. It is important to monitor potassium, magnesium, and calcium levels closely, almost daily, during arsenic trioxide therapy; maintaining these levels near the upper range of normal is important in preventing arrhythmia.

The most recent US Intergroup APL trial incorporated arsenic trioxide in consolidation therapy for APL in first CR. Patients were randomized to receive either 2 cycles of daunorubicin plus ATRA or 2 cycles of arsenic trioxide followed by 2 cycles of daunorubicin plus ATRA for consolidation. Patients were then randomized to receive maintenance with either ATRA alone or in combination with mercaptopurine and methotrexate. The data from the trial are currently being analyzed.

Gemtuzumab ozogamacin is also an effective agent for patients with relapsed APL. In a small series, 91% of patients with a molecular relapse of APL achieved a molecular remission following two doses of gemtuzumab ozogamicin (6 mg/m^2).

Monitoring response to therapy Reverse-transcriptase (RT) PCR for the PML/RAR-α fusion protein can be used to follow response to therapy. The marker clears slowly, with many patients still testing positive following induction therapy. However, patients with persistence of PML/RAR-α at the end of consolidation therapy are at high risk of relapse, as are those with reemergence of the marker following a period without detectable protein. Salvage chemotherapy should be considered for patients with persistent or recurrent confirmed molecular relapse.

SUGGESTED READING

ON ACUTE LEUKEMIAS (GENERAL)

Haferlach T, Kohlmann A, Schnittger S, et al: Global approach to the diagnosis of leukemia using gene expression profiling. Blood 106:1189–1198, 2005.

ON ALL

Boissel N, Auclerc MF, Lheritier V, et al: Should adolescents with acute lymphoblastic leukemia be treated as old children or young adults? Comparison of the French FRALLE-93 and LALA-94 trials. J Clin Oncol 21:774–780, 2003.

Bruggemann M, Ruff T, Florhr T, et al: Clinical significance of minimal residual disease quantification in adult patients with standard risk acute lymphoblastic leukemia. Blood 107:1116–1123, 2006.

Kantarjian H, Thomas D, O'Brien S, et al: Long-term follow-up results of hyperfractionated cyclophosphamide, vincristine, doxorubicin, and dexamethasone (Hyper-CVAD), a dose-intensive regimen, in adult acute lymphocytic leukemia. Cancer 101:2788–2801, 2004.

Kurtzberg J, Ernst TJ, Keating MJ, et al: Phase I study of 506U78 administered on a consecutive 5-day schedule in children and adults with refractory hematologic malignancies. J Clin Oncol 23:3396–3403, 2005.

Mancini M, Scappaticci D, Cimino G, et al: A comprehensive genetic classification of adult acute lymphoblastic leukemia (ALL): Analysis of the GIMEMA 0496 protocol. Blood 105:3434–3441, 2005.

Rowe JM, Buck G, Burnett AK, et al: Induction therapy for adults with acute lymphoblastic leukemia: Results of more than 1,500 patients from the International ALL trial. Blood 106:3760–3767, 2005.

Verhaak R, Goudswaard C, von Putten W, et al: Mutations in nucleophosmin (NPM1) in acute myeloid leukemia (AML): Association with other gene abnormalities and previously established gene expression signatures and their favorable prognostic significance. Blood 106:3747-3756, 2005.

Yanada M, Takeuchi J, Sagiura I, et al: High remission rate and promising outcome by combinations of imatinib and chemotheraapy for newly diagnosed BCR/ABL positive acute lymphoblastic leukemia: A phase II study by the Japan Adult Leukemia Study Group. J Clin Oncol 24:460–466, 2006.

ON AML

Amadori S, Suciu S, Stasi R, et al: Gemtuzumab ozogamcin (Mylotarg) as a single-agent treatment for frail patients 61 years of age and older with acute myeloid leukemia: Final results of AML-15B, a phase 2 study of the European Organisation for Research and Treatment of Cancer and Gruppo Italiano Malattie Ematologiche dell'Adulto Leukemia Groups. Leukemia 19:1768–1773, 2005.

Applebaum FR, Gundacker H, Head DR, et al: Age and acute myeloid leukemia. Blood 107:3481–3485, 2006.

Bachner T, Berdal WE, Schoch C, et al: Double induction containing either two or one course of high dose cytarabine plus mitoxantrone and post remission therapy with either autologous stem-cell transplantation or by prolonged maintenance for acute myeloid leukemia. J Clin Oncol 29:2480–2489, 2006.

Kell WJ, Burnett AK, Chopra R, et al: A feasibility study of simultaneous administration of gemtuzumab ozogamicin with intensive chemotherapy in induction and consolidation in younger patients with acute myeloid leukemia. Blood 102:4277–4283, 2003.

ON APL

Estey E, Garcia-Manero G, Ferrajuli A, et al: Use of all trans-retinoic acid plus arsenic trioxide as an alternative to chemotherapy in untreated acute promyelocytic leukemia. Blood 107:3469–3473, 2006.

Sanz MA, Martin G, Gonzalez M, et al: Risk-adapted treatment of acute promyelocytic leukemia with all-trans-retinoic acid and anthracycline monochemotherapy: A multicenter study by the PETHEMA group. Blood 103:1237–1243, 2004.

Shen ZX, Shi ZZ, Fang J, et al: All-trans-retinoic acid/As2O3 combination yields a high quality remission and survival in newly diagnosed acute promyelocytic leukemia. Proc Natl Acad Sci U S A 101:5328–5335, 2004.

CHAPTER 33

Chronic myelogenous leukemia

Jorge E. Cortes, MD, Richard T. Silver, MD, and Hagop Kantarjian, MD

Chronic myelogenous leukemia (CML) is a clonal myeloproliferative disorder resulting from the neoplastic transformation of the primitive hematopoietic stem cell. The disease is monoclonal in origin, affecting myeloid, monocytic, erythroid, megakaryocytic, B-cell, and, sometimes, T-cell lineages. Bone marrow stromal cells are not involved.

CML accounts for 15% of all leukemias in adults. Approximately 4,500 new cases of CML will be diagnosed in 2007, and it is estimated that 600 patients will die of CML this year. The incidence is 1.7 per 100,000 population. With imatinib (Gleevec) therapy, the annual mortality may be reduced significantly (less than 2%–3% per year).

CML

Epidemiology

Gender The male-to-female ratio is 1.1–1.4:1.

Age According to SEER (Surveillance, Epidemiology, and End Results) and MRC (Medical Research Council, UK) data, the median age of patients with CML is 66 years. However, most patients who are admitted to chemotherapy studies are 50–60 years old, with a median age of ~53 years. Patients in bone marrow transplantation (BMT) studies are even younger, with a median age of ~40 years. Age differences must be considered in all studies because this variable may affect results.

Etiology and risk factors

The etiology of CML is unclear. Some associations with genetic and environmental factors have been reported, but in most cases, no such factors can be identified.

Genetic factors There is little evidence linking genetic factors to CML. Offspring of parents with CML do not have a higher incidence of CML than the general population.

Environmental factors Nuclear and radiation exposures, including therapeutic radiation, have been associated with the development of CML. Exposure to chemicals has not been associated with greater risk except for the use of benzene.

TABLE 1: Criteria for accelerated-phase CML according to MDACC, IBMTR, and WHO

Characteristic	MDACC	IBMTR	WHO
Blasts	≥ 15%	≥ 10%	10%–19%**
Blasts + promyelocytes	≥ 30%	≥ 20%	NA
Basophils	≥ 20%	≥ 20%*	≥ 20%
Platelets	< 100	Unresponsive ↑ or persistent ↓	< 100 or > 1,000 unresponsive
Cytogenetics	CE	CE	CE not at diagnosis
WBC	NA	Difficult to control or doubling in < 5 days	NA
Anemia	NA	Unresponsive	NA
Splenomegaly	NA	Increasing	NA
Other	NA	Chloromas, myelofibrosis	Megakaryocyte proliferation, fibrosis

* Basophils + eosinophils

** Blast phase ≥ 20% blasts (≥ 30% for MDACC and IBMTR)

IBMTR = International Bone Marrow Transplant Registry; MDACC = M. D. Anderson Cancer Center; WHO = World Health Organization; NA = not applicable; CE = clonal evolution

CML

Signs and symptoms

CML usually runs a biphasic or triphasic course. This process includes an initial chronic phase and a terminal blastic phase, which is preceded by an accelerated phase in 60%–80% of patients.

Chronic phase If untreated, chronic-phase CML is associated with a median interval of 3.5–5.0 years before transforming to the more aggressive phases leading to death. During the chronic phase, CML is asymptomatic in 15%–40% of all cases and, in these cases, is discovered on a routine blood examination.

In symptomatic patients, the most common presenting signs and symptoms are fatigue, left upper quadrant pain or mass, weight loss, and palpable splenomegaly. Occasionally, patients with very high WBC counts may have manifestations of hyperviscosity, including priapism, tinnitus, stupor, visual changes from retinal hemorrhages, and cerebrovascular accidents.

Patients in chronic-phase CML do not have an increased risk for infection. Splenomegaly is documented in 30%–70% of patients. The liver is enlarged in 10%–20% of cases.

Accelerated phase This is an ill-defined transitional phase. The criteria (M. D. Anderson Cancer Center [MDACC]) used recently in all the imatinib studies include the presence of ≥ 15% blasts, ≥ 30% blasts and promyelocytes, or ≥ 20%

basophils in the peripheral blood or a platelet count < 100×10^9/L unrelated to therapy. Cytogenetic clonal evolution is also a criterion for acceleration. Other classifications include more subjective criteria (Table 1). The classification used may affect the expected outcome for a group of patients defined as accelerated phase. With imatinib therapy, the estimated 4-year survival rate exceeds 50%. Thus, a new definition of accelerated phase (ie, predictive for short survival) needs to be developed.

The accelerated phase is frequently symptomatic, including the development of fever, night sweats, weight loss, and progressive splenomegaly.

Blastic phase The blastic phase morphologically resembles acute leukemia. Its diagnosis requires the presence of at least 30% of blasts in the bone marrow or peripheral blood. The World Health Organization has proposed to consider blast phase with ≥ 20% blasts, but this classification has not been validated, and recent evidence suggests that patients with 20% to 29% blasts have a significantly better prognosis than those with ≥ 30% blasts. In some patients, the blastic phase is characterized by extramedullary deposits of leukemic cells, most frequently in the CNS, lymph nodes, skin, or bones.

Patients in blastic phase usually die within 3–6 months. Approximately 70% of patients in blastic phase have a myeloid phenotype; 25%, lymphoid; and 5%, undifferentiated. Prognosis is slightly better for patients with a lymphoid blastic phase than for myeloid or undifferentiated cases (median survival 9 vs 3 months).

Patients in blastic phase are more likely to experience symptoms, including weight loss, fever, night sweats, and bone pain. Symptoms of anemia, infectious complications, and bleeding are common. Subcutaneous nodules or hemorrhagic tender skin lesions, lymphadenopathy, and signs of CNS leukemia may also occur.

There is growing evidence suggesting that the most primitive CML progenitor cells are insensitive to imatinib (Gleevec). These cells are quiescent and are responsible for persistence of disease. Recent studies suggest that these cells express Bcr-Abl at significantly higher levels than do normal progenitors, and this results in an increase in phosphorylation of CrkL. In addition, these early progenitors have increased propensity to develop spontaneous mutations of the Abl kinase domain (*Jiang X, Saw KM, Eaves A, et al: Blood [abstract] 106:132a, 2005; Copland M, Hamilton A, Baird JW, et al: Blood [abstract] 106:205a, 2005*). Dasatinib (BMS-354825) has increased activity against earlier leukemic progenitors compared with imatinib, but it does not eradicate the quiescent CML stem cells. However, the combination of dasatinib with BMS-214662, a farnesyl transferase inhibitor, significantly reduces the pool of these primitive cells (*Copland M, Hamilton A, Allan EK, et al: Blood [abstract] 106:204a, 2005*).

Laboratory features

Peripheral blood The most common feature of CML is an elevated WBC count, usually > 25×10^9/L and frequently > 100×10^9/L, occasionally with cyclic variations. The finding of unexplained, persistent leukocytosis (eg, > $12–15 \times 10^9$/L) in the absence of infections or other causes of WBC count elevation should prompt a work-up for CML.

The WBC differential usually shows granulocytes in all stages of maturation, from blasts to mature, morphologically normal granulocytes. Basophils are elevated, but only 10%–15% of patients have ≥ 7% basophils in the peripheral blood. Frequently, eosinophils are also mildly increased. The absolute lymphocyte count is elevated at the expense of T lymphocytes.

The platelet count is elevated in 30%–50% of patients and is higher than $1{,}000 \times 10^9$/L in a small percentage of patients with CML. When thrombocytopenia occurs, it usually signals disease acceleration.

Some patients have mild anemia at diagnosis.

Neutrophil function is usually normal or only mildly impaired, but natural killer (NK) cell activity is impaired. Platelet function is frequently abnormal but usually has no clinical significance.

Bone marrow The bone marrow is hypercellular, with cellularity of 75%–90%. The myeloid-to-erythroid ratio is usually 10–30:1. All stages of maturation of the WBC series are usually seen, but the myelocyte predominates.

Megakaryocytes are increased in number early in the disease and may show dysplastic features. They are usually smaller than the typical normal megakaryocytes. Fibrosis may be evident at diagnosis but increases with disease progression and is usually an adverse prognostic finding.

Other laboratory findings Leukocyte alkaline phosphatase activity is reduced at diagnosis. Serum levels of vitamin B_{12} and transcobalamin are increased, sometimes up to 10 times normal values. Serum levels of uric acid and lactic dehydrogenase (LDH) are also frequently elevated.

Cytogenetic and molecular findings

Philadelphia chromosome CML is characterized by the Philadelphia (Ph) chromosome, which represents a balanced translocation between the long arms of chromosomes 9 and 22, t(9;22)(q34;q11). The c-*abl* proto-oncogene located in chromosome 9q34 encodes for a nonreceptor protein-tyrosine kinase expressed in most mammalian cells. In chromosome 22, the breakpoint occurs within the BCR gene and usually involves an area known as the breakpoint cluster region major *(m-bcr),* located either between exons b3 and b4 or between exons b2 and b3. Therefore, two different fusion genes can be formed, both of them joining exon 2 of *abl* with either exon 2 (b2a2) or exon 3 of *bcr* (b3a2). Among the 5% to 10% of patients who do not have the Ph chromosome detected by karyotyping, 30% to 40% have the molecular rearrangement identified by fluorescent in situ hybridization (FISH)/polymerase chain reaction (PCR). Those patients without this rearrangement are considered to have atypical CML and have a different prognosis and treatment.

Upon translation, a new protein with a molecular weight of 210 kd ($p210^{BCR\text{-}ABL}$) is synthesized, which, compared with the normal c-*abl*, has markedly increased kinase activity and can transform transfected cells and induce leukemia in transgenic mice. Occasionally, the breakpoint can occur in other areas (m-*bcr* and μ-*bcr*), leading to different transcripts (eg, $p190^{BCR\text{-}ABL}$ and $p230^{BCR\text{-}ABL}$, respectively). The mechanism of oncogenesis of $p210^{BCR\text{-}ABL}$ is unclear, but, upon phosphorylation, it can activate several intracellular pathways, including *ras* and the MAP kinase pathway, the Jak-Stat pathway, the PI3 kinase pathway, and the *myc* pathway. Ultimately, this leads to altered adhesion to extracellular matrix and stroma, constitutive activation of mitogenic signals, and inhibition of apoptosis.

Staging and prognosis

Staging systems Several characteristics of CML, including age; spleen size; WBC and platelet counts; and percentage of blasts, eosinophils, and basophils in the peripheral blood, affect the prognosis. Deletions of the derivative chromosome 9 are identified in 10% to 15% of patients and have been associated with an adverse prognosis with most treatment modalities. Imatinib may overcome the adverse prognosis associated with del der(9), although this remains controversial. These factors have been incorporated into several staging systems.

Sokal's classification A frequently used risk classification is Sokal's prognostic risk system. In this system, the hazard ratio function is derived from the following formula: $\lambda_i(+)/\lambda_o(t)$ = Exp 0.0116 (age – 43.4) + 0.0345 (spleen – 7.51) + 0.188 [(platelets/700)^2 – 0.563] + 0.0887 (blasts – 2.10).

This risk classification defines three prognostic groups with hazard ratios of < 0.8, 0.8.–1.2, and > 1.2.

The Hasford classification has been suggested to separate more clearly and without overlap risk groups among patients treated with interferon therapy. The Hasford score is derived from the formula (0.6666 × age [0 when age < 50 years; 1, otherwise] + 0.0420 × spleen size [cm below costal margin] + 0.0584 × blasts [%] + 0.0413 × eosinophils [%] + 0.2039 × basophils [0 when basophils < 3%; 1, otherwise] + 1.0956 × platelet count [0 when platelet count < 1,500 × 10^9/L; 1, otherwise]) × 1000. Based on the score, patients can be classified into three risk groups: low (score ≤ 780), intermediate (score > 780 and ≤ 1480), and high (≥ 1480). This classification may be less predictive in the imatinib era. In an analogous fashion, patients who might be candidates for transplantation can be assessed using the European Bone Marrow Transplant (EBMT) score.

Treatment

CHRONIC PHASE

Conventional chemotherapy

Busulfan (Busulfex, Myleran) and hydroxyurea were the chemotherapeutic agents used most frequently in CML until the development of imatinib. Busulfan is usually given at a dose of 0.1 mg/kg/d until the WBC count decreases by 50%, at which point the dose is reduced by 50%. Therapy is discon-

TABLE 2: Response definitions in CML

Response	Category	Criteria
Hematologic remission	Complete	Normalization of WBC counts to $< 9 \times 10^9$/L with normal differential; normalization of platelet counts to $< 450 \times 10^9$/L; disappearance of all signs and symptoms of disease
Cytogenetic response[b]	Complete[a]	No evidence of Ph chromosome-positive cells
	Partial[a]	5%–34% of metaphases Ph chromosome-positive cells
	Minor	35%–95% of metaphases Ph chromosome-positive cells
	None	Persistence of Ph chromosome in all analyzable cells

[a] Major cytogenetic response includes complete and partial cytogenetic responses.

[b] Response assessed on routine cytogenetic analysis with at least 20 metaphases counted.

tinued when the WBC count drops below 20×10^9/L and is restarted when it rises above 50×10^9/L.

Busulfan is associated with lung, marrow, and heart fibrosis and can cause an Addison-like disease. In 10% of patients, prolonged myelosuppression may be observed.

Hydroxyurea has a lower toxicity profile than does busulfan. The usual dose of hydroxyurea is 40 mg/kg/d; this dose is reduced by 50% when the WBC count drops below 20×10^9/L. The dose is then adjusted individually to keep the WBC count between 2 and 8×10^9/L.

Both busulfan and hydroxyurea can control the hematologic manifestations of CML in more than 80% of patients, although hydroxyurea results in a longer duration of chronic phase and overall survival than does busulfan. Neither drug significantly reduces the percentage of cells bearing the Ph chromosome, and, therefore, transformation to the blastic phase is unchanged. Their use should be limited to temporary control of hematologic manifestations before definitive therapy (eg, imatinib, stem-cell transplantation) is instituted.

Interferon

Recombinant interferon (rIFN-α) can induce a complete hematologic response (Table 2) in 70%–80% of patients with CML, with some degree of suppression of Ph chromosome-positive cells (referred to as a cytogenetic response) in 40%–60% of patients, which is complete in up to 20%–25% of patients. Randomized studies have documented a survival advantage for patients treated with rIFN-α vs those treated with chemotherapy.

In patients who achieve complete cytogenetic responses, they are durable in ≥ 80% of cases. Patients who achieve a complete cytogenetic response have a 10-year survival rate of 75% or more.

Interferon and cytarabine (Ara-C) The combination of IFN-α and low-dose Ara-C has induced major cytogenetic responses in 40%–50% of patients. Two randomized trials confirmed an improved response rate with this combination compared with rIFN-α alone, and one of them also demonstrated a survival advantage. The response to rIFN-α is dose-dependent, and the recommended dose is 5×10^6 U/m²/d. However, higher doses are also associated with increased toxicity, and at least 30% of patients will require dose reductions and/or discontinuation of therapy because of toxicity.

A recent long-term follow-up analysis has confirmed that a fraction of patients (approximately 30% of those achieving complete cytogenetic remission) treated with IFN-α in early chronic phase may achieve a sustained molecular remission and are probably cured. Among the others, 40% to 60% remain free of disease after more than 10 years despite the presence of minimal residual disease. This has been called "operational cure."

New formulations of rIFN-α attached to polyethylene glycol (PEG-IFN) have a longer half-life that allows for weekly administration. It may also be associated with decreased toxicity, allowing for increased dose intensity, but has shown no therapeutic advantage.

Imatinib is a potent inhibitor of the tyrosine kinase activity of BCR-ABL and a few other tyrosine kinases, such as PDGF-R (platelet-derived growth factor-receptor) and c-*kit*. It has demonstrated significant activity in patients with CML in all phases of the disease, whether they have received prior therapy or not. Among patients with chronic-phase CML for whom prior IFN-α therapy failed, 55%–85% of patients achieved a major cytogenetic remission, including 45%–80% with a complete cytogenetic remission. The estimated rate of survival free of transformation to accelerated with blast phase is 69% at 60 months. Among patients treated in early chronic-phase CML who had not received prior therapy, the rate of complete cytogenetic response is 85%–90%, with an overall survival rate at 54 months of 93%, and survival-free of transformation, 93%.

In a randomized trial, imatinib was significantly superior to IFN-α plus Ara-C in hematologic, cytogenetic, and molecular responses and disease progression-free survival, as well as toxicity profile and quality of life. Because of a high rate of crossover

> As with most other tumors, dose intensity plays an important role in the probability of response to imatinib (Gleevec). A recent study analyzed the actual dose intensity of high-dose imatinib (600 mg daily) as the initial therapy for patients in chronic phase. Patients were grouped by the median daily dose (MDD) received during the first 6 months of therapy and then over the second 6 months. Those who received an MDD of less than 600 mg daily had the lowest probability of achieving a major molecular response after 12 and 24 months of therapy (22% and 43%, respectively). In contrast, those who received an MDD of 600 mg during both 6-month periods had the highest probability of major molecular response at 24 months (89%) *(Hughes T, Branford S, Reynolds J, et al: Blood [abstract] 106:51a, 2005)*.

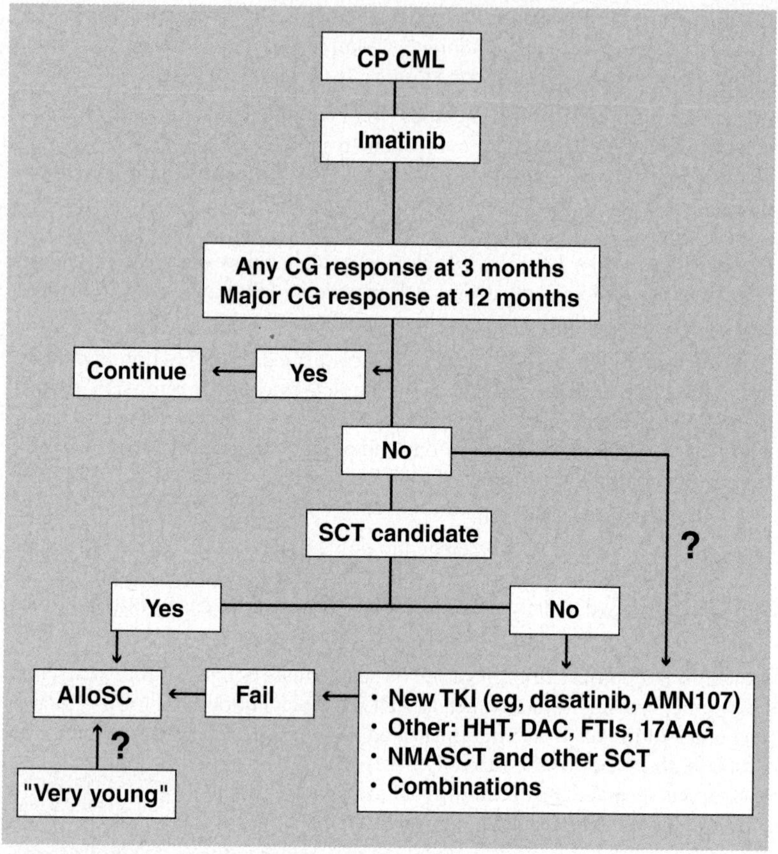

Figure 1: Treatment algorithm including imatinib for chronic-phase CML.

CP = chronic phase; CG = cytogenetic response; SCT = stem–cell transplantation; AlloSC = allogeneic stem–cell; TKI = tyrosine kinase inhibitor; HHT = homoharringtonine; DAC = decitabine; FTIs = farnesyl transferase inhibitors; NMASCT = nonmyeloablative allogeneic stem–cell transplantation

from IFN-α to imatinib, there was no difference in overall survival. However, comparisons with historic controls treated with IFN-α have shown the expected survival benefit with imatinib therapy. Thus, imatinib has become the standard therapy for CML (Figure 1). The proper management of patients receiving imatinib is important.

Dose The standard dose of imatinib is 400 mg daily for chronic phase and 600 mg for accelerated and blastic phases. Dose reductions may be needed in some patients because of toxicity, but doses less than 300 mg daily are not recommended. Available data from the phase I study show a clear decrease in the probability of response with doses lower than 300 mg daily. Several studies have suggested that starting therapy for patients in chronic phase with a higher dose of imatinib (600 or 800 mg daily) may improve the rate of complete cytogenetic and molecular responses with adequate tolerance. A randomized trial is currently ongoing to address whether the standard dose should be changed.

An unanswered question for patients treated with imatinib (Gleevec) is whether therapy can be interrupted after achieving a molecular remission. Several case reports and small series have suggested that discontinuation of therapy results in relapse, even in patients with undetectable Bcr-Abl transcripts. Most patients respond again when treatment is resumed (*Cortes J, O'Brien S, Kantarjian H: Blood 104:2204-2205, 2004*). The one exception may be among patients previously treated with interferon alpha. In a recent report, four of eight such patients remained in complete remission 2 years after discontinuation of therapy, suggesting that the immune modulation resulting from interferon may contribute to preventing recurrence (*Rousselot P, Huguet F, Cayuela JM, et al: Blood [abstract] 106:321a, 2005*).

Toxicity Imatinib is well tolerated. However, a significant fraction of patients develop grade 1–2 adverse events, including nausea, peripheral or periorbital edema, muscle cramps, diarrhea, skin rashes, weight gain, and fatigue. These events frequently are minor and either do not require therapy or respond to adequate early intervention. Fluid retention responds to diuretics when indicated; diarrhea can be managed with loperamide or other agents; nausea usually responds to prochlorperazine, promethazine, or other agents; muscle cramps can be managed with tonic water or quinine; skin rash may be managed with antihistamines and/or corticosteroids (topical and/or systemic).

Myelosuppression is the most common grade 3–4 adverse event. Neutropenia can be seen in up to 45% of patients, thrombocytopenia in up to 25% of patients, and anemia in 10% of patients. Treatment is held for grade ≥ 3 neutropenia (neutrophil count < 10^9/L) or thrombocytopenia (platelet count < 50 × 10^9/L) and restarted when counts recover above these levels. If the recovery takes longer than 2 weeks, the dose may be reduced. Treatment interruptions and dose reductions are not usually recommended for anemia. Myelosuppression is much more likely to occur during the first 2 to 3 months of therapy and is best managed with treatment interruption and close monitoring. Hematopoietic growth factors (granulocyte colony-stimulating factor [G-CSF, filgrastim, Neupogen] and erythropoietin) have been used successfully to manage prolonged or recurrent myelosuppression.

Reduced-intensity transplants are being increasingly used. A recent study reported on 186 patients with CML (118 in first chronic phase, with a median age of 50 years) who received reduced-intensity transplantation. Transplant-related mortality was 23% at 2 years, and the rate of extensive chronic graft-vs-host disease was 24%. The overall and progression-free survival rates at 3 years were 54% and 33%, respectively, for the total group and 69% and 43% for patients in chronic phase (*Crawley C, Szydlo R, Lalancette M, et al: Blood 106: 2969-2976, 2005*).

Monitoring The treatment objective has evolved from hematologic responses (hydroxyurea) to cytogenetic responses (IFN-α), to molecular responses in the imatinib era. All patients have to be evaluated with cytogenetic analysis before the start of therapy, and a baseline quantitative PCR analysis is useful. Conventional cytogenetic analysis is important at baseline and for follow-up because it provides valuable information about the entire karyotype (ie, clonal evolution, cytogenetic abnormalities in Ph chromosome-negative cells) that cannot be obtained with FISH or PCR and has prognostic implications. A cytogenetic analysis every 3 to 6 months during the first year and every 6 to 12 months thereafter is recommended. Quantitative PCR is recommended every 3 to 6 months. It is inappropriate not to follow patients with cytogenetic and molecular analyses.

Duration of therapy At this time, the duration of therapy is unclear. A minority of patients have reached undetectable levels of disease by PCR, and few have discontinued therapy. This has usually resulted in relapse. Thus, until further evidence becomes available, patients should continue therapy indefinitely.

Patients who have at least a minor cytogenetic response after 3 to 12 months of therapy still have a 35%–50% probability of achieving a complete cytogenetic response with continuation of therapy. Thus, these patients should continue therapy unless a more effective, low-risk option is available. Patients who fail to respond or lose their response to therapy may improve with an increased dose of imatinib. Up to 50% of patients may improve their cytogenetic response by doubling the dose from 300 or 400 mg to 600 or 800 mg daily.

Allogeneic BMT

Allogeneic BMT is potentially curative in CML, although relapses and mortality for complications such as chronic graft-vs-host disease (GVHD) may occur many years after transplantation. Results are better for patients in the chronic phase than in either the accelerated or blastic phase. Long-term survival rates of 50%–80% and disease-free survival rates of 30%–70% can be achieved in the chronic phase. The role of BMT is now changing in view of the results obtained with imatinib.

Predictors of response Early BMT within the first 1–3 years after diagnosis may be associated with a better outcome than BMT later in the course of disease. Younger patients also have a better outcome than older patients, with those younger than age 20 to 30 having the best prognosis. The use of the EBMT score helps to separate those patients who may have a better outcome from those who will not.

Conditioning regimens, including total-body irradiation (TBI), have been traditionally used, but non–TBI-containing regimens (eg, with busulfan and cyclophosphamide [Cytoxan, Neosar]) have produced similar results. More recently, conditioning regimens using pharmacologic targeting of busulfan have been associated with decreased regimen-related toxicity while preserving the antileukemia effect.

Also, nonmyeloablative conditioning regimens frequently containing purine analogs (mini-BMT) have been tested recently to expand the use of transplants to older patients or to patients with medical conditions that preclude conventional BMT.

Graft-vs-host disease The major morbidity from BMT is GVHD. T-cell depletion of the graft can reduce the incidence of this complication but at the expense of higher relapse and graft failure rates. (For a full discussion of GVHD, see chapter 36.)

Alternatives to matched-related donors For patients who do not have a matched-related donor, matched unrelated donor (MUD) transplants are reasonable alternatives. The 9-year experience from the National Marrow Donor Program in 1,432 patients reported a 3-year survival rate of 37.5%. Early transplantation results in better outcome, with patients transplanted in chronic phase having a 3-year disease-free survival of 63%. The outcome of patients transplanted in accelerated, blastic, or second chronic phase is inferior.

Relapse after BMT Donor leukocyte infusions are the most effective strategy to treat patients who relapse after BMT. With this strategy, 70%–80% of patients can achieve a cytogenetic complete response; the best results are achieved when patients are treated during cytogenetic or molecular relapse. Imatinib has also been effective for patients who relapse after BMT. A complete hematologic response in > 70% of patients and a cytogenetic response in 58% have been reported, with the best responses obtained in patients relapsing in chronic phase.

Autologous BMT

Although 40%–70% of patients can achieve some degree of suppression of Ph chromosome-positive cells upon engraftment of the autologous transplant, this result is usually short-lived, and most patients relapse within 1 year. Some patients previously refractory to rIFN-α may regain sensitivity after autologous BMT. The role of autologous BMT with cells collected after complete response to imatinib

> A phase I study of AMN 107 has been completed among patients with CML in all phases who received imatinib (Gleevec), which either failed or intolerance was a problem. Among patients in chronic phase, a complete hematologic response (CHR) was achieved in 92% and a cytogenetic response in 53% (complete in 35%). In accelerated phase, hematologic responses were achieved in 72% and cytogenetic, in 48%, and the corresponding figures for myeloid blast phase were 42% and 29%, respectively, and in lymphoid blast phase, 33% and 22%. Treatment was well tolerated overall. The dose-limiting toxicities at 600 mg twice daily were neutropenia and hyperbilirubinemia, and the maximum tolerated dose recommended for phase II studies was 400 mg twice daily. These phase II studies are ongoing (*Kantarjian H, Ottman O, Cortes J, et al: Blood [abstract] 106:15a, 2005*).

> Dasatinib has been used in patients with CML or Ph-positive CML who were resistant or intolerant to imatinib (Gleevec). A total of 84 patients were treated. The rate of complete hematologic response is 50% in accelerated phase, 18% in myeloid blast phase, and 50% in lymphoid blast phase/Ph-positive acute lymphoblastic leukemia (ALL). Responses were observed among a wide spectrum of Bcr-Abl kinase domain mutations. These results led to a series of phase II studies in the different phases of the disease. After only 3 months of therapy, four patients in chronic phase for whom imatinib had failed had already achieved a complete cytogenetic response (CCR) with dasatinib and one a partial cytogenetic response. Similarly, cytogenetic responses were achieved in 13 of 24 patients (54%) in accelerated phase (4 CCR), 13 of 29 (45%) in myeloid blast phase (6 CCR), and 12 of 28 in lymphoid blast phase or Ph-positive ALL (11 CCR; *Sawyers C, Kantarjian H, Shah N, et al: Blood [abstract] 106:16a, 2005*).

> Data from interferon and stem-cell transplant studies suggest that immune modulation is an important element of the long-term control and possible eradication of CML. One approach to pursue immune modulation is through vaccines. One recent study used a vaccine derived from the Bcr-Abl junction peptide vaccine to treat 16 patients with stable residual disease while on imatinib (Gleevec) or IFN-α. Of nine patients receiving imatinib, five achieved a complete cytogenetic response, and three had a complete molecular response. Of six patients treated with IFN-α, cytogenetic response was improved in five patients (*Bocchia M, Gentili S, Abruzzese E, et al: Lancet 365: 657-662, 2005*).

and with imatinib-based therapy after transplantation is currently being investigated.

Treatment recommendations

No compatible related donor Most patients (> 70%) do not have a related HLA-compatible donor. With the approval of imatinib for first-line therapy in CML, it should be considered standard for these patients.

Matched-related or one-antigen-mismatched donor When allogeneic bone marrow from a matched-related (or one-antigen-mismatched) donor is available, it could be considered as the initial option when the 1-year transplant-related mortality is expected to be < 20%. The impressive results with imatinib are changing this algorithm, and it is currently recommended to use imatinib as first-line therapy for all patients. The use of higher doses of imatinib should be considered. If no cytogenetic response is achieved after 6 months of therapy or no major cytogenetic response is seen after 12 months, transplantation can be considered in younger patients with available donors.

MUD Transplant-related mortality is > 20% in most cases. Therefore, it is recommended that imatinib be used for patients who have only an unrelated donor available and whose expected transplant-related mortality is > 20%. MUD BMT should be considered for patients who do not respond to imatinib therapy if they have a full match and their expected mortality is < 40%.

Imatinib failure When to consider failure to imatinib is still a matter of debate. However, most patients will achieve a hematologic response to imatinib within 3 months and a major cytogenetic response by 12 months. Patients not achieving any cytogenetic response after 6 months of therapy have a low probability (less than 15%) of later achieving a complete response. In contrast, patients having at least a minor cytogenetic response at 6 or 12 months still have a 20%–50% probability of achieving a complete cytogenetic response with continuation therapy. Increasing the dose of imatinib (eg, from 400 mg/d to 800 mg/d) may result in a major cytogenetic response in ~40% of patients. Patients in whom imatinib fails to induce a response and who are not candidates for BMT should be offered investigational options. Agents currently being investigated alone or in combination with imatinib include second-generation tyrosine kinase inhibitors, decitabine, homoharringtonine (HHT), and farnesyl transferase inhibitors. Among them, the new tyrosine kinase inhibitors, such as AMN107 and BMS-354825 (dasatinib) are particularly attractive. AMN107 was designed based on the imatinib structure with modifications to improve its binding to BCR-ABL and increase its selectivity; these modifications result in an agent at least one order of magnitude more potent than imatinib against BCR-ABL. Dasatinib is structurally unrelated to imatinib and, in contrast to it, can bind both the inactive and active configurations of BCR-ABL. In addition, dasatinib is a dual inhibitor that blocks Src as well as Abl and is two orders of magnitude more potent than imatinib. Both agents have been shown to inhibit both the wildtype BCR-ABL and nearly all of the clinically significant mutants of Bcr-Abl, except for T315I. The results from the early clinical trials have been impressive.

The most frequently identified mechanism of resistance to imatinib is the development of mutations at the Abl kinase domain. Mutations are identified in 30% to 50% of patients, with the most frequent occurring in the P loop. Not all mutations confer the same level of resistance to imatinib, and some may be overcome by increased concentrations of imatinib. The most resistant mutation is T315I. Although P-loop mutations have been reported to be linked to a poor prognosis, this theory has not been confirmed in all studies and it is probably more appropriate to consider individual mutations rather than "families."

Changing therapy based on molecular responses cannot be justified in most instances at the present time. Even when patients who have not achieved a 3-log reduction in transcript levels after 12 months of therapy have an inferior prognosis compared with those with at least a 3-log reduction, they still have a 92% probability of disease progression-free survival at 3 years, and in most instances, this only represents a loss of cytogenetic response. If the proposed alternative treatment option has any significant risk of mortality, the risk may be unnecessary. The clinical significance of the presence of mutations is still unclear. For example, the poor prognosis proposed for patients with P-loop mutations has not been confirmed by some groups. Thus, it is not clear that changes in therapy should be recommended based on the presence of mutations alone. However, in most instances, mutations are identifed in the context of clinical evidence of failure. In this instance, change in treatment strategy is indicated.

ACCELERATED AND BLASTIC PHASES

Imatinib

Imatinib is also effective for patients with CML in transformation. Seventy-one percent of patients in accelerated phase treated with 600 mg/d of imatinib had a hematologic response. The major cytogenetic response rate was 24%, with a time to disease progression of 12 months at 67%. These results are significantly superior to those with 400 mg/d, making 600 mg/d the standard dose in accelerated phase. In blast phase, 52% of patients achieved a hematologic remission and 31% a sustained remission lasting at least 4 weeks with imatinib. However, the median response duration is only 10 months, even when considering only patients with sustained remission (ie, lasting at least 4 weeks). Patients with clonal evolution have a lower probability of response and shorter survival than patients without clonal evolution when treated with imatinib.

Chemotherapy

Intensive chemotherapy regimens, including high-dose Ara-C and daunorubicin, induce remissions in only 25%–35% of patients in accelerated or blast phase (median survival durations of 8–18 months and 3 months, respectively). However, patients with a lymphoid blastic phase treated with therapy similar to that given for acute lymphocytic leukemia (ie, vincristine, doxorubicin, and dexamethasone, with or without cyclophosphamide) have a complete response rate of 60%–80%. Preliminary observations suggest that imatinib can be safely combined with chemotherapy regimens and may improve the duration of remission. Early results are encouraging, but long-term follow-up is pending.

A recent study combined HCVAD (cyclophosphamide, vincristine, Adriamycin [doxorubicin], and dexamethasone), a regimen used for acute lymphoblastic leukemia (ALL), with imatinib to treat 20 patients with Ph-positive ALL. All 15 patients with active disease achieved a complete response. Of 10 patients who subsequently received BMT, 9 remained in complete remission after a median follow-up of 12 months. Of the 10 patients ineligible for BMT, 1 relapsed after 1 year, 2 older patients died in complete remission, and all others remained in complete remission after a median of 20 months. This study suggests that the addition of imatinib to combination chemotherapy regimens used for ALL is well tolerated and may improve the results of patients with Ph chromosome-positive ALL.

New agents and combination regimens (eg, decitabine, cyclophosphamide, Ara-C, farnesyl transferase inhibitors, and second-generation tyrosine kinase inhibitors) are currently being evaluated. The best results have been obtained with the new tyrosine kinase inhibitors dasatinib and AMN107.

Decitabine is a hypomethylating agent with promising activity in patients in accelerated or blast phase. Decitabine has achieved an objective response in 33% of patients in blast phase and 66% of those in accelerated phase. Lower doses of decitabine achieve optimal demethylation with reduced toxicity and are currently being evaluated.

BMT

Compared with those results in patients in chronic phase, results with allogeneic BMT are worse in patients in accelerated or blastic phase, with 4-year survival rates of only 10%–30%. Patients in accelerated phase (determined on the basis of clonal evolution only) who undergo BMT < 1 year after diagnosis have a 4-year probability of survival of 74%.

SUGGESTED READING

Bocchia M, Gentili S, Abruzzese E, et al: Effect of a p210 multipeptide vaccine associated with imatinib or interferon in patients with chronic myeloid leukaemia and persistent residual disease: A multicentre observational trial. Lancet 365:657–662, 2005.

Branford S, Rudzki Z, Parkinson I, et al: Real-time quantitative PCR analysis can be used as a primary screen to identify patients with CML treated with imatinib who have BCR-ABL kinase domain mutations. Blood 104:2926–2932, 2004.

Cortes J, Giles F, O'Brien S, et al: Result of high-dose imatinib mesylate in patients with Philadelphia chromosome-positive chronic myeloid leukemia after failure of interferon-α. Blood 102:83–86, 2003.

Cortes JE, Talpaz M, Giles F, et al: Prognostic significance of cytogenetic clonal evolution in patients with chronic myelogenous leukemia on imatinib mesylate therapy. Blood 101:3794–3800, 2003.

Cortes J, Talpaz M, O'Brien S, et al: Molecular responses in patients with chronic myelogenous leukemia in chronic phase treated with imatinib mesylate. Clin Cancer Res 11:3425–3432, 2005.

Hughes TP, Kaeda J, Branford S, et al: Frequency of major molecular responses to imatinib or interferon alfa plus cytarabine in newly diagnosed chronic myeloid leukemia. N Engl J Med 349:1423–1432, 2003.

Kantarjian HM, Cortes JE, O'Brien S, et al: Imatinib mesylate therapy in newly diagnosed patients with Philadelphia chromosome-positive chronic myelogenous leukemia: High incidence of early complete and major cytogenetic responses. Blood 101:97–100, 2003.

Kantarjian HM, Cortes JE, O'Brien S, et al: Long-term survival benefit and improved complete cytogenetic and molecular response rates with imatinib mesylate in Philadelphia chromosome-positive chronic-phase chronic myeloid leukemia after failure of interferon-alpha. Blood 104:1979–1988, 2004.

Kantarjian HM, O'Brien S, Cortes J, et al: Imatinib mesylate therapy improves survival in patients with newly diagnosed Philadelphia chromosome-positive chronic myelogenous leukemia in the chronic phase: Comparison with historic data. Cancer 98:2636–2642, 2003.

Kantarjian HM, Talpaz M, O'Brien S, et al: Dose escalation of imatinib mesylate can overcome resistance to standard-dose therapy in patients with chronic myelogenous leukemia. Blood 101:473–475, 2003.

Kantarjian H, Talpaz M, O'Brien S, et al: High-dose imatinib mesylate therapy in newly diagnosed Philadelphia chromosome-positive chronic phase chronic myeloid leukemia. Blood 103:2873–2878, 2004.

Kantarjian H, Talpaz M, O'Brien S, et al: Prediction of initial cytogenetic response for subsequent major and complete cytogenetic response to imatinib mesylate therapy in patients with Philadelphia chromosome-positive chronic myelogenous leukemia. Cancer 97:2225–2228, 2003.

Kantarjian H, Talpaz M, O'Brien S, et al: Survival benefit with imatinib mesylate therapy in patients with accelerated-phase chronic myelogenous leukemia: Comparison with historic experience. Cancer 103:2099–2108, 2005.

Radich JP, Gooley T, Bensinger W, et al: HLA-matched related hematopoietic cell transplantation for chronic-phase CML using a targeted busulfan and cyclophosphamide preparative regimen. Blood 102:31–35, 2003.

Rosti G, Martinelli G, Bassi S, et al: Molecular response to imatinib in late chronic-phase chronic myeloid leukemia. Blood 103:2284–2290, 2004.

Shah NP, Tran C, Lee FY, et al: Overrriding imatinib resistance with a novel ABL kinase inhibitor. Science 305:399–401, 2004.

CHAPTER 34

Chronic lymphocytic leukemia

William G. Wierda, MD, PhD, Nicole Lamanna, MD, Jorge E. Cortes, MD, and Mark A. Weiss, MD

Chronic lymphocytic leukemia (CLL) is a clonal malignancy that results from expansion of the mature lymphocyte compartment. This expansion is a consequence of prolonged cell survival, despite a varied cell turnover. The affected lymphocytes are of B-cell lineage in 95% of cases, and the remaining cases involve T lymphocytes, representing a distinct disorder.

CLL is the most common leukemia in adults in Western countries, accounting for approximately 25%-30% of all leukemias. The proportion of cases diagnosed with the early stages of the disease (Rai stage 0) has risen from 10% to 50%, probably because of earlier diagnosis (routine automated blood counts).

Epidemiology

The incidence of CLL in the general population is 3.6:100,000 population, with an estimated death rate of 1.6:100,000 population. It was estimated that there were 10,020 patients diagnosed with CLL in 2006.

Gender The male-to-female ratio is 2:1. There is little change with age, as the male-to-female ratio is 2.1:1.0 for patients < 65 years old, compared with 1.9:1.0 for those ≥ 65 years old.

Age The median age at diagnosis is 72 years, and CLL is rarely seen before the age of 35 years. Less than 3% of all cases are younger than 45 years at the time of diagnosis.

Race In the American population, the incidence of CLL is similar in different races. However, the incidence is much lower in Asia (Japan, Korea, and China), Latin America, and Africa than in the United States and Western Europe.

CLL

Etiology and risk factors

The etiology of CLL is unclear. However, some factors associated with CLL have been identified.

Genetic factors There is a high familial risk for CLL, with family members of CLL patients having a twofold to sevenfold higher risk of developing the disease. CLL with a familial association tends to occur in younger individuals with subsequent generations, perhaps because of increased screening. Association with certain HLA patterns has not been consistent.

Environmental factors There is no documented association of CLL with exposure to radiation, alkylating agents, or known leukemogenic chemicals. However, exposure to some chemicals used in agriculture may increase the risk of developing CLL.

Viral infections Associations between CLL and several viruses, including human T-cell lymphotrophic viruses I and II (HTLV-I and HTLV-II) and Epstein-Barr virus (EBV), have been suggested. However, no conclusive evidence of a causal relationship exists. Adult T-cell leukemia/lymphoma, a T-cell disorder that can resemble CLL, is caused by HTLV-I.

Monoclonal B lymphocytosis In a recent study, 3.8% of unselected healthy individuals older than age 65 in the general population had monoclonal (by light chain analysis) $CD5^{+}/19^{+}/23^{+}$ B cells. These asymptomatic individuals did not have lymphocytosis or clinical evidence of disease and did not fulfill diagnostic criteria for CLL. Whether or not these individuals will eventually reach diagnostic criteria or develop symptomatic disease is unknown. Nevertheless, this finding indicates that the incidence of a monoclonal lymphoproliferative process is potentially much more common in the aging population than previously appreciated.

Signs and symptoms

In approximately 20% of patients, CLL is asymptomatic at diagnosis and is discovered on a routine blood examination. When symptoms are present, they are nonspecific and include fatigue, weakness, and malaise and, in fact, may not even be attributable to CLL.

Constitutional B symptoms (ie, fever, weight loss, and night sweats) are not common at diagnosis but may signal disease transformation. Patients frequently notice enlarged lymph nodes or abdominal discomfort and early satiety related to splenomegaly.

Patients with CLL have an increased susceptibility to infections, which may be the presenting complaint.

Lymphadenopathy is common at diagnosis. Lymph nodes are usually symmetrical, mobile, and nontender.

Splenomegaly and hepatomegaly The spleen and, less frequently, the liver may be enlarged. Splenomegaly may be massive in advanced cases. Only occasionally is splenomegaly found in the absence of lymphadenopathy, but recognition of such patients may identify a group that may benefit from splenectomy.

Other organs In advanced disease, other organs may be involved, including the GI mucosa, prostate, lungs, pleura, and bones. Rarely is such involvement clinically important unless (Richter's) transformation has occurred.

TABLE 1: Diagnostic criteria for CLL according to the National Cancer Institute (NCI) and International Workshop on CLL (IWCLL)

Cells	NCI	IWCLL
Lymphocytes	≥ 5 x 10^9/L + ≥ 1 B-cell marker (CD19, CD20, CD23) + CD5	≥ 10 x 10^9/L + B-cell phenotype or bone marrow involvement
Atypical cells (eg, prolymphocytes)	< 55%	Not stated
Bone marrow lymphocytes	≥ 30%	> 30%

Laboratory features

Peripheral blood The most consistent feature of CLL is marked lymphocytosis, with median values of 30–50 × 10^9/L. The lymphocytes are small and mature-appearing, with little cytoplasm and clumped chromatin. A few larger nucleolated cells, which represent prolymphocytes, usually constitute < 10% of the total lymphocytes. Diagnostic criteria for CLL defined by the National Cancer Institute (NCI) and International Workshop on CLL (IWCLL) are presented in Table 1.

A positive Coombs' test is seen in as many as 30% of patients at some time during the disease course, although it is uncommon (< 5%) during early stages. Autoimmune phenomena are relatively frequent, with hemolytic anemia (lifetime risk approximately 10%–20%) and thrombocytopenia (lifetime risk approximately 5%–10%) occurring most commonly. Autoimmune neutropenia and other autoimmune sequelae are infrequent but more common than in the general population.

Bone marrow The bone marrow is usually hypercellular but can be normocellular. The most characteristic feature is the presence of at least 30% mature lymphocytes. The lymphocyte infiltration can be interstitial, nodular, mixed interstitial and nodular, or diffuse. Diffuse lymphocyte infiltration is associated with a poor prognosis.

Other laboratory findings Progressive hypogammaglobulinemia is seen in > 50% of patients with CLL, usually affecting IgA first, followed by IgM and IgG. However, 5%–10% of patients may have a small monoclonal peak. Paraproteinemia is more common at disease transformation.

Elevated serum levels of B_2-microglobulin (β2M) have been associated with a poor prognosis. Elevation of serum lactic dehydrogenase (LDH) levels is found in < 10% of patients at diagnosis and may indicate autoimmune hemolytic anemia or (Richter's) transformation to large-cell lymphoma (LCL).

Immunophenotyping More than 95% of all cases have a B-cell phenotype. In these patients, CD19 and/or CD20 are essentially always coexpressed with

CD5, which normally is expressed on T cells and a subset of normal B cells. Other markers, such as CD21 and CD22, may also be expressed. Expression of CD23 helps to differentiate CLL from mantle cell lymphoma, in which cells coexpress CD19 and CD5 but lack CD23. Furthermore, the monoclonal antibody FMC7 (which recognizes an epitope on CD20) rarely reacts with CLL cells but frequently binds the cells of patients with mantle cell lymphoma.

Expression of surface immunoglobulin is usually weak and is lower than in normal B lymphocytes or most other B-cell lymphomas. Expression of CD38 on the surface of CLL cells portends a worse prognosis than that for patients whose cells do not express CD38.

Cytogenetic and molecular findings

Chromosomal abnormalities

A number of recurrent cytogenetic abnormalities have been identified in CLL. Most have not been associated with a specific gene defect or abnormality; however, their detection is prognostically important, and work continues toward identifying the associated gene or genes.

Chromosomal abnormalities occur in 50%–65% of CLL patients with analyzable metaphases. Because of the low mitotic rate in CLL, traditional karyotypic methods frequently fail. Fluorescent in situ hybridization (FISH) has increased the detection of clonal genetic abnormalities in CLL patients. In a landmark study, Dohner et al evaluated 325 patients with CLL. Using a variety of fluorescent probes, they identified chromosomal aberrations in 82%. Among these findings was the recognition that some subtypes (17p and 11q) had markedly shorter time to initiate chemotherapy and shorter overall survival than did other types. In this study, the most frequent change was a deletion in 13q14 (55% of patients). Other typical abnormalities included deletion 11q22–23 (18%), trisomy 12q13 (16%), and deletion 17p13 (7%).

These genetic abnormalities help explain some of the clinical variations seen in CLL. For example, patients with 13q deletions tend to have modest or absent lymphadenopathy, whereas patients with deletion 11q frequently have bulky adenopathy.

Disease progression also is heavily influenced by the underlying genetic abnormality. Time from diagnosis to treatment averaged only 9 months for patients with 17p abnormalities, compared with 92 months for patients with 13q deletions.

Prognostic importance These chromosomal abnormalities were potent predictors of outcome with the following median survivals: deletion 17p, 32 months; deletion 11q, 79 months; trisomy 12, 114 months; and deletion 13q, 133 months.

Molecular abnormalities

No single gene has been implicated in the pathogenesis of CLL. However, several genetic abnormalities have biologic and/or prognostic implications.

The *P53* gene is located on the short arm of chromosome 17 and is deleted in the leukemia clone of up to 10% of patients with CLL. Mutations of *P53* occur in a similar proportion of CLL cases, usually in association with *P53* deletion in the other *P53* allele. The 17p deletion involving *P53* is considered the most significant negative cytogenetic prognostic factor in CLL. The p53 protein normally responds to DNA damage by inducing cell cycle arrest and facilitating DNA repair. It can also induce apoptosis in cells with damaged DNA and in this way mediates the cytotoxicity of many anticancer agents. Resistance to treatment is a particular characteristic of p53 deletion and has been observed for agents including purine analogs.

> Recently, further investigation of the common 13q deletion has revealed the detection of specific microRNA genomic sequence abnormalities expressed in patients with CLL. Further analysis suggests a microRNA signature profile may be associated with Zap-70 expression and mutational status of IgVH as well as disease progression *(Calin GA, Ferracin M, Cimmino A, et al: N Engl J Med 353:1793-1801, 2005).*

Overexpression of *bcl*-2 Abnormalities of the long arm of chromosome 14 frequently involve region 14q32, the site encoding for the immunoglobulin heavy-chain gene. However, gene translocations such as t(11;14)(q13;q32) and t(14;18)(q32;q21), which juxtapose genes *bcl*-1 and *bcl*-2 to the heavy-chain immunoglobulin gene, are relatively uncommon and should prompt consideration of alternative diagnoses (mantle cell or follicular lymphoma). Nevertheless, increased expression of *bcl*-2 mRNA and protein is common in CLL. Since overexpression of *bcl*-2 inhibits apoptosis, it is possible that this gene participates in the pathogenesis of CLL.

Multidrug resistance gene Approximately 40% of patients with CLL have overexpression of the multidrug resistance gene (*MDR1*).

Staging and prognosis

Staging systems Two staging systems of CLL are commonly used: one proposed and later modified by Rai and the other proposed by Binet (Table 2). Both systems include three categories of low, intermediate, and high risk, with median survival durations of approximately 10, 6, and 2 years, respectively.

Other prognostic factors Stage of disease has been considered the main prognostic indicator for CLL. However, other factors have prognostic implications, such as chromosomal aberrations, serum levels of β2M, pattern of bone marrow infiltration, the lymphocyte doubling time, and serum levels of soluble CD23.

Somatic hypermutation (SHM) normally occurs in germinal centers of lymphoid tissues and is a process that introduces mutations in the variable region of immunoglobulin genes. It is responsible for affinity maturation, the process of producing B cells with high-affinity antibody. CLL can be divided into two distinct prognostic groups based on the extent to which the expressed immunoglobulin heavy chain variable (IgV_H) gene has undergone SHM. CLL cases with an IgV_H gene with < 98% homology to germline are considered mutated and those with an IgV_H gene with ≥ 98% homology to germline are considered unmutated.

TABLE 2: Staging systems for CLL

RAI SYSTEM

Rai stage	Modified Rai stage (risk)	Clinical characteristics	Median survival (yr)
0	Low	Lymphocytosis in peripheral blood and bone marrow only	> 10
I	Intermediate	Lymphocytosis and enlarged lymph nodes	6
II		Lymphocytosis and enlarged spleen and/or liver	
III	High	Lymphocytosis and anemia (hemoglobin < 11 g/dL)	2
IV		Lymphocytosis and thrombocytopenia (platelets < 100×10^9/L)	

BINET SYSTEM

Binet stage	Clinical characteristics	Median survival (yr)
A	Hemoglobin level ≥10 g/dL, platelet count ≥100×10^9/L, and < 3 areas involved	> 7
B	Hemoglobin level ≥10 g/dL, platelet count ≥100×10^9/L, and ≥ 3 areas involved	< 5
C	Hemoglobin level < 10 g/dL, platelet count < 100 x 10^9/L, or both (independent of areas involved)	< 2

CLL cases with an unmutated IgV_H gene generally have rapid progression and an unfavorable prognosis, whereas CLL cases with a mutated IgV_H gene generally have slowly progressive disease and a favorable prognosis. Patients with unmutated IgV_H genes have a median survival of 8 years, compared with 24 years for those with mutated IgV_H genes. The biologic differences between these groups are also reflected in the association of unmutated IgV_H genes with other poor prognostic features, such as expression of CD38, and unfavorable cytogenetic abnormalities.

The immunoglobulins expressed by CLL cells are frequently polyreactive autoantibodies. It follows that the cell that gives rise to the CLL B cell may experience persistent antigen stimulation, which contributes to malignant transformation. The role of antigen selection is implicated by the overrepresentation of certain IgV_H genes in CLL. In addition, there is also a biased distribution of these genes between the mutated and unmutated subgroups. The VH3 and VH4 families of genes are frequently found in the subgroup with mutated IgV_H genes, whereas the VH1 family, particularly VH1-69, is more common in the subgroup with unmutated IgV_H genes. Specific genes, such as VH3-21, have also been associated with a poor prognosis, independent of IgV_H mutation status.

ZAP-70 encodes a protein tyrosine kinase normally expressed by T cells and involved in intracellular signaling initiated by T-cell receptor ligation. Expres-

TABLE 3: Suggested indications for therapy for early-stage CLL

Progressive disease-related symptoms (eg, fever, night sweats, weight loss)
Bone marrow involvement with progressive anemia and thrombocytopenia
Progressive or painful splenomegaly
Progressive or bulky lymphadenopathy
Rapidly increasing lymphocytosis
Autoimmune hemolytic anemia or thrombocytopenia

sion of ZAP-70 by CLL B cells (> 20% CLL cells ZAP-70+) is associated with unmutated IgV_H genes, shorter time to initial treatment, and inferior survival compared to ZAP-70 negative (< 20% cases). Detection of ZAP-70 protein by flow cytometry or immunohistochemistry may provide a useful prognostic marker for patients with CLL.

Treatment

TREATMENT RECOMMENDATIONS

Traditionally, the initial therapy for CLL has been chlorambucil (Leukeran) with or without prednisone. However, accumulating data suggest that fludarabine has significantly greater activity than these agents. This agent produces higher overall and CR rates and provides a longer remission duration than does chlorambucil. Newer data suggest that combination chemotherapy, particularly a nucleoside analog combined with an alkylating agent, produces higher response rates, and the addition of monoclonal antibodies to such regimens appears to increase the CR rates. However, to date, a survival advantage has not been demonstrated for administering these regimens as initial therapy.

The development of nonmyeloablative transplants has provided the possibility of allogeneic transplantation for CLL, where the median age of patients is near 70, but this new technique should only be performed in the context of a clinical trial. An effort should be made to enroll patients in clinical trials that offer them the possibility of receiving some of the new alternatives, which may eventually achieve the goal of curing CLL.

EARLY-STAGE DISEASE

Since patients with early-stage CLL have a good long-term prognosis, and early therapy has not changed the outcome of the disease, patients in the early stages should not be treated unless specific indications exist (Table 3). Randomized trials comparing chlorambucil vs no therapy have documented no advantage for patients with early-stage CLL who received immediate therapy with chlorambucil. New alternatives for treatment of high-risk early-stage CLL (ZAP-70–positive, unmutated IgH status) are being investigated (eg, monoclonal antibodies).

TABLE 4: Response criteria in CLL according to the IWCLL

Complete response

Resolution of lymphadenopathy, splenomegaly, hepatomegaly, and constitutional symptoms

Normalization of blood counts:

- Neutrophils > 1.5×10^9/L
- Platelets > 100×10^9/L
- Lymphocytes < 4×10^9/L

Normalization of bone marrow

- < 30% lymphocytes[a]
- Nodular or focal infiltrates[b]

Partial response

Downstaging (from Binet stages C to A or B and from B to A)[b]

or

> 50% decrease in absolute lymphocyte count, splenomegaly, lymphadenopathy, hepatomegaly

- Neutrophils ≥ 1.5×10^9/L
- Platelets ≥ 100×10^9/L
- Hemoglobin > 11 g/dL
- > 50% improvement in peripheral blood counts[a]

[a] National Cancer Institute (NCI) criteria; [b] International Workshop on CLL (IWCLL) criteria

CONVENTIONAL CHEMOTHERAPY

Single-agent chemotherapy

The German CLL Study Group (GCLLSG) reported on a randomized trial of fludarabine (F) vs F plus cyclophosphamide (FC) in younger patients (< 66 years old) with untreated CLL. The FC combination resulted in a higher frequency of responses (94%) and complete responses (24%) than did F alone (83% and 7%, *P* = .001, *P* < .001, respectively). The median progression-free survival was 48 months for FC vs 20 months for F (*P* = .001). There is no difference in overall survival between these groups. There was more grade 3/4 thrombocytopenia and leukopenia in patients who received FC, but infectious complications were not increased (*Eichhorst BF, Busch R, Hapfinger G, et al: Blood 107:885-891, 2006*).

Chlorambucil Historically, the initial agent used for CLL has been chlorambucil, given as either 0.1 mg/kg daily or 20–40 mg/m^2 every 2–4 weeks. Therapy is continued until the signs or symptoms requiring therapy are controlled.

Chlorambucil is frequently combined with oral prednisone (30–100 mg/m^2/d), although there is no clear evidence that the combination improves responses or overall survival over chlorambucil alone. Prednisone is of value, however, in the management of autoimmune cytopenias.

Cyclophosphamide is an alternative to chlorambucil. The usual dose is 0.5–1 g/m^2 every 3–4 weeks alone or together with vincristine and steroids (eg, COP [cyclophosphamide, vincristine (Oncovin), and prednisone] regimen).

TABLE 5: Comparison of fludarabine, CAP, and CHOP treatment for CLL

Patient characteristic	Response rate Fludarabine	CAP	CHOP
Response	71%	58%	72%
Complete response	8%	2%	9%
Median survival	69 months	70 months	67 months

CAP = cyclophosphamide, Adriamycin (doxorubicin), and prednisone; CHOP = cyclophosphamide, low-dose doxorubicin, vincristine (Oncovin), and prednisone

Combination chemotherapy

COP and CHOP Various drug combinations have been used in CLL, mostly in patients with advanced-stage disease. The most frequently employed combinations have been COP and these three drugs plus doxorubicin (CHOP). The dose of doxorubicin used is usually low (25 mg/m^2). A higher dose of doxorubicin (50 mg/m^2) has been employed in some regimens, such as CAP (cyclophosphamide, doxorubicin [Adriamycin], and prednisone).

The group at M. D. Anderson Cancer Center has developed a regimen combining 3 days of fludarabine and cyclophosphamide with one dose of rituximab (Rituxan) given monthly. The overall response rate in previously untreated patients was 95%, and 70% of the patients achieved a complete response. Two-thirds of patients achieved flow cytometric complete responses *(Keating MJ, O'Brien S, Albitar M, et al: J Clin Oncol 23:4079-4088, 2005).*

Response rates have been 40%–85% with these combinations. In randomized studies, COP was no better than chlorambucil plus prednisone. Although CHOP initially achieved better survival than COP (in patients with Binet stage C disease) or chlorambucil plus prednisone, longer follow-up has not confirmed this survival advantage.

Nucleoside analogs

Fludarabine, now frequently the drug of choice for treating CLL, has been demonstrated to be more effective than chlorambucil for the treatment of CLL. When given to previously treated patients at a dose of 25–30 mg/m^2/d for 5 days every 3–4 weeks, this nucleoside analog produced responses in 20%–50% of patients, with 5%–15% of patients achieving a complete response (CR) and an additional 5%–20% a "nodular partial response (PR)," ie, a CR but with the presence of lymphoid nodules in the bone marrow (Table 4). In previously untreated patients, the response rate was 63%–80%, with 8%–35% of patients achieving a CR.

The addition of prednisone or chlorambucil to fludarabine therapy did not improve the response rate and is associated with an increased incidence of opportunistic infections and other toxicities. A large randomized study comparing fludarabine, CAP, and CHOP demonstrated an increased response rate with fludarabine but no difference in survival (Table 5). Randomized trials of fludarabine vs chlorambucil in previously untreated patients showed improvements in response rate (overall and CR), duration of response, and disease progression-free survival with fludarabine but no survival advantage.

Other nucleoside analogs Cladribine (2-chlorodeoxyadenosine, 2-CdA) is also active in CLL when given at doses of 0.1 mg/kg/d (or 4 mg/m^2/d) for 7 days. At therapeutic doses, this agent appears to be associated with more myelosuppression, particularly thrombocytopenia, than fludarabine. This finding limits its utility in treating CLL, but a direct comparison with fludarabine has not been reported.

The third purine analog active against CLL is pentostatin (Nipent). Previously, toxicity limited its use as an antineoplastic agent. More recently, the recognition that safe use of this drug requires concomitant hydration and close attention to renal function (it is both toxic to and cleared by the kidneys) has renewed interest in clinical evaluation with this agent. The group at Memorial Sloan-Kettering Cancer Center has studied pentostatin combined with cyclophosphamide and demonstrated responses in > 70% of previously treated patients (including those whose disease is refractory to fludarabine) with acceptable toxicity.

Rituximab (Rituxan) has subsequently been added to the pentostatin/cyclophosphamide combination, and this three-drug regimen appears to be active and safe in patients with previously treated CLL.

NEW APPROACHES

Recently, three randomized clinical trials for chemotherapy-naive patients with CLL have reported significantly higher complete and overall response rates with fludarbine and cyclophosphamide and longer progression-free survival than with fludarabine alone. These studies included the Eastern Cooperative Oncology Group (ECOG) 2997, British MRC CLL4 trial, and German CLL Study Group CLL4 trials. Greater myelosuppression was seen with the combination, but there was no increase in the incidence of infection.

Combination chemotherapy The combination of fludarabine (30 mg/m^2/d for 3 days) and cyclophosphamide (300 mg/m^2/d for 3 days) has resulted in an improved response (overall and CR) rate vs fludarabine alone. Longer follow-up is needed to assess the effect of this combination on survival.

Using a sequential approach with these two agents, the group at Memorial Sloan-Kettering Cancer Center has shown that consolidation therapy with high-dose cyclophosphamide markedly improves the frequency of a CR over fludarabine alone.

Recent data suggest that the addition of a monoclonal antibody to fludarabine-based therapy may markedly improve CR rates in this disease. A study conducted by the Cancer and Leukemia Group B (CALGB) randomized patients with previously untreated CLL to receive fludarabine or a combination of fludarabine and the anti-CD20 antibody rituximab at standard doses. Patients in both arms subsequently received a consolidation course of rituximab for 4 weeks.

Overall response rates were high in both arms, but there was a significantly higher CR rate (33%) in the concurrent arm than in the arm with fludarabine alone (15%); however, both groups experienced similar response durations and overall survival. The CR rate increased in both groups after consolidation therapy with rituximab. This study illustrated the fact that adding rituximab to fludarabine increases the frequency of a CR both when administered concomitantly and sequentially.

Elter et al recently reported on the use of fludarabine in combination with alemtuzumab (Campath), a humanized monoclonal antibody targeting the panlymphocyte antigen CD52, in 36 patients with relapsed or refractory disease. The overall frequency of response was 83%, with 11 complete responses.

Monoclonal antibody–targeted therapy Monoclonal antibodies have been used in patients with CLL to exploit antibody-mediated cytotoxicity. Alemtuzumab has been approved by the FDA for the treatment of refractory CLL. In a pivotal trial in patients with fludarabine-refractory disease, alemtuzumab resulted in an overall response rate of 33%.

Rituximab also has been investigated and is active both as a single agent and in combination with chemotherapy. Because of rituximab's efficacy without significant toxicity, it is assuming a greater role in the treatment of patients with CLL.

The combination of alemtuzumab and rituximab has been evaluated in patients with relapsed or refractory lymphoid malignancies. Alemtuzumab was given twice weekly at 30 mg IV for 4 weeks. Rituximab (375 mg/m^2)was given concurrently weekly for the 4 weeks. Responses were reported for 48 patients, 32 with CLL, 9 with CLL/PLL (prolymphocytic leukemia), 1 with PLL, 4 with mantle cell lymphoma, and 2 with Richter's transformation. The overall response rate was 52%; CR was noted in 8%, nodular PR in 4%, and PR in 40% of treated patients. Toxicities included infusion-related reactions. Infections occurred in 52% of patients with cytomegalovirus reactivation occurring in 27% of patients. Overall, this was a well-tolerated combination for relapsed patients with CLL.

Achieving minimal residual disease-free status The current formal criteria to assess response are based on physical examination, blood counts, and microscopic evaluation of bone marrow (Table 4). Minimal residual disease (MRD) can be evaluated by more sensitive methods such as polymerase chain reaction (PCR) for the IgV_H gene or 4-color flow cytometry. In a study of 91 previously treated patients who received alemtuzumab (30 mg thrice weekly for up to 16 weeks), 36% achieved CR, and the overall response rate was 54%. Of the 91 patients, 18 achieved MRD-free status by flow-cytometry evaluation of their bone marrow. Survival was significantly longer for patients who achieved MRD-free status. Overall survival for the 18 patients with MRD-free remission was 84% at 5 years.

For patients who have residual disease after purine analog–based therapy, the marrow has been the major site of involvement. Elimination of residual disease, particularly in the marrow, may improve treatment outcome. Because of the significant activity of alemtuzumab at clearing blood and marrow of disease, its ability to eliminate residual disease after chemotherapy is under investigation.

Stem-cell transplantation

Both allogeneic and autologous stem-cell transplantations (SCTs) have been tested in patients with CLL.

Allogeneic SCT is a viable option for younger patients with CLL, particularly if they have not responded to alkylating agents and/or nucleoside analogs and are in an advanced stage of disease. The series reported to date, including a majority of patients with advanced refractory disease, has documented a CR rate in excess of 70%. The response is sustained in most patients, although reported follow-up is typically short. SCT using nonablative conditioning regimens has produced encouraging results and should be considered in the setting of a clinical trial, particularly for patients > 60 years.

Autologous SCT Since the median age of patients with CLL is usually higher than the age considered acceptable for allogeneic SCT, autologous transplants using purged marrow have also been investigated. In general, results have been disappointing, with the best results seen in patients with responsive disease and low tumor burdens–a group that might have fared well without a transplant.

Splenectomy

Splenectomy may be beneficial for patients in whom hypersplenism is the cause of cytopenias (particularly in patients without significant lymphadenopathy) or for palliation when splenomegaly is symptomatic and refractory to chemotherapy. Cytopenias frequently respond to splenectomy. Perioperative mortality varies widely and is largely related to the experience of the surgeon in performing splenectomy in these patients. In experienced hands, splenectomy can be performed with minimal mortality, even in patients with end-stage disease.

Complications

Infections Patients with CLL are prone to multiple infections, and infectious complications are a leading cause of death in patients with CLL. Hypogammaglobulinemia plays a central role in the predisposition of patients to this problem, and prophylactic IV administration of immunoglobulin preparations may reduce the incidence of infections. Cytotoxic therapy further weakens the immune system and may increase the risk of opportunistic infections.

Autoimmune cytopenias frequently complicate CLL and may be precipitated or aggravated by therapy (eg, fludarabine) for CLL. Autoimmune hemolytic anemia can be treated successfully with prednisone in the majority of patients. Combinations of cyclophosphamide with rituximab are beneficial in cases refractory to prednisone, splenectomy, or cyclosporine. Similar approaches may be useful for autoimmune thrombocytopenia. In a study from M. D. Anderson Cancer Center, 31 patients with CLL and autoimmune anemia or thrombocytopenia received cyclosporine (300 mg/day). Sixty-three percent of patients responded, with a median duration of response of 10 months.

No grade 3/4 toxicity was seen.

Pure red cell aplasia and the less commonly amegakaryocytic thrombocytopenia are infrequent complications of CLL, which are mediated by immune mechanisms. Therapy with cyclosporine (3–6 mg/kg/d) is frequently effective.

TRANSFORMATION

Large cell lymphoma (LCL) CLL transforms into LCL in 3%–10% of patients. This phenomenon, known as Richter's transformation, has an aggressive presentation with fever and other B symptoms and progressive lymphadenopathy. Extranodal involvement occurs in approximately 40% of patients. Paraproteinemia, hypercalcemia, and a sharp rise in serum LDH levels can be frequently seen.

The prognosis of patients whose disease progresses to LCL is variable and depends in part on the degree of prior treatment used for the underlying CLL. In treatment-naive patients with LCL, standard therapy with CHOP and rituximab may offer long-term control of the transformed component. In patients who have had significant prior therapy, the disease is often refractory, and combination chemotherapy including SCT is frequently ineffective.

PLL More rarely, CLL can transform into PLL, characterized by a > 55% increase in prolymphocytes. The transformation is frequently accompanied by progression of splenomegaly, cytopenias, and refractoriness to therapy.

Other diseases Anecdotal cases of CLL evolving into acute lymphocytic leukemia, myeloma, low-grade lymphoma, and Hodgkin's lymphoma have been reported. The rarity of these reports makes a true causal connection less likely.

HAIRY-CELL LEUKEMIA

Hairy-cell leukemia (HCL) is an infrequent B-cell malignancy usually associated with pancytopenia and splenomegaly. About 600 cases are reported yearly in the United States. Despite its relative rarity, there are a disproportionate number of highly effective therapies available.

Epidemiology and etiology

The male-to-female ratio of HCL is 4:1. The median age at presentation is 50 years. The etiology is unknown.

Differential diagnosis

HCL can be confused with malignant lymphomas, splenic lymphoma with villous lymphocytes (SLVLs), CLL, other non-Hodgkin's lymphomas in leukemic phase, and occasionally even myelodysplastic syndromes.

Treatment

The indications for treatment of HCL are an absolute neutrophil count (ANC) < 1,000/μL, platelet count < 100 × 10^3/μL, or hemoglobin level < 10 g/dL; leukemic phase of HCL; symptomatic splenomegaly; recurrent infections; or autoimmune complications.

Response criteria The criteria for a CR are normalization of the complete blood cell (CBC) count, with ANC > 1,500/μL, platelet count > 100,000/μL, and hemoglobin level > 12 g/dL; regression of organomegaly to normal; and bone marrow and peripheral blood free of hairy cells. PRs require reduction of the hairy cells in the bone marrow to < 50%, < 5% hairy cells in peripheral blood, > 50% reduction in organomegaly, and normalization of the CBC count.

Splenectomy is reserved for patients with splenic rupture, infarcts, a massively enlarged spleen, severe hypersplenism, or failure to respond to systemic chemotherapy.

Interferon-α (IFN-α), at a dose of 3 mU/d administered by IM or SC injection for 6 months followed by 3 mU/d three times weekly for 12 or 24 months, induces a CR in 8%–10% of patients and a PR in 74%. The median time to response was 6 months in patients achieving a PR and 14 months in those achieving a CR. Patients frequently relapse between 12 and 24 months after discontinuation of therapy. The superiority of purine analog therapy (discussed later) has essentially led most clinicians to abandon the use of IFN for this disease.

Purine analogs The recommended dose of pentostatin is 4 mg/m^2 by IV bolus every other week until a CR is obtained. Usually, patients require a median of 8 courses (range, 4–15). The CR rate varies between 59% and 89% in different studies, and the PR rate varies between 4% and 37%. Responses can last for many years, and patients who relapse often respond to retreatment with pentostatin. In an update of a large randomized trial comparing pentostatin and IFN-α, Flinn et al reported that in 241 patients with HCL treated with pentostatin, the 10-year overall survival rate was 81%, with only two deaths (1%) attributable to HCL.

Cladribine shows activity in treating HCL similar to that of pentostatin. Due to this finding and the fact that cladribine is given as 1 cycle of a 7-day continuous infusion or 5-day bolus, this agent usually is the preferred treatment of this disorder. Piro et al treated 144 HCL patients with cladribine, 0.1 mg/kg/d by continuous IV infusion for 7 days. A total response rate of 97% was obtained, with 85% CRs and 12% PRs. Response was independent of previous treatment with IFN or splenectomy, and three patients whose disease was refractory to pentostatin responded to cladribine. Recovery of CBC counts occurred on average by day 61 (range, 11–268 days).

The largest series reporting long-term follow-up results on patients with HCL treated with cladribine was from the Scripps group. A total of 349 patients, with a median duration of response follow-up of 59 months, were evaluated. Twenty-six percent had relapsed at a median of 29 months, but most of them were patients who had achieved only a PR. The time-to-treatment failure rate at 48 months was only 16% in complete responders.

Recently, Else et al reported on a large series of 219 patients with HCL, comparing their experience with pentostatin and cladribine. Treatment results were similar in terms of frequency of complete responses, relapse, and overall survival. Though the results are excellent, with more than 95% of patients alive at 10 years, the disease-free survival curves do not plateau, indicating these drugs are not curative in HCL.

Immunotoxin The NCI evaluated a recombinant immunotoxin containing an anti-CD22 variable domain fused to a truncated Pseudomonas exotoxin; it was given by IV infusion every other day for a total of three doses. Sixteen patients whose disease was resistant to cladribine were treated; 2 achieved a PR and 11 achieved a CR. Of the 11 patients, 3 who had a CR relapsed and were retreated; all of these patients achieved a second CR.

SUGGESTED READING

Byrd JC, Peterson BL, Morrison VA, et al: Randomized phase II study of fludarabine with concurrent vs sequential treatment with rituximab in symptomatic, untreated patients with B-cell chronic lymphocytic leukemia: Results from Cancer and Leukemia Group B 9712 (CALGB 9712). Blood 101:6–14, 2003.

Calin GA, Ferracin M, Cimmino A, et al: A MicroRNA signature associated with prognosis and progression in chronic lymphocytic leukemia. N Engl J Med 353:1793–1801, 2005.

Crespo M, Bosch F, Villamor N, et al: ZAP-70 expression as a surrogate for immunoglobulin-variable-region mutations in chronic lymphocytic leukemia. N Engl J Med 348:1764–1775, 2003.

Damle RN, Wasil T, Fais F, et al: Ig V gene mutation status and CD38 expression as novel prognostic indicators in chronic lymphocytic leukemia. Blood 94:1840–1847, 1999.

Else M, Ruchlemer R, Osuji N, et al: Long remissions in hairy cell leukemia with purine analogs. Cancer 104:2442–2448, 2005.

Elter T, Borchmann P, Schulz H, et al: Fludarabine in combination with alemtuzumab is effective and feasible in patients with relapsed or refractory B-cell chronic lymphocytic leukemia: Results of a phase II trial. J Clin Oncol 23:7024–7031, 2005.

Hamblin TJ, Davis Z, Gardiner A, et al: Unmutated Ig V(H) genes are associated with a more aggressive form of chronic lymphocytic leukemia. Blood 94:1848–1854, 1999.

Keating MJ, O'Brien S, Albitar M, et al: Early results of a chemoimmunotherapy regimen of fludarabine, cyclophosphamide, and rituximab as intital therapy for chronic lymphocytic leukemia. J Clin Oncol 23:4079–4088, 2005.

Lundin J, Kimby E, Bjorkholm M, et al: Phase II trial of subcutaneous anti-CD52 monoclonal antibody alemtuzumab (Campath-1H) as first-line treatment for patients with B-cell chronic lymphocytic leukemia (B-CLL). Blood 100:768–773, 2002.

Moreton P, Kennedy B, Lucas G, et al: Eradication of minimal residual disease in B-cell chronic lymphocytic leukemia after alemtuzumab therapy is associated with prolonged survival. J Clin Oncol 23:2971–2979, 2005.

Rai KR, Peterson BL, Appelbaum FR, et al: Fludarabine compared with chlorambucil as primary therapy for chronic lymphocytic leukemia. N Engl J Med 343:1750–1757, 2000.

Schetelig J, Thiede C, Bornhauser M, et al: Evidence of a graft-versus-leukemia effect in chronic lymphocytic leukemia after reduced-intensity conditioning and allogeneic stem-cell transplantation: The Cooperative German Transplant Study Group. J Clin Oncol 21:2747–2753, 2003.

Weiss MA, Maslak PG, Jurcic JG, et al: Pentostatin and cyclophosphamide: An effective new regimen in previously treated patients with chronic lymphocytic leukemia. J Clin Oncol 21:1278–1284, 2003.

Wierda W, O'Brien S, Wen S, et al: Chemoimmunotherapy with fludarabine, cyclophosphamide, and rituximab for relapsed and refractory chronic lymphocytic leukemia. J Clin Oncol 23:4070–4078, 2005.

CHAPTER 35

Myelodysplastic syndromes

Jorge E. Cortes, MD, Alan List, MD, and Hagop Kantarjian, MD

Myelodysplastic syndromes (MDS) are a group of hematologic malignancies of the pluripotent hematopoietic stem cells. These disorders are characterized by ineffective hematopoiesis, including abnormalities in proliferation, differentiation, and apoptosis. The overall clinical result is peripheral cytopenias in the setting of a normocellular or hypercellular bone marrow and a high incidence of transformation to acute leukemia.

The incidence of MDS approximates 2 cases per 100,000 population per year, with 30 cases per 100,000 population per year in patients > 70 years old. It is estimated that approximately 15,000 to 20,000 new cases are diagnosed annually in the United States. Unfortunately, there are no accurate statistics on the actual incidence of MDS.

Epidemiology

Gender The overall incidence of MDS is slightly higher in males than in females (1.5–2.0:1).

Age The incidence of MDS increases with age, with a median age at diagnosis of about 70 years. MDS is rare in children; childhood cases are more frequently associated with monosomy of chromosome 7.

Etiology and risk factors

MDS is a clonal disorder of bone marrow stem cells. The vast majority of cases (80%–90%) occur de novo, whereas 10%–20% of cases are secondary. The etiology of de novo MDS is unclear. Exposure to radiation and/or cytotoxic agents is a recognized etiologic factor in secondary disease forms. Cumulative exposure to environmental toxins, genetic differences in leukemogen susceptibility and metabolism, and genomic senescence may contribute to disease pathogenesis in de novo cases.

Genetic factors It has been suggested that a genetic change causes an irreversible alteration in the structure and function of the stem cell, with disruption of a multistep process involving control of cell proliferation, maturation, and interactions with growth factors; mutations of tumor-suppressor genes and proto-oncogenes; and deregulation of apoptosis.

Constitutional childhood disorders, such as Fanconi's anemia, Shwachman-Diamond syndrome, Down's syndrome, neurofibromatosis, and mitochondrial cytopathies, have been associated with MDS and monosomy of chromosome 7.

Environmental factors Exposure to benzene and its derivatives may result in karyotypic abnormalities often seen in MDS and acute myelogenous leukemia (AML). Persons chronically exposed to insecticides and pesticides may have a higher incidence of MDS than the general population.

An increased incidence of MDS has been reported among smokers and ex-smokers, possibly linked to associated exposures to polycyclic hydrocarbons and radioactive polodium present in tobacco smoke.

An association of MDS with magnetic fields, alcohol, or occupational exposure to other chemicals has not been demonstrated.

Antineoplastic drugs Therapy-related myelodysplasia and therapy-related AML are recognized long-term complications of chemotherapy and radiotherapy. Therapy-related MDS usually develops 3–7 years after exposure to chemotherapy and is most frequently related to complete or partial loss of chromosomes 5 or 7 in patients previously treated with alkylating agents. Approximately 80% of cases of AML occurring after exposure to antineoplastic drugs, particularly alkylating agents, are preceded by MDS.

More than 85% of patients who develop chemotherapy-related leukemia or MDS have been exposed to alkylating agents. Patients exposed to nitrosoureas have a relative risk of developing MDS or AML of 14.4 and a 6-year actuarial risk of 4%. The mean cumulative risk of leukemia in patients exposed to epipodophyllotoxins (eg, etoposide and teniposide [Vumon]) is about 5% at 5 years. Most of these therapy-related leukemias are not preceded by a dysplastic phase and are associated with abnormalities in chromosome 11q23.

Autologous bone marrow transplantation (BMT) has also been associated with a 5-year actuarial risk of MDS of 15% (95% confidence interval, 3.4–16.6). Fluorescent in situ hybridization (FISH) analyses of pretreatment bone marrow specimens for informative cytogenetic markers indicate that these secondary myeloid malignancies derive from clones demonstrable before the transplant procedure. Prior therapy with fludarabine, older age, low CD34+ dose, and prolonged platelet reconstitution have been associated with the development of MDS or AML in patients with lymphoid malignancies after autologous stem-cell transplantation (SCT).

TABLE 1: Main features of MDS according to the FAB classification

FAB subgroup	BM blasts (%)	Ringed sideroblasts (%)	PB monocytes ($\times 10^9$/L)	Chromosomal abnormalities (%)	Frequently associated karyotype	Rate of leukemic progression (%)	Median survival (mo)
RA	< 5	< 15	< 1	30	5q-, -7, +8, 20q-	12	32
RARS	< 5	≥ 15	< 1	20	+8, 5q-, 20q-	8	42
RAEB	5-20	Variable	< 1	45	-7, 7q-, -5, 5q-, +8	44	12
RAEB-t	21-30	Variable	Variable	60	-7, 7q-, -5, 5q-, +8	66	5
CMML	1-20	Variable	≥ 1	30	-7, +8, t(5;12), 7q-, 12q-	14	20

BM = bone marrow; CMML = chronic myelomonocytic leukemia; FAB = French-American-British; PB = peripheral blood; RA = refractory anemia; RAEB = refractory anemia with excess blasts; RAEB-t = refractory anemia with excess blasts in transformation; RARS = refractory anemia with ringed sideroblasts

Classification

In 1982, the French-American-British (FAB) group proposed a classification system for MDS that consists of five subgroups, based on the percentage of blast cells in the peripheral blood and bone marrow, the presence of ringed sideroblasts in the bone marrow, and the monocyte count in the peripheral blood (Table 1). The five subgroups are:

- refractory anemia (RA)
- refractory anemia with ringed sideroblasts (RARS)
- refractory anemia with excess blasts (RAEB)
- refractory anemia with excess blasts in transformation (RAEB-t)
- chronic myelomonocytic leukemia (CMML).

The presence of Auer rods in granulocyte precursors classifies a patient as having RAEB-t, even if blasts comprise < 20% of bone marrow cells. The presence of > 30% blast cells in the bone marrow or peripheral blood establishes the diagnosis of AML rather than MDS.

More recently, the World Health Organization (WHO) has proposed a modified classification of hematologic malignancies (Table 2). The following changes have been proposed, based on the effect of cytogenetics and the number of dysplastic lineages on clinical behavior:

- The FAB classification of RAEB-t is eliminated.
- The blast percentage that defines AML is changed to ≥ 20%.
- RA and RARS are defined by dysplasia restricted to the erythroid lineage either with or without ringed sideroblasts, respectively.
- The presence of dysplasia in erythroid and nonerythroid lineages (multilineage dysplasia with or without ringed sideroblasts) and 5q- syndrome are regarded as separate entities of MDS.
- RAEB is divided into two categories distinguished by marrow blast percentage (ie, RAEB-1: 5%–9%; RAEB-2: 10%–19%) or the presence of Auer rods (RAEB-2).
- A category is added to include unclassifiable MDS defined by nonerythroid, single-lineage dysplasia.
- CMML is included in a separate category of myelodysplastic/myeloproliferative diseases that also includes atypical chronic myelogenous leukemia and juvenile myelomonocytic leukemia. CMML is further classified into CMML-1 (≤ 9% blasts), CMML-2 (10%–19% blasts), and CMML-Eos (eosinophils ≥ 1,500/µL).

This proposal represents a step ahead, but there are some aspects that still need to be addressed. For example, some biologic features that have been associated with MDS, such as the presence of spontaneous apoptosis, increased angiogenesis, and infrequent FLT_3 mutations, may define better specific subsets, and the WHO classification does not incorporate unfavorable cytogenetic patterns.

TABLE 2: Criteria for myelodysplastic syndromes according to the WHO classification

Disease	Blood findings	Bone marrow findings
Refractory anemia (RA)	Anemia No or rare blasts	Erythroid dysplasia *only* < 5% blasts < 15% ringed sideroblasts
Refractory anemia with ringed sideroblasts (RARS)	Anemia No blasts	Erythroid dysplasia *only* ≥ 15% ringed sideroblasts < 5% blasts
Refractory cytopenias with multilineage dysplasia (RCMD)	Cytopenias (bicytopenia or pancytopenia) No or rare blasts No Auer rods $< 1 \times 10^9$/L monocytes	Dysplasia in ≥ 10% of cells in 2 or more myeloid cell lines, including erythroids < 5% blasts in marrow No Auer rods < 15% ringed sideroblasts
Refractory cytopenias with multilineage dysplasia and ringed sideroblasts (RCMD-RS)	Cytopenias (bicytopenia or pancytopenia) No or rare blasts No Auer rods $< 1 \times 10^9$/L monocytes	Dysplasia in ≥ 10% of cells in 2 or more myeloid cell lines ≥ 15% ringed sideroblasts < 5% blasts No Auer rods
Refractory anemia with excess blasts-1 (RAEB-1)	Cytopenias < 5% blasts No Auer rods $< 1 \times 10^9$/L monocytes	Unilineage or multilineage dysplasia 5%-9% blasts No Auer rods
Refractory anemia with with excess blasts-2 (RAEB-2)	Cytopenias 5%-19% blasts Auer rods ± $< 1 \times 10^9$/L monocytes	Unilineage or multilineage dysplasia 10%-19% blasts Auer rods ±
Myelodysplastic syndrome, unclassified (MDS-U)	Cytopenias No or rare blasts No Auer rods	Unilineage dysplasia in granulocytes or megakaryocytes < 5% blasts No Auer rods
MDS associated with isolated del(5q)	Anemia < 5% blasts Platelets normal or increased	Normal to increased megakaryocytes with hypolobulated nuclei < 5% blasts No Auer rods Isolated del(5q31.1)

WHO = World Health Organization

Signs and symptoms

Nearly 50% of patients with MDS are asymptomatic at the time of initial diagnosis. Signs and symptoms relate to hematopoietic failure, leading to anemia, thrombocytopenia, or leukopenia.

Symptoms related to anemia may range from fatigue to exertional dyspnea that may exacerbate angina or cause congestive heart failure.

Infection Approximately one-third of patients report recurrent localized or systemic infections as a result of granulocytopenia or dysfunctional granulocytes and monocytes.

Bleeding manifestations, such as petechiae or gross hemorrhage, can occur with thrombocytopenia or platelet dysfunction. However, < 10% of patients present with serious bleeding.

Organomegaly and lymphadenopathy Splenomegaly and/or hepatomegaly may be found in 5%–25% of patients. A large spleen is more frequently seen in CMML.

Acute neutrophilic dermatosis (Sweet's syndrome) and pyoderma gangrenosum may be observed, particularly in patients with CMML or advanced MDS.

Paraneoplastic syndromes Diabetes insipidus, vasculitis, and other rare paraneoplastic syndromes have been described in patients with MDS.

Laboratory features

Peripheral blood

Anemia is the most frequent abnormality in MDS, with > 80% of patients presenting with hemoglobin concentrations < 10 g/dL. The anemia is usually normocytic or macrocytic, but the mean corpuscular volume rarely exceeds 120 μm^3.

Other RBC abnormalities Hypochromic changes and red-shape abnormalities are frequent, including poikilocytosis, anisocytosis, elliptocytosis, macro-ovalocytosis, and sometimes stomatocytes. Stippled and nucleated RBCs can be observed in 10% of cases. Reticulocyte counts are usually reduced.

WBC abnormalities The peripheral WBC count may be normal or low in MDS but is frequently elevated in CMML. The proportion of monocytes may be increased, and a circulating monocyte count of $\geq 1 \times 10^9$/L defines CMML.

Neutropenia is seen in about 50% of patients with MDS at diagnosis, often associated with pseudo–Pelger-Huët anomaly (neutrophils have a condensed chromatin and unilobed or bilobed nuclei with a pince-nez shape), ring-shaped nuclei, hypogranulation, and hypolobulation or other signs of dysgranulopoiesis.

Granulocytes frequently disclose reduced myeloperoxidase activity, increased α-naphthyl acetate esterase activity, and other functional abnormalities.

Chemotactic and bactericidal capability is impaired, which can potentiate the risk of infection, even in the presence of normal WBC counts.

Patients frequently have a decreased number of natural killer cells and helper T lymphocytes.

Platelet abnormalities Thrombocytopenia is present at diagnosis in approximately 30% of patients.

Platelets may be abnormally large; have poor granulation; or have large, fused central granules.

Decreased platelet aggregation is observed when platelets of patients with MDS are challenged with collagen or epinephrine.

Thrombocytosis may be seen in association with the 5q- syndrome.

Bone marrow

Bone marrow aspiration and biopsy should be performed in every patient suspected of having MDS or unexplained persistent cytopenias. The bone marrow is normocellular or hypercellular in 85%–90% of patients with MDS but may be hypocellular for the patients' age in as many as 10%–15%.

Trilineage dyspoiesis The main morphologic feature of MDS is hematopoietic dyspoiesis, although myelodysplastic features do not always involve all three lineages. Cytologic dysplasia must be detected in ≥ 10% of the affected lineages.

Dyserythropoiesis Erythroblasts usually have a megaloblastoid appearance. Iron may be abnormally deposited in mitochondria and is easily stained with Prussian blue, producing a ring-shaped staining pattern around the nucleus. Pathologic sideroblasts have five or more granules/cell.

Dysgranulopoiesis The characteristic findings in dysgranulopoiesis are hypogranulation and hyposegmentation with nuclear morphologic abnormalities.

Excess bone marrow blasts Bone marrow blasts > 5% but < 30% are seen in 30%-50% of patients with MDS; in the context of myelodysplasia, this finding is a feature of MDS.

The FAB group distinguishes three types of blasts on the basis of the maturation as assessed by morphology. Type I blasts have an uncondensed nuclear chromatin, one to three nucleoli, and basophilic cytoplasm without a Golgi zone. Cytoplasmic granules and Auer rods are absent. In type II blasts, the nuclear/cytoplasm ratio is lower than in type I blasts, and few primary granules are seen. Type III blasts have 20 or more azurophilic granules without a Golgi zone.

Dysmegakaryocytopoiesis At least 10 megakaryocytes should be evaluated. Micromegakaryocytes are small cells with a diameter two times smaller than the normal megakaryocyte (< 80 μm). Multiple, dispersed, small nuclei or mononucleated forms, as well as hypogranulated megakaryocytes, also can be found.

Other abnormalities An increase in reticulin and collagen fibers in the bone marrow may be seen in some patients.

Angiogenesis Increased marrow vascularity and increased levels of angiogenic cytokines such as vascular endothelial growth factor (VEGF), and basic fibroblast growth factor (bFGF) have been described in patients with MDS.

Other laboratory findings

Serum iron, transferrin, and ferritin levels may be elevated. As a result of ineffective hematopoiesis, lactic dehydrogenase (LDH) and uric acid concentrations are frequently increased. Monoclonal gammopathy, polyclonal hypergammaglobulinemia, and hypogammaglobulinemia are found occasionally but may be detected in up to 15% of patients with CMML.

Cytogenetic and molecular findings

Chromosomal abnormalities

Clonal cytogenetic abnormalities are found at diagnosis in 50%–60% of patients with de novo MDS and 75%–85% of those with secondary MDS or AML. An interesting feature that distinguishes MDS from AML is the high incidence of complete or partial chromosomal loss or, less frequently, chromosomal gain and the relative rarity of translocations. Among the translocations, unbalanced translocations leading to a loss of chromosomal material are most frequent.

Common cytogenetic abnormalities are listed in Table 1. None of them is specific for MDS, since all can be found in other myeloid disorders.

Some of the most frequent abnormalities are interstitial deletion of the long arm of chromosome 5 (5q-), monosomy of chromosome 7, trisomy of chromosome 8, 20q-, and loss of the Y chromosome. "Complex" cytogenetic abnormalities involving three or more chromosomes occur in approximately 15% of de novo MDS cases and 50% of secondary MDS cases.

Therapy-related MDS Loss of chromosome 7 and/or 7q- has been reported in as many as 50% of patients previously exposed to chemotherapy for other malignancies, most frequently in association with prolonged use of alkylating agents. Other abnormalities commonly associated with prior exposure to alkylating agents include -5 and/or del(5q) in 25% of cases and involvement of chromosomes 17p and 21 in 10%–15%. Complex chromosomal abnormalities may be found in nearly 50% of patients.

Cytogenetics and FAB classification

RA and RARS Approximately 15%–30% of patients with RA and RARS have abnormal karyotypes. The most frequent abnormality in patients with RA is 5q, whereas the most common abnormalities in patients with RARS are 5q-, +8, and 20q- (each occurring in 20% of patients).

RAEB and RAEB-t Nearly 60% of patients with RAEB and RAEB-t have cytogenetic abnormalities, with 5q-, -7, 7q-, and +8 being the most frequent.

CMML Chromosomal abnormalities are found in 25%–30% of patients with CMML; the predominant abnormalities include -7, 7q-, +8, 12q-, and t(5;12). Interestingly, 5q- is seen in < 1% of cases of CMML.

Monosomy of chromosome 7 is found in up to 25% of children with MDS, most frequently as an isolated abnormality. In contrast, older patients most often have monosomy of chromosome 7 associated with other chromosomal abnormalities.

5q- syndrome

The isolated interstitial deletion characteristic of the 5q- syndrome involves a variable segment length that includes the critical deleted region at 5q31, a region known to contain genes coding for granulocyte-macrophage colony-stimulating factor (GM-CSF), macrophage colony-stimulating factor (M-CSF), interleukin (IL)-3, IL-4, IL-5, IL-9, IL-12, M-CSF receptor, platelet-derived growth factor receptor-beta, interferon-regulatory factor-1 (IRF-1), endothelial cell growth factor, glucocorticoid receptor, and early growth response gene-1 (EGR-1). However, the critical gene deletion involved in this syndrome has yet to be identified.

Clinical features This syndrome has characteristic clinical features, including older age, female predominance, diagnosis of RA without excess (< 5%) blasts in 75% of cases, macrocytosis with severe anemia, erythroblastopenia, normal leukocyte counts, normal or increased platelet counts, and hypolobulated megakaryocytes in the bone marrow.

Progression to AML is infrequent (< 20%), and the prognosis is usually good. However, not every patient with del(5q) has this syndrome and its associated good prognosis. Additional cytogenetic abnormalities or the presence of ≥ 5% blasts in the peripheral blood or bone marrow are inconsistent with this diagnosis.

Molecular findings

The *ras* family of genes is most frequently altered in MDS, although other abnormalities involving NF1, FMS, *p53*, TEL, EVI, AXL, TEC, HCK, c-*mpl*, and other genes have also been described.

Mutations in *ras* Mutations in the *ras* family occur in approximately 20%–40% of patients with MDS but are most frequently found in those with CMML. Mutations in *ras* are more common in codons 12, 13, and 61. Mutations in N-*ras* are more common than those in K-*ras* or H-*ras*.

A difference in the surface expression of phosphatidylserine (a marker of apoptosis) on cell membranes among de novo AML, MDS, and secondary AML and normal bone marrow cells has been found (increased in MDS and secondary AML). Epigenetic silencing of the *p15* tumor-suppressor gene by promoter hypermethylation occurs particularly among patients with high-risk MDS and is associated with a poor prognosis. FLT_3 mutations or internal tandem duplications occur much less frequently in MDS (usually < 5%) than in AML.

Staging and prognosis

Prognostic factors

FAB and WHO classifications The FAB classification has a long history of use to evaluate survival and risk for AML transformation (Table 1). The WHO

TABLE 3: International Prognostic Scoring System (IPSS) for MDS

Characteristic	Value	Score
Bone marrow blasts (%)	< 5	0
	5-10	0.5
	11-20	1.5
	21-30	2.0
Karyotype[a]	Good	0
	Intermediate	0.5
	Poor	1.0
Cytopenias	0-1	0
	2-3	0.5
Risk group	**Sum of score**	
Low	0	
Intermediate 1	0.5-1.0	
Intermediate 2	1.5-2.0	
High	≥ 2.5	

[a] Good = diploid, -y, del(5q), del(20 q); Poor = chromosome 7 abnormalities or complex (≥ 3) abnormalities; Intermediate = all others.

classification has similar prognostic implications, based primarily upon the prognostic impact of blast percentage and the number of dysplastic lineages.

> The combination of erythropoietin and filgrastim (Neupogen) has been used to treat many patients with MDS to improve hemoglobin levels. One study included 129 patients, among whom 77% were low- or intermediate-1 risk according to the International Prognostic Scoring System. The erythroid response rate was 39%, including a complete response rate in 22% of patients. The median duration of response was 23 months. The lowest effective maintenance dose for erythropoietin varied from 5,000 to 50,000 U/week (median 30,000 U) and for filgrastim ranged from 0 to 900 µg/week (median 225 µg). Responses were more durable among patients with RA or RARS *(Howe RB, Porwit-MacDonald A, Wanat R, et al: Blood 103:3265-3270, 2004).*

Cytogenetics Patients with complex karyotypes and abnormalities in chromosome 7 have a poor prognosis, whereas those with a normal karyotype, -Y, 5q-, or 20q- have a favorable prognosis.

Peripheral cytopenias (hemoglobin level < 10 g/dL, absolute neutrophil count [ANC] < 1.5×10^9/L, and platelet count < 100×10^9/L) have a cumulative adverse effect on prognosis.

Other prognostic factors Other parameters associated with a poor outcome include CD34 cell expression, high serum LDH levels, expression of the c-*mpl* gene, *ras* mutations, *p*-glycoprotein (Pgp) expression, *p15* inactivation, and *p53* mutations. However, it is unclear whether these factors have independent prognostic value.

International Prognostic Scoring System (IPSS)

An International MDS Risk Analysis Workshop has proposed a system that combines clinical, morphologic, and cytogenetic data to generate a consensus prognostic system.

By multivariate analysis, the most significant independent variables were percentage of bone marrow blasts, cytogenetics, and number of cytopenias (Table 3). It is important to keep in mind, however, that other variables (eg, age and prior therapy) not included in this system may alter the prognosis and influence the results of therapy among patients in similar IPSS groups. Still, this may be the most valuable risk classification for treatment planning.

> Histone deacetylase (HDAC) inhibitors are being investigated in patients with MDS. Valproic acid has been reported to induce the differentiation of several tumor cell lines, and this effect has been presumed to be related to its ability to inhibit HDAC. In a recent study, 18 patients with MDS were treated with valproic acid alone (n = 18) or in combination with all-*trans*-retinoic acid (ATRA; n = 5). Eight patients (44%) responded to valproic acid alone (most hematologic improvement), with a median duration of response of 4 months. None of the patients treated with valproic acid and ATRA from the beginning responded, but two of five who lost their response to valproic acid alone responded again to the combination (*Kuendgen A, Strupp C, Aivado M, et al: Blood 104:1266-1269, 2004*).

Treatment

The treatment of MDS is dictated by the risks imposed by the disease, age, and patient preference. Suggested guidelines are outlined in Table 4 and discussed below.

Supportive care

The use of transfusions affords temporary benefits and is an alternative that can be considered in patients with lower risk MDS or that otherwise can be used in conjunction with more definitive therapy. To delay or prevent end-organ complications, chelation therapy should be considered when red blood cell transfusions exceed 25 U or ferritin levels > 1,800 ng/mL.

> Deferasirox (Exjade, ICL670) is an orally available iron-chelating agent that has been shown to be effective in patients requiring frequent transfusion, including those with MDS. In a study of 184 patients with transfusion-dependent anemia, including 47 with MDS, the mean (±SD) decrease in ferritin levels after administration of deferasirox was 268 ± 2053 ng/mL, with a mean decrease in liver iron concentration of 5.7 ± 6.3 mg Fe/g dw (*Greenberg P, Dine G, Ganser A, et al: Blood 106:757a, 2005*). In addition, daily doses of 20–30 mg/kg of deferasirox were shown to induce iron balance or net negative iron balance is achieved by in regularly transfused patients, including patients with MDS (*Porter J, Borgna-Pignatti C, Baccarani M, et al: Blood 106:755a, 2005*).

Cytokines

Recombinant human erythropoietin (rHuEPO [Epogen, Procrit]) may decrease transfusion requirements in 15%–25% of patients with MDS, usually those with low plasma levels of EPO (< 100 mU/mL). The addition of granulocyte colony-stimulating factor (G-CSF, filgrastim [Neupogen]) or GM-CSF to rHuEPO may increase the response rate, mostly in patients with low transfusion requirements.

TABLE 4: Suggested approach to the treatment of MDS

IPSS risk group	Treatment
Low, intermediate 1	Observation (particularly if mild cytopenia) Supportive care (transfusions, hematopoietic growth factors) Lenalidomide (for patients with 5q- abnormalities) Hypomethylating agents (azacitidine, decitabine) New (investigational) approaches, such as arsenic trioxide, farnesyl transferase inhibitors, histone deacetylase inhibitors, thalidomide, ATG (particularly if hypoplastic and low platelet count)
High, intermediate 2	AML-like chemotherapy Hypomethylating agents (azacitidine, decitabine) SCT (particularly for young patients with HLA-identical siblings; front-line vs in remission?) New (investigational) agents, such as topoisomerase inhibitors (topotecan, rubitecan), farnesyl transferase inhibitors, histone deacetylase inhibitors

AML = acute myelogenous leukemia; ATG = antithymocyte globulin; IPSS = International Prognostic Scoring System; SCT = stem-cell transplantation

Darbepoetin alfa (Aranesp) is a hypersialated form of EPO with an extended half-life. Trials of darbepoetin alfa in MDS have shown comparable activity to recombinant EPO with or without G-CSF with less frequent dosing. Preliminary results of a phase II study investigating the benefit of weekly darbepoetin alfa (at a dose of 300 μg) in 55 lower risk patients with low endogenous EPO levels (< 500 mU/mL) reported a major erythroid response rate of 49%, with few failures salvaged by the addition of G-CSF. These data suggest that response to darbepoetin alfa may be comparable to that expected with the combination of EPO and G-CSF. IL-11 (at low doses of 10 μg/kg/d) has been used in patients with bone marrow failure disorders, including MDS.

G-CSF and GM-CSF may improve neutropenia and decrease infections in up to 70% of patients with MDS, but the effect is usually transient. No increase in the probability of developing AML has been demonstrated with extended use of these cytokines.

Other alternatives

Antithymocyte globulin (ATG [Atgam]) has been associated with response (defined as independence from transfusions) in 34% of patients, which was sustained for a median of 36 months in 81% of them. Also, 48% had sustained platelet improvement and 55% had an increase in neutrophils. Younger patients and those with low platelet counts are more likely to respond than older patients and those with higher platelet counts.

A simple method for predicting response to immunosuppressive therapy in MDS has been proposed. It is based on the age of the patient, the duration of red blood cell transfusion dependence, and the HLA-DR15 status. Younger patients with a shorter duration of transfusion requirements have a higher predicted probability of response (40%–100%), particularly when their status is positive for HLA-DR15.

Cyclosporine significantly increases cell colony growth in laboratory studies of hypoplastic RA. Responses have been reported in a limited number of patients.

Lenalidomide Lenalidomide (Revlimid) is a thalidomide analog that belongs to the immunomodulatory family of drugs. Lenalidomide has numerous properties that make it attractive for the management of neoplastic and inflammatory conditions, including the inhibition of production of cytokines such as tumor necrosis factor-α (TNF-α) and interleukins-1 (IL-1)IL-6, IL-10, and IL-12. Lenalidomide is markedly more potent than thalidomide in inhibiting the secretion of TNF-α. In addition, lenalidomide may potentiate erythropoietin-induced signaling in erythroid progenitors and stimulate stem-cell differentiation to erythroid cells.

Lenalidomide has been recently approved for the treatment of patients with MDS with abnormalities in the long arm of chromosome 5 (5q- abnormalities), whether they are isolated or present together with other cytogenetic abnormalities. In a study of patients with transfusion-dependent MDS with 5q- abnormalities, 75% of patients responded, with 66% of the total population becoming transfusion independent. The response rate was similar regardless of whether the cytogenetic abnormality was isolated or seen in conjunction with other cytogenetic abnormalities, and more than half of the responses were durable for more than 1 year. In addition, a cytogenetic response was observed in 70% of patients. Lenalidomide has also been investigated for patients with MDS without 5q- abnormalities. Erythroid responses were seen in over 40%, with 27% of the total population becoming transfusion independent.

Azacitidine (Vidaza) and 5-Aza-2-deoxycytidine (DAC, decitabine) are hypomethylating agents that have shown activity in MDS. In a randomized trial, 191 patients with MDS (63% RAEB or RAEB-t) were treated with azacitidine or supportive care. Responses were observed in 60% of those treated with azacitidine (complete response [CR]: 6%; partial response [PR]: 10%; improvement: 47%) compared with 5% with supportive care.

In a study of 92 patients with MDS, three different schedules of decitabine were investigated: 20 mg/m² IV over 1 hour daily for 5 days, 10 mg/m² IV over 1 hour daily for 10 days, or 10 mg/m² SQ twice daily for 5 days. The overall response rate was 76%, with the complete response rate being 36%. The complete response rate by schedule was 41%, 28%, and 24%, respectively. Compared with a historic control treated with intensive chemotherapy, those treated with decitabine had a lower induction mortality (15% vs 21%) and improved overall survival. These results suggest that decitabine is an effective agent for the management of patients with MDS (*Kantarjian H, O'Brien S, Giles F, et al: Blood [abstract] 106:708a, 2005*).

There was a significant improvement in probability of transformation to AML and overall survival when the confounding effect of early crossover to azacitidine was eliminated.

Azacitidine has recently been approved by the US Food and Drug Administration for the treatment of patients with all types of MDS. The standard dose is 75 mg/m^2/d subcutaneously for 7 days every 4 weeks for as long as the patient benefits. Responses occur after a median of 3 to 4 cycles, so it is recommended to continue therapy for at least 4 cycles unless there is significant toxicity or progression of disease. The dose may be increased to 100 mg/m^2/d after 2 cycles if no improvement has occurred. Myelosuppression may occur but is not a reason to discontinue therapy. Rather, patients should be supported during myelosuppression and should continue therapy to give patients the best opportunity of response.

In a multicenter phase II study, 66 patients (73% RAEB or RAEB-t) were treated with decitabine. The overall response rate was 49% (CR: 20%; PR: 4%; improvement: 24%). The actuarial median response duration was 31 weeks, and median survival was 22 months. In addition, 31% of patients with cytogenetic abnormalities presented before treatment achieved a cytogenetic response. Cytogenetic response conferred a survival advantage to these patients.

Steroids, androgens, and pyridoxine are rarely effective, although they are often used clinically.

Chemotherapy

The rationale for this strategy stems from the concepts that MDS is a clonal disorder and that MDS and AML are overlapping illnesses with an arbitrary frontier defined by the WHO and FAB classifications (ie, a 20%–30% blast threshold).

The Cancer and Leukemia Group B (CALGB) treated 874 patients with AML and 33 patients with MDS with AML-like chemotherapy. The CR rate was 79% for patients with MDS vs 68% for patients with AML (P= .37), median CR duration was 11 vs 15 months (P= .28), and median survival was 13 vs 16 months. The authors concluded that the FAB distinction between MDS (RAEB and RAEB-t) and AML has minimal therapeutic implications.

Estey et al treated 372 patients with AML, 52 with RAEB, and 106 with RAEB-t with AML-type chemotherapy. CR rates were 62% for patients with RAEB, 66% for those with RAEB-t, and 66% for those with AML (P= .79). Event-free survival was significantly better for patients with AML/RAEB-t than for patients with RAEB. However, when cytogenetics and other prognostic variables were considered in a multivariate analysis, no difference in outcome could be identified among FAB subgroups.

These findings suggest that the prognosis is determined more by cytogenetics and other prognostic features than by the percentage of blasts or FAB classification. However, this finding does not necessarily mean that MDS and AML are biologically equivalent entities.

A recent study investigated a new schedule of administration of tipifarnib (Zarnestra) consisting of an alternate week (1 week on/1 week off) schedule. The starting dose was 100 mg twice daily; the dose was escalated by 100 mg orally twice daily, until grade 2 nonhematologic toxicity was observed, with a total dose of 100 mg per day until the maximum tolerated dose was reached. Of the 63 patients treated, 15 of 61of the evaluable patients (25%) responded (3 complete responses, 12 hematologic improvement), with major platelet responses being the most common (11 patients). The regimen was well tolerated, with 20% of patients reporting no side effects *(Kurzrock R, Verstovsek S, Wright J, et al: Blood [abstract]106:708a, 2005).*

Combination regimens Different combination chemotherapy regimens have been investigated. The combination of cytarabine (Ara-C) and anthracycline is the cornerstone of intensive chemotherapy, leading to CRs in 40%–60% of patients. However, despite the fact that cytogenetic remissions frequently accompany hematologic CRs, the median remission duration and survival times are brief, rarely exceeding 1 year. The death rate during induction therapy is 5%–20%.

Myeloblasts in RAEB-t and secondary AML commonly express the multidrug exporter Pgp, which extrudes anthracyclines and limits their activity. A randomized, controlled trial performed by the Southwest Oncology Group (SWOG) reported a twofold improvement in survival for patients treated with an anthracycline- and Ara-C–containing induction and consolidation regimens with the Pgp antagonist cyclosporine added.

It is possible that certain chemotherapeutic agents may be particularly useful in MDS.

Topotecan (Hycamtin), a topoisomerase I inhibitor, has shown significant activity as a single agent in the treatment of MDS, with a CR rate of 37% in previously treated patients with RAEB/RAEB-t and 27% in patients with CMML. The median CR duration was 7.5 months, and survival was 10.5 months. Topotecan is well tolerated, with a mortality rate during induction therapy of < 5%.

Combinations of topotecan with Ara-C resulted in a 56% CR rate (66% in previously untreated patients). Similar CR rates were observed despite the risk category. This regimen is well tolerated, with an induction mortality rate of 7%. A randomized trial of topotecan and Ara-C vs idarubicin (Idamycin) and Ara-C showed that the topotecan combination was an equivalent regimen, possibly with lower toxicity.

Stem-cell transplantation is a treatment option for some patients with MDS, although its timing remains controversial. A recent analysis used a Markov model to examine three transplantation strategies for newly diagnosed MDS: transplantation at the time of diagnosis, transplantation at the time of progression to leukemia, and transplantation at an interval from diagnosis but prior to leukemic progression. Although transplantation at the time of diagnosis may be superior for patients with intermediate-2 and high-risk IPSS (International Prognostic Scoring System) scores, delayed transplantation was associated with improved life expectancy *(Cutler CS, Lee SJ, Greenberg P, et al: Blood [abstract] 104:579-585, 2004).*

SCT

Allogeneic SCT can be of benefit in a subset of patients with MDS. However, most series have concentrated on younger patients, who constitute a minority of patients with MDS and frequently have favorable cytogenetics and therefore a better prognosis. The best results to date have been reported in patients with a better prognosis (ie, those with RA/RARS). In most series, allogeneic SCT is associated with a long-term remission rate of approximately 40%, a 30% relapse rate, and a 30% rate of transplant-related death.

The timing of transplantation remains controversial. Runde et al reported on a group of 131 patients (median age, 33 years; range, 2–55 years) who underwent allogeneic SCT as front-line therapy without prior induction chemotherapy. The 5-year disease-free survival rate was 34%, overall survival rate was 41%, and transplant-related mortality was 38%. The actuarial probability of relapse at 5 years was 39%, with better results observed in the RA/RARS subgroup.

Patients with adverse cytogenetics have a poor outcome with other treatment modalities, and SCT can be considered for such patients during first CR. However, the long-term outcome for these patients after SCT has not proved to be superior to that after any other approach, although the procedure may prove to be curative in a small percentage of patients. SCT should be considered particularly in the setting of a clinical trial.

New applications for allogeneic SCT (eg, nonmyeloablative) to make this option available to the typical patient with MDS (who is frequently older and has other associated medical problems), as well as matched-unrelated donor SCT, should be investigated further.

Autologous SCT In the majority of patients with MDS, lymphocytes do not appear to be part of the clone, suggesting the presence of normal nonclonal stem cells. De Witte et al described 79 patients with MDS or secondary AML who underwent autologous SCT during first CR. The 2-year survival, disease-free survival, and relapse rates were 39%, 34%, and 64%, respectively. The 2-year survival rate for the MDS group was 40%, and treatment-related mortality was 9%. The best outcome was seen among patients with RA/RARS.

Treatment recommendations

Treatment of patients with MDS is an evolving and controversial issue, and enrollment in a clinical trial should be encouraged. Treatment can be considered according to the IPSS.

Patients with low or intermediate-1 IPSS scores can frequently be treated with supportive measures. Hematopoietic-promoting agents such as EPO, amifostine (Ethyol), ATG, and thalidomide (Thalomid) could be used alone or in combination. Patients with 5q- benefit from lenalidomide, particularly in terms of erythroid response, and this should be considered the treatment of choice. Some patients with MDS without the 5q- abnormality may also benefit from lenalidomide, but the use in this setting is still investigated. Azacitidine is now available and should be considered for all patients. Although decitabine is another good option, it currently is only available through clinical trials.

Patients with high or intermediate-2 IPSS scores have significant risk of mortality from cytopenias or AML evolution. They should be considered for treatment options with the intention to cure, extend survival, or delay the progression of AML. The hypomethylating agents (azacitidine and decitabine) are good alternatives for patients who are not candidates for curative therapy. Investigational agents should be strongly considered.

SCT is an alternative for younger patients with higher risk MDS and an HLA-identical donor, particularly patients with adverse cytogenetic abnormalities. However, the best results to date have been reported in patients with a better prognosis (ie, younger patients and those with RA/RARS). Therefore, allogeneic transplantation and other transplant alternatives should be considered preferentially in a research setting (eg, mixed-unrelated donor and minitransplants).

SUGGESTED READING

Bernard JF, Giraudier S, Rosenthal E, et al: High response rate to darbepoetin alpha in low risk MDS: Results of phase II study. Blood 104:24a, 2004.

Cortes J: CMML: A biologically distinct myeloproliferative disease. Curr Hematol Rep 2:202–208, 2003.

Ho AY, Pagliuca A, Kenyon M, et al: Reduced-intensity allogeneic hematopoietic stem cell transplantation for myelodysplastic syndrome and acute myeloid leukemia with multilineage dysplasia using fludarabine, busulphan, and alemtuzumab (FBC) conditioning. Blood 104:1616–1623, 2004.

Howe RB, Porwit-MacDonald A, Wanat R, et al: The WHO classification of MDS does make a difference. Blood 103:3265–3270, 2004.

Jadersten M, Montgomery SM, Dybedal I, et al: Long-term outcome of treatment of anemia in MDS with erythropoietin and G-CSF. Blood 106:803–811, 2005.

Kuendgen A, Strupp C, Aivado M, et al: Treatment of myelodysplastic syndromes with valproic acid alone or in combination with all-trans-retinoic acid. Blood 104:1266–1269, 2004.

Kurzrock R, Kantarjian HM, Cortes JE, et al: Farnesyltransferase inhibitor R115777 in myelodysplastic syndrome: Clinical and biologic activities in the phase I setting. Blood 102:4527–4534, 2003.

List A, Kurtin S, Roe DJ, et al: Efficacy of lenalidomide in myelodysplastic syndromes. N Engl J Med 352:549–557, 2005.

Malcovati L, Porta MG, Pascutto C, et al: Prognostic factors and life expectancy in myelodysplastic syndromes classified according to WHO criteria: A basis for clinical decision making. J Clin Oncol 23:7594–7603, 2005.

Musto P, Lanza F, Balleari E, et al: Darbepoetin alpha for the treatment of anemia in low - intermediate risk myelodysplastic syndromes. Br J Haematol 128:208–209, 2004.

Saunthararajah Y, Nakamura R, Wesley R, et al: A simple method to predict response to immunosuppressive therapy in patients with myelodysplastic syndrome. Blood 102:3025–3027, 2003.

CHAPTER 36

Hematopoietic cell transplantation

Stephen J. Forman, MD

Hematopoietic cell transplantation (HCT) is the IV infusion of hematopoietic progenitor cells designed to establish marrow and immune function in patients with a variety of acquired and inherited malignant and nonmalignant disorders. They include hematologic malignancies (eg, leukemia, lymphoma, and myeloma), nonmalignant acquired bone marrow disorders (aplastic anemia), and genetic diseases associated with abnormal hematopoiesis and function (thalassemia, sickle cell anemia, and severe combined immunodeficiency). HCT also is used in the support of patients undergoing high-dose chemotherapy for the treatment of solid tumors for which hematologic toxicity would otherwise limit drug administration (eg, breast, germ-cell, and ovarian cancers).

Types of transplantation

Since the advent of HCT in the 1960s, several different methods of transplantation have evolved. At present, the hematopoietic cells used for HCT are obtained from either bone marrow or peripheral blood. The decision to use a certain type of HCT is dictated by the patient's disease and condition and the availability of a donor. In some cases, more than one approach is possible. Table 1 summarizes the advantages and disadvantages of each stem-cell source.

Allogeneic BMT, matched related This method involves procurement of bone marrow from an HLA-identical sibling of the patient. In some cases, a partially matched sibling or family donor (one antigen mismatch) can be used for bone marrow transplantation (BMT).

Allogeneic BMT, matched unrelated Given that there are a limited number of alleles of the HLA system, typing of large numbers of individuals has led to the observation that full matches for patients exist in the general population. Tissue typing is performed on the patient's blood, and a search of the computer files of various international registries is made to determine whether a patient has a match with an unrelated individual.

Haploidentical transplantation involves the transplantation of large numbers of T-cell–depleted stem cells from a donor, usually a sibling or a parent, who is half matched to the patient. Although these are the most difficult transplantations to perform successfully, there is great interest in this approach because most patients will have a donor in their family who is at least a 50% HLA match. Although most transplants will engraft and few patients will have significant graft-vs-host disease (GVHD), the relapse rate is high and the process of immune reconstitution is slow, with patients often having troublesome infections for a long time after transplantation.

Autologous BMT This form of transplantation entails the use of the patient's own bone marrow, which is harvested and then cryopreserved prior to administration of chemotherapy and/or high-dose radiation therapy. Following completion of therapy, the marrow cells are then thawed and reinfused into the patient to reestablish hematopoiesis.

Autologous peripheral blood stem-cell transplantation With the recognition that the marrow stem cells circulate in the peripheral blood, methods have been devised to augment the number of these cells in the patient's circulation. The blood is then collected on a cell separator and frozen, similar to autologous marrow, to be utilized after high-dose chemotherapy and/or radiation therapy. This is now the most common source of stem cells used in the autologous setting.

Syngeneic transplantation In this form of transplantation, marrow or peripheral blood stem cells are procured from an individual who is a genetic identical twin to the patient.

Donor leukocyte infusion This method involves the infusion of mononuclear cells from the marrow donor into the recipient to treat relapse after transplantation. The cells can mediate an antitumor effect, known as a graft-vs-tumor effect (often in association with concomitant GVHD), and can achieve remission of the malignancy.

Nonmyeloablative or reduced-intensity transplantation This approach uses lower doses of chemotherapy, with or without total-body irradiation (TBI) and immunosuppression, to facilitate engraftment of donor stem cells. Donor stem cells obtained from either the peripheral blood or marrow are then infused into the patient, leading to hematopoietic engraftment. The major therapeutic effect that results from this type of transplantation is a graft-vs-tumor effect, as the nonmyeloablative regimen has limited long-term antitumor efficacy. Some disorders such as chronic myelogenous leukemia (CML), acute myelogenous leukemia (AML), low-grade lymphoma, and multiple myeloma are particularly sensitive to this approach. This type of transplant allows older patients to undergo the procedure, as the transplant-related mortality is greatly reduced with this approach.

Cord blood transplantation The blood in the umbilical cord of newborn babies contains large numbers of stem cells, which have been shown to be capable of long-term engraftment in children and some adults after transplantation. Similar to unrelated-donor registries, cord blood banks have been developed to store cord blood cells that can be utilized for unrelated-donor transplantation. Given the immunologic immaturity of cord blood cells, these transplants can be accomplished even when there are disparities (mismatching) in the HLA typing between the donor and recipient. Cord blood transplants are generally used in situations where an adult unrelated donor cannot be identified through the international registries.

TABLE 1: Stem-cell sources for allogeneic BMT

Type	Advantages	Disadvantages
Allogeneic		
Sibling donor 6/6 HLA match or 5/6	Match able to be identified rapidly (2 weeks)	GVHD (25%-40%) for non–T-cell-depleted marrow grafts
	Low rate of graft rejection (2%-5%)	Only 30% of patients will have sibling donor
Matched unrelated donor	Extends donor availability (60%-70% of patients will have potential match)	Takes time to find donor (6 weeks to > 6 months)
	Greater graft-vs-tumor effect	Higher graft failure rates (5%-10%)
		Higher GVHD rates (50%-60%)
Umbilical cord donor	Lesser degrees of match can be used	Limited number of cells (reduced applicability to large recipient)
		Slower engraftment
	Much lower rate of GVHD (10%-20%) despite one and two antigen mismatches	Higher rate of graft failure (10%)
		No chance for second infusion for graft failure or DLI for relapse
Haploidentical family donor	Almost all patients have a sibling, parent, or child who is haploidentical. These donors can be used if patients have relapsed or there is refractory disease and no better donor has been identified	Needs much more profound immunosuppression (T-cell depletion of donor product included) to achieve engraftment
		High risk of infectious complications
		Graft failure rate of 10%-15%
Syngeneic Identical twin	No need for immunosuppression	No graft-vs-tumor effect
	No GVHD	

BMT = bone marrow transplantation; DLI = donor lymphocyte infusion; GVHD = graft-vs-host disease

Allogeneic transplantation

HLA typing

Finding a related donor As noted previously, matched related allogeneic BMT involves a donor who is an HLA-matched sibling of the recipient. The formula for calculating the chances of a particular person having an HLA-matched sibling is $1 - (0.75)^N$, where N denotes the number of potential sibling donors. In general, a patient with one sibling has a 25% chance of having a match. The average American family size usually limits the success of finding a family donor to approximately 30% of patients.

HLA typing is performed on blood samples obtained from the patient and potential donor. Serologic methods have been used to detect the identity of the class I and II antigens; molecular methods are now utilized for more refined matching of both classes. A match is noted when the major class I antigens (A and B loci), as well as class II antigens (DR), are the same as those of the donor. Each sibling receives one set of antigens (A, B, DR) from each parent (chromosome 6). Genotypic identity can be confirmed by testing the parents and determining the inheritance of each set of antigens.

Finding an unrelated donor In cases in which the patient needs an allogeneic transplant and a donor cannot be found within the family, the identification of a matched-unrelated donor is accomplished by searching the computer files of the National Marrow Donor Program, as well as other international registries. As there are multiple alleles of any given HLA locus, serologic identity does not necessarily imply genotypic identity, such as is the case among sibling donor-recipient pairs. The development of oligonucleotide probes has greatly increased the precision of HLA typing and has allowed for more specific selection of bone marrow donors by matching molecular alleles of the class I and II antigens.

Advantages and disadvantages

The major advantages of an allogeneic graft include the absence of malignant cells contaminating the graft; the potential for an immunologic anticancer graft-vs-tumor effect; and the ability to treat malignant and nonmalignant disorders of the bone marrow, including genetic and immunologic diseases.

The disadvantages of an allogeneic transplant include the difficulty in finding an appropriate HLA-matched donor and the development of GVHD after BMT, which contributes to the morbidity and mortality of the procedure.

Autologous transplantation

Advantages and disadvantages

In autologous transplantation, the reinfused stem cells come from either the patient's own bone marrow or peripheral blood. These cells do not cause GVHD, and, thus, autologous transplantation is associated with less morbidity and mortality than allogeneic BMT and increases the number of patients who can undergo the procedure, as well as the upper age limit.

The disadvantages of autologous BMT include the likelihood of tumor cell contamination within the graft in many diseases, which can cause relapse; the lack of a significant therapeutic graft-vs-tumor effect; and the limited ability to use autologous stem cells in the treatment of patients not in remission or with inherited nonmalignant lymphohematopoietic diseases. Table 2 summarizes the advantages and disadvantages of these two approaches.

TABLE 2: Comparison of allogeneic vs autologous stem-cell transplantation

Allogeneic

Advantages

No tumor contamination of the graft and no prior marrow injury from chemotherapy (less risk of later myelodysplasia)

Graft-vs-tumor effect

Can be used for patients with marrow involvement by tumor or with bone marrow dysfunction, such as aplastic anemia, hemoglobinopathies, or prior pelvic irradiation

Disadvantages

Dose-intensive regimen limited by toxicity (usually limited to patients < age 55)

Takes time to identify donor if no sibling donor available/limited availability of donor for some ethnic groups

Higher early treatment-related mortality from graft-vs-host disease and infectious complications (20%-40% depending on age and donor source)

Autologous

Advantages

No need to identify donor if peripheral blood marrow uninvolved by tumor at time of collection

No immunosuppression = less risk of infections

No graft-vs-host disease

Dose-intensive therapy can be used for older patients (usually up to age 70)

Low early treatment-related mortality (2%-5%)

Disadvantages

Not feasible if peripheral blood stem cells/marrow involved

Possible marrow injury leading to late myelodysplasia (either from prior chemotherapy or transplant regimen)

No graft-vs-tumor effect

Not all patients can be mobilized to give adequate cell doses for reconstitution

Modifications of the stem-cell graft

The disadvantages of both allogeneic and autologous transplantations have led to the development of modifications of the stem-cell graft.

Removing T cells from donor marrow With regard to allogeneic BMT, it is known that contaminating T cells from the donor mediate the onset and persistence of acute and chronic GVHD. T cells have been removed from the donor marrow to prevent the development of severe GVHD. However, this approach has increased the incidence of both graft rejection and relapse of malignancy. Some investigators are exploring planned add-back of donor T cells after hematopoietic recovery to help prevent relapse.

Primed peripheral blood stem cells from marrow donors have reduced transplant-related complications without a substantial increase in acute GVHD. Thus far, the data show that this approach induces more rapid engraftment. Most studies have reported an increase in chronic GVHD.

Eliminating tumor cells from autologous grafts Although autologous peripheral blood stem-cell transplantation has led to more rapid restoration of hematopoiesis, it is associated with a higher relapse rate than is allogeneic BMT. Attempts to deplete the autologous graft of tumor cells have included in vitro purging with monoclonal antibodies and/or chemotherapeutic agents and the enrichment of stem cells over various separation columns.

Post-transplantation immunomodulation For patients undergoing autologous transplantation, several post-transplantation immunomodulating strategies, such as rituximab (Rituxan) after autologous transplantation for B-cell lymphoma, are being tested to determine whether they will decrease relapse by augmenting immunologic antitumor responses following transplantation. In some diseases such as myeloma, post-transplant treatment with medication such as dexamethasone and with thalidomide (Thalomid) helps prolong remission.

Collection of the graft

Allogeneic bone marrow cells Current techniques for harvesting bone marrow involve repeated aspirations from the posterior iliac crests, designed to obtain adequate numbers of cells that can lead to hematopoiesis. While the donor is under general or spinal anesthesia, between 1 to 3×10^8 cells/kg of the recipient's body weight are procured. The procedure has no long-term side effects and poses little risk if care is taken to ensure that the donor has no confounding medical conditions. In most cases of ABO incompatibility, the marrow can be treated to remove RBCs to prevent lysis after infusion.

Autologous peripheral stem cells Collection of circulating peripheral blood progenitor cells is performed via an apheresis technique. Although this procedure can be accomplished in an individual with a baseline blood count, the number of cells and the efficiency of collection are increased if the cells are procured during WBC recovery following chemotherapy or after the administration of hematopoietic growth factors.

The most effective strategy appears to be the collection of cells after both chemotherapy and administration of growth factors. In most circumstances, adequate numbers of cells can be collected utilizing granulocyte colony-stimulating factor (G-CSF, filgrastim [Neupogen]) to prime the patient prior to one to three apheresis procedures.

> Although busulfan-based regimens are the most commonly used worldwide for allogeneic transplantation, the oral administration of the drug leads to unpredictable absorption, which has been correlated with relapse (low absorption) and increased toxicity (increased absorption). Recent studies with an intravenous formulation of the drug have shown much more predictable pharmacokinetics, less toxicity, and good survival when utilized in the transplantation regimen.

Currently, the adequacy of the number of hematopoietic stem cells is assessed by determining the number of cells that have the CD34 antigen (stem-cell) marker. Usually, a minimum of 2×10^6 CD34 cells/kg of body weight is required to ensure engraftment.

The use of autologous stem cells continues to undergo refinement. Approaches under study include ex vivo expansion to augment the number of progenitor cells, as well as techniques that separate hematopoietic cells from any potential contaminating tumor cells. In addition, hematopoietic stem cells are the usual targets of marrow-based gene therapy utilizing viral vectors for transduction of cells prior to cryopreservation.

Indications for transplantation

The expanded methods of stem-cell transplantation have complicated the choice for patients and their physicians among the different types of transplantation in some instances. Therefore, the decision requires evaluation of the patient and the disease involved. In general, for disorders that require replacement of an abnormally functioning hematopoietic system, such as thalassemia and aplastic anemia, an allogeneic transplantation is performed. However, as genetic therapy for hematopoietic stem cells becomes more of a reality, even patients with these diseases may be candidates for autologous transplantation after gene modification (adenosine deaminase deficiency, chronic granulomatous disease).

Hematologic malignancies The most common use of allogeneic BMT has been for the eradication of hematologic malignancies, such as leukemia and non-Hodgkin lymphoma. For some disorders (aplastic anemia, myelodysplasia, leukemia in relapse, and CML), allogeneic transplantation is the only significant therapeutic option, whereas for other diseases (AML in remission, lymphoma, Hodgkin lymphoma, and multiple myeloma), either autologous or allogeneic marrow grafting may be possible.

Nonmyeloablative or reduced-intensity transplantation approaches are being studied worldwide, which has facilitated transplantation for many people who otherwise would not have been candidates due to concomitant medical problems or older age. The results indicate that malignancies that are not rapidly progressive are the most responsive. Thus, patients with low-grade lymphoma, AML, myeloma, myelodysplasia, and CML are probably good candidates for this type of allogeneic transplantation, whereas those with advanced disease such as leukemia in relapse or high-grade lymphoma benefit less, as the allogeneic antitumor effect requires time to develop and achieve remission of the disease. Table 3 shows the relative sensitivity of different hematologic malignancies to a graft-vs-malignancy effect that could be mediated by a nonmyeloablative transplant.

Solid tumors In general, only autologous transplantation is utilized for some solid tumors, such as breast, germ-cell, and ovarian cancers. Studies and longer follow-up of recently completed trials continue to determine whether there is a benefit to the use of transplant-based approaches in the treatment of high-risk

TABLE 3: Disease sensitivity to a graft-vs-malignancy effect
Most sensitive
Chronic myelogenous leukemia
Low-grade lymphoma
Mantle cell lymphoma
Chronic lymphocytic leukemia
Intermediate
Acute myelogenous leukemia
Intermediate-grade lymphoma
Multiple myeloma
Least sensitive
Acute lymphoblastic leukemia
High-grade lymphoma
Hodgkin lymphoma (?)
Renal cell carcinoma

(stages II, IIIA, IIIB) breast cancer. Allogeneic transplant studies in patients with renal cell cancer suggest that a graft-vs-tumor effect can be elicited against this tumor as well.

Timing of transplantation

The Goldie-Coldman model proposes that the probability that a tumor contains treatment-resistant cells is a function of its size and inherent mutation rate. This finding suggests that the likelihood of cure is greatest when marrow transplantation is performed early in the natural history of an inherently chemosensitive tumor. Studies to date indicate that patients undergoing transplantation late in their disease course have inferior disease-free survival, compared with those who undergo transplantation early.

Phases of transplantation

PREPARATIVE PHASE

In the first phase of marrow transplantation, the preparative phase, patients receive high-dose chemotherapy and/or radiation therapy (sometimes referred to as a conditioning regimen).

Allogeneic transplantation The conditioning regimen used in the allogeneic setting has both a therapeutic component designed to eliminate tumor cells and an immunosuppressive component to prevent host immune responses from rejecting the transplanted donor graft. The doses of radiation therapy and chemotherapy employed take advantage of the steep dose-response curve that exists for many malignancies. The doses have been established based on the limitations of other nonhematopoietic organs, such as the liver and lungs.

Typically, preparative regimens for full allogeneic BMT consist of TBI and/or chemotherapeutic agents (cyclophosphamide, busulfan [Busulfex, Myleran], and

TABLE 4: Acute and long-term toxicities of common preparative agents used for BMT

Agent	Acute toxicity	Long-term toxicity
Total-body irradiation	Nausea, vomiting, enteritis, mucositis	Cataracts, sterility, pneumonitis, myelodysplasia
Cyclophosphamide	Nausea, vomiting, hemorrhagic cystitis, cardiac toxicity	Sterility, leukemia
Etoposide	Skin rash, hypotension, acidosis, mucositis	Leukemia
Carmustine (BiCNU)	Seizures, nausea, vomiting, headaches	Interstitial pneumonitis
Busulfan	Seizures, nausea, vomiting, veno-occlusive disease	Alopecia, pulmonary fibrosis
Cisplatin	Renal impairment, hearing loss, tinnitus	Hearing loss, tinnitus, neuropathy
Thiotepa	Nausea, vomiting, CNS changes, veno-occlusive disease	—
Paclitaxel	Allergic reactions	Neuropathy
Fludarabine	Hemolytic anemia, CNS changes	Prolonged immune suppression, EBV-related lympho-proliferative disorder
Melphalan	Nausea, pulmonary	Peripheral neuropathy

BMT = bone marrow transplantation; EBV = Epstein-Barr virus

etoposide). The most commonly used regimens are (1) TBI (1,200–1,400 cGy administered in multiple fractions over a period of days) and cyclophosphamide (60 mg/kg for 2 days); (2) fractionated TBI and etoposide (60 mg/kg); and (3) busulfan (16 mg/kg over 4 days) and cyclophosphamide (60 mg/kg for 2 days).

Autologous transplantation For patients undergoing autologous transplantation, stem cells are reinfused following high-dose therapy to reestablish hematopoiesis as rapidly as possible. The regimens used for autologous BMT depend on the disease being treated. High-dose melphalan (Alkeran; 200 mg /m^2) is the most commonly used regimen for myeloma and BEAM (BiCNU, etoposide, cytosine arabinoside, and melphalan) or CBV (cyclophosphamide, BiCNU, and etoposide) are the two most commonly used regimens for lymphoma.

Toxicities of preparative regimens The acute toxicities of irradiation and chemotherapy include nausea and vomiting, which can be managed by prophylactic use of antiemetics, particularly serotonin antagonists. Busulfan can cause seizures; prophylactic phenytoin is effective in preventing this complication. Both cyclophosphamide and etoposide require forced hydration to reduce toxicities. Table 4 lists the acute and long-term toxicities of the major agents used in BMT preparative regimens.

TRANSPLANT PHASE

After completion of the preparative regimen, there is a day or more wait before reinfusion of marrow or peripheral blood stem cells. This delay allows for elimination of any active drug metabolites so that the reinfused cells are not injured by any remaining drug.

Minimal toxicities are associated with the infusion. They include headache, nausea, and dizziness. Dizziness is related more to the cryoprotectant dimethyl sulfoxide (DMSO) used to store cells from most patients undergoing autologous transplantation.

SUPPORTIVE CARE PHASE

Following administration of the preparative regimen and during and after marrow transplantation, all patients require strict attention to infectious disease-related complications secondary to neutropenia. The duration of neutropenia following transplantation increases the risk of complicating infections. Patients undergoing full allogeneic transplantation usually require more stringent isolation, whereas patients undergoing autologous transplantation need less rigorous protection. With the availability of more effective antiemetics (eg, ondansetron [Zofran] and granisetron [Kytril]), portions of the transplantation can now be performed in the outpatient setting.

Following allogeneic transplantation, various complications may develop that require treatment. For some complications, prophylactic measures can be instituted to prevent their occurrence.

Neutropenic sepsis

Nearly all patients undergoing transplantation will develop fever, often with positive blood cultures, within 7 days of becoming neutropenic. Sepsis usually is caused by enteric bacteria or those found on the skin, and antibiotic choices are based on initial assessment and the results of blood cultures. The antibiotics chosen are continued until the neutrophil count begins to rise (> 500 k/μL). Most patients undergoing allogeneic transplantation usually receive bowel decontamination (eg, with a fluoroquinolone, such as levofloxacin [Levaquin], 500 mg/d PO) in the post-transplantation phase to reduce the risk of serious infection during neutropenia.

Prevention of fungal infections For patients who are expected to have prolonged neutropenia, various methods of antifungal prophylaxis are used, including PO fluconazole (Diflucan; 200 mg bid) or voriconazole (Vfend; 200 mg IV or PO bid). The use of liposomal amphotericin B (AmBisome or Abelcet) or caspofungin (Cancidas) formulations has improved safety and lowered toxicity of antifungal therapy and is particularly worthwhile in patients with renal compromise.

Mucositis, nausea, and anorexia

Regimen-related toxicity often results in severe oral mucositis, nausea, and anorexia. Patients often require supplemental parenteral nutrition to maintain adequate caloric intake during this period. Because of the mucositis, enteral feedings are usually not employed, and total parenteral nutrition is maintained until patients are able to eat. Studies are exploring novel agents that could prevent severe mucositis or accelerate healing with keratinocyte growth factor (KGF), which has been shown to decrease this complication following TBI-based autologous transplant regimens.

Oral HSV reactivation

Nearly all patients who are seropositive for herpes simplex virus (HSV) will have a reactivation of the virus, which can accentuate the pain and oral discomfort following BMT. To prevent this problem, most transplant programs utilize acyclovir at a dose of 250 mg/m^2 tid during the neutropenic phase.

Transfusion

All patients will require both RBCs and platelets in proportion to the duration of the pancytopenia. Platelets are kept over 10,000–20,000/µL because of complicating bleeding from mucositis, although, in some instances, a lower threshold is feasible. Patients no longer receive granulocyte transfusions unless they have uncontrolled sepsis with positive blood cultures. For patients who are negative for cytomegalovirus (CMV) and who have a CMV-negative donor, CMV-negative cell support is generally provided (see section on "CMV infection").

All blood products are irradiated to prevent engraftment of lymphoid cells and are often filtered to reduce CMV or alloimmunization and febrile reactions. Most patients receive single-donor platelet pheresis products, which may need to be HLA-matched if patients show evidence of refractoriness to the transfusion (ie, if platelet levels fail to rise after transfusion).

Sinusoidal obstruction syndrome (veno-occlusive disease)

In the first few weeks after BMT, sinusoidal obstruction syndrome, characterized by hepatomegaly, jaundice, and fluid retention, develops in 5%–20% of patients. It is caused by damaged endothelial cells, sinusoids, and hepatocytes and is related to the intensity of the cytoreductive therapeutic regimen.

The diagnosis of sinusoidal obstruction syndrome is usually made on clinical grounds, based on the occurrence (usually within 8–10 days after starting the cytoreductive regimen) of the triad of hepatomegaly, weight gain, and jaundice. Patients also exhibit renal sodium retention, and prognosis is related to the degree of liver and kidney dysfunction and the level of bilirubin. The use of regimens that contain busulfan has been associated with the highest incidence of veno-occlusive disease, which has decreased with targeted oral or intravenous busulfan dosing.

Treatment Once veno-occlusive disease has occurred, treatment is primarily supportive, consisting of careful management of fluid overload, kidney dysfunction, and other attendant complications. In few cases, the early use of thrombolytic agents can reverse established veno-occlusive disease. Based on

TABLE 5: Clinical classification of acute GVHD according to organ injury

Stage key	0	1	2	3	4
Skin	No rash	Maculopapular rash, less than 25% of body surface	Maculopapular rash, 25%-50% of body surface	Rash on greater than 50% of body surface or generalized erythroderma	Generalized or erythroderma with bullous formation and/or desquamation
Lower GI (diarrhea)	Less than or equal to 500 mL/d or less than 280 mL/m^2	Greater than 500 but ≤ 1,000 mL/d or 280 to 555 mL/m^2	Greater than 1,000 but ≤ 1,500 mL/d or 556 to 833 mL/m^2	> 1,500 mL/d or > 833 mL/m^2	Severe abdominal pain with or without ileus, or stool with frank blood or melena
Upper GI	No protracted nausea and vomiting	Persistent nausea, vomiting, or anorexia plus biopsy showing a GVHD of the stomach or duodenum			
Liver (total bilirubin)	Less than 2.0 mg/dL	2.0-3.0 mg/dL	3.1-6.0 mg/dL	6.1-15.0 mg/dL	> 15 mg/dL

Overall clinical grading of severity of acute GVHD–1994 Keystone Consensus Criteria

Grade	Skin		Liver		Gut		Karnofsky performance scale (KPS)
I	1-2	&	0	&	0		
II	3	or	1	or	1		
III	0-4	or	2-3	or	2-4		
IV	4	or	4	or	0-4	or	KPS score ≤ 30% or decrease ≥ 40% from baseline KPS score

GVHD = graft-vs-host disease

TABLE 6: Prophylaxis of acute graft-versus-host disease

Day	Cyclosporine	Methotrexate
–2	5 mg/kg IV daily	
+1	5 mg/kg IV daily	15 mg/m^2 IV single dose
+3	5 mg/kg IV daily	10 mg/m^2 IV single dose
+4	3 mg/kg IV daily	
+6	3 mg/kg IV daily	10 mg/m^2 IV single dose
+11	3 mg/kg IV daily	10 mg/m^2 IV single dose
+15	2.75 mg/kg IV daily	
+36	10 mg/kg PO daily	
+84	8 mg/kg PO daily	
+98	6 mg/kg PO daily	
+120	4 mg/kg PO daily	
+180	off	

early phase II studies, defibrotide is now being tested in phase III trials as an agent that can help reverse the syndrome.

Acute GVHD

GVHD is a clinical syndrome that results from the infusion of immunocompetent lymphocytes accompanying the marrow graft that are capable of recognizing minor HLA-related antigens in the host and initiating an immunologic reaction. This syndrome may arise after allogeneic transplantation or rarely after transfusion of cellular blood products in patients who are immunodeficient and share HLA loci that allow engraftment of transfused cells. For unknown reasons, the primary organs affected by acute GVHD are the skin, liver, and GI tract.

The syndrome usually occurs within 15–60 days after transplantation and can vary in severity. Table 5 shows a commonly used grading system for GVHD. This system has both therapeutic and prognostic importance.

Prophylaxis All patients undergoing non–T-cell-depleted transplantation require some form of GVHD prophylaxis. The most common regimens involve a combination of methotrexate and cyclosporine or tacrolimus [Prograf]. The combination of tacrolimus and sirolimus (Rapamune) has been studied and appears to be an effective approach for the prevention of GVHD. These medications, in the absence of GVHD, are tapered over 6–12 months after BMT. Table 6 shows a common regimen used to prevent GVHD after an allogeneic sibling transplantation. The regimens of sirolimus and tacrolimus are tapered in a similar manner. Side effects of tacrolimus and cyclosporine include renal toxicity, hypertension, magnesium wasting, seizures, and microangiopathy. Sirolimus, an oral agent, can cause hemolytic uremic syndrome in association with tacrolimus and requires careful dose and drug level monitoring. It can also raise blood triglyceride levels.

Treatment Despite prophylaxis, many allogeneic transplant recipients still develop some degree of GVHD and require increasing doses of prednisone (1–2 mg/kg/d). For patients who do not respond to steroids, antithymocyte globulin (Atgam; 10 mg/kg/d for 5–10 days) has been used. Daclizumab (Zenapax; 1 mg/kg on days 1, 4, 8, 15, and 22), pentostatin (Nipent), and etanercept (Enbrel) are likely more effective agents than antithymocyte globulin.

Chronic GVHD

Chronic GVHD may occur within 3–6 months in patients who have undergone allogeneic BMT. It is often preceded by acute GVHD, which may or may not have resolved. Although chronic GVHD is also related to infusion of T cells with the marrow graft, it resembles other autoimmune connective tissue diseases, such as scleroderma, Sjögren's syndrome, biliary cirrhosis, and bronchiolitis obliterans. Patients with chronic GVHD often have accompanying cytopenias and immune deficiency as well as abnormalities of the oral mucosa, conjunctiva, and gastrointestinal tract.

Treatment Chronic GVHD is generally treated with prolonged courses of steroids, cyclosporine, tacrolimus, and, occasionally, azathioprine and other modalities, such as psoralen-ultraviolet A light (PUVA) for skin and mouth GVHD. Thalidomide (Thalomid), mycophenolate mofetil (CellCept), sirolimus, and photopheresis have also been employed, with varying response rates. Like that for acute GVHD, the prognosis for chronic GVHD is related to the extent of organ compromise and response to treatment.

GVHD and relapse Although, in general, GVHD has contributed to significant morbidity and mortality in patients undergoing allogeneic BMT, it is also associated with reduced relapse rates, primarily in patients with hematologic malignancies.

Late infections

Late infections after BMT are caused by impaired cellular and humoral immunity. The most common late pathogens include *Pneumocystis carinii*, varicella zoster, and encapsulated bacteria.

***Pneumocystis* prophylaxis** All patients undergoing allogeneic transplantation require prophylaxis against *P carinii*. This can be accomplished with one double-strength trimethoprim-sulfamethoxazole tablet bid twice a week once hematopoiesis has been restored. Alternatively, atovaquone (Mepron; 750 mg bid) has been utilized.

Treatment of herpes zoster Approximately 40% of patients will develop herpes zoster (either dermatomal or disseminated), which is often treated with oral or IV acyclovir. A patient may complain of severe localized pain for several days before the rash develops. The use of valacyclovir (Valtrex) for 1 year after BMT can reduce or delay the risk of reactivation of herpes zoster after allogeneic BMT.

Bacterial prophylaxis Many patients with chronic GVHD develop an accompanying severe immunodeficiency syndrome that leaves them susceptible to infection with encapsulated bacteria, primarily in the sinuses and lungs. In some cases, prolonged prophylaxis with trimethoprim-sulfamethoxazole or penicillin is necessary, as well as immunoglobulin replacement.

CMV infection

Historically, CMV interstitial pneumonia has been responsible for approximately 15%–20% of patient deaths following allogeneic BMT. CMV pneumonia occurs 7–10 weeks after BMT and is due to reactivation of latent CMV or is acquired from donor marrow or transfusions. Active CMV infection, GVHD, and the inability to develop a virus-specific immune response that limits viral infection are risk factors for CMV pneumonia.

Diagnosis Infection is diagnosed by the combination of an abnormal chest x-ray, hypoxemia, and the detection of CMV in bronchoalveolar lavage or lung biopsy specimens, as well as the absence of other pathogens.

Treatment The only consistent treatment has been the combination of ganciclovir, 5 mg/kg bid for 3 weeks, and IV immunoglobulin, given every other day. Although the reason for the synergy between these agents is unclear, neither one alone is effective in reversing pneumonia once it has developed.

Prevention in CMV-seronegative patients The most successful means of preventing CMV infection in CMV-seronegative patients who have a seronegative donor is to limit their exposure to the virus by providing CMV-negative blood and platelet support. As most patients who undergo marrow transplantation are CMV-seropositive, this strategy has limited application. However, the presence of leukocytes in blood products increases the transmission of CMV. Thus, the use of CMV-seronegative blood products in CMV-seronegative recipients decreases the incidence of primary CMV infection. Also, CMV status should be determined in all patients prior to BMT to plan for post-transplantation transfusion strategies.

Prevention in CMV-seropositive patients The most effective strategy for preventing reactivation of CMV infection in patients who are CMV-seropositive is the preemptive use of ganciclovir, either prophylactically in all CMV-sero-positive patients or at the first sign of CMV after transplantation (as indicated by blood culture, shell viral culture, or antigen or polymerase chain reaction [PCR] detection of the virus). The timing and duration of prophylaxis are somewhat controversial.

Ganciclovir has been the most effective agent for both strategies, as it significantly reduces both viral reactivation and associated disease. However, if one waits until after viral reactivation to initiate ganciclovir therapy, there are some patients who will not benefit from a prophylactic strategy, namely those in whom reactivation occurs simultaneously with disease. Ganciclovir has many side effects, including neutropenia and elevated creatinine levels, and thus exposes a large number of patients to potential toxicity.

The required duration of ganciclovir treatment is also unclear, but it would appear that several weeks is necessary to protect the patient from viral reactivation and the development of pneumonitis within the first 3 months after BMT. Monitoring for CMV of all patients after completion of antiviral therapy is necessary, as some patients, particularly those with GVHD are at risk for infection due to an inadequate immune response against CMV. Some patients have developed late CMV pneumonia after drug discontinuation, which is probably related to ganciclovir inhibition of the development of CMV-specific cytolytic T cells. Nevertheless, the use of ganciclovir has reduced the problems related to CMV pneumonia and should be a part of every management strategy for preventing complications following allogeneic transplantation. Currently, newer antiviral drugs such as miribavir are being tested and appear to have good antiviral activity with less toxicity.

Other post-transplantation therapies

Growth factors have found their most significant use in the acceleration of hematopoietic recovery after autologous reinfusion of stem cells. Clinical trials in allogeneic transplantation have not yet shown an advantage to their use, probably due to the immunosuppressive medications such as methotrexate used to prevent GVHD. Studies do support the use of G-CSF or GM-CSF after autologous marrow transplantation, although the impact of these growth factors on acceleration of hematopoietic recovery, beyond that achieved with the use of primed autologous stem cells, is not clear.

Epoetin alfa (Epogen, Procrit) or darbepoetin alfa (Aranesp) is sometimes used effectively in patients who have persistent anemia after transplantation.

Management of relapse

Despite the intensity of the preparative regimen, some patients relapse after allogeneic BMT. For patients with CML, withdrawal of immunosuppression to allow for an augmented graft-vs-tumor effect sometimes leads to remission. Other patients with CML may respond to post-transplantation interferon or reintroduction of drugs such as imatinib (Gleevec), which appears to be a useful approach. Intriguingly, infusion of donor lymphoid cells in patients with CML is an effective means of inducing hematologic and cytogenetic responses in those who have relapsed after transplantation; this approach has led to complete and durable remissions.

Some patients with AML have responded to either infusion of donor stem cells or the combination of chemotherapy and donor stem cells. Patients with acute lymphoblastic leukemia have had the lowest response rate to this strategy. Patients who develop myelodysplasia after autologous transplantation can sometimes be treated with reduced-intensity allogeneic transplant to restore normal hematopoiesis and cure the myelodysplastic syndrome.

Long-term problems

For patients undergoing autologous stem-cell transplantation, the major long-term problem is the risk of relapse and myelodysplasia, but changes in libido, sexual dynsfunction, and infertility also should be addressed to help patients achieve good long-term quality of life. Patients undergoing allogeneic transplantation also have similar long-term issues but also have major long-term effects related to chronic GVHD and the complications related to immunosuppression, especially infection. In addition, patients undergoing allogeneic transplantation are at higher risk for second malignancies, and thus aggressive screening studies should be part of the care of all long-term survivors of transplantation.

Second malignancy after hematopoietic cell transplantation

Patients undergoing transplantation are at risk for developing a second cancer. For those undergoing autologous transplantation, particularly for treatment of lymphoma and Hodgkin lymphoma, the most common cancer is myelodysplasia/AML, which occurs in up to 10% of patients, usually within 3 to 7 years after transplantation.

Risk factors for the development of myelodysplasia/AML after transplantation include the number of prior chemotherapy and radiation therapy treatments, specific drugs such as alkylating agents or topoisomerase inhibitors, difficulty in mobilizing stem cells, persistent cytopenias after transplantation, and use of TBI in the transplant preparative regimen. All patients should undergo cytogenetic screening of the marrow prior to stem-cell collection and should be followed for this complication after recovery from transplantation.

Patients undergoing either autologous and allogeneic transplantation are also at risk for the development of solid tumors, up to 20 years after transplantation. The risk is greater in patients receiving an allogeneic transplant. The most common tumors are related to the skin, but both common (breast, lung, and colon) and less common (sarcoma) tumors have been seen. As part of their long-term follow-up, all patients require screening for this complication to diagnose the cancer in its earliest stage.

SUGGESTED READING

Antin JH, Kim HT, Cutler C, et al: Sirolimus, tacrolimus, and low-dose methotrexate for graft-versus-host disease prophylaxis in mismatched related donor or unrelated donor transplantation. Blood 102:1601–1605, 2003.

Arvin AM: Varicella-zoster virus: Pathogenesis, immunity, and clinical management in hematopoietic cell transplant recipients. Biol Blood Marrow Transplant 6:219–230, 2000.

Attal M, Harousseau JL, Facon T, et al: Single versus double autologous stem-cell transplantation for multiple myeloma. N Engl J Med 349:2495–2502, 2003.

Bethge WA, Hegenbart U, Stuart MJ, et al: Adoptive immunotherapy with donor lymphocyte infusions after allogeneic hematopoietic cell transplantation following nonmyeloablative conditioning. Blood 103:790–795, 2004.

Blume KG, Forman SJ, Appelbaum FR (eds): Hematopoietic Cell Transplantation, 2nd ed. Malden, Massachusetts, Blackwell Science, 2004.

Cutler C, Kim HT, Hochberg E, et al: Sirolimus and tacrolimus without methotrexate as graft-versus-host disease prophylaxis after matched related donor peripheral blood stem cell transplantation. Biol Blood Marrow Transplant 10:328–336, 2004.

de Lima M, Giralt S: Allogeneic transplantation for the elderly patient with acute myelogenous leukemia or myelodysplastic syndrome. Semin Hematol 43:107–117, 2006.

Deeg HJ, Gooley TA, Flowers ME, et al: Allogeneic hematopoietic stem cell transplantation for myelofibrosis. Blood 102:3912–3918, 2003.

Fung HC, Cohen S, Rodriguez R, et al: Reduced-intensity allogeneic stem cell transplantation for patients whose prior autologous stem cell transplantation for hematologic malignancy failed. Biol Blood Marrow Transplant 9:649–656, 2003.

Gopal AK, Gooley TA, Maloney DG, et al: High-dose radioimmunotherapy versus conventional high-dose therapy and autologous hematopoietic stem cell transplantation for relapsed follicular non-Hodgkin lymphoma: A multivariable cohort analysis. Blood 102:2351–2357, 2003.

Harousseau JL, Moreau P: Evolving role of stem cell transplantation in multiple myeloma. Clin Lymphoma Myeloma 6:89–95, 2005.

Hertzberg M, Grigg A, Gottlieb D, et al: Reduced-intensity allogeneic haemopoietic stem cell transplantation induces durable responses in patients with chronic B-lymphoproliferative disorders. Bone Marrow Transplant Mar 27, 2006 [Epub ahead of print].

Laughlin MJ, Eapen M, Rubinstein P, et al: Outcomes after transplantation of cord blood or bone marrow from unrelated donors in adults with leukemia. N Engl J Med 351:2265–2275, 2004.

Lavoie JC, Connors JM, Phillips GL, et al: High-dose chemotherapy and autologous stem cell transplantation for primary refractory or relapsed Hodgkin lymphoma: Long-term outcome in the first 100 patients treated in Vancouver. Blood 106:1473–1478, 2005.

Ljungman P, Urbano-Ispizua A, Cavazzana-Calvo M, et al: Allogeneic and autologous transplantation for haematological diseases, solid tumours, and immune disorders: Definitions and current practice in Europe. Bone Marrow Transplant 37:439–449, 2006.

Maloney DG, Molina AJ, Sahebi F, et al: Allografting with nonmyeloablative conditioning following cytoreductive autografts for the treatment of patients with multiple myeloma. Blood 102:3447–3454, 2003.

McSweeney PA, Niederwieser D, Shizuru JA, et al: Hematopoietic cell transplantation in older patients with hematologic malignancies: Replacing high-dose cytotoxic therapy with graft-vs-tumor effects. Blood 97:3390–3400, 2001.

Nademanee A, Forman S, Molina A, et al: A phase 1/2 trial of high-dose yttrium-90-ibritumomab tiuxetan in combination with high-dose etoposide and cyclophosphamide followed by autologous stem cell transplantation in patients with poor-risk or relapsed non-Hodgkin lymphoma. Blood 106:2896–2902, 2005.

Richardson PG, Murakami C, Jin Z, et al: Multi-institutional use of defibrotide in 88 patients after stem cell transplantation with severe veno-occlusive disease and multisystem organ failure: Response without significant toxicity in a high-risk population and factors predictive of outcome. Blood 100:4337–4343, 2002.

Syrjala KL, Langer SL, Abrams JR, et al: Late effects of hematopoietic cell transplantation among 10-year adult survivors compared with case-matched controls. J Clin Oncol 23:6596–6606, 2005.

Tauro S, Craddock C, Peggs K, et al: Allogeneic stem-cell transplantation using a reduced-intensity conditioning regimen has the capacity to produce durable remissions and long-term disease-free survival in patients with high-risk acute myeloid leukemia and myelodysplasia. J Clin Oncol 23:9387–9393, 2005.

Van Besien K: The evolving role of autologous and allogeneic stem cell transplantation in follicular lymphoma. Blood Rev Feb 28, 2006 [Epub ahead of print].

Zaia JA: Prevention of cytomegalovirus disease in hematopoietic stem cell transplantation. Clin Infect Dis 35:999–1004, 2002.

CHAPTER 37

Pain management

Sharon M. Weinstein, MD, Penny R. Anderson, MD, Alan W. Yasko, MD, and Lawrence Driver, MD

PAIN

Most patients with advanced cancer and up to 60% of patients with any stage of the disease experience significant pain. The World Health Organization (WHO) estimates that 25% of all cancer patients die with unrelieved pain.

The cause of cancer pain should be treated whenever possible. By doing so, one can frequently achieve rapid, lasting pain relief and may prevent the problems associated with untreated progressive disease, such as spinal cord compression and pathologic fracture. Also, the need for pain medications may be diminished, thus reducing side effects and drug interactions.

In most cancer patients, pain can be relieved adequately, and yet it is undertreated for a multitude of reasons. The problem is not trivial, as unrelieved pain is known to be a risk factor for suicide in cancer patients. Current efforts are being directed toward standardizing pain treatment and separating issues of pain treatment from those of substance abuse.

The effective management of cancer patients with pain is best accomplished with coordination of the services of multidisciplinary professionals, community volunteers, and the family.

Pathophysiology

Pathophysiologic classification of pain forms the basis for therapeutic choices. Pain states may be broadly divided into those associated with ongoing tissue damage (nociceptive) and those resulting from nervous system dysfunction in the absence of ongoing tissue damage (non-nociceptive or neuropathic).

Damage to the nervous system may result in pain in an area of altered sensation. Such pain is typically described as burning or lancinating. Patients may report bizarre complaints, such as painful numbness, itching, or crawling sensations. The postamputation phenomenon of phantom pain (pain referred to the lost body part) may be disabling.

Psychological factors Psychological factors may affect the reporting of pain. Chronic unrelieved pain has psychological consequences, but this does not support a psychiatric basis for the pain complaint. "Psychogenic pain" or somatoform pain disorder is rare in cancer patients.

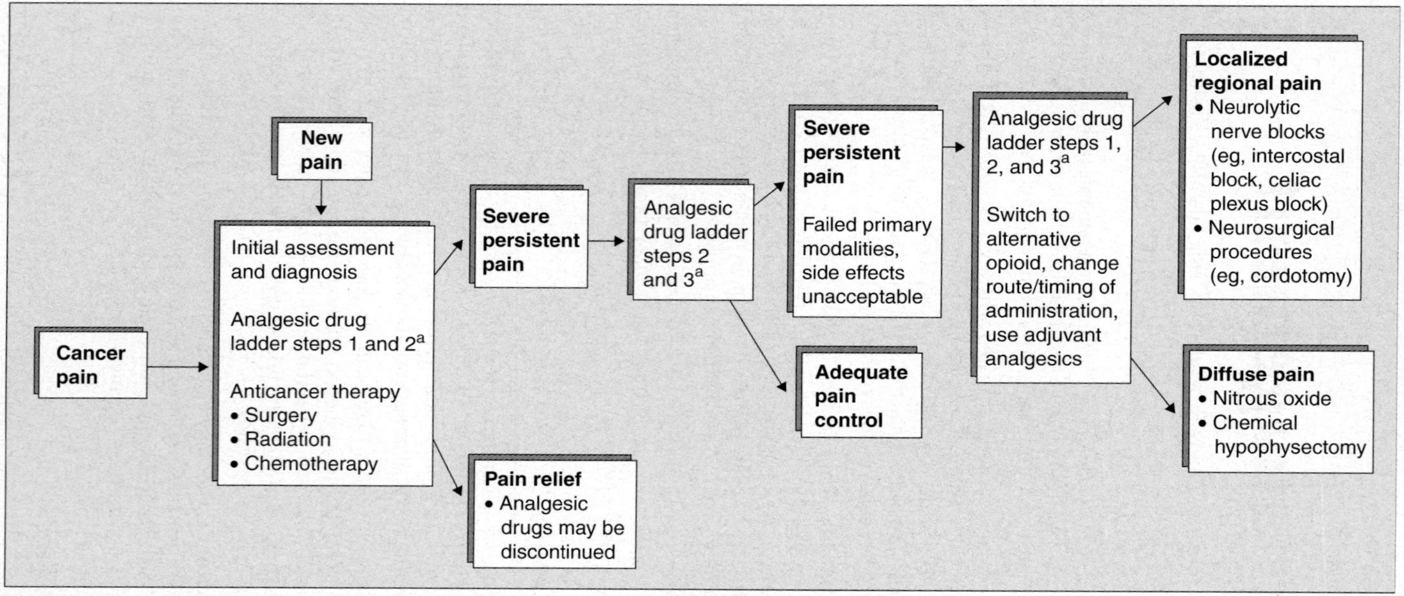

FIGURE 1: Algorithm for the integration of pharmacologic management approaches to cancer pain

[a] Step 1 - Nonopioid ± adjuvant, Step 2 - Opioid + nonopioid ± adjuvant, Step 3 - Strong opioid ± nonopioid ± adjuvant

Adapted from Foley KM, Arbit E, in DeVita VT, Hellman S, Rosenberg SA (eds): Cancer: Principles & Practice of Oncology, 3rd ed, vol 2, pp 2064-2087. Philadelphia, JB Lippincott, 1989.

Pain syndromes

Cancer pain syndromes vary by tumor type and are related to patterns of tumor growth and metastasis. Pain may also be related to antineoplastic therapy or may be unrelated to either the neoplasm or its treatment.

Elements of management

Elements of cancer pain management include a proper medical evaluation, psychosocial assessment, formulation of the pain "diagnosis," and consideration of pharmacologic and nonpharmacologic treatments. Ongoing care is needed to monitor the efficacy of analgesics and the evolution of different symptoms during treatment or disease progression.

The steps in medical decision-making are to:

- determine whether primary antineoplastic therapy is indicated for palliation
- tailor pharmacologic analgesic therapy to individual needs
- consider concurrent nonpharmacologic analgesic methods
- monitor response and modify treatment accordingly (Figure 1).

The patient is the focus of care, although family members and others often participate in treatment decisions and require emotional support.

Medical evaluation

Pain history Begin with a thorough history. As there are no objective means with which to verify the presence of pain, one must believe a patient's complaint. The physiologic signs of acute pain—elevated blood pressure and pulse rate—are unreliable in subacute or chronic pain.

Most cancer patients report more than one site of pain. A detailed history of each type of pain should be elicited (Table 1). As the chief complaint resolves, what was initially a secondary problem may require attention.

Pain rating scales should be used to establish a baseline against which the success of treatment may be judged (Figure 2). Behavioral observations may be used to assess patients who are unable to communicate. Although there are standardized tools for preverbal children, they are not available for impaired adults. Thus, it is sometimes necessary to treat pain presumptively.

Physical examination includes careful neurologic testing, especially if neuropathic pain is suspected. Pain in an area of reduced sensation, allodynia (ie, when normal stimuli are reported as painful), and hyperpathia or summation of painful stimuli indicate a neuropathic process. The assessment should evaluate the putative mechanisms that may underlie the pain.

Review of disease extent and current conditions The extent of disease and current medical conditions must be determined.

Diagnostic tests should be reviewed and supplemented as necessary.

TABLE 1: Features of the pain history—"PQRST"

P	Provocative factors, palliative factors
Q	Quality (characteristics)
R	Region, pattern of radiation, referral
S	Severity, intensity (use pain rating scales [Figure 2])
T	Temporal factors: onset, duration, time to maximum intensity, frequency, daily variation

Treatment and drug history Cancer treatment and prior analgesic interventions, along with their outcomes, should be recorded. Psychological dependency on any drug, including alcohol, must be identified.

Psychosocial assessment

To establish trust, the evaluating clinician should explore with the patient the significance of the pain complaint. The impact of pain and other symptoms on functional status must be understood to establish treatment goals. Suffering may be attributable to many factors besides physical complaints. The clinician should ask about such psychological factors as financial worries, loss of independence, family problems, social isolation, and fear of death. Often, cancer patients meet diagnostic criteria for the psychiatric diagnosis of adjustment disorder with anxiety and/or depressed mood.

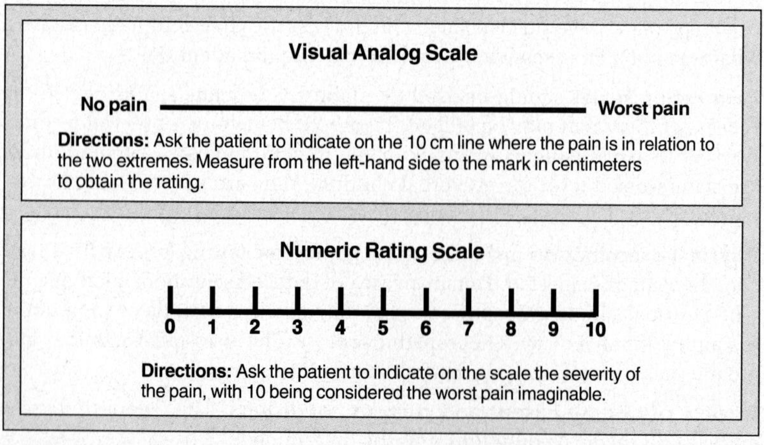

FIGURE 2: Pain rating scales used to establish a baseline against which treatment results are judged; the numeric scale is also administered verbally.

Patient subgroups

To help define therapeutic goals, the patient's age and prognosis may be considered. Adjustments in drug doses are usually needed for elderly patients, who are more sensitive to analgesics and their side effects. Adolescents may require relatively larger doses of opioids. Pain in children is underreported and should be specifically elicited using age-appropriate assessment tools.

Pharmacologic treatment

The WHO has devised a three-step analgesic ladder outlining the use of nonopioid analgesics, opioid analgesics, and adjuvant medications for progressively severe pain. According to this schema, a nonopioid analgesic, with or without an adjuvant agent, should be tried first (step 1). If pain persists or increases on this regimen, the patient should be switched to an opioid plus a nonopioid agent, with or without an adjuvant medication (step 2). If pain continues or intensifies despite this change in therapy, a strong opioid analgesic should be prescribed, with or without a nonopioid and/or an adjuvant agent (step 3).

Nonopioid analgesics

Nonopioid analgesics are associated with ceiling effects, and exceeding the maximum dose ranges can result in organ toxicity. Potential side effects, such as hematologic, renal, and GI reactions, may be of clinical concern in cancer patients (Table 2). Cyclo-oxygenase-2 (COX-2) inhibitors are many times more potent against COX-2 than COX-1. Clinicians are advised to watch the emerging literature regarding the safety of these agents.

Opioid analgesics

General guidelines for the use of opioid therapy are outlined in Table 3.

Dosage Opioid agonists do not exhibit ceiling effects. Dosing is guided by efficacy and limited by side effects (Table 4). Dosages of tablets combining a nonsteroidal anti-inflammatory drug (NSAID) or acetaminophen and an opioid are limited according to the nonopioid component.

Routes of administration The oral route should be used when possible, though some patients may express a preference for an alternative route. If so, or if the oral route is not feasible or systemic side effects are uncontrollable, alternative routes are indicated, such as transdermal, transmucosal, rectal, and neuraxial infusion. Such alternative routes of administration of certain opioid agonists (see Table 5) may improve patients' quality of life and may be particularly useful for treating certain types of cancer pain.

Side effects of opioids can usually be anticipated and treated. In particular, with regular opioid dosing, laxatives should be prescribed for constipation.

Physical dependence and tolerance to some effects develop with chronic opioid use. Tolerance to respiratory depression, sedation, and nausea is likely to de-

TABLE 2: Nonopioid analgesics and NSAIDs useful for treating cancer pain

Generic name (usual dosage range)	Maximum dose/day	Adverse effects/ comments
Acetaminophen (325-975 mg q4-6h)	4,000 mg	Hepatic and renal impairment
Acetylsalicylic acid (aspirin, ASA) (325-975 mg q4-6h)	4,000 mg	Dyspepsia and GI ulceration, antiplatelet effect, bleeding
Celecoxib	400 mg	[a]
Choline magnesium trisalicylate (500-1,500 mg q8-12h)	4,500 mg	Dyspepsia, reduced antiplatelet effect, hypermagnesemia in renal failure
Choline salicylate (435-870 mg q3-4h)	5,220 mg	Dyspepsia, reduced antiplatelet effect
Magnesium salicylate (300-600 mg q4h)	4,800 mg	Same as choline salicylate
Salsalate (1,000-1,500 mg q8-12h)	4,000 mg	Same as choline salicylate
Sodium salicylate (325-650 mg q3-4h)	5,200 mg	Same as choline salicylate
Ibuprofen (200-800 mg q4-6h)	2,400 mg	[b]Dermatitis +
Ketoprofen (25-75 mg q6-8h)	300 mg	[b]Headache +++
Ketorolac tromethamine (oral: 10 mg q4-6h; parenteral: 60 mg, then 15-30 mg q6h)	Oral: 40 mg Parenteral: 120 mg	[b]Limit duration of therapy; headache +++, GI bleeding [b]Limit therapy to 5 days; headache +++, GI bleeding
Meclofenamate sodium (50-100 mg q4-6h)	400 mg	[b]Headache +, dermatitis +
Mefenamic acid (250 mg q6h)	1,000 mg	[b]Limit therapy to 7 days
Naproxen sodium (220-550 mg q8-12h)	1,375 mg	[b]Headache +
Naproxen (250-500 mg q8-12h)	1,500 mg	[b]Headache +

[a] Monitor emerging literature regarding safety concerns.

[b] Minor adverse reactions include dyspepsia, heartburn, nausea, vomiting, anorexia, diarrhea, constipation, flatulence, bloating, epigastric pain, abdominal pain, dizziness, and drowsiness. Major adverse reactions that may appear at any time include renal failure, hepatic dysfunction, bleeding, and gastric ulceration.

+ Each plus sign represents a 5% incidence of the reported adverse effect.

Adapted with permission from American Pain Society: Principles of Analgesic Use in the Treatment of Acute Pain and Cancer Pain, 5th ed. Skokie, Illinois, American Pain Society, 2003.
NSAIDs = nonsteroidal anti-inflammatory drugs

TABLE 3: Guidelines for the use of opioid analgesics

Start with an analgesic with the potential to provide relief

Know the essential pharmacology of the analgesic:

- Analgesic type
- Pharmacokinetics
- Influences of coadministered drugs, disease, or age on analgesic disposition and response
- Equianalgesic starting dose for the drug and route to be used
- Route of administration and a dosage form to fit the patient's needs

Individualize/titrate the dosage

Administer analgesics regularly after the initial dose titration

Provide for breakthrough pain

Use drug combinations that enhance analgesia

Recognize and treat side effects

Make conversions from one route to another or from one agent to another using known equianalgesic doses

Manage physical dependence (ie, prevent withdrawal)

Adapted with permission from Inturrisi C: Cancer 63(suppl):2308–2320, 1989.

TABLE 4: Opioid agonist analgesics for mild to moderate pain

Drug	Equianalgesic dose to 650 mg of aspirin[a]	Dose interval	Half-life (h)	Comments
Codeine	32-65 mg	q4-6h	2-3	b,c
Hydrocodone	—	q3-4h	4	b
Oxycodone	2.5 mg	q3-6h	—	b

[a] The equianalgesic dose should not be interpreted as the starting, standard, or maximum dose but rather as a guide for switching drugs or changing routes of administration.

[b] Doses of products containing aspirin or acetaminophen should be monitored for safety.

[c] Doses above 65 mg provide diminished incremental analgesia with increasing doses, but side effects may worsen.

Adapted with permission from American Pain Society: Principles of Analgesic Use in the Treatment of Acute Pain and Cancer Pain, 3rd ed. Skokie, Illinois, American Pain Society, 1992.

TABLE 5: Opioid agonist analgesics for severe pain

Drug	Equianalgesic dose to 10 mg of IV morphine		Half-life	
	Oral	Parenteral	(h)	Comments
Fentanyl, oral transmucosal	[a]	NA	[a]	For breakthrough cancer pain
Fentanyl, transdermal	NA	NA	—	[b, c] Patch sizes of 12, 25, 50, 75, 100 μg/h; slow onset to effect, necessitating "breakthrough" analgesics
Hydromorphone	4 mg	1.5 mg	2-3	[b]
Levorphanol	4 mg	2 mg	12-16	[b]
Methadone	20 mg	10 mg	15-36	[b,d] Risk of delayed toxicity due to accumulation; reduce dose or lengthen dose interval if over-sedation occurs after 4-5 days; may schedule as prn initially
Morphine sulfate, controlled release	30 mg	NA	3	[b] Mg-for-mg conversion from immediate-release form; do not crush or chew tablets
Morphine sulfate, immediate release	30 mg	10 mg	3	[b]

velop. Tolerance to analgesia is not a major clinical problem and can usually be managed by changing the dose or substituting another agent.

Most current definitions of addiction imply a behavioral syndrome of compulsive, harmful use but do not require the existence of physical dependence or tolerance. Aberrant drug-taking is not likely to occur in patients without a history of substance abuse.

Precautions during chronic therapy During chronic opioid therapy, certain precautions should be observed:

- Normeperidine is a toxic metabolite of meperidine that accumulates with repetitive dosing; thus, use of meperidine for chronic pain should be limited. Propoxyphene is also relatively contraindicated due to accumulation of norpropoxyphene.

Drug	Equianalgesic dose to 10 mg of IV morphine		Half-life	
	Oral	Parenteral	(h)	Comments
Oxycodone, controlled release	15 mg	NA	—	b, e
Oxycodone, immediate release	15 mg	NA	2-3	b
Oxymorphone	NA	1 mg	2-3	b

Adapted with permission from American Pain Society: Principles of Analgesic Use in the Treatment of Acute Pain and Cancer Pain, 5th ed. Skokie, Illinois, American Pain Society, 2003.

NA = not available

[a] See package insert for dosing instructions.

[b] Common side effects include constipation, nausea, and sedation. Uncommon side effects include itching, dry mouth, and urinary retention. Rare side effects are hypotension and inappropriate antidiuretic hormone secretion.

[c] Patch duration = 72 hours but may be 48 hours for some patients.

Equianalgesic conversion for fentanyl:

Parenteral morphine dose (mg/24 h)	Transdermal fentanyl (μg/h)
8-22	25
23-37	50
38-52	75
53-67	100
68-82	125
83-97	150

[d] Consult pain expert if converting to/from methadone in high-dose patients.

[e] Available alone and in combination with aspirin or acetaminophen; at higher doses, use as a single agent.

- Placebo use is discouraged, as it does not help distinguish the pathophysiology of pain.
- Physical withdrawal symptoms can be avoided by tapering doses.
- A change in mental status should not be attributed to opioid therapy until medical and neurologic factors have been fully evaluated.
- Mixed agonist-antagonist drugs and partial agonist drugs are not recommended for cancer pain.

Adjuvant medications Neuropathic pain may be less responsive to standard analgesics alone. Adjuvants, such as antidepressants, anticonvulsants, benzodiazepines, local anesthetics, neuroleptics, psychostimulants, antihistamines, corticosteroids, levodopa, calcitonin, and bisphosphonates, are useful for particu-

TABLE 6: Adjuvant drug therapy for cancer pain

Antidepressants
Anticonvulsants
Anxiolytics
Muscle relaxants
Topical local anesthetics
Amphetamines
Phenothiazines
Bisphosphonates
Corticosteroids

lar indications (Table 6). These agents may be administered via oral and other routes. Topical local anesthetic preparations (Table 7) and neurolytic blocks (Table 8) should also be considered.

Surgery for bone metastasis

Surgical intervention is warranted for bone metastases to stabilize a pathologic fracture or preempt an impending fracture. The objectives of surgery are to palliate pain, reduce patient anxiety, improve patient mobility and function, facilitate nursing care, and control local tumor when nonsurgical therapies fail. In general, surgery involves excision of all gross tumor followed by stabilization of the bone, prior to or after fracture, by means of an internal fixation or prosthetic device.

Indications

No strict criteria have been established for surgical treatment. Clinical parameters, such as the patient's general medical condition, performance status, nature of the primary tumor, effectiveness of other therapies, extent of extraskeletal disease, and degree of osseous involvement, as well as the patient's life expectancy, must be considered before surgery.

> There are no clearly defined criteria for the presence of an impending fracture of a long bone. Current guidelines, derived from retrospective clinical studies, include lytic lesions > 2.5 cm in diameter, cortical destruction > 50%, and pain despite local irradiation. In the proximal femur, an avulsion fracture of the lesser trochanter places the hip at high risk for fracture, and operative intervention should be considered.

Fracture and long bone pain In general, the presence of a pathologic fracture, an impending fracture, or a painful lesion in a long bone despite radiotherapy should be considered indications for surgery. A pathologic fracture can result from structural insufficiency and can develop in the absence of viable tumor following treatment with irradiation and/or systemic therapy.

Other considerations Patients deemed to be candidates for surgery should have an expected longevity of > 1 month. All patients

TABLE 7: Anesthetic/neurosurgical approaches for controlling cancer pain

Procedure	Usual indication(s)	Examples
Local anesthetic blocks with or without steroids	Diagnostic blocks Prognostic blocks Acute pain, muscle spasm Premorbid chronic pain Postsurgical syndromes Herpes zoster	Trigger point injection Intercostal block Epidural steroids
Neurolytic/neuroablative blocks and ablative neurosurgery	Localized refractory pain that is expected to persist, usually in the presence of a short life expectancy; pain localized to a region that is associated with a low risk of neurologic complications	Alcohol celiac plexus block Phenol intercostal block Percutaneous cordotomy Midline myelotomy
Spinal analgesics	Refractory pain, usually in the lower body but may be widespread or diffuse	Externalized epidural catheter Intrathecal catheter with fully implanted pump

TABLE 8: Neurolytic procedures[a] that may be considered early in certain pain situations

Procedure	Indication
Celiac plexus neurolysis	Abdominal pain, back pain
Superior hypogastric plexus neurolysis	Pelvic pain
Phenol saddle block	Perineal pain with urinary diversion
Thoracic subarachnoid neurolysis	Focal chest wall pain
Intercostal neurolysis	Focal chest wall pain
Lumbar subarachnoid neurolysis	Unilateral leg pain

[a] The risk-benefit ratio of these procedures in the specified settings is sufficiently favorable and well established to warrant early consideration.

should be medically able to withstand the planned surgical procedure. The surgical goals should be achievable with reasonable certainty, and the potential benefits should outweigh the operative risks. All surgical interventions should be performed with the intent to provide benefit that will outlast the patient's anticipated survival.

Lesion site Major long bones (femur, tibia, and humerus), the vertebrae, and periacetabular regions demand specific attention, as optimal patient function and mobility are predicated on a stable, painless extremity. Osseous destruction sufficient to compromise the mechanical integrity of these bones should be addressed surgically. Lesions in the weight-bearing bones of the lower extremity (femur and tibia) are particularly vulnerable to fracture.

Lesions in the humerus should be treated surgically when the upper extremities serve a weight-bearing function (eg, assisted ambulation using a walker, crutches, or cane). Early surgical intervention, aggressive rehabilitation, and vigilant postoperative surveillance may optimize patient outcome.

Role of radiation therapy

Cancer pain can often be relieved by radiation therapy delivered by localized external-beam irradiation (also known as involved-field irradiation), wide-field external-beam irradiation (eg, hemibody irradiation [HBI]), or systemic treatment with radioactive isotopes (eg, strontium-89 chloride [Metastron], samarium SM 153 lexidronam [Quadramet], phosphorus-32, and iridium-131). Since the most common cause of cancer pain is bone metastasis, this discussion will focus on the use of irradiation in its treatment. Other examples of cancer pain due to primary or metastatic cancer that are amenable to irradiation include headache from CNS involvement, pain due to localized neural involvement (eg, brachial plexus or sciatic nerve), visceral pain (eg, liver or adrenal), pain due to effusions (eg, pericardial or pleural), and pain due to obstruction (eg, urethral, esophageal).

Systemic radiotherapy

Strontium-89 is a systemic radionuclide that has clinical efficacy in the palliation of pain from bone metastases. Reduction of pain due to bone metastases has been observed most frequently in patients with metastases from prostate cancer.

The primary toxicity of strontium-89 is myelosuppression, particularly thrombocytopenia. Therefore, it should not be administered to patients with thrombocytopenia or significant bone marrow suppression. Strontium-89 levels in bone are regulated much like calcium, and strontium-89 has less hematologic toxicity than phosphorus-32.

Samarium-153 is a β-emitting radioisotope that is bound to a phosphonate that preferentially localizes in active bone, specifically in sites of metastatic disease. Mild-to-moderate myelosuppression was noted in the samarium-153 group, yet a potential advantage of samarium-153 over strontium-89 is the decreased incidence and severity of hematologic toxicity noted with samarium-153.

Physical treatments

Cancer patients may benefit from formal rehabilitation evaluation and treatment. Physical modalities, such as massage, ultrasonography, hydrotherapy, transcutaneous electrical nerve stimulation (TENS), electroacupuncture, and trigger-point manipulation, are indicated for musculoskeletal pain. Also, any of these techniques may enhance exercise tolerance in a patient undergoing rehabilitation. Skillful soft-tissue manipulation is probably underutilized. Electrical stimulation may also be applied to the peripheral nerves, spinal cord, and even deep brain structures.

Management of psychological, sociocultural, and spiritual factors

The appropriate treatment of cancer pain must extend beyond the physical complaint. Psychological, sociocultural, and spiritual factors significantly affect the patient's quality of life. Thus, the clinician must always care for the whole person. A multifactorial approach to pain management recognizes the complexity of the human being, especially one with a terminal illness.

Although the physician's initial therapeutic goal is to cure the disease, cancer is often incurable. Caring entails recognizing the whole person as a physical, intellectual, social, emotional, and spiritual being. Empathic caring helps the patient perceive the value in life despite the gravity of the situation.

Psychological factors, such as anxiety and depression, must be thoroughly addressed, as revealed by emerging evidence from the disciplines of psycho-oncology and psychoneuroimmunology. Attitude and state of mind affect the individual's perception of pain and response to it in myriad ways and may affect the duration of survival.

A detailed discussion of pharmacologic and nonpharmacologic approaches to anxiety and depression in cancer patients may be found in chapter 39. In addition, patients may regain a much needed sense of control by using psychological techniques, such as imagery, hypnosis, relaxation, biofeedback, and other cognitive or behavioral methods.

Sociocultural influences affect the patient's experience and expression of pain. This is especially true for the patient whose cancer does not respond to therapy and progresses to end-stage disease.

Pain may be an unwelcome reminder of the presence and progression of cancer. Concomitant fear, anger, frustration, disappointment, and other negative emotions may hold the patient hostage to physical pain.

Existential distress may bridge an undesirable transition from hopeful coping with pain to hopeless suffering from it. As patients are confronted with personal mortality, the limits of their life spans move from an abstract concept to a real issue. Self-image changes, and patients may develop emotional and psychic turmoil, which may compromise their medical condition and treatment.

Achieving relief of psychic suffering may enable the patient to transcend physical pain, enhancing the effects of pain medications and other treatments. Prayer, meditation, counseling, clergy visits, and support groups may all be beneficial. Relieving suffering means allowing the patient and family to realize improved quality of life and even find contentment or peace in the face of failing health and imminent death. Palliative care of the family includes bereavement counseling in anticipation of and after the loss of a loved one.

Ongoing care

The goals of pain management must be frequently reviewed and integrated into the overall management plan. Communication among the professional staff, patient, and family is essential. A sensitive, frank discussion with the patient regarding his or her wishes should guide medical decision-making during all phases of the illness.

SUGGESTED READING

ON CANCER PAIN MANAGEMENT

American Pain Society: Principles of Analgesic Use in the Treatment of Acute Pain and Cancer Pain, 5th ed. Skokie, Illinois, American Pain Society, 2003.

Breitbart W: Suicide, in Holland J, Rowland J (eds): Handbook of Psychooncology. New York, Oxford University Press, 1999.

Chochinov HM, Breitbart W (eds): Ethical and Spiritual Issues: Handbook of Psychiatry in Palliative Medicine, Part VI, pp 337–396. New York, Oxford University Press, 2000.

Doyle D, Hanks G, Cherny NI, et al (eds): Oxford Textbook of Palliative Medicine, 3nd ed. New York, Oxford University Press, 2005.

World Health Organization: Cancer Pain Relief and Palliative Care in Children. Geneva, Switzerland, World Health Organization, 1998.

ON ANESTHETIC AND SURGICAL APPROACHES

Weinstein SM: Management of spinal cord and cauda equina compression, in Berger A, Portenoy RK, Weissman DE (eds): Principles and Practice of Palliative Care and Supportive Oncology. Philadelphia, JB Lippincott, 2002.

ON RADIATION THERAPY IN CANCER PAIN MANAGEMENT

Gaze MN, Kelly CG, Kerr GR, et al: Pain relief and quality of life following radiotherapy for bone metastases: A randomized trial of two fractionation schedules. Radiother Oncol 45:109–116, 1997.

Rose CM, Kagan AR: The final report of the expert panel for the radiation oncology bone metastasis work group of the American College of Radiology. Int J Radiat Oncol Biol Phys 40:1117–1124, 1998.

CHAPTER 38

Management of nausea and vomiting

Steven M. Grunberg, MD, and Marisa Siebel, MD

Although marked progress in controlling chemotherapy-induced emesis has occurred over the past 10 to 20 years, nausea and vomiting remain among the most distressing side effects of cancer chemotherapy. With the increased use of chemotherapy in primary and adjuvant treatment settings, the need for improved control of emesis remains an important consideration in both medical oncology and supportive care.

Over the past few years, several major oncology groups have published consensus reports or guidelines on the prevention of chemotherapy-induced emesis. However, the introduction of several new agents may change these paradigms. In addition, an understanding of the neuropharmacology of this problem is useful in planning patient care.

NAUSEA

Pathophysiology of emesis

Although the mechanism by which cancer chemotherapy induces emesis is still not completely understood, a physiologic basis for our current understanding of this complex problem has now emerged.

Stimulation of neurotransmitter receptors

The emetic reflex arc is activated by stimulation of receptors in the CNS and/or GI tract. These receptor areas relay information to the vomiting center in the medulla, which then coordinates the act of vomiting. The chemoreceptor trigger zone (CTZ), also located in the medulla, serves as a "chemosensor" and is exposed to blood and CSF. These areas are rich in a variety of neurotransmitter receptors.

Dopamine For many years, the dopamine receptors were the main focus of interest in antiemetic research. Available antiemetics, such as phenothiazines (chlorpromazine and prochlorperazine) and substituted benzamides (metoclopramide), were known to affect these receptors, as were butyrophenones (haloperidol and droperidol).

Serotonin The role of the neurotransmitter serotonin (5-hydroxytryptamine [5-HT]) has also been elucidated. The improved antiemetic activity of higher doses of metoclopramide was not explained by its dopamine-binding properties but by the fact that it also affects serotonin receptors. This led to the development of several highly specific compounds that interact solely with serotonin receptors, specifically the type 3, or 5-HT_3, receptor subtype. Four compounds from this family are currently available in the United States. The 5-HT_3 receptor, which is found in both the GI tract and CNS, is an important mediator of the emetic reflex arc. Recent work has suggested that mutation of the 5-HT_{3B} receptor subunit may affect antiemetic efficacy.

Substance P Tachykinins, such as substance P, play an important role in emesis, as well as in pain and a variety of inflammatory conditions. These neurotransmitters are 11–amino acid molecules that bind to specific receptors. Substance P binds to the neurokinin type 1, or NK_1, receptor.

Several NK_1 receptor antagonists have been synthesized and used both preclinically and in clinical trials in patients receiving cancer chemotherapy. Results indicate that these agents are effective against a broad range of causes of emesis, particularly delayed emesis. One member of this family, aprepitant (Emend), has been approved for clinical use.

Emetic problems

Emesis related to chemotherapy

Both nausea and vomiting are seen in patients receiving cancer chemotherapy. Nausea occurs at a slightly higher frequency than vomiting and is more difficult to control. The control of vomiting is strongly correlated with the control of nausea, although some patients experience nausea without vomiting.

The three most common emetic patterns in patients receiving chemotherapy are outlined below.

Acute chemotherapy-induced emesis is defined as nausea or vomiting that occurs within the initial 24 hours of chemotherapy administration. The time of greatest risk is from 1 to 6 hours after chemotherapy with most agents.

Delayed emesis is emesis that begins ≥ 24 hours after chemotherapy. Delayed emesis is particularly likely to occur in patients who have received cisplatin, carboplatin (Paraplatin), or cyclophosphamide. Recent data indicate that this problem may begin somewhat earlier than 24 hours in some patients.

Anticipatory emesis is defined as a conditioned vomiting response following inadequate antiemetic protection with prior courses of chemotherapy.

Emesis unrelated to chemotherapy

Patients receiving anticancer drugs may also develop emesis for other reasons. Emesis can be induced by concomitant medications (such as analgesics, anti-infectives, or bronchodilators) or by tumor-related complications (such as intestinal obstruction or brain metastases). In these instances, adjustment of medication or treatment of tumor-related complications is more important than selecting an antiemetic agent.

Patient characteristics and emesis

History of poor emetic control Poor control of emesis with past courses of chemotherapy predisposes a patient to unsatisfactory antiemetic results with any subsequent treatment, regardless of the emetic stimulus or antiemetic employed. Both delayed and conditioned anticipatory emesis are more likely to occur in these patients, and there is likely to be greater difficulty in controlling acute emesis.

History of alcohol intake Emesis is easier to control in patients with a history of chronic, high alcohol intake (> 100 g/d of alcohol [approximately five alcohol units or drinks]). In a prospective evaluation of 52 patients receiving high-dose cisplatin and an effective combination antiemetic regimen, 93% of those with a history of high alcohol intake had no emesis, as opposed to 61% of those without such a history. This difference in emesis control is independent of the patient's current alcohol intake.

Age Most trials have found that it is easier to control emesis in older patients than in younger ones. Younger patients have a predilection for developing acute dystonic reactions when dopamine-blocking antiemetics are administered (see section on "Antiemetic agents for high-emetic-risk chemotherapy"). Younger patients also have a greater tendency to develop anticipatory emesis than do older patients.

Gender It is more difficult to control emesis in women than in men given the same chemotherapy and antiemetic regimen.

Motion sickness Patients with a history of motion sickness are more likely to develop chemotherapy-induced nausea and vomiting than are those without such a history.

The above predisposing factors appear to be additive. One can identify patients at particularly high risk of emesis, such as younger women without a history of high alcohol intake. Awareness of these factors is helpful in monitoring individual patients and interpreting the results of clinical trials.

Chemotherapeutic agents and emesis

Emetic potential The most accurate predictor of the risk of emesis is the chemotherapeutic agent that a patient is receiving. Several different classifications of commonly used chemotherapy agents have been devised. Table 1 is based on the consensus report of the Multinational Association of Supportive Care in Cancer (MASCC) as updated in June 2004.

The emetic potential of a chemotherapeutic combination is determined by identifying the most emetic agent in the combination. Other agents in a combination may also increase the risk.

In general, agents that have the highest *incidence* of emesis also induce the most *severe* emesis. Differences occur among patients and even between identical treatment courses in the same patient. Both the dose and route of administration of the chemotherapeutic agent can affect the incidence of nausea and vomiting.

TABLE 1: Emetic potential of chemotherapy agents

Level	Frequency of emesis (%)[a]	Agent
High	> 90	Carmustine Cisplatin Cyclophosphamide (≥ 1,500 mg/m^2) Dacarbazine Hexamethylmelamine Mechlorethamine Procarbazine Streptozocin
Moderate	30-90	Carboplatin Cyclophosphamide (< 1,500 mg/m^2) Cytarabine (> 1,000 mg/m^2) Daunorubicin Doxorubicin Epirubicin Idarubicin Ifosfamide Irinotecan Oxaliplatin Temozolomide
Low	10-30	Capecitabine Cytarabine (≤ 100 mg/m^2) Docetaxel Etoposide Fluorouracil Gemcitabine Methotrexate (> 50 mg/m^2) Mitomycin Mitoxantrone Paclitaxel Pemetrexed Topotecan
Minimal	< 10	Bleomycin Busulfan Chlorambucil 2-Chlorodeoxyadenosine Fludarabine Hydroxyurea Melphalan Thioguanine Vinblastine Vincristine Vinorelbine

[a] Proportion of patients experiencing emesis in the absence of effective antiemetic prophylaxis

Time of onset of emesis In patients receiving initial chemotherapy of high emetic risk, nausea or vomiting typically begins between 1-2 hours after chemotherapy. Cyclophosphamide and carboplatin may be associated with a late onset of emesis (ie, 8-18 hours following chemotherapy administration).

Antiemetic agents for high-emetic-risk chemotherapy

Careful antiemetic research has shown that numerous agents are safe and effective. Dosage and administration schedules for some of these agents are given in Table 2. Antiemetic therapy is commonly administered either orally or intravenously.

Among the best studied agents are ondansetron (Zofran), granisetron (Kytril), dolasetron (Anzemet), palonosetron (Aloxi), metoclopramide, haloperidol, dexamethasone, aprepitant (Emend), lorazepam, dronabinol (Marinol), prochlorperazine, and chlorpromazine.

The combination of a single prechemotherapy dose of a 5-HT_3 antagonist and dexamethasone is the most commonly used therapy to prevent emesis in patients receiving chemotherapy of high emetic risk (both cisplatin and noncisplatin) as listed in Table 1. Addition of aprepitant may increase the rate of antiemetic protection.

Serotonin antagonists: Ondansetron, granisetron, dolasetron, and palonosetron

Ondansetron, granisetron, dolasetron, and palonosetron are highly selective 5-HT_3 receptor antagonists. All are effective in controlling emesis induced by a variety of chemotherapeutic agents. Oral and IV routes of administration available for ondansetron, granisetron, and dolasetron are equally effective, as demonstrated in large randomized trials. In addition, single-dose regimens given before chemotherapy are as effective as more cumbersome multiple- or continuous-dose regimens.

All four serotonin receptor antagonists are similar with regard to efficacy and side effects, although palonosetron has a significantly longer half-life. Choice of one agent over another may therefore reflect economic or convenience factors as well as therapeutic index. Doses of these agents are given in Table 2.

Side effects Ondansetron, granisetron, dolasetron, and palonosetron have all demonstrated excellent safety characteristics over a large dosing range. Toxicities have been minor and have included headache, mild transient elevation of hepatic enzyme levels, constipation, and, with some agents, minor prolongation of cardiac conduction intervals.

Dystonic reactions and akathisia (restlessness), which may be treatment-limiting with antiemetic agents known to block dopamine receptors, are not seen with serotonin antagonists, even when given on consecutive days. This finding is of particular importance for younger patients, in that several regimens used to treat malignancies in this age group utilize a schedule of daily chemotherapy.

TABLE 2: Dosage and administration schedules of antiemetic agents for acute emesis for chemotherapy of high emetic risk

	Dosage[a]	
Antiemetic agent	**Oral**	**Intravenous**
Dolasetron	100 mg once	100 mg (1.8 mg/kg) once
Granisetron	1 or 2 mg once	1 mg (0.01 mg/kg) once
Ondansetron	16-24 mg once or 8 mg bid	8 mg (0.15 mg/kg) once
Palonosetron	Not available	0.25 mg once
Dexamethasone	20 mg once	20 mg once over 5 min
Metoclopramide	Not recommended	2-3 mg/kg q2h
Haloperidol	1-2 mg q4-6h	1-3 mg q4-6h
Dronabinol	5 mg/m^2 q4h	Not available
Prochlorperazine	Not recommended	10-20 mg q3-4h
Lorazepam[b]	0.5-2.0 mg	0.5-2.0 mg q4-6h
Aprepitant	125 mg	Not available

[a] All agents are to be administered prior to chemotherapy, usually 30 minutes beforehand, although the serotonin antagonists can be effective if administered as late as immediately before the start of chemotherapy. Recommended dosages have been found to be effective in clinical trials and may vary from those given in package inserts.

[b] Lorazepam is indicated only as an adjunct to antiemetics in this setting.

Efficacy The serotonin antagonists have been reported to achieve complete control of emesis in 30%-50% of patients receiving cisplatin. These agents have also proved to be at least as effective against all other chemotherapeutic agents, with complete control rates of about 70%.

Many trials have examined the benefit of adding corticosteroids to a serotonin antagonist. Typically, the complete control of emesis is improved by 10%-20% in patients receiving highly emetic chemotherapy. Both the American Society of Clinical Oncology (ASCO) and MASCC guidelines recommend that a corticosteroid be added whenever a serotonin antagonist is indicated (ie, in all patients receiving chemotherapy of high emetic risk).

Dexamethasone

The antiemetic mechanism of action of dexamethasone remains unclear. Several randomized trials and a recent meta-analysis have all confirmed its effectiveness in controlling emesis and its safety. Other corticosteroids are also effective; however, dexamethasone is the most widely studied steroid and is available in oral and parenteral dosage forms as an inexpensive generic product. Dexamethasone is an excellent agent for use in combination antiemetic regimens and as a single agent for patients receiving chemotherapy of low emetic risk (< 30% incidence).

Dose Dexamethasone doses have generally ranged from 4 to 20 mg/d. In a randomized trial in patients receiving chemotherapy of high emetic risk, a single 20-mg dose was superior in completely controlling both nausea and vomiting. Thus, the 20-mg dose is recommended in this setting. For patients receiving chemotherapy of moderate emetic risk, a single 8-mg dose may be sufficient.

Side effects Toxicities associated with short courses of dexamethasone used for antiemetic therapy have been mild and generally consist of insomnia and mild epigastric burning. Care using this agent in patients with diabetes is particularly warranted.

Metoclopramide

Metoclopramide has proved to be safe and effective when given in high IV doses. Metoclopramide was thought to function as an antiemetic through blockade of dopamine receptors. However, high concentrations of this agent effectively block 5-HT_3 receptors as well.

Efficacy In patients receiving cisplatin, high-dose metoclopramide is an active antiemetic agent. However, randomized trials comparing metoclopramide with serotonin antagonists in high-risk settings have shown advantages for the latter agents. Metoclopramide is a second-choice agent, after the serotonin antagonists, in these settings.

Side effects Commonly observed side effects with metoclopramide include mild sedation, dystonic reactions, akathisia, anxiety, and depression. Dystonic reactions are age-related and route-related. In a report summarizing the experience of nearly 500 patients receiving metoclopramide, the incidence of trismus or torticollis was only 2% in those older than age 30; in contrast, a 27% occurrence was reported in younger patients. Also, such reactions are more common when metoclopramide is administered by the oral route or is given over several consecutive days.

Acute dystonic reactions are not allergic in nature. In general, dystonic reactions and akathisia can be prevented or easily controlled by administering diphenhydramine, benztropine (Cogentin), or a benzodiazepine. These reactions should not be viewed as a contraindication to further use of dopamine-blocking drugs.

Haloperidol

Haloperidol exerts its antiemetic action through dopaminergic blockade. A formal study comparing haloperidol with metoclopramide in patients receiving cisplatin found both agents to be effective, although metoclopramide afforded better emetic control.

Dose Haloperidol doses of 1-3 mg given IV q4-6h have been used.

Side effects Toxicities of haloperidol include sedation, dystonic reactions, akathisia, and occasional hypotension.

Lorazepam

Although lorazepam and other benzodiazepines are potent anxiolytic agents that can be useful additions to antiemetic therapy, they should not be used as single agents for chemotherapy-induced emesis. Lorazepam has been shown to achieve a high degree of patient acceptance and subjective benefit but only minor objective antiemetic activity. However, the anxiolytic properties of benzodiazepines may be particularly useful in the treatment of anticipatory nausea and vomiting.

Dose Lorazepam is usually given in doses of 0.5-1.5 mg/m^2 IV or 1-2 mg PO. These doses, especially the higher IV administrations, can be associated with marked sedation lasting for several hours.

Dronabinol and other cannabinoids

Many trials have tested the antiemetic effects of dronabinol (delta-9-tetrahydrocannabinol [THC]), a component of marijuana. Dronabinol has modest antiemetic activity, similar to that seen with oral prochlorperazine.

Semisynthetic cannabinoids (such as nabilone) have been tested but appear to have no clear advantage over dronabinol. The modest antiemetic activity and significant toxicity of cannabinoids make them a second choice for the control of chemotherapy-related emesis.

Dose Dronabinol has been tried in many doses and schedules. The most useful doses have ranged from 5 to 10 mg/m^2 PO q3-4h.

Side effects are frequently associated with cannabinoids and are particularly bothersome in older adults. They include dry mouth, sedation, orthostatic hypotension, ataxia, dizziness, euphoria, and dysphoria.

Phenothiazines

Although phenothiazines were the first effective antiemetics, the results of antiemetic trials with this class of agents against highly emetogenic chemotherapy have been poor. Randomized trials have found standard-dose prochlorperazine, given orally or intramuscularly, to be less effective than metoclopramide or dexamethasone and equivalent to or less effective than dronabinol. IV administration is more effective than oral administration but can rarely cause profound hypotension (unlike serotonin antagonists or metoclopramide). Phenothiazines are seldom used as first-line antiemetic agents for highly or moderately emetogenic chemotherapy.

Side effects of phenothiazines include sedation, akathisia, hypotension, and dystonic reactions.

Aprepitant

Aprepitant is the first NK_1 antagonist antiemetic. NK_1 antagonists have demonstrated activity against a wide range of emetogenic stimuli. Although less effective than serotonin antagonists as single agents against acute emesis, NK_1 antagonists have shown superior activity against delayed emesis, suggesting the value of combination therapy.

TABLE 3: Antiemetic regimens for acute emesis by emetic risk

Risk level	Recommended antiemetic regimen[a]
High (cisplatin)	Serotonin antagonist *plus* Dexamethasone (12 mg) *plus* Aprepitant (125 mg)
High/moderate	Serotonin antagonist *plus* Dexamethasone (20 mg)
Low	Single agent, such as corticosteroid or serotonin antagonist
Minimal	No preventive agent is recommended for general use

[a] See Table 2 for doses.

In a multicenter, randomized, double-blind, phase III trial, 866 breast cancer patients being treated with cyclophosphamide with or without doxorubicin or epirubicin (Ellence) were randomized to receive either a regimen of aprepitant (125 mg), ondansetron (8 mg bid), and dexamethasone (12 mg) on day 1 with aprepitant (80 mg qd) on days 2 to 3 or a standard regimen of ondansetron (8 mg bid) on days 1 to 3 and dexamethasone (20 mg) on day 1. Of the 857 evaluable patients, 50.8% in the aprepitant arm, vs 42.5% ($P = .015$) in the standard regimen arm, achieved a complete response. In addition, more patients in the aprepitant arm achieved a complete response during both acute (75.7% vs 69.0%, $P = .034$) and delayed (55.4% vs 49.1%, $P = .064$) phases. Both treatments were generally well tolerated.

Combination antiemetic regimens

Table 3 summarizes recommended antiemetic regimens, according to the emetic potential of the chemotherapy regimen.

Serotonin antagonist plus dexamethasone Combinations of a 5-HT_3 antagonist and dexamethasone form the basis of the most effective regimens for controlling acute chemotherapy-induced emesis. Use of these two agents combined has proved to be more effective than either agent alone. Addition of an NK_1 antagonist (aprepitant) results in increased activity against acute cisplatin-induced emesis.

Treatment of emesis

ACUTE EMESIS

A management strategy to prevent acute chemotherapy-induced emesis is outlined in Table 3. All patients should receive education and reassurance, as well as antiemetics tailored to the chemotherapy regimen. For regimens that commonly cause emesis (> 30%), antiemetic combinations are recommended; for regimens of low risk (10%-30% incidence), a single agent will usually suffice. As stated in Table 3, chemotherapy of minimal risk typically does not require preventive treatment.

The rationale for treating high-risk patients receiving either cisplatin or other chemotherapy with the same serotonin antagonist doses is based on our current understanding of the neuropharmacology of emesis. Once all of the relevant receptors ($5\text{-}HT_3$) are saturated by the antiemetic, dose escalation will not be helpful. However, to achieve maximal benefit, it is necessary to give a dose that achieves this saturation. Thus, the lowest fully effective dose is the proper one for any chemotherapy-associated emetic setting in which a serotonin antagonist is to be given.

DELAYED EMESIS

Delayed emesis is defined as nausea or vomiting beginning or persisting ≥ 24 hours after chemotherapy administration. The pathophysiology of this problem is unclear, but it is particularly common after high-dose cisplatin (≥ 50 mg/m^2), carboplatin (≥ 300 mg/m^2), cyclophosphamide (≥ 600 mg/m^2), or doxorubicin (≥ 50 mg/m^2).

In one natural history study, 89% of patients experienced some delayed emesis from 24 to 120 hours after receiving high-dose cisplatin, with a peak incidence occurring between 48 and 72 hours. With anthracyclines or cyclophosphamide, the rate of delayed emesis without preventive antiemetics is about 30%.

Some observations suggest that delayed emesis may begin earlier. When combination antiemetic regimens for acute emesis "fail," the initial emetic episode is often at 17 to 23 hours following chemotherapy. In some trials, antiemetics to prevent delayed emesis have been initiated at 16 to 17 hours.

Treatment options The combination of oral dexamethasone and metoclopramide has been found to be superior to dexamethasone alone or placebo in a double-blind, randomized trial. The combination of dexamethasone and aprepitant has also demonstrated efficacy. The recommended doses and schedules for the prevention of delayed emesis are given in Table 4.

The majority of trials examining the role of $5\text{-}HT_3$ antagonists as single agents in the control of delayed emesis have been disappointing. The $5\text{-}HT_3$ receptor may be less involved in the pathophysiology of delayed emesis. Regimens combining a serotonin antagonist with dexamethasone can lessen delayed emesis (see Table 4 for dosages) and are comparable to metoclopramide and dexamethasone in activity but are markedly more costly. In moderate-risk settings, dexamethasone alone may be sufficient for many patients.

TABLE 4: Treatment regimens for delayed emesis

Risk level	Duration	Agent	Dose and schedule
High	Days 2-4	Aprepitant	80 mg PO qd x 2
		plus	
		Dexamethasone	8 mg PO qd
		Serotonin antagonist	
		Ondansetron	8 mg PO bid
		Dolasetron	100 mg PO bid
		Granisetron	1 mg PO bid
		Palonosetron[a]	0.25 mg IV day 1 only
		plus	
		Dexamethasone	8 mg PO bid
		Metoclopramide	30-40 mg PO bid
		plus	
		Dexamethasone	8 mg PO bid
Moderate	Days 2-3	Serotonin antagonist or dexamethasone or metoclopramide as single agent or in combination at dose and schedule above	
Low		No preventive regimen is recommended for general use	
Minimal		No preventive regimen is recommended for general use	

[a] Palonosetron has only been studied when given on day 1 with a single dose of dexamethasone (20 mg IV)

Perhaps the greatest single problem in antiemetic prescribing is the omission of dexamethasone in the prevention of acute and especially delayed emesis.

ANTICIPATORY EMESIS

This problem is defined as nausea or vomiting beginning before the administration of chemotherapy in patients with poor emetic control during previous chemotherapy. As this problem is a conditioned response, the hospital environment or other treatment-related associations may trigger the onset of emesis unrelated to chemotherapy. Strong emetic stimuli combined with poor emetic control increase the likelihood that anticipatory emesis will occur.

Treatment approach Behavioral therapy involving systematic desensitization can be helpful in managing anticipatory emesis. Also, benzodiazepines appear to be useful. However, the best approach to anticipatory emesis is prevention, which underscores the need to provide the most effective and appropriate antiemetic regimens with the initial course of emesis-producing chemotherapy.

SUGGESTED READING

Gralla R, Lichinitser M, Van Der Vegt S, et al: Palonosetron improves prevention of chemotherapy-induced nausea and vomiting following moderately emetogenic chemotherapy: Results of a double-blind randomized phase III trial comparing single doses of palonosetron with ondansetron. Ann Oncol 14:1570–1577, 2003.

Italian Group for Antiemetic Research: Dexamethasone, granisetron, or both for the prevention of nausea and vomiting during chemotherapy for cancer. N Engl J Med 332:1–5, 1995.

Koeller JM, Aapro MS, Gralla RJ, et al: Antiemetic guidelines: Creating a more practical treatment approach. Support Care Cancer 10:519–522, 2002.

Kris MG, Gralla RJ, Clark RA, et al: Incidence, course, and severity of delayed nausea and vomiting following the administration of high-dose cisplatin. J Clin Oncol 3:1379–1384, 1985.

Poli-Bigelli S, Rodrigues-Pereira J, Carides AD, et al: Addition of the neurokinin 1 receptor antagonist aprepitant to standard antiemetic therapy improves control of chemotherapy-induced nausea and vomiting: Results from a randomized, double-blind, placebo-controlled trial in Latin America. Cancer 97:3090–3098, 2003.

Tremblay PB, Kaiser R, Sezer O, et al: Variations in the 5-hydroxytryptamine type 3B receptor gene as predictors of the efficacy of antiemetic treatment in cancer patients. J Clin Oncol 21:2147–2155, 2003.

Warr DG, Hesketh PJ, Gralla RJ, et al: Efficacy and tolerability of aprepitant for the prevention of chemotherapy-induced nausea and vomiting in patients with breast cancer after moderately emetogenic chemotherapy. J Clin Oncol 23:2822-2830, 2005.

CHAPTER 39

Depression, anxiety, and delirium

Alan Valentine, MD

Psychiatric disorders are common in the setting of malignant disease, occurring in almost 50% of patients. Many cancer patients cope well with their disease. For those who do not, untreated psychological and neuropsychiatric disorders can seriously compromise quality of life and treatment compliance. Although there is a wide variety of presentations, three behavioral syndromes that are often encountered in clinical practice will be discussed here: depression, anxiety, and delirium.

Depression

"Depression" exists on a continuum ranging from an emotion common in daily life (sadness) to a syndrome of severe physical and psychological symptoms consistent with a defined psychiatric disorder (major depressive disorder).

In cancer patients, identical symptoms may be caused or influenced by physical (eg, tumor site, pain), psychological (eg, stress, premorbid function, maturity), and social (eg, finances, interpersonal relationships) factors. Depression occurs more frequently in the setting of severe illness; several studies of cancer inpatients report a prevalence of 25%–42%.

SIGNS AND SYMPTOMS/DIAGNOSIS

Patients with depressive syndromes experience specific symptoms that vary in intensity and severity.

Psychological symptoms include dysphoria (sadness), anhedonia (pervasive loss of pleasure in activities), feelings of guilt or low self-esteem, and thoughts of death or suicide.

Somatic symptoms include sleep disturbance, change in appetite, loss of libido, fatigue, diminished concentration, and psychomotor agitation or withdrawal.

Focus of diagnostic evaluation Although the diagnosis of major depressive disorder requires that multiple symptoms (including dysphoria or anhedonia) must be present for at least 2 weeks, patients who do not meet these criteria may be in significant distress. The diagnosis of depression in medically ill patients is complicated by the fact that somatic symptoms of depression may also be caused by factors related to disease and treatment. For this reason, when evaluating the depressed cancer patient, special attention should be paid to psychological symptoms, which are less likely to be directly related to treatment.

ETIOLOGY

Psychological causes

Isolated symptoms Isolated depressive symptoms, if temporally related to an identifiable stressor, may be classified as adjustment disorders. In the setting of malignancy, obvious stressors include the initial diagnosis, treatment failure, or disease progression. Patients may also face potential psychosocial stressors, including changes in independence, body image, finances, and family function, as well as issues related to death and dying.

Persistent symptoms Persistent mood symptoms may indicate the presence of an evolving major depressive disorder. Major depressive disorder is common in the general population (point prevalence, ~6%) and is a recurrent disease. Patients with a history of mood disorder are at risk for relapse in the face of a cancer diagnosis.

Disease- and treatment-related causes

Presenting symptom of malignancy Depression may be a presenting symptom of some primary malignancies, including primary pancreatic and gastric carcinomas. Primary and metastatic brain tumors may cause frontal lobe syndromes or personality changes that mimic depression and other psychiatric disorders.

Drugs Many drugs used in general medical practice are associated with psychiatric syndromes. The most common of these drugs are β-blockers, antihypertensives, barbiturates, opioids, and benzodiazepines.

In contrast, few drugs used as primary and supportive therapies for cancer are commonly associated with depression. The exceptions to this rule are corticosteroids, cytokines (especially interferon-alfa [IFN-α; Intron A, Roferon-A] and interleukin-2 [aldesleukin, Proleukin]), and whole-brain radiation therapy. Depressive syndromes may also be seen with certain chemotherapeutic agents, including asparaginase (Elspar) and procarbazine (Matulane). Patients treated with tamoxifen may complain of depression or "chemobrain." The latter term usually refers to cognitive slowing.

MANAGEMENT

Management of depressive syndromes involves accurate diagnosis, use of antidepressant medication, and psychotherapy. Patients should be assessed for somatic and psychological symptoms of depression. The clinician should always ask about suicidal thoughts or intent. Metabolic and thyroid function should be evaluated and medications reviewed.

The diagnosis and treatment of depression in patients with cancer require a high index of suspicion and regular, careful follow-up. Ideally, only patients with clinically significant or progressive symptoms would be offered antidepressant therapy. When the diagnosis of depression is in doubt, it may be best to seek psychiatric consultation or to have a low threshold for initiation of treatment to minimize the risk of missing a reversible disorder.

TABLE 1: Selected antidepressants used in cancer patients

Drug	Starting dose	Maintenance dose	Comments
Selective serotonin reuptake inhibitors			
Sertraline	25-50 mg qAM	50-150 mg/d	Usually well tolerated; possible nausea
Fluoxetine	10-20 mg qAM	20-60 mg/d	Long half-life; possible nausea, sexual dysfunction
Paroxetine	20 mg/d qAM	20-60 mg/d	Possible nausea, sedation
Escitalopram	10 mg/d	10-20 mg/d	Usually well tolerated; possible nausea, sexual dysfunction, fatigue
Tricyclic antidepressants			
Nortriptyline	25-50 mg qhs	50-200 mg/d	Moderate sedation; useful for neuropathic pain
Amitriptyline	25-50 mg qhs	50-200 mg/d	Maximal sedation; anticholinergic effects; useful for neuropathic pain
Desipramine	25-50 mg qAM or hs	50-200 mg/d	Modest sedation; anticholinergic effects; useful for neuropathic pain
Other agents			
Venlafaxine	18.75-37.5 mg	75-225 mg/d	Possible nausea; may be useful for neuropathic pain, hot flashes
Bupropion	50-75 mg	150-450 mg/d	Activating; no reports of sexual dysfunction; risk of seizures in predisposed patients
Methylphenidate	5 mg (2.5 mg qAM, noon)	10-60 mg/d	Activating; rapid effect possible; monitor blood pressure
Mirtazapine	15 mg qhs	15-45 mg qhs	Sedating, variable appetite-stimulant, antiemetic effects
Duloxetine	20-30 mg	60 mg/d	Possible efficacy for neuropathic pain

Antidepressants

Selected antidepressants used in cancer patients are listed in Table 1. No antidepressant has been shown to be more effective than any other in the cancer setting. Often, the choice of an antidepressant is based on side-effect profile. In the general population, antidepressants often take at least 2 weeks or longer to produce initial relief of symptoms. There is some anecdotal evidence that a more rapid effect is seen in cancer patients. As a general rule, antidepressant therapy should continue for 4-6 months after symptoms stabilize.

Selective serotonin reuptake inhibitors (SSRIs), such as fluoxetine (Prozac, Sarafem), sertraline (Zoloft), paroxetine (Paxil), and escitalopram (Lexapro), are often used in patients with cancer because of their benign side-effect profile. In particular, their lack of anticholinergic and α-adrenergic–blocking properties makes them attractive options for patients with a serious medical illness.

Unlike the tricyclic agents (discussed below), the SSRIs are not lethal in overdose, making them a safe choice in the treatment of patients experiencing suicidal ideations.

Side effects Mild nausea and anxiety are common side effects of all SSRIs, which vary in severity from patient to patient. Sexual dysfunction may occur with fluoxetine and paroxetine. Sedation may occur with paroxetine.

Dosage In ambulatory patients with normal metabolic function, SSRIs can be started at the same doses used in general psychiatry (ie, 20 mg/d qAM for fluoxetine, 50 mg/d qAM for sertraline, 20 mg/d qAM for paroxetine). These doses can be increased if there is no response within 2-3 weeks.

Hospitalized or elderly patients, those with compromised renal or hepatic function, and those receiving highly emetogenic treatments should be started at one-half or even one-quarter of these starting doses, which can then be increased if tolerated.

Tricyclic antidepressants (TCAs) These older antidepressants (eg, amitriptyline, nortriptyline, and desipramine) remain effective options for the treatment of depression in cancer patients. The sedative properties of TCAs can be useful in the treatment of insomnia associated with depression. In addition, TCAs are useful adjuncts in the treatment of neuropathic pain.

TCAs have the advantage of established therapeutic blood levels, although the applicability of these levels to cancer patients is uncertain.

Side effects The common side effects of TCAs include sedation, dry mouth, orthostatic hypotension, constipation, and blurred vision. These side effects are related to anticholinergic, α-adrenergic–blocking, and antihistaminic properties of TCAs and are often the reason these drugs are not used as the first line of treatment in depressed medically ill patients. TCAs must be used cautiously in patients with active suicidal ideations and in those with cardiac conduction abnormalities.

Dosage Initial dosing of TCAs should be conservative (25-50 mg PO qhs for nortriptyline, 25-50 mg qhs for amitriptyline, 25-50 mg qAM or hs for desipramine), with escalation of doses if tolerated every 4-7 days. Therapeutic response is sometimes seen at doses lower than those used in the general population, that is, lower than 75-150 mg/d for nortriptyline, 150-300 mg/d for amitriptyline, and 200-300 mg/d for desipramine.

Atypical and newer antidepressants Bupropion (Wellbutrin) is activating, which may be of potential benefit in patients with psychomotor slowing. Another advantage is that it is not associated with sexual dysfunction. However, bupropion has been associated with seizures and therefore should be used with caution (if at all) in patients who suffer from seizures or who have a history of seizures.

Venlafaxine (Effexor), nefazodone (Serzone), and mirtazapine (Remeron) are newer agents with selective effects on serotonin and norepinephrine metabolism. They should be started at low doses to establish whether they can be tolerated. Venlafaxine may be effective against treatment-induced hot flashes. Mirtazapine has sedative, appetite-stimulant, and antiemetic effects, which can be very useful in selected cases.

Duloxetine (Cymbalta) is approved for treatment of diabetic neuropathy and may have applications in the depressed cancer patient with neuropathic pain.

Psychostimulants

Psychostimulants that have direct or indirect dopamine-agonistic properties, such as dextroamphetamine, methylphenidate, and pemoline, have an established role in the treatment of depression in the medically ill. Psychostimulants are activating agents useful in patients with psychomotor retardation, deconditioning, or apathy states associated with depression, as well as in those with CNS disease or treatment side effects.

The antidepressant effects of psychostimulants may be seen more quickly than those of first-line antidepressants. Improvements in mood, physical activity, well-being, and appetite are sometimes observed within 24-48 hours of the initiation of psychostimulant treatment.

Side effects Like other activating agents, psychostimulants may cause insomnia, anxiety, palpitations, and GI upset. Hypertension or hypotension may also occur.

Dosage Initial dosing should be conservative (eg, 5 mg/d in two divided doses every morning and noon for methylphenidate, 5 mg/d qAM for dextroamphetamine). If tolerated, stimulant doses can be increased until a therapeutic effect is achieved or side effects develop.

Psychotherapy

Although antidepressants alone are effective in the treatment of depression, patients often require and benefit from psychotherapy.

In some cases, such therapy can be limited to support while response to medication is monitored. Other patients may require cognitive-behavioral interventions to help them deal with misperceptions about their disease status or to resolve preexisting issues.

For some patients, group therapy can be helpful, although others find it difficult to interact with patients who are equally or more severely ill.

Anxiety

Like depression, the term "anxiety" refers to both a subjective emotion and a constellation of signs and symptoms that can be of physical or psychological origin.

Especially in seriously ill patients, subjective anxiety may be the first sign of a serious or catastrophic physiologic derangement (eg, sepsis or pulmonary embolus). It is also common at disease milestones, especially at initial diagnosis, time of recurrence, and progression to the terminal phase. In patients whose disease is stable or in remission, anxiety frequently occurs before or at the time of routine reevaluation.

SIGNS AND SYMPTOMS/DIAGNOSIS

Psychological symptoms Patients who experience anxiety typically complain of feeling worried, irritable, and frightened. They may appear depressed; there is considerable comorbidity between the two syndromes. Patients are often hyperalert and hypervigilant. The affective state is labile; individuals may cry suddenly or experience paroxysmal temper outbursts. Thought processes are ruminative; individuals cannot distract themselves from worry.

If anxiety proceeds to panic, patients may experience feelings of impending doom or annihilation. Occasionally, distress is so intense that patients experience suicidal thoughts. The hyperaroused state makes sleep difficult and impairs appetite. Physical and psychological fatigue and exhaustion may follow.

Physical symptoms Numerous physical symptoms may be experienced, especially as anxiety becomes more severe.

Cardiovascular signs and symptoms include palpitations and tachycardia, as well as subjective chest tightness or pain.

Respiratory symptoms include dyspnea; patients may hyperventilate and feel light-headed or dizzy.

GI symptoms are common and include difficulty in swallowing, abdominal cramping, nausea, diarrhea, and constipation.

Patients may become diaphoretic. Preexisting pain may be aggravated.

ETIOLOGY

Psychological causes

For many patients, the diagnosis of cancer is extremely stressful. Anxiety is often a function of fear. Patients anticipate the possibility of pain, suffering, or death. Concerns about loss of control and independence, finances, and family obligations also contribute.

Painful or unpleasant diagnostic or therapeutic procedures and medications may lead to anxiety, which can become conditioned. For example, conditioned anxiety states, such as anticipatory nausea, develop in some individuals after such treatments as chemotherapy and confinement for bone marrow transplantation.

Patients who achieve remission often worry about possible recurrence. Associated anxiety may become more pronounced shortly before clinic visits or tests.

Anxiety may also become more pronounced when active treatment ends. In some cases, the process of diagnosis and treatment is so psychologically difficult that a post-traumatic stress disorder develops.

Generalized anxiety disorder and panic disorder are relatively common in the general population. Affected individuals are at risk for exacerbation of the anxiety disorder in the face of a cancer diagnosis. Individuals who have specific phobias (eg, to blood, needles, or hospitals) will likely suffer intense anxiety at diagnosis or during treatment and may require referral to a mental health specialist.

Especially in the elderly, anxiety may mask an underlying mood disorder, usually depression.

Disease- and treatment-related causes

Toxic metabolic states Hypoxia should be the initial metabolic consideration in anxious patients. Possible causes include anemia and pulmonary edema.

Anxiety may be the initial manifestation of pulmonary embolus.

Electrolyte disturbances may cause anxiety, especially if they are severe or occur in the setting of CNS impairment.

Endocrine disturbances (eg, hyperthyroidism, hypercalcemia, and hyperadrenalism) also can cause anxiety. These endocrine disturbances may be preexisting conditions, a function of disease, and/or a side effect of treatment.

Anxiety may be an early sign of sepsis.

Drugs Several medications commonly used in oncology may cause anxiety of variable severity. For example, corticosteroids can produce anxiety that varies from mild nervousness to frank agitation resembling mania.

Antiemetics, including promethazine, prochlorperazine, and metoclopramide, are associated with akathisia, a sense of internal restlessness and anxiety that compels patients to move in order to achieve relief. The anxiety can be quite severe; patients suffering from severe akathisia have attempted suicide. Antipsychotic medications (eg, haloperidol and chlorpromazine) also can cause akathisia.

Anticholinergic medications (eg, benztropine [Cogentin]), opioids, and benzodiazepine anxiolytics can cause paradoxical reactions that include anxiety; this is especially true in geriatric patients and in those with CNS impairment.

Drug toxicity (eg, from immunosuppressants, bronchodilators, psychostimulants) and drug withdrawal states (eg, from opioids, benzodiazepines, and alcohol) often produce anxiety, which may evolve into delirium.

Disease factors The most important of these factors is inadequate pain relief, which may cause or exacerbate anxiety and depression. Hormone-secreting tumors (eg, pheochromocytomas, small-cell lung tumors, and some thyroid carcinomas) also may cause paroxysmal symptoms of anxiety or panic.

MANAGEMENT

The initial approach to anxious patients depends on the severity of anxiety and their medical status. In all cases, the multiple possible medical causes of anxiety should be considered and addressed or corrected. In some cases, it is not possible to remove offending medications (ie, corticosteroids), and symptomatic relief must be provided while these agents continue to be used.

Psychotherapy

Supportive therapy for anxious patients is universally appropriate. Anxious patients benefit from reassurance that they are not alone, that help is available, and that action will be taken to help them deal with the cause of their distress.

Patients suffering from phobic or conditioned anxiety states, as well as those with anxious depression, may benefit from specialized treatment, including cognitive therapy, guided imagery, self-relaxation training, and biofeedback. These techniques, which may require referral to a specialist, provide patients with a sense of control and teach skills that can be applied to minimize future threats.

Anxiolytics

Antidepressants are becoming mainstays of pharmacologic treatment of chronic anxiety disorders, including generalized anxiety disorder, panic disorder, and social phobia. Use of these medications avoids the issues of side effects and tolerance associated with benzodiazepines. The antidepressants are also attractive in this setting because anxiety and depression are frequently comorbid conditions.

Currently, paroxetine and escitalopram have FDA indications for the management of generalized anxiety disorder, as does venlafaxine. Most of the SSRIs have been used successfully in the treatment of panic disorder. Typically, it

TABLE 2: Selected benzodiazepines used to treat anxiety in cancer patients

Drug	Dose range (prn or scheduled)	Comments
Lorazepam	0.5-2.0 mg PO/IM/IVP/IVPB q4-12h	Versatile; favorable metabolic profile useful in the severely ill; can be administered via continuous infusion in rare cases
Alprazolam	0.25-1.0 mg PO q6-24h	Potent, rapid onset and cessation of effects; tolerance may develop quickly; antidepressant effects
Diazepam	2-10 mg PO/IM/IV q6-24h	Useful for general/persistent anxiety but problematic in elderly or seriously ill patients
Clonazepam	0.5-2.0 mg PO q6-24h	Useful for general/persistent anxiety, episodic anxiety, and aggressive behavior in some CNS-impaired patients

IVP = IV push; IVPB = IV piggyback

takes 2 to 4 weeks before the antianxiety effects of these medications are noted. It may be useful or necessary to use a short-acting benzodiazepine as adjunctive therapy until the antidepressant takes effect. Typical dose ranges for these agents follow: paroxetine, 20-60 mg/d; escitalopram, 10-20 mg/d; sertraline, 50-150 mg/d; and extended-release venlafaxine, 75-225 mg/d (see Table 1).

Benzodiazepines are the mainstays of pharmacologic treatment of anxiety. These medications are generally safe and effective. Selected benzodiazepines that are commonly used to treat anxiety in cancer patients are listed in Table 2. Issues related to dependence or oversedation are usually not of major concern.

Benzodiazepines have variable hypnotic, antiemetic, and muscle-relaxant effects useful in other aspects of supportive care of cancer patients. Caution is required when these agents are used in the settings of serious illness (because of the risk of additive sedation with other medications), advanced age, or CNS impairment (because of the risk of disinhibition or delirium).

Short-acting benzodiazepines, such as lorazepam and alprazolam, have a rapid onset but relatively short duration of action, making them useful for treating intermittent paroxysmal anxiety or panic attacks. For the same reason, they are also useful in patients with severe medical illness.

Typical doses are 0.5-1.0 mg PO/IM/IVP/IVPB (lorazepam) every 4 to 12 hours or 0.25-0.5 mg PO (alprazolam) every 6 to 8 hours as needed. For patients with persistent anxiety, these medications can be given on a regular schedule.

In cases of extremely severe anxiety, lorazepam may be administered via continuous infusion. Its lack of active metabolites makes it a good choice in patients with hepatic or renal compromise.

Tolerance develops more rapidly to short-acting benzodiazepines than to their longer-acting counterparts. Therefore, if short-acting agents are used for any length of time, they should be discontinued gradually.

Longer-acting benzodiazepines, such as diazepam and clonazepam, are useful for persistent anxiety. Their longer duration of action is such that they do not "wear off" quickly, leaving patients unprotected. Tolerance does not develop as quickly to these agents, and patients with generalized anxiety disorders may be maintained on them for years.

Clonazepam is typically given at a dose of 0.5-1.0 mg every 6 to 8 hours on a scheduled basis, whereas the diazepam dose typically starts at 2-10 mg every 6 to 24 hours. Higher doses are often required.

These drugs have multiple active metabolites that can adversely affect the elderly and patients with renal or hepatic impairment. In such patients, it is best to "start low and go slow."

Other medications At low doses, antipsychotic medications, such as thioridazine, haloperidol, olanzapine (Zyprexa), quetiapine (Seroquel), and risperidone (Risperdal), may be used as anxiolytics. These agents are most appropriate for patients with a history of, or at high risk for, adverse reactions to benzodiazepines.

Opioid analgesics are effective anxiolytics in some terminally ill patients, especially those patients in whom compromised respiratory function is a cause of anxiety.

Delirium

Delirium (also known as encephalopathy and acute confusional state) is the most common mental disorder of purely organic origin in the cancer setting. This syndrome is characterized by diffuse brain dysfunction, caused by one or more pathologic factors related to the disease or its treatment.

The prevalence of delirium is a function, in part, of the severity of medical illness. In some surveys, 15%-30% of cancer inpatients and up to 85% of those who are terminally ill experience delirium. The overall prevalence of delirium in the inpatient setting is expected to increase with the aging of the general population.

SIGNS AND SYMPTOMS/DIAGNOSIS

The onset of delirium is acute, within hours to days, and is characterized by alterations in arousal, perception, and cognition. There may be a prodromal phase of irritability or anxiety.

Alterations in arousal Delirious patients demonstrate a sensorium (or level of alertness) that varies from hyperalert and vigilant to obtunded or stuporous. Psychomotor activity varies in a similar way; a hyperactive or hypoactive delirium may be encountered.

Alterations in perception/cognition Delirious patients may have perceptual difficulties, with illusions and hallucinations, which they cannot distinguish from reality. Patients may also experience delusions, often of the paranoid type. Typically, patients have lucid intervals (minutes to hours) during which their mental status appears to be appropriate and intact. Cognition is impaired because patients cannot attend to and register new information.

Other signs/symptoms Typically, delirious patients have a disordered sleep/wake cycle, which may be a function of the delirium or a preceding cause. Autonomic dysfunction may be encountered in patients with hyperaroused states.

Left untreated, delirium may resolve spontaneously or evolve into another neuropsychiatric disorder. Failure of delirium to resolve with aggressive management may signal a preterminal event.

ETIOLOGY

Disease- and treatment-related causes

As with anxiety states, delirium can have many possible causes in cancer patients. Often, the etiology is multifactorial, and in up to 50% of cases, a definite etiology cannot be identified.

Direct and indirect disease effects Primary and metastatic brain tumors will occasionally present as delirium, as will leptomeningeal carcinomatosis and paraneoplastic syndromes. Most, but not all, patients with these diseases also have frank neurologic signs.

Toxic metabolic abnormalities Hypoxia, which often causes anxiety, may also produce delirium, especially as a function of a rapidly evolving insult.

Severe electrolyte disturbances, especially sodium and potassium, may cause delirium, as may altered serum calcium and magnesium levels.

Other common toxic metabolic causes of delirium include liver and renal failure, systemic or CNS infection, and severe nutritional deficiencies.

Cancer therapies Corticosteroids, which are ubiquitous in cancer treatment, produce a wide variety of psychiatric side effects, including an agitated psychotic state that resembles delirium.

Irradiation of the brain occasionally causes delirium, which typically begins during or immediately after the completion of treatment. This side effect is thought to be due to edema and raised intracranial pressure. It is usually controlled or prevented by corticosteroid therapy.

Chemotherapeutic and biotherapeutic agents Many chemotherapeutic and biotherapeutic agents have been associated with delirium or encephalopathic states, although some are more often responsible than others. They include ifosfamide (Ifex), methotrexate, and cytarabine (cerebellar syndrome). Interleukin-2, alone or in combination with IFN-α, may cause agitated delirium. Toxic levels of immunosuppressants (eg, tacrolimus [Prograf]) and antiviral agents also have been associated with encephalopathies.

Other drugs Benzodiazepines, opioid analgesics, and anticholinergic medications (eg, benztropine) can induce delirium in certain situations. Usually, this problem occurs when high doses of these agents are used in seriously ill patients. However, the elderly and patients with CNS compromise are vulnerable to this adverse effect when given low doses, especially at night.

Severe alcohol withdrawal is a common cause of hyperactive delirium.

MANAGEMENT

Evaluation

Initial management of delirium involves a search for a reversible cause. In all cases, physical and neurologic examinations are indicated. An exhaustive

TABLE 3: Selected medications used to treat delirium in cancer patients

Drug	Dose range	Comments
Antipsychotics		
Haloperidol	0.5-2.0 mg PO/IM/IVPB/SC q4-12h	IV route twice as potent as PO route and has fewer side effects; 2.0–5.0-mg bolus/continuous infusion for severe agitation
Chlorpromazine	25-100 mg PO/IM/IVP/IVPB q4-12h	Very sedating; may be administered as continuous infusion; monitor blood pressure
Risperidone	0.5-3.0 mg PO q12-24h	Useful in elderly patients; may pose lower risk of parkinsonian effects; not useful for severe agitation
Olanzapine	2.5-5.0 mg PO q8-12h	Zydis formulation is an orally disintegrating tablet that is easily swallowed
Quetiapine	25-250 mg PO/d	Fairly sedating, especially attractive for sleep-deprived patients
Benzodiazepine		
Lorazepam	0.5-4.0 mg PO/IM/IVP/IVPB q4-12h	Most effective when used with an antipsychotic; when used alone can exacerbate delirium; may be administered as a continuous infusion
Anesthetic		
Propofol	10-50 mg IV qh	Rapid onset, short duration of action; not an antipsychotic; dose can be titrated to desired level of sedation

IVP = IV push; IVPB = IV piggyback

work-up for all possible causes is usually not necessary. The patient's clinical situation and known history should provide guidance. Attention should be paid to the patient's metabolic and respiratory status. Evaluation of hepatic and renal function should be completed.

The role of prescribed and illicit medications, chemotherapeutic agents, and biotherapeutic agents should be considered.

Diagnostic tests Diagnostic imaging of the brain (eg, CT, MRI) may be indicated. In some cases, electroencephalography may help establish the presence of an encephalopathic state. Assessment of CSF is appropriate for patients with suspected CNS infection or leptomeningeal carcinomatosis.

Behavioral management

The patient's safety must be secured. Depending on individual circumstances, this may require close observation, use of physical restraints, or neuroleptic medications. Unless there is a medical contraindication, restraints should not be used without medications to assist in calming the patient.

Ideally, patients should be managed in a setting of moderate environmental stimulation. Both sensory overstimulation and deprivation are disadvantageous. Because delirious patients are often anxious or frightened, the presence of family members can provide reassurance.

Antipsychotics

If more conservative measures are ineffective, pharmacotherapy is required to treat delirium. Antipsychotic medications treat sensory and cognitive misperceptions as well as provide anxiolysis and some degree of sedation. Table 3 lists selected drugs often used to treat delirium in cancer patients.

Haloperidol is a potent antipsychotic that may be administered by PO, IM, IV, or SC routes (with the SC route often used for terminal delirium). The IV formulation is twice as potent as the PO preparation.

Side effects Haloperidol is usually well tolerated, although it does carry a risk of producing akathisia and parkinsonian side effects. These side effects can be treated with benztropine, benzodiazepines, or other medications. The risk of these adverse reactions can be minimized by IV administration.

Dosage Elderly patients or patients with end-stage disease usually require very modest doses (0.5-1.0 mg PO or IV at night or twice daily) to control delirium. Especially in hyperactive delirium, higher and more frequent dosing is usually required (eg, 2-5 mg PO/IVPB every 6 hours). Total doses of ≥ 100 mg/d may be administered via continuous infusion in unusual cases.

Chlorpromazine is a potent antipsychotic that is more sedating than haloperidol and may be administered by the same routes. Typically, chlorpromazine is given at a dose of 25-50 mg PO/IVPB every 6 to 12 hours. Rapid calming of an agitated patient may require IM or IV doses of 50-100 mg. Chlorpromazine can be given by IV infusion if necessary.

Chlorpromazine has significant anticholinergic and α-adrenergic–blocking effects, which can be problematic if used in seriously ill patients or elderly patients vulnerable to hypotensive episodes.

Risperidone is given orally. At doses of 0.5-3.0 mg once or twice daily, it is useful in treating low-intensity delirium or delusional symptoms, especially in elderly patients, in whom it may have fewer adverse effects than oral haloperidol. Risperidone is not useful for treating acute agitation.

Olanzapine has been shown to be effective in the management of delirious cancer patients. Though it is not available for parenteral administration, the Zydis formulation of olanzapine is an orally disintegrating tablet that easily dissolves in the mouth and may be useful for some agitated patients and those with swallowing difficulties.

Quetiapine is fairly sedating and is an attractive option for treatment of low-intensity delirium, especially when given at night to control behavior and promote sleep.

Other agents

Benzodiazepines are used as adjuncts in the control of hyperactive delirium. They are the treatment of choice for alcohol withdrawal delirium. Lorazepam, 0.5-4.0 mg IV or IM, may be given with haloperidol to rapidly control acute agitation. It is sometimes effective to alternate doses of lorazepam and haloperidol every 30 minutes until the patient falls asleep.

Benzodiazepines do not have antipsychotic properties and, if used by themselves, will exacerbate disinhibition and cognitive impairment of a delirious patient, unless a sufficiently large dose is given to cause sleep.

Propofol is a short-acting anesthetic that is effective in achieving rapid sedation. It is often administered as a continuous IV infusion in the ICU setting. Propofol does not have antipsychotic properties.

SUGGESTED READING

ON DEPRESSION

Jacobsen PB, Donovan KA, Weitzner MA: Distinguishing fatigue and depression in patients with cancer. Semin Clin Neuropsychiatry 8:229–240, 2003.

Spiegel D, Giese-Davis J: Depression and cancer: Mechanisms and disease progression. Biol Psychiatry 54:269–282, 2003.

Trask PC: Assessment of depression in cancer patients. J Natl Cancer Inst 32:80–92, 2004.

ON ANXIETY

Stark D, Kiely M, Smith A, et al: Anxiety disorders in cancer patients: Their nature, associations, and relation to quality of life. J Clin Oncol 20:3137–3148, 2002.

ON DELIRIUM

Centeno C, Sanz A, Bruera E: Delirium in advanced cancer patients. Palliat Med 18:184–194, 2004.

Fann JR, Sullivan AK: Delirium in the course of cancer treatment. Semin Clin Neuropsychiatry 8:217–228, 2003.

Gaudreau J-D, Gagnon P, Harel F, et al: Psychoactive medications and risk of delirium in hospitalized cancer patients. J Clin Oncol 23:6712–6718, 2005.

ON PSYCHOTROPIC DRUGS

Buclin T, Mazzocato C, Berney A, et al: Psychopharmacology in supportive care of cancer: A review for the clinician, IV. Other psychotropic agents. Support Care Cancer 9:213–222, 2001.

Fisch MJ, Kim HF: Use of atypical antipsychotic agents for symptom control in patients with advanced cancer. J Support Oncol 2:447–452, 2004.

Joshi N, Breitbart WS: Psychopharmacologic management during cancer treatment. Semin Clin Neuropsychiatry 8:241–252, 2003.

CHAPTER 40

Hematopoietic growth factors

Sally Yowell Barbour, PHARMD, and Jeffrey Crawford, MD

For years, chemotherapy-associated myelosuppression has represented a major limitation to a patient's tolerance of anticancer therapy. In addition, the clinical consequences of chemotherapy-induced myelosuppression (such as febrile neutropenia, dose reductions, or lengthy dose delays) may have had significant negative effects on quality of life or even response to treatment.

Before the widespread availability of agents to stimulate host hematopoiesis, administration of antibiotics, transfusion of blood products, and reductions or delays in chemotherapy dose have been the major means of combating the myelotoxicity of chemotherapy. It is now possible to stimulate clinically relevant production of several formed elements of the blood: neutrophils, erythrocytes, and platelets.

This chapter summarizes data supporting the clinical activity of several hematopoietic growth factors. A thorough knowledge of these data will help clinicians to make judicious, informed decisions about how to use these agents most responsibly.

Hematopoietic growth factors

Over the past several years, a great deal of progress has been made in understanding the process of hematopoiesis by which mature cellular elements of blood are formed. Hematopoietic growth factors are a family of regulatory molecules that play important roles in the growth, survival, and differentiation of blood progenitor cells, as well as in the functional activation of mature cells.

Table 1 lists the recombinant human hematopoietic growth factors (also known as hematopoietic cytokines) that have been approved by the US Food and Drug Administration (FDA) for clinical use: granulocyte colony-stimulating factor (G-CSF, filgrastim [Neupogen]); pegfilgrastim [Neulasta]; yeast-derived granulocyte-macrophage colony-stimulating factor (GM-CSF, sargramostim [Leukine, Prokine]); recombinant human erythropoietin (epoetin alfa, EPO [Epogen, Procrit]); darbepoetin alfa (Aranesp); and interleukin-11 (IL-11, oprelvekin [Neumega]). In addition, several other hematopoietic cytokines are under clinical development.

The commercial availability of these recombinant human hematopoietic growth factors has led to their wide clinical application in oncology practice. However,

TABLE 1: FDA-approved indications for hematopoietic growth factors/cytokines

Growth factor/ cytokine	Generic name	Trade name(s)	Distributor(s)/ manufacturer(s)	Indication(s)
G-CSF	Filgrastim Pegfilgrastim	Neupogen Neulasta	Amgen Amgen	Cancer patients receiving myelosuppressive chemotherapy Patients with nonmyeloid malignancy following BMT For mobilization of PBPCs Patients with severe chronic neutropenia Following induction chemotherapy in AML
GM-CSF	Sargramostim	Leukine Prokine	Immunex	Following autologous BMT BMT engraftment delay or failure Following induction chemotherapy in older patients with AML Allogeneic BMT For mobilization of PBPCs and for use after PBPC transplantation
EPO[a]	Epoetin alfa	Epogen Procrit	Amgen Ortho Biotech	Anemia in chronic renal failure patients (predialysis or dialysis) Anemia in zidovudine-treated HIV-infected patients Anemia in patients with nonmyeloid malignancy receiving chemotherapy Anemia in patients scheduled for elective, noncardiac, nonvascular surgery
	Darbepoetin alfa	Aranesp	Amgen	Anemia in chronic renal failure patients Anemia in patients with nonmyeloid malignancy receiving chemotherapy
IL-11	Oprelvekin	Neumega	Genetics Institute	Following myelosuppressive chemotherapy in patients with nonmyeloid malignancy who are at high risk for severe thrombocytopenia

[a] FDA alert issued March 9, 2007, to provide new safety information about erythropoiesis-stimulating agents. See box on opposite page.

AML = acute myelogenous leukemia; BMT = bone marrow transplantation; PBPC = peripheral blood progenitor cell

GROWTH FACTORS

the substantial costs of colony-stimulating factor utilization as supportive care for patients receiving myelosuppressive chemotherapy make it imperative to identify the optimal settings in which their use can make a significant difference in patient outcomes.

FDA issued an alert on March 9, 2007, to provide new safety information for erythropoiesis-stimulating agents (ESAs) [Aranesp (darbepoetin alfa), Epogen (epoetin alfa), and Procrit (epoetin alfa)]. FDA and Amgen, the manufacturer of Aranesp, Epogen, and Procrit have changed the full prescribing information for these drugs. Changes are summarized below; for the complete announcement, go to: http://www.fda.gov/cder/drug/ and search "ESA".

Avoid serious cardiovascular and arterial and venous thromboembolic events by using the lowest dose of [Aranesp/Epogen/Procrit] that will gradually raise the hemoglobin concentration to the lowest level sufficient to avoid the need for blood transfusion; [Aranesp/Epogen/Procrit] and other ESAs increased the risk for death and for serious cardiovascular events when dosed to achieve a target hemoglobin level of greater than 12 g/dL.

Use of ESAs to achieve a target hemoglobin of 12 g/dL or greater in cancer patients:

- Shortened the time to tumor progression in patients with advanced head and neck cancer receiving radiation therapy;
- Shortened overall survival and increased deaths attributed to disease progression in patients with metastatic breast cancer receiving chemotherapy;
- Increased the risk of death in patients with active malignant disease not under treatment with chemotherapy or radiation therapy. ESAs are not indicated for this patient population.

This chapter discusses the appropriate uses of only the FDA-approved hematopoietic growth factors/cytokines: G-CSF, GM-CSF, EPO, darbepoetin alfa, and IL-11. For a more detailed review of recommendations for the use of myeloid CSFs, readers are referred to the evidence-based, clinical practice guidelines developed in 1994 (last updated in 2006) by the American Society of Clinical Oncology (ASCO). The ASCO guidelines were formulated to encourage reasonable use of CSFs when their efficacy has been well documented but to discourage excess use when marginal benefit is anticipated. These clinical practice guidelines have been published and are most easily accessed at the official web site of ASCO (www.asco.org). In addition, the National Comprehensive Cancer Network (NCCN) (www.nccn.org) has published for the first time guidelines on the use of colony-stimulating factors.

Myeloid growth factors

Three myeloid growth factors are currently licensed for clinical use in the United States: G-CSF, pegfilgrastim, and GM-CSF.

G-CSF (filgrastim) is lineage-specific for the production of functionally active neutrophils. G-CSF has been extensively evaluated in several clinical scenarios. G-CSF was first approved in 1991 for clinical use to reduce the incidence of febrile neutropenia in cancer patients receiving myelosuppressive chemotherapy.

This broad initial indication has since been expanded even further, to include many other areas of oncologic practice, such as stimulation of neutrophil recovery following high-dose chemotherapy with stem-cell support. In addition, G-CSF is indicated to increase neutrophil production in endogenous myeloid disorders, such as congenital neutropenic states.

Pegylated G-CSF (pegfilgrastim) When polyethylene glycol was attached to the protein backbone of filgrastim, a new molecule (pegfilgrastim) with a longer half-life than the standard human G-CSF was created. Pegfilgrastim was approved in 2002 to reduce febrile neutropenia. It has been studied and shown to be equally efficacious to filgrastim, with the advantage of once-per-cycle dosing and self-regulating features of clearance of the drug during neutrophil recovery. Findings have suggested that pegfilgrastim is more effective than G-CSF in preventing febrile neutropenia, but further study is required. The use of pegfilgrastim in cycles < 3 weeks has not been approved; however, it has been studied in 2-week regimens and appears to be safe and effective. In addition, pegfilgrastim is not currently approved in bone marrow transplantation (BMT) or in pediatrics, but studies are under way.

GM-CSF (sargramostim), primarily a myeloid-lineage–specific growth factor, stimulates the production of neutrophils, monocytes, and eosinophils. It has been extensively evaluated and received a more narrow FDA approval in 1991 for clinical use in patients with nonmyeloid malignancies undergoing autologous BMT. Since that initial indication, GM-CSF has also been approved for an expanded range of conditions, such as mitigation of myelotoxicity in patients with leukemia who are undergoing induction chemotherapy.

To date, no large-scale randomized trials have directly compared the efficacy of these two CSFs in the same clinical setting. Future comparative trials may help to determine the optimal clinical utility of these CSFs in different clinical situations.

INDICATIONS

Uses to support chemotherapy

CSFs have been used to support both conventional and intensified doses of chemotherapy. The use of CSFs in this setting can be defined as prophylactic or therapeutic.

Prophylactic use is defined as the administration of a growth factor to prevent febrile neutropenia. "Primary prophylaxis" denotes the use of CSF following the first cycle of multicourse chemotherapy *prior to* any occurrence of febrile neutropenia. The term "secondary prophylaxis" is reserved for the use of CSFs to prevent a subsequent episode of febrile neutropenia in a patient who has already experienced infectious complications in a previous chemotherapy cycle.

Primary prophylaxis G-CSF has been evaluated in at least three major randomized clinical trials in cancer patients receiving chemotherapy. The use of G-CSF as primary prophylaxis reduced the incidence of febrile neutropenia by approximately 50% in these trials, in which the incidence of febrile neutropenia in the control group was high (≥ 40%). More recently studies have evaluated the value of CSFs in patients receiving less myelosuppressive regimens.

Several studies presented at the 2004 meetings of ASCO and the Multinational Association of Supportive Care in Cancer (MASCC) provide evidence to support the use of CSFs in less myelosuppressive regimens. At the ASCO meeting, Timmer-Bonte and colleagues reported the results of a prospective, randomized study evaluating the impact of filgrastim in patients with small-cell lung cancer receiving CAE (cyclophosphamide, Adriamycin [doxorubicin], and etoposide) chemotherapy and prophylactic antibiotics. The incidence of febrile neutropenia in the first cycle and overall was 23% and 30%, respectively, for those receiving antibiotics and 10% and 18%, respectively, for those receiving filgrastim.

Originally presented at the 2004 MASCC meeting, a study by Schwartzberg and colleagues evaluated a single dose of pegfilgrastim vs placebo 24 hours after chemotherapy in 950 patients with breast cancer receiving docetaxel (100 mg/m^2). This regimen was specifically chosen to try to assess the potential benefit of growth factor in a setting associated with approximately a 20% risk of febrile neutropenia. The placebo group experienced a 17% incidence of febrile neutropenia, compared with a 1% incidence in the pegfilgrastim group. The results from these three studies suggest a benefit to pegfilgrastim at least as great or greater than that seen in the previous clinical trials that evaluated filgrastim in treatment settings where the risk of febrile neutropenia was higher. The results of this study were pivotal in the new labeling of pegfilgrastim and recommendations for prophylactic use with regimens associated with a 17% risk of febrile neutropenia. Furthermore, pharmacoeconomic sensitivity analyses have suggested that CSF use may be cost-effective if the anticipated risk of febrile neutropenia is > 20%.

The 2006 update of the ASCO guidelines has established the threshold for use of prophylactic growth factor at 20%. In addition, the recently published NCCN guidelines have recommended CSFs be used in regimens with a 20% risk of neutropenic fever (Table 2). In addition, certain patient risk factors for neutropenia have been identified and should be considered in conjunction with the regimen (Table 3).

Secondary prophylaxis Available data indicate that the use of CSFs as secondary prophylaxis in patients who have had a prior episode of febrile neutropenia can decrease the likelihood of febrile neutropenia in subsequent cycles of chemotherapy. It is important to recognize that this conclusion has never been specifically proven in any randomized clinical trial. Rather, it has been derived from analyses of subsets of patients who crossed over from the placebo arms of the initial randomized clinical trials, as well as large clinical experience.

Thus, in clinical settings where maintenance of chemotherapy dose appears to be important, secondary prophylaxis with CSF to prevent new episodes of neutropenic fever is appropriate. CSF support can also be considered to maintain standard dose delivery of chemotherapy when the maintenance of dose may impact outcome.

TABLE 2: Chemotherapy regimens with 20% risk of neutropenic fever

Bladder	TC, MVAC
Breast	AC → T, AT, TAC
NHL	VAPEC-B
Ovarian	Topotecan, paclitaxel, docetaxel
Sarcoma	MAID
SCLC	CAE, topotecan
Testicular	VIP

AC → T = Adriamycin (doxorubicin]) cyclophosphamide, Taxotere (docetaxel); AT = Adriamycin (doxorubicin), Taxol (paclitaxel); CAE = cyclophosphamide, Adriamycin (doxorubicin), etoposide; NHL = non-Hodgkin lymphoma; MAID = mesna, Adriamycin (doxorubicin), ifosfamide, dacarbazine; MVAC = methotrexate, vinblastine, Adriamycin (doxorubicin) cisplatin; SCLC = small-cell lung cancer; TAC = Taxotere (docetaxel), Adriamycin (doxorubicin), cyclophosphamide; TC = Taxol (paclitaxel), cisplatin; VAPEC-B = vincristine, Adriamycin (doxorubicin), prednisolone, etoposide, cyclophosphamide, bleomycin; VIP = vinblastine, ifosfamide, Platinol (cisplatin)
Adapted from NCCN Myeloid Growth Factors in Cancer Treatment, v2.2005. (www.nccn.com)

Therapeutic use is defined as the administration of a growth factor at the time when neutropenia or neutropenic fever is documented in a patient who had not been receiving CSFs previously.

Clinical trials do not support the routine use of CSFs as an adjunct to antibiotics in the treatment of all patients with uncomplicated febrile neutropenia. However, in certain high-risk patients who have features predictive of poor outcome (eg, sepsis syndrome, pneumonia, fungal infection), use of a CSF with antibiotics may be justified. To conduct appropriate clinical trials to test the hypothesis that CSF support may improve the outcomes of subsets of patients, selection of patients based on risk-stratification criteria that have been validated to predict poor outcomes or delayed recovery from neutropenia will be critical. Certain trials performed with more selective entry criteria (such as absolute neutrophil count (ANC) < 100 cells/μL) have, in fact, shown statistically significant benefits from the use of CSFs as an adjunct to antibiotics in these high-risk patients with febrile neutropenia. Continued analyses of these data and the performance of larger scale, confirmatory studies are needed to further assess the therapeutic use of CSFs.

There are no indications for CSF use to treat uncomplicated neutropenia without fever. A large-scale randomized clinical trial noted no difference in patients who had CSF support in whom afebrile neutropenia was detected vs those patients whose hematologic status was allowed to recover spontaneously without CSF support. Thus, low neutrophil counts alone do not represent a reason to prescribe CSF support. One effective way to use CSFs is prophylactically, 24 hours after chemotherapy is completed.

TABLE 3: Selected risk factors for neutropenia

Treatment related	
	History of severe neutropenia with similar chemotherapy
	Planned relative dose intensity > 80%
	Preexisting neutropenia (absolute neutrophil count < 1,000 cells/mL)
	Extensive prior chemotherapy
Patient related	
	Poor performance status (Eastern Cooperative Oncology Report [ECOG] > 2)
	Poor nutritional status (eg, low albumin)
	Age > 65 years
	Female gender
	Decreased immune function
Cancer related	
	Bone marrow involvement with tumor
	Elevated lactic dehydrogenase level (lymphoma)
Conditions associated with increased risk of serious infection	
	Open wounds
	Active tissue infection
Comorbidities	
	Chronic obstructive pulmonary disease
	Cardiovascular disease
	Diabetes mellitus
	Low basebline hemoglobin level
	Liver disease (elevated levels of bilirubin, alkaline phosphatase)

Adapted from NCCN Myeloid Growth Factors in Cancer Treatment, v2.2005. (www.nccn.com)

Use to increase dose intensity of chemotherapy

The available evidence indicates that CSF use can permit chemotherapy dose maintenance or allow modest increases in dose intensity in clinical scenarios where the main toxicity is neutropenia. Recently, delivery of dose-dense chemotherapy every 2 weeks with G-CSF support has improved survival compared with standard every-3-week dosing in women with breast cancer receiving adjuvant cyclophosphamide and doxorubicin, followed by paclitaxel. This promising dose-dense approach warrants study in other settings. Outside this setting of dose-dense adjuvant chemotherapy, the study of dose density/intensity should be limited to clinical trials.

Meanwhile, in patients with potentially curable disease for which chemotherapy dose delivery may be critical, the use of CSF support to maintain dose intensity may be appropriate. In settings where dose is not a critical determinant of outcomes, modification of chemotherapy dose and implementation of reasonable supportive care measures remain sound alternatives.

Use following stem-cell transplantation

Autologous stem-cell and/or BMT High-dose chemotherapy with autologous hematopoietic stem-cell support has been used in the treatment of several malignancies, based on the notion that dose intensity may be an important determinant of response in chemosensitive malignancies. The prolonged period of myelosuppression following such cell-supported high-dose therapy, with its attendant increased risk of infectious and bleeding complications, has been deemed justifiable in such diseases as Hodgkin's lymphoma, other lymphomas, multiple myeloma, high-risk or relapsed germ-cell cancers, and sarcomas, for which other, less toxic therapeutic options yield suboptimal outcomes.

Several randomized trials have documented that CSFs can effectively reduce the duration of neutropenia, infectious complications, and hospitalization in patients who are receiving high-dose cytotoxic treatment with autologous BMT. GM-CSF was the first hematopoietic growth factor evaluated and approved for clinical use in this setting. G-CSF has subsequently been approved for this indication as well. Pegfilgrastim is under study.

Allogeneic BMT Similar beneficial effects of CSFs have been seen following allogeneic BMT, and the routine use of hematopoietic growth factors is appropriate in this setting. There has been no evidence of any increase in graft-vs-host disease, graft rejection, or relapse with the use of CSFs.

Delayed or inadequate neutrophil engraftment CSFs can also be useful in patients who have delayed or inadequate neutrophil engraftment following progenitor cell transplantation.

Mobilization of peripheral blood progenitor cells

CSFs have been used successfully to enhance mobilization of peripheral blood progenitor cells (PBPCs) into the peripheral blood. Available data suggest that mobilization of PBPCs may decrease the costs of harvesting cells and post-transplantation supportive care. Reinfusion of mobilized PBPCs following high-dose chemotherapy results in more rapid hematopoietic recovery than does autologous BMT. CSFs have also been utilized to mobilize donor PBPCs for allogeneic transplantation.

Administration of CSFs can enhance hematopoietic recovery following PBPC transplantation.

Use in myeloid malignancies

Acute myelogenous leukemia Since myeloid leukemia cells express receptors for CSFs, there has been a concern that leukemia cells might be stimulated after chemotherapy. However, given the high incidence of infectious complications following induction therapy for acute myelogenous leukemia (AML), especially in older patients, studies have evaluated CSFs in this setting. Data from several such studies demonstrate that CSFs, when given after the completion of induction chemotherapy, can shorten the duration of neutropenia and may reduce infectious complications. There does not appear to be any detrimental effect, on either response rate or regrowth of leukemia, by CSF administration following induction therapy.

GM-CSF has been approved for use in patients with AML (≥ 55 years old) following induction therapy to shorten the time to neutrophil recovery and to reduce severe, life-threatening infections. Clinical data on the use of CSFs in younger patients (< 55 years old) are currently limited. G-CSF has also proved to be effective in mitigating the myelotoxicity of leukemia therapy without increasing the risk of leukemic relapse or impairing response rates.

Myelodysplastic syndrome Patients with myelodysplastic syndrome (MDS) are prone to infections related to neutropenia and functional abnormalities of mature neutrophils. Although no data supporting the safety of long-term CSF use are available, short-term use of CSFs may be appropriate in severely neutropenic patients who experience recurrent infections. CSFs have not been shown to have a significant impact on clinical outcomes in patients with MDS or other marrow dysfunction states overall, perhaps reflecting abnormalities in the underlying stem-cell pool, which is unable to respond optimally to pharmacologic doses of CSFs.

Severe chronic neutropenia (ie, an ANC < 500 cells/µL) resulting from congenital, cyclic, or idiopathic neutropenia is often associated with recurrent infections. G-CSF is effective in normalizing neutrophil levels and significantly reducing the incidence of infections in > 90% of patients with these conditions.

TOXICITY

G-CSF (filgrastim and pegfilgrastim)

G-CSF has been a remarkably well-tolerated growth factor overall, based on extensive clinical experience with this cytokine over the past decade.

Bone pain The predominant side effect observed with the use of filgrastim and pegfilgrastim is mild to moderate bone pain, which typically occurs in the lower back, pelvis, or sternum in about one-third of patients. Bone pain is usually seen at the initiation of G-CSF therapy or at the very beginning of neutrophil recovery. In randomized studies, no difference in the incidence, severity, or duration of bone pain was noted between filgrastim and pegfilgrastim.

Uncommon side effects Other uncommon side effects include exacerbation of preexisting psoriasis, Sweet's syndrome (neutrophilic dermatitis), and cutaneous vasculitis. Chronic administration of G-CSF to patients with congenital or idiopathic neutropenia has been associated with splenomegaly.

Laboratory abnormalities observed with the rise in WBC count that occurs during G-CSF administration include elevations in serum lactic dehydrogenase (LDH) levels, uric acid, and alkaline phosphatase levels. Finally, a modest decrease in platelet count without significant clinical sequelae has been reported occasionally with G-CSF use. Antibody formation to either preparation with resultant neutropenia has not been seen in large clinical trials.

GM-CSF

Yeast-derived GM-CSF is generally well tolerated at recommended doses. In the transplant setting, no excessive toxicity is seen in patients treated with this form of GM-CSF, as compared with controls.

Constitutional symptoms In phase I-II trials in other settings, the most commonly reported side effects of GM-CSF have included constitutional symptoms, such as fever, bone pain, myalgia, headaches, and chills. These side effects have been dose- and schedule-dependent and are seen more frequently when GM-CSF is administered at higher doses and by continuous IV infusion than when given at recommended doses by the SC route.

Uncommon side effects Other less frequently observed side effects of GM-CSF include diarrhea, anorexia, facial flushing, dyspnea, and edema. Other side effects that have been reported with *Escherichia coli*-derived GM-CSF, such as the first-dose phenomenon and capillary leak syndrome, have rarely been observed with sargramostim.

Laboratory abnormalities, such as elevation of LDH levels, uric acid, and alkaline phosphatase levels; decreases in serum cholesterol and albumin; and occasional thrombocytopenia, have been reported with GM-CSF.

DOSE, ROUTE, AND SCHEDULE OF ADMINISTRATION

Recommended doses The recommended dose of the filgrastim version of recombinant human G-CSF is 5 μg/kg/d. This dose is clinically well tolerated and is effective in reducing the duration of neutropenia. The dose should begin 24 hours after chemotherapy and continue until the ANC is > 10,000 cells/μL. However, in clinical practice, dosing is commonly stopped when adequate neutrophil recovery has occurred.

G-CSF is used at a higher dose (10 μg/kg/d) for mobilization of progenitor cells and following BMT. Outside the context of stem-cell mobilization and transplantation, however, there are no data indicating that doses in excess of 5 μg/kg/d are indicated.

Pegfilgrastim is given as a fixed 6-mg dose. This dose has been shown to be effective regardless of age and weight in adults. It is given only once per cycle 24 hours after chemotherapy. For patients who develop febrile neutropenia after administration of pegfilgrastim, further dosing with daily filgrastim is not likely to be beneficial and is not recommended.

The recommended dose of yeast-derived GM-CSF following autologous BMT is 250 μg/m^2/d given by a 2-hour IV infusion. In phase I-II studies in the chemotherapy setting, activity has been observed at doses ranging from 250 to 750 μg/m^2/d. In patients with MDS, neutrophil responses have been seen at much lower doses (30 to ≤ 250 μg/m^2/d).

Although recommended doses in patients receiving chemotherapy are 5 μg/kg/d for G-CSF and 250 μg/m^2/d for GM-CSF, rounding these doses to the nearest vial size is appropriate for cost savings and convenience. In patients with MDS, the dose can be titrated to the smallest effective level to avoid untoward side effects.

Route of administration The SC route is the preferred route of administering filgrastim, pegfilgrastim, and sargramostim, for convenience. However, IV infusion is an acceptable route for filgrastim and sargramostim, if clinically indicated.

Timing of administration To obtain the greatest benefit from CSFs, the appropriate timing of administration is 24-48 hours following the completion of chemotherapy. CSF therapy should be continued until neutrophil recovery is adequate. The discontinuation of CSF therapy after neutrophil recovery is sometimes followed by a decline in ANC, especially in patients with compromised bone marrow reserve. This fall in neutrophil count can be precipitous with G-CSF and appears to be somewhat less pronounced following discontinuation of GM-CSF. Therefore, blood counts should be checked before initiating the next cycle of chemotherapy.

Initiation of the next cycle of chemotherapy is not recommended for at least 24 hours after the completion of CSF therapy because of the potential concern that progenitor cells, which are rapidly dividing following CSF administration, may be sensitized to chemotherapy. Future trials should help to determine the optimal interval that should be allowed between CSF discontinuation and initiation of the next chemotherapy cycle. There remains some theoretic concern that serial exposure of cycling progenitor cells to chemotherapy may accelerate cumulative marrow damage.

Because of the same concern, concurrent administration of CSFs with chemotherapy or radiotherapy is not recommended outside the context of clinical trials. Trials using GM-CSF concurrently with radiotherapy to the chest area have shown excessive hematologic toxicity, especially thrombocytopenia. It has been speculated that CSF-mobilized progenitor cells in the great vessels may be sensitized to radiation delivered to the chest.

Erythropoietin

Erythropoietin, an RBC lineage-specific glycoprotein hormone, was the first hematopoietic growth factor to become commercially available for clinical use in the United States. Recombinant human EPO has been approved for the treatment of anemia of chronic renal failure in predialysis or dialysis patients, anemia associated with zidovudine (Retrovir) therapy in patients infected with human immunodeficiency virus (HIV), anemia in cancer patients receiving chemotherapy for nonmyeloid malignancies, and anemia in patients scheduled for elective, noncardiac, nonvascular surgery.

In 2001, darbepoetin alfa was approved by the FDA to allow a new option of treatment of anemia associated with chronic renal failure. In 2002, darbepoetin alfa was approved by the FDA for the treatment of chemotherapy-induced anemia in patients with nonmyeloid malignancies. Darbepoetin alfa is a hyperglycosylated molecule based on the protein backbone structure of human erythropoietin. The increased level of glycosylation allows a longer duration of the drug in the circulation of humans after administration (with an up to three times longer half-life than EPO).

CHEMOTHERAPY-INDUCED ANEMIA

The anemia caused by chemotherapy is due mainly to drug effects on bone marrow precursor cells and is proportional to chemotherapy dose intensity. In addition, with platinum agents, anemia may be related to renal effects of these drugs on the production of EPO. Based on these observations, multicenter trials in the United States and Europe have examined the efficacy of recombinant human EPO in correcting the anemia of cancer caused by chemotherapy.

DOSE AND SCHEDULE OF ADMINISTRATION

The original FDA-approved recommended initial dose of EPO in cancer patients is 150 U/kg SC 3 times a week. This dose can be increased to 300 U/kg 3 times weekly if an adequate response (ie, a decrease in transfusion requirements or a rise in hemoglobin value [≥ 1 g/dL]) does not occur after 4 weeks of therapy. However, very few oncologists use the thrice-weekly regimen of EPO dosing anymore. A more common practice, based on data from several clinical trials and recently FDA-approved dose, is to administer EPO at a dose of 40,000 U SC *once weekly,* with an increase to 60,000 U once weekly if there is no adequate response after 4 weeks. This dose is well tolerated and appears to be equivalent in clinical effectiveness to three-times-weekly dosing while increasing patient convenience. EPO is approved by the FDA for once-weekly administration in the surgery population. A recent pharmacokinetic/pharmacodynamic study in healthy volunteers demonstrated that once-weekly EPO doses of 600 U/kg resulted in similar increases in hemoglobin value as did 150 U/kg 3 times weekly.

Darbepoetin alfa has a longer half-life than EPO and requires less frequent dosing. The current FDA-approved recommended initial dose of darbepoetin alfa in cancer patients is 2.25 μg/kg SC once a week or 500 μg once every 3 weeks. The weekly dose can be increased to 4.5 μg/kg once a week at 6 weeks if hemoglobin values increase less than 1 g/dL. No dose increase is recommended for the 500-μg-every-3-weeks regimen. In the community oncology setting, the dose of darbepoetin alfa often used is 200 μg every 2 weeks or 300 μg every 3 weeks, with an increase to 300 μg every 2 weeks at 6 weeks or 500 μg every 3 weeks, respectively, if hemoglobin values increase less than 1 g/dL. Additional dosing schedules have been studied (ie., loading doses, etc.) with both agents.

A patient who does not respond after 8 weeks of EPO or 12 weeks of darbepoetin alfa therapy (despite a dose increase) is unlikely to respond to higher doses. The dose of EPO/darbepoetin alfa should be reduced appropriately (25%-40%) if there is a rapid rise in hemoglobin value (ie, > 1 g/dL after 2 weeks) or if hematocrit values exceed 40% and should be titrated to maintain the desired hemogloblin value (ie, decrease dose or prolong dosing interval). In patients treated with 500 μg every 3 weeks, once Hgb reaches 11g/dL, the dose should be reduced to 300 μg every 3 weeks. If response is suboptimal, the clinician should consider rechecking levels of nutritional cofactors (eg, iron, total iron-binding capacity, ferritin) or evaluate other reasons for lack of response (eg, underlying infection, inflammatory process, occult blood loss, other vitamin deficiencies). Patients (especially premenopausal women) may require supplemental iron to avoid depletion of marginal iron stores and to adequately support erythropoiesis stimulated by EPO. Recent data support the use of intravenous iron products for supplementation, as oral agents are relatively ineffective and often poorly tolerated.

EMERGING SAFETY ISSUES

Recent reports of four new studies in patients with cancer found a higher chance of serious and life-threatening side effects and/or death with the use of erythropoiesis stimulating agents (ESAs). These research studies were evaluating an unapproved dosing regimen, a patient population for which ESAs are not approved, or a new unapproved ESA. For more information and the most up-to-date announcements regarding use of ESAs in patients with cancer, see the box on page 903 and go to http://www.fda.gov/cder/drug/ and search "ESA."

Cytokines with thrombopoietic activity

Although G-CSF and GM-CSF have significantly reduced neutropenia in patients receiving chemotherapy, thrombocytopenia still remains a frequent dose-limiting toxicity of several chemotherapeutic regimens. Several hematopoietic cytokines with thrombopoietic activity have been evaluated in clinical trials. They include IL-1, IL-3, IL-6, IL-11, thrombopoietin (TPO), megakaryocyte growth and development factor (MGDF), and hybrid/synthetic cytokines, such as PIXY321 (a GM-CSF/IL-3 fusion protein) or SC71858 (promegapoietin, a synthetic cytokine comprising mutated versions of IL-3 and TPO).

Most of these cytokines have shown modest thrombopoietic activity and have the potential to induce nonspecific biologic activities, including some undesirable effects. To date, IL-11 is the only thrombopoietic cytokine that has received FDA approval for clinical use.

Interleukin-11

IL-11 is a pleiotropic cytokine with thrombopoietic activity. In vitro, IL-11 acts synergistically with other hematopoietic growth factors, such as TPO, IL-3, and stem-cell factor (c-*kit* ligand), to promote the proliferation of hematopoietic progenitor cells and to induce maturation of megakaryocytes.

IL-11 was approved by the FDA to prevent severe thrombocytopenia and to reduce the need for platelet transfusions following myelosuppressive chemotherapy in patients with nonmyeloid malignancies who are at risk of severe thrombocytopenia based on the results of a randomized clinical trial of IL-11 in cancer patients who required at least one platelet transfusion after a chemotherapy cycle. In this trial, the use of IL-11 as secondary prophylaxis reduced the need for platelet transfusions in a subsequent cycle of chemotherapy.

However, it should be recognized that severe thrombocytopenia requiring platelet transfusions is an uncommon acute problem with initiation of standard-dose chemotherapy. Nonetheless, thrombocytopenia can represent a cumulative problem with the many chemotherapeutic regimens often used to treat solid tumors, especially in patients with more heavily pretreated marrows.

Major bleeding is a rare complication related to chemotherapy-induced thrombocytopenia. Therefore, the appropriate use of thrombopoietic agents will require careful attention to several endpoints, including the need for platelet transfusions, ability to deliver chemotherapy without treatment-limiting thrombocytopenia, the safety profile of the thrombopoietic agent, and the associated health care costs.

Dose and schedule of administration The recommended dose of IL-11 for prophylaxis in adults is 50 μg/kg SC once daily. Therapy is started from 6 to 24 hours after the completion of chemotherapy and is continued until the postnadir platelet count is ≥ 50,000 cells/μL. Dosing beyond 21 days per treatment cycle is not recommended.

Adverse reactions Patients treated with IL-11 commonly experience mild to moderate fluid retention, as manifested by peripheral edema and/or dyspnea. In some patients, preexisting pleural effusions have increased during IL-11 administration. Therefore, patients with a history of pleural or pericardial effusions or ascites should be carefully monitored during IL-11 therapy. In addition, fluids and electrolytes should be monitored carefully in patients requiring the use of a diuretic.

Moderate decreases in hemoglobin values (thought to be related to dilutional anemia) have also been observed in patients receiving IL-11. The fluid retention and anemia are reversible within several days after IL-11 is discontinued.

IL-11 should be used with caution in patients with a history of cardiac arrhythmia, since palpitations, tachycardia, and atrial arrhythmia (atrial fibrillation or flutter) have been reported in some patients receiving this agent.

TPO

TPO is a lineage-dominant hematopoietic cytokine that regulates proliferation and maturation of cells of the megakaryocyte/platelet lineage. Preclinical studies have clearly shown that TPO cells are the key regulators of megakaryocyte mass and platelet production. Mice with induced genetic defects in TPO or its receptor, c-*mpl*, have > 90% loss of platelet production capacity.

The results of initial clinical trials of TPO are encouraging and suggest an important role for this agent in the treatment of cancer patients undergoing myelosuppressive treatment. No recombinant version of TPO has yet been approved by the FDA, showing the difficulty in developing thrombopoietic growth factors.

Development of TPO and related molecules has been complicated by the development of antibodies directed against some—but not all—of the recombinant human versions of this molecule. Clinical development of MGDF, a highly truncated recombinant version of TPO, was halted due to the occurrence of neutralizing antibodies directed against TPO. These potentially dangerous antibodies could prolong thrombocytopenia. However, similar antibodies have not been detected with the full-length version of recombinant human TPO.

For that reason, further clinical trials of TPO continue. This promising agent does not produce the edema or other nonspecific side effects that occur with IL-11, and, thus, further data from larger trials of TPO are awaited.

SUGGESTED READING

Auerbach M, Ballard H, Trout JR, et al: Intravenous iron optimizes the response to recombinant human erythropoietin in cancer patients with chemotherapy-related anemia: A multicenter, open-label, randomized trial. J Clin Oncol 22:1301–1307, 2005.

Bennett CL, Luminari S, Nissenson AR, et al: Pure red-cell aplasia and epoetin therapy. N Engl J Med 351:1403–1408, 2004.

Citron ML, Berry DA, Cirrincione C, et al: Randomized trial of dose-dense versus conventionally scheduled and sequential versus concurrent combination chemotherapy as postoperative adjuvant treatment of node-positive primary breast cancer: First report of Intergroup Trial C9741/Cancer and Leukemia Group B trial 9741. J Clin Oncol 21:1431–1439, 2003.

Crawford J, Cella D, Cleeland CS, et al: Relationship between changes in hemoglobin level and quality of life during chemotherapy in anemic cancer patients receiving epoetin alfa therapy. Cancer 95:888–895, 2002.

Glaspy JA: Hematopoietic management in oncology practice. Part 1: Myeloid growth factors. Oncology 17:1593–1603, 2003.

Glaspy JA: Hematopoietic management in oncology practice. Part 2: Erythropoietic factors. Oncology 17:1724–1730, 2003.

Holmes FA, O'Shaughnessy JA, Vukelja S, et al: Blinded, randomized, multicenter study to evaluate single administration pegfilgrastim once per cycle versus daily filgrastim as an adjunct to chemotherapy in patients with high-risk stage II or stage III/IV breast cancer. J Clin Oncol 20:727–731, 2002.

Ozer H, Armitage JO, Bennett CL, et al: 2000 update of recommendations for the use of hematopoietic colony-stimulating factors: Evidence-based, clinical practice guidelines. American Society of Clinical Oncology Growth Factors Expert Panel. J Clin Oncol 18:3558–3585, 2000.

Rossert J, Casadevall N, Eckardt KU: Anti-erythropoietin antibodies and pure red cell aplasia. J Am Soc Nephrol 15:398–406, 2004.

Vogel CL, Wojtukiewicz MZ, Carroll RR, et al: First and subsequent cycle use of pegfilgrastim prevents febrile neutropenia in patients with breast cancer: A multicenter, double-blind, placebo-controlled phase III study. J Clin Oncol 23:1178-1184, 2005.

CHAPTER 41

Fatigue and dyspnea

Sriram Yennurajalingam, MD, and Eduardo Bruera, MD

Fatigue and dyspnea are two of the most common symptoms associated with advanced cancer. Fatigue is also commonly associated with cancer treatment and occurs in up to 90% of patients undergoing chemotherapy. Both symptoms have many possible underlying causes. In most patients, the etiology of fatigue or dyspnea is multifactorial, with many contributing interrelated abnormalities. In one study of patients with advanced cancer, fatigue was found to be significantly correlated with the intensity of dyspnea. This chapter will discuss the mechanisms, clinical features, assessment, and management of both of these troublesome and often undertreated symptoms in cancer patients.

Fatigue

Fatigue has been defined as easy tiring and decreased capacity to maintain performance. It results in physical and/or mental weariness following exertion and is transient in most of us. In cancer patients, fatigue is often severe; has a marked anticipatory component; and results in lack of energy, malaise, lethargy, and diminished mental functioning that profoundly impairs quality of life. It may be present early in the course of the illness, may be exacerbated by treatments, and is present in almost all patients with advanced cancer.

Fatigue is sometimes referred to as asthenia, tiredness, lack of energy, weakness, and exhaustion. Not all these terms have the same meaning to all patient populations. Moreover, different studies of fatigue and asthenia have looked at different outcomes, ranging from physical performance to the purely subjective sensation.

MECHANISM

The mechanisms of cancer-related fatigue are not well understood. Substances produced by the tumor are postulated to induce fatigue. Blood from a fatigued subject when injected into a rested subject has produced manifestations of fatigue. The host production of cytokines in response to the tumor can also have a direct fatigue-inducing effect. Muscular or neuromuscular junction abnormalities are a possible cause of chemotherapy- or radiotherapy-induced fatigue. In summary, fatigue is the result of many syndromes–not just one. Multiple mechanisms are involved in causing fatigue in most patients with advanced cancer.

CLINICAL FEATURES

The causes of fatigue in an individual patient are often multiple with many interrelated factors. Figure 1 summarizes the main contributors to fatigue in cancer patients.

Cachexia Cancer cachexia results from a complex interaction of host and tumor products. Host cytokines such as tumor necrosis factor, interleukin-1 (IL-1), and IL-6 are capable of causing decreased food intake, loss of body weight, a decrease in synthesis of both lipids and proteins, and increased lipolysis. Tumors are also capable of producing lipolytic factors (lipolytic factor, toxohormone L-2) and proteolytic by-products (proteolysis-inducing factor). The metabolic abnormalities involved in the production of cachexia and the loss of muscle mass resulting from progressive cachexia may cause profound weakness and fatigue. However, many abnormalities described in Figure 1 are capable of causing profound fatigue in the absence of significant weight loss.

Immobility has been shown to cause deconditioning and decreased endurance to both exercise and normal activities of daily living. On the other hand, overexertion is a frequent cause of fatigue in noncancer patients. It should also be considered in younger cancer patients who are undergoing aggressive antineoplastic treatments such as radiation therapy and chemotherapy and who are nevertheless trying to maintain their social and professional activities.

Psychological distress In patients without cancer who present with fatigue, the final diagnosis is psychological in almost 75% of patients (depression, anxiety, and other psychological disorders). The frequency of major psychiatric disorders in cancer patients is low. However, symptoms of psychological distress or adjustment disorders with depressive or anxious moods are much more frequent. Patients with an adjustment disorder or a major depressive disorder can have fatigue as their most prevalent symptom.

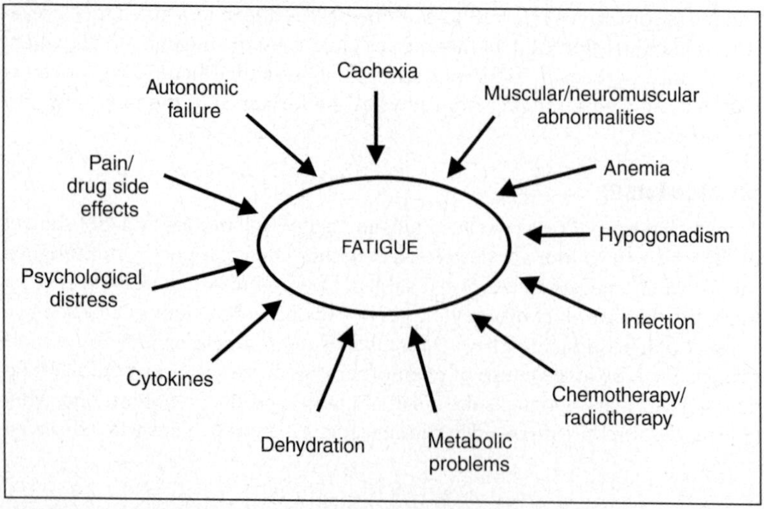

FIGURE 1: Contributors to fatigue in cancer patients

Anemia related to advanced cancer or chemotherapy has been associated with fatigue, and its treatment results in improvement of fatigue and quality of life in these patients. In terminally ill patients with advanced cancer, treatment of anemia may not resolve the symptom adequately due to the multifactorial nature of the etiology of fatigue. It may be the result of the more intense nature of the other contributory factors.

Autonomic failure Autonomic insufficiency is a frequent complication of advanced cancer. Autonomic failure has also been documented in patients with a subset of severe chronic fatigue syndrome. Although the association between fatigue and autonomic dysfunction has not been established in cancer patients, it should be suspected in patients with severe postural hypotension or other signs of autonomic failure.

Hypogonadism Research has shown that both intrathecal and systemic opioid therapy, as well as cachexia and some antineoplastic therapies, can result in hypogonadotropic hypogonadism. This can lead to fatigue, depression, and reduced libido.

Chemotherapy These treatments are common causes of fatigue in cancer patients. Chemotherapy and radiotherapy for malignancy cause a specific fatigue syndrome. Combined therapy with the two modalities appears to cause worse fatigue than either modality given alone. The pattern of fatigue reported by patients with cancer who receive myelosuppressive chemotherapy is cyclical. It begins within the first few days after therapy is started, peaks around the time of the WBC nadir, and diminishes in the week thereafter, only to recur again with the next cycle of chemotherapy. Fatigue tends to worsen with subsequent cycles of chemotherapy, which suggests a cumulative dose-related toxic effect. Compared with women with no history of cancer, former patients with breast cancer who had received adjuvant chemotherapy reported more fatigue and worse quality of life due to this symptom. Similar results have been noted in breast cancer patients who have been treated with high-dose chemotherapy and autologous stem-cell support and in patients treated for lymphoma.

Radiotherapy Radiation therapy tends to cause a different pattern of fatigue. It is often described as a "wave" that starts abruptly within a few hours after treatment and subsides shortly thereafter. Fatigue has been noted to decrease in the first 2 weeks after localized treatment for breast cancer but then to increase as radiation therapy persists into week 4. It then decreases again 3 weeks after radiation therapy ceases. The mechanism for fatigue in these situations is not well understood.

Surgery is another common cause of fatigue in patients with cancer. In addition, commonly used medications such as opioids and hypnotics may cause sedation and fatigue.

Other Comorbid conditions not necessarily related to cancer, such as renal failure or congestive heart failure, may coexist and contribute to the problem. Other conditions include the chronic stress response (possibly mediated through hypothalamic-pituitary axis), disrupted sleep or circadian rhythms, and

TABLE 1: Assessment of fatigue

Functional capacity	
	Treadmill performance (time, speed)
	Number of errors (eg, driving, pilots)
Task-related fatigue (eg, treadmill, driving)	
	VAS (visual analog scales), numerical scale
	Pearson and Byars Fatigue Feeling Checklist
Performance status	
	ECOG (Eastern Cooperative Oncology Group)
	Karnofsky performance status
	Edmonton Functional Assessment Tool (EFAT)
Subjective assessment of fatigue	
	VAS, numerical scale
	Brief Fatigue Inventory
	Piper Fatigue Self-Report Scale

hormonal changes (eg, premature menopause and androgen blockade secondary to cancer treatment).

ASSESSMENT

Since fatigue is essentially a subjective sensation, it is by nature difficult to assess. There is agreement that self-assessment should be the "gold standard." Due to the complex nature of the symptoms of fatigue, an effort to identify a set of diagnostic criteria similar to those for depression has been attempted. This syndromal approach has been useful to assess the presence or absence of the clinical syndrome of fatigue.

Table 1 summarizes the four most common measurable indices to assess fatigue. The first category in Table 1 looks at the objective function that the patient is capable of performing when subjected to a standard task. These functional tasks have limited value in cancer care, however, as they are very difficult for the advanced cancer patient to perform.

The second category in Table 1 attempts to assess the subjective effects of standard tasks.

The third category in Table 1 has been the most commonly used in oncology. The two most common scales (ECOG [Eastern Cooperative Oncology Group] and Karnofsky performance status) consist of a physician's rating of the patient's functional capabilities after a regular medical consultation. A physiotherapist performs the Edmonton Functional Assessment Tool and attempts to determine the functional status, as well as all the obstacles to clinical performance in these patients.

The fourth category in Table 1 is the most relevant for both clinical management and clinical trials in fatigue. Visual analog scales (VAS), numerical scales,

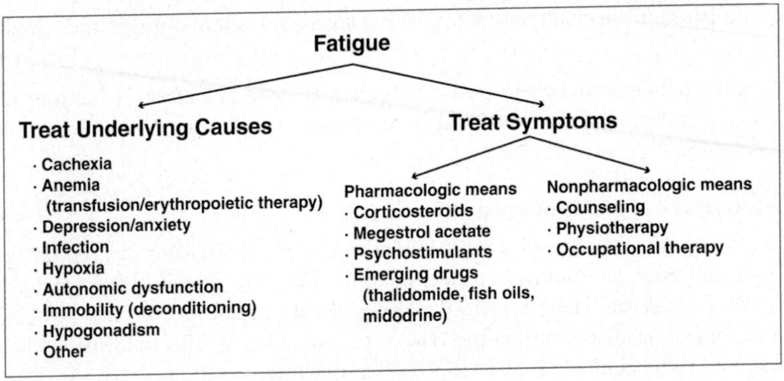

FIGURE 2: Therapeutic approach to managing fatigue

the Brief Fatigue Inventory, and the Piper Fatigue Self-Report Scale have been validated. In addition, there are validated functional assessments in most quality-of-life questionnaires.

In addition to the assessment of the intensity of fatigue, the clinical assessment of these patients requires clinicians to determine the impact of all factors on the presence of fatigue.

MANAGEMENT

To treat fatigue optimally, it is vital to identify and prioritize the different underlying factors in each individual patient. A thorough history, including recent treatment history, physical examination, and medication review, in addition to simple laboratory investigations will help identify possible underlying causes. Figure 2 outlines a therapeutic approach to fatigue management in cancer patients. Whenever possible, an attempt should be made to treat these contributing factors. It is impossible to be certain whether one of these identified problems is a major contributor to fatigue or is simply a coexisting problem in a given patient. Therefore, it is of great importance to measure the intensity of fatigue and the patient's performance before and after treating any contributing factor. If the level of fatigue does not improve after correction of these abnormalities, it is clear then that further treatment will not result in improvement in the future.

In patients with cancer treatment-related fatigue, it is important to exclude specific causes, such as hypothyroidism, hypogonadism, and anemia, and to consider other potential adverse effects of treatment. If specific problems are identified, they should be appropriately managed. For instance, patients with anemia may experience symptomatic improvement with the administration of erythropoietic therapy (epoetin alfa [Epogen, Procrit] and darbepoetin alfa [Aranesp]) at the dose and frequency interval that best fit the patient's need. Epoetin alfa may be administered weekly by subcutaneous injection; darbepoetin alfa has a longer half-life, requiring less frequent dosing. Dosages and schedules of both agents may be increased if necessary. (See section on "Dose and schedule of administration" in chapter 40 for specific information about dosages and schedules.)

In most patients, there will be no identified reversible causes. A number of effective pharmacologic and nonpharmacologic symptomatic treatments are available for these patients.

Pharmacologic treatments

Corticosteroids There is substantial evidence that corticosteroids can reduce fatigue and other symptoms in cancer patients. They are probably best retained for short-term use. Their beneficial effects generally last between 2 and 4 weeks, and longer term use carries the risk of serious adverse effects. Most studies have used the equivalent of 40 mg/d of prednisone.

Progestational agents In recent studies of terminally ill patients, megestrol (60–480 mg/d) has been shown to have a rapid (less than 1 week) beneficial effect on appetite, fatigue, and general well-being.

Psychostimulants Psychostimulants (eg, methylphenidate, 5–10 mg in the morning and at noon or 5 mg as needed) may be of use in treating fatigue in patients with advanced cancer. The safety and efficacy of long-term use of methylphenidate for fatigue have not been established.

A National Cancer Institute-sponsored trial on the use of modafinil (Provigil) for treatment of cancer-related fatigue is under way. In addition, dexmethylphenidate (D-MPH, Focalin) has been found to be more effective than placebo in the treatment of fatigue and impaired memory after chemotherapy in adults with cancer in a randomized phase III trial.

In addition to these agents, a number of other drugs have been tried in preliminary studies in patients with fatigue. Early positive results have been observed with both thalidomide (Thalomid) and fish oils. In addition, there are donezepil for fatigue associated with opioid sedation and midodrine (ProAmatine) in cases of autonomic failure.

Nonpharmacologic treatment

Physiotherapy and occupational therapy Physiotherapy may encourage increased activity where appropriate and provide active range of motion to prevent painful tendon retraction. Recent evidence suggests that aerobic exercise may reduce fatigue during chemotherapy. Assessment of the home environment by an occupational therapist can be useful. The provision of ramps, walkers, wheelchairs, elevated toilets, and hospital beds may allow the patient to remain at home in a safe environment. Education regarding the pattern of fatigue during treatment has been helpful. Counseling for stress management, depression, and anxiety may reduce distress and fatigue as well as improve mood.

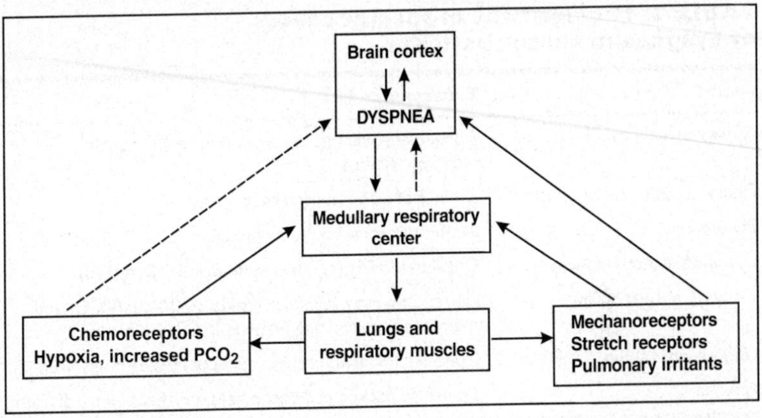

FIGURE 3: Mechanisms of dyspnea

Dyspnea

Dyspnea has been defined as an uncomfortable awareness of breathing. It is a subjective sensation and does not necessarily correlate with clinical findings in a given patient. It occurs in up to 75% of patients with advanced cancer, and good symptom control is less frequently achieved, even by experienced palliative care teams, than with other symptoms of terminal cancer such as pain or nausea.

MECHANISMS

The pathophysiology of dyspnea is complex and has not been completely elucidated. The respiratory center in the medulla controls breathing, but dyspnea is the result of cortical stimulation. Abnormalities of blood gases detected by both lung and central chemoreceptors and stimulation of lung and respiratory muscle mechanoreceptors stimulate the respiratory center. Mechanoreceptors respond to stretch and irritants and also have a demonstrated effect on the brain cortex, causing dyspnea. In addition, it is possible that both the chemoreceptors and the medullary respiratory center stimulate the cerebral cortex, directly contributing to the sensation of dyspnea. Figure 3 summarizes the mechanisms of dyspnea.

CLINICAL FEATURES

There are many causes of dyspnea in patients with advanced cancer, such as pulmonary embolism, lung metastasis, pleural effusion, congestive heart failure, anemia, psychological distress, pneumonia, muscle weakness, and preexisting pulmonary disease.

TABLE 2: Management of specific causes of dyspnea in cancer patients

Cause	Treatment
Airway obstruction by tumor	Corticosteroids (eg, dexamethasone 6-8 mg qid), radiation therapy
Pleural or pericardial effusion	Drain if effusion is significant
Pneumonia	Antibiotics (oral route preferred)
Carcinomatous lymphangitis	Corticosteroids (eg, dexamethasone 6-8 mg qid)
Congestive heart failure	Diuretic therapy (eg, furosemide 10-20 mg IV/SC) and angiotensin-converting enzyme (ACE) inhibitors
Underlying asthma, COPD	Optimize bronchodilators, corticosteroids if required
Anemia	Transfuse packed red blood cells, erythropoietic therapy

COPD = chronic obstructive pulmonary disease

Direct tumor effects Dyspnea may be the result of direct primary or metastatic tumor effects such as airway obstruction, atelectasis, parenchymal lung involvement, phrenic nerve palsy, carcinomatous lymphangitis, or superior vena caval obstruction.

Indirect tumor effects Indirect cancer effects include pneumonia, anemia, pleural effusion, and pulmonary embolism. Cardiac complications of cancer such as congestive heart failure, pericarditis, or pericardial effusion may contribute to the problem. Intra-abdominal disorders such as gross ascites or hepatomegaly may cause elevation of the diaphragm and may interfere with respiratory function. Generalized muscle weakness due to cachexia or fatigue may exacerbate breathlessness. Preexisting lung diseases including asthma or chronic obstructive pulmonary disease (COPD) may contribute to the problem.

Treatment side effects Contributing treatment side effects include pneumonitis or fibrosis following chemotherapy or radiotherapy.

Psychological conditions Anxiety, depression, or somatization will alter a patient's perception of dyspnea. Anxiety has been found to be an independent correlate with the intensity of dyspnea in cancer patients with moderate to severe dyspnea. Any of these factors may occur in isolation or in combination, and care is needed during assessment, as there are often many contributors in an individual patient.

ASSESSMENT

Dyspnea is a subjective sensation, and researchers have found much variability in the expression of dyspnea in individuals with similar levels of functional abnormalities. In addition, patients' perception of dyspnea can be influenced by their beliefs and intrapsychic and cultural factors. The presence or absence of physical signs such as tachypnea, wheezing, or use of accessory muscles is not a reliable indicator of the degree of distress felt by patients. The intensity of dyspnea can be easily assessed using verbal, numeric, or visual analog scales similar to those used in pain or nausea. Recently, maximal inspiratory pressure has been found to be an independent correlate of the intensity of dyspnea. Physical examination, chest x-ray, and pulse oximetry should be performed. Other investigations such as CBC, echocardiogram, or pulmonary function tests may be indicated.

In a prospective study, a multivariate analysis of 74 patients with cancer showed that dyspnea was significantly associated with fatigue ($P = .001$), pain ($P = .01$), depression ($P = .0003$), and FEV_1 ($P = .004$). Two types of dyspnea were observed. In the first type, dyspnea occurred in short periods of about 5 minutes (breakthrough dyspnea); in the second type, dyspnea was continuous. Breakthrough dyspnea may require a different treatment algorithm from continuous dyspnea and may be difficult to control (*Reddy S, Elsayem A, Palmer L, et al: J Clin Oncol [abstract] 23[suppl]:733s, 2005*).

MANAGEMENT

Specific causes

Underlying specific causes will require treatment as indicated in Table 2.

Symptomatic management

The three modalities of symptomatic treatment in cancer-related dyspnea are oxygen therapy, drug therapy, and counseling.

Oxygen therapy In hypoxemic cancer patients with dyspnea, oxygen has been shown to provide significant symptomatic relief. Oxygen can be administered by nasal cannula at 2–6 L/min or by mask and titrated to maintain an O_2 saturation at > 90%. Care must be taken in patients with COPD. Oxygen is not useful in patients with dyspnea and an O_2 saturation > 90%.

Drug therapy There is substantial evidence that systemic opioids have a beneficial effect on cancer-related dyspnea. This is possible without inducing respiratory depression. The optimal type, dose, and mode of administration have not been determined. If the patient is already on opioids, the breakthrough dose can be used to manage dyspnea as well as pain. If not, morphine can be started at 5–10 mg PO (or 2.5–5.0 mg SC) q4h with additional prn doses of 2.5–5.0 mg PO (or 2.5 mg SC) every hour for breakthrough dyspnea. Nebulized opiates are not recommended, as there is insufficient evidence to support their use.

Benzodiazepines have not been found to be effective in the general management of dyspnea, but they may be useful for treatment of episodes associated with anxiety attacks. Regular use of benzodiazepines should be avoided where possible to limit side effects such as confusion or falls.

A number of conditions that cause dyspnea in cancer patients respond to corticosteroid medication, including superior vena caval obstruction, carcinomatous lymphangitis, and COPD. However, corticosteroids may adversely affect muscle function, and the diaphragm may be more susceptible than other muscles. This may be of importance because of the frequency of muscle weakness and fatigue in patients with advanced cancer.

Counseling Dyspnea is a variable symptom and is exacerbated by physical activities. Patients and families should be educated so they can identify factors likely to worsen dyspnea. Devices such as bathroom aids and wheelchairs can help reduce physical activity, and the addition of portable oxygen can enable the patient to remain active and autonomous. Medication used for symptomatic relief such as opioids can be administered 30–45 minutes prior to dyspnea-causing maneuvers. The family should be educated that dyspnea is subjective and that tachypnea and use of accessory muscles do not necessarily indicate that the patient is suffering. The aim of treatment is to relieve the patient's subjective dyspnea, not to abate physical signs of respiratory distress.

SUGGESTED READING

ON FATIGUE

Bruera E, Driver L, Barnes EA, et al: Patient-controlled methylphenidate for the management of fatigue in patients with advanced cancer: A preliminary report. J Clin Oncol 21:4439–4443, 2003.

Bruera E, Strasser F, Shen L, et al: The effect of donezepil on sedation and other symptoms in patients receiving opioids for cancer pain: A pilot study. J Pain Symptom Manage 26:1049–1054, 2003.

Cleary J: The reversible causes of asthenia in cancer patients, in Portenoy R, Bruera E (eds): Topics in Palliative Care, vol 2, pp 183–202. New York, Oxford University Press, 1998.

Dimeo F, Stieglitz R, Novelli-Fischer U, et al: Effects of physical activity on the fatigue and psychological status of cancer patients during chemotherapy. Cancer 85:2273–2277, 1999.

Hann DM, Garovoy N, Finkelstein B, et al: Fatigue and quality of life in breast cancer patients undergoing autologous stem-cell transplantation: A longitudinal comparative study. J Pain Symptom Manage 17:311–319, 1999.

Howell SJ, Radford JA, Adams JE, et al: Randomized placebo-controlled trial of testosterone replacement in men with mild Leydig cell insufficiency following cytotoxic chemotherapy. Clin Endocrinol 55:315–324, 2001.

Munch TN, Zhang T, Willey J, et al: The association between anemia and fatigue in patients with advanced cancer receiving palliative care. J Palliat Med 8:1144–1149, 2005.

Neuenschwander H, Bruera E: Pathophysiology of cancer asthenia, in Portenoy R, Bruera E (eds): Topics in Palliative Care, vol 2, pp 171–181. New York, Oxford University Press, 1998.

Reddy S, Elsayem A, Palmer L, et al: The characteristics and correlates of dyspnea in advanced cancer patients [abstract]. J Clin Oncol 23(suppl):733s, 2005.

Sadler IJ, Jacobsen PB, Booth-Jones M, et al: Preliminary evaluation of a clinical syndrome approach to assessing cancer-related fatigue. J Pain Symptom Manage 23:406–416, 2002.

Seidenfeld J, Piper M, Flamm C, et al: Epoetin treatment of anemia associated with cancer therapy: A systematic review and meta-analysis of controlled clinical trials. J Natl Cancer Inst 93:1204–1214, 2001.

ON DYSPNEA

Allard P, Lamontagne C, Bernard P, et al: How effective are supplementary doses of opioids for dyspnea in terminally ill cancer patients? A randomized continuous sequential clinical trial. J Pain Symptom Manage 17:256–265, 1999.

Bruera E, Schmitz B, Pither J, et al: The frequency and correlates of dyspnea in patients with advanced cancer. J Pain Symptom Manage 19:357–362, 2000.

Mancini I, Body JJ: Assessment of dyspnea in advanced cancer patients. Support Care Cancer 7:229–232, 1999.

Ripamonti C, Fulfaro F, Bruera E: Dyspnea in patients with advanced cancer: Incidence, causes, and treatments. Cancer Treat Rev 42:60–80, 1998.

CHAPTER 42

Anorexia and cachexia

Charles Loprinzi, MD, and Aminah Jatoi, MD

Many patients with advanced cancer undergo a wasting syndrome associated with cancer anorexia/cachexia and asthenia. In a study that looked at symptoms in cancer patients being entered on a palliative care service, anorexia/cachexia and asthenia were more common problems than were pain or dyspnea. Patients who exhibit such symptoms generally have a short survival, respond poorly to cytotoxic agents, and suffer from increased toxicity from these agents.

In addition, cancer anorexia/cachexia is oftentimes associated with weakness, fatigue, and a poor quality of life. This problem not only affects the patient but also frequently has an impact on family members, as the patient is no longer able to participate fully in eating as a social activity.

Diagnostic criteria

Although some authors have tried to define criteria for diagnosing cancer cachexia, in general, it is not difficult to identify affected patients. In North Central Cancer Treatment Group (NCCTG) research trials involving more than 2,500 patients, simple criteria for anorexia/cachexia have been used:

- a 5-lb weight loss in the preceding 2 months and/or an estimated daily caloric intake of < 20 calories/kg
- a desire by the patient to increase his or her appetite and gain weight
- the physician's opinion that weight gain would be beneficial for the patient

Management

Nutritional counseling

Nutritional counseling, as provided by written materials, dietitians, physicians, and nurses, has been recommended, although its value has not been well demonstrated. Recommendations typically include eating frequent, small meals (as opposed to large meals), consuming larger quantities of food in the morning than in the evening, and avoiding spicy foods. Patients may do better if they are not exposed to the aroma of cooking. Although the benefits of such nutritional counseling are clearly limited, it does appear reasonable to provide.

> A recent placebo-controlled trial from the North Central Cancer Treatment Group showed that etanercept, a tumor necrosis factor alpha inhibitor, was ineffective in the treatment of the cancer anorexia/weight loss syndrome *(Jatoi A, Dakhil SR, Kugler JW, et al: J Clin Oncol [abstract] 24[18S]:476s, 2006).*

Appetite stimulants

Corticosteroids were the first agents to undergo placebo-controlled, double-blind evaluation for possible use in cancer cachexia. The first such trial, conducted in the 1970s by Moertel and colleagues at the Mayo Clinic, demonstrated that corticosteroids can stimulate appetite in patients with advanced, incurable cancer. Several subsequent placebo-controlled trials, using various steroid preparations and doses, have confirmed these results.

Dexamethasone (3-8 mg/d) is a reasonable option for clinical use. Known detriments to corticosteroid use include the well-known toxicities associated with chronic administration, including myopathy, peptic ulcer disease, infection, and adrenal suppression. Many patients with advanced cancer anorexia and cachexia, however, do not survive long enough to suffer from these toxicities.

Progestational agents Several placebo-controlled, double-blind clinical trials have demonstrated that progestational agents, such as megestrol acetate and medroxyprogesterone acetate, can lead to appetite stimulation and weight gain in patients with anorexia and cachexia. These trials also demonstrated that the effect of these drugs is seen in a matter of days and that they are effective antiemetics.

Although high doses of progestational agents can cause adrenal suppression because of their mild corticosteroid-type activity (a phenomenon not well understood by many clinicians), they do not appear to cause many of the side effects attributable to classic corticosteroids (such as peptic ulcer disease, myopathy, and opportunistic infections). In lieu of this adrenal suppression, however, stress doses of corticosteroids may be necessary in patients with trauma or infection or in surgical patients while on progestational agents. On the other hand, progestational agents increase the risk of thromboembolic phenomena–a side effect that is not seen with classic corticosteroids.

A dose-response study with megestrol acetate demonstrated a positive correlation between appetite stimulation and increased megestrol acetate doses, as doses ranged from 160 to 800 mg/d. Nonetheless, given that appetite stimulation has been demonstrated with megestrol acetate doses as low as 240 mg/d, much lower doses are used by many physicians, based primarily on cost considerations.

In the United States, a liquid formulation of megestrol acetate is considerably less expensive than the tablet form, and, milligram for milligram, the liquid preparation is more bioavailable. It is reasonable to start with 400 mg/d of liquid megestrol acetate, titrating this dose upward (maximum, 800 mg/d) or downward based on clinical response or the emergence of side effects.

A randomized, prospective clinical trial comparing the utility of megestrol acetate (800 mg/d) with dexamethasone (0.75 mg qid) demonstrated similar effects of these medications on patients' appetites but different toxicity profiles. Whereas megestrol acetate was associated with a higher incidence of thromboembolic phenomena, dexamethasone was associated with more myopathy, cushingoid body changes, and peptic ulcers.

Other agents Various other drugs have been evaluated definitively for the treatment of cancer anorexia and cachexia and have demonstrated little or no benefit. These drugs include fluoxymesterone, pentoxifylline, hydrazine sulfate, dronabinol (Marinol), cyproheptadine, and eicosapentaenoic acid (EPA). Of note, however, the antiserotonergic drug cyproheptadine does appear to be a relatively strong appetite stimulant in patients with the carcinoid syndrome, presumably because it directly counteracts the large amounts of serotonin secreted in these patients.

> A double-blind clinical trial comparing an eicosapentaenoic acid (EPA)-enhanced nutritional supplement vs megestrol acetate vs both agents was recently published by the North Central Cancer Treatment Group (NCCTG). Megestrol acetate produced better results with regard to appetite stimulation than the EPA-enhanced nutritional supplement, and EPA did not appear to provide any additional benefits when compared with megestol acetate (*Jatoi A, Rowland K, Loprinzi CL, et al: J Clin Oncol 22:2469-2476, 2004*).

EPA has been tested extensively for cancer anorexia and cachexia. Although preliminary studies had claimed improvement in appetite, body composition, and survival with EPA, these favorable findings have not been borne out in subsequent phase III trials. A total of three recently completed phase III trials have shown that EPA does relatively little for cancer anorexia and cachexia when tested in the setting of either EPA vs placebo or EPA vs megestrol acetate (see sidebar).

A number of other drugs have been evaluated in a pilot fashion for the treatment of cancer anorexia and cachexia. They include branched-chain amino acids, thalidomide (Thalomid), metoclopramide, oxandrolone (Oxandrin), and adenosine triphosphate. It is hoped that new information will be available in the near future to shed light on the possible therapeutic roles of these agents.

Enteral or parenteral nutrition

Despite the demonstrated efficacy of corticosteroids and progestational agents in patients with cancer anorexia and cachexia, these drugs do not have a major long-term impact on the vast majority of such patients. Consequently, other treatment approaches, such as enteral or parenteral nutritional methods, have been studied extensively. Several randomized trials failed to demonstrate that these nutritional approaches improve either quantity or quality of life. As a result, experts generally agree that the routine use of parenteral or enteral nutrition cannot be justified in patients with advanced cancer anorexia and cachexia.

There are, however, relatively rare circumstances in which parenteral nutrition may play a role in patients with advanced cancer. Such circumstances have been documented by case reports and small case series of patients. For example, patients with GI insufficiency due to surgery, radiation therapy, or abdominal carcinomatosis (without impending failure of other organs) may be appropriate candidates for parenteral nutrition.

Prophylactic therapy

Given the positive impact of corticosteroids and progestational agents on cancer anorexia and cachexia and the fact that many patients with advanced cancer die with, and/or of, inanition, the potential prophylactic use of these agents was evaluated. A double-blind trial was conducted in which patients with newly diagnosed extensive-stage small-cell lung cancer were randomized to receive megestrol acetate or placebo along with standard chemoradiation therapy. This trial was unable to demonstrate any beneficial effect of megestrol acetate on treatment response, quality of life, or survival.

Thus, patients should not be treated prophylactically for cancer anorexia and cachexia outside a clinical trial. Rather, such treatment should be reserved for patients in whom anorexia and cachexia are patient-determined, symptomatic clinical problems.

Nutrition as it relates to end-of-life care

Anorexia and cachexia are major problems for many oncology patients as they approach the final stage of life. Family members are generally more distressed than the patients if/when appetite stimulants do not provide relief. Questions commonly arise about giving enteral or parenteral nutrition or "forcing" patients to consume more calories in the belief that they would feel better, get stronger, and live longer. A small measure of appropriate education, noting that the intake of more calories does not appear to have a clinical benefit, provides substantial relief. It is worthwhile to note that patients randomized to receive total parenteral nutrition or appetite stimulants (such as megestrol acetate) do not live any longer than do control patients and that "force-feeding" is not in the patients' best interests.

SUGGESTED READING

Agteresch HJ, Rietveld T, Kerkhofs LG et al: Beneficial effects of adenosine triphosphate on nutritional status in advanced lung cancer patients: A randomized clinical trial. J Clin Oncol 20:371–378, 2002.

Bruera E, Strasser F, Palmer JL, et al: Effect of fish oil on appetite and other symptoms in patients with advanced cancer and anorexia/cachexia: A double-blind, placebo-controlled study. J Clin Oncol 21:129–134, 2003.

Jatoi A, Dakhil SR, Kugler JW, et al: A placebo-controlled trial of etanercept, a tumor necrosis factor (TNF) inhibitor, in patients with the cancer anorexia/weight loss syndrome. J Clin Oncol 24(18S):476s, 2006.

Jatoi A, Loprinzi CL: Adenosine triphosphate: Does it help cancer patients 'get bigger and stronger?' J Clin Oncol 20:362–363, 2002.

Jatoi A, Rowland K, Loprinzi CL, et al: An eicosapentaenoic acid supplement versus megestrol acetate versus both for patients with cancer-associated wasting: A North Central Cancer Treatment Group and National Cancer Institute of Canada collaborative effort. J Clin Oncol 22:2469–2476, 2004.

Jatoi A, Windschitl HE, Loprinzi CL, et al: Dronabinol vs megestrol acetate vs both for cancer-associated anorexia: A North Central Cancer Treatment Group Study. J Clin Oncol 20:567–573, 2002.

Loprinzi CL, Kugler JW, Sloan JA, et al: Randomized comparison of megestrol acetate versus dexamethasone versus fluoxymesterone for the treatment of cancer anorexia/cachexia. J Clin Oncol 17:3299–3306, 1999.

Mann M, Koller E, Murgo A, et al: Glucocorticoid-like activity of megestrol. Arch Intern Med 157:1651–1656, 1997.

Moertel CG, Schutt AJ, Reitemeier RJ, et al: Corticosteroid therapy of preterminal gastrointestinal cancer. Cancer 33:1607–1609, 1974.

Tchekmedyian S, Fesen M, Price LM, et al: Ongoing placebo-controlled study of oxandrolone in cancer-related weight loss. Int J Radiat Oncol Biol Phys 57(2 suppl):S283–S284, 2003.

CHAPTER 43

Long-term venous access

Stephen P. Povoski, MD

VENOUS ACCESS

The use of multidrug chemotherapy and bone marrow transplantation in cancer treatment has made the utilization of reliable, long-term venous access (LTVA) an essential component of cancer therapy. The placement of LTVA devices not only permits the delivery of these complex therapeutic regimens but also drastically improves patients' quality of life.

Indications

No definitive guidelines are available for utilization of central venous access. There are several important factors to consider when deciding upon LTVA device placement:

- the frequency and duration of therapy
- the frequency of blood draws
- the nature of therapy (eg, delivering vesicating agents into a central vein decreases the risk of extravasation)
- the need for supportive therapies (eg, total parenteral nutrition or systemic antibiotics)
- the need for stem-cell collection, plasmapheresis, and bone marrow reinfusion
- patient preference.

Patient selection

LTVA should always be considered an elective procedure. Therefore, before an LTVA device is placed, the patient should have recovered from acute infections and the treatment of complications. If there is an absolute need for immediate central venous access before such times, a temporary percutaneous central venous access catheter can be placed. A history of vascular access catheter insertion, deep venous thrombosis of an upper extremity or central vein, thoracic surgery, neck surgery, irradiation, or mediastinal and thoracic disease should alert the surgeon to possible changes in normal venous drainage.

Physical examination, documenting the integrity of the skin, changes in the skin secondary to previous surgical treatment and reconstruction, sites of previous central venous access catheter insertions, evidence of venous obstruction (presence of venous collaterals in the skin of the chest, unilateral arm swelling, or superior vena cava syndrome), and pulmonary reserve, should be performed in every patient. If there is any evidence of venous obstruction or a history of multiple central venous access catheters, the physical examination should be complemented with a formal venous imaging study.

Duplex Doppler ultrasonography can visualize the patency and flow of the neck and arm veins. Intrathoracic veins and the right atrium are not well visualized by duplex Doppler ultrasonography but are better visualized with transesophageal echocardiography. This can be utilized preoperatively or intraoperatively.

CT and MRI are useful for documenting the presence of thrombosis and the patency of major intrathoracic veins.

Venography is still the gold standard for studying venous anatomy. Venography should be performed whenever the clinical situation warrants it and noninvasive venous imaging studies fail to provide a definitive diagnosis. This can be utilized preoperatively or intraoperatively.

Chest radiography can disclose important information (such as the presence of pleural effusions, lung metastases, mediastinal adenopathy, and mediastinal tumors) that can modify selection of a site for LTVA placement.

Contraindications and precautions

Neutropenia A neutrophil count < 1,000/mm^3 is a relative contraindication to the placement of an LTVA device, since patients with neutropenia may have a higher incidence of septic episodes. The use of prophylactic antibiotics may reduce the incidence of infection in patients with a low absolute neutrophil count (ANC).

Thrombocytopenia and platelet dysfunction are frequently encountered in the cancer patient. Preoperative platelet transfusion to approximately 50,000/mL may allow the catheter to be safely placed with a reduction in the risk of bleeding complications. In those patients with thrombocytopenia refractory to platelet transfusions, venous cutdown may be a safer approach for catheter placement.

Clotting factor abnormalities Many cancer patients have abnormalities in their clotting factors secondary to malnutrition or chemotherapy. Correction with vitamin K or fresh frozen plasma may be necessary.

Active infection The presence of an active infection represents an absolute contraindication to the placement of an LTVA device. In those patients with an active infection who require long-term antibiotic treatment, a temporary central venous access catheter or a peripherally inserted central venous catheter is preferable.

LTVA device selection

Two types of LTVA devices are available. There are tunneled external catheters that have skin surface access (Hickman, Broviac, Groshong, Quinton). Likewise, there are subcutaneous implanted ports (Port-A-Cath, Infusaport). Both types of central venous access devices are available with different lumen diameters and numbers. Peripherally placed central venous access devices, such as the PAS (peripherally accessed system) port or PICC (peripherally inserted central catheter), have become popular because of their ease of placement. PICC devices can be placed by specially trained nursing personnel. Important differences between tunneled external catheters and subcutaneous implanted ports are outlined in Table 1.

General considerations An important general consideration in the selection of an appropriate LTVA device is that the infusion flow resistance depends on the catheter length and lumen diameter. Likewise, catheters with a split valve at the tip (Groshong catheter) are less reliable for blood drawing.

Frequency of device access Subcutaneous implanted ports are preferred in patients who require intermittent device access for treatment or blood drawing. Tunneled external catheters are preferred in patients who require continuous or frequent device access for treatment, blood drawing, or delivery of supportive therapies (parenteral nutrition, blood product transfusion, pain medication) or who are receiving therapy that would be potentially toxic if extravasated into the subcutaneous tissue. Peripherally placed devices are used mainly in patients who require single, continuous, infusional therapy (systemic antibiotics, hydration, pain medication), as is seen frequently for palliation.

TABLE 1: Differences between tunneled external catheters and subcutaneous implanted ports

Characteristic	Tunneled external catheters	Subcutaneous implanted ports
Lumen	Single, dual, and triple lumen	Single and dual lumen only
Maintenance training	Usually daily; requires patient required	Monthly; no patient training
Activity	Some restrictions (eg, swimming)	No restrictions
Blood draw	Very reliable	Moderately reliable
Cost	Higher maintenance cost	Higher initial cost
Access	External	Percutaneous Huber needle
Flow gauge	Determined by the lumen diameter	Determined by the Huber needle gauge
Complication rate (for infections)	Higher	Lower
Removal	Can usually be done in the office or at the bedside	May require a second surgical procedure

Number of lumens The choice of the number of lumens should be based on the intensity and complexity of the therapy.

Specially designed catheters There are specially designed catheters for hemodialysis or apheresis treatment. These catheters are shorter in length and have a lumen that is larger in diameter and is staggered at the tip to prevent recirculation. These catheters have a higher incidence of kinking, and, thus, care should be taken to avoid sharp angles at the skin exit site. In patients who already have an LTVA device in place and require short-term access for apheresis or stem-cell collection, consideration should be given to placing a temporary percutaneous hemodialysis or apheresis catheter rather than replacing the existing LTVA device.

Insertion technique

Placement of LTVA devices is best performed in a surgical suite or an appropriate interventional radiology suite to minimize the incidence of infections. Most procedures are performed on an outpatient basis or immediately prior to a scheduled admission. Local anesthesia and short-acting barbiturates and sedatives are safe and provide excellent patient comfort and sedation. The use of intraoperative fluoroscopy is strongly recommended to document appropriate device placement and to prevent potential complications.

The most common technique used in LTVA device placement is the percutaneous method of Seldinger, using the subclavian or internal jugular vein. Alternatively, a venous cutdown of the cephalic, external jugular, internal jugular, or saphenous vein can provide appropriate access for central venous device placement.

Placement of tunneled external catheters

For the percutaneous approach, the patient is placed supine and in the Trendelenburg position. Patients who cannot tolerate the Trendelenburg position frequently can have their device placed through a venous cutdown approach. A rolled sheet placed vertically in the small of the back is preferred by some to rotate the tips of the shoulders posteriorly. The region of the anterior chest, neck, and shoulders is prepared and draped in a sterilized fashion. The skin overlying the anticipated venipuncture site is infiltrated with a local anesthetic.

Vein penetration The venipuncture needle is carefully and slowly advanced, bevel up, into the vein, while the attached syringe is aspirated (without Luer-lock). If the vein is unable to be accessed after multiple attempts with the venipuncture needle, the contralateral side should not be approached during the same session without documenting the absence of complications.

Guidewire placement Once easy flow of blood into the syringe confirms vein penetration, the bevel is rotated downward, the syringe is disconnected without allowing introduction of air through the venipuncture needle, and a flexible J guidewire is advanced through the venipuncture needle.

Fluoroscopy should be used to confirm the placement of the tip of the guidewire within the right atrium. Atrial arrhythmia may be seen when the guidewire is advanced into the right atrium. If pulsatile blood flow is noted upon introducing the venipuncture needle (indicating an arterial puncture), the venipuncture needle should be withdrawn and local pressure applied for 5-10 minutes (see section on "Complications"). Resistance to the advancement of the guidewire is usually due to misdirection of the guidewire into a secondary vein or migration of the guidewire outside the vein. Fluoroscopy will confirm the guidewire's position. If the guidewire is suspected to be outside the vein, the venipuncture needle and the guidewire should be removed together, as a unit, to prevent shearing of the guidewire. If the guidewire is suspected to be in the wrong vein tributary, the venipuncture needle can be removed and a 16-gauge angiocatheter can be placed over the guidewire prior to readjusting the position of the guidewire.

Catheter placement The anticipated skin exit site and subcutaneous tunnel for the external catheter are infiltrated with a local anesthetic. The catheter is then advanced along the subcutaneous tunnel from the anticipated skin exit site to the venipuncture site. The catheter is measured and custom cut to reach the junction between the superior vena cava and right atrium (approximately at the fourth anterior intercostal space). The catheter cuff is positioned midway in the subcutaneous tunnel.

The dilator and peel-away introducer sheath are slowly and carefully advanced over the guidewire under fluoroscopy. The guidewire is gently and slightly withdrawn and advanced while the dilator and peel-away introducer sheath are advanced over the guidewire to confirm that they are indeed threading over the guidewire and that the guidewire has not migrated outside the vessel. The dilator and guidewire are then withdrawn from the peel-away introducer sheath. The catheter is then advanced through the peel-away introducer sheath and the tip of the catheter is advanced to the junction of the superior vena cava and right atrium.

Difficulties in advancing the catheter through the peel-away introducer sheath usually imply that the peel-away introducer sheath is bent. This occurs most frequently during the subclavian vein approach if the venipuncture is attempted too medially and through the costoclavicular ligament. If the catheter cannot be advanced through the peel-away introducer sheath, repeat venipuncture in a more lateral position may be necessary. The catheter should never be handled with sharp instruments. Only nontoothed forceps should be used, if needed.

Confirmation of catheter position Prior to removal of the peel-away introducer sheath, the catheter position should be confirmed by fluoroscopy. Failure to position the fluoroscopic beam perpendicular to the patient will give a false impression of the catheter's position.

At the completion of catheter placement, the entire catheter should be examined with fluoroscopy to confirm its position and to rule out any kinking that would prevent normal functioning. Catheter infusion (looking for impedance to inflow/infusion) and withdrawal (looking for interruption of flow on blood return) should be tested in the surgical suite prior to heparinization of the catheter lumen. A chest x-ray should be obtained in the recovery room to rule out complications and as a record of catheter position. Lastly, ultrasonography may be used during catheter placement to aid in vein localization for venous access and to determine the position of the catheter tip.

Placement of subcutaneous implanted ports

The procedure for placing a subcutaneous implanted port is similar to that for a tunneled external catheter, except for the creation of a subcutaneous port pocket. To prevent wound disruption, the subcutaneous port pocket should permit no tension in the placement of the port. The port is sutured to the muscular fascia to prevent port migration and is placed over the rib cage to provide easy access.

Device care

Subcutaneous implanted ports require flushing with a heparin solution (2-3 mL; 100 U/mL) after each use or monthly during periods of nonuse. During continuous infusion therapy, the noncoring (Huber) access needle should be replaced every third to fifth day.

Tunneled external catheters require more frequent care. The exit site is cleaned with an antiseptic agent, and an occlusive dressing is applied. This is generally done daily; however, some now advocate only biweekly cleanings and dressing changes. Hickman catheters are generally flushed daily with a heparin solution (2-3 mL; 100 U/mL) or after each use, and protective caps are replaced biweekly. However, some now advocate only biweekly flushing with a heparin solution (2-3 mL; 100 U/mL). Groshong catheters generally only require weekly flushing with 5 mL of a saline solution.

Complications

During device insertion

Complications during device placement are generally related to the method of insertion and the experience of the operator.

Pneumothorax is the most common complication of the percutaneous insertion technique, especially via the subclavian vein approach. The incidence of pneumothorax has been reported in most series to be approximately 1%-5%. It appears to be more frequently seen in nutritionally compromised and emaciated patients. Its incidence has also been thought to be related to the number of attempts required to access the vein and to the experience of the operator. Utilization of a venous cutdown approach eliminates the risk of pneumothorax.

Pneumothorax is usually recognized on a postoperative upright chest x-ray. The ability to detect a small pneumothorax on chest x-ray can be aided by performing an expiratory film. Delayed pneumothorax can develop several hours to several days after attempted percutaneous device insertion. If the pneumothorax is small (< 5%), the patient can be followed with subsequent chest x-rays, and the air occupying the pneumothorax can be left in place to be reabsorbed. Use of 100% oxygen can aid in reabsorption of a pneumothorax. Patients with a larger pneumothorax are generally treated by placement of a chest tube that is connected to a closed suction system or a Heimlich valve (one-way valve).

Iatrogenic arterial puncture occurs most frequently with the percutaneous internal jugular approach and less frequently with the percutaneous subclavian vein approach. Pulsatile flow confirms an arterial puncture. In this instance, the venipuncture needle should be removed and the vessel compressed for 5-10 minutes. If an arterial puncture is initially unrecognized and the guidewire is passed into the vessel, a position of the guidewire to the left of the thoracic spine on fluoroscopy should alert the operator's suspicions for the occurrence of this complication. In a patient with a persistent left vena cava, the guidewire will also be seen to the left of the spine on fluoroscopy. An intraoperative venogram may help to confirm the diagnosis.

Hemothorax as a result of injury to major vessels is seen less than 1% of the time. It can be life-threatening, however, when it does occur. During the percutaneous approach, injury to one of the major vessels with the venipuncture needle, guidewire, or dilator and peel-away introducer sheath may result in a hemothorax. Careful attention to insertion technique and use of fluoroscopy will help to prevent this complication. Utilization of a venous cutdown approach is much less likely to injure a major vessel.

Most patients who develop a hemothorax can be treated with a large-bore, laterally placed chest tube connected to a closed suction system. Many of these closed suction systems have a blood re-infusion collecting system. Thoracotomy may be indicated in certain circumstances [in patients with ongoing bleeding (> 500 mL/hr) or with a massive hemothorax (> 1,500 mL)].

Local hematomas can occur more frequently in thrombocytopenic patients or coagulopathic patients. They are best treated by local compression. Adequate replacement of platelets and clotting factors prior to device placement can help prevent these complications.

Catheter tip malposition is usually recognized and corrected at the time of catheter placement with the use of intraoperative fluoroscopy. However, catheters situated in the azygos vein or the right internal mammary vein can look strikingly similar to catheters situated in the superior vena cava in an anterior-posterior projection under intraoperative fluoroscopy. Frequently, these catheters do not withdraw blood easily and the catheter tip does not move with the cardiac rhythm. Lateral rotation of the intraoperative fluoroscope and utilization of intraoperative venography can help to differentiate this sometimes subtle finding.

Other device-related complications

Catheter compression, fracture, and embolization can occur when a catheter placed by the percutaneous subclavian approach is inserted too medially along the clavicle at the medial costoclavicular ligament. In such cases, the catheter may become chronically compressed between the clavicle and the first rib. This can be recognized radiographically as a "pinch-off sign." Chronic compression of the catheter may result in structural fatigue of the catheter wall that may eventually cause fracturing and distal embolization of the catheter. This can be prevented by ensuring that the venipuncture site is situated more laterally on the clavicle as well as 1-2 cm below the clavicle. If this problem is recognized during catheter placement, the catheter should be removed and then placed through a different venipuncture site.

Device malfunction can be divided into two types: (1) inability to withdraw blood from a device and (2) inability to infuse into a device. Inability to withdraw blood from a device, despite retaining the ability to infuse into the device, is most frequently caused by a fibrin sheath at the tip of the catheter that produces a one-way valve effect. Less frequently, it is due to a catheter tip positioned against the side wall of the vein. In patients with this problem, a Valsalva maneuver or repositioning of the patient can sometimes result in a successful blood withdraw.

Inability both to withdraw blood from and infuse into a device can result from many mechanical causes, such as catheter tip malposition, catheter kinking, catheter intraluminal thrombosis, intraluminal precipitation of medications, or venous thrombosis. A simple chest x-ray can identify some of these mechanical causes. Venography and venous duplex Doppler ultrasound imaging are also useful.

Thrombolytic therapy, using tissue plasminogen activator (tPA) or alteplase (recombinant tPA), can help to restore the ability to withdraw blood from a device or to clear a device from intraluminal thrombosis or intraluminal precipitation of medications. Usually 1-2 mg of tPA in 1-2 cc of sterile water is instilled into the device, left in place for 1-2 hours, and then aspirated. Alternatively, 2.5-cc aliquots (diluted to 1 mg/mL) of alteplase can be used in a similar fashion. This may be repeated daily for several days until total patency is restored. Likewise, chemical occlusion of a device resulting from precipitation of chemotherapeutic agents, poorly soluble salts (calcium, magnesium, or phosphates), or antibiotics (amikacin [Amikin], vancomycin) can be successfully treated with instillation of 0.2-1.0 mL of 0.1 N hydrochloric acid. The solution is irrigated in and out of the device for 2 minutes, left in place for 1 hour, and then aspirated. This may be repeated daily for several days until total patency is restored. No side effects or metabolic acidosis has been associated with hydrochloric acid at these doses.

External catheter damage External catheters can be damaged at the site of a catheter clamp or at a suture site. The use of needleless connections for infusions and irrigations should prevent needle damage to external portions of the catheter. Most external catheters have repair kits to replace any damaged external portion of the catheter.

Drug extravasation into the subcutaneous tissues can occur with subcutaneous implanted ports when there is inappropriate placement or accidental dislodgment of the Huber access needle from the implanted port. This may result in chemical cellulitis, tissue necrosis, and loss of soft tissue in the area of extravasation. Clinical signs of extravasation include pain, burning, soft-tissue swelling, skin erythema, and skin vesicle formation at the infusion site. If drug extravasation is suspected, the infusion should be stopped and the Huber access needle should be immediately withdrawn. Management depends on the type of drug infused and the amount of drug extravasated.

Venous thrombosis occurs more commonly than believed. The incidence of venous thrombosis varies in multiple studies, ranging from 0% to 65%. The incidence of venous thrombosis is higher in patients in whom the catheter tip is placed in the innominate vein or proximal superior vena cava as compared with the distal superior vena cava/right atrial junction. Ideally, the catheter tip should be positioned at the superior vena cava/right atrial junction and should be free floating. The incidence of venous thrombosis is higher in patients with multiple-lumen catheters than in those with single-lumen catheters. The incidence of venous thrombosis is higher in patients in whom the device was placed percutaneously than in those who underwent a venous cutdown approach. PICCs have been recently shown to be associated with a significant risk of upper extremity deep vein thrombosis. Preexisting hypercoagulable states predispose patients to the development of venous thrombosis.

Ipsilateral arm swelling, pain, and development of collateral veins in the skin overlying the chest wall should alert the clinician to the possibility of venous thrombosis. Venography, venous duplex Doppler ultrasound imaging, and CT/MRI scan can establish the diagnosis and the site of the obstruction.

Previous studies have suggested that the use of antithrombotic prophylaxis reduces the risk of central venous catheter-associated thrombosis in cancer patients. However, two recent double-blind, placebo-controlled, randomized trials assessing antithrombotic prophylaxis have now failed to show any such risk reduction within the time frame of those studies.

In one such trial by Verso et al, patients undergoing central venous catheter placement received either 6 weeks of subcutaneous low molecular weight heparin (LMWH; n = 155) or 6 weeks of subcutaneous placebo (n = 155). The overall incidence of central venous catheter-associated thrombosis was assessed at 6 weeks with upper extremity venography. Venography-proven thrombosis was observed in 14.2% (22 of 155) of the LMWH group and in 18.1% (28 of 155) of the placebo group ($P = 0.35\%$). Symptomatic thrombosis was observed in 1.0% of the LMWH group and in 3.1% of the placebo group. They concluded that the incidence of venography-proven thrombosis was lower than previously reported and that routine antithrombotic prophylaxis in cancer patients with central venous catheters should be reconsidered.

In one other such trial by Couban et al, patients undergoing central venous catheter placement received either 9 weeks of a 1-mg daily dose of warfarin (n = 130) or 9 weeks of a daily placebo (n = 125). The overall incidence of central venous catheter-associated thrombosis was assessed clinically, as defined as symptomatic central venous catheter-associated thrombosis. All symptomatic cases were then confirmed radiographically, first by compression ultrasonography, and then by venography, if ultrasonography results were normal. There was no statistically significant difference in the incidence of symptomatic central venous catheter-associated thrombosis between the two groups, with 4.6% (6 of 130) observed in the warfarin group and 4.0% (5 of 125) observed in the placebo group. They concluded that the incidence of symptomatic thrombosis was lower than previously reported and that administration of 1 mg/d of warfarin was not effective antithrombotic prophylaxis in cancer patients with central venous catheters. However, with the low rate of symptomatic central venous catheter-associated thrombosis, a much larger trial is required to address the issue definitively.

As a last point with regard to low-dose warfarin antithrombotic prophylaxis in cancer patients with central venous catheters, recent data have also shown a high incidence of INR (international normalized ratio) abnormalities in patients receiving 5-FU–based chemotherapy regimens who were maintained on 1 mg/d of warfarin, noted in 55 of 427 patients (12.8%), as reported by Magagnoli et al. In this regard, they recommended that such patients should undergo periodic monitoring of the prothrombin time and INR.

Treatment should be directed toward prevention of pulmonary embolism, avoidance of clot propagation, prevention of the postphlebitic syndrome, and preservation of the LTVA device, if possible. With these objectives in mind, the LTVA device should be removed only if it is no longer necessary or if initial therapy for venous thrombosis fails. The patient can be initially treated with systemic heparinization or subcutaneous low-molecular-weight heparin followed by conversion to oral anticoagulation with warfarin. The LTVA device may be kept in place as long as the patient is asymptomatic and there is no contraindication to anticoagulation. Anticoagulant therapy should be continued for at least 3 months.

Device-related infections

Device-related infections can be divided into device-related bacteremia and site infections. Site infections consist of subcutaneous catheter tunnel infections and subcutaneous port pocket infections.

In general, device-related infections are thought to be greater for tunneled external catheters than subcutaneous implanted ports and greater for multiple-lumen catheters than single-lumen catheters. However, considerable controversy on this topic exists in the literature, since various studies examining device-related infection rates differ significantly with respect to patient characteristics, device maintenance schedules, and diagnostic criteria for defining a device-related infection. Differing device-use patterns and patient medical illness acuity are thought to explain the difference in device-related infection rates between tunneled external catheters and subcutaneous implanted ports and between multiple-lumen catheters and single-lumen catheters. Device-related infections of PICCs seem to occur more often in oncology patients than in non-oncology patients. Therefore, PICCs should be used with caution in oncology patients, except in cases of end-stage palliative comfort care.

It is controversial whether utilization of perioperative antibiotics for LTVA device placement decreases the incidence of device-related infections. Some studies have evaluated the addition of antibiotics (such as vancomycin) to the standard heparin-flush solution administered through LTVA devices to prevent device-related infections. Such results should be viewed with caution, however, in light of the increased incidence of vancomycin-resistant organisms in the hospital inpatient population.

Device-related bacteremia

Device-related bacteremia is a potentially life-threatening complication, especially in the immunocompromised patient. The infection generally is caused by gram-positive cocci (coagulase-negative staphylococci) or enteric gram-negative bacilli (*Enterobacteriaceae, Escherichia coli,* and *Pseudomonas* species). Less frequently, device-related bacteremia is caused by fungi (*Candida* species). The incidence of fungal infection is significantly higher in immunocompromised patients.

Criteria for diagnosis of device-related bacteremia vary among institutions. Some institutions utilize quantitative analysis of blood culture results, whereas others utilize qualitative analysis of blood culture results. Quantitative analysis involves comparing the number of colony-forming units seen in blood drawn through the device to blood drawn through the periphery. Usually, a 5- to 10-fold increase in the number of colony-forming units from blood drawn from the device as compared with concomitant peripheral cultures (or in the absence of positive peripheral cultures, > 1,000 colony-forming units from blood drawn from the device) signifies device-related bacteremia.

Qualitative analysis involves comparing positivity and negativity of blood cultures drawn from both the device and the periphery. Usually, simultaneous positive blood cultures drawn from both the device and the periphery, along with clinical relevance, signifies device-related bacteremia.

Management If device-related bacteremia is suspected, appropriate systemic antibiotic coverage should be instituted after device and peripheral blood cultures are obtained. Antibiotic selection should be reassessed after organism identification and antibiotic sensitivities are available. Up to 70% of cases of device-related bacteremia can be successfully treated with a course of appropriate systemic antibiotics. The indications for device removal are the persistence of positive blood cultures after an appropriate course of systemic antibiotics, hypotension or severe systemic compromise, infections caused by *Candida* species, or recurrent infections caused by the same organism after successful systemic antibiotic therapy. (See chapter 46 on "Infectious Complications.")

Site infections

Site infections consist of subcutaneous catheter tunnel infections and subcutaneous port pocket infections. They can be superficial or deep. These infections are usually caused by gram-positive cocci (coagulase-negative staphylococci). Swelling, tenderness, and warmth over the site usually indicate a site infection. In the neutropenic patient, fever is often the only symptom. Swab culture of the skin exit site of the external catheter or the skin around the Huber access needle overlying the implanted port can sometimes identify the offending organism.

Management Local care at the skin exit site of the tunneled external catheter or removal of the Huber access needle from the subcutaneous implanted port and systemic antibiotics can be effective for most superficial site infections. Deep-seated subcutaneous catheter tunnel infections and subcutaneous port pocket infections may require device removal for successful eradication of the infection. Site infections caused by *Candida* species usually require device removal.

SUGGESTED READING

Abdullah BJ, Mohammad N, Sangkar JV, et al: Incidence of upper limb venous thrombosis associated with peripherally inserted central catheters (PICC). Br J Radiol 78:596–600, 2005.

Cheong K, Perry D, Karapetis C, et al: High rate of complications associated with peripherally inserted central venous catheters in patients with solid tumours. Intern Med J 34:234–238, 2004.

Couban S, Goodyear M, Burnell M, et al: Randomized placebo-controlled study of low-dose warfarin for the prevention of central venous catheter-associated thrombosis in patients with cancer. J Clin Oncol 23:4063–4069, 2005.

Estes JM, Rocconi R, Straughn JM, et al: Complications of indwelling venous access devices in patients with gynecologic malignancies. Gynecol Oncol 91:591–595, 2003.

Labourey JL, Lacroix P, Genet D, et al: Thrombotic complications of implanted central venous access devices: Prospective evaluation. Bull Cancer 91:431–436, 2004.

Magagnoli M, Masci G, Castagna L, et al: Prophylaxis of central venous catheter-related thrombosis with minidose warfarin: Analysis of its use in 427 cancer patients. Anticancer Res 25:3143–3147, 2005.

Povoski SP: External jugular vein cutdown approach for chronic indwelling central venous access in cancer patients: A potentially useful alternative. World J Surg Oncol 2:7, 2004.

Povoski SP, Zaman SA: Selective use of preoperative venous duplex ultrasound and intraoperative venography for central venous access device placement in cancer patients. Ann Surg Oncol 9:493–499, 2002.

Timoney JP, Malkin MG, Leone DM, et al: Safe and cost effective use of alteplase for the clearance of occluded central access devices. J Clin Oncol 20:1918–1922, 2002.

Verso M, Agnelli G, Bertoglio S, et al: Enoxaparin for the prevention of venous thromboembolism associated with central vein catheter: A double-blind, placebo-controlled, randomized study in cancer patients. J Clin Oncol 23:4057–4062, 2005.

CHAPTER 44

Prevention and management of radiation toxicity

Nicos Nicolaou, MD

RADIATION TOXICITY

The aim of radiation oncology is the achievement of uncomplicated locoregional control of malignancy by the use of radiation therapy (RT). Accomplishing this goal requires precise knowledge of tumoricidal and tolerance doses of the various normal tissues at risk within the RT field.

Types of RT injury

Radiation injuries can be divided into functional impairment and oncogenesis. There are also different phases of RT injury.

Early effects are usually seen during treatment or within the first few weeks after its completion. These reactions are common, can be significant and symptomatic, but eventually seem to heal completely. Nevertheless, despite what may appear to be total recovery, significant residual damage is often present.

Intermediate effects typically occur several weeks to months after the completion of RT.

Late effects are usually rare and are encountered many months to years after RT. Functional impairments may take a long time to become apparent; an example is memory problems in children who have received cranial irradiation. Oncogenesis is usually a late effect of RT.

Tolerance doses of radiation

Numerous studies have attempted to specify RT tolerance doses for the various tissues and structures of the body. The minimal tolerance dose (TD 5/5) and maximal tolerance dose (TD 50/5) refer to a severe complication rate of 5% and 50%, respectively, within 5 years of RT completion (Table 1). These tolerance doses have been valuable but were drastically revised recently because of the advent of combined-modality therapy (see section on "Combined chemotherapy and irradiation") and altered RT fractionation regimens.

Chemoradiosensitivity of normal tissues Cell-cycle kinetics, mitotic behavior, and differentiation determine the chemoradiosensitivity of normal tissues.

TABLE 1: Normal tissue tolerance to therapeutic irradiation

Organ	TD 5/5 volume[a]			TD 50/5 volume[a]			Selected endpoint
	1/3	2/3	3/3	1/3	2/3	3/3	
Kidneys	5,000	3,000[b]	2,300		4,000[b]	2,800	Clinical nephritis
Bladder		8,000	6,500		8,500	8,000	Symptomatic bladder contracture and volume loss
Bone							
Femoral head			5,200			6,500	Necrosis
TMJ	6,500	6,000	6,000	7,700	7,200	7,200	Marked limitation of joint function
Rib cage	5,000			6,500			Pathologic fracture
Skin			$100\ cm^2$ / 5,000			$100\ cm^2$ / 6,500	Telangiectasis
Skin	$10\ cm^2$ / 7,000	$30\ cm^2$ / 6,000	$100\ cm^2$ / 5,500			$100\ cm^2$ / 7,000	Necrosis/ulceration
Oral mucosa			$50\ cm^3$ / 6,000			$50\ cm^3$ / 7,500	Ulcer/fibrosis
Brain	6,000	5,000	4,500	7,500	6,500	6,000	Necrosis/infarction
Brainstem	6,000	5,300	5,000			6,500	Necrosis/infarction
Optic nerve			5,000			6,600	Blindness
Chiasma			5,000			6,500	Blindness
Spinal cord	5 cm / 5,000	10 cm / 5,000	20 cm / 4,700	5 cm / 7,000	10 cm / 7,000		Myelitis/necrosis
Cauda equina			6,000			7,500	Clinically apparent nerve damage
Brachial plexus	6,200	6,100	6,000	7,700	7,600	7,500	Clinically apparent nerve damage
Eyes (lens)			1,000			1,800	Cataract requiring intervention
Eyes (retina)			4,500			6,500	Blindness
Ears (middle/external)	3,000	3,000	3,000[b]	4,000	4,000	4,000[b]	Acute serous otitis
Ears (middle/external)	5,500	5,500	5,500[b]	6,500	6,500	6,500[b]	Chronic serous otitis

[a] There is insufficient information for recommendations where no values are provided. Clinical judgment and experience are used in these instances, and extrapolation from available information is made.

[b] < 50% of volume does not make a significant change.

Adapted from Emami B, Lyman J, Brown A, et al: Int J Radiat Oncol Biol Phys 21:109-122, 1991; Rubin P, Casarett GW: Clinical Radiation Pathology. Philadelphia, WB Saunders, 1968.

Organ	TD 5/5 volume[a] 1/3	2/3	3/3	TD 50/5 volume[a] 1/3	2/3	3/3	Selected endpoint
Parotid[b]		3,200[b]	3,200[b]		4,600[b]	4,600[b]	Xerostomia
Larynx	7,900[b]	7,000[b]	7,000[b]	9,000[b]	8,000[b]	8,000[b]	Cartilage necrosis
Larynx		4,500	4,500[b]			8,000[b]	Laryngeal edema
Lungs	4,500	3,000	1,750	6,500	4,000	2,450	Pneumonitis
Heart	6,000	4,500	4,000	7,000	5,500	5,000	Pericarditis
Esophagus	6,000	5,800	5,500	7,200	7,000	6,800	Clinical stricture/ perforation
Stomach	6,000	5,500	5,000	7,000	6,700	6,500	Ulceration/ perforation
Small intestine	5,000		4,000[b]	6,000		5,500	Obstruction/ perforation/fistula
Colon	5,500		4,500	6,500		5,500	Obstruction/ perforation/ ulceration/fistula
Rectum			6,000			8,000	Severe proctitis/ necrosis/fistula/ stenosis
Liver	5,000	3,500	3,000	5,500	4,500	4,000	Liver failure
Testes			± 500			2,000	Sterility
Ovaries			± 300			1,200	Sterility
Vagina			$\frac{5\ cm^3}{9{,}000}$			10,000	Ulcer/fistula
Pituitary			4,500				Hypopituitarism
Thyroid			4,500			7,000	Hypothyroidism
Muscle			5,000				Clinical myositis
Muscle			10,000				Atrophy
Cartilage (child)			1,000			3,000	Growth arrest
Bone (child)			$\frac{10\ cm^3}{2{,}000}$			$\frac{10\ cm^3}{2{,}000}$	Growth arrest

TMJ = temporomandibular joint

TD 5/5 (minimal tolerance dose) and TD 50/5 (maximal tolerance dose) refer to the RT doses required to produce a severe complication rate of 5% and 50%, respectively, within 5 years of RT completion. These RT dose values are used for guidance only and are not absolute. They are modified appropriately depending on the prevailing circumstances.

1/3, 2/3, and 3/3 refer to the approximate volume of organ that is irradiated.

The dividing cell is more vulnerable to RT than the quiescent cell, especially one that is functionally mature.

Dose-limiting organs and tissues have been divided into three classes according to their RT tolerance doses and importance to survival:

- Class I organs are those in which irreparable damage leads to death or severe morbidity.
- Class II organs are those in which damage is associated with moderate morbidity.
- Class III organs are those in which damage produces minimal morbidity.

Combined chemotherapy and irradiation

In combined-modality therapy, several temporal strategies with different rationales are utilized: concurrent RT and chemotherapy, local RT followed by chemotherapy, chemotherapy followed by local RT, and alternating chemotherapy and RT cycles.

POTENTIAL INTERACTIONS

When used in combination, RT and chemotherapy can act independently, with each mode acting in isolation in different parts of the body. The combined use of the two modalities can also result in increased or decreased therapeutic activity, as well as various possible adverse interactions:

- Damaging effects of RT on the target organ can be increased by chemotherapy. Some chemotherapeutic agents are RT enhancers or reactivators, which, when used concurrently with RT, can produce reactions in various tissues at much lower RT doses than expected.
- Damaging effects of chemotherapy on the target organ can be increased by RT.
- Independent injuries can be caused by the individual treatment modality in the same organ, which can combine to increase the resulting dysfunction. Subclinical residual injury from one treatment modality may be uncovered by the subsequent use of a seemingly safe dose of another modality.
- An injury can be produced that is not commonly seen with either modality alone.

The inherent difficulty in understanding these consequences is further complicated by the number of chemotherapeutic agents generally combined in treatment protocols and the variety of conventional or altered RT delivery techniques.

Quantification of treatment toxicity

In addition to therapeutic efficacy, quantification of RT toxicity is crucial for evaluating new regimens and selecting therapy for individual patients. The optimal therapeutic ratio requires not only complete tumor clearance but also minimal residual injury to surrounding vital normal tissues.

Morbidity scoring schemes developed by the Radiation Therapy Oncology Group (RTOG), European Organisation for Research and Treatment of Cancer (EORTC), and the National Cancer Institute (NCI) are used most commonly. The late effects of normal tissues (LENT) scoring system was adopted by the RTOG and EORTC in 1995. It graded toxicity according to four parameters, denoted by the acronym SOMA: subjective (symptoms reported), objective (signs on examination), management (instituted), and analytic (tissue function assessed by objective diagnostic tools).

In 1997, the NCI with other American (eg, RTOG) and international cooperative groups, the pharmaceutical industry, and the World Health Organization (WHO) revised and expanded the Common Toxicity Criteria (CTC) by integrating systemic agent, radiation, and surgical criteria into a comprehensive and standardized system. The CTC v. 2.0 replaced the previous NCI, CTC, and RTOG Acute Radiation Morbidity Scoring Criteria.

The third version of the CTC has been renamed Common Terminology Criteria for Adverse Events v. 3.0 (CTCAE v. 3.0). The purpose of renaming it was to move away from the term "toxicity," which implies causation and does not fit the jargon commonly used across all modalities. It is anticipated that after October 2003, all NCI-sponsored trials will use CTCAE v. 3.0, which represents the first comprehensive multimodality grading system to include both acute and late effects. The new system is designed for application to all modalities.

TOXIC EFFECTS AND THEIR MANAGEMENT

The incidence and severity of normal tissue toxicity from RT depend on a wide variety of factors, including total dose, fraction size, interval between fractions, quality and type of RT, dose rate, intrinsic radiosensitivity, and specific tissue irradiated. The most common toxic effects seen in different organ systems are outlined here and in Table 2, along with recommended treatments. Where appropriate, the specific effects of chemoradiation therapy are discussed separately.

Head and neck

ORAL MUCOSA

Acute effects Oral mucositis results from radiation-induced mitotic death of the basal cells of the oral mucosal epithelium. It appears about 2 weeks after

TABLE 2: Possible irradiation side effects and treatment

Organ	RT side effects	Treatment
Skin	Erythema and dry desquamation	Nonionic moisturizers (eg, Lotionsoft applied tid); topical 1% hydrocortisone cream or ointment applied tid prn, especially for pruritus; Aquaphor; TheraCare cream; vitamin A and E ointment or cream; Biafine, gentle washing; avoid skin irritants
	Moist desquamation	Normal saline compresses or modified Burow's solution soaks before applying creams; polymyxin B/neomycin cream applied tid; Nu-Gel protective wound dressings; antifungal agents for *Candida*, eg, ketoconazole cream; silver sulfadiazine, vitamin A and E ointment
	Ulceration/necrosis	Exclude and treat infections; normal saline compresses; modified Burow's solution soaks; polymyxin B/neomycin cream applied tid; debridement of necrotic tissue, vitamin E (1,000 IU/d) and pentoxifylline (400 mg PO bid-tid); flexible hydroactive dressings (eg, DuoDerm); debriding with fibrinolysin and desoxyribonuclease (eg, Elase)
	Chronic skin changes (eg, skin dryness)	Moisturizers; sun blocks
Oral and oropharyngeal mucosa	Mucositis	Saline/bicarbonate solution oral lavage qid; equal parts of topical viscous lidocaine/diphenhydramine/simethicone mixture for analgesia to swish in mouth or for gargling (5-10 mL qid prn); RadiaCare oral wound rinse; systemic analgesics prn; antifungals; ketoconazole (200 mg/d PO), itraconazole (100-200 mg /d PO), or fluconazole (100-200 mg/d PO) may be helpful; sucralfate suspension (1 g/10 mL), swish and swallow (10 mL PO qid), Gelclair
Esophagus	Esophagitis	Equal parts of topical viscous lidocaine/diphenhydramine/simethicone mixture for analgesia (5-10 mL PO qid); systemic analgesics prn; nasogastric, gastrostomy, or jejunostomy feeding tube; sucralfate, omeprazole, metoclopramide, or ranitidine sometimes useful, especially in the presence of GE reflux
Salivary glands	Sialadenitis/parotitis	Aspirin/NSAIDs
	Xerostomia	Sialogogues; pilocarpine (5 mg PO tid-qid), during and post RT; fluoride gel applications to prevent dental caries; artificial saliva (eg, Salivart, Moi-Stir); amifostine (200 mg/m^2 infused IV over 3 min before daily RT), to protect salivary glands (only in head and neck cancer patients receiving postresection adjuvant RT); Evoxac (30 mg PO tid)

Organ	RT side effects	Treatment
Salivary glands	Thick saliva	Papain enzyme, guaifenesin (Mucinex), and scopolamine patch
Ears	Otitis externa	Hydrocortisone/neomycin/polymyxin B ear drops tid
	Serous otitis media	Decongestants; myringotomy; phenylephrine otic solution
Mandible	Temporomandibular joint fibrosis	Daily stretching exercises
	Osteoradionecrosis	Complete any necessary dental work (especially extractions) before RT; hyperbaric oxygen; eliminate infection with antibiotics; pentoxifylline; perform sequestrectomy only if all else fails
Lungs	Radiation pneumonitis	Prednisone (30-60 mg/d PO for 2-3 weeks), with appropriate tapering
	Pulmonary fibrosis	Supportive measures (eg, oxygen/bronchodilators), pentoxifylline
Bladder	Acute cystitis	Phenazopyridine (100-200 mg PO tid prn), for dysuria; flavoxate hydrochloride (200 mg PO tid prn), for urinary frequency/urgency; oxybutynin chloride (5 mg PO tid prn), for frequency/urgency
Prostate	Obstructive urinary symptoms	Terazosin hydrochloride or doxazosin mesylate (1-2 mg/d PO); tamsulosin (0.4 mg/d PO); finasteride (5 mg/d PO)
Bowel	Diarrhea	Low-residue diet; loperamide or diphenoxylate (1-2 tabs PO qid prn); exclude *Clostridium difficile* infection; psyllium PO sometimes helpful; cholestyramine (4-8 g PO qid); octreotide (0.1 mg SC tid)
	Proctitis	Anusol-HC cream and Nupercainal ointment perianally or Anusol suppositories per rectum tid prn; psyllium PO sometimes helpful; glucocorticoid retention enemas (eg, Cortenema); mesalamine suppositories (eg, Rowasa); sulfasalazine
Breasts	Erythema and dry desquamation	Nonionic moisturizers (eg, Lotionsoft, TheraCare, Aquaphor applied tid); topical 1% hydrocortisone cream applied tid prn; Biafine; gentle washing; avoid skin irritants
	Moist desquamation	Normal saline compresses or modified Burow's solution soaks before application of creams; polymyxin B/neomycin cream applied tid; Nu-Gel or Telfa protective, nonadherent wound dressings; antifungal agents for *Candida;* silver sulfadiazine to prevent infections; vitamin A and E ointment to promote healing

Spielberger et al compared the effect of palifermin with placebo on the development of oral mucositis in 212 patients with hematologic cancers treated with fractionated total-body irradiation plus high-dose chemotherapy for autologous hematopoietic stem-cell transplantation. The incidence of oral mucositis of WHO grade 3 or 4 was 63% in the palifermin group (6 days' duration) and 98% in the placebo group (9 days' duration; $P < .001$). Compared with placebo, palifermin was associated with significant reductions in the incidence of grade 4 oral mucositis (20% vs 62%; $P < .001$), patient-reported soreness of the mouth and throat (area-under-the-curve score, 29.0 vs 46.8; $P < .001$), the use of opioid analgesics (median, 212 mg of morphine equivalents; $P < .001$), and the incidence of use of total parenteral nutrition (31% vs 55%; $P < .001$; *Spielberger R, Stiff P, Bensinger W, et al: N Engl J Med 351:2590-2598, 2004*).

initiation of RT and can progress from patchy to confluent mucositis.

Regular lavage of the oral cavity with bicarbonate of soda or normal saline solutions (mix 1 tsp of baking soda or 1 tsp of salt with 1 qt of water) is soothing, promotes oral hygiene, and restores normal oral pH. Topical anesthetic mixtures, such as viscous lidocaine, diphenhydramine, and simethicone (in equal parts) and RadiaCare oral wound rinse, may relieve oral discomfort.

Sucralfate suspension (1 g/10 mL) protects the oral mucosa by a coating action; a 10-mL oral dose should be swished and swallowed four times daily. This agent may have a prophylactic benefit and may also aid in the healing process. Fentanyl transdermal patches (Duragesic) or oral transmucosal fentanyl (Actiq) may be necessary for pain control to promote oral intake.

Candida species can colonize the damaged mucosa and exacerbate the mucositis. Oral candidiasis is treated with topical or systemic antifungal agents, such as nystatin (100,000–200,000 U PO qid); ketoconazole (Nizoral, 200 mg/d PO); fluconazole (Diflucan, 100–200 mg/d PO); clotrimazole troches dissolved orally bid-qid; and itraconazole (Sporanox, 100 mg PO bid).

Antibiotics are necessary when superimposed bacterial infection may be present; they may include clindamycin (Cleocin), penicillin V, ciprofloxacin (Cipro), or clarithromycin (Biaxin). Mucosal healing is complete within 2–3 weeks after completion of RT.

Late effects can be characterized by pallor and thinning of the oral mucosa with loss of pliability, submucosal ulceration, and necrosis with exposure of underlying bone and soft tissue. Few interventions are of value once chronic damage has occurred.

Soft-tissue necrosis may be painful and may require systemic or topical anesthetics, eg, viscous lidocaine mixed with equal parts of simethicone and diphenhydramine. Scrupulous hygiene is essential, and antibiotics are used when infection is present. Surgical intervention involves grafting of tissue. Hyperbaric oxygen may promote healing of soft-tissue necrosis.

Effects of chemoradiation therapy The acute ulceration of mucosal epithelium that results from chemoradiation therapy of the head and neck is most severe when both modalities are given simultaneously. Drugs that tend not to produce mucositis, such as cisplatin, are preferable. Percutaneous endoscopic gastrostomy (PEG) tubes are essential to administer nutrition, hydration, and medications during definitive chemoradiation therapy for head and neck malignancies.

Recombinant human keratinocyte growth factor (rHuKGF) effectively reduced the duration of severe oral mucositis in patients undergoing a preparative regimen of total-body irradiation, etoposide, and cyclophosphamide before autologous peripheral stem-cell transplantation (SCT) from 7.7 days to 4.0 days ($P = .001$).

SALIVARY GLANDS

Acute effects Tenderness and marked swelling of the salivary glands (sialadenitis/parotitis) may occur within a few hours after they are first irradiated and usually subside within a few days. These effects can be treated with aspirin or nonsteroidal anti-inflammatory drugs (NSAIDs).

Xerostomia Saliva becomes thickened and output decreases during RT, eventually leading to xerostomia. Commencing treatment with a salivary gland stimulant, such as pilocarpine tablets (Salagen, 5 mg PO tid-qid), maintains salivary output during irradiation and lessens morbidity. After completion of RT, pilocarpine stimulates the remaining salivary glands to increase saliva output.

Significant preservation of salivary gland function was found when oral pilocarpine was used concomitantly with curative RT in a phase III randomized study (RTOG 9709), compared with patients for whom pilocarpine was omitted during RT. This finding indicates a prophylactic effect on irradiated salivary glands by pilocarpine.

Amifostine (Ethyol) is now approved by the US Food and Drug Administration (FDA) as a salivary gland radioprotector in head and neck cancer patients who have undergone a complete resection of their cancer and will be receiving adjuvant RT that includes the parotid salivary glands. Amifostine (200 mg/m^2) is administered daily as a 3-minute IV infusion 15–30 minutes before standard RT (1.8–2.0 Gy) to reduce the incidence of moderate to severe xerostomia in patients in whom the radiation field includes the parotid glands.

Glyceride, baking soda, guaifenesin (Mucinex), scopolamine patch, and carbonated drinks may improve the acute problems caused by thickened saliva. Always ensure that patients being treated with RT are adequately hydrated. Dehydration makes saliva thicker and reduces output. Papain, the proteolytic enzyme found in papayas, helps dissolve thick saliva.

Chronic effects Xerostomia may persist for months to years, with recovery depending on the volume irradiated, the total RT dose, and individual patient variation. Xerostomia is treated with saliva substitutes and sialogogues, including water and glycerin preparations, commercially prepared "artificial saliva" (eg, Salivart, Xero-Lube, Moi-Stir), and salivary gland stimulants (eg, bromhexine and pilocarpine tablets).

> Cevimeline (Evoxac) is being assessed for efficacy and safety in the treatment of radiation therapy–induced xerostomia. It is presently FDA approved for Sjögren syndrome. The dose is 30 mg PO tid.

Daily pilocarpine (15–30 mg in divided doses) may be administered following RT to increase salivary output. Early improvement may be observed, but up to 12 weeks of uninterrupted therapy may be necessary to assess whether a beneficial response will be achieved.

TASTE BUDS

Some patients experience loss of food flavor during the acute mucosal reaction to RT, due to damage of the taste bud cells. These cells are capable of repopulating within 4 months after treatment, but some degree of permanent impairment may remain. Sour and bitter tastes are suppressed to a greater extent than are sweet and salty tastes. Xerostomia and mucositis also contribute to the dysgeusia.

EXTERNAL AND MIDDLE EAR

Inflammatory changes in the external auditory meatus and middle ear occur during RT or soon thereafter and may be manifested by pain, infection, or decreased hearing. Hydrocortisone/neomycin/polymyxin B ear drops or benzocaine/antipyrine/phenylephrine otic solution (Tympagesic) may be used for otitis externa. Decongestants and/or antihistamines, eg, pseudoephedrine/triprolidine, pseudoephedrine/guaifenesin, astemizole (Hismanal), and fexofenadine (Allegra), are useful for otitis media, but occasionally myringotomy is performed to relieve discomfort. Possible superimposed infections are treated also with oral antibiotics, eg, clarithromycin and amoxicillin/potassium clavulanate (Augmentin).

PHARYNX AND ESOPHAGUS

Pharyngitis and esophagitis with resultant dysphagia develop 2–3 weeks after RT commencement. Dysphagia usually resolves 2–3 weeks after the completion of irradiation (see also section on the esophagus in "Gastrointestinal system" later in this chapter).

Oral topical (see previous section on "Oral mucosa") or systemic analgesics are used to provide relief and enable adequate nutrition. Sucralfate suspension is useful as a mucosal protective coating agent and may promote healing. A nasogastric, gastrostomy, or jejunostomy tube may be necessary for nutritional support.

SKELETON AND SOFT TISSUES

Mandible Irradiation can diminish the ability of bone to withstand trauma and avoid infection, with resultant osteoradionecrosis (a hypovascular, hypocellular dissolution of bone). Important risk factors include poor nutrition and oral hygiene, trauma (especially dental extractions), continued tobacco and alcohol consumption, RT quality, total dose, overall duration, and frequency (daily vs bid). To decrease the risk of these adverse effects, any necessary dental work (especially extractions) should be performed at least 10 days prior to the initiation of RT.

Dental extractions performed after RT must be done judiciously, since they may initiate osteoradionecrosis. Hyperbaric oxygen may be useful prior to teeth extractions from heavily irradiated bones. It is also used to aid healing in established cases of osteoradionecrosis. Pentoxifylline improves blood flow.

Infection can expand the area of necrosis and cause severe pain. Antibiotics (eg, clarithromycin, ciprofloxacin, and amoxicillin/potassium clavulanate) are often necessary and require long-term administration. Sequestrectomy is performed only if all conservative measures have failed.

Okunieff et al studied the effects of pentoxifylline (400 mg po tid) on 30 patients with irradiation-induced fibrosis at 1 to 29 years after 40 to 84 Gy of radiotherapy. The primary outcome measurement was change in physical impairments secondary to irradiation, including active and passive range of motion (AROM and PROM), muscle strength, limb edema, pain, and plasma levels of tumor necrosis factor-alpha and fibroblast growth factor 2 (FGF2). After 8 weeks of pentoxifylline intervention, 20 of 23 patients with impaired AROM and 19 of 22 with impaired PROM improved; 11 of 19 patients with muscle weakness showed improved motor strength; 5 of 7 patients with edema had decreased limb girth; 9 of 20 patients had decreased pain. Pretreatment FGF2 levels dropped from an average of 44.9 pg/mL to 24.0 pg/mL after 8 weeks of treatment (*Okunieff P, Augustine E, Hicks, JE, et al: J Clin Oncol 22:2207-2213, 2004*).

Teeth Loss of adequate saliva for food lubrication and buffering of acids can lead to multiple problems, including dental caries. Optimal oral and periodontal hygiene must be maintained indefinitely. Daily topical fluoride applications, preferably a fluoride gel held in contact with the teeth by a tray, are extremely effective. Attempts should be made to replace or increase salivary flow (see previous section on "Salivary glands").

Temporomandibular joint (TMJ) Masticatory muscle and TMJ fibrosis can result in trismus. Stretching exercises may alleviate this problem. The Therabite jaw motion rehabilitation system provides anatomically correct motion of the jaw to patients experiencing hypomobility of the mandible. It consists of a mouthpiece and lever that exerts appropriate force to increase the interdental gap.

Soft tissues Soft-tissue necrosis is rare but may occur after insertion of an ill-fitting prosthesis or treatment with a high local dose of radiation, as is delivered by an interstitial implant. Conservative management includes oral hygiene, antibiotics, pentoxifylline, and hyperbaric oxygen.

Irradiation of the neck, by itself, produces little or no impairment of function but in the postoperative setting may exacerbate surgically induced limitations of head and neck motion by up to 20%. Physical therapy prevents contractures. Patients should stretch the affected area prophylactically several times a day. This practice is especially useful in preventing trismus.

LARYNX

Edema of the arytenoids may occur after a course of RT to the larynx. It may be managed conservatively by resting the voice and administering antibiotics and steroids. Pentoxifylline may also be tried. Edema persisting for more than 3 months following RT may be due to recurrent or persistent tumor.

HYPERBARIC OXYGEN THERAPY

Hyperbaric oxygen (HBO) has been used for more than half a century to treat associated late complications of irradiation. The European Society for Therapeutic Radiotherapy and Oncology and the European Committee for Hyperbaric Medicine organized a consensus conference in 2001 to deal with the indications of HBO for the treatment and prevention of late complications from irradiation. A systematic literature search was performed at the time. The review was updated recently to include the years 1960 and 2004. Hyperbaric oxygen treatment involving complications to the head and neck, pelvis, and nervous system and the prevention of complications after surgery in irradiated tissues was studied. Despite the small number of controlled trials, HBO was recommended for the treatment of mandibular osteoradionecrosis in combination with surgery and hemorrhagic cystitis resistant to conventional treatments. The most significant level of evidence seemed to be for the prevention of osteoradionecrosis after dental extractions.

Bui et al investigated the efficacy of HBO in 45 patients with late irradiation-induced side effects, most of whom had failed to respond to previous interventions. Improvement of principal presenting symptoms after HBO was noted in 75% of head and neck, 100% of pelvic, and 57% of "other" subjects (median duration of response was 62, 72, and 69 weeks, respectively). Bone and bladder symptoms were most likely to benefit from HBO (response rate, 81% and 83%, respectively). Half of subjects with soft-tissue necrosis or mucous membrane side effects improved with HBO. A low response rate was seen with salivary (11%), neurologic (17%), and upper gastrointestinal symptoms (22%). The incidence of relapse was low (22%), and minor HBO-related complications occurred in 31% of patients.

Komaki et al randomized two groups of 62 patients in total with inoperable nonmetastatic non–small-cell lung cancer: arm 1 and arm 2 received concurrent cisplatin-based chemotherapy and radiotherapy (RT), but arm 2 received amifostine (Ethyol) also. Amifostine reduced the severity and incidence of acute esophageal, pulmonary, and hematologic toxicity resulting from the chemotherapy and RT. Maximal esophageal toxicity was mild (grade 1) in 23%, moderate (grade 2) in 42%, and severe (grade 3/4) in 35% of patients in arm 1; the corresponding rates for arm 2 patients were 48%, 35%, and 16%, respectively (*P* = .021). Severe pneumonitis occurred in 16% of patients in arm 1 and in 0% of the arm 2 patients (*P* = .020, chi-square test). Neutropenic fever occurred in 39% of arm 1 patients and 16% of arm 2 patients (*P* = .046, chi-square test; *Komaki R, Lee JS, Milas L, et al: Int J Radiat Oncol Biol Phys 58:1369-1377, 2004*).

Lungs

Radiation pneumonitis When doses of thoracic RT exceed tolerance levels, pulmonary reactions are expressed clinically as a pneumonitic process 1–3 months after the completion of therapy. This process can prove lethal if both lungs are involved or if threshold doses of chemotherapeutic drugs have been exceeded. Recovery from acute pneumonitis usually occurs, and the second phase of fibrosis follows almost immediately, with eventual progression to the late fibrotic phase.

Acute symptoms include low-grade fever, congestion, cough, dyspnea, pleuritic chest pain, and hemoptysis. Evidence of consolidation may be found in the region corresponding to the pneumonitis. The acute pneumonitic phase is relatively short-lived but can be severe. Chest x-ray and CT show a diffuse infiltrate corresponding to the RT field.

Management Optimal management is clearly prevention. Corticosteroids can foster recovery from acute RT pneumonitis; a dose of 30–60 mg of prednisone is administered daily for 2–3 weeks and then tapered. Antibiotics for proven infection and supplemental oxygen may be necessary.

In recent phase III randomized trials of lung cancer patients treated with chemoradiation therapy, amifostine significantly reduced acute pneumonitis from 23% to 3.7% ($P = .037$), without any reduction in tumoricidal activity.

Pulmonary fibrosis develops insidiously in the previously irradiated field and stabilizes after 1–2 years, with most patients being asymptomatic. Symptoms are proportional to the extent of lung parenchyma involved and the preexisting pulmonary reserve and are generally minimal if fibrosis is limited to < 50% of one lung. If fibrosis exceeds this limit, dyspnea associated with progressive chronic cor pulmonale may become clinically manifest.

Radiologic changes consistent with fibrosis are usually seen. Retraction of the involved lung with elevation of the hemidiaphragm are the two predominant findings. CT scanning is currently favored for imaging this region. Pulmonary function tests may show mild deterioration as fibrosis develops. Significant changes are not seen when small volumes of lung tissue are irradiated, due to functional compensation from adjacent lung regions. Diffusion capacity studies provide the best assessment of whole lung function.

Management Radiation-induced fibrosis presently appears to be irreversible. Management consists of supportive measures, such as oxygen, bronchodilators (ie, albuterol), and ipratropium (Atrovent). Counseling on the risks of smoking is imperative. Pentoxifylline with vitamin E has recently been shown to cause regression of RT-induced fibrosis.

Effects of chemoradiation therapy The pneumonitis and fibrosis associated with RT can also be seen with several chemotherapeutic drugs, including bleomycin, methotrexate, mitomycin (Mutamycin), nitrosoureas, alkylating agents, and vinca alkaloids. Obviously, these agents can potentiate the damaging effects of RT on the lungs.

Cardiovascular system

PERICARDIAL DISEASE

Acute pericarditis is a rare complication of RT that usually follows irradiation of a radiosensitive mass contiguous to the heart. Signs and symptoms are similar to those of acute, nonspecific pericarditis and include chest pain, fever, and, often, electrocardiographic (ECG) abnormalities.

Pericardial effusion Chronic pericardial effusion may be asymptomatic or lead to cardiac tamponade, which must then be relieved by pericardiocentesis or pericardiectomy.

Pericardial constriction can occur as a final stage of either of the two pericardial syndromes or may develop insidiously without an obvious antecedent event.

MYOCARDIAL DISEASE

Pancarditis Patients treated with RT alone can develop cardiomyopathy and present with severe signs and symptoms of pericardial disease, along with constriction and severe heart failure. Pathologically, there are alterations in the pericardium and myocardium. This condition has been termed "pancarditis." Radiation myocardiofibrosis may occur to a minor degree in asymptomatic patients.

Radiation cardiomyopathy is uncommon with modern treatment techniques unless tolerance doses are exceeded. Simultaneous or sequential chemotherapy (especially with the anthracyclines) aggravates the condition. The interaction between the two modalities appears to be additive. Risk factors for anthracycline cardiotoxicity are other types of heart disease, such as valvular, coronary, or myocardial lesions and hypertension, as well as age > 70 years.

Management The best treatment is clearly prevention. In patients treated with RT and concomitant or sequential doxorubicin, downward adjustment of tolerance doses is appropriate. Dexrazoxane (Zinecard) is a cardioprotective agent used in the prevention and reduction of cardiotoxicity that can be associated with doxorubicin. Dexrazoxane has been shown to reduce doxorubicin-induced cardiomyopathy and allows administration of higher doses of doxorubicin in randomized trials. No evidence has shown an adverse effect of dexrazoxane on the antitumor activity of doxorubicin.

CORONARY ARTERY DISEASE

Radiation-induced coronary artery disease has the same clinical manifestations as are observed in patients who have not received RT. Treatment, including coronary artery bypass surgery, is also the same.

VALVULAR DEFECTS AND CONDUCTION ABNORMALITIES

Other cardiac problems attributed to RT include valvular defects (due to myocardial fibrosis adjacent to valves) and conduction abnormalities (due to ischemic fibrosis of the conduction system).

Skin

Acute effects The acute skin reaction occurs during the first 7–10 days following RT and begins with erythema, progressive pigmentation, epilation, and desquamation as the dose increases. Dry desquamation may then progress to moist desquamation, which usually heals by 50 days following RT; however, it may not heal completely and even may progress to necrosis.

Management Symptomatic treatment that controls pain, keeps the radiation field clean, and removes the crust suffices until epithelial remodeling and reepithelialization restore the skin to normal. Daily normal saline compresses or modified Burow's solution soaks are useful. Topical hydrocortisone creams and nonionic moisturizers, such as Lotionsoft, TheraCare, Biafine, and Aquaphor, are used to alleviate pruritus and the acute inflammatory response to irradiation, whereas antibiotic agents and silver sulfadiazine are prescribed to prevent infection in areas of moist desquamation.

Patients should be advised to wash their skin gently and dry it by dabbing. Irritating skin products should be avoided. Nu-Gel protective wound dressings can also be used; they provide a soothing sensation when cooled. Telfa nonadhesive pads are used to protect the wound. Vitamin A and E ointment or cream promotes healing. Silver sulfadiazine cream and antibiotic creams prevent infection.

Late effects occur many weeks following RT. A variable period during which the skin appears normal follows the acute reaction. Scaling, atrophy, telangiectasis, subcutaneous fibrosis, and necrosis can then develop and progress for long periods. Telangiectasis develops in an atrophic dermis under a thin epidermis as an area of reddish discoloration displaying multiple, prominent, thin-walled, dilated vessels. Fibrosis is characterized by progressive induration, edema, and thickening of the dermis and subcutaneous tissues and is most severe in areas where there was an earlier moist desquamation.

Management Permanent use of skin moisturizers may be necessary, and irradiated skin must always be protected from the sun. Medical management of chronic ulcers is directed at relieving symptoms and treating infections while attempting to promote healing. Surgical management consists of excision and grafting of the irradiated area. Laser treatment of telangiectasis improves cosmesis. Pentoxifylline (400 mg PO bid-tid) increases blood velocity and may promote healing. One clinical trial showed striking regression of chronic radiotherapy-induced fibrosis in patients after they were treated for at least 6 months with pentoxifylline (400 mg bid) and tocopherol (vitamin E), 1,000 IU/d.

Effects of chemoradiation therapy An additive response between chemotherapy and RT should be anticipated. An increased erythematous response is seen in breast cancer patients receiving combined therapy that includes methotrexate.

The most consistent aggravated skin responses occur in patients with anal, vulvar, or penile carcinoma who receive RT and fluorouracil (5-FU). The first reaction, which occurs following the initial infusion of 5-FU during the first week of RT, is mild. The acute moist reaction produced after the second infusion of 5-FU and the higher accumulated RT doses is more severe. It involves the entire field but heals after a few weeks. Similar reactions are noted in patients with head and neck cancer who receive chemoradiation therapy.

Central nervous system

BRAIN

Acute effects are rare during conventionally fractionated brain RT. Acute encephalopathic changes have been noted in conjunction with several cytotoxic agents, including cisplatin, asparaginase (Elspar), ifosfamide (Ifex), methotrexate, cytarabine (Ara-C), interferon, and interleukin-2 (IL-2 [Proleukin]). Clinical changes include alteration of mental status or level of consciousness, focal worsening of neurologic signs, and/or generalized seizures. These changes are commonly thought to be due to RT-induced edema and are usually treated adequately with concomitant corticosteroid administration.

Subacute or early delayed reactions Two types of subacute or early delayed reactions have been observed after RT.

Somnolence syndrome is noted 2–6 months after RT and is characterized by somnolence, anorexia, and irritability without accompanying focal neurologic abnormalities. The syndrome is usually transient (resolving within 2–5 weeks), associated with an uneventful recovery, and thought to be due to demyelination following a temporary inhibition of myelin synthesis. The somnolence syndrome is commonly seen after cranial RT for childhood acute lymphocytic leukemia (ALL). Similar transitory, self-limited changes of fatigue and/or exacerbation of focal neurologic signs are noted following full cranial or local RT for primary CNS tumors.

Focal neurologic signs seen after the treatment of CNS tumors may be related to intralesional reactions and are probably indicative of tumor response and/or perilesional reactions, such as edema or demyelination. These signs may be associated with imaging changes, such as focal enhancement, indicating areas of blood-brain barrier disruption and inhomogeneity in the white matter. New RT techniques appear to be frequently associated with subacute CNS reactions.

Clinical deterioration and MRI changes representing intralesional necrosis with diffuse pontine swelling have occurred in up to 40% of patients 1–6 months after hyperfractionated RT for brainstem gliomas. High-dose, volume-limited stereotactic radiosurgery is followed by transient white matter alterations, often apparent on MRI. These abnormalities generally begin ≥ 6 months after RT and are usually self-limited. Similar phenomena have been reported following interstitial brain implants.

Late effects Various late CNS effects have been described following RT.

Focal radiation necrosis Localized necrosis develops between 6 months and 2 years following irradiation. New anatomically related functional/irritative signs and symptoms are seen, associated with increasing intracranial pressure.

CT changes are usually confined to the high-dose volume and include low-density white matter changes with irregular enhancement, often associated with surrounding diffuse edema and a variable degree of mass effect. MRI shows similar local changes associated with more extensive areas of white matter alterations, including edema. Differentiating necrosis from tumor recurrence/progression is usually difficult. ^{18}F-fluorodeoxyglucose (FDG)-PET scans indicate hypometabolic findings.

Corticosteroids and surgical resection of focal areas of radiation necrosis can result in clinical improvement of neurologic deficits.

Postirradiation diffuse white matter injury Low-density changes diffusely involving one or both cerebral hemispheres may be evident within several months following full-brain RT. It is common to see white matter alterations extending peripherally beyond the high-dose RT volume.

MRI is more sensitive than CT to white matter changes and shows injury initially limited to periventricular white matter and later extending to include most of the rest of the cerebral white matter. Ventricular dilatation and cortical atrophy are seen with more severe white matter injury.

Symptoms vary widely from mild lassitude or personality changes to marked, incapacitating dementia. Progressive memory loss precedes frank dementia in cases with pronounced ipsilateral or diffuse bilateral changes.

Combined-therapy diffuse white matter injury/leukoencephalopathy In its milder forms, this syndrome is characterized by transient lassitude, dysarthria, or seizures temporally related to the administration of prophylactic cranial RT and methotrexate in children with ALL. The syndrome appears to be continuous, with more severe CNS damage (including progressive degrees of ataxia, confusion, and memory loss) ultimately leading to dementia or death. More recently, similar clinical events of varying severity have been noted 12–18 months after treatment in adults surviving intensive chemotherapy and prophylactic cranial irradiation (PCI) for small-cell lung carcinoma (SCLC).

Imaging findings are similar to those previously noted for postirradiation diffuse white matter injury. Dystrophic calcifications (mineralizing microangiopathy) are noted as late changes in leukoencephalopathy and are most often limited to the basal ganglia and gray-white matter interface.

Neuropsychologic effects Intellectual impairment has been reported increasingly among long-term cancer survivors. Cognitive changes in children are marked by memory deficits and learning disabilities. Memory deficits are apparent by 6 months, whereas a decline in global IQ is more often noted beyond 1–2 years after treatment. Neurocognitive impairment is most pronounced in children < 4–7 years old. Deterioration in IQ is statistically significant primarily in children following full-brain or supratentorial RT for primary CNS tumors.

Retrospective studies have reported neurotoxicity in approximately 19% of long-term survivors of SCLC who received PCI and chemotherapy. Problems include memory loss, confusion, dementia, ataxia, psychomotor retardation, and optic atrophy. Discernible intellectual decline is first seen at 4–6 months after therapy and becomes more pronounced 2–3 years later. These studies did not assess neuropsychologic function before RT was administered. Other studies that have assessed similar patients' neuropsychologic function before and after PCI have not found any evidence of neurotoxicity.

Cerebrovascular effects Arterial cerebrovasculopathy is an infrequent effect that occurs almost exclusively following RT to the parasellar region. Single- or multiple-vessel narrowing/obliteration results in deficits typical of stroke. Vasculopathy is usually related to RT for optic chiasmatic/hypothalamic gliomas in children.

Radiation-induced neurologic tumors Most RT-induced gliomas occur in patients who were irradiated as children and young adults. The 30-year cumulative risk for these tumors is about 0.8%.

SPINAL CORD

Transient radiation myelopathy has an incidence of approximately 15%, with a latency period of 1–29 months after RT, and is seen especially in patients who have received mantle-field RT for Hodgkin lymphoma. This syndrome is due to transient demyelination in the posterior columns and/or lateral spinothalamic tracts within the RT field.

Patients experience sudden electric-like shocks radiating from the spine to the extremities on neck flexion (Lhermitte's sign); these shocks are usually symmetric and unrelated to a specific dermatome. Neurologic examination is otherwise normal. The clinical picture reverses spontaneously after an average of about 5 months.

Delayed radiation myelopathy Patients present with a several-month history of progressive neurologic signs and symptoms, such as paresthesias and decreased pain and temperature sensation. A bimodal frequency distribution of latency has been reported, with peaks at 13 and 26 months, possibly corresponding to white matter parenchymal and vascular damage, respectively. Symptoms usually progress over 6 months and involve all spinal cord systems but may develop acutely following infarction of the spinal cord.

Temporary remissions have been reported following treatment with steroids or hyperbaric oxygen, but about 50% of patients die of secondary complications. Larger daily RT fractions, decreased number of treatments, treatment of larger lengths of spinal cord, and high total doses increase the risk of RT-induced myelopathy.

Effects of chemoradiation therapy Although experimental data are sparse, simultaneous administration of RT and chemotherapeutic agents known to be neurotoxic (eg, methotrexate, cisplatin, vinblastine, and cytarabine) may further reduce spinal cord tolerance. Intrathecal chemotherapy can produce myelopathy; thus, its use in combination with RT clearly must be approached with caution. Studies of hyperfractionated RT regimens have shown the spinal cord to be the dose-limiting organ. The interval between RT fractions should be at least 6 hours and preferably longer.

Eyes and adnexa

OCULAR ADNEXA AND ANTERIOR SEGMENT

Acute effects include transient skin erythema, conjunctivitis, epilation of hair follicles in the irradiated field, and chemosis. The cornea develops epithelial edema, leading to punctate epithelial keratopathy. Perilimbal injection may be seen with mild keratouveitis. Treatment involves artificial tear drops and topical steroids. Antibiotic eyedrops may be added to prevent or treat infection.

Late effects result in chronic structural changes, such as trichiasis, closure of eyelid puncta, and ectropion or entropion. Skin changes can progress in some areas to pallor, atrophy, telangiectasis, and loss of the eyelashes. Keratitis sicca (dry eye syndrome) may be caused by damage to the lacrimal, goblet, meibomian, and accessory lacrimal glands, which are essential to adequate tear film production. Epiphora may be due to excessive tearing from reflex aqueous production in response to keratitis sicca but may also herald closure of the nasolacrimal drainage system.

Management of epiphora is directed toward determining the cause of the chronic tearing and treating the underlying pathology. Keratitis is managed with aggressive lubrication (Celluvisc, Lacrilube, Lacinsent), eye patching, and antibiotic drops to prevent recurrent corneal erosions.

LENS

Radiation induces cataracts by damaging the germinal zone of the lens epithelium; this damage usually presents as subcapsular opacifications. The frequency, latency, and progression of lens opacities are a function of RT dose and fractionation. Prevention of damage with customized lens shields during RT is clearly the best management.

RETINA

Radiation-induced retinopathy is caused by an occlusive microangiopathy, which is manifested by cotton wool exudates, microaneurysms, telangiectasis, retinal hemorrhage, macular edema, proliferative neovascularization, vitreous hemorrhage, and pigmentary changes. Central retinal artery and vein occlusion has been described. Incomplete perfusion of the capillary bed, as shown by fluorescein angiography, is the most consistent finding. Visual symptoms depend on the retinal area that has been damaged. Radiation-induced and diabetic retinopathies are similar pathologically.

Argon panretinal photocoagulation has resulted in regression of fibrovascular neovascularization. Focal and grid macular treatment can stabilize the progression of visual loss in some patients with macular edema.

OPTIC NERVE

Radiation optic neuropathy (RON) presents as sudden, painless, monocular loss of vision. Visual-field abnormalities usually associated with RON include optic nerve fiber bundle defects and central scotomas.

Effective treatment for RON has not been identified. Prevention is most important and is accomplished by avoiding large single fractions in stereotactic radiosurgery and short intense schedules comprising large fractions.

SECONDARY NEOPLASMS

Children with heritable retinoblastoma have a cancer diathesis, and RT further increases this risk. The most common tumor occurring within the RT field is osteosarcoma of the facial bones. Other secondary neoplasms reported include soft-tissue sarcomas, brain tumors, leukemia, and melanoma.

Bladder, urethra, and ureter

Bladder injury may be either global or focal. Symptoms of global injury include urinary frequency, urgency, decrease in bladder capacity, and cystitis. Symptoms of focal injury include bleeding, ulceration, stone formation, and fistulas.

Acute RT cystitis presents with symptoms of dysuria and urinary frequency and urgency. The incidence varies widely, depending on factors related to radiation timing, dose, and volume. Acute symptoms subside within several weeks following RT.

Management is generally symptomatic. Phenazopyridine (Pyridium) is used as a topical analgesic for dysuria. Oxybutynin (Ditropan), an antispasmodic that relaxes bladder smooth muscle by inhibiting the muscarinic effects of acetylcholine, is useful in relieving symptoms of urinary frequency and urgency. Flavoxate (Urispas) and hyoscyamine counteract bladder muscle spasm.

Terazosin (Hytrin) and doxazosin (Cardura), both at 1–2 mg PO daily, may be used in prostate cancer patients who develop obstructive urinary symptoms during pelvic RT. Tamsulosin (Flomax) and finasteride (Proscar) are also used in these patients.

Late effects The interval between RT and the onset of late complications is several months to years, with a median of approximately 13–20 months. Most bladder complications occur within 2–3 years of therapy and include decreased bladder capacity, hematuria from telangiectasis, chronic irritative or obstructive urinary symptoms, and fistulas.

Urethral strictures occur more frequently when there is a history of transurethral resection of the prostate. Defects in urethral resistance are less common than strictures. Severe sphincteric insufficiency may be managed with periurethral injection of polytetrafluoroethylene collagen. Patient-controlled low pressure sphincters may be placed surgically. Urethral strictures are most often managed with simple endoscopic incision or open surgical repair.

Ureteral injury is rarely seen and is reported primarily following pelvic RT and chemotherapy. The length of the ureter irradiated, the presence of tumor, and surgical manipulation all affect tolerance of the ureter to RT.

Management The assessment and management of bladder dysfunction after RT, with or without chemotherapy, require adequate evaluation, including radiography and urodynamics to determine the precise cause of the dysfunction. Drugs to increase bladder storage include propantheline (Pro-Banthine), oxybutynin, and imipramine. Drugs to increase outlet resistance include ephedrine, pseudoephedrine, and phenylpropanolamine. Severe reductions in bladder capacity that do not respond to pharmacotherapy may be managed with bladder augmentation using a segment of intestine.

Severe hemorrhage caused by RT complications should be treated with cystoscopy and selective cauterization of bleeding sites, followed by irrigation with various agents, such as alum, silver nitrate, or dilute formalin.

Female reproductive system

VULVA

Acute effects Acutely, the vulva demonstrates erythema, which progresses to confluent moist desquamation that is radiation volume- and dose-dependent. The reaction is greatest in the intertriginous areas. Acute effects resolve 2–6 weeks after completion of RT. Skin edema of the vulva and mons pubis may develop 1–3 months after treatment. It is usually painless but can be severe and become chronic. Streptococcal lymphangitis may also develop.

Late effects develop 6–12 months following RT and include vulvar skin thinning, atrophy, dryness, pain, pruritus, and telangiectasis. Epilation is usually complete, and increased skin pigmentation may also develop. Fibrosis of the underlying subcutaneous tissues can result in dyspareunia if it involves the clitoris or vaginal introitus. Painful late ulceration with chronic serous drainage 1–2 years after RT may also occur.

Management The key to management of vulvar skin reactions is aggressive, individualized personal hygiene. Twice-daily sitz baths and gentle skin cleansing should be followed by complete drying of the vulvar region. The best method for drying the skin is a small fan or hair dryer (cool setting). This regimen should be closely followed until the skin is completely healed.

Topical steroid and antibiotic creams are applied for symptomatic relief and to prevent infection, respectively (see previous section on "Skin"). Whirlpool baths may be beneficial. Ulceration or necrosis requires debridement, which should continue until granulation tissue has formed. Myocutaneous flaps may be necessary.

Atrophic vulvar skin, once healed, may benefit from topical estrogen or testosterone creams. Daily dilatation to prevent fibrotic stenosis of the introitus may be necessary.

VAGINA

Acute effects Erythema, moist desquamation, confluent mucositis, severe congestion, and submucosal hemorrhage can be seen acutely and may resolve within 2–3 months after irradiation. Some patients demonstrate progressive vascular damage and ischemia, which result in epithelial sloughing, ulcer formation, and necrosis. These changes may require 4–8 months to heal.

Late effects include thinning and atrophy of the vaginal epithelium with development of telangiectasis. Reduced vaginal capacity due to fibrosis and decreased lubrication results in dyspareunia. Thin, filmy adhesions or synechiae develop and can become permanent, with fusion of the vaginal walls (agglutination) if not managed appropriately. Vaginal ulceration or necrosis may develop several months following RT.

Management Acute RT vaginitis is managed with vaginal douching (using a mixture of 1 part hydrogen peroxide to 10 parts water 2–3 times daily until resolution). Daily vaginal dilatation is required once the acute reaction has resolved, to prevent vaginal stenosis. Intravaginal estrogen cream appears to stimulate epithelial regeneration and may be used twice weekly to promote healing, prevent vaginal mucosal atrophy, and improve lubrication and elasticity.

Fistula formation may be treated with periodic debridement and antibiotics. Urinary and fecal diversion is sometimes required, with delayed reanastomosis and myocutaneous grafting for repair.

CERVIX AND UTERUS

Superficial ulceration of the cervix is an inevitable consequence of RT for carcinoma of the cervix that may persist for months, resulting in a thin, clear vaginal discharge.

Cervical os stenosis occurs 3–6 months following high-dose brachytherapy for cervical and endometrial carcinomas.

Rare complications Rarely, hematometra can develop due to residual functioning endometrium, which responds to hormonal stimulation. There is consequent retention of hemorrhagic debris because of obliteration of the endocervical canal or cervical os stenosis. True necrosis of the endometrial cavity also occurs rarely following RT for endometrial carcinoma. An uncommon complication of pelvic RT is development of high-grade endometrial carcinoma or uterine sarcoma many years after therapy.

Management Cervicitis, ulceration, and necrosis of the cervix are managed with douching (1 part hydrogen peroxide to 10 parts water 2–3 times daily until resolution) and debridement as necessary. Dilatation of the stenotic cervical os may be necessary to prevent hematometra or, in the case of uterine necrosis, to allow drainage of necrotic material.

OVARIES AND REPRODUCTIVE/ENDOCRINE FUNCTION

Hormonal changes Premenopausal women with intact ovaries exposed to sufficiently high RT doses experience premature menopause. In a North Central Cancer Treatment Group (NCCTG) randomized trial, venlafaxine (Effexor) was found to substantially reduce hot flashes in women with breast cancer experiencing menopausal symptoms and in whom estrogen and progesterone preparations were contraindicated.

Ovarian carcinoma following pelvic RT for carcinoma of the cervix is extremely uncommon.

Sexual dysfunction is a frequent occurrence following surgery, RT, and chemotherapy for pelvic malignancies and results in psychosexual problems.

Management The ovaries can be protected by moving them away from areas that are to be irradiated. A sexual function history should be obtained from all patients at 3 months after RT using one of the several available psychologic instruments. Interventions include improving personal hygiene, hormones, vaginal lubrication, and routine use of a vaginal dilator. Hormonal replacement is accomplished with oral conjugated estrogens or estradiol patches (Estraderm) and progesterone as necessary.

Male reproductive system

Testicular dysfunction following RT includes azoospermia, oligospermia, and hormonal changes. Recovery of sperm count may take months to years. Oligospermia occurs after low doses of RT. It may therefore be precipitated by exposure to scattered RT from other treatment sites, as well as by total-body RT used as a conditioning regimen for bone marrow transplantation (BMT). Sterility develops at higher RT doses. Erectile dysfunction is seen in patients receiving high RT doses to the pelvis, as for prostate cancer.

Management The best management is prevention by appropriate RT field tailoring and shielding. Sperm-banking should always be carried out if there are fertility concerns. Sildenafil (Viagra), vardenafil (Levitra), and tadalafil (Cialis) are available for impotent patients.

Gastrointestinal system

LIVER

Radiation- and chemotherapy-induced liver disease The chief hepatic toxicity of chemotherapy and RT is subacute, beginning 7–90 days after completion of therapy. There are many similarities between radiation-induced liver disease (RILD) and combined modality-induced liver disease (CMILD). Pathologically, the common lesion for both is veno-occlusive disease (VOD).

RILD occurs approximately 4–8 weeks after the completion of RT. Symptoms include fatigue, rapid weight gain, increased abdominal girth, and right upper quadrant discomfort. Patients are rarely jaundiced and may develop ascites and hepatomegaly with elevated alkaline phosphatase levels out of proportion to other hepatic enzymes. CT scan shows low density in the irradiated region of the liver.

CMILD differs from RILD in some respects, with the most distinctive differences being the faster onset of the former and the early expression of jaundice. Liver enzymes are mildly increased, and bilirubin levels are significantly elevated. As CMILD produces no distinctive changes on imaging studies, the diagnosis is one of exclusion.

CMILD is most commonly seen in the setting of allogeneic BMT, which requires aggressive preparative techniques involving administration of both high-dose chemotherapy and total-body RT. Patients present 1–4 weeks post transplantation with at least two of the following conditions: jaundice, weight gain, right upper quadrant pain, hepatomegaly, ascites, and encephalopathy.

Chronic RILD The liver usually heals after the subacute RT injury, but chronic fibrosis may develop depending on the degree of RT and chemotherapy injury. When fully expressed, the damage resembles finely nodular cirrhosis both pathologically and clinically. Irradiation to parts of the liver can cause localized fibrosis with no clinical sequelae of hepatic insufficiency if the consequent hypertrophy/hyperplasia of the untreated organ provides sufficient functional compensation.

Management No established therapies exist for RILD, although the use of anticoagulants and steroids has been suggested. The majority of patients with this syndrome also respond to conservative diuresis. There are also no established therapies for CMILD.

ESOPHAGUS

Acute effects Symptoms of gastroesophageal reflux with dysphagia develop approximately 2 weeks following initiation of RT. Early RT esophagitis is generally the dose-limiting reaction in aggressive multimodality therapy, as is used for esophageal and lung cancers. Decreased mucosal thickness may progress to frank ulceration, which may heal with fibrosis and cause benign strictures. In phase III randomized trials, amifostine significantly decreased severe esophagitis in lung cancer patients treated with chemoradiation therapy from 26.0% to 6.5% ($P = .038$).

Analgesics, topical anesthetics (see previous section on "Oral mucosa"), sucralfate, H_2-receptor blockers (ranitidine, cimetidine, famotidine), omeprazole (Prilosec), metoclopramide, or antacids are used for symptomatic relief. Sucralfate slurry may also be used prophylactically, before and after RT daily to reduce the severity of esophagitis, and may promote healing (see also the pharynx and esophagus section under "Head and neck ").

Late effects Formation of benign strictures and changes in motility secondary to muscle and/or nerve damage cause chronic dysphagia. Strictures develop a median of 6 months after RT and generally are not seen before 3 months. Strictures are dilated with Maloney or Savory dilators. Prokinetic drugs, such as metoclopramide, can lessen gastroesophageal reflux by increasing lower esophageal sphincter pressure and the rate of gastric emptying. Cisapride (Propulsid) also increases GI motility.

Effects of chemoradiation therapy Cisplatin, 5-FU, dactinomycin (Cosmegen), doxorubicin, bleomycin, and methotrexate can augment the acute effects of RT on the esophagus, but the effect of these agents on late complications is not yet well established.

STOMACH

Acute effects Acute nausea and vomiting can occur shortly after the daily delivery of RT. Gastric secretions are suppressed acutely but recover later. Erosive and ulcerative gastritis can develop 2–3 weeks after RT begins but is generally transient and abates rapidly after the completion of RT.

Use of antiemetics (eg, ondansetron [Zofran], metoclopramide, prochlorperazine, granisetron [Kytril], dronabinol [Marinol], lorazepam, and chlorpromazine) and a decrease in the RT daily dose per fraction may ameliorate acute nausea and vomiting. Antiemetics begun within an hour before RT delivery may prevent the nausea and vomiting that may occur shortly after such therapy.

Late effects of irradiation on the stomach include the following conditions:

Dyspepsia arises at 6 months after RT (range, 2–20 months) as vague gastric symptoms.

Gastritis develops at 12 months after RT (range, 1–48 months) and is accompanied by radiologic evidence of spasm or stenosis of the antrum. The pathologic basis is fibrosis of the submucosal tissue, leading to mucosal fold smoothening and atrophy.

Ulceration typically arises at 5 months after RT (range, 1–72 months). Radiation-induced ulcers are indistinguishable from peptic ulcers. Spontaneous healing may occur but can be accompanied by submucosal fibrosis, which can produce antral fibrosis. Progressive stomach contracture results in early satiety, anorexia, and weight loss.

Ulcer with perforation may develop at 2 months after RT (range, 1–30 months).

Late RT toxicities have been treated with H_2-receptor antagonists and sucralfate. Surgery (eg, partial gastrectomy) is utilized for perforation, bleeding, or gastric outlet obstruction.

SMALL AND LARGE INTESTINES

The tolerance of the small and large intestines is a major dose-limiting factor in the treatment of many cancers of the abdomen and pelvis.

Acute effects Nausea, vomiting, early satiety, anorexia, and fatigue are frequent acute effects. Nausea and vomiting may develop shortly after RT delivery, necessitating the use of prophylactic antiemetics. Acute proctocolitis in patients undergoing pelvic RT is extremely common, manifesting clinically as watery bowel movements with rectal urgency and tenesmus. Patients receiving RT following low anterior resection experience frequent small stools since the rectal vault capacity is markedly diminished. Hematochezia occurs infrequently and is often due to hemorrhoidal irritation.

Radiation enteritis develops if significant volumes of small bowel are irradiated. Symptoms appear 2–3 weeks after the initiation of RT, and the enteritis increases in severity until several days after treatment is discontinued. Loose to watery diarrhea with voluminous frequent stools and cramping abdominal pain are characteristic of fully developed enteritis.

Management Diarrhea is treated with a low-residue diet and loperamide or diphenoxylate, 1–2 tablets PO qid prn. Psyllium is sometimes helpful, as is cholestyramine (Questran, Prevalite). *Clostridium difficile* infection should be ruled out. Octreotide (Sandostatin; a long-acting analog of somatostatin) at 0.1 mg SC tid was compared with diphenoxylate in a randomized trial and was found to be more effective in controlling diarrhea induced by pelvic irradiation.

Similarly, proctitis may be treated according to the prevailing problem. Anusol-HC cream or Anusol suppositories are effective for alleviation of local symptoms of proctitis, such as tenesmus. Oral sucralfate may promote healing of proctitis. Mesalamine suppositories and glucocorticoid retention enemas may be used for unresponsive proctitis and sulfasalazine for associated bleeding. (For management of nausea and vomiting, see previous section on "Stomach.")

Late small bowel effects The median onset of late small bowel RT effects is 1–5 years following the completion of RT and may be hastened by concomitant chemotherapy. Obstruction, the most common late effect, is preceded by sporadic or gradually increasing episodes of acute colicky abdominal discomfort. Perforation presents with an acute abdomen. Occasionally, late bowel damage is manifested by massive bleeding. Radiographic findings include fibrosis and ischemia. Spasm is seen, with altered bowel transit times, ulceration, thickened folds, narrowed bowel segments, and marked mesenteric adhesions.

Malabsorption is a common sequela of the late changes of RT and can include bile salt wasting from extensive ileal involvement. Stasis predisposes to bacterial overgrowth. Enterocolonic fistulae can also cause massive intraluminal bacterial overgrowth with severe steatorrhea and vitamin B_{12} deficiency.

Late large bowel injury becomes manifest earlier than late injury to the small bowel (within 2 years of treatment; median, 6–18 months). Fistulae occur more often in the rectum than elsewhere in the gut and are confined almost exclusively to cases in which brachytherapy was used for gynecologic cancer. They usually occur along the anterior rectal wall posterior to the vaginal fornix.

Other chronic symptoms include strictures, tenesmus, bleeding, cramps, obstipation, diarrhea, and rectal urgency; surgical intervention is sometimes necessary if these symptoms become severe enough. Radiographically, the most frequent appearance of large bowel injury is a smooth, elongated narrowing. Alternatively, submucosal changes can give the appearance of a nodular or thumbprinting effect on the large bowel wall. Mesenteric shortening can produce retraction of the transverse colon.

Ulceration is frequent and sometimes simulates diverticulitis. Bleeding can occur from sites of ulceration and telangiectasis.

Management Mild cases of chronic RT injury to the small and large intestines can be managed by a low-residue diet, stool softeners, psyllium, loperamide, or diphenoxylate. Fiber laxatives give a firmer consistency to the stool and soften it. Cholestyramine can improve diarrhea due to small bowel injury by binding bile salts that are irritative to irradiated bowel. Bleeding from sites of ulceration and telangiectasis can be treated by endoscopic laser therapy. Patients with malabsorption may benefit from pancreatic enzymes (eg, Pancrease) or lactase enzymes (eg, LactAid). Flatulence may be treated with simethicone. Pentoxifylline increases blood velocity and may promote healing. Again, mesalamine suppositories and glucocorticoid enemas may be helpful, as may sulfasalazine.

Surgical management for late bowel complications is controversial. Some investigators favor an aggressive approach, with lysis of all adhesions to free up the full length of the small bowel and resection of all severely involved segments. Others advocate a much more conservative approach of bypassing injured bowel by the simplest procedure possible.

Effects of chemoradiation therapy Dactinomycin or concurrent doxorubicin enhances the risk of late intestinal complications. Bolus infusion of 5-FU, which is included in most chemoradiation therapy regimens, has not been shown to increase the risk of late intestinal complications. High-dose infusional 5-FU, however, may enhance the risk of late intestinal complications.

Thyroid

HYPOTHYROIDISM

Primary hypothyroidism may be seen in patients who have received therapeutic RT doses to the cervical area. Subclinical hypothyroidism is the most common finding, with clinical hypothyroidism seen less frequently. The cumulative risk of developing overt or subclinical hypothyroidism is approximately 50%, and half of this risk manifests within 5 years of therapy. The use of iodinated radiographic contrast agents prior to RT, especially the ethiodized oil emulsion used in lymphangiography in Hodgkin lymphoma and other lymphomas, has been proposed as a contributing factor.

Hypothyroidism has been documented after irradiation to the craniospinal axis for CNS tumors, after total-body RT for BMT, and after RT for Hodgkin lymphoma or head and neck malignancies.

Hypothyroidism may develop as the result of thyrotropin (thyroid-stimulating hormone [TSH]) deficiency or hypothalamic injury following RT for pituitary adenomas, brain tumors, or head and neck cancers. Thyrotropin deficiency may be the sole manifestation of pituitary injury or may be accompanied by loss of corticotropin, gonadotropins, and growth hormone.

HYPERTHYROIDISM

Thyrotoxicosis (Graves' disease) may also develop after external irradiation of the thyroid, as seen in patients with Hodgkin lymphoma. These patients develop hypothyroidism after several months.

THYROID ENLARGEMENT, NODULARITY, AND DEVELOPMENT OF NEOPLASMS

Hashimoto's thyroiditis has been observed after RT of the thyroid in patients with Hodgkin lymphoma. Persistently elevated TSH levels result in hyperstimulation of the thyroid gland with development of nodules (adenomas or carcinomas). The actuarial risk of developing thyroid cancer after RT has been reported to be 1.7, as compared with an expected risk of 0.07% in the normal population matched for age and sex. The relative risk of developing thyroid cancer after RT for Hodgkin lymphoma is approximately 15.6 (95% confidence interval [CI], 6.3–32.5), and the absolute risk is 33.9 cases per 100,000 person-years.

Management Serum TSH levels and free thyroxine (FT_4) should be determined annually, and levothyroxine sodium should be prescribed for subclinical hypothyroidism. Cancer risk may also be reduced by limiting the effects of TSH on RT-damaged thyroid follicles. (For further discussion of thyroid nodules and thyroid carcinomas, see chapter 5.)

Hematopoietic stem-cell compartment

Acute effects Lymphopenia occurs almost immediately after RT because lymphocytes are exquisitely sensitive and die in interphase. Neutropenia occurs in the first week after irradiation of large volumes of bone marrow, followed by thrombocytopenia in 2–3 weeks and anemia in 2–3 months.

A rapid depletion of vital stem cells occurs within 1 week following appropriate total-body doses. The microvasculature usually survives the conventional doses used for total-body RT and allows the implantation and proliferation of transferred stem cells, resulting in recovery. Acute effects are not usually seen unless a substantial portion of bone marrow is treated. RT is usually not commenced if the absolute neutrophil count is $< 1.5 \times 10^3/\mu L$, with the platelet count $< 75 \times 10^3/\mu L$. A hemoglobin value of 10 g/dL is desirable during RT. Adequate oxygenation increases tumor radiosensitivity.

Permanent ablation or hypoplasia The capacity of the unexposed bone marrow to compensate by accelerating its rate of hematopoiesis is sufficient when the RT field involves < 10%–15% of the bone marrow. When 25%–50% of bone marrow is irradiated, permanent ablation or hypoplasia also occurs at similar dose levels as for small fields. The unirradiated marrow becomes hyperactive to meet the demands for hematopoiesis.

When 50%–75% of the bone marrow is irradiated, hematopoietic activity increases in the unexposed marrow segments, followed by extension of functioning marrow into previously quiescent areas. Although hematopoietic stem cells are exquisitely radiosensitive, it is damage to the bone marrow stroma that primarily accounts for chronic RT injury. Irreversible injury after RT is a consequence of irreparable damage to the microvasculature, manifested by irrevocable bone marrow fibrosis.

Management Treatments for bone marrow injury include transfusions of erythrocytes, platelets, and possibly granulocytes in patients who have severe neutropenia (< 200/μL) and documented infections that have not responded to appropriate antibiotics. Administration of growth factors is a common supportive measure in patients with RBC or WBC deficiencies. Epoetin alfa (Epogen, Procrit) has been used for anemia, granulocyte colony-stimulating factor (G-CSF, filgrastim [Neupogen]) has been used for neutropenia, and oprelvekin (Neumega) has been given for thrombocytopenia. The American Society of Hematology (ASH) and the American Society of Clinical Oncology (ASCO) recommend epoetin alfa for anemia, with hemoglobin levels < 10 g/dL, related to cancer treatment. The use of epoetin alfa for anemia (10–12 g/dL) should be determined by clinical circumstances. Darbepoetin alfa (Aranesp) is longer acting, allowing less frequent dosing. Peripheral blood stem-cell transfusions are effectively used as an alternative to autologous BMT. Allogeneic BMT is an obvious approach to restoring marrow function in patients with chronic marrow failure.

Effects of chemoradiation therapy When RT and chemotherapy are administered concurrently and sufficient time is allowed for recovery of peripheral blood cell counts (1–2 months), the increased marrow toxicity of the second modality reflects the irreparable damage caused by the first modality. The potential effects of chemoradiation therapy are much more complicated when both modalities are used simultaneously.

Bone

Inhibition or impairment of skeletal growth is an important dose-limiting toxicity of ionizing radiation, especially in children. Few attempts have been made to quantify RT-related growth arrest or to develop consistent methods for assessing its impact on function and cosmesis. Consequently, the impact of various treatments and the influence of clinical interventions once complications have developed have been difficult to evaluate.

Axial skeletal growth arrest may be terminated by irradiation, resulting in disproportionate sitting and standing heights.

Scoliosis can be caused by partial RT of vertebral bodies, soft-tissue asymmetry caused by surgery, and RT-induced hypoplasia of the rib cage and pelvis. Failure to correct leg-length discrepancies can also cause back problems, including scoliosis.

Slipped capital femoral epiphysis has also been reported as a complication of hip RT in children.

Abnormalities of craniofacial growth can cause significant cosmetic and functional deformities.

Management Careful RT technique to exclude the epiphyseal growth plates can minimize the risk of serious late effects. Early intervention can prevent secondary progressive injury and improve the functional result of treatment in the fully grown individual.

Mild asymptomatic scoliosis may be treated conservatively. Physical therapy and exercise programs can be helpful. In cases of severe back pain and spinal curvatures – 20°, braces may improve support. Surgical intervention with placement of a Harrington rod is recommended only for severe cases.

Appropriate shoe lifts can correct leg-length discrepancies. Prompt recognition of capital femoral epiphysis slippage is extremely important. Surgical treatment typically consists of pinning, but severe cases may require osteotomy and osteoplasty.

Nerves and muscles

PERIPHERAL NERVES

Peripheral nerve damage from RT is rare, but latency is important in its evaluation. Peripheral nerve damage has been seen following intraoperative RT and appears to be the dose-limiting toxicity in many cases. Cranial nerve injury is not usually seen.

Brachial plexopathy increases in incidence when large daily RT doses are used and is sometimes reported after axillary RT (eg, for breast cancer). Breast cancer patients who have received chemotherapy have a higher incidence of brachial plexopathy than those receiving RT only.

Sacral plexus injuries after RT for carcinoma of the cervix have also been reported occasionally.

MUSCLES

Late complications include limb contracture, edema, decreased range of motion, pain, and decreased muscle strength. They may be of minor or severe functional importance. Latency is important in the evaluation of muscle injury since progression may continue for as long as 10 years after RT. Chemotherapy does not seem to have a major impact on the incidence of late soft-tissue injury but does increase the rate of acute reactions.

Management is aimed at decreasing the size of the RT field, thereby sparing more functional healthy tissue, as long as cure is not compromised. Vigorous physical therapy and rehabilitation during and especially after RT are important. Muscle relaxants, eg, cyclobenzaprine (Flexeril), and anxiolytics, such as lorazepam, are useful for muscle spasms. Pentoxifylline may be tried to improve blood flow velocity and promote healing.

Neuroendocrinologic system

Growth hormone deficiency, the most common RT-induced endocrine disturbance, is most evident in the growing child as a reduction in growth velocity. In the postpubertal individual, growth hormone deficiency is associated with a relative decrease in muscle mass and an increase in adipose tissue.

Gonadotropin deficiency Young children may fail to enter puberty, and females may experience primary amenorrhea. Adult deficiency may be associated with infertility, sexual dysfunction, and decreased libido.

Early sexual maturation Precocious puberty may be seen in patients who have received cranial RT.

TSH deficiency Excessive weight gain and lethargy can be seen with complete TSH deficiency of long duration. Children may have poor linear growth and delayed puberty.

Adrenocorticotropic deficiency and hyperprolactinemia may also be seen.

Kidneys

A number of overlapping clinical syndromes are recognized, depending on the renal volume irradiated and the RT dose delivered.

Radiation nephropathy Acute radiation nephropathy (up to 6 months) following RT is rarely symptomatic; the glomerular filtration rate may be decreased. Signs and symptoms in the subacute period (6–12 months) include dyspnea on exertion, headaches, ankle edema, lassitude, anemia, hypertension, elevated blood urea levels, and urinary abnormalities. Benign or malignant hypertension is seen in the chronic period (generally after 18 months), depending on the severity of renal damage.

Chronic radiation nephropathy, in its mildest forms, may not be diagnosed for many years after RT. The only abnormalities may be proteinuria and azotemia with urinary casts or mild hypertension. A contracted kidney is seen on IV pyelography. Death may occur from chronic uremia or left ventricular failure, pulmonary edema, pleural effusion, and hepatic congestion.

Other syndromes More recently, hyper-reninemic hypertension has been described following unilateral renal RT, as has the nephrotic syndrome.

Management Hypertension and peripheral and pulmonary edema should be treated actively with appropriate medications, and anemia should be corrected. Renal tubular function may show some recovery. Dialysis and transplantation are sometimes necessary.

Effects of chemoradiation therapy Combined-modality treatment appears to intensify RT-induced renal changes.

SUGGESTED READING

Benson AB III, Ajani JA, Catalano RB, et al: Recommended guidelines for the treatment of cancer treatment-induced diarrhea. J Clin Oncol 22:2918–2926, 2004.

Brizel DM, Wasserman TH, Henke M, et al: Phase III randomized trial of amifostine as a radioprotector in head and neck cancer. J Clin Oncol 18:3339–3345, 2000.

Epstein JB, Schubert MM: Oropharyngeal mucositis in cancer therapy. Oncology 17:1767–1779, 2003.

Komaki R, Lee JS, Milas L, et al: Effects of amifostine on acute toxicity from concurrent chemotherapy and radiotherapy for inoperable non-small cell lung cancer: Report of a randomized comparative trial. Int J Radiat Oncol Biol Phys 58:1369–1377, 2004.

Okunieff P, Augustine E, Hicks JE, et al: Pentoxifylline in the treatment of radiation-induced fibrosis. J Clin Oncol 22:2207–2213, 2004.

Pasquier D, Hoelscher T, Schmutz J, et al: Hyperbaric oxygen therapy in the treatment of radiation induced lesions in normal tissues: A literature review. Radiother Oncol 72:1–13, 2004.

Rubin P, Constine LS, Fajardo LF, et al: Late effects of normal tissues (LENT) scoring system. Int J Radiat Oncol Biol Phys 31:1041–1042, 1995.

Schuchter LM, Hensley ML, Meropol NJ, et al: 2002 Update of recommendations for the use of chemotherapy and radiotherapy protectants: Clinical Practice Guidelines of the American Society of Clinical Oncology. J Clin Oncol 20:2895–2903, 2002.

Trotti A, Byhardt R, Stetz J, et al: Common toxicity criteria: Version 2.0: An improved reference for grading the acute effects of cancer treatment: Impact on radiotherapy. Int J Radiat Oncol Biol Phys 47:13–47, 2000.

Trotti A, Colevas AD, Setser A, et al: CTCAE v3.0: Development of a comprehensive grading system for the adverse effects of cancer treatment. Semin Radiat Oncol 13:176–181, 2003.

Yarbro JW, Mastrangelo MJ, Curran WJ: The Fourth International Cytoprotection Investigators Congress. Semin Oncol 31(suppl 18), 2004.

CHAPTER 45

Oncologic emergencies and paraneoplastic syndromes

Carmen P. Escalante, MD, Ellen Manzullo, MD, and Mitchell Weiss, MD,

SUPERIOR VENA CAVA SYNDROME

Superior vena cava syndrome (SVCS) is a common occurrence in cancer patients and can lead to life-threatening complications such as cerebral or laryngeal edema. Although most commonly resulting from external compression of the vena cava by a tumor, SVCS can also stem from nonmalignant causes in cancer patients.

EMERGENCIES

Etiology

Malignant causes

Primary intrathoracic malignancies are the cause of SVCS in approximately 87%–97% of cases. The most frequent malignancy associated with the syndrome is lung cancer, followed by lymphomas and solid tumors that metastasize to the mediastinum.

Lung cancer SVCS develops in approximately 3%–15% of patients with bronchogenic carcinoma, and it is four times more likely to occur in patients with right- vs left-sided lesions.

Metastatic disease Breast and testicular cancers are the most common metastatic malignancies causing SVCS, accounting for > 7% of cases. Metastatic disease to the thorax is responsible for SVCS in ~3%–20% of patients.

Nonmalignant causes

Thrombosis The most common nonmalignant cause of SVCS in cancer patients is thrombosis secondary to venous access devices (see chapter 43).

Other nonmalignant causes include cystic hygroma, substernal thyroid goiter, benign teratoma, dermoid cyst, thymoma, tuberculosis, histoplasmosis, actinomycosis, syphilis, pyogenic infections, radiation therapy, silicosis, and sarcoidosis. Some cases are idiopathic.

Signs and symptoms

Classic symptoms Patients with SVCS most often present with complaints of facial edema or erythema, dyspnea, cough, orthopnea, or arm and neck edema. These classic symptoms are seen most commonly in patients with complete obstruction, as opposed to those with mildly obstructive disease.

Other associated symptoms may include hoarseness, dysphagia, headaches, dizziness, syncope, lethargy, and chest pain. The symptoms may be worsened by positional changes, particularly bending forward, stooping, or lying down.

Common physical findings The most common physical findings include edema of the face, neck, or arms; dilatation of the veins of the upper body; and plethora or cyanosis of the face. Periorbital edema may be prominent.

Other physical findings include laryngeal or glossal edema, mental status changes, and pleural effusion (more commonly on the right side).

Diagnosis

It is important to establish the diagnosis and underlying etiology of SVCS, since some malignancies may be more amenable to specific treatment regimens than others. In the majority of cases, the diagnosis of SVCS is evident based on clinical examination alone.

The following diagnostic procedures may aid in establishing the diagnosis of SVCS and its etiology: chest x-ray, bronchoscopy, limited thoracotomy or thoracoscopy, contrast and radionuclide venography, Doppler ultrasonography, CT (especially contrast-enhanced spiral CT), and MRI.

Prognosis

The prognosis of SVCS depends on the etiology of the underlying obstruction. A review by Schraufnagel showed the average overall survival after the onset of SVCS to be 10 months, but there was wide variation (± 25 months) depending on the underlying disease, with an average survival of 7.6 months. This duration was not significantly different from the survival duration of 12.2 months in patients presenting with SVCS as the primary manifestation of the disease. Thoracic malignancy, the most common cause of SVCS, had a poor prognosis of < 5 months.

Treatment

Treatment includes radiotherapy, chemotherapy, thrombolytic therapy and anticoagulation, expandable wire stents, balloon angioplasty, and surgical bypass.

Most patients derive sufficient relief from obstructive symptoms when treated with medical adjuncts, such as diuretics and steroids (see section on "Adjunctive medical therapy"), so they can tolerate a work-up to determine the etiology of SVCS. In some instances, it is appropriate to delay treatment for 1–2 days if necessary to establish a firm tissue diagnosis.

Radiotherapy and chemotherapy

Both radiotherapy and chemotherapy are treatment options for SVCS, depending on the tumor type. The specific drugs and doses used are those active against the underlying malignancy.

Life-threatening symptoms, such as respiratory distress, are indications for urgent radiotherapy. A preliminary determination of the treatment goal (potentially curative or palliative only) is necessary prior to the initiation of treatment, even in the emergent setting.

Radiation therapy is the standard treatment of non–small-cell lung cancer (NSCLC) with SVCS. Recent studies suggest that chemotherapy may be as effective as radiotherapy in rapidly shrinking SCLC. Chemoradiation therapy may result in improved ultimate local control over chemotherapy alone in SCLC and non-Hodgkin lymphoma. Retrospective reviews of patients with SCLC have reported equivalent survival in patients with or without SVCS treated definitively with chemoradiation therapy.

Reasonable palliative courses can range from 2,000 cGy in 1 week to 4,000 cGy in 4 weeks. Curative regimens can range from 3,500 to 6,600 cGy based on histology. If indicated, more rapid palliation may be achieved by delivering daily doses of 400 cGy up to a dose of 800–1,200 cGy, after which the remainder of the appropriate total dose can be given in more standard daily fractions of 180 to 200 cGy. Some European investigators have used doses as high as 600 cGy 1 week apart in elderly patients.

Anticoagulation and thrombolysis

Anticoagulation for SVCS has become increasingly important due to thrombosis related to intravascular devices. In certain situations, the device remains in place. Both streptokinase and urokinase have been used for thrombolysis, although urokinase has been more effective in lysing clots in this setting. Urokinase is given as a 4,400-U/kg bolus followed by 4,400 U/kg/h, whereas streptokinase is administered as a 250,000-U bolus followed by 100,000 U/h. The use of thrombolytic therapy is controversial for catheter-related thrombosis, however.

Stenting

Placement of an expandable wire stent across the stenotic portion of the vena cava is an appropriate therapy for palliation of SVCS symptoms when other therapeutic modalities cannot be used or are ineffective. Use of stents is limited when intraluminal thrombosis is present.

Other interventional treatments

Balloon angioplasty and surgical bypass have also been used in appropriate patients but are rarely indicated. Balloon angioplasty may be considered in

The Institut Catala d'Oncologia in Barcelona, Spain, published its results using endovascular stent insertion for the treatment of malignant superior vena cava syndrome. Stenting was performed in all 52 patients with lung cancer. Phlebographic resolution of the obstruction was achieved in 100% of cases, and symptomatic improvement was achieved in more than 80% of patients. There was one major complication due to bleeding during anticoagulation. Reobstruction of the stent occurred in 17% of cases, mostly due to disease progression. Improvement of the obstruction allowed for delivery of full-dose systemic therapy for patients for whom this approach was indicated (*Urruticoechea A, Mesia R, Dominguez J, et al: Lung Cancer 43:209-214, 2004*).

patients with SVCS, significant clinical symptoms, and critical superior vena cava obstruction demonstrated by angiography. Surgical bypass is usually limited to patients with benign disease; however, for a select group of patients with SVCS, bypass may be an important aspect of palliative treatment. Other palliative efforts may be considered prior to bypass in this patient population.

Adjunctive medical therapy

Medications that may be used as adjuncts to the treatments described above include diuretics and steroids.

Diuretics may provide symptomatic relief of edema that is often immediate although transient. The use of diuretics is not a definitive treatment, and resulting complications may ensue, such as dehydration and decreased blood flow. Loop diuretics, such as furosemide, are often used. Dosage depends on the patient's volume status and renal function.

Steroids may be useful in the presence of respiratory compromise. They are also thought to be helpful in blocking the inflammatory reaction associated with irradiation.

Dosage depends on the severity of clinical symptoms. For severe and significant respiratory symptoms, hydrocortisone, 100–500 mg IV, may be administered initially. Lower doses every 6–8 hours may be continued. Tapering of the steroid dosage should begin as soon as the patient's condition has stabilized. Prophylactic gastric protection is advised during steroid administration.

VENOUS THROMBOEMBOLIC COMPLICATIONS OF CANCER

Deep vein thrombosis (DVT) and pulmonary embolism (PE) are common and potentially serious clinical challenges. In the United States, the estimated incidence of DVT and PE is approximately 450,000 and 355,000 cases per year, respectively. The actual incidence is likely much higher than presently documented due to often vague complaints and symptoms. PE may be associated with increased mortality and contributes to approximately 240,000 deaths annually in the United States.

Armand Trousseau noted the association between thrombosis and cancer more than 125 years ago. The risk of venous thromboembolism (VTE) in cancer patients depends upon the type and extent of the malignancy, the type of cancer treatment, the existence and nature of comorbidities, and changes in hemostasis of the blood, which have been noted in more than 90% of cancer patients. The prevalence of clinically noted venous thrombosis in cancer patients is 15%; patients undergoing surgery, hormonal therapy, and chemotherapy have the highest risk. Venous thrombosis is the second leading cause of death in cancer patients.

Etiology of VTE in cancer patients

The etiology of VTE in cancer patients may be attributed to several factors, including hypercoagulable states, surgical interventions, chemotherapy, indwelling central venous catheters, and prolonged immobilization.

The mechanisms by which tumors cause a hypercoagulable state are not completely understood, but they may be attributed to abnormalities of blood composition (increased plasma levels of clotting factors, cancer procoagulant A, tissue factor, and cytokines) and increased release of plasminogen activator. Postoperative VTE was more common in patients with malignant disease (36%) than in those patients with benign disease (20%), according to recent analyses of several clinical trials in surgical patients.

Patients undergoing chemotherapy are at increased risk of venous thrombosis secondary to endothelial cell damage from drug toxicity. In the recent ATAC (Arimidex, Tamoxifen, Alone or in Combination) trial, the aromatase inhibitor anastrozole (Arimidex) was compared with tamoxifen for 5 years in 9,366 postmenopausal women with localized breast cancer. Forty-eight patients (1.6%) receiving anastrozole developed DVT events, compared with 74 patients (2.4%) in the tamoxifen arm ($P = .02$). Anastrozole was associated with significant reductions in DVT events and should be considered for initial treatment in this population.

Indwelling central venous catheters predispose patients to upper extremity thrombosis and thrombosis of the axillary/subclavian vein. The catheters are also prone to occlusion. Increased venous stasis owing to immobility also promotes blood pooling into the intramuscular venous sinuses of the calf and may lead to thrombosis formation.

TUMOR TYPE ASSOCIATED WITH VTE

Several tumor types have been associated with higher rates of VTE, including those arising from the pancreas, lungs, and other mucin-secreting tumors. In general, tumor types associated with an increased incidence of thromboembolic events reflect the frequency of the tumors in the general population: In women, the most common tumors are breast, lung, gynecologic, and GI tumors; in men, prostate, lung, and GI tumors are most common.

Treatment

Several classes of agents have been used for prevention and treatment of VTE. Nonpharmacologic approaches to prophylaxis may include intermittent pneumatic compression, elastic stockings, and inferior vena cava filters. Commonly used pharmacologic agents for thromboprophylaxis and treatment of VTE include unfractionated heparin (UFH; standard, low-dose, or adjusted-dose), oral anticoagulants such as warfarin, and low molecular weight heparin (LMWH).

Initial treatment of DVT and PE includes inpatient UFH or LMWH and, more recently, outpatient LMWH for low-risk patients with DVT. (Although patients with PE have been treated with LMWH as outpatients, it is not the standard of care in the United States.)

UFH generally is administered as a bolus of 5,000 U followed by a continuous drip, usually initiated between 750–1,000 U/h. A baseline partial thromboplastin time (PTT) and prothrombin time (PT) are drawn prior to the initiation of treatment. PTT is then rechecked approximately 4–6 hours after treatment is begun, and the UFH is titrated to approximately 1.5 to 2 times control in most patients. Warfarin is usually begun on day 1 or 2 of treatment; therapy is monitored to maintain an international normalized ratio (INR) between 2.0 and 3.0. (Patients with prosthetic valves require a higher INR.) It is standard practice to maintain UFH for 4–5 days while the warfarin is titrated to therapeutic levels. Most patients are maintained on warfarin for 3–6 months depending upon underlying risk factors. There is controversy regarding the duration of anticoagulation, and some investigators maintain that patients with active cancer should continue anticoagulation for as long as the cancer remains active. Patients with recurrent VTE are usually maintained on anticoagulants for the rest of their lives.

Patient response to warfarin depends on numerous factors, such as age, diet, alcohol consumption, and liver and GI function, as well as concomitant medications.

Recent studies have demonstrated the safety and efficacy of LMWH in the treatment and management of VTE. Several studies have demonstrated no appreciable differences in recurrent thromboembolism and an increased risk of bleeding with UFH and LMWHs. Because LMWHs do not require a continuous drip and frequent serum testing, some low-risk patients are now treated as outpatients. Studies are ongoing in the cancer patient population.

In the United States, enoxaparin (Lovenox) has received US Food and Drug Administration (FDA) approval for prevention and treatment of DVT. Tinzaparin (Innohep) also has FDA approval for the treatment of DVT. Dalteparin (Fragmin), another LMWH agent indicated for prophylaxis, has been approved by the FDA for cardiac use.

LMWH doses vary by product and are not equivalent. Enoxaparin is generally administered twice a day for treatment of VTE, whereas the indications for tinzaparin and dalteparin are for once-daily dosing. The commonly administered dose for treatment of DVT with enoxaparin is 1 mg/kg SC (subcutaneous) every 12 hours. Tinzaparin is given via SC injection at a dose of 175 IU/kg body weight once daily, and the dalteparin dose is 200 IU/kg SC once daily. Therapy with LMWH is continued for a minimum of 5 days. Generally, laboratory monitoring is unnecessary, although for individuals with renal insufficiency or those with < 50 kg body weight or obesity, plasma antifactor Xa concentrations may need to be monitored.

In an international study comparing the long-term treatment benefits of dalteparin vs warfarin in cancer patients with VTE, long-term dalteparin substantially reduced the rate of recurrent VTE, compared with warfarin therapy, without an increase in bleeding.

DIFFICULTIES IN ANTICOAGULATION

Often, therapeutic challenges arise in patients on anticoagulation therapy for VTE who require surgical interventions and, therefore, temporary discontinuation of their anticoagulation treatment.

Preoperative guidelines The timing of discontinuation of anticoagulation depends upon the type of treatment and the surgical intervention planned. For patients on continuous-drip heparin, the drip may be discontinued 4–6 hours prior to the procedure. A PTT (partial thromboplastin time) should be drawn prior to the procedure to check for total reversal of the treatment. In cases where only partial reversal is noted or an emergency arises, fresh frozen plasma may be administered for rapid reversal.

Patients on warfarin may be advised to discontinue their medication 2–3 days prior to the planned procedure. This approach allows for a gradual reduction in the anticoagulation effect. An INR should be checked prior to the procedure. If partial reversal is noted or an emergency arises, vitamin K and/or fresh frozen plasma may be administered for acute reversal.

Postoperative guidelines Timing of postoperative therapy depends on the type of procedure undertaken and its associated risk of bleeding. Direct communication between the surgeon and the physician managing the anticoagulation treatment is necessary. When the surgeon believes that the risk of bleeding is at an acceptable level, anticoagulation should be restarted. It may be prudent to utilize UFH or LMWH prior to the initiation of warfarin, especially if a substantial risk of bleeding remains.

High-risk patients For high-risk patients (prosthetic valve, recurrent VTE), it may be reasonable to switch from warfarin to either UFH or LMWH, with appropriate discontinuation prior to the procedure. Both UFH and LMWH have shorter reversal times than does warfarin, although LMWHs are not fully reversible. Another option is to continue warfarin until shortly before the procedure, reversing treatment with vitamin K and/or fresh frozen plasma. The risk/benefit ratio should be considered when reviewing the options for the individual patient.

Surgery has long been known to be a risk factor for VTE. The nature of surgery in part determines the relative risk: Patients undergoing orthopedic surgery are at a particularly high risk. The risk is modified by the presence of other factors, such as underlying malignancy, age, obesity, and history of previous thromboembolism. Recent meta-analyses of clinical trials have shown there is a high overall risk of DVT during general surgery, based on rates observed in control subjects; there is a confirmed incidence of DVT of 25% noted by the fibrinogen uptake test. The risk is even higher (29%) in surgical patients with malignancy. Risk is also increased in those individuals with multiple risk factors (eg, age > 65 years, obesity, bed rest > 5 days). A comparison of commonly used prophylaxis in 160 clinical trials indicates that overall, low-dose UFH and LMWH are the most effective agents in reducing the incidence of DVT after general surgery. A higher dosage of the prophylactic agent may be needed for adequate prevention in patients with malignant disease.

Treatment alternatives for recurrence There are several treatment options for patients with recurrent VTE. Patients who develop recurrence of thrombosis while on therapeutic doses of anticoagulation should be considered for inferior vena cava filter placement. The filter will not prevent new clots from forming, but it does provide a physical barrier to prevent propagation of clots to the pulmonary bed. Alternatively, an inferior vena cava filter can be placed to avoid the need for long-term anticoagulant therapy if there are contraindications to anticoagulation. Or, another LMWH may be utilized prior to placement of an inferior vena cava filter, since there may be other complications related to filter placement (ie, postphlebitis syndrome, clotting of the filter).

Depending upon patient prognosis and tumor factors, other comorbidities, and propensity for bleeding, continued therapy with warfarin or LMWH may also be considered in addition to filter placement.

SPINAL CORD COMPRESSION

Spinal cord compression develops in 1%–5% of patients with systemic cancer. It should be considered an emergency, as treatment delays may result in irreversible paralysis and loss of bowel and bladder function.

Etiology

Compression of the spinal cord is due predominantly to extradural metastases (95%) and usually results from tumor involvement of the vertebral column. A tumor may occasionally metastasize to the epidural space without bony involvement.

Site of involvement The segment most often involved is the thoracic spine (70%), followed by the lumbosacral (20%) and cervical spine (10%).

Most common malignancies Spinal cord compression occurs in a variety of malignancies; the most common are lung, breast, unknown primary, prostate, and renal cancers.

Signs and symptoms

Early signs More than 90% of patients present with pain localized to the spine or radicular in nature (ie, not due to bony involvement but rather to neural compression). Pain, which is usually secondary to bony involvement, is often exacerbated with movement, recumbency, coughing, sneezing, or straining. The majority of patients experience pain for weeks to months before neurologic symptoms appear.

Intermediate signs If cord compression goes untreated, weakness often develops next. It may be preceded or accompanied by sensory loss.

Late signs Symptoms of autonomic dysfunction, urinary retention, and constipation are late findings. Once autonomic, motor, or sensory findings appear, spinal cord compression usually progresses rapidly and may result in irreversible paralysis in hours to days if untreated.

Physical findings may include tenderness to palpation or percussion over the involved spine, pain in the distribution of the involved nerve root, muscle weakness, spasticity, abnormal muscle stretch reflexes and extensor plantar responses, and sensory loss. Sensory loss occurs below the involved cord segment and indicates the site of compression. In patients with autonomic dysfunction, physical findings include a palpable bladder or diminished rectal tone.

Diagnosis

The first step in the diagnosis of spinal cord compression is an accurate neurologic history and examination.

X-rays More than 66% of patients with spinal cord compression have bony abnormalities on plain radiographs of the spine. Findings include erosion and loss of pedicles, partial or complete collapse of vertebral bodies, and paraspinous soft-tissue masses. Normal spine films are not helpful for excluding epidural metastases.

MRI The standard for diagnosing and localizing epidural cord compression is MRI. Gadolinium-enhanced MRI has been especially helpful in assessing cord compression secondary to spinal epidural abscesses, as gadolinium enhances actively inflamed tissues and defines anatomic boundaries. An abnormal signal within the disk space suggests the possibility of infection.

Primary or secondary neoplasms involving the vertebral bodies generally demonstrate a long T1, resulting in decreased signal intensity on a T1-weighted image, and a long T2, with increased signal intensity on the T2-weighted image.

CT and myelography If MRI is unavailable, a CT scan and/or myelogram may be used to diagnose and localize epidural cord compression.

Prognosis

Treatment outcome correlates with the degree and duration of neurologic impairment prior to therapy. In a prospective analysis of 209 patients treated for spinal cord compression with radiotherapy and steroids, Maranzano and Latini reported that of patients who were ambulatory, nonambulatory, or paraplegic prior to treatment, 98%, 60%, and 11%, respectively, were able to ambulate following therapy. Treatment outcome in the most radiosensitive malignancies (eg, lymphoma) was superior to that in the less sensitive cancers (renal cell carcinoma). Almost all ambulatory patients treated with either irradiation alone or laminectomy followed by postoperative irradiation remained ambulatory after treatment, whereas ~ 10% of patients whose lower extremities were paralyzed could walk after treatment.

Treatment

The goals of treatment of spinal cord compression are recovery and maintenance of normal neurologic function, local tumor control, stabilization of the spine, and pain control. Choice of treatment depends on clinical presentation, availability of histologic diagnosis, rapidity of the clinical course, type of malignancy, site of spinal involvement, stability of the spine, and previous treatment.

In general, radiation therapy has been the treatment of choice for these patients. This is based upon the belief that radiotherapy is as effective as surgery in terms of pain relief and maintaining neurologic function. In other words, the potential complications and convalescence associated with surgery can be avoided in this group of patients with a limited life expectancy.

This approach has been further investigated in a randomized clinical trial recently reported by Patchell et al. A total of 101 patients with spinal cord compression caused by metastatic cancer were randomized to undergo either surgery followed by adjuvant radiation therapy (n = 50) or radiation therapy alone (n = 51). Radiotherapy for both groups consisted of 10 fractions of 300 cGy each. The primary endpoint was the ability to walk.

The study was stopped after an interim analysis of the 101 patients revealed that 42 of 50 patients (84%) in the surgery group were able to walk after treatment, compared with 29 of 51 patients (57%) in the radiotherapy group ($P = .001$). Additionally, patients treated with surgery retained the ability to walk significantly longer than those patients treated with radiation therapy alone (median, 122 days vs 13 days; $P = .003$). Of the 32 patients who entered the trial unable to walk, 10 of 16 (62%) in the surgery arm regained the ability to walk, compared with 3 of 16 (19%) in the radiotherapy arm ($P = .01$). Based on the results of this trial, decompressive surgery followed by adjuvant radiation therapy should be considered in the treatment of patients with spinal cord compression.

The ability to regain ambulatory function after surgery had been recognized prior to this study. This finding represented the rationale for strong consideration of surgery in this group of patients. The authors advocated the wider use of surgery in most patients with spinal cord compression. Still, there are reasons to consider radiotherapy alone as appropriate initial treatment. They include the disappointing results in the radiotherapy-alone arm in this study compared with the experiences of previous studies and the possible reluctance to consider spinal surgery by patients and/or physicians (based upon limited life expectancy). These issues should, of course, be thoroughly reviewed during the process of informed consent.

Steroids

Dexamethasone should be administered if the patient's history and neurologic examination suggest spinal cord compression. There is controversy as to whether an initial high dose of IV dexamethasone (100 mg) followed by 10 mg of dexamethasone every 6 hours is necessary. Some studies have suggested lower doses are just as effective.

> The University Hospital Hamburg reported its prospective evaluation of 10 vs 20 fractions of radiation therapy for metastatic spinal cord compression. A total of 214 patients were irradiated with 30 Gy in 10 fractions (n=110) or 40 Gy in 20 fractions (n=104). Motor function improved in 43% of patients treated with 30 Gy and in 41% of patients treated with 40 Gy (P = .799). There was no significant difference in post-treatment ambulatory rates (60% and 64%, respectively; P = .708). As expected, being ambulatory prior to the initiation of treatment was associated with better functional outcome after irradiation (P = .035). Acute toxicity was mild, and no late toxicity was observed during the 12-month follow-up (*Rades D, Fehlauer F, Stalpers LJ, et al: Cancer 101:2687-2692, 2004*).

Radiation therapy

Radiation therapy alone is still usually the standard initial treatment for most patients with spinal cord compression due to a radiosensitive malignancy. Treatment outcome is contingent upon both the relative radiosensitivity of the malignancy and the neurologic status of the patient at the time radiotherapy is initiated.

Radiation portal In general, the treatment volume should include the area of epidural compression (as determined by MRI or myelography) plus two vertebral bodies above and below. Consideration should be given to including adjacent areas of abnormalities if feasible. Careful matching techniques should be employed in patients treated to adjacent vertebral levels, a situation that is not uncommon.

Radiation dose and fractionation The chosen regimen should take into account such factors as field size and normal tissue tolerance. Smaller fields are appropriately treated to 2,000–3,000 cGy over 1 or 2 weeks, respectively. Larger fields may occasionally necessitate longer courses, such as 4,000 cGy over 4 weeks, to minimize side effects.

Recently, the University Hospital Hamburg has reported their results on five fractionation schemes of radiation therapy for spinal cord compression. In this retrospective review, 1,304 patients were treated from January 1992 through December 2003. Radiation schedules included 1 x 8 Gy (n = 261), 5 x 4 Gy (n = 279), 10 x 3 Gy (n = 274), 15 x 2.5 Gy (n = 233), and 20 x 2 Gy (n = 257). Improvement in motor function was noted in 26% (1 x 8 Gy), 28% (5 x 4 Gy), 27% (10 x 3 Gy), 31% (15 x 2.5 Gy), and 28% (20 x 2 Gy). Motor function improvement and post-treatment ambulatory rates were not significantly different throughout all groups.

On multivariate analysis, age, performance status, pretreatment ambulatory status, and length of time motor deficits were present prior to the initiation of radiotherapy were all significantly associated with improved functional outcome, whereas the schedule of radiation therapy was not a significant indicator. Recurrence rates at 2 years were 24%, 26%, 14%, 9%, and 7%, respectively. There was mild acute toxicity and no late toxicity. The authors concluded that shorter fractionation schemes should be considered for those patients with poor predicted survival.

TABLE 1: Symptoms associated with hypercalcemia by organ system

General	CNS	Cardiac	GI	Renal
Dehydration	Weakness	Bradycardia	Nausea and vomiting	Polyuria
Anorexia	Hypotonia	Short QT interval	Constipation	Nephrocalcinosis
Pruritus	Proximal myopathy	Prolonged PR interval	Ileus	–
Weight loss	Mental status changes	Wide T wave	Pancreatitis	–
Fatigue	Seizure Coma	Atrial or ventricular arrhythmia	Dyspepsia	–

Retreatment may be entertained, particularly when no effective alternative exists. Usually, doses of 2,000 cGy over 2 weeks can be used for retreatment. It is important, however, to counsel the patient regarding the risk of radiation neuropathy. Furthermore, only those patients who had a lasting response to the initial treatment should be reirradiated, as tumors that were refractory to the first course or that recur within 3 months are unlikely to respond to subsequent courses.

Surgery

Vertebral body resection for a tumor anterior to the cord and posterior laminectomy for a tumor posterior to the cord may be appropriate treatment options for relieving spinal cord compression in patients who require spinal stability, have undergone previous radiotherapy in the area of the compression, require a tissue diagnosis of malignancy, or experience progression of the cord compression despite optimal treatment with steroids and irradiation.

In general, surgical decompression should be strongly considered in patients whose cord compression is caused by a relatively radioresistant cancer and who have a severe neurologic deficit (such as bowel or bladder dysfunction). Unfortunately, many patients in this situation are not candidates for aggressive surgery. In these cases, radiotherapy is offered, albeit with limited expectations for neurologic recovery.

Chemotherapy

Chemotherapy may be an effective treatment of spinal cord compression in select patients with a chemosensitive metastatic tumor. It also may be considered in combination with other treatment modalities, such as radiotherapy, or as an alternative if those modalities are not suitable options for relieving spinal cord compression.

HYPERCALCEMIA

Hypercalcemia is the most common metabolic emergency seen in individuals with cancer, occurring in an estimated 10%–20% of patients.

Etiology

The malignancies most commonly associated with hypercalcemia include myeloma, lung cancer (epidermoid tumors more often than small-cell tumors), and renal cancer. In some cases, the pathogenesis of hypercalcemia may relate to the release of parathyroidlike hormones, prostaglandins, and osteoclast-activating factor.

Signs and symptoms

Symptoms of hypercalcemia may involve various organ systems, including the central nervous, cardiac, GI, and renal systems (Table 1).

Bony metastasis vs paraneoplastic syndrome The signs and symptoms of hypercalcemia secondary to bony metastases are often indistinguishable from those of hypercalcemia as a paraneoplastic syndrome. The laboratory findings may vary. A tumor secreting an immunoreactive parathyroid hormone (iPTH)-like substance will have increased levels of cyclic adenosine monophosphate (cAMP), low levels of serum phosphorus, and variable levels of iPTH, depending on the specificity of the assay. Many patients with bony metastases also exhibit features consistent with "ectopic" hyperparathyroidism.

Diagnosis

An accurate history and physical examination are often the most helpful diagnostic tools to exclude correctable nonmalignant causes of hypercalcemia. Hypercalcemia in association with occult malignancies is rare. The presence of weight loss, fatigue, or muscle weakness should increase clinical suspicion of malignancy as the cause of hypercalcemia.

Laboratory findings In patients with hypercalcemia of malignancy, serum iPTH levels, determined by a double-antibody method, are extremely low or undetectable; levels of inorganic phosphorus are low or normal; and levels of 1,25-dihydroxyvitamin D are low or normal.

Use of additional tests to identify the underlying malignancy responsible for the hypercalcemia often depends on the history and physical findings.

Treatment

Asymptomatic patients with minimally elevated calcium levels (< 12.0 mg/dL) may be treated as outpatients, with close monitoring of calcium levels and symptoms. Encouragement of oral hydration, mobilization, and elimination of drugs that contribute to hypercalcemia are essential. Patients who are symptomatic

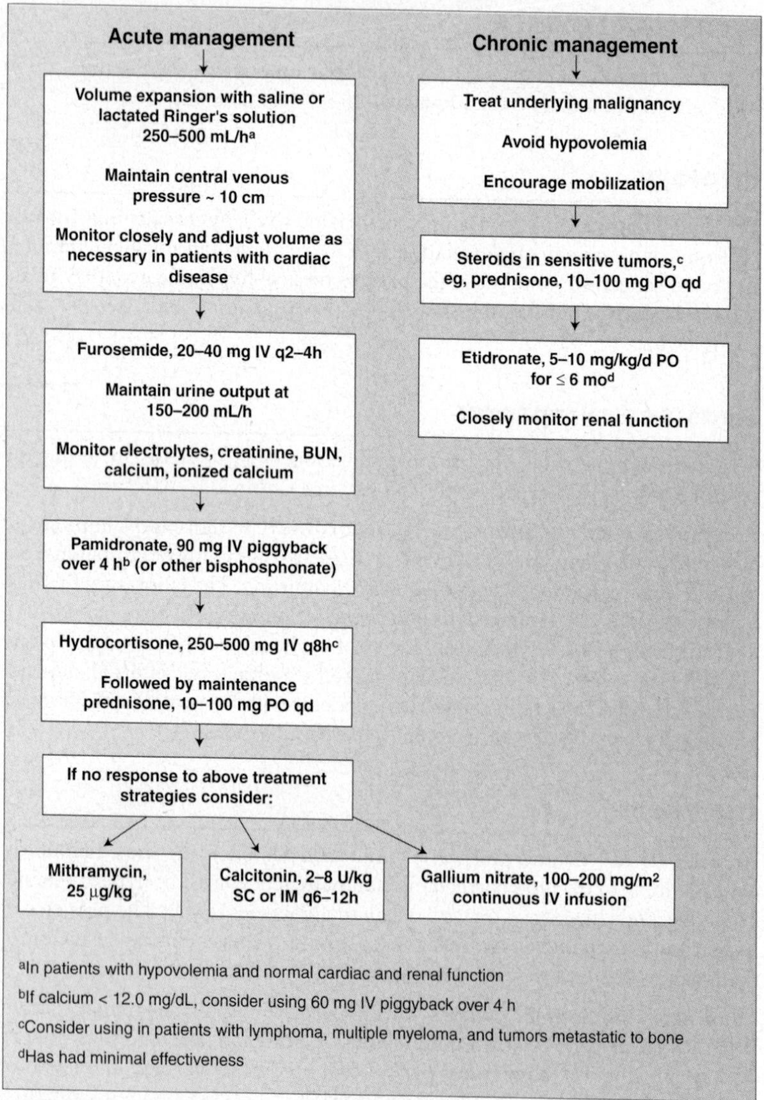

Acute management
Volume expansion with saline or lactated Ringer's solution 250–500 mL/h[a]
Maintain central venous pressure ~ 10 cm
Monitor closely and adjust volume as necessary in patients with cardiac disease
Furosemide, 20–40 mg IV q2–4h
Maintain urine output at 150–200 mL/h
Monitor electrolytes, creatinine, BUN, calcium, ionized calcium
Pamidronate, 90 mg IV piggyback over 4 h[b] (or other bisphosphonate)
Hydrocortisone, 250–500 mg IV q8h[c]
Followed by maintenance prednisone, 10–100 mg PO qd
If no response to above treatment strategies consider:
Mithramycin, 25 μg/kg
Calcitonin, 2–8 U/kg SC or IM q6–12h
Gallium nitrate, 100–200 mg/m²
continuous IV infusion
Chronic management
Treat underlying malignancy
Avoid hypovolemia
Encourage mobilization
Steroids in sensitive tumors,[c] eg, prednisone, 10–100 mg PO qd
Etidronate, 5–10 mg/kg/d PO for ≤ 6 mo[d]
Closely monitor renal function
[a]In patients with hypovolemia and normal cardiac and renal function
[b]If calcium < 12.0 mg/dL, consider using 60 mg IV piggyback over 4 h
[c]Consider using in patients with lymphoma, multiple myeloma, and tumors metastatic to bone
[d]Has had minimal effectiveness

FIGURE 1: Algorithm for the treatment of hypercalcemia of malignancy

or have calcium levels ≥ 12.0 mg/dL should be considered for inpatient management if medically appropriate. An algorithm for the acute and chronic treatment of hypercalcemia of malignancy is shown in Figure 1.

Volume expansion (eg, lactated Ringer's solution, 0.9% NaCl) Volume expansion and natriuresis increase renal blood flow and enhance calcium excretion secondary to the ionic exchange of calcium for sodium in the distal tubule. The volume required depends on the extent of hypovolemia, as well as the patient's cardiac and renal function. Often, infusion rates of 250–500 mL/h are needed. Typically, the onset of action is 12–24 hours.

Loop diuretics There is much controversy over the effectiveness of loop diuretics in the treatment of hypercalcemia. In theory, furosemide-induced natriuresis should enhance urinary calcium excretion. However, in most cases of significant hypercalcemia, hypovolemia is present. Thus, once euvolemia has been achieved with saline infusion, diuretics may be useful in preventing hypervolemia. Diuretic dosages depend on the patient's underlying renal function, and the dosing frequency should be based on hourly urine output. In patients with normal renal function, furosemide, 20–40 mg IV, may be initiated after volume expansion is achieved, with subsequent doses given when urine output is < 150–200 mL/h.

Bisphosphonates (etidronate, clodronate, pamidronate, and zoledronic acid [Zometa]) bind avidly to hydroxyapatite crystals and inhibit bone resorption. Their antiresorptive effects may be mediated by the inhibition of osteoclasts and activation by cytokines. Bisphosphonates also inhibit recruitment and differentiation of osteoclast precursors. They are poorly absorbed from the GI tract, have a very long half-life in bone, and appear to accumulate at sites of active bone turnover.

Pamidronate has been shown to be effective in restoring normocalcemia in 60%–100% of patients with hypercalcemia secondary to malignancy. The recommended dose is 90 mg IV over 4 hours. The single IV dose over 4 hours, lack of renal toxicity, and superiority over etidronate make pamidronate a logical choice for bisphosphonate therapy for hypercalcemia of malignancy. Side effects include low-grade fever and mild hypocalcemia and hypomagnesemia. Clodronate, another bisphosphonate indicated for cancer-associated hypercalcemia, is dosed at 300 mg IV daily for 5 consecutive days (infused over at least 2 hours) or 800–3,200 mg/d orally. Zoledronic acid (4 mg IV) is a newer bisphosphonate that can be infused quicker and has fewer systemic side effects than other bisphosphonates.

Corticosteroids In certain malignancies, such as lymphomas and hormone-sensitive breast cancers, corticosteroids may be of some value in producing a direct antitumor effect. In the majority of solid tumors, however, steroids are of limited or no value.

The onset of action is 3–5 days. Doses of prednisone (or its equivalent) may range from 10 to 100 mg/d.

Calcitonin inhibits bone degradation by binding directly to receptors on the osteoclast. It has few serious side effects (rare hypersensitivity) and can be given to patients with organ failure.

Calcitonin's onset of action is 2–4 hours, but its hypocalcemic effect is of short duration and peaks at 48 hours. There is little response to continued treatment. Doses range from 2 to 8 U/kg SC or IM (intramuscular) every 6–12 hours.

Plicamycin (Mithracin) has direct osteoclast inhibitory effects and may also block the effects of vitamin D or parathyroid hormone. It reportedly is effective in ~80% of patients with hypercalcemia secondary to malignancy.

The onset of action of plicamycin is 24–48 hours. The duration of normocalcemia varies, but retreatment is required in 72–96 hours in most patients. The usual dose is 25 μg/kg (range: 10 to 50 μg/kg).

Significant toxicity increases with multiple injections and includes renal and liver toxicity. Thrombocytopenia is a common side effect.

Gallium nitrate (Ganite) directly inhibits osteoclasts and increases bone calcium without producing cytotoxic effects on bone cells. It successfully restores normocalcemia in 75%–85% of patients.

Gallium nitrates's onset of action is 24–48 hours. The dose range is 100-200 mg/m^2 given by continuous IV infusion for 5 days.

A study by Bertheault-Cvitkovic et al suggested that gallium nitrate may be superior to pamidronate for the acute normalization of cancer-related hypercalcemia. In other comparative trials, gallium nitrate proved to be more effective than both calcitonin and etidronate in patients with hypercalcemia that is secondary to malignancy.

There are some disadvantages to gallium nitrate therapy, including the need for inpatient care and daily IV infusions and potential nephrotoxicity. It has been recommended that the drug not be used in patients with creatinine levels > 2.5 mg/dL.

HYPERURICEMIA

Compared with hypercalcemia, hyperuricemia is a less common metabolic emergency in cancer patients.

Etiology and risk factors

Hyperuricemia occurs most often in patients with hematologic disorders, particularly leukemias, high-grade lymphomas, and myeloproliferative diseases (polycythemia vera). It may occur secondary to treatment of the malignancy.

Drugs Hyperuricemia is also associated with certain cytotoxic agents (eg, tiazofurin and aminothiadiazoles). Various other drugs can contribute to hyperuricemia by increasing uric acid production or decreasing its excretion. Diuretics (thiazides, furosemide, and ethacrynic acid [Edecrin]) cause acute uricosuria, and hyperuricemia may occur secondary to volume contraction. Antituberculous drugs, such as pyrazinamide and ethambutol (Myambutol), as well as nicotinic acid (niacin) are also associated with hyperuricemia.

Extensive or aggressive tumors Patients with extensive, anaplastic, or rapidly proliferating tumors are at greatest risk for hyperuricemia. These patients include patients with bulky lymphomas and sarcomas, those with chronic myelocytic leukemia or chronic lymphocytic leukemia and extreme leukocytosis, and those undergoing remission-induction chemotherapy for acute leukemia.

Renal impairment Individuals with preexisting renal impairment are also at risk of becoming hyperuricemic.

Signs and symptoms

Patients with clinical syndromes caused by hyperuricemia present with significant elevations of serum uric acid. Gouty arthritis may be seen occasionally, but the most significant complication is renal dysfunction, particularly acute renal failure. Clinical symptoms associated with renal dysfunction vary depending on the degree of dysfunction and the timing of its development. In patients with acute renal failure, clinical symptoms may include abnormal mental status, nausea and vomiting, fluid overload, pericarditis, and seizures.

Diagnosis

The diagnosis of hyperuricemia is based on laboratory findings of high serum uric acid levels, hyperuricosuria, and increased serum creatinine and urea nitrogen levels.

Prognosis

Prognosis often depends on the etiology of the hyperuricemia.

Treatment

Prophylactic measures against the development of hyperuricemia should be undertaken prior to the initiation of chemotherapy. Drugs that increase serum urate levels or produce acidic urine (eg, thiazides and salicylates) should be discontinued if possible. Alkalinization of the urine should be initiated to maintain a urine pH > 7.0. Usually, sodium bicarbonate solution (50–100 mmol/L) is added to IV fluids and then adjusted so that an alkaline urinary pH is maintained. The carbonic anhydrase inhibitor acetazolamide (Diamox) may be used to increase the effects of alkalinization. It is important to remember that alkalinization is secondary to the overall goal of decreasing urinary uric acid concentration by increasing urinary volume.

Allopurinol, a xanthine oxidase inhibitor, is the mainstay of drug treatment and may be started 1–2 days prior to cytotoxic treatment. Dosages range from 300–600 mg/d, and therapy is usually continued for 1-2 weeks or until the danger of hyperuricemia has passed.

Rasburicase (Elitek) is an antihyperuricemia drug. It has been approved by the FDA for malignancy-associated hyperuricemia in pediatric patients but is also used in adults. The usual pediatric dose is 0.15 or 0.2 mg/kg IV over 30 minutes for 5 days. The usual adult dosage is 0.15–0.2 mg/kg/d in limited studies.

Acute oliguria In patients who develop acute oliguria, ureteral obstruction by urate calculi should be considered. This condition should be evaluated by ultrasonography or CT. Administration of IV contrast agents for pyelography should be avoided, as they may increase the risk of acute tubular necrosis.

Dialysis Patients with advancing renal insufficiency and subsequent renal failure may benefit from peritoneal dialysis or hemodialysis. Dialysis has been shown to be effective in reversing renal failure caused by urate deposition.

TUMOR LYSIS SYNDROME

Tumor lysis syndrome occurs due to the rapid release of intracellular contents into the bloodstream, leading to life-threatening concentrations. If the resulting metabolic abnormalities remain uncorrected, patients may develop renal failure and sudden death.

Etiology and risk factors

Tumor lysis syndrome most commonly develops during the rapid growth phase of high-grade lymphomas and leukemia in patients with high leukocyte counts; it is less common in patients with solid tumors. The syndrome is often iatrogenic, caused by cytotoxic chemotherapy. Because of clinicians' increased awareness of the tumor lysis syndrome during the past decade and the use of adequate prophylaxis prior to the initiation of chemotherapy, there are fewer cases currently. Occasionally, the syndrome occurs following treatment with irradiation, glucocorticosteroids, tamoxifen, or interferon.

Patients at risk The typical patient at risk for tumor lysis syndrome tends to be young (< 25 years of age) and male and has an advanced disease stage (often with abdominal disease) and a markedly elevated lactic dehydrogenase level.

Other predisposing factors include volume depletion, concentrated acidic urine pH, and excessive urinary uric acid excretion rates.

Signs and symptoms

The syndrome is characterized by hyperuricemia, hyperkalemia, hyperphosphatemia, hypocalcemia, and, often, oliguric renal failure.

Diagnosis

The diagnosis of tumor lysis syndrome is based on the development of increased levels of serum uric acid, phosphorus, and potassium; decreased levels of serum calcium; and renal dysfunction following chemotherapy.

Prognosis

Prognosis varies depending on the adequate correction of metabolic abnormalities and the underlying etiology of tumor lysis.

TABLE 2: Criteria for the diagnosis of SIADH

Criterion	Definition
Hyponatremia	Serum sodium level < 135 mEq/L
Hypo-osmotic plasma	Plasma osmolality < 280 mOsm/kg
Hyper-osmotic urine	Urinary osmolality > 500 mOsm/kg
Hypernatremic urine	Urinary sodium level > 20 mEq/L (without diuretic therapy)

Treatment

Prophylactic measures Patients at risk for tumor lysis syndrome should be identified before the initiation of chemotherapy and should be adequately hydrated and given agents to alkalinize the urine. Treatment with allopurinol (IV or PO) may be instituted to minimize hyperuricemia. The recommended dosage of IV allopurinol ranges from 200 to 400 mg/m^2/d. This regimen should be started 24–48 hours before the initiation of cytotoxic treatment. The dose may be equally divided into 6-, 8-, or 12-hour increments, but the final concentration should not exceed 6 mg/mL. (For oral dosages of allopurinol and IV doses of rasburicase, see the section on "Hyperuricemia, treatment" earlier in this chapter.)

Serum electrolytes, uric acid, phosphorus, calcium, and creatinine levels should be checked repeatedly for 3–4 days after chemotherapy is initiated, with the frequency of monitoring dependent upon the clinical condition and the risk profile of the patient.

Established tumor lysis Once tumor lysis is established, treatment is directed at vigorous correction of electrolyte abnormalities, hydration, and hemodialysis (as appropriate in patients with renal failure).

SYNDROME OF INAPPROPRIATE SECRETION OF ANTIDIURETIC HORMONE

The syndrome of inappropriate secretion of antidiuretic hormone (SIADH) is a paraneoplastic condition that is associated with malignant tumors (particularly SCLC), CNS disease (eg, infection, intracerebral lesions, head trauma, and subarachnoid hemorrhage), and pulmonary disorders (eg, tuberculosis, pneumonia, and abscess).

Signs and symptoms

Hyponatremia is the most common presenting sign of SIADH. Patients who experience a rapid fall in plasma sodium levels are usually the most symptomatic.

Other presentations Patients with SIADH can also experience malaise, altered mental status, seizures, coma, and, occasionally, death. Focal neurologic findings can occur in the absence of brain metastases.

Diagnosis

To make a diagnosis of SIADH, certain criteria must be met (Table 2). In addition to those criteria, patients should have normal renal, adrenal, and thyroid function, along with normal extracellular fluid status.

Drug history It is important to obtain a full list of the medications that the patient is taking, since certain drugs can impair free water excretion either by acting on the renal tubule or by inducing pituitary arginine vasopressin (AVP). These drugs include morphine, cyclophosphamide, vincristine, chlorpropamide (Diabinese), amitriptyline, and clofibrate (Atromid-S).

Treatment

The major focus of treatment for SIADH related to malignancy is successful treatment of the underlying cancer.

Acute treatment is indicated in patients who are symptomatic and who have severe hyponatremia (eg, serum sodium level < 125 mEq/L). The goals of therapy in these patients are to initiate and maintain rapid diuresis with IV furosemide (1 mg/kg body weight) and to replace the sodium and potassium lost in the urine. Usually, the latter goal can be achieved by administering 0.9% saline with added potassium.

This rapid correction should not exceed a 20-mEq/L rise in serum sodium concentration during the first 48 hours. Patients who experience too rapid a rise in serum sodium concentration may suffer neurologic damage and central pontine myelinolysis.

Chronic treatment The mainstay of chronic therapy is water restriction to 500–1,000 mL/d. When this measure alone is unsuccessful, demeclocycline (Declomycin), 300–600 mg PO bid, may be used in patients without liver disease. The onset of action may be > 1 week.

LAMBERT-EATON SYNDROME

The Lambert-Eaton syndrome is strongly associated with SCLC. It is caused by antibodies that interfere with the release of presynaptic acetylcholine at the neuromuscular junction.

Signs and symptoms

Fatigue/muscle weakness This syndrome is characterized by fatigue and proximal muscle weakness, particularly of the pelvic girdle and thighs.

Autonomic symptoms Many patients with this disorder have autonomic symptoms, one of the most common of which is dry mouth.

Other symptoms Other possible symptoms include diplopia or blurred vision, ptosis, dysarthria, dysphagia, and paresthesias.

Diagnosis

Patients with the Lambert-Eaton syndrome show an improvement in muscle strength with exercise.

Electromyographic (EMG) studies are helpful in making the diagnosis. These studies reveal an increase in the muscle action potential with repeated nerve stimulation at rates faster than 10 per second.

Edrophonium test In addition, in contrast to individuals with myasthenia gravis, patients with the Lambert-Eaton syndrome have a poor response to the edrophonium test.

Treatment

Chemotherapy is the first line of treatment, since 90% of patients with SCLC will respond to this measure. In fact, recovery from the Lambert-Eaton syndrome has been noted in some patients treated with chemotherapy.

Other therapies For patients in whom chemotherapy fails to improve symptoms or control the tumor, guanidine has been reported to be useful, as has 3,4-diaminopyridine.

Guanidine is taken orally beginning with a dosage of 5–10 mg/kg/d divided throughout the waking hours. The dosage may be increased to a maximum of 30 mg/kg/d on the basis of the patient's clinical response. However, side effects may be severe at dosages > 1 g/d. Also, the dose of guanidine should not be increased more often than every 3 days, since the maximum response to a dose may not be seen for 2–3 days. At dosages of 5–25 mg 3-4 times per day, 3,4-diaminopyridine can significantly improve symptoms. Side effects of this drug include perioral and acral paresthesias, insomnia, and epigastric distress.

In addition, plasmapheresis, steroids, immunosuppression, and IV gamma globulin are all of potential benefit.

POLYMYOSITIS/DERMATOMYOSITIS

The relationship between polymyositis/dermatomyositis and malignancy was established long ago. The most commonly associated malignancies are breast, lung, and ovarian cancers. An increased incidence of cancer patients with dermatomyositis (10%) has been observed, but the association of cancer with polymyositis is less clear.

Signs and symptoms

Muscle weakness Patients with this syndrome typically experience proximal muscle weakness that progresses over weeks to months. Weakness in the hips, thighs, and shoulder girdle may cause patients to have difficulties in getting out of a chair, climbing stairs, or combing their hair. Patients also may experience dysphagia as well as weakness of the flexor muscles of the neck.

In the majority of cases, the distal muscles of the extremities are not involved. Also, most patients do not have involvement of the extraocular muscles.

Rashes Patients with dermatomyositis can have involvement of the eyelids, forehead, cheeks, chest, elbows, knees, and knuckles with the classic heliotrope rash. A more diffuse rash may also occur.

Diagnosis

Muscle enzymes and erythrocyte sedimentation rate Patients with polymyositis/dermatomyositis usually have an elevation in their serum muscle enzyme levels and erythrocyte sedimentation rate (ESR).

EMG studies and muscle biopsies In addition, EMG tracings are abnormal, and muscle biopsies reveal minimal inflammatory changes, along with muscle fiber necrosis, in patients with polymyositis/dermatomyositis.

Treatment

Steroids In addition to treatment of the underlying malignancy, patients with polymyositis or dermatomyositis are treated with high-dose oral steroids (eg, prednisone, 60–80 mg/d). Other supportive measures, such as range-of-motion exercises, are also prescribed.

Immunosuppressives In patients who do not respond to steroid therapy, immunosuppressive therapy is often added. This type of therapy needs to be tailored to the individual patient, and consultation with a rheumatologist should be considered.

Therapy for skin disease The skin disease of dermatomyositis can be treated with a variety of measures, such as topical corticosteroids, antimalarials, photoprotection, and, at times, low-dose methotrexate.

SUGGESTED READING

ON SUPERIOR VENA CAVA SYNDROME

Kramer GW, Gans S, Ullmann E, et al: Hypofractionated external beam radiotherapy as retreatment for symptomatic non-small-cell lung carcinoma: An effective treatment? Int J Radiat Oncol Biol Phys 58:1388–1393, 2004.

Urruticoechea A, Mesia R, Dominguez J, et al: Treatment of malignant superior vena cava syndrome by endovascular stent insertion: Experience on 52 patients with lung cancer. Lung Cancer 43:209–214, 2004.

ON VENOUS THROMBOEMBOLIC COMPLICATIONS

Howell A, Cuzick J, Baum M, et al: Results of the ATAC (Arimidex, Tamoxifen, Alone or in Combination) trial after completion of 5 years' adjuvant treatment for breast cancer. Lancet 365:60–62, 2005.

Lee AY, Levine MN, Baker RI, et al; Randomized Comparison of Low-Molecular Weight Heparin Versus Oral Anticoagulant Therapy for the Prevention of Recurrent Venous Thromboembolism in Patients with Cancer (CLOT) investigators: Low–molecular-weight heparin versus a coumarin for the prevention of recurrent venous thromboembolism in patients with cancer. N Engl J Med 349:146–153, 2003.

Kearon C, Ginsberg JS, Kovacs MJ, et al: Comparison of low-intensity warfarin therapy with conventional-intensity warfarin therapy for long-term prevention of recurrent venous thromboembolism. N Engl J Med 349:631–639, 2003.

ON SPINAL CORD COMPRESSION

Metser U, Lerman H, Blank A, et al: Malignant involvement of the spine: Assessment of 18F-FDG PET/CT. J Nucl Med 45:279–284, 2004.

Patchell RA, Tibbs PA, Regine WF, et al: Direct decompressive surgical resection in the treatment of spinal cord compression caused by metastatic cancer: A randomised trial. Lancet 366:643–648, 2005.

Rades D, Stalpers LJ, Veninga T, et al: Evaluation of five radiation schedules and prognostic factors for metastatic spinal cord compression. J Clin Oncol 23:3366–3375, 2005.

ON HYPERCALCEMIA

Atula ST, Tahtela RK, Nevalainen JI, et al: Clodronate as a single-dose intravenous infusion effectively provides short-term correction of malignant hypercalcemia. Acta Oncol 42:735–740, 2003.

ON HYPERURICEMIA/TUMOR LYSIS SYNDROME

Jeha S, Kantarjian H, Irwin D, et al: Efficacy and safety of rasburicase, a recombinant urate oxidase (Elitek), in the management of malignancy-associated hyperuricemia in pediatric and adult patients: Final results of a multicenter compassionate use trial. Leukemia 19:34–38, 2005.

ON SYNDROME OF INAPPROPRIATE SECRETION OF ANTIDIURETIC HORMONE

Flombaum CD: Metabolic emergencies in the cancer patient. Semin Oncol 27:322–334, 2000.

ON LAMBERT-EATON SYNDROME

Dropcho EJ: Remote neurologic manifestations of cancer. Neurol Clin 20:85–122, 2002.

Wirtz PW, Smallegange TM, Wintzen AR, et al: Differences in clinical features between the Lambert-Eaton myasthenic syndrome with and without cancer: An analysis of 227 published cases. Clin Neurol Neurosurg 104:359–363, 2002.

ON POLYMYOSITIS/DERMATOMYOSITIS

Sparsa A, Liozon E, Herrmann F, et al: Routine vs extensive malignancy search for adult dermatomyositis and polymyositis: A study of 40 patients. Arch Dermatol 138:885–890, 2002.

Wakata N, Kurihara T, Saito E, et al: Polymyositis and dermatomyositis associated with malignancy: A 30-year retrospective study. Int J Dermatol 41:729–734, 2002.

CHAPTER 46

Infectious complications

James Ito, Jr., MD

Infections are among the most common, potentially serious complications of cancer and its treatment. This chapter discusses infections from a syndromic approach: that is, infections present as a complex of signs and symptoms to the clinician. The syndromes addressed include febrile neutropenia, pneumonia, catheter-associated infections, and gastrointestinal infections (*Clostridium difficile*-associated diarrhea and typhlitis). Special sections focus on fungal and viral infections.

INFECTION DURING FEBRILE NEUTROPENIA

It has long been recognized that the incidence of infection is high in patients who develop a fever during neutropenia and that empiric antimicrobial therapy is warranted in such patients.

Definitions

Fever is usually defined as a temperature ≥ 38.3°C.

Neutropenia is defined as a neutrophil count of 500/μL, although patients with a neutrophil count between 500 and 1,000/μL in whom a decrease is anticipated are considered to be neutropenic. Patients with a neutrophil count < 100/μL are at greatest risk for infection, as are those with a rapid decrease in neutrophil count and those with protracted neutropenia.

Etiology

Bacteria Infections occurring during episodes of febrile neutropenia are caused predominantly by aerobic gram-negative bacilli (especially *Escherichia coli, Klebsiella pneumoniae*, and *Pseudomonas aeruginosa*) and gram-positive cocci (coagulase-negative staphylococci, β-hemolytic streptococci, viridans streptococci, enterococci, and *Staphylococcus aureus*). In recent years, gram-positive infections have become more prominent with the increasing use of indwelling IV catheters.

Fungi Fungal infections usually occur after a patient has received broad-spectrum antimicrobial therapy and/or steroids. The most common fungal pathogens are *Candida* species (predominantly *C albicans* and *C tropicalis*) and

Aspergillus species. Less common are *Fusarium, Scedosporium*, and *Zygomycetes* infections (see also section on "Fungal infections").

Viruses Viral infections occurring during neutropenia are caused predominantly by herpesviruses and respiratory viruses. The herpesviruses include herpes simplex virus (HSV), varicella zoster virus (VZV), cytomegalovirus (CMV), and Epstein-Barr virus (EBV). The respiratory viruses include adenovirus, respiratory syncytial virus, parainfluenza virus, influenza A and B viruses, and rhinovirus (see also section on "Viral infections").

Signs and symptoms

The most remarkable aspect of the febrile, neutropenic patient is the lack of physical findings. This is due to the neutropenia and the absence of an inflammatory response at the infection site. The patient may have only a fever with or without chills or rigors. Even if the patient has pneumonia, there may be few respiratory symptoms. Likewise, a perirectal abscess may be relatively asymptomatic.

Diagnosis

An initial evaluation and diagnostic work-up of any fever in a neutropenic patient should begin immediately but should not delay the initiation of empiric therapy (see below). A complete history (exposures, past infections, rashes, cough, abdominal pain, diarrhea) should be taken and a physical examination (skin lesions, exit site and tunnel of right atrial catheter, oropharynx, abdomen, perineum) should be performed.

Diagnostic work-up should include:

- at least two sets of blood cultures: one from a peripheral vein and one from each port of a central venous catheter. If fever persists in the face of negative cultures, blood cultures for fungi and acid-fast bacilli should be considered.
- culture of any drainage from a catheter exit site
- stool examination for *C difficile* and other bacterial/protozoal agents
- urine culture and urinalysis
- chest radiograph
- aspiration or biopsy of any skin lesions.

CT If indicated by signs or symptoms, CT scans of the brain (followed by lumbar puncture), chest, abdomen, and pelvis can be performed.

Laboratory tests Determination of serum transaminases, CBC, and serum creatinine is also recommended.

Treatment

INITIAL EMPIRIC ANTIBIOTIC THERAPY

Initial antibacterial therapy in the febrile, neutropenic patient should be broad-spectrum and should be based on the prevalence and susceptibility of bacterial isolates seen in the individual hospital setting (Figure 1). When choosing an antibiotic, the clinician also should take into consideration the patient's allergies, renal and hepatic function, and other drugs he or she is receiving that may interact with the empiric antimicrobial agent.

The choice of initial empiric antibiotic therapy for the febrile, neutropenic patient is dictated in part by the susceptibility pattern of blood isolates seen at a particular cancer center. If the prevalence of extended-spectrum βeta-lactamase (ESBL) gram-negative bacteria is high, for example, one probably would not want to use a third-generation cephalosporin such as ceftazidime as initial empiric monotherapy. (Some data suggest that prolonged use of ceftazidime monotherapy in this setting promotes the emergence of ESBL bacteria.) City of Hope has been using ceftazidime as initial monotherapy for the past 15 years, however, without a significant rise in the incidence of resistant gram-negative infections, and this experience has been shared by other centers. Finally, any special circumstance, such as the suspicion of an indwelling IV catheter-associated infection, may influence the antibiotic choice.

Either single antibiotics or antibiotic combinations can be used for initial empiric therapy (see Table 1 for dosage regimens).

Monotherapy

Ceftazidime, cefepime (Maxipime), imipenem-cilastatin (Primaxin), or meropenem (Merrem), when used as monotherapy, avoids the potential for nephrotoxicity. However, none of these antibiotics covers coagulase-negative staphylococci, methicillin-resistant *S aureus* (MRSA), vancomycin-resistant or vancomycin-susceptible enterococci, some strains of penicillin-resistant *Streptococcus pneumoniae,* and viridans streptococci. Also, ceftazidime does not cover anaerobes well, and imipenem-cilastatin may have CNS toxicity at high doses.

Duotherapy

Aminoglycoside plus antipseudomonal β-lactam The aminoglycoside could be gentamicin, tobramycin, or amikacin (Amikin). The β-lactam could be ticarcillin (Ticar) or piperacillin (Pipracil), either alone or with a β-lactamase inhibitor (piperacillin/tazobactam [Zosyn]); mezlocillin (Mezlin); ceftazidime; or cefoperazone (Cefobid).

Advantages of the combination of an aminoglycoside and an antipseudomonal β-lactam include possible synergistic effects against gram-negative bacilli and decreased emergence of resistant strains. The major disadvantages of the combination are potential nephrotoxicity, ototoxicity, hypokalemia, and the need to monitor drug levels of the aminoglycoside. Also, gram-positive coverage is not ideal.

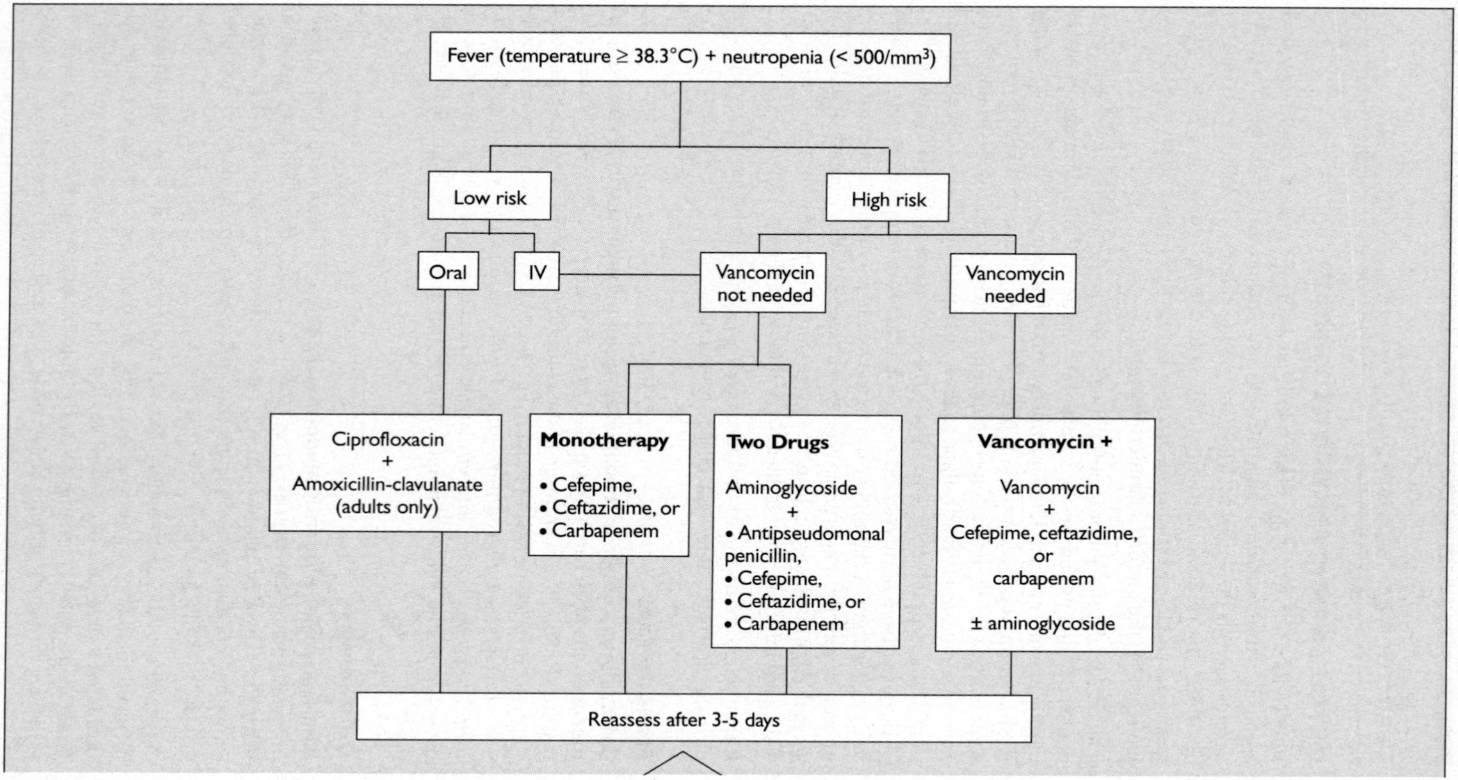
Fever (temperature ≥ 38.3°C) + neutropenia (< 500/mm³)
Low risk
High risk
Oral
IV
Vancomycin not needed
Vancomycin needed
Ciprofloxacin + Amoxicillin-clavulanate (adults only)
Monotherapy
• Cefepime,
• Ceftazidime, or
• Carbapenem
Two Drugs
Aminoglycoside +
• Antipseudomonal penicillin,
• Cefepime,
• Ceftazidime, or
• Carbapenem
Vancomycin +
Vancomycin + Cefepime, ceftazidime, or carbapenem
± aminoglycoside
Reassess after 3-5 days

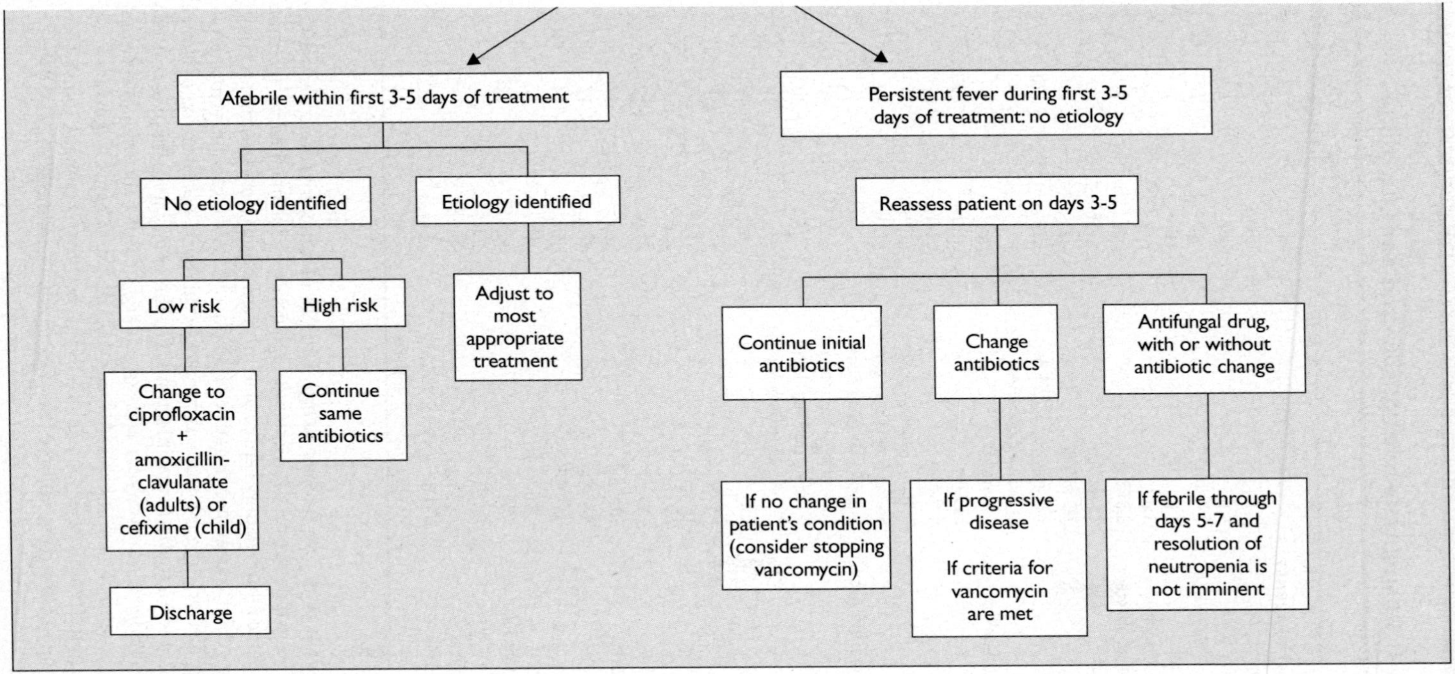

FIGURE 1: Guide to the initial management of the febrile neutropenic patient

Adapted, with permission, from Hughes WT, et al: 2002 guidelines for the use of antimicrobial agents in neutropenic patients with cancer. Clin Infect Dis 34:730-751, 2002.

TABLE 1: Dosing schedules of selected antimicrobials

Drug	Dose	Frequency	Route
Antibacterial agents			
Ceftazidime	2 g	q8h	IV
Cefepime	2 g	q8h	IV
Imipenem-cilastatin	500 mg	q6h	IV
Meropenem	1 g	q8h	IV
Piperacillin sodium	3 g	q4h	IV
Piperacillin/tazobactam	3.375 g	q6h	IV
Vancomycin	15 mg/kg	q12h	IV
	7.5 mg/kg	q6h	IV
	125 mg (for *C difficile*-associated diarrhea)	q6h	PO
Quinupristin/dalfopristin	7.5 mg/kg	q8h	IV
Linezolid	600 mg	q12h	IV/PO
Daptomycin	4 mg/kg	q24h	IV
Tigecycline	100 mg (loading dose)	q12h	IV
	50 mg (maintenance)	q12h	IV
Gentamicin/tobramycin	2 mg/kg (loading dose)		IV
	1.5 mg/kg (maintenance)	q8h	IV
Amikacin	8 mg/kg (loading dose)		IV
	7.5 mg/kg (maintenance)	q8h	IV
Cefazolin	2 g	q6h	IV
Nafcillin	2 g	q4h	IV
Ciprofloxacin	400 mg	q12h	IV
	750 mg	bid	PO
Levofloxacin	500 mg	q24h	IV/PO
Metronidazole	500 mg	q6h	IV
Clindamycin	900 mg	q8h	IV
TMP-SMZ	15 mg/kg/d	q6h	IV
Erythromycin	1 g	q6h	IV
Amoxicillin/clavulanate	500 mg	q8h	PO
Ampicillin/sulbactam	3 g	q6h	IV
Clarithromycin	500 mg	bid	PO
Azithromycin	500 mg (day 1), 250 mg	q24h	PO
	500 mg (day 1), 250 mg	q24h	IV

Vancomycin plus one or two drugs The use of vancomycin as part of the initial regimen is controversial. Certainly, a majority of documented bacteremias in neutropenic febrile patients are caused by gram-positive organisms, and most of them are due to coagulase-negative staphylococci. Also, vancomycin is probably the preferred drug for viridans streptococcal sepsis and the drug of choice for MRSA and *Corynebacterium* infections. On the other hand, there is concern for the overuse of vancomycin and the emergence of vancomycin-resistant enterococci (and now *S aureus*). A study by the European Organization for Research and Treatment of Cancer (EORTC) and the National Cancer Institute of Canada did not support the use of vancomycin in initial empiric therapy.

Drug	Dose	Frequency	Route
Antifungal agents			
Amphotericin B			
Therapy	0.5-1.0 mg/kg	daily	IV
Prophylaxis	0.1-0.2 mg/kg	daily	IV
Fluconazole	400 mg	daily	IV or PO
Itraconazole capsules	200 mg (loading dose)	tid × 4 d	PO
	200 mg (maintenance)	bid	PO
Itraconazole oral solution	(see capsules above)		
Itraconazole injection	200 mg (loading dose)	bid × 4 doses	IV
	200 mg (maintenance)	daily	IV
Amphotericin B			
Lipid complex	5 mg/kg	daily	IV
Cholesteryl sulfate	3-6 mg/kg	daily	IV
Liposome	3-5 mg/kg	daily	IV
Caspofungin	70 mg (loading dose)		IV
	50 mg (maintenance)	daily	IV
Voriconazole	6 mg/kg (loading dose) × 2	q12h	IV
	4 mg/kg (maintenance)	q12h	IV
	200 mg (maintenance) for > 40 kg	q12h	PO
	100 mg (maintenance) for ≤ 40 kg	q12h	PO
Micafungin	50 mg (for prophylaxis)	q24h	IV
	150 mg (treatment)	q24h	IV
Anidulafungin	200 mg (loading dose)		IV
	100 mg (maintenance)	daily	IV
Posaconazole	200 mg (prophylaxis)	tid	PO
	400 mg (treatment)	bid	PO
Antiviral agents			
Acyclovir			
For HSV	5 mg/kg	q8h	IV
For VZV	10 mg/kg	q8h	IV
For HSV encephalitis	15 mg/kg	q8h	IV
Ganciclovir	5 mg/kg (induction)	q12h	IV
	5 mg/kg (maintenance)	daily	IV
Valganciclovir	900 mg (induction)	q12h	PO
Foscarnet	60 mg/kg (induction)	q8h	IV for 14 d
	90 mg/kg (maintenance)	daily	IV
Cidofovir	5 mg/kg	q wk × 2	IV
	then	q2wk	
Amantadine, rimantadine	100 mg	bid	PO
Zanamivir	5 mg	bid	inhalation
Oseltamivir	75 mg	bid	PO

HSV = herpes simplex virus; TMP-SMZ = trimethoprim-sulfamethoxazole; VZV = varicella zoster virus

It should be noted that the Centers for Disease Control and Prevention (CDC) advises against the use of vancomycin in initial empiric therapy for a febrile, neutropenic patient "unless initial evidence indicates that the patient has an infection caused by gram-positive micro-organisms (eg, at an inflamed exit site of Hickman catheter) and the prevalence of infections caused by MRSA in the hospital is substantial."

Thus, it is recommended (in the 2002 guidelines for the use of antimicrobial agents in neutropenic patients with unexplained fever developed by the Infectious Diseases Society of America) that vancomycin be added to the initial regimen (eg, with ceftazidime) in selected patients, including:

- patients with clinically obvious, serious catheter-related infections
- patients undergoing intensive chemotherapy that produces substantial mucosal damage (ie, high-dose cytarabine [Ara-C], which increases the risk of penicillin-resistant streptococcal infections, particularly those due to viridans streptococci)
- patients receiving prophylaxis with quinolones before the onset of the febrile episode
- patients who have known colonization with pneumococci that are resistant to penicillin and cephalosporins or MRSA
- patients with a blood culture positive for gram-positive bacteria before final identification and susceptibility testing
- patients with hypotension or other evidence of cardiovascular impairment.

Double β-lactam therapy usually consists of a third-generation cephalosporin (ceftazidime or cefoperazone) and a ureidopenicillin (piperacillin, ticarcillin, or mezlocillin). The advantages of this regimen are low toxicity (mainly renal) and theoretical synergism. However, it is more costly (compared with monotherapy) and has the possibility of antagonism.

CHANGES IN INITIAL THERAPY

Defervescence If the fever subsides after 3 days of empiric therapy and a specific organism is identified, broad-spectrum antibiotic coverage can be modified to provide optimal treatment. Antibiotics can be discontinued after 7 days if all evidence of infection has been eradicated.

If no organism is isolated, treatment with the initial regimen should be continued for a minimum of 7 days. If the patient is clinically well, the regimen can be switched to an oral antibiotic, such as cefixime (Suprax) or a quinolone.

Persistent, unresponsive fever If the fever persists after 4-7 days of antibiotic therapy, reassessment is recommended. If no infectious etiology is determined, a change in or addition to the antibiotic regimen is recommended.

If vancomycin was not part of the initial empiric regimen, many physicians would consider adding it. However, because of the recent recommendation by the CDC against empiric vancomycin use, it probably should not be added unless there is a strong clinical or microbiologic reason to do so. Instead, cefazolin or nafcillin could be added for better gram-positive coverage. If the initial regimen did not provide anaerobic coverage, metronidazole could be added. Finally, if fever and neutropenia persist despite 3-5 days of antibiotic therapy, an antifungal agent (caspofungin [Cancidas], liposomal amphotericin B [AmBisome], amphotericin B lipid complex [Abelcet], itraconazole [Sporanox], voriconazole [Vfend]), or even fluconazole ([Diflucan] if the risk of mold infection is low) should be added. If the patient is already on antifungal prophylaxis with an azole or echinocandin, a polyene (an amphotericin B lipid

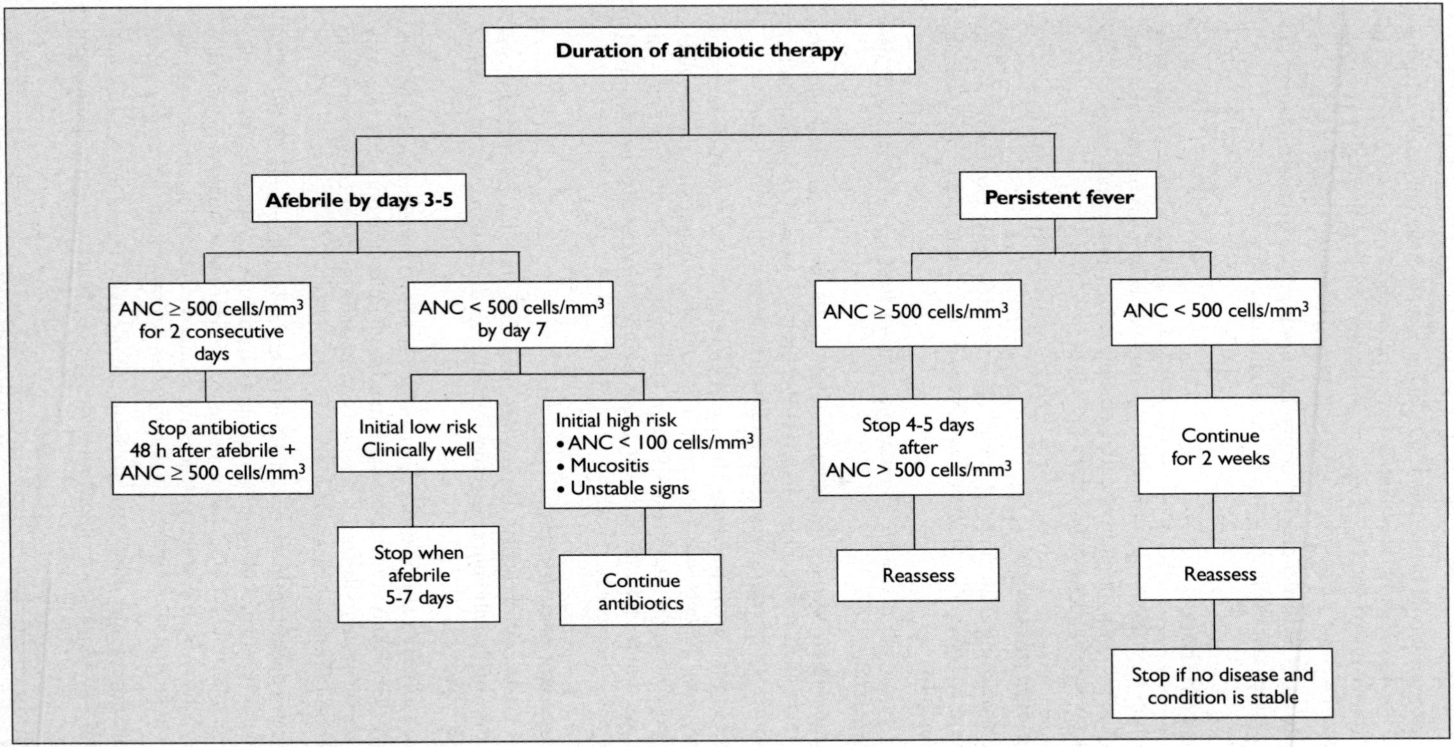

FIGURE 2: Duration of antibiotic therapy ANC = absolute neutrophil count

Adapted, with permission, from Hughes WT, et al: 2002 guidelines for the use of antimicrobial agents in neutropenic patients with cancer. Clin Infect Dis 34:730-751, 2002.

formulation) should be started. If the patient is receiving a polyene as prophylaxis, the dose should be escalated, or, alternatively, a change can be made to an extended-spectrum azole (eg, voriconazole). Another alternative is to add an echinocandin (caspofungin) to the increased dosage of the polyene.

Duration of antimicrobial therapy The most important determinant of the duration of therapy is the absolute neutrophil count (Figure 2).

Prevention

Attempts to prevent infection in the neutropenic host focus on two broad areas: preventing acquisition of pathogenic organisms and suppressing or eradicating endogenous microbial flora.

Hygienic measures

Hand-washing The simplest, most effective, and least expensive way to prevent acquisition of potential pathogens is to institute strict hand-washing precautions.

Diet A cooked diet with elimination of fresh fruit and vegetables is also recommended.

Water and air Water purification systems (to eliminate *Legionella* organisms) and high-efficiency particulate air (HEPA) filtration systems (to eliminate fungal spores) can decrease rates of acquisition of these pathogens.

"Protective" environments The use of more "protective" environments for neutropenic patients is controversial. The total protective environment, which consists of a totally sterile environment and an aggressive antimicrobial regimen, can reduce the rate of infection but does not contribute to increased survival and is also costly.

Antibiotic prophylaxis

Prophylactic antimicrobial therapy generally falls into three categories: oral nonabsorbable antibiotics, selective decontamination regimens, and systemic prophylaxis.

Nonabsorbable antibiotics Although the use of oral nonabsorbable antibiotics has demonstrated some reduction in infection rates, this option has become less popular due to its cost, side effects, unpalatability, poor compliance, and selection of resistant organisms.

Selective decontamination with trimethoprim-sulfamethoxazole (TMP-SMZ), ie, establishment of "colonization resistance" by preserving anaerobic flora while reducing aerobic bacteria, has not resulted in clear-cut reductions in infection rates. Moreover, the disadvantages of prolonged neutropenia and emergence of resistant organisms make this regimen less desirable than others.

Fluoroquinolones More recently, many studies have touted the value of antibacterial prophylaxis with fluoroquinolones (eg, ciprofloxacin [Cipro], ofloxacin

[Floxin], and levofloxacin [Levaquin]) in neutropenic patients. However, no single study (except for a recent meta-analysis of 52 trials) has demonstrated a survival advantage. Thus, neither the National Comprehensive Cancer Network (NCCN) nor the Infectious Diseases Society of America (IDSA) guidelines recommend using antibacterial prophylaxis in neutropenic patients. The NCCN guideline recommends that bacterial prophylaxis (fluoroquinolones) be considered for high-risk patients (neutropenia < 100 μL for ≥ 7 days). Despite this lack of a strong recommendation, fluoroquinolone (mainly levofloxacin) prophylaxis is widely used at many cancer centers; the obvious downside of this trend is the emergence of resistant bacteria, which has already been observed in many institutions. (See the sidebar on page 1022 for another consequence of the overuse of levofloxacin.)

***Pneumocystis carinii* pneumonia** In patients at risk for *P carinii* pneumonia (patients undergoing allogeneic hematopoietic cell transplantation [HCT], those with lymphoma, or those receiving steroids), TMP-SMZ, administered for only 2 or 3 days per week, can reduce the incidence of infection.

Antifungal prophylaxis

Fluconazole, itraconazole, and micafungin (Mycamine) have all been shown to lower the incidence of invasive fungal infection when used as prophylaxis in the HCT setting. In a retrospective study, low-dose conventional amphotericin B has also been associated with a lower incidence of infection. Fluconazole, however, has no activity against molds. Itraconazole is limited by its gastrointestinal and hepatic toxicity. Antifungal prophylaxis should be reserved for those patients at highest risk for invasive fungal infection–ie, HCT and high-risk leukemia patients undergoing high-dose chemotherapy (see also “Prevention” section under “Fungal infections”).

Antiviral prophylaxis

Acyclovir Patients at risk for mucositis (ie, those undergoing induction therapy for leukemia or lymphoma or HCT) who have evidence of prior HSV infection (positive serology) can receive prophylaxis with twice-daily IV acyclovir (see Table 1 for dose).

Ganciclovir has been shown to be an effective “preemptive” and prophylactic antiviral in preventing CMV interstitial pneumonia in allogeneic HCT recipients who show evidence of CMV in bronchoalveolar lavage fluid or blood (see section on “Viral infections”).

PNEUMONIA

A significant number of infections in cancer patients are due to pneumonia. For example, 25% of documented infections in patients with nonlymphocytic leukemia are caused by pneumonia. Also, 50% of allogeneic HCT recipients will develop pneumonia.

TABLE 2: Altered host defenses and associated respiratory pathogens in immunocompromised patients with cancer

Granulocytopenia	
Gram-negative bacilli: *Pseudomonas aeruginosa, Klebsiella pneumoniae, Escherichia coli, Enterobacter* species	
Gram-positive cocci: *Staphylococcus aureus, Staphylococcus epidermidis*, group D streptococci, α-hemolytic streptococci	
Gram-positive bacilli: *Bacillus* species, *Clostridium* species	
Fungi: *Aspergillus* species, *Zygomycetes, Fusarium* species, *Trichosporon beigelii, Candida* species, *Torulopsis glabrata*	
Cellular (T-lymphocyte) immune defects	
Bacteria: *Mycobacterium* species, *Nocardia asteroides, Legionella* species, *Listeria monocytogenes, Salmonella* species	
Viruses: Cytomegalovirus, varicella zoster virus, herpes simplex virus, Epstein-Barr virus	
Protozoa: *Pneumocystis carinii, Toxoplasma gondii*	
Fungi: *Cryptococcus neoformans, Histoplasma capsulatum, Coccidioides immitis*	
Helminths: *Strongyloides stercoralis*	
Humoral (B-lymphocyte) immune deficiency	
Bacteria: *Streptococcus pneumoniae, Haemophilus influenzae*	
Impaired tracheobronchial clearance	
Bacteria and fungi colonizing the lower respiratory tract	
Invasive procedures: Mechanical disruption of epithelial barriers	
Bacteria and fungi colonizing the respiratory tract and skin	
Altered neurologic function	
Bacteria and fungi colonizing the oropharynx and upper respiratory tract	

Adapted, with permission, from Walsh TJ, Rubin R, Pizzo PA: Respiratory diseases in patients with malignant neoplasms, in Shelhamer J, Pizzo PA, Parillo JE, et al (eds): Respiratory Disease in the Immunosuppressed Host, p 640. Philadelphia, JB Lippincott, 1991.

Etiology and risk factors

Some of the risk factors that predispose cancer patients to pneumonia are cellular and humoral immune deficiencies, neutropenia, impaired tracheobronchial clearance, use of antibiotics and steroids, and surgery.

Etiologic agents The etiologic agents responsible for pneumonia in the cancer patient run the gamut of most bacterial, fungal, and viral organisms.

Noninfectious processes mimicking pneumonia Numerous noninfectious processes can mimic pneumonia in cancer patients. They include congestive heart failure, aseptic emboli, metastatic disease, adult respiratory distress syndrome, hemorrhage, radiation injury, hypersensitivity disorders and reactions, and trauma.

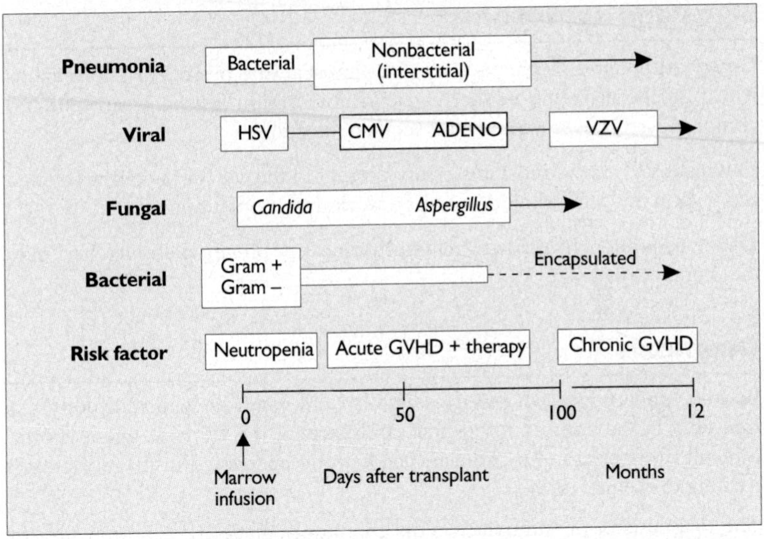

FIGURE 3: Timing of infectious syndromes after bone marrow transplantation

ADENO = adenovirus; CMV = cytomegalovirus; GVHD = graft-vs-host disease; HSV = herpes simplex virus; VZV = varicella zoster virus

Adapted, with permission, from Meyers JD: Infections in marrow recipients, in Mandell GL, Doublas RG, Bennett JE (eds): Principles and Practice of Infectious Diseases, 2nd ed, pp 1674-1676. New York, Wiley, 1985.

Pinpointing the pathogen Certain characteristics of each cancer patient may help predict the specific etiologic agent.

Type of immunosuppression One characteristic that is particularly useful is the type of immunosuppression that the patient is experiencing. This depends on the type of neoplastic disease (eg, lymphoma, leukemia) and, more importantly, the type of therapy (eg, chemotherapy, radiation therapy, allogeneic HCT). For example, certain gram-negative and gram-positive bacteria are more prevalent during neutropenia, whereas other bacteria (*S pneumoniae*, *Haemophilus influenzae*) are more common with a humoral immune deficiency, such as occurs after splenectomy (see Table 2).

Timing of pneumonia Another important characteristic is the timing of the pneumonia; in other words, the phase of the immunosuppression can help predict the etiology. For example, an interstitial pneumonia occurring during the first 30 days after allogeneic HCT would not be expected to be due to CMV (Figure 3).

Other factors Finally, other factors such as the duration of neutropenia, prior antimicrobial therapy, other agents (such as steroids) used, and the specific local microbiota help in prediction. For example, if an allogeneic HCT patient receiving steroids for graft-vs-host disease (GVHD) develops nodular infiltrates after weeks of broad-spectrum antibacterial antibiotics, an *Aspergillus* species would be highly suspected.

Signs and symptoms

Cough Although a productive cough is almost always present in a normal host with pneumonia, often neither a cough nor sputum is seen in an immunocompromised cancer patient with such an infection.

Fever, however, is almost invariably present in the cancer patient with pneumonia and, by itself, should prompt a work-up for pneumonia.

Other possible symptoms include shortness of breath, pleuritic chest pain, and hemoptysis.

Diagnosis

Because pneumonia can progress rapidly and result in high morbidity and mortality in the compromised host, and because the etiologic agent is often difficult to ascertain, the clinician needs to be aggressive in diagnosing and treating these infections.

The diagnosis of pneumonia is most commonly made by a simple chest radiograph. However, there are rare occasions when a pulmonary infiltrate or small nodular lesion is seen only on a CT scan.

Etiologic diagnosis

An etiologic diagnosis is made by the following procedures: sputum (expectorated or induced), bronchoscopy with bronchoalveolar lavage and transbronchial biopsy, transthoracic needle biopsy/aspiration, and open lung biopsy.

Sputum An adequate sputum specimen is difficult to obtain from cancer patients, especially during neutropenia.

Bronchoscopy with bronchoalveolar lavage is a much more sensitive technique than sputum analysis but may miss the organism when the pulmonary disease is peripheral or nodular.

Transthoracic needle biopsy/aspiration under CT guidance may be helpful if the lesion is proximal but may be contraindicated in a severely thrombocytopenic patient. This procedure is indicated when there is a focal/nodular lesion in the periphery.

Open lung biopsy is the most definitive diagnostic procedure but also the most invasive. It is still not clear whether the information obtained by open biopsy improves overall survival. The less invasive thoracoscopic open lung biopsy is becoming more popular than open lung biopsy.

Smears and cultures Both fluid and tissue specimens should be sent for bacterial smears (including acid-fast bacilli and modified acid-fast bacilli) and cultures (including those for anaerobes, acid-fast bacilli, and *Legionella* organisms), fungal smears (potassium hydroxide) and cultures, cytology (for viral inclusions and silver stains for fungi and *P carinii*), and histopathology.

Treatment

The therapeutic approach to pneumonia in the cancer patient should take into consideration the category of immunosuppression (neoplastic disease and immunosuppressive therapy), as well as the timing of onset and pattern of the pneumonia.

EMPIRIC ANTIBIOTIC THERAPY

In neutropenic patients experiencing their first fever and localized pulmonary infiltrates, one can justify initiating empiric therapy similar to that used for febrile, neutropenic patients (see previous discussion), since the majority of pneumonias in this setting are caused by gram-negative bacteria. However, in other situations, such as pneumonia that has a later onset, develops after empiric antibiotics have been initiated, is more aggressive or severe, occurs in a more severely compromised host (eg, a patient who has had allogeneic HCT), or is characterized by a diffuse or interstitial infiltrate, one should proceed to immediate bronchoscopy with bronchoalveolar lavage (and possibly transbronchial biopsy).

ADDITIONS TO EMPIRIC THERAPY

If no diagnosis is forthcoming after bronchoscopy and bronchoalveolar lavage, additions to empiric therapy should be made.

Anaerobic, gram-positive, and *Legionella* coverage Certainly, anaerobic coverage should be considered, as well as gram-positive coverage. *Legionella* coverage should be added, especially if warranted by the epidemiologic setting.

Antifungal and antituberculous therapy Finally, antifungal therapy should be initiated if there is no response to antibacterial therapy and especially if there are nodular or cavitary lesions. In addition, if such lesions are present and/or the epidemiologic setting is compatible, antituberculous therapy should be added.

Further diagnostic procedures If bronchoscopy with bronchoalveolar lavage does not reveal an etiology and the pneumonia is progressing despite empiric therapy, consideration should be given to transthoracic needle biopsy/aspiration and open lung biopsy. As mentioned previously, if there is a peripheral, focal lesion, transthoracic needle biopsy/aspiration can be attempted.

The ultimate diagnostic procedure is open biopsy, but because its contribution to increased survival is unknown, the decision to proceed with this most invasive procedure must be undertaken carefully.

SPECIFIC ANTIMICROBIAL THERAPY

The specific antimicrobial therapy suggested for each etiology is listed in Table 3.

TABLE 3: Probable causes of and treatments for pulmonary infiltrates in granulocytopenic patients

Pattern of infiltrate	Probable organisms	Treatment
Localized		
Early[a]	*Klebsiella* species, other Enterobacteriaceae, *Pseudomonas aeruginosa*	Empiric antibacterial therapy
Refractory[b]	Resistant Enterobacteriaceae and resistant *P aeruginosa*	Modify according to susceptibility
	Pseudomonas maltophilia	
	Pneumocystis carinii[c]	TMP-SMZ
	Legionella species[c]	Macrolide (clarithromycin, azithromycin) with or without rifampin
	Mycoplasma species	Macrolide (clarithromycin, azithromycin)
	Mycobacterium tuberculosis[c]	Isoniazid, rifampin, and pyrazinamide
	Nocardia asteroides[c]	TMP-SMZ, minocycline, imipenem
	Cryptococcus neoformans[c]	Amphotericin B formulation
	Histoplasma capsulatum[d]	Amphotericin B formulation
	Aspergillus species[e]	Voriconazole, amphotericin B formulation, caspofungin, itraconazole[f]
Late[a,b]	*Aspergillus* species	Voriconazole, amphotericin B formulation, caspofungin, itraconazole[f]
	P carinii[c]	TMP-SMZ
	Trichosporon beigelii	Amphotericin B formulation[f]
	Scedosporium	Amphotericin B formulation, voriconazole
	Fusarium species	Amphotericin B formulation[f]
	Zygomycetes	Amphotericin B formulation
	Candida species	Amphotericin B formulation, fluconazole, itraconazole, caspofungin, voriconazole
	Resistant Enterobacteriaceae and resistant *P aeruginosa*	Modify according to susceptibility
	Xanthomonas maltophilia	TMP-SMZ
	Legionella species[c]	Macrolide (clarithromycin, azithromycin)

Prevention

Methods to prevent pulmonary infections fall into the following categories: colonization prevention, antimicrobial prophylaxis (and preemptive treatment), vaccination, and immunomodulation.

Hand-washing The simplest method of colonization prevention is hand-washing.

Other colonization prevention methods, such as protective environments, are discussed in the previous section.

Air and water With regard to pulmonary pathogens, HEPA-filtered rooms can eliminate *Aspergillus* spores from the immediate environment. Water supplies can be checked for *Legionella* contamination and/or adequate disinfection maintained (eg, chlorination, copper/silver ionization, temperature [60°C]).

Pattern of infiltrate	Probable organisms	Treatment
Late	*N asteroides*[c]	TMP-SMZ, minocycline, imipenem
	M tuberculosis[c]	Isoniazid, rifampin, and pyrazinamide
	H capsulatum[d]	Amphotericin B formulation
	Coccidioides immitis[d]	Amphotericin B formulation
Diffuse	*P carinii*[c]	TMP-SMZ
	Legionella species[c]	Macrolide (clarithromycin, azithromycin) with or without rifampin
	Chlamydia pneumoniae	Macrolide (clarithromycin, azithromycin) or tetracycline
	M tuberculosis[c]	Isoniazid plus rifampin
	H capsulatum[d]	Amphotericin B formulation
	Strongyloides stercoralis[d]	Thiabendazole
	Cytomegalovirus	Ganciclovir plus IV immune globulin, foscarnet
	If diagnostic procedure is not possible	Empiric therapy with macrolide and TMP-SMZ

TMP-SMZ = trimethoprim-sulfamethoxazole

Adapted, with permission, from Walsh TJ, Pizzo PA: Ann Intern Med 117:424–428,1992.

a The terms "early" and "late" refer to the time of development of pulmonary infiltrates during the course of granulocytopenia.

b Serial chest radiographs and, where appropriate, a baseline and follow-up CT scan of refractory and late focal infiltrates are recommended.

c Granulocytopenic patients who have concomitant defective cell-mediated immunity or who are receiving corticosteroids are at particularly high risk for these infections.

d Granulocytopenic patients from endemic areas who have concomitant defective cell-mediated immunity or who are receiving corticosteroids are at particularly high risk for these infections.

e Granulocytopenic patients with a previous episode of pulmonary aspergillosis have a high risk of developing recurrent pulmonary aspergillosis early in the course of subsequent cytotoxic chemotherapy.

f These pulmonary fungal infections often develop in patients who are already receiving empiric amphotericin B (0.5 mg/kg/d). These pulmonary mycoses may be more responsive to higher doses of amphotericin B (1.0-1.5 mg/kg/d). Refractory infections may require investigational antifungal triazoles or lipid formulations of amphotericin B, depending on the organism.

Antimicrobial prophylaxis is discussed in the previous section.

Active immunization The influenza and pneumococcal (killed) vaccines should be administered to cancer patients.

Immunomodulation Immunomodulators, such as granulocyte colony-stimulating factor (G-CSF, filgrastim [Neupogen]) and granulocyte-macrophage colony-stimulating factor (GM-CSF, sargramostim [Leukine]), may help reduce infection by decreasing the duration of neutropenia. (For more on growth factors, see chapter 40.)

CATHETER-ASSOCIATED INFECTIONS

Chronic indwelling right atrial catheters are commonly placed in cancer patients, as they permit frequent, long-term vascular access for drug and blood product administration, hyperalimentation, and blood drawing.

Hickman and Broviac catheters have an exit site on the skin surface, are anchored with a subcutaneous Dacron felt cuff, and have a subcutaneous tunnel entering the venous system (via the subclavian, external jugular, internal jugular, cephalic, saphenous, or femoral veins), where they lead into the superior or inferior vena cava or right atrium. These catheters can have single, double, or triple lumens. Another type of catheter has a totally implanted port (Port-A-Cath) that is accessed percutaneously.

There are four types of catheter-associated infections: exit-site infections, tunnel infections, catheter-associated bacteremia/fungemia, and septic thrombophlebitis.

There are approximately 0.4 infections per 100 catheter-days and 0.26 bacteremias per 100 catheter-days.

Etiology

It is assumed that catheter-associated infections are caused by tracking of organisms from the skin along the catheter, contamination of the lumen during manipulation, or direct seeding during bacteremia/fungemia.

Staphylococci By far, the most common micro-organisms associated with catheter-associated infections are coagulase-negative staphylococci. The next most common pathogen is coagulase-positive *S aureus*.

Less common pathogens include gram-negative bacilli, gram-positive bacilli (such as *Corynebacterium* JK and *Bacillus* species), fungi (especially *Candida* species), and rapidly growing mycobacteria.

Signs and symptoms

Exit-site infections may be manifested by local erythema, warmth, and tenderness. Purulent drainage may be present.

Tunnel infections are characterized by tenderness along the subcutaneous track.

Catheter-associated bacteremia/fungemia usually displays no local findings. A fever may be the only sign, but other signs and symptoms of sepsis or even full-blown septic shock syndrome may be present.

Septic thrombophlebitis Likewise, septic thrombophlebitis may have no findings, except those associated with sepsis or venous thrombosis (edema).

Diagnosis

In any cancer patient with a right atrial catheter who becomes febrile or is shown to be bacteremic or fungemic, a catheter-associated infection should be suspected.

Cultures A catheter-associated infection is more likely when blood cultures from the catheter sampling are positive and those from the peripheral vein are negative. A catheter infection should be assumed when the organism isolated is a coagulase-negative *Staphylococcus, Corynebacterium, Bacillus,* or *Candida* species or a mycobacterium.

If signs are consistent with an exit-site or tunnel infection, an attempt should be made to culture any exit-site drainage.

Treatment

Catheter removal

Although it was once believed that all catheters had to be removed to eradicate infection, it is now clear that many catheters can be salvaged. An exception to this guideline would be if the organism isolated is *Corynebacterium* JK, a *Bacillus* species, a *Candida* organism, or a rapidly growing mycobacterium. Some physicians would add to this list *S aureus*, vancomycin-resistant enterococci, *P aeruginosa*, polymicrobial bacteremia, and *Fusarium* species. The catheter also should be removed in patients with septic thrombophlebitis or evidence of septic emboli. A tunnel infection or pocket-space abscess should prompt catheter removal as well. Finally, fever or bacteremia that persists (> 72 hours) after therapy has been initiated necessitates removal of the catheter if there is no other source of infection.

Antibiotic therapy

Empiric therapy If a catheter-associated infection is suspected, vancomycin should be initiated empirically. If the patient is known to be colonized with vancomycin-resistant enterococci, empiric therapy with quinupristin/dalfopristin (Synercid) or linezolid (Zyvox) should be considered.

Two new antimicrobial agents with activity against methicillin-resistant *Staphylococcus aureus* (MRSA) and vancomycin-resistant enterococci (VRE) have recently been approved: daptomycin (Cubicin) and tigecycline (Tygacil). Both drugs have activity against MRSA and VRE, but they are approved only for MRSA infections. Although some of these new agents have shortcomings (eg, activity of daptomycin is neutralized by surfactant in the lungs and emergence of resistance while on this antibiotic), they enlarge our armamentarium for fighting these resistant gram-positive infections.

Specific therapy When a micro-organism has been isolated and tested for sensitivity, specific antimicrobial therapy should be added. If the catheter is left in place, a minimum of 14 days of parenteral (not oral) therapy should be administered through the catheter (rotating through each port), and follow-up cultures should be obtained.

Search for infectious metastasis

Whether or not the catheter is removed, if the patient remains febrile, a search for sources of metastatic infection (lungs, liver, spleen, brain, heart valves) should be initiated.

Fibrinolytics and anticoagulants

The use of fibrinolytics and anticoagulation is controversial. Anticoagulation is indicated in cases of septic thrombophlebitis when the deep venous system is involved.

C DIFFICILE–ASSOCIATED DIARRHEA

Although many infectious complications involve the GI tract and abdomen in cancer patients, *C difficile*–associated diarrhea and typhlitis are the most important clinically.

Diarrhea is common in the cancer patient during chemotherapy. One of the most common causes of diarrhea is antibiotic-associated colitis. By far, the predominant etiology of antibiotic-associated colitis is *C difficile*.

Etiology and risk factors

Reports of outbreaks of hypervirulent, resistant strains of *Clostridium difficile* have occurred in Canada and the United States recently. The increased severity of disease and the higher mortality rates are being attributed to hyperproduction of toxins A and B (*Warny M, Pepin J, Fang A, et al: Lancet 366:1079-1084, 2005*). The relapse rates are also higher than previously observed. Poorer responses to therapy have been noted (*Pepin J, Valiquette L, Alary ME, et al: CMAJ 171:466-472, 2004*). The use of fluoroquinolones, to which *C difficile* appears to be resistant, has emerged as the major risk factor for disease (*Pepin J, Saheb N, Coulombe MA, et al: Clin Infect Dis 41:1254-1260, 2005*).

Antibiotics The major risk factor for *C difficile*–associated diarrhea is treatment with antibiotics, especially broad-spectrum β-lactams with activity against enteric bacteria and clindamycin (Cleocin). Antibiotic therapy causes a disruption in the normal bacterial flora of the colon. This disruption allows for colonization with *C difficile*, a spore-forming anaerobe present in the hospital environment, via the oral-fecal route. Pathogenic strains then produce toxins that cause diarrhea and pseudomembranous colitis.

Other risk factors include surgery (primarily colonic, gastric, and pelvic), colon carcinoma, leukemia, and uremia. Obviously, the hospitalized cancer patient undergoing chemotherapy and/or surgery and receiving broad-spectrum antibiotics is most vulnerable to this infection.

Signs and symptoms

Infection with *C difficile* can be asymptomatic. When signs and symptoms do occur, they may range from mild to moderate diarrhea with lower abdominal pain, to antibiotic-associated colitis without pseudomembranous formation, to pseudomembranous colitis, to fulminant colitis. Fulminant colitis may be associated with toxic megacolon and even perforation of the viscus and peritonitis. On occasion, a patient may present with just abdominal pain or fever and no diarrhea.

Pseudomembranes may be absent in mild disease but usually are present in severe disease and are easily recognized on sigmoidoscopic or colonoscopic examination as adherent yellow plaques that may coalesce over large areas.

Diagnosis

The development of diarrhea or even abdominal pain or fever in a cancer patient should prompt a work-up for *C difficile*–associated diarrhea.

Stool cytotoxin test The laboratory diagnosis of *C difficile* infection depends on the demonstration of *C difficile* toxins in the stool. The gold standard is the stool cytotoxin test, a tissue-culture assay that demonstrates cell rounding by *C difficile* toxin B.

Enzyme immunoassay Another test that can demonstrate *C difficile* toxins (A and/or B) in the stool is an enzyme immunoassay. It is less expensive and faster than the cytotoxin test and does not need to be performed by specially trained laboratory personnel.

Stool culture Although a stool culture for *C difficile* may also be obtained, it has less significance in making the diagnosis.

Treatment

INITIAL MANAGEMENT

The initial step in the management of *C difficile*–associated diarrhea is to discontinue antibiotic therapy. Patients may not require any other therapy. However, stopping antibiotics in a cancer patient may not be possible or the patient may be severely ill from the colitis. In these instances, specific anti–*C difficile* therapy is required.

Specific antibiotic therapy

Metronidazole and vancomycin Metronidazole (250 mg PO qid) and vancomycin (125 mg PO qid), both given for 10 days, are the drugs of choice. Metronidazole is preferred because it is less expensive and the use of vancomycin may promote the emergence of vancomycin-resistant enterococci.

For the patient who cannot tolerate oral medications, IV metronidazole (500 mg q6h) can be given. IV vancomycin should not be used, as high intraluminal levels cannot be attained.

Other agents that might be used for treatment include bacitracin (25,000 U PO qid) and cholestyramine (4 g PO qid).

TREATMENT OF RELAPSE

Relapse occurs in 10%-20% of patients. Mild cases may not need to be treated. If treatment is indicated, a repeat 7- to 14-day course of either metronidazole or vancomycin may be administered. If the infection persists after repeated therapy, longer courses (4-6 weeks) followed by a gradual tapering of the dose may be helpful.

Prevention

Contact isolation Patients with *C difficile*–associated diarrhea and those who are known carriers should be placed in "contact isolation"; ie, the use of gloves, gowns, and careful hand-washing should be instituted.

Disinfection During outbreaks, the use of sodium hypochlorite to disinfect contaminated surfaces has been recommended.

Antibiotic prophylaxis of high-risk patients or carriers is not recommended.

TYPHLITIS

Typhlitis (necrotizing enterocolitis) occurs in patients who are severely neutropenic, usually in the setting of chemotherapy. Pathologically, the areas of involvement include the cecum and terminal ileum. Typhlitis is a broad-spectrum disease characterized by bowel wall edema, diffuse or patchy necrosis involving the mucosa alone or the full thickness of the bowel wall, mucosal ulcerations, hemorrhage, inflammatory infiltrates, and infiltration of the bowel wall by bacteria or fungi. Mild cases are self-limiting when treated with bowel rest/antibiotics. Death may occur in severe cases.

Signs and symptoms

Signs and symptoms of typhlitis can be nonspecific but usually include fever, abdominal pain (typically in the right lower quadrant), and abdominal distention. The patient may have diarrhea (sometimes bloody), nausea, and vomiting or may demonstrate signs and symptoms consistent with those of acute appendicitis.

Physical findings There may be abdominal guarding and rebound tenderness, diminished bowel sounds, or even a mass in the right lower quadrant of the abdomen.

Diagnosis

Radiographs or CT scans of the abdomen may demonstrate a thickened cecum, mass, or even gas within the colon wall.

Treatment

Mortality from typhlitis is high (> 50%) and therapy is controversial. However, broad-spectrum antibiotics covering both gut aerobes and anaerobes and resection of necrotic bowel are recommended.

FUNGAL INFECTIONS

Fungal infections are a leading cause of morbidity and mortality in cancer patients. These infections pose a formidable management challenge, in that diagnosis is often difficult to make at an early stage and, therefore, appropriate treatment may be delayed.

Etiology and risk factors

***Candida* species** The most common fungal infections in cancer patients are caused by *Candida* species. Of the candidal pathogens found in these patients, *C albicans* is the most common. However, more recently other *Candida* species, such as *C tropicalis, C glabrata, C parapsilosis, C krusei,* and *C lusitaniae,* have become more prevalent. This finding is significant, as many of these species (*C krusei, C glabrata, C lusitaniae*) can be resistant to fluconazole and less susceptible to amphotericin B.

Major risk factors for candidal infections include neutropenia, a breakdown in physical defense barriers (such as mucositis induced by chemotherapy and radiation therapy), broad-spectrum antibiotics, immune dysfunction (caused by chemotherapy and steroids), surgery (especially GI surgery), long-term indwelling vascular catheters, and poor nutritional status/total parenteral nutrition.

***Aspergillus* species** is a less common cause of infection in cancer patients than candidal organisms but is more virulent. The most common of the *Aspergillus* species is *A fumigatus*, followed by *A flavus, A niger,* and *A terreus.*

Risk factors for *Aspergillus* infections include severe immunosuppression (primarily allogeneic HCT), steroid therapy, GVHD, and environmental exposure.

Other fungi Other emerging fungal pathogens in the cancer patient include *Fusarium, Trichosporon, Zygomycetes,* and *Scedosporium* species; *Malassezia furfur;* and the dematiaceous/pigmented fungi (eg, *Bipolaris spicifera, Cladosporium bantianum).*

Finally, the endemic fungi, *Coccidioides immitis* and *Histoplasma capsulatum,* are often more virulent and aggressive than other fungi in the immunocompromised host.

Signs and symptoms

Candidiasis

Candidiasis can present as a wide spectrum of diseases, from mucosal infection to disseminated and invasive disease.

Local mucosal infection Oropharyngeal candidiasis can present as classic thrush with beige plaques. It may be painful, as there may be a concurrent mucositis due to the ablative chemotherapy. Oropharyngeal candidiasis may extend into the esophagus as esophagitis, which may manifest as odynophagia. Epiglottitis may present as odynophagia and laryngeal stridor.

Disseminated infection Candidemia may present simply as an asymptomatic fever or may result in a full-blown septic shock syndrome (acute disseminated candidiasis). In contrast, chronic disseminated candidiasis, which involves the chronic, indolent infection of different organs, such as the liver, spleen, and kidneys, may be manifested by fever alone.

Aspergillosis

Invasive aspergillosis most commonly involves the lungs and sinuses. However, it can also disseminate to the brain (and may be the most common cause of brain abscesses in HCT patients). Less commonly, aspergillosis can disseminate to other organs, including the skin.

Pulmonary aspergillosis Signs and symptoms of invasive pulmonary aspergillosis include pleuritic pain, pulmonary hemorrhage, hemoptysis, and cavitation. The chest radiograph or CT scan may demonstrate pulmonary nodular infiltration and/or cavitary lesions.

Sinusitis Patients with sinusitis may have few signs (swelling) or symptoms (pain), especially if they are neutropenic.

Brain abscess Patients with brain abscesses may have headaches and neurologic signs consistent with the specific site of the lesion.

Skin involvement may present as necrotizing skin nodules or ulcers.

Other infections

***Fusarium* infections** The signs and symptoms of *Fusarium* infections are similar to those of aspergillosis; ie, pulmonary infiltrates, sinusitis, and cutaneous lesions are prominent.

***Trichosporon* infections** are similar to *Candida* infections in that they can cause disseminated disease in multiple organs.

***Zygomycetes* infections** cause sinopulmonary disease.

***Scedosporium* species** are similar to *Aspergillus* species in their structure and predilection for the respiratory tract.

C immitis* and *H capsulatum also target the lungs but can disseminate to other organs.

Diagnosis

In the arena of diagnostic tests for invasive aspergillosis, only recently has the *Aspergillus* galctomannan enzyme immunoassay been available in the United States. It was reported that antifungal therapy decreases the sensitivity of this assay and thus limits its usefulness in high-risk patients on antifungal prophylaxis (*Marr KA, Laverdiere M, Gugel A, et al: Clin Infect Dis 40:1762-1769, 2005*). There are also two other diagnostic tests now available: the glucan assay (for [1,3]-β-D-glucan) and the *Aspergillus* DNA polymerase chain reaction. Unfortunately, there is a paucity of data and lack of experience with these assays to determine their utility in diagnosing and predicting invasive fungal infection in patients at highest risk.

Diagnosis of fungal infection in the cancer patient requires documentation by culture or histologic examination.

Candidiasis Although the diagnosis of oropharyngeal candidiasis often is made on clinical grounds, the lesions should be scraped for microscopic examination and culture. Biopsy of esophageal lesions via endoscopy should be performed to confirm *Candida* (as opposed to HSV or CMV) as the etiology of the infection.

A positive blood culture for *Candida* (especially a species other than *C albicans)* should never be considered a "contaminant" and often implies a right atrial catheter infection. Less likely to result in positive blood cultures are chronic, deep-seated infections, such as hepatosplenic candidiasis. Such infections require biopsy for confirmation.

***Aspergillus* species,** like other species, such as *Zygomycetes* and dematiaceous fungi, is rarely found in the bloodstream and requires tissue sampling for diagnosis. Occasionally, bronchoalveolar lavage fluid or sinus drainage will yield *Aspergillus*, but often a lung biopsy is required. Recently, an *Aspergillus* galactomannan enzyme immunoassay test has become available for the diagnosis of invasive aspergillosis. Unfortunately, it is not clear that it is a sufficiently sensitive (especially in patients receiving antifungal agents) or predictive test for the disease.

***Fusarium*, *Scedosporium*, and *Trichosporon* species,** in contrast to *Aspergillus* species, are often found in the bloodstream.

Skin lesions Any skin lesion should be suspected of being of fungal origin and should be biopsied, cultured, and examined histologically.

Search for sites of infection When a fungal infection is suspected or documented, a search for possible sites of infection should ensue. For a blood culture that grows a *Candida* species, the intravascular catheter should, in most cases, be removed for diagnostic as well as therapeutic reasons, and the catheter tip should be cultured. A CT scan of the abdomen should be obtained. In cases of suspected *Aspergillus* infection, in addition to a CT scan of the chest, a CT scan of the brain and sinuses should be performed.

Treatment

ANTIFUNGAL AGENTS

There are now three major groups of antifungal agents: 1) the polyenes (amphotericin B deoxycholate and its lipid formulations [amphotericin B lipid complex, liposomal amphotericin B, amphotericin B cholsteryl sulfate]); 2) the azoles (fluconazole, itraconzaole, voriconazole, posaconazole); and 3) the echinocandins (caspofungin, micafungin, anidulafungin).

Amphotericin B deoxycholate has been the standard therapy for invasive fungal infection for 50 years. It is fungicidal and has a broad spectrum of activity against yeasts and molds, including the *Zygoycetes.* It is thought to be less active against *C guillermondii* and *C lusitaniae.* However, it is limited by its nephrotoxicity and infusional toxicity. The lipid formulations are less nephrotoxic but much more expensive than the other formulations.

The azoles are not nephrotoxic. The first-generation azoles (fluconazole and itraconazole) are considered fungistatic, whereas the extended-spectrum azoles (voriconazole and posaconazole) are considered more fungicidal. Fluconazole is well absorbed orally and can be administered orally or intravenously but is not active against molds and certain *Candida* species (*C krusei*). Itraconazole is hepatoxic and is not well absorbed when orally adminstered. Voriconazole is well absorbed orally and can also be administered intravenously. It is broadly active against most *Candida* species and most molds, with the exception of the *Zygomycetes.* Posaconazole can only be orally administered and is well absorbed. It is broadly active against most *Candida* species and most molds, including the *Zygomycetes.*

The echinocandins are the least toxic of the antifungal agents. They can only be administered intravenously. They are said to be fungicidal against yeasts but fungistatic against molds.

Candidiasis

Local mucosal candidiasis In patients with local mucosal candidiasis (including esophagitis), oral fluconazole or itraconazole can be used. If the patient has difficulty in taking oral medication, IV fluconazole should be used. If the patient was receiving prophylactic fluconazole when candidiasis developed, there is a high likelihood that the causative *Candida* species may be azole-resistant, and either an echinocandin (caspofungin, micafungin, or anidulafungin) or a lipid formulation of amphotericin B should be used.

Candidemia If candidemia is documented, the intravascular catheter should be removed. This step should be followed by the administration of an antifungal for at least 2 weeks after the last positive blood culture is obtained and all signs and symptoms have resolved. Although fluconazole has been shown to be an effective and safe agent in the treatment of candidemia, there are certain circumstances in which an alternative (an echinocandin or a lipid formulation of amphotericin B) might be preferable. These situations would include hemodynamic instability, neutropenia, or high suspicion of azole resistance (eg, a patient who is colonized with a resistant *Candida* species or has been on recent fluconazole prophylaxis or treatment).

Disseminated, deep-seated candidiasis (eg, hepatosplenic infection). Although the standard of therapy for deep-seated candidiasis has been long-term therapy with amphotericin deoxycholate, it has been limited by nephrotoxicity. Thus, the lipid formulations of amphotericin B have allowed higher cumulative doses with a lower nephrotoxic potential. The azoles (fluconazole, voriconazole) have the advantage of convenient (ie, oral) administration and good absorption, with little toxicity. The echinocandins also have been shown to be effective against this infection.

> Micafungin (Mycamine), the second echinocandin agent, was approved by the FDA in 2005 and joins caspofungin in our antifungal armamentarium. Although it was approved for treatment of esophageal candidiasis and prophylaxis of *Candida* infections in patients undergoing hematopoietic cell transplantation (HCT), it has activity against *Aspergillus* species and only missed showing significant ($P = .07$) protection against aspergillosis by a thin margin because of the short duration of prophylaxis (*van Burik JA, Ratanatharathorn V, Stepan DE, et al: Clin Infect Dis 39:1407-1416, 2004*). This agent may become the antifungal prophylactic drug of choice for hospitalized high-risk HCT recipients. Posaconazole, another extended-spectrum azole joining voriconazole, has recently become available, and its advantages are broad activity against molds (including the *Zygomycetes*) and its oral administration. Posaconazole may be the ideal prophylactic agent in the outpatient HCT setting. Finally, the echinocandin anidulafungin also has been recently approved, demonstrating superior activity over fluconazole in invasive candidiasis.

Aspergillosis

Antifungal therapy Amphotericin B deoxycholate (1.0-1.5 mg/kg/d) had been the standard therapy for invasive aspergillosis. However, voriconazole led to better responses, improved survival, and fewer adverse events than did amphotericin B when used as initial therapy in patients with invasive aspergillosis. Thus, voriconazole is the standard therapy for invasive aspergillosis. In addition, new antifungals and new formulations of amphotericin B have been approved for use in invasive aspergillosis in patients who are intolerant of or refractory to conventional amphotericin B. They include amphotericin B lipid complex, amphotericin B cholesteryl sulfate, liposomal amphotericin B, itraconazole oral solution, IV itraconazole, and caspofungin. All of these formulations are less nephrotoxic than amphotericin B deoxycholate.

Surgical removal of infected sites In addition to antifungal therapy, it is important to attempt surgical removal of infected sites, if at all feasible. Sinus surgery should be performed. Resection of pulmonary lesions should be attempted if there are only one or two limited, discrete lesions.

Infections with other fungi

Although amphotericin B is the drug of choice for most invasive fungal infections, there are exceptions. *Scedosporium* and *Fusarium* species are often resistant to amphotericin B, and voriconazole may be the drug of choice for these infections. Voriconazole, however, is not active against *Zygomycetes* species, and if an infection with this organism is suspected or documented, amphotericin B deoxycholate, an amphotericin B lipid formulation, or posaconazole should be used. The dematiaceous/pigmented fungi also may be better treated with itraconazole. For *Trichosporon* infections, voriconazole may be more effective than amphotericin B.

Prevention

Because invasive fungal infection occurs with high frequency in the setting of HCT, most prophylactic studies have been performed in HCT recipients. Thus, the following recommendations apply mainly to this group, although prophylaxis can be justified when the incidence of these infections in any population is high enough.

Fluconazole Two randomized, placebo-controlled studies using prophylactic fluconazole (400 mg/d) have demonstrated a decrease in invasive and superficial *C albicans* infections. One study showed a reduction in mortality. As fluconazole is not active against *C krusei, C glabrata,* or *Aspergillus* species, there is concern that its prophylactic use will increase the incidence of these resistant fungi. Some authors have reported such an occurrence.

Micafungin has recently been approved for use as an antifungal (candidiasis) prophylactic agent in HCT. There was also a trend toward protection against *Aspergillus* infection with micafungin, although it was not significant.

Itraconazole has been shown to be an effective antifungal prophylactic agent in HCT, but no survival benefit has been demonstrated, possibly because of the toxic GI effects and hepatotoxicity associated with this agent.

Low-dose amphotericin B was observed, in a retrospective study, to decrease the incidence of *Candida* infection. However, this regimen only delayed the onset of *Aspergillus* infections.

Other prophylactic regimens have been used in small numbers of patients, with varying degrees of success. They include aerosolized amphotericin B, intranasal amphotericin B, and amphotericin B lipid complex. Voriconazole (vs fluconazole) is currently being studied as a prophylactic agent in HCT. The prophylactic regimen of the future may be an echinocandin (eg, micafungin) initially (while patients are hospitalized) followed by an oral azole (eg, posaconazole) administered to those outpatients who remain at high risk for mold infections.

HEPA filtration Other than using prophylactic antifungals, there is little that can be done to prevent fungal infections in cancer patients. The one possible exception is the use of HEPA filtration, which can eliminate *Aspergillus* spores from the environment. However, most patients emerge from this environment still possessing the same risk factors (steroids, GVHD) for aspergillosis.

VIRAL INFECTIONS

Opportunistic viral infections are a particular problem in cancer patients who undergo HCT and those with hematologic cancers. Accurate diagnosis of viral infections is important, as treatment is available for many of them.

Etiology

As mentioned previously, viral infections in cancer patients are caused predominantly by herpesviruses (HSV, VZV, CMV, and EBV). The herpesvirus infections usually are reactivations of latent infections. Respiratory viruses that infect cancer patients include respiratory syncytial virus, influenza viruses A and B, parainfluenza virus, rhinovirus, and adenovirus.

Signs and symptoms

Although all of the herpesviruses can cause fever and a septic picture, HSV usually presents as mucositis or a vesicular rash, VZV presents as a vesicular rash in a dermatomal distribution, and CMV, in the HCT setting, presents as interstitial pneumonia. When HSV or VZV disseminates, each virus can cause disseminated cutaneous lesions or visceral (liver, lung, brain) involvement. VZV infection can present with GI symptoms, such as epigastric or general abdominal pain.

Diagnosis

To make a specific viral etiologic diagnosis, tissue or fluid must be obtained from the infected site and processed for histologic/cytologic examination and culture.

Vesicular skin lesions When a cancer patient presents with a vesicular rash, it is invariably due to either HSV or VZV. If the distribution of lesions is in a dermatomal pattern, a clinical diagnosis of VZV can be made. However, if there is cutaneous dissemination, the vesicular lesions should be aspirated (and sent for viral culture) or scraped down to the base, smeared on a glass slide, and sent for direct fluorescent antibody staining (for HSV and VZV).

Visceral involvement When there is visceral involvement with either HSV, VZV, or CMV, biopsy material is examined for inclusions and is submitted for culture.

Respiratory infection For the respiratory viruses, diagnosis is usually made by examination of bronchoalveolar lavage fluid (obtained by bronchoscopy) or biopsy (obtained by transbronchial, percutaneous thoracic, thoracoscopic, or open lung biopsy). In the special case of CMV interstitial pneumonitis in the HCT setting, diagnosis of infection (prior to disease onset) can be made by detection of antigens or virus in the bloodstream, in addition to evidence of the virus in bronchoalveolar lavage fluid.

Antibody testing is of little use in the diagnosis of viral infection in the cancer patient.

Treatment

HSV infection Localized HSV infection is usually treated with acyclovir, 5 mg/kg IV q8h. If there is dissemination, a dose of 10 mg/kg q8h can be used, and if there is CNS involvement, up to 15 mg/kg IV q8h can be utilized. If acyclovir-resistant HSV is suspected, foscarnet (Foscavir) can be used (see Table 1 for doses). However, this is a nephrotoxic drug.

VZV infection is usually treated with acyclovir, administered at a dose of 10 mg/kg IV q8h.

CMV infection is treated with ganciclovir or foscarnet. Ganciclovir is the drug of choice but is toxic to bone marrow.

In the HCT setting, "preemptive" treatment (treatment to prevent disease after evidence of infection is obtained) consists of ganciclovir, 5 mg/kg IV bid for 7 days followed by 5 mg/kg/d IV for another 3-5 weeks. Actual treatment of CMV interstitial pneumonia consists of ganciclovir, 5 mg/kg IV q12h, along with immunoglobulin, 500 mg/kg IV every other day for 21 days (induction phase). Maintenance therapy (for as long as immunosuppression is present) consists of ganciclovir, 5 mg/kg/d IV for 5 days each week, and immunoglobulin, 500 mg/kg IV every week.

Foscarnet can be used instead of ganciclovir if there is marrow toxicity but poses a potential risk of nephrotoxicity.

Respiratory viral infection Among the respiratory viruses, there is specific antiviral therapy only for respiratory syncytial virus and influenza A. Ribavirin (Virazole), 1.1 g/d by aerosol (20 mg/mL), has been used for respiratory syncytial virus and rimantadine (Flumadine) or amantadine (Symmetrel), both 100 mg PO bid, for influenza A. Zanamivir (Relenza) and oseltamivir (Tamiflu, 75 mg PO bid) can be used for both influenza A and B. Finally, cidofovir (Vistide) has been used (but not FDA approved) for adenovirus infection.

Prevention

Herpesvirus infections

Acyclovir HSV and VZV reactivate with great frequency in cancer patients undergoing chemotherapy and/or radiation therapy. This finding is especially true in the HCT population, in which 80% of HSV-seropositive patients and up to 40% of VZV-seropositive patients have a reactivation of HSV or VZV. Therefore, in HSV-seropositive HCT patients, prophylactic acyclovir is indicated. However, prophylaxis may only delay the onset of infection. Any HSV infection that occurs during acyclovir prophylaxis should be considered resistant to acyclovir. Acyclovir has also been shown to reduce the incidence of CMV infection after HCT.

Ganciclovir is the drug of choice for prophylaxis against CMV in the HCT setting, however. It can be used as preemptive therapy, as previously described, but can also be used universally as true prophylaxis to reduce the incidence of CMV infection. However, because of its marrow toxicity (ie, neutropenia) and high cost, ganciclovir cannot be strongly recommended as universal prophylaxis.

CMV-seronegative blood support In the small group of HCT recipients who are CMV-seronegative, the use of CMV-seronegative blood support has been shown to reduce CMV infection dramatically.

Varicella zoster immune globulin In any susceptible cancer patient exposed to VZV, varicella zoster immune globulin should be administered within 96 hours of exposure.

Varicella virus vaccine (Varivax) should not be given to those with hematologic malignancies, malignant neoplasms, or immunodeficiencies, with the exception of those with childhood leukemia in remission for 1 year, when selected criteria are met.

Influenza

Influenza vaccine Although the efficacy of the influenza vaccine is unknown in the HCT setting, it should be administered to all cancer patients.

Rimantadine, amantadine, zanamivir, or oseltamivir can be given prophylactically during an outbreak of influenza.

SUGGESTED READING

ON FEVER AND NEUTROPENIA

Baden LR: Prophylactic antimicrobial agents and the importance of fitness. N Engl J Med 353:1052–1054, 2005.

Freifeld AG, Baden LR, Brown AE, et al: National Comprehensive Cancer Network practice guidelines in oncology: fever and neutropenia - v.1.2006. Available at: http://www.nccn.org/professionals/physicians_gls/PDF/fever.pdf. Accessed August 2006.

Gafter-Gvili A, Fraser, A, Paul M, et al: Meta-analysis: Antibiotic prophylaxis reduces mortality in neutropenic patients. Ann Intern Med 142:979–995, 2005.

Hughes WT, Armstrong D, Bodey GP, et al: 2002 guidelines for the use of antimicrobial agents in neutropenic patients with cancer. Clin Infect Dis 34:730–751, 2002.

Rolston KV: Management of infections in the neutropenic patient. Annu Rev Med 55:519–526, 2004.

Rolston KV: Challenges in the treatment of infections caused by gram-positive and gram-negative bacteria in patients with cancer and neutropenia. Clin Infect Dis 40(suppl 4):S246–S252, 2005.

Wingard JR: Empirical antifungal therapy in treating febrile neutropenic patients. Clin Infect Dis 39(suppl 1):S38–S43, 2004.

ON PNEUMONIA

Rolston KV: The spectrum of pulmonary infections in cancer patients. Curr Opin Oncol 13:218–223, 2001.

ON CATHETER-ASSOCIATED INFECTIONS

Mermel LA, Farr BM, Sherertz RJ, et al: Guidelines for the management of intravascular catheter-related infections. Clin Infect Dis 32:1249–1272, 2001.

O'Grady NP, Alexander M, Dellinger EP, et al: Guidelines for the prevention of intravascular catheter-related infections. Centers for Disease Control and Prevention. MMWR Recomm Rep 51(RR-10):1–29, 2002.

Sheretz RJ: Update on vascular catheter infections. Curr Opin Infect Dis 17:303–307, 2004.

ON *C DIFFICILE*–ASSOCIATED DIARRHEA

Riley TV: Nosocomial diarrhoea due to *Clostridium difficile.* Curr Opin Infect Dis 17:323–327, 2004.

ON FUNGAL INFECTIONS

De Pauw B: Preventive use of antifungal drugs in patients treated for cancer. J Antimicrob Chemother 53:130–132, 2004.

Klastersky J: Empirical antifungal therapy. Int J Antimicrob Agents 23:105–112, 2004.

Leather HL, Wingard JR: Prophylaxis, empirical therapy, or pre-emptive therapy of fungal infections in immunocompromised patients: Which is better for whom? Curr Opin Infect Dis 15:369–375, 2002.

Pappas PG, Rex JH, Sobel JD, et al: Guidelines for treatment of candidiasis. Clin Infect Dis 38:161–189, 2004.

Rubin ZA, Somani J: New options for the treatment of invasive fungal infections. Semin Oncol 31(2 suppl 4):91–98, 2004.

Stevens DA, Kan VL, Judson MA, et al: Practice guidelines for diseases caused by *Aspergillus.* Clin Infect Dis 30:696–709, 2000.

CHAPTER 47

Fluid complications

Frederic W. Grannis, Jr., MD, Carey A. Cullinane, MD, and Lily Lai, MD

MALIGNANT PLEURAL EFFUSION

Malignant pleural effusions complicate the care of approximately 150,000 people in the United States each year. The pleural effusion is usually caused by a disturbance of the normal Starling forces regulating reabsorption of fluid in the pleural space, secondary to obstruction of mediastinal lymph nodes draining the parietal pleura. Tumors that metastasize frequently to these nodes, eg, lung cancer, breast cancer, and lymphoma, cause most malignant effusions. It is, therefore, puzzling that small-cell lung cancer infrequently causes effusions. Primary effusion lymphomas caused by human herpesvirus 8 and perhaps Epstein-Barr virus (EBV) are seen in patients with AIDS.

Pleural effusion restricts ventilation and causes progressive shortness of breath by compression of lung tissue as well as paradoxical movement of the inverted diaphragm. Pleural deposits of tumor cause pleuritic pain.

Pleural effusions commonly occur in patients with advanced-stage tumors, who frequently have metastases to brain, bone, and other organs, physiologic deficits, malnutrition, debilitation, and other comorbidities. Because of these numerous clinical and pathologic variables, it is difficult to perform meaningful trials in patients with pleural effusions. For the same reason, it is often difficult to predict a potential treatment outcome for the specific patient with multiple interrelated clinical problems. Altundag and colleagues from M. D. Anderson Cancer Center performed a retrospective study of patients with "wet" IIIB non–small-cell lung cancer. Of the 37 patients who had no detectable distant metastasis at the time of diagnosis, 12 (32%) experienced improved survival. They concluded that selected patients with wet IIIB disease may benefit from aggressive local treatment strategies.

> Pokieser of Vienna, Austria, studied 3,856 patients with breast cancer retrospectively and noted that the site of first recurrence was a malignant effusion in 5.34%. In comparison to a control group, patients with invasive ductal carcinoma in the inner quadrants had a significantly higher incidence of malignant pleural and pericardial effusions (*Pokieser W, Cassik P, Fischer G, et al: Breast Cancer Res Treat 83:139-142, 2004*).

Diagnosis

The new onset of a pleural effusion may herald the presence of a previously undiagnosed malignancy or, more typically, complicate the course of a known tumor.

Thoracentesis The first step in management in almost all cases is thoracentesis. An adequate specimen should be obtained and sent for cell count; determination of glucose, protein, lactic dehydrogenase (LDH), and pH; and appropriate cultures and cytology. A negative cytology result is not uncommon and does not rule out a malignant etiology.

The Light criteria (LDH > 200 U/L; pleural-serum LDH ratio > 0.6, and pleural-serum protein ratio > 0.5) help categorize pleural effusions as exudates. The majority of undiagnosed exudates are eventually diagnosed as malignant, whereas < 5% of transudates are shown to be caused by cancer.

Because it is sometimes difficult to prove the malignant nature of an effusion, many molecular tests on pleural fluid have been investigated. Multiple reports measure pleural tumor marker proteins, cadherins, matrix metalloproteins, cytokines, telomerase, mRNA, exosomes, and serum and pleural DN methylation patterns, but to date, no test or panel of tests can reliably diagnose malignant effusions.

Pleural biopsy If cytology of an exudative effusion is negative and malignant disease is still suspected (approximately 50% of cases), blind pleural biopsy has a low diagnostic yield that can be improved by CT or ultrasonographic guidance.

Thoracoscopy Thoracoscopic examination is emerging as a reliable diagnostic technique with a low complication rate. It allows comprehensive visualization of one pleural cavity, coupled with the opportunity to biopsy areas of disease. This method provides a definitive diagnosis and allows the pathologist to suggest possible sites of primary disease based on the histopathology. Furthermore, this technique permits the diagnosis and staging of malignant mesothelioma if it is the cause of the effusion. Thoracoscopy also offers the opportunity for simultaneous treatment.

Bronchoscopy may be helpful when an underlying lung cancer is suspected, especially if there is associated hemoptysis, a lung mass, atelectasis, or a massive effusion. It may also be useful when there is a cytologically positive effusion with no obvious primary tumor.

Prognosis

Prognosis of patients with malignant pleural effusion varies by primary tumor. For example, median survival for patients with lung cancer is 3 months, whereas it is 10 months for patients with breast cancer. Median survival is also shorter in patients with encasement atelectasis (3 months).

Treatment

INITIAL TREATMENT

Because the specific clinical circumstances may vary markedly in different patients, treatment must be individualized to provide the best palliation for each patient. In general, malignant pleural effusion should be treated aggressively as soon as it is diagnosed. In most cases, effusion will rapidly recur after treatment by thoracentesis or tube thoracostomy alone. If the clinician decides to administer systemic chemotherapy for the underlying primary malignancy, in tumors such as breast cancer, lymphoma, and small-cell lung cancer, it is important to monitor the patient carefully for recurrent effusion and treat such recurrences immediately.

If a malignant pleural effusion is left untreated, the underlying collapsed lung will become encased by tumor and fibrous tissue in as many as 10%–30% of cases. Once this encasement atelectasis has occurred, the underlying lung is "trapped" and will no longer reexpand after thoracentesis or tube thoracostomy. Characteristically, the chest x-ray in such cases shows resolution of the pleural effusion after thoracentesis, but the underlying lung remains partially collapsed. This finding is often misinterpreted by the inexperienced clinician as evidence of a pneumothorax, and a chest tube is placed. The air space persists and the lung remains unexpanded, even with high suction and pulmonary physiotherapy. Allowing the chest tube to remain in place can worsen the situation, resulting in bronchopleural fistulization and empyema.

Physical techniques

To avoid encasement atelectasis, pleural effusion should be treated definitively at the time of initial diagnosis. Multiple physical techniques of producing adhesions between the parietal and visceral pleurae, obliterating the space, and preventing recurrence have been used. They include open or thoracoscopic pleurectomy, gauze abrasion, or laser pleurodesis. Surgical methods have not been demonstrated to have any advantage over simpler chemical pleurodesis techniques in the treatment of malignant effusions. Gauze abrasion can easily be employed when unresectable lung cancer with associated effusion is found at the time of thoracotomy.

A randomized, prospective study from Ljubljanska, Slovenia, of 87 patients with malignant pleural effusion secondary to breast cancer showed that the thoracoscopic mechanical abrasion pleurodesis was equivalent to talc pleurodesis in those with normal pleural fluid pH and superior in patients with a low pH.

Chemical agents

Multiple chemical agents have been used.

Tetracycline Tetracycline pleurodesis results in a lower incidence of recurrence when compared with tube thoracostomy alone but often causes severe pain.

Doxycycline and minocycline are probably equivalent in efficacy to tetracycline.

Bleomycin Intrapleural bleomycin, in a dose of 60 U, has been shown to be more effective than tetracycline and is not painful, but it is costly. Absorption of the drug can result in systemic toxicity. Combined use of tetracycline and bleomycin has been demonstrated to be more efficacious than the use of either drug singly.

Kwek, from Massachusetts General Hospital, reported that PET scans performed on nine patients, an average of 22 months following talc pleurodesis, showed focal nodular fluorodeoxyglucose (FDG) uptake in the pleura (mean standard error of mean 5.4; range: 1.2-16; *Kwek BH, Aquino SL, Fischman AJ: Chest 125:2356-2360, 2004*).

Talc pleurodesis was first introduced by Bethune in the 1930s. Talc powder (Sclerosol Intrapleural Aerosol) has demonstrated efficacy in numerous large studies, preventing recurrent effusion in 70%–92% of cases. Talc is less painful than tetracycline. Cost is minimal, but special sterilization techniques must be mastered by the hospital pharmacy. Talc formulations may have significant differences in the size of particles. Smaller particles may be absorbed and disseminated systemically.

Talc can be insufflated in a dry state at the time of thoracoscopy or instilled as a slurry through a chest tube. The dose should be restricted to no more than 5 g. A prospective phase III intergroup trial of 501patients randomized to receive thoracoscopic talc vs talc slurry pleurodesis showed similar efficacy in each arm, with increased respiratory complications (14% vs 6%) but less fatigue and higher patient ratings in the insufflation group.

Multiloculated effusions may follow talc use. It is important to ensure that talc does not solidify and form a concretion in the chest tube, thus preventing the drainage of pleural fluid and complete reexpansion of the lung following pleurodesis. Such an event is more likely when small-bore chest tubes are used.

Pleurodesis technique With talc pleurodesis, a 24- to 32-French tube has customarily been inserted through a lower intercostal space and placed on underwater seal suction drainage until all fluid is drained and the lung has completely reexpanded. Because severe lung damage can be produced by improper chest tube placement, it is imperative to prove the presence of free fluid by a preliminary needle tap and to enter the pleural space gently with a blunt clamp technique, rather than by blind trocar insertion. If there is any question about the presence of loculated effusion or underlying adhesions, the use of CT or sonography may enhance the safety of the procedure. In the case of large effusions, especially those that have been present for some time, the fluid should be drained slowly to avoid reexpansion pulmonary edema.

Significant complications can occur with both thoracentesis and chest tube thoracostomy. These procedures should not be performed by inexperienced practitioners without training and supervision.

Premedications If doxycycline or talc is to be used, the patient should be premedicated with narcotics. Intrapleural instillation of 20 mL of 1% lidocaine before administration of the chemical agent may help reduce pain.

Following instillation of the chemical agent, the chest tube should remain clamped for at least 2 hours. If high-volume drainage persists, the treatment can be repeated. The chest tube can be removed after 2 or 3 days if drainage is < 300 mL/day.

Follow-up x-rays at monthly intervals assess the adequacy of treatment and allow early retreatment in case of recurrence.

Alternative approaches Use of fluid-sclerosing agents and outpatient pleurodesis has been advocated by some investigators and has the potential for reducing hospital stay and treatment cost. Patz performed a prospective, randomized trial of bleomycin vs doxycycline (72% bleomycin vs 79% doxycycline) pleurodesis via a 14-French catheter and found no difference in efficacy.

Other approaches that must be considered experimental at this time include quinacrine, iodopovidone, and silver nitrate and use of various biologic agents, including *Corynebacterium parvum,* OK-432, tumor necrosis factor, interleukin-2 (Proleukin), interferon-α (Intron A, Roferon-A), interferon-β (Betaseron), and interferon-γ (Actimmune).

TREATMENT OF ENCASEMENT ATELECTASIS

If encasement atelectasis is found at thoracentesis or thoracoscopy, tube thoracostomy and pleurodesis are futile and contraindicated.

Surgical decortication has been advocated for this problem. This potentially dangerous procedure may result in severe complications, however, such as bronchopleural fistula and empyema.

Pleuroperitoneal shunts The Royal Brompton Hospital, London, group reported experience with pleuroperitoneal shunts in 160 patients with malignant pleural effusion and a trapped lung. Effective palliation was achieved in 95% of patients; 15% of patients required shunt revisions for complications.

Intermittent thoracentesis, as needed to relieve symptoms, may be the best option in patients with a short anticipated survival.

Catheter drainage Another new option is to insert a tunneled, small-bore, cuffed, silicone catheter (PleurX pleural catheter, Denver Biomaterials, Inc., Denver, Colorado) into the pleural cavity. The patient or family members may then drain fluid, using vacuum bottles, whenever recurrent effusion causes symptoms.

Kakuda reported on placement of 61 PleurX pleural catheters in 50 patients with malignant pleural effusions at City of Hope. Thirty-four percent had lung cancer and 24% had breast cancer. There were no operative deaths. In cases where the catheter was placed under thoracoscopic control, 27 of 38 patients (68%) had encasement atelectasis visualized. Eighty-one percent had a good result with control of effusion, with subsequent catheter removal (19%) or intermittent drainage for > 1 month or until death (62%). Five percent of patients had major complications, including empyema and tumor implant.

Putnam prospectively compared PleurX catheter drainage with doxycycline pleurodesis and found the two to be equally effective.

Chemotherapy options depend on the cell type of the tumor and the general condition of the patient. Although intrapleural chemotherapy offers the possibility of high-dose local therapy with minimal systemic effects, only a few, small pilot studies utilizing mitoxantrone (Novantrone), doxorubicin, and hyperthermic cisplatin have been published.

Ang and colleagues from Singapore reported longer mean survival (12 vs 5 months) when systemic chemotherapy was given to 71 patients who initially presented with malignant pleural/pericardial effusions. New studies in this area are much needed.

In Taiwan, Su et al treated 27 patients with non–small-cell lung cancer presenting with a malignant pleural effusion with a regimen of intrapleural cisplatin and gemcitabine, followed by radiotherapy (7,020 cGy in 39 fractions), and completed with IV docetaxel. Only two patients experienced recurrent pleural effusion. The median disease-free and overall survival rates were 8 and 16 months, respectively, and 63% of patients were alive at 1 year.

Radiation therapy may be indicated in some patients with lymphoma but has limited effectiveness in other tumor types, particularly if mediastinal adenopathy is absent.

Chylothorax (in the absence of trauma) is usually secondary to cancer, most frequently lymphoma. An added element of morbidity is conferred by the loss of protein, calories, and lymphocytes in the draining fluid. Chylothorax secondary to lymphoma is usually of low volume and responds to talc pleurodesis in combination with radiotherapy or chemotherapy.

PERICARDIAL EFFUSION

Pericardial effusion develops in 5%–15% of patients with cancer and is sometimes the initial manifestation of malignancy. Most pericardial effusions in cancer patients result from obstruction of the lymphatic drainage of the heart secondary to metastases. The typical presentation is that of a patient with known cancer who is found to have a large pericardial effusion without signs of inflammation. Bloody pericardial fluid is not a reliable sign of malignant effusion.

The most common malignant causes of pericardial effusions are lung and breast cancers, leukemias (specifically acute myelogenous, lymphoblastic, and chronic myelogenous leukemia [blast crisis]), and lymphomas.

Not all pericardial effusions associated with cancer are malignant, and cases with negative cytology may represent as many as half of cancer-associated pericardial effusions. Such effusions are more common in patients with mediastinal lymphoma, Hodgkin lymphoma, or breast cancer. Other nonmalignant causes include drug-induced or postirradiation pericarditis, tuberculosis, collagen diseases, uremia, and congestive heart failure. Many effusions that initially have negative cytology will become positive over time.

> Martinoni from Milan, Italy, reported on the use of intrapericardial administration of thiotepa (15 mg on days 1,3, and 5) following placement of a pericardial drainage catheter in 33 patients with malignant pericardial effusion. There were three recurrent effusions (9.1%). The medial survival was 115 days. They concluded that this protocol is safe, well tolerated, and improves quality and duration of life (*Martinoni A, Cipolla CM, Cardinale D, et al: Chest 126:1412-1416, 2004*).

Tamponade occurs when fluid accumulates faster than the pericardium can stretch. Compression of all four heart chambers ensues, with tachycardia and diminishing cardiac output. Fluid loading can counteract intrapericardial pressure temporarily. Reciprocal filling of right- and left-sided chambers with inspiration and expiration, secondary to paradoxical movement of the ventricular septum, is a final mechanism to maintain blood flow before death.

Diagnosis

A high index of suspicion is required to make the diagnosis of pericardial effusion.

Signs and symptoms Dyspnea is the most common symptom. Patients may also complain of chest pain or discomfort, easy fatigability, cough, and orthopnea or may be completely asymptomatic. Signs include distant heart sounds and pericardial friction rub. With cardiac tamponade, progressive heart failure occurs, with increased shortness of breath, cold sweats, confusion, pulsus paradoxus > 13 mm Hg, jugular venous distention, and hypotension.

Chest x-ray Chest radiographic evidence of pericardial effusion includes cardiomegaly with a "water bottle" heart; an irregular, nodular contour of the cardiac shadow; and mediastinal widening.

ECG The ECG shows nonspecific ST- and T-wave changes, tachycardia, low QRS voltage, electrical alternans, and atrial dysrhythmia.

Pericardiocentesis and echocardiography An echocardiogram not only can confirm a suspected pericardial effusion but also can document the size of the effusion and its effect on ventricular function. A pericardial tap with cytologic examination (positive in 50%–85% of cases with associated malignancy) will confirm the diagnosis of malignant effusion or differentiate it from other causes of pericardial effusion. Serious complications, including cardiac perforation and death, can occur during pericardiocentesis, even when performed with echocardiographic guidance by experienced clinicians.

Tumor markers or special staining and cytogenetic techniques may improve the diagnostic yield, but ultimately an open pericardial biopsy may be necessary. Szturmowicz from Warsaw, Poland, studied pericardial fluid carcinoembryonic antigen (CEA) and CYFRA 21-1 levels in 84 patients with pericardial effusion. There were significant differences in patients with malignant vs benign effusions with both tests. Using cutoff points of > 100 ng/mL for CYFRA 21-1 and > 5 ng/mL for CEA, 14 of 15 patients with malignant pericardial effusion with negative cytologic results had a positive result on one or both tests.

CT and MRI as diagnostic adjuncts may provide additional information about the presence and location of loculations or mass lesions within the pericardium and adjacent structures.

Cardiac catheterization may occasionally be of value to rule out superior vena caval obstruction, diagnose microvascular tumor spread in the lungs with secondary pulmonary hypertension, and document constrictive pericarditis before surgical intervention. Pericardial fluid has been aspirated in experimental animals by femoral vein catheterization and needle puncture of the right atrial appendage from within. This technique has not been used in humans.

Pericardioscopy allows visualization and biopsy at the time of subxiphoid or thoracoscopic pericardiotomy and can improve the diagnostic yield.

Prognosis

In general, cancer patients who develop a significant pericardial effusion have a high mortality, with a mean time to death of 2.2–4.7 months. However, about 25% of selected patients treated surgically for cardiac tamponade enjoy a 1-year survival.

Treatment

GENERAL CONCEPTS

As is the case with malignant pleural effusion, it is difficult to evaluate treatments for pericardial effusion because of the many variables. Since malignant pericardial effusion is less common than malignant pleural effusion, it is more difficult to collect data in a prospective manner. Certain generalizations can, however, be derived from available data:

- All cancer patients with pericardial effusion require a systematic evaluation and should not be dismissed summarily as having an untreatable and/or terminal problem.
- Ultimately, both the management and natural course of the effusion depend on (1) the underlying condition of the patient, (2) the extent of clinical symptoms associated with the cardiac compression, and (3) the type and extent of the underlying malignant disease.

GENERAL TREATMENT APPROACHES

Asymptomatic, small effusions may be managed with careful follow-up and treatment directed against the underlying malignancy. On the other hand, cardiac tamponade is a true oncologic emergency. Immediate pericardiocentesis, under echocardiographic guidance, may be performed to relieve the patient's symptoms. A high failure rate is anticipated because the effusion rapidly recurs unless steps are taken to prevent it. Therefore, a more definitive treatment plan should be made following the initial diagnostic/therapeutic tap.

In patients with symptomatic, moderate-to-large effusions who do not present as an emergency, therapy should be aimed at relieving symptoms and preventing recurrence of tamponade or constrictive pericardial disease. Patients with tumors responsive to chemotherapy or radiation therapy may attain longer remissions with appropriate therapy.

There are two theoretical mechanisms for control of pericardial effusion: creation of a persistent defect in the pericardium allowing fluid to drain out and be reabsorbed by surrounding tissues or sclerosis of the mesothelium resulting in the formation of fibrous adhesions that obliterate the pericardial cavity.

Postmortem studies have demonstrated that both of these mechanisms are operative. The fact that effusions can recur implies that there is either insufficient damage to the mesothelial layer or that rapid recurrence of effusion prevents coaptation of visceral and parietal pericardium and prevents the formation of adhesions. This, in turn, would suggest that early closure of the pericardial defect can result in recurrence.

TREATMENT METHODS

Various methods can be used to treat malignant pericardial effusion.

Observation Observation alone may be reasonable in the presence of small asymptomatic effusions.

Pericardiocentesis is useful in relieving tamponade and obtaining a diagnosis. Echocardiographic guidance considerably enhances the safety of this procedure. Ninety percent of pericardial effusions will recur within 3 months after pericardiocentesis alone.

Pericardiocentesis and percutaneous tube drainage can now be performed with low risk and are recommended by some clinical groups. Problems that may occur include occlusion or displacement of the small-bore tubes, dysrhythmia, recurrent effusion, and infections. Mayo Clinic cardiologists recommend initial percutaneous pericardiocentesis with extended catheter drainage as their technique of choice.

Intrapericardial sclerotherapy and chemotherapy following percutaneous or open drainage have been reported to be effective treatments by some groups. Problems include pain during sclerosing agent treatments and recurrence of effusions. Good results have been reported with instillation of a number of agents, including bleomycin (10 mg), cisplatin (30 mg), mitomycin C (2 mg), thiotepa (1.5 mg), and mitoxantrone (10–20 mg). Agents are selected based on their antitumor or sclerosing effect.

Pericardiocentesis and balloon pericardial window After percutaneous placement of a guidewire following pericardiocentesis, a balloon dilating catheter can be placed across the pericardium under fluoroscopic guidance and a window created by balloon inflation.

At the National Taiwan University, cardiologists performed percutaneous double-balloon pericardiotomy in 50 patients with cancer and pericardial effusion and followed their course

> At City of Hope, Cullinane et al reported on 62 patients with malignant disease who had surgical pericardial window for management of pericardial effusion. Windows were created either thoracoscopically (32) or by subxiphoid (12) or limited thoracotomy (18) approaches. Primary tumors included non–small-cell lung cancer (NSCLC), breast, hematologic, and other solid-organ malignancies. Three recurrent effusions (4.8%) required reoperations. Eight patients (13%) died during the same admission as their surgical procedure. Median survival was much shorter for patients with NSCLC (2.6 mo) than for patients with breast cancer (11 months) or hematologic malignancy (10 months). Surgical pericardial window is a safe and durable operative procedure that may provide extended survival in certain subgroups of cancer patients *(Cullinane CA, Paz, IB, Smith D: Chest 125:1328-1334, 2004).*

using serial echocardiograms. Success without recurrence was achieved in 88%. Fifty percent of patients died within 4 months, and 25% survived to 11 months.

Subtotal pericardial resection is seldom performed today. Although it is the definitive treatment, in that there is almost no chance of recurrence or constriction, higher morbidity and longer recovery time render this operation undesirable in patients who have a short anticipated survival. Its use is restricted to cancer patients with recurrent effusions who are in good overall condition and are expected to survive for up to 1 year.

Limited pericardial resection (pericardial window) via anterior thoracotomy or a thoracoscopic approach has a lower morbidity than less invasive techniques, but recovery is delayed. There is a low risk of recurrence. Cardiac herniation is possible if the size of the opening in the pericardium is not carefully controlled.

Subxiphoid pericardial resection can be performed with the patient under local anesthesia and may be combined with tube drainage and/or pericardial sclerosis. Our group and others have noted recurrences following this technique.

Subxiphoid pericardioperitoneal window through the fused portion of the diaphragm and pericardium has been developed to allow continued drainage of pericardial fluid into the peritoneum. Experience with the procedure is limited, but recurrences may be less frequent than those associated with subxiphoid drainage alone.

Technical factors Prior pleurodesis for malignant pleural effusion makes an ipsilateral transpleural operation difficult or impossible. In lung cancer patients, major airway obstruction may preclude single-lung anesthesia and, thus, thoracoscopic pericardiectomy. Prior median sternotomy may prohibit the use of a subxiphoid approach.

Complications A 30-day mortality rate of 10% or higher has been reported for all of these modalities but is related more to the gravity of the underlying tumor and its sequelae. A small percentage of patients will develop severe problems with pulmonary edema or cardiogenic shock following pericardial decompression. The mechanisms of these problems are poorly understood. Late neoplastic pericardial constriction can occur following initially successful partial pericardiectomy.

Radiotherapy

External-beam irradiation is utilized infrequently in this clinical setting but may be an important option in specialized circumstances, especially in patients with radiosensitive tumors who have not received prior radiation therapy. Responses ranging from 66% to 93% have been reported with this form of treatment, depending on the type of associated tumor.

Systemic therapy

Chemotherapy Systemic chemotherapy is effective in treating pericardial effusions in patients with lymphomas, hematologic malignancies, or breast cancer. Long-term survival can be attained in these patients. If the pericardial effusion is small and/or asymptomatic, invasive treatment may be omitted in some of these cases. Data regarding the effectiveness of systemic chemotherapy or chemotherapy delivered locally in prevention of recurrent pericardial and pleural effusion are limited. New studies in this area are badly needed.

Biologic therapy with various agents is in the early stages of investigation.

MALIGNANT ASCITES

Malignant ascites results when there is an imbalance in the secretion of proteins and cells into the peritoneal cavity and absorption of fluids via the lymphatic system. Greater capillary permeability as a result of the release of cytokines by malignant cells increases the protein concentration in the peritoneal fluid. Recently, several studies have demonstrated higher levels of vascular endothelial growth factor (VEGF), a cytokine known to cause capillary leak, in the sera and effusions of patients with malignancies.

Signs and symptoms

Patients with malignant ascites usually present with anorexia, nausea, respiratory compromise, and immobility. Complaints of abdominal bloating, heaviness, and ill-fitting clothes are common. Weight gain despite muscle wasting is a prominent sign.

Diagnosis

A malignant etiology accounts for only 10% of all cases of ascites. Nonmalignant diseases causing ascites include liver failure, congestive heart failure, and occlusion of the inferior vena cava or hepatic vein. About one-third of all patients with malignancies will develop ascites. Malignant ascites has been described with many tumor types but is most commonly seen with gynecologic neoplasms (~50%), GI malignancies (20%–25%), and breast cancer (10%–18%). In 15%–30% of patients, the ascites is associated with diffuse carcinomatosis of the peritoneal cavity.

Physical examination does not distinguish whether ascites is due to malignant or benign conditions. Patients may have abdominal fullness with fluid wave, anterior distribution of the normal abdominal tympany, and pedal edema. Occasionally, the hepatic metastases or tumor nodules studding the peritoneal surface can be palpated through the abdominal wall, which has been altered by ascitic distention.

RADIOLOGIC STUDIES

Radiographs Ascites can be inferred from plain radiographs of the abdomen. Signs include a ground-glass pattern and centralization of the intestines and abdominal contents.

After paracentesis, 78% of all patients reported relief of their symptoms, especially in the areas of abdominal bloating, anorexia, dyspnea, insomnia, and fatigue. In addition, overall quality of life improved after paracentesis (*Easson A, Bezjak A, Ross S, et al: J Clin Oncol [abstract] 23[suppl]:545s, 2005*).

Ultrasonography Abdominal ultrasonography has been shown to be the most sensitive, most specific method for detecting and quantifying ascites. It also permits delineation of areas of loculation.

CT Abdominal and pelvic CT is effective in detecting ascites. In addition, CT scans may demonstrate masses, mesenteric stranding, omental studding, and diffuse carcinomatosis. Intravenous and oral contrasts are necessary, thus increasing the degree of invasiveness of this modality.

Paracentesis After the diagnosis of peritoneal ascites has been made on the basis of the physical examination and imaging, paracentesis should be performed to characterize the fluid. The color and nature of the fluid often suggest the diagnosis. Malignant ascites can be bloody, opaque, chylous, or serous. Benign ascites is usually serous and clear.

Analysis of the fluid should include cell count, cytology, LDH level, proteins, and appropriate evaluation for infectious etiologies. In addition, the fluid can be sent for the determination of tumor markers, such as CEA, CA-125, *p53*, and human chorionic gonadotropin-β (hCG-β). The hCG-β level is frequently elevated in malignancy-related ascites and has been combined with cytology to yield an 89.5% efficiency in diagnosis. The use of DNA ploidy indices allowed a 98.5% sensitivity and a 100% sensitivity in the identification of malignant cells within ascitic fluid. The use of the telomerase assay, along with cytologic evaluation of the ascitic fluid contents, has a 77% sensitivity in detecting malignant ascites.

Laparoscopy Several studies have utilized minimally invasive laparoscopy as the diagnostic tool of choice. The fluid can be drained under direct visualization, the peritoneal cavity can be evaluated carefully, and any suspicious masses can be biopsied at the time of the laparoscopy.

Prognosis

The presence of ascites in a patient with malignancy often portends end-stage disease. Median survival after the diagnosis of malignant ascites ranges from 7 to 13 weeks. Patients with gynecologic and breast malignancies have a better overall prognosis than patients with GI malignancies.

Treatment

Medical therapy

Traditionally, the first line of treatment is medical management. Medical therapies include repeated paracentesis, fluid restriction, diuretics, chemotherapy, and intraperitoneal sclerosis.

Repeated paracentesis, probably the most frequently employed treatment modality, provides significant symptomatic relief in the majority of cases. The procedure is minimally invasive and can be combined with abdominal ultrasonography to better localize fluid collections. High-volume paracentesis has been performed without inducing significant hemodynamic instability and with good patient tolerance.

> Success at removing peritoneal fluid in patients was markedly better with ultrasonographic assistance, as demonstrated in a randomized trial. Ultrasonography improved the physician's ability to aspirate ascites from 67% (27 of 44 patients) to 95% (40 of 42 patients; *Nazeer SR, Dewbre H, Miller AH: Am J Emerg Med 23:363-367, 2005*).

Significant morbidity occurs with repeated taps and becomes more severe with each tap necessary to alleviate symptoms. Ascitic fluid contains a high concentration of proteins. Routine removal of ascites further depletes protein stores. The removal of large volumes of fluid also can result in electrolyte abnormalities and hypovolemia. In addition, complications can result from the procedure itself. They include hemorrhage, injury to intra-abdominal structures, peritonitis, and bowel obstruction. Contraindications to repeated paracentesis are viscous loculated fluid and hemorrhagic fluid.

With the placement of an intraperitoneal port, used also for the instillation of intraperitoneal chemotherapy, removal of ascitic fluid is possible without the need for repeated paracentesis. Other possible catheters for use in repeated paracentesis include PleurX and Tenckoff catheters (used for intraperitoneal dialysis). Placement of a semipermanent catheter minimizes the risk of injury to intra-abdominal structures. However, the benefits are tempered by increased infectious risks as well as the possibility of a nonfunctioning catheter requiring removal and replacement.

Diuretics, fluid and salt restriction Unlike ascites from benign causes such as cirrhosis and congestive heart failure, malignant ascites responds poorly to fluid restriction, decreased salt intake, and diuretic therapy. The most commonly used diuretics (in patients who may have some response to diuretic treatment) are spironolactone (Aldactone) and amiloride (Midamor). Patients with massive hepatic metastases are most likely to benefit from spironolactone.

The onset of action for spironolactone is delayed (3–4 days), whereas the effects of amiloride are seen after 24 hours. The most common complications associated with these diuretics are painful gynecomastia, renal tubular acidosis, and hyperkalemia.

Chemotherapy, both systemic and intraperitoneal, has had some success in the treatment of malignant ascites. The most commonly used agents are cisplatin and mitomycin (Mutamycin). Intraperitoneal hyperthermic chemotherapy has been used with some efficacy in GI malignancies to decrease recurrence of ascites as well as to prevent the formation of ascites in patients with peritoneal carcinomatosis.

Sclerotherapy Sclerosing agents include bleomycin (60 mg/50 mL of normal saline), tetracycline (500 mg/50 mL of normal saline), and talc (5

Intraperitoneal application of a new class of bispecific antibodies (trifunctional antibodies) was shown to be effective in obliterating ascites. When given as intraperitoneal applications, the antibodies bind to EpCAM- or HER2/neu-antigen on tumor cells and initiate tumor cell killing by T cells, macrophages, NK cells, and dendritic cells. All patients who received the treatment had disappearance of ascites accumulation (*Heiss MM, et al: Int J Cancer 117:435-443, 2005*).

g/50 mL of normal saline). Responses are seen in ~30% of patients treated with these agents.

Theoretically, intraperitoneal chemotherapy and sclerosis obliterate the peritoneal space and prevent future fluid accumulation. If sclerosis is unsuccessful, it may produce loculations and make subsequent paracentesis difficult.

Other systemic therapies There are several reports of the use of gold-198 or phosphorus-32 in patients with peritoneal effusions, with response rates of 30%–50%. Experimental models and early clinical trials have shown that an intraperitoneal bolus of tumor necrosis factor (45–350 μg/m^2) given weekly may be effective in resolving malignant ascites. Other cytokines, including interferon-α, had varying success. A randomized, prospective trial definitively addressing the role of cytokines and other biologic treatments in the management of malignant ascites has yet to be completed.

Surgery

Limited surgical options are available to treat patients who have refractory ascites after maximal medical management, demonstrate a significant decrease in quality of life as a result of ascites, and have a life expectancy of > 3 months.

Peritoneovenous shunts have been used since 1974 for the relief of ascites associated with benign conditions. In the 1980s, shunting was applied to the treatment of malignant ascites.

The LeVeen shunt contains a disc valve in a firm polypropylene casing, whereas the Denver shunt has a valve that lies within a fluid-filled, compressible silicone chamber. Both valves provide a connection between the peritoneal cavity and venous system that permits the free flow of fluid from the peritoneal cavity when a 2- to 4-cm water pressure gradient exists.

Success rates vary with shunting, depending on the nature of the ascites and the pathology of the primary tumor. Patients with ovarian cancer, for example, do very well, with palliation achieved in ≥ 50% of cases. However, ascites arising from GI malignancies is associated with a poorer response rate (10%–15%).

Patient selection Candidates for shunt placement should be carefully selected. Cardiac and respiratory evaluations should be performed prior to the procedure. Shunt placement is *contraindicated* in the presence of the following:

- a moribund patient whose death is anticipated within weeks
- peritonitis
- major organ failure
- adhesive loculation
- thick, tenacious fluid.

Complications of shunting Initial concerns about the use of a shunt in the treatment of malignant ascites centered around intravascular dissemination of tumor. In practice, there has been little difference in overall mortality in patients with and without shunts.

The efficacy of peritoneovenous shunts in patients with malignant ascites was evaluated retrospectively. Overall, the morbidity rate was 36%, the occlusion rate was 12%, and postoperative survival after placement of the shunt was a mean of 54.5 days. A decrease in body weight and abdominal girth was shown. Most patients did not require further care for their ascites (*Tomiyama K, et al: Anticancer Res 26:2393-2395, 2006*).

Disseminated intravascular coagulation During the early experience with shunting, particularly in cirrhotic patients, symptomatic clinical disseminated intravascular coagulation (DIC) developed rapidly and was a major source of morbidity and mortality. However, overwhelming DIC occurs infrequently in the oncologic population.

The pathophysiology of DIC has been studied extensively and is thought to be multifactorial. The reinfusion of large volumes of ascitic fluid may cause a deficiency in endogenous circulating coagulation factors by dilution. Secondarily, a fibrinolytic state is initiated by the introduction of soluble collagen (contained within the ascitic fluid) into the bloodstream, leading to a DIC state. Infrequently, full-blown DIC results and requires ligation of the shunt or even shunt removal. Discarding 50%–70% of the ascitic fluid before establishing the peritoneovenous connection may prevent this complication but may increase the risk of early failure due to a reduced initial flow rate.

Commonly, coagulation parameters are abnormal without signs or symptoms. In some institutions, these laboratory values are so consistently abnormal that they are used to monitor shunt patency. Abnormalities most commonly seen include decreased platelets and fibrinogen and elevated prothrombin time, partial thromboplastin time, and fibrin split products.

Other common complications include shunt occlusion (10%–20%), heart failure (6%), ascitic leak from the insertion site (4%), infection (< 5%), and perioperative death (10%–20% when all operative candidates are included).

Shunt patency may be indirectly correlated with the presence of malignant cells. One study found that patients with positive cytology results had a 26-day shunt survival, as compared with 140 days in patients with negative cytology results. Other studies have failed to demonstrate a correlation between ascites with malignant cells and decreased survival.

Clearly, shunting is not a benign procedure, but in carefully selected patients who have not responded to other treatment modalities and who are experiencing symptoms from ascites, it may provide needed palliation. Because of the limited effectiveness of peritoneovenous shunts, patients should be carefully selected prior to shunt placement.

Radical peritoniectomy Other surgical procedures used to treat malignant ascites have been proposed. They include radical peritoniectomy combined with intraperitoneal chemotherapy. This is an extensive operation with significant morbidity, although initial results appear to demonstrate that it decreases the production of ascites. To date, no randomized trial has demonstrated that radical peritoniectomy increases efficacy or survival.

SUGGESTED READING

ON MALIGNANT PLEURAL EFFUSION

Altundag O, Stewart DJ, Stevens C, et al: The risk of distant metastases in patients with non-small cell lung cancer (NSCLC) with cytologically proven malignant pleural effusion, stage IIIB: A retrospective analysis (abstract). J Clin Oncol 23(suppl):853s, 2005.

Antunes G, Neville E, Duffy J, et al: British Thoracic Society Guidelines for the management of malignant pleural effusions. Thorax 58(suppl 2):1129–1138, 2003.

Cardillo G, Facciolo R, Carbone L, et al: Long-term follow-up of video-assisted talc pleurodesis in malignant recurrent pleural effusions. Eur J Cardiothorac Surg 21:302–305, 2002.

Crnjac A, Sok M, Kamenik M: Impact of pleural effusion pH on the efficacy of thoracoscopic mechanical pleurodesis in patients with breast carcinoma. Eur J Cardiothorac Surg 26:432–436, 2004.

Dresler CM, Olak J, Herndon JE 2nd, et al: Phase III intergroup study of talc poudrage vs talc slurry sclerosis for malignant pleural effusion. Chest 127:909–915, 2005.

Haddad FJ, Younes RN, Gross JL, et al: Pleurodesis in patients with malignant pleural effusions: Talc slurry or bleomycin? Results of a prospective randomized trial. World J Surg 28:749–753, 2004.

Lee YC, Baumann MH, Maskell NA, et al: Pleurodesis practice for malignant pleural effusions in five English-speaking countries: Survey of pulmonologists. Chest 124:2229–2238, 2003.

Paschoalini Mda S, Vargas FS, Marchi E, et al: Prospective randomized trial of silver nitrate vs talc slurry in pleurodesis for symptomatic malignant pleural effusions. Chest 128:684–689, 2005.

Shaw P, Agarwal R: Pleurodesis for malignant pleural effusions. Cochrane Database Syst Rev 1:CD002916, 2004.

Ukale V, Agrenius V, Hillerdal G, et al: Pleurodesis in recurrent pleural effusions: A randomized comparison of a classical and a currently popular drug. Lung Cancer 43:323–328, 2004.

ON PERICARDIAL EFFUSION

Dosios T, Theakos N, Angouras D, et al: Risk factors affecting the survival of patients with pericardial effusion submitted to subxiphoid pericardiostomy. Chest 124:242–246, 2003.

Maisch B, Seferovic PM, Ristic AD, et al: Guidelines on the diagnosis and management of pericardial diseases executive summary: The Task Force on the Diagnosis and Management of Pericardial Diseases of the European Society of Cardiology. Eur Heart J 25:587–610, 2004.

McDonald JM, Meyers BF, Guthrie TJ, et al: Comparison of open subxiphoid pericardial drainage with percutaneous catheter drainage for symptomatic pericardial effusion. Ann Thorac Surg 76:811–816, 2003.

Szturmowicz M, Tomkowksi W, Fijalkowska A, et al: Diagnostic utility of CYFRA 21-1 and CEA assays in pericardial fluid for the recognition of neoplastic pericarditis. Int J Biol Markers 20:43–49, 2005.

Tomkowski WZ, Wisniewska J, Szturmowicz M, et al: Evaluation of intrapericardial cisplatin administration in cases with recurrent malignant pericardial effusion and cardiac tamponade. Support Care Cancer 12:53–57, 2004.

Tsang TS, Enrique-Sarano M, Freeman WK, et al: Consecutive 1,127 therapeutic echocardiographically guided pericardiocenteses: Clinical profile, practice patterns, and outcomes spanning 21 years. Mayo Clin Proc 77:429–436, 2002.

ON MALIGNANT ASCITES

Becker G, Galandi D, Blum HE: Malignant ascites: Systematic review and guideline for treatment. Eur J Cancer 42:589–597, 2006.

Bieligk SC, Calvo BF, Coit DG: Peritoneovenous shunting for nongynecologic malignant ascites. Cancer 91:1247–1255, 2001.

Smith EM, Jayson GC: The current and future management of malignant ascites. Clin Oncol 15:59–72, 2002.

APPENDIX I

Performance scales

Karnofsky performance index

Definition		
Able to carry on normal activity and to work	100	Normal; no complaints; no evidence of disease
	90	Able to carry on normal activity; minor signs or symptoms of disease
	80	Normal activity with effort; some signs or symptoms of disease
Unable to work; able to live at home, care for most personal needs; a varying amount of assistance is needed	70	Cares for self; unable to carry on normal activity or to do active work
	60	Requires occasional assistance but is able to care for most needs
	50	Requires considerable assistance and frequent medical care
Unable to care for self; requires equivalent of institutional or hospital care; disease may be progressing rapidly	40	Disabled; requires special care and assistance
	30	Severely disabled; hospitalization is indicated, although death is not imminent
	20	Very sick; hospitalization necessary; active supportive treatment necessary
	10	Moribund; fatal processes progressing rapidly
	0	Dead

From Karnofsky DA, Abelmann WH, Craver LF, et al: The use of the nitrogen mustards in the palliative treatment of carcinoma. Cancer 1:634–656, 1948.

The Karnofsky performance index and WHO (Zubrod) scale (on the following page) are included here because they are commonly used as proxy measures for quality of life. Because they measure only one dimension of the construct, they would not be considered quality-of-life measures by today's standards. However, given their historic relevance and current high frequency of usage as proxy measures, we have included them here.

WHO (Zubrod) scale

This scale is used to measure performance of which the patient is *capable.* For example, a patient in the hospital for metabolic studies may be fully capable of performing normal activities but will remain in bed through his or her own choice. Such a patient should be coded 0, "normal."

0	Normal activity
1	Symptoms but nearly fully ambulatory
2	Some bed time but needs to be in bed < 50% of normal daytime
3	Needs to be in bed > 50% of normal daytime
4	Unable to get out of bed

From Zubrod CG, Schneiderman M, Frei E III, et al: Appraisal of methods for the study of chemotherapy of cancer in man: Comparative therapeutic trial of nitrogen mustard and triethylene thiophosphoramide. J Chron Dis 11:7–33, 1960.

APPENDIX 2

Cancer information on the Internet

J. Sybil Biermann, MD

The Internet has become nearly indispensable for finding the latest information on cancer diagnosis, treatment, and prevention. This chapter highlights several websites that cater to oncology professionals, researchers, and patients.

Cancer.gov, the National Cancer Institute's website

One of the most comprehensive websites for evidence-based cancer information is supported and maintained by the National Cancer Institute (NCI). The site provides a wide variety of resources to help meet the user's informational needs, including summaries on cancer treatment, prevention, and supportive care, as well as information on ongoing clinical trials, a bibliographic cancer database, funding opportunities, research programs, and cancer incidence and mortality data.

The NCI's vast website provides information suitable to clinical practitioners, researchers, patients, and the general public. Among the cancer resources available from the home page (http://cancer.gov) are:

- peer-reviewed, frequently updated summaries on cancer treatment, screening, prevention, genetics, and supportive care (http://cancer.gov/cancerinfo/pdq/);
- a registry of approximately 25,000 clinical studies sponsored by the National Institutes of Health, other Federal agencies, and private industries and conducted in all 50 states and in more than 120 countries (http://www.clinicaltrials.gov), plus up-to-date information for locating these trials;
- a comprehensive database of NCI-supported basic and clinical research programs (http://researchportfolio.cancer.gov/);
- a directory of NCI research tools and funding opportunities (human, animal, and genomic) for cancer researchers (http://cancer.gov/researchandfunding);
- statistical databases and resources, including cancer incidence by gender, race, ethnicity, and type of cancer; 5-year survival rates; frequen-

cies of childhood cancers; and cancer mortality in the United States by gender and race (http://cancer.gov/statistics).

- patient information: NCI Fact Sheets; extensive, peer-reviewed, and frequently updated patient information sheets.

PubMed

PubMed (http://pubmed.gov/), a service of the National Library of Medicine (NLM), provides access to over 12 million MEDLINE citations in abstract form dating back to the mid-1960s. New features at PubMed are icons that alert researchers to whether the full text of a MEDLINE citation is available and a growing list of biomedical books that can be read and searched online.

In addition, PubMed offers selected cancer topic searches (http://www.cancer.gov/search/pubmed/) for more than 100 different cancer topics. They are prepared literature searches of the NLM's PubMed database, with specifiable date ranges. Users also have a "search cancer subset" option, to retrieve only cancer-related citations from the PubMed database.

Cancer Information Service (CIS)

CIS is a nationwide network of 14 regional offices supported by the NCI. Through its toll-free phone service, CIS provides accurate, up-to-date information on cancer to the public. The phone number is 1-800-4-CANCER. The service responds to calls in English and Spanish.

Reliable information on cancer causes and prevention and a collection of recently issued *NCI Cancer Facts* fact sheets and the new *What You Need To Know About*™ series of patient guides are also available online by following links from the CIS home page (http://cis.nci.nih.gov/).

Cancer.org, the American Cancer Society's website

This large, complex website is most easily searched by specifying key words, such as "breast cancer" or "survival rates," in the search form on the home page (www.cancer.org). Basic resources including the American Cancer Society's *Cancer Facts & Figures 2006* are also now readily available from the home page. Estimates of the numbers of new cancer cases and deaths for the current year are presented according to gender, site, and stage. Also presented is information on cancer mortality, the probability of developing cancer at certain ages, and cancer survival in adults and children.

New resources on the site include sections for survivors and supporters. Most of the information available is intended for patients, especially those who have been newly diagnosed with cancer, and the general public, with several notable exceptions.

Resources for professionals are neatly organized under a "Professionals" heading. This section includes free continuing medical education (CME) and research funding information.

Surveillance, Epidemiology, and End Results (SEER)

The NCI's SEER program collects and publishes cancer incidence and survival data from population-based cancer registries covering approximately 26% of the US population. Trends in age-adjusted SEER cancer incidence and mortality, by race and gender, are presented, as well as 5-year survival rates, by race and gender, and much more. The home page is http://seer.cancer.gov/.

Centers for Disease Control and Prevention

The Centers for Disease Control and Prevention (CDC) maintains several websites for both health professionals and researchers, as well as the public.

Links to CDC statistical reports and online databases are available in the "data warehouse" section of the National Center for Health Statistics website (www.cdc.gov/nchs/datawh.htm). Information on CDC cancer prevention programs may be accessed at the National Center for Chronic Disease Prevention and Health Promotion's website (www.cdc.gov/nccdphp/).

Cancernetwork.com

Another excellent source of reliable cancer information is cancernetwork.com (www.cancernetwork.com). The site features:

- free access to the full text of over 6,000 peer-reviewed medical journal articles from the pages of *ONCOLOGY* and news reports from *Oncology News International;*
- selected text of this handbook;
- the complete proceedings of over 80 cancer symposia, conferences, and workshops focusing on new treatments held around the world;
- a worldwide calendar of oncology meetings and CME courses;
- over 800 direct links to cancer support and research organizations, cancer centers, medical schools, hospices, governmental resources of cancer information and guidelines, and alternative medicine sites;
- free CME based on review articles, cancer-related news stories, and background material online.

CenterWatch

CenterWatch (www.centerwatch.com) offers a worldwide directory of more than 41,000 active industry and government-sponsored trials with independent review board (IRB) approval. Each listing contains a brief summary of the study, the general inclusion/exclusion criteria, and contact information. The database is easily searched, even by a newcomer, and the website has become a major influence for patient recruitment into active clinical trials.

Coalition of National Cancer Cooperative Groups

The Coalition of National Cancer Cooperative Groups was founded in 1997 by the Cancer and Leukemia Group B (CALGB), Eastern Cooperative Oncology Group (ECOG), North Central Cancer Treatment Group (NCCTG), National Surgical Adjuvant Breast and Bowel Project (NSABP), Pediatric Oncology Group (POG), and Radiation Therapy Oncology Group (RTOG). The Coalition's website (http://www.cancertrialshelp.org/medicalCommunity/medicalCommunity.jsp) provides details on the Coalition's initiatives in many areas and features a new software tool, TrialCheck^{SM}, for locating ongoing clinical trials among the Coalition's cooperative groups.

Other Internet sources of cancer information

- The American Society for Therapeutic Radiology and Oncology (ASTRO) has created www.rtanswers.org, a website to explain to cancer patients and their families how radiation therapy is used to safely and effectively treat cancer. The site discusses treatment steps and what patients can expect during treatment. It also offers a "Doctor Finder" feature to allow patients to find a radiation oncologist in their area.
- The American Society of Clinical Oncology (ASCO) website, located at www.asco.org, contains cancer information for patients, including information on treatment, support groups, and other resources. Health care professionals can access information on ASCO policies, clinical guidelines, publications, and a searchable database of abstracts from ASCO's annual scientific meetings dating back to 1995. People Living with Cancer (www/plwc.org) provides patient education materials, a "find an oncologist" function, and an extensive database of patient support organizations.
- An exhaustive collection of articles and reviews on hematologic malignancies, mostly in Adobe Acrobat format and all intended for a professional audience, may be found at the American Society of Hematology's (ASH) website (www.hematology.org). The site also offers a direct link to the Society's official journal, *Blood,* where the full text of all articles dating back to January 1996 can be downloaded and printed.
- The National Comprehensive Cancer Network (NCCN) website, at www.nccn.org, provides access to the NCCN's current Clinical Practice Guidelines, links to ongoing clinical trials at member institutions, and a directory of physicians for referrals. Recent additions include treatment guidelines for patients in both Spanish and English as well as NCCN drugs and biologic companions.
- MdLinx (http://mdlinx.com/HemeOncLinx/) provides daily summaries of hematology/oncology articles culled from a wide variety of professional publications. Articles can be accessed by linkage from the web page. Registered users (registration is free) can also have synopses sent daily to e-mail accounts on general or specified topics within hematology and oncology.

- OncoLink (www.oncolink.com) is a popular website maintained by the University of Pennsylvania, offering a broad variety of news articles, fact sheets, and annotated links to cancer-related information at other websites. The site includes multimedia slide shows, video films, and audio lectures on a wide range of topics.
- Other cancer society and organization websites worth visiting include those of the American Association for Cancer Research (www.aacr.org), the Leukemia & Lymphoma Society (www.leukemia-lymphoma.org), the American College of Radiology (www.acr.org), and the Oncology Nursing Society (www.ons.org). Among European sites, the sites maintained by the International Union Against Cancer (www.uicc.org), CancerBACUP (www.cancerbacup.org.uk), and the European Organisation for Research and Treatment of Cancer (http://www.eortc.be/) are extensive, information-rich resources designed primarily for health care professionals.
- Links to the web pages of state and other regional cancer registries may be found at www.askcnet.org/dataq/cancer.htm. This site also includes links to cancer registries around the world. Other places to look for cancer registries and statistical data in the United States and Canada are the websites maintained by the North American Association of Central Cancer Registries (www.naaccr.org) and the International Agency for Research on Cancer (www.iarc.fr).
- Alternative therapies: An excellent resource for information on commonly used herbs and botanicals is the Memorial Sloan-Kettering Cancer Center site (www.mskcc.org/mskcc/html/11570.cfm). General information on health-related frauds can be found at www.quackwatch.org.

APPENDIX 3

Cancer Drugs and Indications Newly Approved By U.S. Food and Drug Administration, May 2005 – April 2007

Anastrozole (Arimidex): Conversion to regular approval for the adjuvant treatment of postmenopausal women with hormone receptor-positive early breast cancer. Issued September 2005.

Bevacizumab (Avastin): Treatment of metastatic colon cancer. Issued June 2006.

Bortezomib (Velcade): Treatment of previously treated mantle cell lymphoma. Issued December 2006.

Capecitabine (Xeloda): Single-agent adjuvant treatment of Dukes' stage C colon cancer in patients who have undergone complete resection of the primary tumor and for whom fluoropyrimidine therapy alone would be preferred. Issued June 2005.

Cetuximab (Erbitux): For use in combination with radiation therapy for the treatment of patients with unresectable squamous cell cancer of the head and neck and for patients whose disease has metastasized despite use of standard chemotherapy. Issued March 2006.

Dasatinib (Sprycel): Treatment of chronic myelogenous leukemia and Philadelphia-chromosome positive acute lymphoblastic leukemia. Issued June 2006.

Decitabine (Dacogen): Treatment of myelodysplastic syndromes. Issued May 2006.

Docetaxel (Taxotere): In combination with cisplatin and fluorouracil prior to radiotherapy for treatment of inoperable locally advanced squamous cell carcinoma of the head and neck. Issued October 2006.

Erlotinib (Tarceva): Treatment of locally advanced or metastatic non–small-cell lung cancer following failure of at least one prior chemotherapy regimen. Issued November 2004; In combination with gemcitabine for first-line treatment of locally advanced, unresectable, or metastatic pancreatic cancer. Approved for this indication November 2005.

Exemestane (Aromasin): Adjuvant treatment of postmenopausal women with estrogen receptor positive early breast cancer who have received 2 or 3 years of tamoxifen therapy and are switched to exemestane for completion of 5 years of adjuvant hormonal therapy. Issued October 2005.

Gefitinib (Iressa): AstraZeneca and FDA approved new labeling for gefitinib limiting its use to cancer patients who are currently benefiting or have previously benefited from treatment with this agent. Distribution limited under a risk-management plan called Iressa Access Program. Issued June 2005.

Gemcitabine (Gemzar): In combination with carboplatin for treatment of ovarian cancer. Issued July 2006.

Lapatinib (Tykerb): Treatment in combination with capecitabine of advanced or metastatic breast cancer (HER2-positive). Issued March 2007.

Lenalidomide (Revlimid): Treatment of patients with deletion 5q cytogenetic abnormality subtype of myelodysplastic syndrome. Issued December 2005. Treatment of multiple myeloma. June 2006.

Letrozole (Femara): Adjuvant treatment of postmenopausal women with hormone-receptor-positive early breast cancer. Issued January 2006.

Nelarabine (Arranon): Accelerated approval for the treatment of refractory or relapsed T-cell acute lymphoblastic leukemia and T-cell lymphoblastic lymphoma. Patients must have had failure of at least two prior chemotherapy regimens. Issued October 2005.

Panitumumab (Vectibix): Treatment of colorectal cancer that has metastasized following standard chemotherapy. Issued September 2006.

Pegaspargase (Oncaspar): Treatment of acute lymphoblastic leukemia in adults and children. Issued July 2006.

Rituximab (Rituxan): First-line treatment of diffuse large B-cell, CD20 positive, non-Hodgkin's lymphoma in combination with CHOP or other anthracycline-based chemotherapy regimens. Issued February 2006.

Sorafenib (Nexavar): Treatment of advanced renal cell carcinoma in adults. Issued December 2005.

Sunitinib maleate (Sutent): Treatment of gastrointestinal stromal tumor (GIST) after disease progression or intolerance to imatinib mesylate (Gleevec). Also accelerated approval for the treatment of advanced renal cell carcinoma based on partial response rates and response duration. Issued January 2006. Approved for first-line treatment of advanced renal cell carcinoma. Issued February 2007.

Thalidomide (Thalomid): Treatment of multiple myeloma. Issued May 2006.

Topotecan (Hycamtin): Treatment of cervical cancer. Issued June 2006.

Trastuzumab (Herceptin): Expanded use of trastuzumab post surgery in combination with other cancer drugs for treatment of HER-2 positive early breast cancer. Issued November 2006.

Vorinostat (Zolinza): Treatment of cutaneous manifestations of progressive, recurrent cutaneous T-cell lymphoma. Issued October 2006.

APPENDIX 4

Chemotherapeutic agents and their uses, dosages, and toxicities

Chris H. Takimoto, MD, PhD, and Emiliano Calvo, MD, PhD

CHEMO AGENTS

Abbreviations: ALL = acute lymphoblastic leukemia; AML = acute myelogenous leukemia; AUC = area under the curve; BMT = bone marrow transplantation; CLL = chronic lymphocytic leukemia; CML = chronic myelogenous leukemia; CMML = chronic myelomacrocytic leukemia; EGFR = epidermal growth factor receptor; 5-FU = fluorouracil; GFR = glomerular filtration rate; GIST = gastrointestinal stromal tumor; HL = Hodgkin lymphoma; MDS = myelodysplastic syndromes; MOPP = mechlorethamine, Oncovin, procarbazine, and prednisone; NHL = non-Hodgkin lymphoma; NSCLC = non–small-cell lung cancer; SCLC = small-cell lung cancer; SIADH = syndrome of inappropriate antidiuretic hormone secretion; WBC = white blood cell

The chemotherapeutic agents included in this Appendix are classified by mechanism of action and are organized as follows: alkylating agents; antimetabolites; natural products; and targeted agents (monoclonal antibodies and molecularly targeted therapies). FDA-approved uses and dose-limiting effects are set in italic type for emphasis. For a complete discussion of these mechanisms of action, see chapter 3 on “Principles of oncologic pharmacotherapy.”

Alkylating agents

Drug and its uses	Dosages	Toxicities
Nitrogen mustards		
Chlorambucil *CLL, HL, NHL,* ovarian cancer, choriocarcinoma, lymphosarcoma	0.1-0.2 mg/kg PO daily for 3-6 wk as required (usually 4-10 mg/d) or intermittent 0.4 mg/kg every 3-4 wk; increase by 0.1 mg/kg until control of disease or toxicity	*Bone marrow depression,* gonadal dysfunction, leukemia, hyperuricemia, pulmonary fibrosis
Cyclophosphamide *AML, ALL, CLL, HL, and NHL, multiple myeloma, mycosis fungoides, neuroblastoma, ovarian and breast cancers, retinoblastoma,* lung, testicular, and bladder cancers, sarcoma	40-50 mg/kg IV in divided doses over 2-5 d to start, followed by 10-15 mg/kg IV every 7-10 d; or 3-5 mg/kg IV twice weekly; or 1-5 mg/kg/d PO	*Bone marrow depression,* hemorrhagic cystitis, immunosuppression, alopecia, stomatitis, SIADH
Estramustine *Prostate, renal cell carcinomas*	14 mg/kg/d PO in 3-4 equally divided doses; 300 mg/d IV for 3-4 wk, followed by 300-450 mg/wk IV over 3-8 wk	*Bone marrow depression,* ischemic heart disease, thromboembolism, thrombophlebitis gynecomastia, nausea and vomiting, hepatotoxicity
Ifosfamide *Germ-cell testicular cancer,* sarcoma, NHL, lung cancer	1.2 $g/m^2/d$ via slow IV infusion for 5 consecutive days; repeat every 3 wk; give with mesna	*Bone marrow depression, hemorrhagic cystitis,* confusion, somnolence
Mechlorethamine *HL NHL, CML, CLL, mycosis fungoides, bronchogenic carcinoma,* lymphosarcoma, polycythemia vera, malignant effusions (intracavitary)	0.4 mg/kg ideal body weight given as single dose or in divided doses of 0.1-0.2 mg/kg/d	*Bone marrow depression, nausea and vomiting,* local phlebitis, severe skin necrosis if extravasated, gonadal dysfunction
Melphalan *Multiple myeloma, breast and ovarian cancers, sarcoma,* testicular and lung cancers	Continuous therapy: 6 mg PO daily for 2-3 wk, no therapy for 2-4 wk, then maintenance with 2-4 mg PO daily Pulse: 10 mg/m^2 PO daily for 4 d every 4-6 wk	*Bone marrow depression,* anorexia, nausea and vomiting, gonadal testicular dysfunction, leukemia

CHEMO AGENTS

Alkylating agents

Drug and its uses	Dosages	Toxicities
Aziridine		
Thiotepa *Ovarian, breast, and superficial bladder cancers,* HL, CML, CLL, bronchogenic carcinoma, malignant effusions (intracavitary), BMT for refractory leukemia, lymphomas	IV: 0.3-0.4 mg/kg by rapid IV infusion Intravesical: 60 mg/60 mL sterile water instilled and retained in bladder for 2 h; repeat weekly for 4 wk Intracavitary: 0.6-0.8 mg/kg	*Bone marrow depression,* nausea and vomiting, mucositis, skin rashes
Alkyl sulfonate		
Busulfan *CML,* BMT for refractory leukemia, lymphomas	2-8 mg PO daily for remission induction; adjust dosage to WBC count; 1-3 mg PO daily for maintenance; withhold induction if WBC count < 15,000/µL; resume therapy when WBC count > 50,000/µL	*Bone marrow depression, pulmonary fibrosis,* aplastic anemia, amenorrhea, gynecomastia, skin hyperpigmentation
Nitrosoureas		
Carmustine *Brain tumor, multiple myeloma, HL, NHL,* melanoma, BMT for refractory solid tumors and lymphomas	150-200 mg/m^2 IV every 6-8 wk	*Delayed bone marrow depression,* nausea and vomiting, reversible hepatotoxicity, local phlebitis, pulmonary and renal damage (high dose)
Gliadel wafers *Glioblastoma multiforme*	Up to 8 wafers placed in the brain cavity created by tumor removal	Fever, pain, and abnormal healing
Lomustine *Brain tumors, HL,* GI carcinomas, NSCLC	130 mg/m^2 PO every 6 wk; adjust dose in combination chemotherapy	*Delayed bone marrow depression,* nausea and vomiting, reversible hepatotoxicity, pulmonary and renal damage, neurologic reactions, leukemia
Streptozocin *Pancreatic islet-cell,* carcinoid, colon, hepatoma, NSCLC, HL	Daily: 500 mg/m^2 IV for 5 d every 6 wk until maximum benefit or toxicity Weekly: 1,000 mg/m^2 IV weekly for first 2 wk, then escalate dose to response or toxicity, not to exceed a single dose of 1,500 mg/m^2	*Renal damage,* nausea and vomiting, diarrhea, altered glucose metabolism, liver dysfunction

Alkylating agents

Drug and its uses	Dosages	Toxicities
Platinum complexes		
Carboplatin *Ovarian cancer,* endometrial, head and neck, lung, testicular, and breast cancers, relapsed acute leukemia, NHL	Single agent: 360 mg/m^2 IV every 4 wk Combination: 300 mg/m^2 IV every 4 wk Calvert formula: Total dose (mg) = Target AUC × (GFR + 25)	*Bone marrow depression,* nausea and vomiting, peripheral neuropathy ototoxicity
Cisplatin *Testicular, ovarian, bladder,* uterine, cervical, and lung cancers, squamous cell cancer of the head and neck, sarcoma, NHL	50 mg/m^2 IV or more every 3 wk; or 20 mg/m^2 IV daily for 4-5 d every 3-4 wk; give vigorous hydration before and after chemotherapy	*Renal damage,* nausea and vomiting, electrolyte disturbance, peripheral neuropathy, bone marrow depression, ototoxicity, radiosensitizer
Oxaliplatin *Colorectal,* ovarian cancers	85 mg/m^2 oxaliplatin and 200 mg/m^2 leucovorin (lv) IV infusion over 120 min on d 1 followed by 400 mg/m^2 5-FU IV bolus, then 600 mg/m^2 5-FU by IV infusion over 22 h. On d 2, 200 mg/m^2 IV over 120 min IV, followed by 400 mg/m^2 5-FU IV bolus, 600 mg/m^2 5-FU IV infusion over 22 h. Repeat every 2 wk	*Bone marrow depression, diarrhea,* nausea and vomiting, neuropathies exacerbated by cold exposure, pharyngolaryngeal dysesthesia
Nonclassic alkylators		
Altretamine *Ovarian,* lung, breast, and cervical cancers, NHL	4-12 mg/kg/d or 260 mg/m^2, PO divided in 3-4 doses for 14-21 d of a 28-d regimen	*Nausea and vomiting,* bone marrow depression, paresthesias, CNS toxicity
Dacarbazine *Malignant melanoma, HL,* soft-tissue sarcomas, neuroblastoma	Melanoma: 2.0-4.5 mg/kg/d IV for 10 d every 4 wk; or 250 mg/m^2/d IV for 5 d every 3 wk HL: 375 mg/m^2 IV on d 1, repeated every 15 d (single agent); 150 mg/m^2/d IV for 5 d every 4 wk (combination therapy)	*Bone marrow depression,* nausea and vomiting, flu-like syndrome, transient hepatotoxicity, local irritation, facial flushing, alopecia
Procarbazine *HL* NHL, brain tumors, lung cancer	Single agent: 4-6 mg/kg/d PO until maximum response HL (MOPP): 100 mg/m^2/d PO for 14 d	*Bone marrow depression,* nausea and vomiting, lethargy, depression, paresthesias, headache, flu-like symptoms
Temozolomide *Anaplastic astrocytoma (relapsed),* renal cell cancer, melanoma	150 mg/m^2/d PO for 5 d every 28 d	*Bone marrow depression,* nausea and vomiting

Antimetabolites

Drug and its uses	Dosages	Toxicities
Folate analog		
Methotrexate *Breast, head and neck, GI, and lung cancers, ALL, CNS leukemia (intrathecal), gestational trophoblastic tumors, NHL (advanced stage),* Burkitt lymphoma, osteosarcoma, mycosis fungoides	Numerous dosing schedules with combination therapy: Low dose: 2.5-5.0 mg PO daily; or 5-25 mg/m^2 PO, IM, IV twice weekly; or 50 mg/m^2 IV every 2-3 wk High dose: 1-12 g/m^2 IV with leucovorin rescue every 1-3 wk Intrathecal: 5-10 mg/m^2 (up to 15 mg) every 3-7 d	*Mucositis, GI ulceration (may produce hemorrhage or perforation), bone marrow depression, pulmonary fibrosis (previously irradiated area),* nerve root irritation and convulsion (intrathecal), liver cirrhosis and osteoporosis (chronic therapy), renal damage (high dose), diarrhea, skin erythema
Pemetrexed *Mesothelioma, NSCLC*	500 mg/m^2 IV over 10 min every 21 d	*Bone marrow depression.* stomatitis/pharyngitis, rash/skin desquamation
Purine analogs		
Fludarabine *CLL,* AML, NHL (low-grade)	25 mg/m^2/d IV over 30 min for 5 d; repeat every 28 d	*Bone marrow depression,* nausea and vomiting, fever, malaise, pulmonary infiltrates, tumor lysis syndrome, CNS effects (high dose)
Mercaptopurine *ALL, CML, AML*	1.5-2.5 mg/kg/d PO (100-200 mg in average adult) until response or toxic effects are seen; may increase dose to 5 mg/kg/d; adjust for maintenance dose; reduce dose by 50%-75% if given with allopurinol or if renal or hepatic insufficiency ensues	*Bone marrow depression,* nausea and vomiting, anorexia, diarrhea, cholestasis
Thioguanine *AML,* ALL, CML, advanced colorectal cancer, multiple myeloma	2 mg/kg/d PO until response or toxic effects are seen; may cautiously increase to 3 mg/kg/d	*Bone marrow depression,* liver damage, stomatitis
Adenosine analogs		
Cladribine *Hairy-cell leukemia,* NHL, mycosis fungoides, AML, CML, CLL	0.09 mg/kg/d (4 mg/m^2/d) by continuous IV infusion for 7 consecutive days	*Bone marrow depression,* febrile episodes, rash, infections, septicemia
Pentostatin *Hairy-cell leukemia,* ALL, CLL, lymphoblastic lymphoma, mycosis fungoides	4 mg/m^2 IV over 30 min every other wk or for 3 consecutive wk; give vigorous hydration before and after chemotherapy	*Nephrotoxicity, CNS depression,* bone marrow depression, nausea and vomiting, conjunctivitis

Antimetabolites

Drug and its uses	Dosages	Toxicities
Pyrimidine analogs		
Capecitabine *Breast cancer (relapsed), colorectal cancer, and other GI malignancies*	1,250 mg/m^2 bid PO with food (2 wk on drug, 1 wk of rest)	*Diarrhea*, stomatitis, nausea and vomiting, fatigue, hand-foot syndrome, bone marrow depression (minimal)
Cytarabine *AML*, ALL, CML, NHL, CNS leukemia (intrathecal)	<u>AML induction:</u> 100 mg/m^2/d by continuous IV infusion on days 1-7; or 100 mg/m^2 IV every 12 h on days 1-7 <u>Relapsed ALL:</u> 3 g/m^2 IV over 1-3 h every 12 h for 4 doses	*Bone marrow depression*, nausea and vomiting, diarrhea, arachnoiditis (intrathecal), stomatitis, hepatic dysfunction, fever, conjunctivitis, confusion, somnolence, cerebellar toxicity
DepoCyt (liposomal cytarabine) *CNS leukemia/lymphoma*	<u>Intrathecal:</u> DepoCyt, 50 mg over 1-5 min every 14 d, with dexamethasone, 4 mg PO bid × 5 d	
Floxuridine *GI adenocarcinomas metastatic to liver*, including oral, pancreatic, biliary, colon, and hepatic cancers, and metastatic breast cancer	0.1-0.6 mg/kg/d over several days via continuous arterial infusion supplying well-defined tumor; treatments given over 1-6 wk	*Stomatitis and GI ulcers, bone marrow depression*, abdominal pain, nausea and vomiting, diarrhea, liver dysfunction (transient)
Fluorouracil *Colon, rectal, stomach, pancreatic, breast*, head and neck, renal cell, prostate, and ovarian cancers, squamous cell carcinomas of esophagus, basal and squamous cell carcinoma of skin (topical), hepatic cancer (intra-arterial)	Numerous dosing schedules with combination therapy: <u>Loading dose:</u> 300-500 mg/m^2; or 12 mg/kg IV daily for 3-5 d, followed by weekly maintenance <u>Maintenance:</u> 10-15 mg/kg IV weekly, as toxicity permits <u>Infusion:</u> 20-25 mg/kg by continuous IV infusion over 24 h daily for 4-5 d, every 4 wk	*Stomatitis and GI ulcers (infusion) bone marrow depression (bolus), diarrhea*, nausea and vomiting, esophagitis, angina, cerebellar ataxia, radiosensitizer
Gemcitabine *Pancreatic, lung, breast, ovarian*, and bladder cancers	1,000 mg/m^2 IV over 30 min, once weekly for up to 7 wk (or until toxicity necessitates reducing or withholding a dose), followed by 1 wk of rest <u>Subsequent cycles</u>: Infusions once weekly for 3 consecutive wk out of every 4 wk	*Bone marrow depression*, transient fever, flu-like syndrome, skin rash, mild nausea and vomiting
Substituted urea		
Hydroxyurea *CML, acute leukemia (emergent treatment), head and neck cancer, ovarian cancer, melanoma*, essential thrombocytosis, polycythemia vera	<u>Intermittent:</u> 80 mg/kg PO every third day <u>Continuous:</u> 20-30 mg/kg PO daily	*Bone marrow depression*, mild nausea and vomiting, skin rashes, radiosensitizer

Natural products

Drug and its uses	Dosages	Toxicities
Antitumor antibiotics		
Bleomycin *Testicular cancer, HL reticulum cell sarcoma, lymphosarcoma, squamous cell cancer of the head and neck, skin, cervix, vulva, and penis*	10-20 U/m^2 given IV, IM, or SC weekly or twice weekly; maximum total dose, 400 U; a 2-U test dose should be given because of a possible anaphylactoid reaction	*Pneumonitis and pulmonary fibrosis,* fever and allergic reactions, anaphylaxis, hyperpigmentation, Raynaud's phenomenon, alopecia
Dactinomycin *Testicular cancer, gestational trophoblastic tumors, Wilms' tumor, rhabdomyosarcoma, Ewing's sarcoma*	0.010-0.015 mg/kg IV daily for 5 d every 3 wk (usual adult dose, 0.5 mg) or 2 mg/m^2 IV as a single dose every 3-4 wk	*Stomatitis, bone marrow depression,* anorexia, nausea and vomiting, diarrhea, alopecia, skin changes, anaphylactoid reaction
Daunorubicin *AML, ALL*	Remission induction: 30-45 mg/m^2/d IV for 3 d in combination therapy; total cumulative dose, 550 mg/m^2	*Bone marrow depression,* cardiotoxicity, alopecia, nausea and vomiting, diarrhea, stomatitis, fever, dermatitis at previously irradiated sites, red urine, anaphylactoid reaction
DaunoXome (liposomal daunorubicin) *Kaposi's sarcoma*	Liposomal preparation: 40 mg/m^2 IV every 2 wk	
Doxorubicin *ALL, AML, breast, ovarian,* bladder cancers, HL, NHL, SCLC, gastric cancer, sarcoma, Wilms' tumor, neuroblastoma, thyroid cancer	60-90 mg/m^2 single IV injection every 21 d, 20-30 mg/m^2/d IV for 3 d every 3-4 wk, or 20 mg/m^2 IV weekly; total cumulative dose of 550 mg/m^2; reduce dose for liver dysfunction	*Bone marrow depression, cardiotoxicity, stomatitis (continuous infusion),* alopecia, nausea and vomiting, diarrhea, fever, dermatitis at previously irradiated sites, red urine, anaphylactoid reaction
Doxil (liposomal doxorubicin) *Ovarian cancer (refractory to paclitaxel- and platinum-based regimens), Kaposi's sarcoma*	50 mg/m^2 IV every 4 wk 20 mg/m^2 IV every 3 wk	*Bone marrow depression,* hand-foot syndrome
Epirubicin *Breast cancer*	100 mg/m^2 IV on day 1 or 60 mg/m^2 IV on days 1 and 8 in combination therapy	*Bone marrow depression, cardiotoxicity, stomatitis,* alopecia
Idarubicin AML, CML (blast phase), ALL	12 mg/m^2/d IV for 3 d every 3 wk in combination therapy	*Bone marrow depression,* nausea and vomiting, stomatitis, alopecia, cardiotoxicity

Natural products

Drug and its uses	Dosages	Toxicities
Mitoxantrone *AML, prostate,* ALL, CML, breast and ovarian cancers	Remission induction: 12 mg/m^2/d IV for 3 d, in combination with Ara-C	*Bone marrow depression,* cardiotoxicity, alopecia, stomatitis, nausea and vomiting, blue urine and sclera
Mitomycin *Gastric, colorectal, pancreatic adenocarcinomas,* NSCLC, breast, uterine, cervical, and head and neck cancers	20 mg/m^2 IV every 6-8 wk as a single agent or 5-10 mg/m^2 IV every 6 wk in combination therapy	*Bone marrow depression (cumulative),* nausea and vomiting, anorexia, alopecia, stomatitis, fever, pulmonary fibrosis
Valrubicin *Bladder*	800 mg IV once a wk for 6 wk	*Local bladder symptoms*
Epipodophyllotoxins		
Etoposide *Testicular cancer (refractory), SCLC,* HL, NHL, AML, gestational trophoblastic tumors	Testicular: 50-100 mg/m^2/d IV for 5 d or 100 mg/m^2/d IV on days 1, 3, and 5 Lung: 35-50 mg/m^2/d IV for 5 d or 100 mg/m^2/d PO for 5 d For both indications, given with combination therapy and repeated every 3-4 wk	*Bone marrow depression,* nausea and vomiting, diarrhea, fever, hypotension with rapid infusion, alopecia, rash
Teniposide *Relapsed ALL in children,* SCLC	ALL: 100 mg/m^2 once or twice weekly or 20-60 mg/m^2/d for 5 d in combination with Ara-C Lung: 80-90 mg/m^2/d for 5 d as a single agent	*Bone marrow depression,* nausea and vomiting, alopecia, hypotension with rapid infusion, increased liver enzymes
Microtubule agents		
Docetaxel *Breast (relapsed), NSCLC prostate,* ovarian, pancreatic, head and neck, esophagus, stomach, cervical, Kaposi's sarcoma, uterine, and bladder cancers	60-100 mg/m^2 IV over 1 h every 21 d or up to 42 mg/m^2 IV every wk	*Bone marrow depression,* fluid retention, hypersensitivity reaction, paresthesias, rash, alopecia, myalgias
Paclitaxel *Ovarian cancer, (relapsed), NSCLC (in combination with cisplatin), Kaposi's sarcoma, breast cancer (relapsed),* head and neck, gastric, colon, esophagus, uterine, prostate, bladder cancers and melanomas	135-175 mg/m^2 by IV infusion (ranging from 3-96 h) every 3 wk or 80 mg/m^2 IV every wk	*Bone marrow depression* peripheral neuropathy, alopecia, mucositis, anaphylaxis, dyspnea, myalgias

Natural products

Drug and its uses	Dosages	Toxicities
Vinblastine *HL, NHL, gestational trophoblastic tumors, testicular and breast cancers, mycosis fungoides, Kaposi's sarcoma, histiocytosis X,* bladder and renal cancers, NSCLC, CML (blast crisis)	4-12 mg/m^2 IV as a single agent every 1-2 wk; titrate dose to myelosuppression; adjust for hepatic insufficiency	*Bone marrow depression,* nausea and vomiting, ileus, alopecia, stomatitis, myalgias, vesication
Vincristine *ALL, HL, NHL, rhabdomyosarcoma, neuroblastoma, Wilms' tumor,* multiple myeloma, sarcomas, breast cancer	0.4-1.4 mg/m^2 IV weekly; maximum total dose, 2 mg/wk; reduce dose for hepatic insufficiency	*Peripheral neuropathy,* ileus, abdominal pain, SIADH, bone marrow depression (mild)
Vinorelbine *NSCLC,* breast, ovarian, head and neck cancers, HL	30 mg/m^2 IV over 10 min; repeat weekly	*Peripheral neuropathy, bone marrow depression,* nausea and vomiting, hepatic dysfunction
Camptothecin analogs		
Irinotecan *Colorectal cancer,* lung, ovarian, and cervical cancers	125 mg/m^2 IV over 90 min once weekly for 4 wk; then 2 wk rest; or 350 mg/m^2 every 21 d	*Bone marrow depression, diarrhea,* nausea and vomiting anorexia, weight loss
Topotecan *Cervical cancer, ovarian cancer (relapsed),SCLC (relapsed),* MDS, CMML	1.5 mg/m^2 IV over 30 min for 5 consecutive days at 21-d intervals	*Bone marrow depression,* fever, flu-like symptoms, nausea and vomiting
Enzyme		
Asparaginase *ALL,* CML, AML	6,000 IU/m^2 IM 3 times weekly for 9 doses or 100 IU/kg/d IV for 10 continuous days, starting on day 22 of treatment; usually given with vincristine and prednisone	*Allergic reactions (fever, chills skin rash, anaphylaxis),* nausea and vomiting, anorexia, liver dysfunction, CNS depression, coagulopathy, hyperglycemia

Targeted therapies: Monoclonal antibodies

Drug and its uses	Dosages	Toxicities
Alemtuzumab *Chemotherapy-refractory B-cell CLL*	Rapid daily dose escalation, until tolerated, from 3 mg/d, and then 10 mg/d, to the recommended maintenance dose of 30 mg IV over 120 min, three times per wk on alternate days for up to 12 wk	*Pancytopenia*, infusion reaction, opportunistic infections, skin rash, nausea/vomiting
Bevacizumab *Colorectal cancer*	5 mg/kg IV over 60-90 min every 14 d	Asthenia, headache, epistaxis, proteinuria, GI perforations/ wound-healing complications, hypertension/hypertensive crisis
Cetuximab *EGFR-expressing colorectal cancer, head and neck cancer*	400 mg/m^2 IV over 120 min, loading dose, and 250 mg/m^2 IV over 60 min every 7 d, as maintenance	*Skin rash, infusion reaction,* asthenia, diarrhea, nausea
Panitumumab *EGFR-expressing colorectal cancer*	6 mg/kg IV over 60 minutes every 14 days	Skin rash, hypomagnesemia, paronychia, fatigue, infusion reactions, nausea/vomiting, diarrhea
Rituximab *CD20-positive B-cell NHL*	375 mg/m^2 IV infusion (50-100 mg/h) once weekly	Infusion reactions, asthenia, headache, skin rash/pruritus, leukopenia/infection, nausea, tumor lysis syndrome
Trastuzumab *HER2-overexpressing breast cancer*	4 mg/kg IV over 90 min, loading dose, and 2 mg/kg IV over 30 min every 7 d, as maintenance	Cardiac failure, infusion reaction, diarrhea

Molecularly targeted therapies

Drug and its uses	Dosages	Toxicities
Bortezomib *Multiple myeloma*	1.3 mg/m^2 days 1, 4, 8, and 11 every 3 wk	*Diarrhea, peripheral neuropathy,* asthenia, fever, anorexia, nausea and vomiting, rash, headache, thrombocytopenia
Dasatinib *CML, ALL*	140 mg/d (divided doses; 70 mg BID)	Fluid retention events (eg, pleural effusion); GI events: diarrhea, nausea, abdominal pain, vomiting; bleeding events; hematologic toxicities: neutropenia, thrombocytopenia, anemia
Erlotinib *NSCLC, pancreas*	150 mg/d PO	*Acne-form skin rash, diarrhea,* anorexia, fatigue, dyspnea
Gefitinib *NSCLC*	250 mg/d PO	*Acne-form skin rash, diarrhea,* transaminitis, asthenia, mild nausea and vomiting
Imatinib *CML, GIST*	400 mg/d PO in chronic-phase CML and GIST and 600 mg/d PO for CML in accelerated phase or blast crisis	Nausea and vomiting, edema and fluid retention, myalgias, diarrhea, myelosuppression, transaminitis
Lapatinib *HER2-positive metastatic breast cancer*	1,250 mg PO qd × 21 days in combination with capecitabine 2,000 mg/m^2/d PO (divided doses) on days 1-14 of a repeating 21-day cycle	*Diarrhea*, hand-foot syndrome, nausea, rash, vomiting, fatigue
Sorafenib *Renal cell cancer*	400 mg bid PO	Diarrhea, nausea, stomatitis, asthenia, cardiac ischemia, hand-foot syndrome, hypertension, bleeding, anorexia
Sunitinib *Renal cell cancer, GIST*	50 mg/d PO for 4 wk, then 2-wk rest period	Diarrhea, nausea, stomatitis, asthenia, skin discoloration, hand-foot syndrome, hypertension, bleeding, anorexia

Index

A

Acute leukemias (*see also* Leukemia)
- acute lymphoblastic leukemia (ALL)
  - diagnosis, 764
  - epidemiology, 761
  - prognostic factors, 767
  - relapse, treatment of, 777
  - signs and symptoms, 762
  - treatment, 768–769
- acute myelogenous leukemia (AML)
  - diagnosis, 764
  - epidemiology, 761
  - etiology and risk factors, 761
  - pathology and cytogenetics, 764
  - refractory or relapsed disease, 782
  - signs and symptoms, 762
  - treatment, 768, 777
- acute promyelocytic leukemia
  - treatment of, 785

Adrenocortical carcinoma
- etiology, 310
- signs and symptoms, 310
- treatment, 311

AIDS-related malignancies (*see also* Kaposi's sarcoma)
- anal carcinoma, 650
  - etiology and risk factors, 651
  - pathology, 651
  - screening and diagnosis, 651
  - signs and symptoms, 651
  - staging and prognosis, 651
  - treatment, 652
- cervical carcinoma, 647
  - epidemiology, 648
  - etiology and risk factors, 648
  - pathology, 649
  - screening and diagnosis, 649
  - signs and symptoms, 648
  - staging and prognosis, 649
  - treatment, 650
- Hodgkin lymphoma, 653
- leiomyosarcoma, pediatric, 653
- lung cancer, 653
- non-Hodgkin lymphoma, 640
  - epidemiology, 641
  - etiology and risk factors, 641
  - pathology, 642
  - screening and diagnosis, 642
  - signs and symptoms, 642
  - staging and prognosis, 643
  - treatment, 645
    - primary CNS lymphoma, 647
    - systemic, 645
- skin cancers, nonmelanomatous, 653

Anal canal carcinoma (*see also* AIDS-related malignancies)
- diagnosis, 366
- epidemiology, etiology, and risk factors, 365
- pathology, 367
- signs and symptoms, 366
- staging, 367
- treatment, 367

Anorexia and cachexia
- diagnostic criteria, 929
- management, 929
- nutrition, end-of-life care, 932

Anxiety
- etiology, 891
- management, 892
- signs and symptoms/diagnosis, 890

Ascites, malignant
- diagnosis, 1045
- prognosis, 1046
- signs and symptoms, 1045
- treatment, 1046

B

Bile duct cancer
- adjuvant chemotherapy, 335
- adjuvant radiation therapy, 334
- diagnosis, 330
- epidemiology, 328
- etiology and risk factors, 328
- pathology, 332
- signs and symptoms, 329
- staging and prognosis, 332
- surgery, 333
- unresectable disease, treatment of, 335

Biliary tract cancers (*see* Bile duct cancer; Gallbladder cancer)

Bladder cancer (*see* Urothelial cancer)

Bone marrow transplantation (*see* Hematopoietic cell transplantation)

Bone sarcomas (*see* Sarcomas, bone)

Brain tumors
- diagnosis, 611
- epidemiology, 609
- etiology and risk factors, 609
- pathology, 612

screening for metastatic, 611
signs and symptoms, 610
staging and prognosis, 615
treatment
definitive, 616
supportive, 616
Breast cancer
chemoprevention, 184
chemotherapy regimens, 205, 215, 231
epidemiology, 163
etiology and risk factors, 165
genetic cancer risk assessment, 168
prevention, 183
risk reduction, lifestyle changes, 183
screening and diagnosis, 173
signs and symptoms, 172
staging and prognosis, 189
Breast cancer, stages 0 and I, 193
follow-up of long-term survivors, 208
stage 0 breast cancer, 193
ductal carcinoma in situ, 194
epidemiology, 194
pathology, 195
risk of invasive cancer, 195
signs and symptoms, 194
treatment options, 195
adjuvant radiation therapy, 197
adjuvant tamoxifen therapy, 198
breast-conserving surgery, 195
sentinel node biopsy, 195
lobular carcinoma in situ, 193
epidemiology and etiology, 193
pathology, 194
risk of invasive cancer, 194
signs and symptoms, 193
treatment options, 194
stage I breast cancer, 198
pathology of invasive cancer, 198
treatment, 199
breast-conservation therapy, 199
mastectomy options, 204
medical, 204
radiation therapy after breast-conserving surgery, 203
surgical and radiation, 199
Breast cancer, stage II, 211
follow-up of long-term survivors, 225
treatment, 211
breast-conservation therapy, 211
endocrine (hormonal) therapy, 217
HER2-positive tumors, 223
medical, 214
toxic effects, 224
postmenopausal women, 220
premenopausal women, 217
radiation therapy after breast-conserving surgery, 212
after mastectomy, 213
surgical and radiation, 211
Breast cancer, stages III and IV, 229
follow-up of long-term survivors, 248
locally advanced disease
diagnosis, 229
treatment, 231
locoregional recurrence, 230
adjuvant systemic therapy for, 240
treatment of, after early invasive cancer or DCIS, 237
metastatic disease, 241
distant, 230
medical treatment, 241
adjunctive bisphosphonate therapy, 246
intermediate- or high-risk patients, 243
low-risk patients, 241
monoclonal antibody therapy, 245
radiation therapy, 247
surgery, 247

C

Cachexia (*see* Anorexia and cachexia)
Cancer pain
care, ongoing, 872
elements of management, 861
pain syndromes, 861
pathophysiology, 859
patient subgroups, 863
pharmacologic treatment, 863
physical treatments, 870
psychological, sociocultural, and spiritual factors, management of, 871
radiation therapy, role of, 870
surgery for bone metastasis, 868
Carcinoid tumors, GI tract, 306
diagnosis, 307
prognosis, 308
signs and symptoms, 307
treatment, of bulky disease, 308
of symptoms, 309
Carcinoma of an unknown primary site (*see* Unknown primary cancer)
Cervical carcinoma (*see also* AIDS-related malignancies)
chemoradiation therapy
for locally advanced disease, 453
chemotherapy

for advanced/recurrent disease, 466
epidemiology, 441
etiology and risk factors, 441
pathology, 445
radiation therapy
adjuvant, following radical hysterectomy, 461
definitive, 457
for recurrent or metastatic disease, 464
for stages I–IV disease, 451
techniques, 453
screening and diagnosis, 443
signs and symptoms, 443
staging and prognosis, 447
surgical treatment of
early-stage disease, 450
recurrent or metastatic disease, 462
treatment, 450
Chronic lymphocytic leukemia (*see also* Leukemia)
complications, 816
transformation, 817
cytogenetic and molecular findings, 808
epidemiology, 805
etiology and risk factors, 805
laboratory features, 807
signs and symptoms, 806
staging and prognosis, 809
treatment, 811
chemotherapy, conventional, 812
early-stage disease, 811
new approaches, 814
Chronic myelogenous leukemia (*see also* Leukemia)
accelerated and blastic phases, treatment of, 801
chronic phase, treatment of, 793
cytogenetic and molecular findings, 792
epidemiology, 789
etiology and risk factors, 789
laboratory features, 791
signs and symptoms, 790
staging and prognosis, 793
treatment, 793
Colony-stimulating factors (*see* Hematopoietic growth factors)
Colorectal cancer
adjuvant therapy
for colon cancer, 354
for rectal cancer, 358
advanced colon cancer, treatment of, 361
advanced rectal cancer, treatment of, 365
chemoprevention, 345
epidemiology, 339
etiology and risk factors, 340
follow-up of long-term survivors, 365
localized disease, primary treatment of, 352
pathology, 351
screening and diagnosis, 347
signs and symptoms, 347
staging and prognosis, 351
treatment, 352

D

Delirium
etiology, 895
management, 896
signs and symptoms/diagnosis, 894
Depression
etiology, 886
management, 886
signs and symptoms/diagnosis, 885
Ductal carcinoma in situ (*see* Breast cancer, stage 0)
Dyspnea
assessment, 924
clinical features, 923
management, 925
mechanisms, 923

E

End-of-life care (*see* Anorexia and cachexia)
Endocrine malignancies (*see* Adrenocortical carcinoma; Pancreatic endocrine tumors; Parathyroid cancer; Pheochromocytoma; Thyroid cancer)
Endometrial cancer
epidemiology, 471
etiology and risk factors, 471
pathology, 475
recurrent or metastatic disease, treatment of, 486
screening and diagnosis, 474
signs and symptoms, 474
staging and prognosis, 475
treatment, 476
adjuvant radiation therapy, 479
adjuvant systemic therapy, 484
definitive radiation treatment, 484
surgery, 476

Esophageal cancer
advanced disease
chemotherapy in, 266
treatment of, 265
diagnosis, 253
epidemiology, 251
etiology and risk factors, 252
localized disease, treatment of, 257
pathology, 254
screening and surveillance, 254
signs and symptoms, 252
staging and prognosis, 256
treatment, 257

F

Fatigue
assessment, 920
clinical features, 918
management, 921
mechanism, 917
Fluid complications (*see* Ascites, malignant; Pleural effusion, malignant; Pericardial effusion)

G

Gallbladder cancer
diagnosis, 329
epidemiology, 328
etiology and risk factors, 328
pathology, 332
signs and symptoms, 329
staging and prognosis, 332
surgery, 333
Gastric cancer
adjuvant therapy, 282
advanced disease, medical treatment of, 283
epidemiology, 273
etiology, risk factors, and prevention, 274
localized disease, primary treatment of, 278
neoadjuvant therapy, 280
pathology, 276
screening and diagnosis, 275
signs and symptoms, 275
staging and prognosis, 277
treatment, 278
unresectable tumors, treatment of, 283
Gastrointestinal cancer (*see* Anal canal carcinoma; Bile duct cancer; Carcinoid tumors, GI tract; Colorectal cancer; Esophageal cancer; Gallbladder cancer; Gastric cancer; Hepatocellular cancer; Pancreatic cancer; Pancreatic endocrine tumors)
Gestational trophoblastic diseases
clinical presentation, 492
diagnostic studies, 493
metastatic disease
low-risk, 495
high-risk, 495
salvage therapy, 496
treatment, 494

H

Hairy-cell leukemia (*see also* Leukemia)
differential diagnosis, 818
epidemiology and etiology, 817
treatment, 818
Head and neck tumors
anatomy, 39
epidemiology, 35
etiology and risk factors, 37
follow-up of long-term survivors, 55
pathology, 43
recurrent cancer, 79
screening and diagnosis, 39
signs and symptoms, 39
staging and prognosis, 45
treatment approaches, 46
treatment of the neck, 55
tumor regions, 57
glottis, 72
hypopharynx, 66
larynx, 67
lips, 59
mouth floor, 61
nasopharynx, 75
oral cavity, 57
oropharynx, 63
subglottis, 73
supraglottis, 71
tongue, 60
tongue base, 64
tonsil and tonsillar pillar, 65
unknown head and neck primary site, 74
Hematopoietic cell transplantation
allogeneic transplantation, 841
autologous transplantation, 842
collection of the graft, 844
indications for, 845
modifications of the stem-cell graft, 843
phases of, 846
post-transplantation therapies, other, 854
relapse, management of, 854

second malignancy after, 855
timing of, 846
types of, 839
Hematopoietic growth factors, 901
cytokines with thrombopoietic activity, 913
erythropoietin, 911
adverse reactions, 913
anemia, treatment of, 912
dose and schedule of administration, 912
safety issues, emerging, 913
myeloid growth factors, 903
dose, route, and schedule of administration, 910
indications for, 904
toxicity of, 909
Hepatobiliary cancer (*see* Bile duct cancer; Gallbladder cancer; Hepatocellular cancer)
Hepatocellular cancer
adjuvant and palliative therapies, 324
cryotherapy and radiofrequency ablation, 326
epidemiology, 319
etiology and risk factors, 320
pathology, 321
screening and diagnosis, 320
signs and symptoms, 320
staging and prognosis, 322
surgery, 323
Hodgkin lymphoma
diagnosis, 668
epidemiology, 667
etiology and risk factors, 667
pathology, 669
radiation therapy, 677
side effects and complications of, 678
relapsed disease, management of, 686
signs and symptoms, 668
stage I/II disease, treatment of, 675
stage III/IV disease, treatment of, 681
combination chemotherapy, 681
long-term toxicities, 684
staging and prognosis, 670
treatment, 674

I

Infections in cancer patients
catheter-associated, 1020
diagnosis, 1021
etiology, 1020
signs and symptoms, 1020
treatment, 1021
Clostridium difficile-associated diarrhea, 1022
diagnosis, 1023
etiology and risk factors, 1022
prevention, 1024
signs and symptoms, 1023
treatment, 1023
febrile neutropenia, infection during, 1003
definitions, 1003
diagnosis, 1004
etiology, 1003
prevention, 1012
signs and symptoms, 1004
treatment, 1005
fungal, 1025
diagnosis, 1027
etiology and risk factors, 1025
prevention, 1030
signs and symptoms, 1026
treatment, 1028
pneumonia, 1013
diagnosis, 1016
etiology and risk factors, 1014
prevention, 1018
signs and symptoms, 1016
treatment, 1017
typhlitis, 1024
diagnosis, 1024
signs and symptoms, 1024
treatment, 1025
viral, 1031
diagnosis, 1031
etiology, 1031
prevention, 1032
signs and symptoms, 1031
treatment, 1032
Internet, cancer resources, 1055

K

Kaposi's sarcoma
epidemiology, 631
etiology and risk factors, 632
pathology, 634
screening and diagnosis, 633
signs and symptoms, 633
staging and prognosis, 634
treatment, 635
Kidney cancer
diagnosis, 433
epidemiology, 432
etiology and risk factors, 432
pathology, 434

signs and symptoms, 433
staging and prognosis, 434
treatment, 436

L

Leukemia (*see* Acute leukemias; Chronic lymphocytic leukemia; Chronic myelogenous leukemia; Hairy-cell leukemia)
Liver cancer (*see* Hepatocellular cancer)
Lobular carcinoma in situ (*see* Breast cancer, stage 0)
Lung cancer (*see* Lung cancer, non–small-cell; Lung cancer, small-cell; Mesothelioma; Thymoma)
Lung cancer, non–small-cell (*see also* Mesothelioma; Thymoma)
diagnosis and staging evaluation, 112
epidemiology, 103
etiology and risk factors, 104
follow-up of long-term survivors, 142
intraoperative staging, 116
pathology, 117
pulmonary evaluation, 116
screening and prevention, 105
signs and symptoms, 108
staging and prognosis, 110
treatment, 118
adjuvant therapy, 121
neoadjuvant chemotherapy or chemoradiation therapy, 123
palliation of local and distant symptoms, 139
photodynamic therapy, 137
stage I/II disease, medically inoperable, 124
stage IIIA/IIIB disease, 125
stage IV disease, 128
surgical approach, 118
tumor biology, 110
Lung cancer, small-cell
follow-up of long-term survivors, 154
pathology and pathophysiology, 146
staging and prognosis, 145
treatment, 146
disease limited to lung parenchyma, surgery for, 146
disease limited to the thorax, 147
extensive disease, 151
palliation of local and distant symptoms, 153
Lymphoma (*see* AIDS-related malignancies; Hodgkin lymphoma; Non-Hodgkin lymphoma)

M

MDS (*see* Myelodysplastic syndromes)
Melanoma
ABCDs of moles and melanomas, (color atlas), 555
adjuvant therapy for, 543
advanced disease, treatment of, 545
color atlas of skin lesions, 559
cutaneous, surgical treatment of, 537
diagnosis, 527
epidemiology, 523
etiology and risk factors, 524
noncutaneous, surgical treatment of, 542
pathology, 530
staging and prognosis, 531
treatment, 537
Mesothelioma
diagnosis, 155
epidemiology, 155
etiology and risk factors, 155
pathology, 156
staging and prognosis, 156
treatment, 156
Myelodysplastic syndromes
classification, 824
cytogenetic and molecular findings, 828
epidemiology, 821
etiology and risk factors, 821
laboratory features, 826
signs and symptoms, 825
staging and prognosis, 829
treatment, 831
Myeloma, multiple
epidemiology, 741
etiology and risk factors, 742
laboratory and pathologic features, 745
refractory or relapsing disease, treatment of, 752
remission maintenance, 751
screening and diagnosis, 744
signs and symptoms, 743
smoldering myeloma, 755
staging and prognosis, 746
treatment, 748
for newly diagnosed patients, 748
treatment response criteria, 747

N

Nausea and vomiting
acute emesis, treatment of, 882
anticipatory emesis, treatment of, 883
antiemetic agents, 877

aprepitant, 880
combination regimens, 881
dexamethasone, 878
dolasetron, 877
dronabinol and other cannabinoids, 880
granisetron, 877
haloperidol, 879
lorazepam, 880
metoclopramide, 879
ondansetron, 877
palonosetron, 877
phenothiazines, 880
chemotherapeutic agents and emesis, 875
delayed emesis, treatment of, 882
emetic problems, 874
pathophysiology, 873
patient characteristics and emesis, 875
Non-Hodgkin lymphoma
B-cell lymphomas
cutaneous, 733
B-cell pseudolymphoma, 736
Burkitt and Burkitt-like lymphoma, 719
chronic lymphocytic leukemia/small lymphocytic lymphoma, 712
epidemiology, 689
etiology and risk factors, 691
follicular lymphoma, 704
follow-up of long-term survivors, 737
HIV-related lymphomas, 736
large B-cell lymphoma
diffuse, 714
of the leg, 735
primary mediastinal, 723
large cell lymphoma
anaplastic, CD30+ cutaneous type, 731
anaplastic, T-/null cell, primary systemic type, 726
large T-cell lymphoma
CD30– cutaneous, 732
lymphomatoid papulosis, 731
lymphoplasmacytic lymphoma/ Waldenström's macroglobulinemia, 714
mantle cell lymphoma, 718
marginal zone lymphoma
nodal, 713
splenic, 712
mycosis fungoides/Sézary syndrome, 729
pathology, 697
plasmacytoma, 736
screening and diagnosis, 695
signs and symptoms, 694
staging and prognosis, 699
T-cell lymphoma
adult, 728
angioimmunoblastic, 725
cutaneous, 729
γ/δ, 733
enteropathy-type intestinal, 727
extranodal NK, nasal and nasal-type, 727
hepatosplenic, 726
peripheral, not otherwise characterized, 724
pleomorphic, with small/medium cells, 733
subcutaneous panniculitis-like, 733
treatment, 703
complications, 737
Nonmelanoma skin cancer (*see* Skin cancer, nonmelanoma)
Non–small-cell lung cancer (*see* Lung cancer; Lung cancer, non–small-cell)

O

Oncologic emergencies
hypercalcemia, 991
diagnosis, 991
etiology, 991
signs and symptoms, 991
treatment, 991
hyperuricemia, 994
diagnosis, 995
etiology and risk factors, 994
prognosis, 995
signs and symptoms, 995
treatment, 995
Lambert-Eaton syndrome, 998
diagnosis, 999
signs and symptoms, 998
treatment, 999
polymyositis/dermatomyositis, 999
diagnosis, 1000
signs and symptoms, 1000
treatment, 1000
spinal cord compression, 986
diagnosis, 987
etiology, 986
prognosis, 987
signs and symptoms, 986
treatment, 988
superior vena cava syndrome, 979
diagnosis, 980

etiology, 979
prognosis, 980
signs and symptoms, 980
treatment, 980
syndrome of inappropriate secretion of antidiuretic hormone, 997
diagnosis, 998
signs and symptoms, 997
treatment, 998
tumor lysis syndrome, 996
diagnosis, 996
etiology and risk factors, 996
prognosis, 996
signs and symptoms, 996
treatment, 997
venous thromboembolic complications of cancer, 982
anticoagulation, difficulties in, 985
etiology, 983
treatment, 983
tumor type associated with, 983
Ovarian cancer
advanced disease, treatment of, 511
chemotherapy, 512–513, 514–515
consolidation therapy, 514
radiotherapy, 516–517
surgery, 511
early disease, treatment of, 508
radiation therapy, 510
surgery, 509
systemic chemotherapy, 509
epidemiology, 499
etiology and risk factors, 500
NIH screening guidelines, 505
pathology, 504
screening and diagnosis, 503
signs and symptoms, 502
staging and prognosis, 506
treatment, 508

P

Pain, 861 (*see also* Cancer pain)
Palliative and supportive care (*see* Anorexia and cachexia; Anxiety; Delirium; Depression; Dyspnea; Fatigue; Hematopoietic growth factors)
Pancreatic cancer
etiology and risk factors, 288
incidence and epidemiology, 287
metastatic adenocarcinoma, treatment of, 298
neoadjuvant and adjuvant therapies, 295
pathology, 291
resectable disease, surgical treatment of, 292
screening and diagnosis, 289
signs and symptoms, 288
staging and prognosis, 291
surgical palliation, 294
treatment, 292
unresectable disease, treatment of, 297
Pancreatic endocrine tumors
signs and symptoms, 302
treatment, 304, 306
chemotherapy, 305
of symptoms, 306
radiation therapy, 305
surgery, for gastrinoma-ZES, 304
for insulinomas, 304
tumor localization, 303
types of, 302
Parathyroid cancer
epidemiology and etiology, 97
pathology, 97
signs and symptoms, 97
treatment, 97
Performance scales
Karnofsky performance index, 1053
WHO (Zubrod) scale, 1054
Pericardial effusion
diagnosis, 1041
prognosis, 1042
treatment, 1042
Pharmacotherapy, oncologic
alkylating agents, 28, 1063
altretamine, 1065
busulfan, 1064
carboplatin, 1065
carmustine (BiCNU), 1064
chlorambucil, 1063
cisplatin, 1065
cyclophosphamide, 1063
dacarbazine, 1065
estramustine, 1063
ifosfamide, 1063
lomustine, 1064
mechlorethamine, 1063
melphalan, 1063
nitrogen mustards, 28, 1063
nitrosoureas, 29, 1064
oxaliplatin, 1065
platinum agents, 29, 1065
procarbazine, 1065
streptozocin, 1064
temozolomide, 1065
thiotepa, 1064
antimetabolites, 30, 1066

analogs, 31
camptothecin, 31, 1070
capecitabine, 1067
cladribine, 1066
cytarabine (Ara-C), 1067
liposomal preparation, 1067
floxuridine, 1067
fludarabine, 1066
fluorouracil (5-FU), 1067
gemcitabine, 1067
hydroxyurea, 1067
mercaptopurine, 1066
methotrexate, 1066
pemetrexed, 1066
pentostatin (deoxycoformycin), 1066
thioguanine, 1066
cellular kinetics, 23
combination regimens
principles of, 24
molecularly targeted therapies, 28, 32, 1072
bortezomib, 1072
erlotinib, 1072
gefitinib, 1072
imatinib, 1072
sorafenib, 1072
sunitinib, 1072
monoclonal antibodies, 31, 1071
alemtuzumab, 1071
bevacizumab, 1071
cetuximab, 1071
rituximab, 1071
trastuzumab, 1071
natural products, 30, 1068
anthracyclines, 30
antitumor antibiotics, 30
asparaginase, 1070
bleomycin, 1068
dactinomycin (actinomycin D), 1068
daunorubicin, 1068
liposomal preparation, 1068
docetaxel, 1069
doxorubicin, 1068
liposomal preparation, 1068
epipodophyllotoxins, 30, 1069
epirubicin, 1068
etoposide, 1069
idarubicin (demethoxydaunorubicin), 1068
irinotecan, 1070
mitomycin, 1069
mitoxantrone, 1069
paclitaxel, 1069
taxanes, 31
teniposide, 1069
topotecan, 1070
valrubicin, 1069
vinblastine, 1070
vinca alkaloids, 31
vincristine, 1070
vinorelbine, 1070
pharmacokinetic and pharmacodynamic variability, 26
tumor growth kinetics, 23
Pheochromocytoma (*see also* Pancreatic cancer), 311
diagnosis, 312
epidemiology and etiology, 312
signs and symptoms, 312
treatment, 313
Plasma cell dyscrasias (*see also* Myeloma, multiple)
amyloidosis, 758
heavy-chain diseases, 759
monoclonal gammopathy of unknown significance, 756
POEMS syndrome, 758
solitary extramedullary plasmacytoma, 756
solitary plasmacytoma of bone, 756
Waldenström's macroglobulinemia, 756
Pleural effusion, malignant
diagnosis, 1035
encasement atelectasis, treatment of, 1039
prognosis, 1036
treatment, initial, 1036
Prostate cancer
advanced systemic disease
chemotherapy for androgen-independent disease, 397
defining, 392
first-line therapies for, 393
newer therapies, 398
palliative radiation therapy, 399
second-line hormonal therapies, 396
clinically localized disease
adjuvant therapy post prostatectomy, 384
definitive radiation therapy, 385
impotence, medications and devices to manage, 389
neoadjuvant hormonal therapy, 383
radical prostatectomy, 381
laparoscopic, 382
treatment of, 380
epidemiology, 373

etiology and risk factors, 374
locally advanced disease (T3, T4)
radical prostatectomy with or without adjuvant therapy, 391
treatment of, 390
node-positive disease, 391
pathology, 377
prevention, 378
prognosis and natural history, 379
recurrence, detection and treatment of, 389
treatment recommendations for postprostatectomy, 385
screening and diagnosis, 375
signs and symptoms, 375
Psychiatric disorders (*see* Anxiety; Delirium; Depression)

Q

Quality of life
performance scales, 1053–1054

R

Radiation therapy
brachytherapy, 16
conformal radiation therapy, 19
CT simulation, 18
electron beams, 13
ionizing radiation, 11
intensity-modulated radiation therapy, 19
photon-tissue interactions, 12
pretreatment procedures, 15
proton therapy, 20
radiation absorption, measuring, 13
stereotactic radiosurgery, 20
tomotherapy, 20
treatment machines, 13
treatment planning and delivery, 15
Radiation toxicity
chemotherapy plus irradiation, 950
quantification of treatment toxicity, 951
radiation therapy tolerance doses of, 947
toxic effects, management of, 951
bladder, 966
bone, 975
brain, 962
cardiovascular system, 959
cervix and uterus, 968
ear, external and middle, 956
esophagus, 970
hematopoietic stem-cell compartment, 974
hyperbaric oxygen therapy, 958
intestines, 971
kidneys, 977
larynx, 957
lens, 965
liver, 969
lungs, 958
male reproductive system, 969
nerves and muscles, 976
neuroendocrinologic system, 976
ocular adnexa and anterior segment, 965
optic nerve, 966
oral mucosa, 951
ovaries and reproductive/endocrine function, 968
pharynx and esophagus, 956
retina, 965
salivary glands, 955
skeleton and soft tissues, 956
skin, 960
spinal cord, 964
stomach, 971
taste buds, 956
thyroid, 973
ureter, 966
urethra, 966
vagina, 968
vulva, 967
types of radiation therapy injury, 947
Rectal cancer (*see* Colorectal cancer)
Renal cell carcinoma (*see* Kidney cancer)
Renal pelvic cancer (*see* Urothelial cancer)

S

Sarcomas, bone
advanced osteosarcoma, treatment of, 574
chemotherapy
for advanced Ewing's sarcoma, 575
for Ewing's sarcoma, 575
for osteosarcoma, 571
epidemiology, 565
etiology and risk factors, 566
metastatic disease, surgical treatment of, 571
pathology, 568
screening and diagnosis, 567
signs and symptoms, 566
staging and prognosis, 569
treatment, primary, 569
Sarcomas, soft-tissue
adjuvant chemotherapy, 591
epidemiology, 577
etiology and risk factors, 577

local recurrence, treatment of, 595
localized disease, treatment of, 584
pathology, 579
pulmonary metastasis, limited, treatment of, 596
screening and diagnosis, 582
signs and symptoms, 578
staging and prognosis, 580
treatment, 584
unresectable locally advanced or metastatic disease, chemotherapy for, 596
Skin cancer, melanoma (*see* Melanoma)
Skin cancer, nonmelanoma
recurrent disease, management of, 552
treatment, 551
Small-cell lung cancer (*see* Lung cancer, small-cell)
Stomach cancer (*see* Gastric cancer)
Surgical oncology, principles of biopsy
of lymph nodes, 1
of sentinel nodes, 7
of tissue-based mass, 2
lymphadenectomy, 6
no touch technique, 5
palliation, 8
pathologic confirmation of the diagnosis, 4
preoperative evaluation, 3
resection, 5
wide excision, 5

T

Testicular cancer
epidemiology, 401
etiology and risk factors, 402
follow-up of long-term survivors, 418
nonseminomas
adjuvant chemotherapy for, 414
stage II disease, medical treatment of, 414
stage III disease, treatment of, 415
surveillance, 411
pathology, 406
salvage chemotherapy, 416
screening and diagnosis, 404
seminomas
stage I or II disease, radiation therapy for, 411
stage III disease, treatment of, 415
signs and symptoms, 403
stage I or II disease, surgical treatment of, 409
staging evaluation, 405
staging systems, 407
treatment, 409
Thymoma
diagnosis, 157
epidemiology, 157
etiology and associated syndromes, 157
pathology, 158
staging and prognosis, 159
treatment, 159
unresectable disease, treatment of, 160
Thyroid cancer
diagnostic work-up, 86
epidemiology, 85
etiology and risk factors, 86
I-131, radioactive, 93
medical therapy, 96
radiation therapy, external, 95
screening, 89
signs and symptoms, 86
staging and prognosis, 90
surgery, 91
treatment, 90
tumor types, 83
Toxicity (*see* Radiation toxicity)

U

Unknown primary cancer
adenocarcinoma, treatment of, 661
chemotherapy, empiric, 665
clinical evaluation, 660
epidemiology, 657
pathologic evaluation, 658
poorly differentiated carcinoma, treatment of, 663
signs and symptoms, 658
squamous cell carcinoma, treatment of, 662
treatment, 661
Ureteral cancer (*see* Urothelial cancer)
Urothelial cancer
advanced disease, chemotherapy for, 432
diagnosis, 424
epidemiology, 423
etiology and risk factors, 423
localized disease
treatment of, 427
pathology, 425
radiation therapy, 429
signs and symptoms, 424
staging and prognosis, 425

treatment, 427
Uterine corpus tumors (*see also* Endometrial cancer; Uterine sarcomas; Gestational trophoblastic tumors)
Uterine sarcomas (*see also* Endometrial cancer)
adjuvant therapies, 491–492
patterns of spread, 490
surgery, 490

V

Venous access, long-term
complications, 940
contraindications and precautions, 936
device care, 940
device selection, 937
indications, 935
infections, device-related, 944 (*see also* Infections in cancer patients)
insertion technique, 938
patient selection, 935

W

World Wide Websites
Cancer.gov, 1055
Cancer Information Service, 1056
Cancernetwork.com, 1057
Cancer.org, 1056
CDC, 1057
CenterWatch, 1057
Coalition of National Cancer Cooperative Groups, 1058
Others, 1058
PubMed, 1056
SEER, 1057